Medical Aspects of Disability

A Handbook for the Rehabilitation Professional

4th Edition

Steven R. Flanagan, MD, is Professor and Chairman of the Department of Rehabilitation Medicine, New York University School of Medicine, and the Medical Director of the Rusk Institute of Rehabilitation Medicine, New York University Langone Medical Center. He received his Bachelor of Science from Fairfield University in 1984, and his medical degree from the University of Medicine and Dentistry of New Jersey in 1988. He completed his residency training in Physical Medicine and Rehabilitation at Mount Sinai School of Medicine in 1992. He has served on medical advisory boards of many national and international committees, including the Brain Trauma Foundation and the Indian Head Injury Foundation. He is Chair-elect of the CNS Council of the American Academy of Physical Medicine and Rehabilitation and serves as a peer reviewer for several medical journals. He has presented at scientific meetings both nationally and internationally, most notably on topics pertaining to brain injury rehabilitation. He has authored numerous chapters and publications and has participated in both federal- and industry-sponsored research.

Herb Zaretsky, PhD, is currently Clinical Professor of Rehabilitation Medicine at the New York University School of Medicine and has also served for many years as the Administrator, Department of Rehabilitation Medicine, Rusk Institute, New York University Langone Medical Center. He received his PhD from Adelphi University. He has published extensively in the field of rehabilitation in such areas as psychological aspects of disability, geriatric rehabilitation, learning and conditioning with the neurologically impaired and spinal cord injured, rehabilitation psychology and long-term care of the chronically ill, chronic pain management, and behavioral medicine applications to rehabilitation. He is a Fellow of the American Psychological Association (APA), past President of APA's Division of Rehabilitation Psychology, and a recipient of the APA's Distinguished Contributions to Rehabilitation Psychology Award. He is a long-serving member of the Board of Directors of the national and international Commission on Accreditation of Rehabilitation Facilities (CARF) and was formerly Chair of the CARF Board. He is currently President of the Board of Directors of the American Cancer Society's (ACS) Eastern Division (New York State and New Jersey), a national Division Delegate of the ACS's National Assembly, and the recipient of the St. George Medal, a national award from ACS in recognition of outstanding contributions to the control of cancer.

Alex Moroz, MD, FACP, is the Director of Residency Training and Medical Education at the Department of Rehabilitation Medicine, New York University School of Medicine, and Director of the Musculoskeletal Rehabilitation Unit at Rusk Institute. He is a full-time Assistant Professor of Rehabilitation Medicine and is an experienced educator in the field of disability and rehabilitation. He developed a curriculum in Medical Aspects of Disability for nonphysician health care providers and taught a graduate-level three-credit course with the same name at the City University of New York during 1999 and 2000. Since joining the faculty at the New York University School of Medicine, he has expanded and improved the postgraduate training program for physicians specializing in rehabilitation and disability, and received recognition awards for his teaching excellence from the graduating residents in 2001 and 2008. He was invited to develop a national self-study curriculum for practicing rehabilitation physicians in the area of neurodegenerative disorders and stroke from 2002 to 2003 and was chosen to facilitate the development of the 2009 Study Guide. He is a founding member of the interdisciplinary Disability Council at New York University.

Medical Aspects of Disability

A Handbook for the
Rehabilitation Professional

4th Edition

Steven R. Flanagan, MD

Herb Zaretsky, PhD

Alex Moroz, MD, FACP

Editors

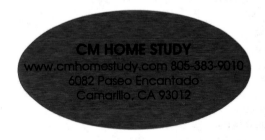

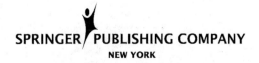

SPRINGER PUBLISHING COMPANY
NEW YORK

Springer Publishing Company, LLC
11 West 42nd Street
New York, NY 10036
www.springerpub.com

Acquisitions Editor: Sheri W. Sussman
Senior Editor: Rose Mary Piscitelli
Cover design: David Levy
Composition: Ashita Shah at Newgen Imaging Systems Ltd
ISBN: 978-0-8261-2783-9
E-book ISBN: 978-0-8261-2784-6
12 13 / 5 4 3

The author and the publisher of this Work have made every effort to use sources believed to be reliable to provide information that is accurate and compatible with the standards generally accepted at the time of publication. Because medical science is continually advancing, our knowledge base continues to expand. Therefore, as new information becomes available, changes in procedures become necessary. We recommend that the reader always consult current research and specific institutional policies before performing any clinical procedure. The author and publisher shall not be liable for any special, consequential, or exemplary damages resulting, in whole or in part, from the readers' use of, or reliance on, the information contained in this book. The publisher has no responsibility for the persistence or accuracy of URLs for external or third-party Internet Web sites referred to in this publication and does not guarantee that any content on such Web sites is, or will remain, accurate or appropriate.

Library of Congress Cataloging-in-Publication Data
Medical aspects of disability : a handbook for the rehabilitation professional / Steven R. Flanagan, Herb Zaretsky, Alex Moroz, editors.
—4th ed.
    p. ; cm.
 Includes bibliographical references and index.
 ISBN 978-0-8261-2783-9
1. Medical rehabilitation. 2. Chronic diseases. 3. Disability evaluation. I. Flanagan, Steven R.
II. Zaretsky, Herb III. Moroz, Alex.
 [DNLM: 1. Disabled Persons—rehabilitation. 2. Disability Evaluation.
3. Rehabilitation—methods. WB 320 M48872 2010]
 RM930.M42 2010
 617'.03—dc22   2010012543

Printed in the United States of America by Hamilton Printing

Special discounts on bulk quantities of our books are available to corporations, professional associations, pharmaceutical companies, health care organizations, and other qualified groups.
If you are interested in a custom book, including chapters from more than one of our titles, we can provide that service as well.

For details, please contact:
Special Sales Department, Springer Publishing Company, LLC
11 West 42nd Street, 15th Floor, New York, NY 10036-8002
Phone: 877-687-7476 or 212-431-4370; Fax: 212-941-7842
Email: sales@springerpub.com

To my family, friends, and especially Lou for their understanding, support, and inspiration.

Steven R. Flanagan

To my wife, Diane, for her love, inspiration, extraordinary support, and cherished friendship; to my daughter, Lauren; my son, Andrew; my son-in-law, Lee; and to my grandchildren, Alec, Will, and Jake—each of whom is a constant source of joy and love in my life.

Herb Zaretsky

To Justin the Fair, to Ryan the Noble, to Marina the Guide, to Vitya the Giver, to Eduard the Youngheart, and to my students and residents.

Alex Moroz

The editors also wish to acknowledge the tireless dedication and invaluable assistance of Linda Yuen-Moy in the timely preparation of this textbook.

The Editors

Contents

PART III: SPECIAL TOPICS

Contributors

Steven B. Abramson, MD, Professor of Medicine and Pathology, New York University School of Medicine, New York, NY

Jung Ahn, MD, Clinical Professor of Rehabilitation Medicine, New York University School of Medicine, New York, NY

Salman Anwar, MD, Clinical Research Fellow, NYU Aging and Dementia Research Center, New York University Langone Medical Center, New York, NY

Stefanie Auer, PhD, Scientific Director, M.A.S. Alzheimerhilfe, Department of Clinical Medicine and Preventive Medicine, Danube University Krems, Krems, Austria

Reema Batra, MD, Assistant Professor of Medicine, New York University School of Medicine, New York, NY

Jeffrey Berliner, DO, Assistant Professor, Spinal Cord Injury Medicine, Department of Physical Medicine and Rehab, TIRR/Memorial Hermann Hospital, Houston, TX

Frederick A. Bevelaqua, MD, Clinical Assistant Professor of Medicine, New York University School of Medicine, New York, NY

Gary R. Bond, PhD, Professor, Department of Psychiatry, Dartmouth Psychiatric Research Center, Lebanon, NH

Brian J. Boon, PhD, President/CEO, Commission on Accreditation of Rehabilitation Facilities, Tucson, AZ

Ludmilla Bronfin, MD, Assistant Professor of Neurology, New York University School of Medicine, New York, NY

Susanne M. Bruyère, PhD, CRC, Professor of Disability Studies, Director, Employment and Disability Institute, Cornell University, ILR School, Ithaca, NY

Tamara Bushnik, PhD, Director of Research, Associate Professor of Rehabilitation Medicine, Rusk Institute of Rehabilitation Medicine, New York University School of Medicine, New York, NY

Jeffrey M. Cohen, MD, Clinical Professor of Rehabilitation Medicine, New York University School of Medicine, New York, NY

Marissa Cohler, MD, New York University School of Medicine, New York, NY

Roy Gordan Cole, OD, FAAO, Director of Vision Program Development, The Jewish Guild for the Blind, Adjunct Professor of Ophthalmology, Columbia University Medical Center, New York, NY

John R. Corcoran, PT, DPT, MS, Cert. MDT, Clinical Assistant Professor of Rehabilitation Medicine, New York University School of Medicine, New York, NY

Adrian Cristian, MD, Chief, Rehabilitation Medicine, James J. Peters VA Medical Center, Associate Professor, Department of Rehabilitation Medicine, Mount Sinai School of Medicine, New York, NY

Teina Daley, OTR/L, CHT, James J. Peters Veterans Medical Center, Bronx, NY

Tara Denham, PT, MA, Clinical Instructor of Rehabilitation Medicine, New York University School of Medicine, New York, NY

W. Scott Dewey, PT, CHT, OCS, Clinical Coordinator, Burn Rehabilitation, U.S. Army Burn Center, Ft. Sam Houston, TX

Jeanne Dzurenko, BSN, MPH, RN, Director of Nursing, Rusk Institute of Rehabilitation Medicine, New York University Langone Medical Center, New York, NY

Joan E. Edelstein, MA, PT, FISPO, CPed, Special Lecturer, Columbia University, New York, NY

Michal Eisenberg, MD, Assistant Professor, Departments of Neurology and Rehabilitation Medicine, New York University School of Medicine, New York, NY

Mary C. Ellis, PT, AVP Clinical Services, Clinical Director, Spinal Cord Program, National Rehabilitation Hospital, Washington, DC

Nancy Eng, PhD, CCC-SLP, Associate Professor, Department of Communication Sciences, Hunter College, New York Downtown Hospital, Department of Rehabilitation Medicine, New York, NY

Emile H. Franssen, MD, Research Associate Professor, Department of Psychiatry, New York University School of Medicine, New York, NY

Robert T. Fraser, MD, PhD, CRC, Professor and Director of Neurological, Vocational Services, Departments of Rehabilitation Medicine, Neurology, Neurosurgery, University of Washington, Seattle, WA

Susan Garritan, PT, PhD, CCS, Clinical Assistant Professor of Rehabilitation Medicine, New York University School of Medicine, New York, NY

Christopher G. Gharibo, MD, Assistant Professor of Anesthesiology, New York University Langone Hospital for Joint Diseases, New York, NY

Joan T. Gold, MD, Clinical Professor of Rehabilitation Medicine, New York University School of Medicine, New York, NY

Thomas P. Golden, MS, CRC, Associate Director, Employment and Disability Institute Extension, Faculty, School of Industrial and Labor Relations, Cornell University, Ithaca, NY

Ilana Grunwald, PhD, Clinical Assistant Professor of Rehabilitation Medicine, New York University School of Medicine, New York, NY

Kristofer J. Hagglund, PhD, ABPP, Professor and Associate Dean, School of Health Professions, Director, Public Health Program, University of Missouri, Columbia, MO

Andrew J. Haig, MD, Professor, Physical Medicine and Rehabilitation, University of Michigan, Ann Arbor, MI

Monwara Hassan, MD, Instructor, Mount Sinai Medical School, New York, NY

Joseph E. Herrera, DO, FAAPMR, Assistant Professor of Rehabilitation Medicine, Director of Sports Medicine, Mount Sinai School of Medicine, New York, NY

Mary Hibbard, PhD, ABPP (RP), Professor of Rehabilitation Medicine, New York University School of Medicine, New York, NY

Brian Im, MD, Instructor of Rehabilitation Medicine, New York University School of Medicine, New York, NY

Patrick Inniss, PhD, Director of Social Work, St. Luke's Roosevelt Hospital, New York, NY

Glenn R. Jacobowitz, MD, Associate Professor of Surgery, Vice Chief, Division of Vascular Surgery, New York University Langone Medical Center, New York, NY

Parul Jajoo, DO, FAAPMR, Assistant Professor, Pain Department, St. Luke's Roosevelt Hospital, New York, NY

Imran A. Jamil, MD, Assistant Director, Clinical Research Preceptorship Program, Aging and Dementia Clinical Research Center, Center for Brain Aging, New York University School of Medicine, New York, NY

Erica K. Johnson, PhD, CRC, Instructor and Clinical Director, Graduate Program in Rehabilitation Counseling, Western Washington University, Bellingham, WA

Sunnie Kenowsky, DVM, Co-Director, Zachary and Elizabeth M. Fisher Alzheimer's Disease Education and Resources Program, New York University Langone Medical Center, New York, NY

M. Fahad Khan, MD, MHS, Department of Anesthesiology, New York University School of Medicine, New York, NY

Marina Kukla, MS, Clinical Psychology Doctoral Student, Indiana University–Purdue University, Indianapolis, IN

Sicy H. Lee, MD, Clinical Assistant Professor of Medicine, New York University School of Medicine, New York, NY

Patricia Kerman Lerner, MA, CCC, Fellow, ASHA, Clinical Assistant Professor of Rehabilitation Medicine, New York University School of Medicine, New York, NY

Jerome Lowenstein, MD, Professor of Medicine, New York University School of Medicine, New York, NY

Jung Woo Ma, MD, Department of Rehabilitation Medicine, Mount Sinai School of Medicine, New York, NY

David G. Marrero, PhD, Director, Diabetes Translational Research, J.O. Ritchey Professor of Medicine, Division of Endocrinology & Metabolism, Indiana University School of Medicine, Indianapolis, IN

John W. Miller, MD, PhD, Professor of Neurology and Neurosurgery, Director, UW Regional Epilepsy Center, University of Washington, Seattle, WA

Ana Mola, MA, RN, ANP-BC, Program Director, Joan and Joel Smilow Center for Cardiopulmonary Rehabilitation and Prevention, New York University Langone Medical Center, New York, NY

Alex Moroz, MD, FACP, Director of Residency Training and Medical Education, Assistant Professor of Rehabilitation Medicine, New York University School of Medicine, New York, NY

Richard J. Morris, PhD, Meyerson Distinguished Professor of Disability and Rehabilitation, Director, School of Psychology Program, University of Arizona, Tucson, AZ

Yvonne P. Morris, PhD, Licensed Psychologist, Tucson, AZ

Pete-Gaye Nation, MD, Long Island Jewish Medical Center, Department of Rehabilitation Medicine, New York, NY

Kotresha Neelakantappa, MD, FACP, Clinical Assistant Professor of Medicine, Cornell University Medical College, Chief of Nephrology, New York Methodist Hospital, Brooklyn, NY

Bryan O'Young, MD, Clinical Associate Professor of Rehabilitation Medicine, Rehabilitation Medicine, New York, NY

Kate Parkin, PT, MA, Clinical Assistant Professor of Rehabilitation Medicine, New York University School of Medicine, New York, NY

Bruce G. Raphael, MD, Clinical Professor of Medicine, Division Head of Benign Hematology, Department of Hematology/Oncology, New York University School of Medicine, New York, NY

Ira Rashbaum, MD, Clinical Professor of Rehabilitation Medicine, New York University School of Medicine, New York, NY

Barry Reisberg, MD, Professor of Psychiatry, Director, Fisher Alzheimer's Disease Program, Clinical Director, Aging & Dementia Clinical Research Center, New York University Langone Medical Center, New York, NY

Mariano J. Rey, MD, FACC, Co-Director, Joan and Joel Smilow Center for Cardiopulmonary Rehabilitation and Prevention, Senior Associate Dean for Community Health Affairs, New York University Langone Medical Center, New York, NY

Bruce P. Rosenthal, OD, FAAO, Chief of the Low Vision Programs, Lighthouse International, Adjunct Professor, Department of Ophthalmology, Mount Sinai Hospital, New York, NY

Negin Salimi, DO, Department of Rehabilitation Medicine, New York University School of Medicine, New York, NY

David Salsberg, PsyD, DABPS, Clinical Instructor of Rehabilitation Medicine, New York University School of Medicine, New York, NY

Jennifer Sayanlar, DO, North Shore Long Island Jewish Medical Center, Great Neck, NY

Robert A. Schulman, MD, Clinical Assistant Professor of Rehabilitation Medicine and Rehabilitation Medicine in Complementary and Integrative Medicine, Weill Cornell Medical College, New York, NY

Liduïn E. M. Souren, RN, MSN, Research Assistant Professor, Department of Psychiatry, New York University School of Medicine, New York, NY

Adam B. Stein, MD, Chairman, Department of Physical Medicine and Rehabilitation, The North Shore-Long Island Jewish Health System, Great Neck, NY

Dale C. Strasser, MD, Associate Professor, Department of Rehabilitation Medicine, Emory University Medical School, Atlanta, GA

Patrick T. Swift, PhD, Clinical Assistant Professor, Neurology and Rehabilitation Medicine, New York University School of Medicine, New York, NY

Sara A. Van Looy, BA, Research Assistant, Employment and Disability Institute, Cornell University, New York, NY

Fran R. Wallach, MD, Associate Professor of Medicine, Division of Infectious Diseases, Mount Sinai School of Medicine, New York, NY

Jonathan H. Whiteson, MD, Assistant Professor of Rehabilitation Medicine, New York University School of Medicine, New York, NY

Steven E. Wolf, MD, Betty and Bob Kelso Distinguished Chair in Burns and Trauma, Professor and Vice Chair for Research, Department of Surgery, University of Texas Health Science Center, San Antonio, TX

Alan W. Young, DO, Clinical Assistant Professor of Rehabilitation Medicine, University of Texas Health Science Center, San Antonio, TX

Mark Young, MD, Chair of Physical Medicine and Rehabilitation at the Workforce and Technology Center, Maryland Rehabilitation Center, Professor, Department of Orthopedic Sciences, New York College of Podiatric Medicine, New York, NY

Introduction

The manner in which health care will be delivered in the future remains uncertain in nearly all fields of medicine, particularly Physical Medicine and Rehabilitation (PM&R). Despite increasing efforts to establish evidence-based practices in PM&R, economic and political forces continually challenge the delivery of care to people with disabilities. This fourth edition of *Medical Aspects of Disability* has been substantially updated from previous editions to reflect advancements in medical care for specific disabling conditions as well as changes in forces that impact the delivery of that care. Chapters in the fourth edition have either been substantially updated by previous authors or completely rewritten by new contributors, including Social Work in Physical Medicine, Stroke, The Computer Revolution—Disability and Assistive Technology, Chronic Pain, Traumatic Brain Injury, Complementary and Alternative Medicine, Rehabilitation in Burns, Disabling Conditions Seen in AIDS and HIV Infection, and Spinal Cord Injury. While some previous chapters were eliminated, several new topics were added to reflect the changing face of rehabilitation medicine and disability, including The History of Rehabilitation, Geriatric Rehabilitation, Challenges and Opportunities for Quality in Rehabilitation, Limb Deficiency, Organ Transplantation and Rehabilitation, Musculoskeletal Disorders, and Future Directions of Rehabilitation Research. Our contributors are among the most widely respected authorities in their respective fields so that we can present our readers the most useful and updated information on the vast array of disabling conditions afflicting millions of people and how they are best addressed and impacted by our current health care system. Our primary goal in this latest edition is to provide health care professionals, teachers, and students a useful and updated handbook that addresses the many conditions and topics that impact people with physical, developmental, and cognitive disabilities. In that sense, the editors are confident that this newly revised and updated fourth edition will be a valuable resource.

Steven R. Flanagan, MD

Medical Aspects of Disability

**A Handbook for the
Rehabilitation Professional**

4th Edition

1

Introduction

Kate Parkin, PT, MA, John R. Corcoran, PT, DPT, MS, Cert. MDT, and Tara Denham, PT, MA

THE HISTORY OF REHABILITATION

The history of rehabilitation is fraught with acrimony, contention, and eventual triumph. Prior to the evolution of physical medicine and rehabilitation (PM&R) as an organized field and profession, individuals unfortunate enough to be suffering from a physical affliction were left to their own measure and often labeled as a cripple, an invalid, or worse.

The first known medical document was discovered in Egypt and dates back to 2000 BC. This document is known as the Edwin Smith Surgical Papyrus (named after the American Egyptologist who purchased the treatise in 1862). The treatise describes the general sentiment of how most disabilities were treated, which could be summarized as sparse at best. For spinal cord injuries, treatment options were nonexistent and this injury was often deemed "an ailment not to be treated" (Donovan, 2007). Unfortunately, treatments for spinal cord injuries and other causes of disabilities did not advance for thousands of years. Most patients with disabilities were treated by their families or in religious establishments until the latter part of the 20th century (Ohry, 2004). In fact, General George Patton (1885–1945), who is famous for many highly successful campaigns in World War II, sustained a spinal cord injury shortly after returning from the war. It is said that he was well aware (likely from seeing injured soldiers first hand) that there were no cures or efficacious treatments available and thus he refused all treatments. Patton died in the hospital (Donovan, 2007). It was Alexander Fleming's discovery of penicillin that greatly decreased deaths from infections, including those seen in spinal cord injury care, and a host of other disabilities that revolutionized all of medicine, including PM&R (Donovan, 2007).

Ancient Egyptians had a life expectancy of only 36 years and high-speed injuries were nonexistent. However, the ancient Egyptians, Greeks, and Romans sustained many fractures and slowly advanced various treatment options. Once again, the initial data come to us from the Edwin Smith Papyrus that outlines several fracture treatments. Compound fractures were considered to have a poor prognosis, but simple fractures of the upper extremity were often reduced by traction and had a favorable prognosis (Brorson, 2009).

It was not until the early 1900s that rehabilitation as a profession and field of study started to become more organized and gain some traction, even though it was initially viewed in large part as quackery (Opitz, Folz, Gelfman, & Peters, 1997). The struggle for legitimacy continued during much of the early years as the field developed. For a fascinating and complete account of the political, social, and medical aspects of the rise of the field of PM&R, the reader is referred to a 1997 edition of the *Archives of Physical Medicine and Rehabilitation* (Folz, Opitz, Peters, & Gelfman, 1997; Gelfman, Peters, Opitz, & Folz, 1997; Opitz et al., 1997; Peters, Gelfman, Folz, & Opitz, 1997).

In studying the history of rehabilitation there are two prominent figures to be considered, Frank H. Krusen, MD, and Howard A. Rusk, MD. Drs. Krusen and Rusk were essential in creating the scope of the field as it is known today. Dr. Krusen's (1898–1973) interest in rehabilitation was shaped by personal experience. While working in his first year of surgical residency training, he was infected with tuberculosis (Opitz et al., 1997). He spent 5 months in a sanitarium, during which time he recognized that he and other patients were becoming physically deconditioned, causing them to become increasingly more dependent on the institution for care. It was then that he came up with the idea of physical rehabilitation with an emphasis on social reintegration, physical reconditioning, and vocational rehabilitation as essential components of convalescence, ultimately becoming his life's work.

The American Medical Association (AMA) did not initially view physical rehabilitation favorably. It was not until 1939 that the first scientific paper on rehabilitation was accepted in a medical journal (Opitz et al., 1997). Dr. Krusen experienced great resistance from several groups that organized against him. His most significant opponents were in the fields of orthopedics and pediatrics as well as in the National Foundation for Infantile Paralysis (whose director, Catherine Worthingham, PhD, PT, was a past president of American Physical Therapy Association) (Gelfman et al., 1997). Many were concerned about the use of the word "rehabilitation" in this developing specialty because it was felt to have a place in many other disciplines. Orthopedists and pediatricians were worried about encroachment on their practice whereas physical therapists were concerned that rehabilitation physicians would impinge on their autonomy as independent practitioners (Gelfman et al., 1997). However, Dr. Krusen's intellect, organizational skills, political ties, and interpersonal skills eventually triumphed over these groups, and on September 5, 1944, the American Congress on Physical Therapy changed its name to the American Congress of Physical Medicine (Folz et al., 1997). The medical journal by the Congress also changed its name from the *Archives of Physical Therapy* to the *Archives of Physical Medicine* (Folz et al., 1997).

Dr. Howard Archibald Rusk (1901–1989) had a similar insight as Dr. Krusen. Although he is often mistaken as a physiatrist, Howard Rusk was an internist who organized comprehensive medical rehabilitation departments in Army Air Corps hospitals during World War II (Gelfman et al., 1997). While working in medical rehabilitation, he noticed that the soldiers were becoming deconditioned and bored during their convalescence. Rusk organized academic class work and physical exercise during the soldiers' hospitalization. He also emphasized interdisciplinary teams and psychosocial functioning in addition to physical and vocation rehabilitation (Gelfman et al., 1997). Through his work, soldiers regained physical fitness and were able to return to active duty at a faster pace while experiencing significantly lower rates of hospital readmission. He also included military training as part of the academic course work provided to the soldiers to enhance their performance when they returned to active duty. For example, he organized replicas of German planes to cycle over the soldiers' hospital beds to assist in identifying them when they returned to the battlefield (Rusk, 1977).

Rusk was also a pioneer in the concept and implementation of early mobilization after illness or injury. He conducted experiments to analyze the impact of returning to activity quickly after surgery and the initial findings were favorable. This success spurred further research.

When he completed his military service, he petitioned the AMA to start residencies in medical rehabilitation. The AMA deferred to the Council on Physical Medicine because of the similarities of the two fields (Gelfman et al., 1997). Dr. Krusen also recognized the close association and with their backing, the AMA Council on Physical Medicine approved a motion to change the residencies to a combination of PM&R (Gelfman et al., 1997). Dr. Rusk, who is generally recognized as the "father of comprehensive rehabilitation," went on to teach and train physicians across the United States and throughout the world, including Russia, Korea, China, and Vietnam.

Just as World War II shaped Rusk's views and thoughts on rehabilitation, the wars in Afghanistan and Iraq have also profoundly influenced the field in recent times. With many soldiers returning from combat with amputations and traumatic brain injuries (TBI), there has been an increase in research and development in these areas. As described throughout this textbook, the reader will learn of recent advances in the care and rehabilitation for people with conditions such as limb loss and TBI resulting from these conflicts.

"Physical rehabilitation in its essence is the preservation and restoration of function" (anonymous) (Haig, Nagy, Lebreck, & Stein, 1995). A significant portion of the U.S. population lives with physical disabilities. Rehabilitation is a process aimed at enabling people with disabilities to reach and maintain their optimal physical, sensory, intellectual, psychological, vocational, social, and functional potential. Rehabilitation provides people with disabilities the tools they need to attain greater independence. The World Health Organization (WHO) estimates that 10% of the world's population experience some form of disability or impairment. The number of people with disabilities is increasing due to population growth, aging, emergence of chronic diseases, increasing motor vehicle use, and medical advances that preserve and prolong life. The most common causes of impairment and disability include chronic diseases such as diabetes, cardiovascular disease, cancer, traumatic injuries, mental impairments, birth defects, malnutrition, HIV/AIDS, and other communicable diseases. These conditions are creating overwhelming demands for health and rehabilitation services (World Health Organization, 2005). Managing these conditions is one of the biggest challenges our health care system faces as we move through the 21st century. People are living longer yet the percentage of them living with chronic diseases has increased significantly over the last two decades. "Over 133 million Americans have at least one chronic disease. With proper care, the onset and progression of these diseases can be better contained and controlled for many years. In addition to the suffering and early death they can cause, these chronic conditions cost a staggering $1.7 trillion yearly" (www.barackobama.com, 2009a).

As the health care system changes and the ability to provide care across a long continuum is being remolded, effective communication between rehabilitation team members becomes increasingly more essential. Thus, the medical rehabilitation model consists of a core group of medical professionals who comprise a comprehensive team to evaluate and treat people to best meet their needs, with communication between members occurring on a regular basis. The interdisciplinary team involves a large number of disciplines that are lead by rehabilitation physicians (Figure 1.1). The physician usually determines which team members should be involved in the care of a particular patient, noting that all disciplines are not always required or involved at the same time. Each discipline plays an integral role in the patient's recovery and includes:

- Child life therapist
- Creative art therapist
- Horticultural therapist
- Nutritionist
- Occupational therapist
- Pastoral care
- Patient
- Physiatrist/physician
- Physical therapist
- Psychologist
- Rehabilitation engineer
- Rehabilitation nurse
- Social worker
- Speech and language pathologist
- Therapeutic recreational specialist
- Vocational counselor.

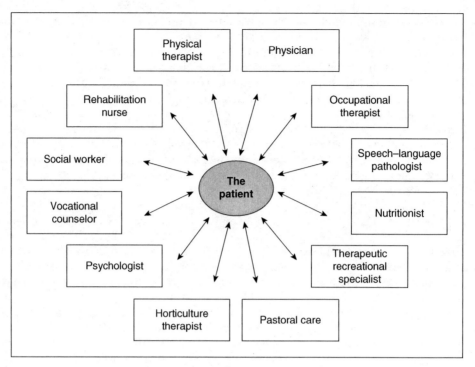

FIGURE 1.1   Patient-centered interdisciplinary team approach.

Below is a brief description of the most common team members.

The patient is by far the most important member of the interdisciplinary team and should be involved in all decisions regarding his/her care. If the patient (or the designee, if the patient is incapable of participation) is not included or is not in agreement with the plan of treatment, rehabilitation is unlikely to succeed.

Occupational therapists (OT) are professionals who help promote health and enhance independence in the performance of activities of daily living (ADLs) for people with disabilities. Occupational therapists assess people's skills and limitations regarding ADLs and use meaningful and purposeful activities in addition to specialized equipment and adaptive aids to promote independent function.

Physical therapists (PT) are professionals who provide services to patients with physical impairments, functional limitations, disabilities, or changes in function and health resulting from injury or disease. PTs assess and treat bed mobility, the ability to move from place to place (e.g., wheelchair to bed), ambulation skills, balance, strength, range of motion, and function.

Physiatrists are physicians specializing in the field of PM&R and leading the rehabilitation team. After reviewing the history and performing the physical examination, the physiatrist prescribes the rehabilitation program and provides medical treatment to people with disabilities.

Psychologists are clinicians who assess patients' cognitive status and mental health. Psychologists help emotionally distressed patients adjust to life that has changed due to injury or illness and provide therapy to improve cognitive performance when necessary.

Therapeutic recreational specialists (TRS) are trained and certified to provide treatment, education, and recreational services to help people with illnesses and disabilities develop leisure activities that enhance their health, functional abilities, independence, and quality of life.

Rehabilitation nurses (RN) are clinicians responsible for monitoring patients' medical status including, but not limited to, vital signs, skin integrity, and sleep status. Rehabilitation nurses also evaluate the patient's mental state, medication usage and effectiveness, pain, and bowel and bladder function and provide essential education to both patients and their families.

Speech-language pathologists (SLP) are clinicians who assess the patient's ability to communicate by both spoken and written language in addition to evaluating swallowing ability, which is often impaired following brain injury. They provide treatment to improve both communication skills and ability to safely swallow food and liquids.

Social workers (SW) assess patients' psychosocial status, including their living situations, support system, and financial status. They assist patients by helping them cope with social issues that impact their life, particularly as they pertain to their disability, in addition to dealing with their personal and professional relationships.

Vocational rehabilitation counselors (CRC) assess a patient's ability to return to work or to previous activities enjoyed. Vocational counselors determine the jobs that are best suited to their patients via interviews, evaluation of their abilities, and selected tests.

PATIENT EXPERIENCE

A patient's experience varies depending on the setting in which rehabilitation is being provided. For example, services provided acutely after injury, in an acute inpatient rehabilitation hospital, subacute rehabilitation facility, or outpatient venue have unique characteristics and regulations that dictate the type and intensity of treatment provided. Services can also vary within each setting with individual rehabilitation centers often offering highly specialized programs to meet the needs of the patients they serve. After the onset of an adverse medical event, a patient will usually be taken to an acute care hospital. After to once patients are medically stabilized, they leave the acute care hospital and may be transferred to an acute rehabilitation facility if they can participate and benefit from intensive therapy. A common element for patients destined for acute rehabilitation is that their lives have been altered physically, psychologically, and often spiritually by the experience.

Imagine for a moment that your ability to walk, dress, and even comprehend a loved one's speech has been suddenly lost because of an acute medical event such as stroke or TBI. Now you find yourself in a medical center with a team of individuals working with you to restore what previously was taken for granted.

The above scenario is quite typical for patients in need of acute rehabilitation following a sudden illness or injury and outlines some key points. In most acute inpatient rehabilitation facilities, bedside rounds attended by representatives of the team occur daily. This is a time to review daily progress, receive updates on medical status and medication changes, review issues that occurred overnight, and answer questions from the patient or their significant others. This is also an opportunity to get the patient's feedback, review team goals, discuss discharge planning, and get information on the patient's preferences.

The team conference is a gathering of the various disciplines that are working with patient, and typically occurs weekly in acute inpatient settings. This conference, usually lead by the physician, will include updates on the patient's medical condition, functional changes, progress toward patient goals, unusual occurrences, discharge planning, and modification of desired or expected goals. In addition to setting individual goals that are specific to each discipline, the team will create and review goals that cross disciplines, such as community mobility that requires the use of mass transportation. Discussions will also focus on planning for discharge, which may include the need for continued medical, nursing, and rehabilitation care. Potential barriers to discharge will be reviewed, including access to and within the patient's home and the availability of others to assist in their care once in the community. Ongoing rehabilitation is often needed after discharge, which may be provided at home, as an outpatient, or at a subacute facility. Subacute rehabilitation is provided in a skilled nursing facility (SNF), but at a lower intensity with about 1 hour of therapy given daily, as opposed to acute rehabilitation where at least 3 hours of daily therapy is provided.

Family meetings are typically arranged by the social worker or case coordinator and include the physician and many of the team members. The psychologist is often present at these meetings as family dynamics are often explored. When possible and appropriate, the patient is included in this meeting. This is a good opportunity to problem solve discharge planning issues and make arrangements for the next level of care. Many factors are considered, such as the availability and adequacy of family and community support and the provision of continued needed care.

Conditions seen for rehabilitation include, but are not limited to, persons who have suffered from the following:

- Traumatic brain injury
- Stroke
- Multiple sclerosis
- Limb loss
- Sports injury
- Vestibular disorders
- Spinal cord injuries
- Developmental delay
- Parkinson's disease
- Muscular dystrophy
- Cerebral palsy
- Amyotrophic lateral sclerosis.

Patients requiring rehabilitation often have complex medical, psychological, and social needs that warrant a coordinated and interdisciplinary approach. The definition of the interdisciplinary team "refers to activities performed towards a common goal by individuals from a group of different disciplines" (Melvin, 1980). The members of the interdisciplinary team need to be skilled not only in their specific discipline, but in others as well to be effective interdisciplinary team members. The goal should be "to accomplish an outcome which is greater than each functioning separately" (Keith, 1991). This also requires considerable education for the patient, their families, and significant others.

CONTINUUM OF CARE

As health care reform progresses, the delivery of services provided throughout the continuum of care is changing. The current model in the United States can provide all aspects of rehabilitation care in various settings, noting that the intensity of services in these practice settings varies. All rehabilitation professionals are available throughout the continuum of care that is described below. National, state, and local laws determine who is authorized to provide these services.

Acute Care

It is provided in a hospital setting. The patient is typically admitted following an acute injury, medical occurrence, or for a surgical procedure. Length of acute hospitalization is often only a few days, and patients are routinely discharged to another level of care or to their homes when medically stable.

Inpatient Acute Licensed Rehabilitation Program

Patients admitted to acute rehabilitation facilities require around-the-clock medical care but do not require the level of medical service provided in an acute care hospital. These patients are usually transferred to acute rehabilitation after medical stability has been achieved in an acute hospital. These patients should tolerate at least 3 hours of therapy services daily (inclusive of PT, OT, and/or SLP), require both acute nursing care and physician availability 24 hours a day, and have the ability to make timely functional improvements.

Subacute Rehabilitation

Subacute rehabilitation provides care that is less intense than in acute rehabilitation, but patients continue to manifest potential to improve their functional skills through rehabilitation. Patients are generally required to tolerate only 1–2 hours of daily therapy, but must still require acute nursing care 24 hours a day and periodic physician care.

Skilled Nursing Facility

These facilities have distinct beds that allow patients the opportunity to recuperate for an extended period of time with some therapy services on a daily basis. These designated beds can also be within a freestanding acute licensed rehabilitation hospital, a freestanding long-term care facility, or a freestanding skilled rehabilitation hospital. Patients treated in this setting have fewer acute medical needs than either acute or subacute rehabilitation. It is typically targeted at older, postacute patients who may not be able to tolerate the intensity of acute rehabilitation but who have the capacity for functional recovery.

Home-Based Therapy

Home therapy is provided to patients who need continued rehabilitation but no longer require care within a hospital, a subacute facility, or a SNF. Patients are typically considered homebound and are therefore incapable of participating in outpatient rehabilitation programs.

Outpatient Therapy

Outpatient services are provided to those patients who no longer require hospital-based therapies and who are not homebound. Services are designed to provide either general rehabilitation to a wide group of individuals or more specialized care to specific groups of patients. Depending on the individual needs of the person being served and the specific discipline prescribed, outpatient therapy is typically provided two to three times per week per discipline. The number of sessions and frequency of treatment depend on the amount of treatment needed and the patient's progress.

Wellness and/or Prevention Centers

These are centers that are often within community fitness centers, health clubs, or a health care facility. Their goal is to educate, instruct, and promote the practices of wellness and prevention of illness or injury. A physiatrist and other rehabilitation professionals often refer individuals to these centers after they have had a course of a more traditional rehabilitation.

Comprehensive Day Treatment Programs

Comprehensive day rehabilitation programs have the goal of preventing long-term institutionalization while providing a daily program of activities. Some comprehensive day rehabilitation programs provide restorative services and are geared toward achieving specific therapeutic endpoints within a defined period of time, with the goal of living a more independent life in the community. Some common types of day treatment programs include brain injury day treatment programs, adult day treatment programs, and dementia day treatment programs. These programs often provide some degree of respite for full time care providers of severely disabled individuals. If these programs were otherwise not available it would require many individuals be institutionalized due to the level of care they require.

World Health Organization (WHO)

In addition to the various settings designed to assist the patients in recovery, there are also organizations that work on a large scale to improve the lives of people who require rehabilitation services. One such organization is the World Health Organization (WHO). WHO's role in the area of disability and rehabilitation is to enhance the quality of life and promote and protect the rights and dignity of people with disabilities through local, national, and global efforts. It is estimated that 650 million people live with disabilities around the world. To enhance the quality of life and to promote and protect the rights and dignity of people with disabilities the key focus is the following:

- Advocacy
- Data collection
- Medical care and rehabilitation
- Community-based rehabilitation
- Assistive devices/technologies
- Capacity building
- Policies
- Partnerships (World Health Organization, 2005).

DISABLEMENT MODELS

The WHO and other groups have been instrumental in creating models to understand function and disability, which are better known as "disablement models." One of the earliest theories in rehabilitation, and the most familiar, concerns the consequences of disease and injury, that is, disablement, and how they integrate the medical and social models of practice. In the *medical model*, disability is viewed as a "characteristic or attribute of the person, which is directly caused by disease, trauma, or other health condition and requires some type of intervention provided by professionals to 'correct' or 'compensate' for the problem." In the *social model*, disability is viewed as a "socially created problem and not as an attribute of the person." In the social model of disability, the underlying problem is created by an unaccommodating or inflexible environment brought about by the attitudes or features of the social and physical environment itself, which calls for a political and physical response or solution (Jette, 2006). The combination of the medical and social model subsequently is the biopsychosocial model. It attempts to integrate both models of disability. This is the key framework of the disablement model that is widely used today.

Rehabilitation medicine experts have been struggling with the concepts and language that describe disablement for decades. Nagi in the 1960s and the WHO in the 1980s were among the major contributors to the literature of rehabilitation medicine (Table 1.1).

TABLE 1.1 *Disablement Concepts and Definitions*

Nagi	ICF
Active pathology—interruption or interference with normal processes and effort of the organism to regain normal state	*Health conditions*—diseases, disorders, and injuries
	Body function—physiological functions of body systems
Impairment—anatomical, physiological, mental, or emotional abnormalities	*Body structures*—anatomical parts of the body
	Impairments—problems in body functions or structure
Functional limitation—limitation in performance at the level of the whole organism or person	*Activity*—the execution of a task or action by an individual
Disability—limitation in performance of socially defined roles and tasks within a sociocultural and physical environment	*Activity limitation*—difficulties an individual may have in executing activities
	Participation—involvement in a life situation
	Participation restriction—problems an individual may experience in involvement in life situations

Reprinted from *International Classification of Functioning, Disability and Health: ICF.* Geneva, Switzerland: World Health Organization, 2001, with permission of the World Health Organization.

> Nagi's disablement model has its origins in the early 1960s as part of a study of disability commissioned for the Social Security Administration (SSA) and his work on conceptual issues related to rehabilitation. Nagi designed a framework that differentiated between four distinct yet related phenomena that he considered basic to the field of rehabilitation. He referred to these as active pathology, impairment, functional limitation, and disability. His conceptual framework has become known as Nagi's disablement model.
>
> Jette, 2006

The World Health Assembly developed a common language and framework to understand and describe similar concepts of rehabilitation. The WHO's model of the International Classification of Impairments, Disabilities and Handicaps (ICIDH) (Jette, 2006) was completed in the early 1980s and differentiated health conditions into *impairments, disabilities,* and *handicaps.* Each model works to try to provide a language and a structure to define disablement (Figure 1.2).

The WHO model, currently known as the International Classification of Functioning Disability and Health (ICF), was not endorsed by the World Health Assembly at the United Nations until 2001, after major revisions from the initial document were made. The intent in the development of the ICF as a disablement model was to provide professionals in the field of rehabilitation medicine a universal, standardized disablement language. One of its goals is to provide a scientific basis for understanding and studying health and health-related disability throughout the world. This common language was designed to help with research, care, and provision of services throughout the world.

RESEARCH

This is an exciting time for research in rehabilitation. Many challenging unanswered questions need to be resolved. It is always a challenge to conduct a well-designed study, and in rehabilitation, there are several added hurdles. First, there are many team members with overlapping responsibilities. Second, there are many types of disabilities and a multitude of different treatments occurring simultaneously (e.g., surgical, pharmaceutical, various

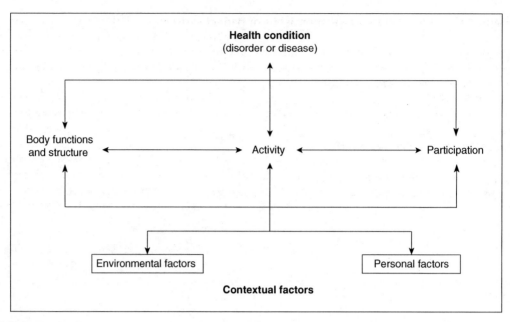

FIGURE 1.2   The International Classification of Functioning, Disability and Health (ICF). Reprinted from *International Classification of Functioning, Disability and Health: ICF*. Geneva, Switzerland: World Health Organization, 2001, with permission of the World Health Organization.

therapies, and medical management). In addition, it is also difficult to isolate how much of an impact rehabilitation has versus the effect of time alone on recovery.

Length of stay defines how long a patient remains in the hospital. Currently, there is a lack of good quality scientific data to show what the ideal length of stay should be to most efficiently benefit individuals with various conditions. A patient's progress and change in functional status give important individual information when determining length of stay. However, the ideal length of stay for various conditions and presentations is largely unknown.

Until optimal length of stay data are clearly delineated, it is likely that inpatient rehabilitation lengths of stay will continue to decrease. Whereas it is certainly initially less costly to have shorter lengths of stays, it remains unclear whether patients receive maximum benefit or if an early discharge potentially leads to greater disability and cost over time. The current fiscal climate appears to beckon for continued length of stay reductions and this will likely continue until research can show that there is a point of diminishing returns.

Disease-specific research in rehabilitation also holds great promise. For example, what is the etiology of Parkinson's disease and multiple sclerosis? Can these and other conditions be prevented? If we understand the disease process better, we can develop more effective interventions or prevent them altogether. There are many exciting research questions to answer in the next decade. The answer to these and many other questions will have a profound influence on rehabilitation care and quality of life for generations to come.

A specific type of research relates to outcomes achieved by a group of patients receiving care from a defined group of health practitioners. Outcome data are becoming a more common means of assessing the effectiveness of health care including medical rehabilitation. Outcome measures allow an organization to measure its performance over time and compare its performance with others in the region and the nation.

Many types of outcomes, such as patient satisfaction, can be assessed. These data points are used to analyze how patients report their overall satisfaction with those health care professionals and organizations that provided their care. For example, Press Ganey ® is a popular and widely used patient satisfaction tool. This and other similar tools have been found to be valid and reliable and allow comparisons of patient satisfaction between medical centers throughout the country that use the same tool. However, one difficulty with these types of data is that they are obtained by patients voluntarily agreeing to complete a survey, which often includes a majority of those that are either highly satisfied or highly dissatisfied, potentially skewing the results.

Another commonly used outcome assessment is the Functional Independence Measure (FIM®), which measures patient's progress and burden of care. The FIM® is considered a PM&R industry standard and measures a patient's improvement (or regression) across several standardized domains such as length of inpatient rehabilitation, abilities in locomotion, transfers, dressing, bathing, cognition, and bowel and bladder function. FIM® data can be combined among specific diagnostic groups within a particular rehabilitation organization that can be compared with similar patients in other organizations. This type of benchmarking provides a means to compare the magnitude of outcomes a particular rehabilitation organization has on a specific group of patients against others in their immediate area, their state, or even the country. This information can then be used to highlight exemplary care or identify problem areas that may be addressed through quality improvement initiatives.

Outcome data have lead to a critical assessment of inpatient length of stay. Length of stay for inpatient rehabilitation has continually decreased over the last two decades. For example, in the early 1990s many patients had more than 30 days of continual inpatient care. Today, the average patient stays only 2 weeks. As mentioned previously, there is every indication that the length of stay will continue to decrease until acute rehabilitation organizations can show a shorter length of stay leads to a worse outcome as compared to a longer length of stay.

ACCREDITATION

The accreditation process is a systematic means of evaluating a program against specific standards from an outside body. During the accreditation process, an outside agency is hired to review either an entire medical center or specific programs within the medical center. There are several accreditation bodies that pertain to rehabilitation. Two of the largest and most renowned are the Committee for the Accreditation of Rehabilitation Facilities (CARF®) and the Joint Commission©.

CARF takes a consultative approach to accreditation and focuses primarily on the patient's experience. The CARF survey ensures the health and safety of the persons served (the term used to denote patients or clients) are maintained and that the persons served are benefiting from the service. CARF also looks to establish exemplary care by sharing best practice ideas and innovations across multiple rehabilitation centers. The CARF accreditation process is a systematic means of ensuring quality, value, and optimal outcomes (*CARF Medical Rehabilitation Standards Manual July 2010–June 2011*, 2010).

CARF surveys are voluntary in that each rehabilitation organization desiring accreditation must request it. Once requested, CARF provides a set of standards that must be met to become accredited and informs the organization in advance of when the survey will occur. All CARF surveyors are actively employed experts in the field. Numerous standards are analyzed in terms of conformance (meeting the intent of the standards). In addition, feedback is given to raise the level of quality of the program. One of CARF's tenements is transparency and the sharing of ideas and resources. Therefore, if an exemplary practice is being implemented in a medical center, CARF will ask permission to share this practice at a national conference and/ or other rehabilitation centers that may benefit from it. The goal of CARF is for organizations to achieve exemplary status where persons served are receiving maximal benefit from the services.

The Joint Commission has a larger scope and looks not only at the rehabilitation services of a medical center but the entire hospital as well. The Joint Commission will come unannounced to a facility and conduct an extensive and systematic review to ensure patient safety and quality of care.

The process of preparing for accreditation itself tends to improve quality. A detailed review of current practices and comparison to the standards outlined by the accreditation bodies helps to identify areas of deficiency and areas of strength in an organization.

The State Department of Health is a regulatory body with great scope and its own standards. The State Department of Health can come unannounced to conduct an investigation of a hospital or section of a hospital. This can be in response to a patient complaint, a patient procedure error, an unexpected medical error, billing inquires, part of a quality check, or other indicators that a particular state monitors.

NEW AREAS OF REHABILITATION AND CURRENT CONCEPTS

Assistive Devices/Technologies

Assistive devices and technologies such as wheelchairs, prostheses, mobility aides, hearing aids, visual aids, and specialized computer software and hardware improve mobility, hearing, vision, and communication capacities. With the aid of these technologies, people with a loss in functioning are able to enhance their abilities and are better able to live independently and participate in their communities.

In many low-income and middle-income countries, only 5–15% of people who require assistive devices and technologies have access to them because their production is low and often of limited quality. There is a scarcity of personnel trained to manage the provision of such devices and technology, especially at the provincial and district levels. In many settings, where access might be possible, costs are prohibitive (Eldi & Parkin, 2005).

The Assistive Technology Act of 1998, defines these devices as "any item, piece of equipment, or produce system, whether acquired commercially, modified, or customized, that is used to increase, maintain, or improve the functional capabilities of individuals with disabilities" (Eldi & Parkin, 2005). Accessing this equipment and technology is often a critical component to successfully reintegrating many individuals to their communities, home, school, and work lives.

> The Convention on the Rights of Persons with Disabilities (Articles 20 and 26), The World Health Assembly resolution WHA58.23, and the United Nations Standard Rules on the Equalization of Opportunities for Persons with Disabilities all highlight the importance of assistive devices. States are requested to promote access to assistive devices and technologies at an affordable cost and facilitate training for people with disabilities and professionals and staff working in habilitation and rehabilitation services. (www.who.int/violence_injury_prevention, 2009b)

DISASTERS, DISABILITY, AND REHABILITATION

"Disasters have an impact on disability, by disproportionately affecting persons with existing disabilities and by creating a new generation of persons with disabilities who will be in need of rehabilitation services. In settings where resources are limited, the impact of disasters on these groups of people can be long term and far reaching" (World Health Organization, 2005). Local and institutional emergency preparedness has become more of a recognized need, in which rehabilitation professionals must be actively involved.

As these issues arise, the impact on individuals with disabilities can be addressed by rehabilitation professionals who are readily available to aide them. Some issues preferentially affecting those with a disability during a disaster may include the following:

■ Persons with disabilities are often more at risk of injury or abandonment

■ Many persons with disabilities lose their assistive devices, including artificial limbs, crutches, hearing aids, and glasses.

Rehabilitation infrastructure is often disrupted during a disaster because care providers are often diverted, cannot reach the individuals in need whom they care for, or are injured themselves. Therefore, individuals with special needs are left in even greater need.

Future of Rehabilitation

It is difficult to predict the future of rehabilitation but trends that are apparent today are likely to change the landscape of future practice. It is clear, for example, that there will be a greater demand for provision of care that is based on scientific evidence, as third-party payers are increasingly demanding proof of treatment efficacy. It will also become necessary to clearly demonstrate the optimal time period for rehabilitation, otherwise length of treatment will likely continue to decrease. In addition, acute inpatient rehabilitation is labor intensive with many disciplines providing care. Unless it can be shown that more team members with specific skills sets can improve outcomes it is unlikely that the model will remain the way it is (Strasser, 1997).

However, there is hope and many exciting new initiatives are taking hold. For example, safe patient handling programs are a new frontier for rehabilitation. Rehabilitation professionals often have a high rate of injury secondary to the physical tasks required to assist disabled patients (e.g., lifting patients and helping them move). One way of improving this is by using specialized equipment to lift and move patients without the risk of injury to the staff. This initiative has benefits for patients as well. Some medical centers are using ceiling harnesses to safely keep patients upright, which also allows safe, early ambulation and mobilization. The patients who would normally take several staff members to walk with are now able to bear weight and practice functional skills without the risk of injury from a fall.

Robotics is an area that has seen tremendous growth recently. The implantation of cerebral electrodes in the patient with a spinal cord injury is being studied now with great promise to decrease the burden of care on themselves and their support systems (Gelfman et al., 1997). Prosthetic limbs have also seen tremendous advancements thanks in large part to new computer-controlled technology that can readily adapt to a changing environment and the unique demands of various situations (Blakeslee, 2009).

After thousands of years of slow advancement, rehabilitation has recently shown tremendous growth. The rehabilitation team is active in many different models throughout the world today. Patients are benefiting from advancing technologies, accrediting bodies, research studies, and the use of a common language. Rehabilitation is a field rich with history, exciting in the moment, and full of possibilities.

REFERENCES

Blakeslee, S. (2009, July 20). Researchers train minds to move matter. *The New York Times*, p. 6.

Brorson, S. (2009). Management of fractures of the humerus in ancient Egypt, Greece and Rome. *Clinical Orthopaedics and Related Research, 467*, 1907–1914.

CARF Medical Rehabilitation Standards Manual July 2010–June 2011. (2010). Tucson, Arizona: Commission on Accreditation of Rehabilitation Facilities.

Donovan, W. H. (2007). Spinal cord injury—past, present and future. *The Journal of Spinal Cord Medicine, 30*, 85–100.

Eldi, H., & Parkin, C. (2005). *Expanding assistive technology services for the departments of physical therapy and occupational therapy at NYU Medical Center*. Unpublished manuscript.

Folz, T. J., Opitz, J. L., Peters, D. J., & Gelfman, R. (1997). The history of physical medicine and rehabilitation as recorded in the diary of Dr. Frank Krusen: Part 2. Forging ahead (1943–1947). *Archives of Physical Medicine & Rehabilitation, 78*, 446–450.

Gelfman, R., Peters, D. J., Opitz, J. L., & Folz, T. J. (1997). The history of physical medicine and rehabilitation as recorded in the diary of Dr. Frank Krusen: Part 3. Consolidating the position (1948–1953) *Archives of Physical Medicine & Rehabilitation, 78,* 556–561.

Haig, A. J., Nagy, A., Lebreck, D. B., & Stein, G. L. (1995). Outpatient planning for persons with physical disabilities: A randomized prospective trial of physiatrist alone versus a multidisciplinary team. *Archives of Physical Medicine and Rehabilitation, 76,* 341–348.

Jette, A. M. (2006). Toward a common language for function, disability, and health. *Physical Therapy, 86,* 726–734.

Keith, R. (1991). The comprehensive treatment team in rehabilitation. *Archives of Physical Medicine and Rehabilitation, 72,* 269–274.

Melvin, J. L. (1980). Interdisciplinary and multidisciplinary activities and the ACRM. *Archives of Physical Medicine & Rehabilitation, 61,* 379–380.

Ohry, A. (2004). Clinical commentary—people with disabilities before the days of modern rehabilitation medicine: Did they pave the way? *Disability & Rehabilitation, 26,* 546–548.

Opitz, J. L., Folz, T. J., Gelfman, R., & Peters, D. J. (1997). The history of physical medicine and rehabilitation as recorded in the diary of Dr. Frank Krusen: Part 1. gathering momentum (the years before 1942). *Archives of Physical Medicine & Rehabilitation, 78,* 442–445.

Peters, D. J., Gelfman, R., Folz, T. J., & Opitz, J. L. (1997). The history of physical medicine and rehabilitation as recorded in the diary of Dr. Frank Krusen: Part 4. Triumph over adversity (1954–1969). *Archives of Physical Medicine & Rehabilitation, 78,* 562–565.

Rusk, H.A. (1977). *A World to Care For – The Autobiography of Howard A. Rusk, M.D.* Random House, Inc. and the Reader's Digest Association, Inc. New York

Strasser, D. C. (1997). Linking treatment to outcomes through teams: Building a conceptual model of rehabilitation effectiveness. *Topics in Stroke Rehabilitation, 4,* 15–27.

World Health Organization. (2005). *Disability and rehabilitation WHO action plan 2006–2011.* Retrieved 2009, from www.who.int/disabilities/publications/en/index

www.barackobama.com. (2009a).

www.who.int/violence_injury_prevention. (2009b).

2

Disabling Conditions Seen in AIDS and HIV Infection

Jennifer Sayanlar, DO, Fran R. Wallach, MD, and Adam B. Stein, MD

A clinician should view human immunodeficiency virus (HIV) infection as a spectrum of illness ranging from the primary infection to a relatively asymptomatic stage that in turn progresses to an advanced stage known as the acquired immunodeficiency syndrome (AIDS). HIV is caused by one of two human retroviruses HIV-1 or HIV-2. HIV-1 is the more common causal agent worldwide and tends to lead to more rapid immune deficiency. Both viruses can be transmitted through sexual exposure, through contact with blood or other body fluids, vertically from mother to child, or via breast milk.

The Centers for Disease Control and Prevention estimate that there are approximately 1.1 million people living with HIV/AIDS in the United States, with more than 50,000 new infections occurring annually (Bradley & Verma, 1996). Major risk groups continue to be men who have sex with men and injection drug users, but high-risk heterosexual contacts accounted for 32% of transmitted HIV infections in 2007 (CDC, 2009). The burden of HIV infections falls disproportionally on minority populations, with African Americans comprising 51% of the total cases, on the basis of the 2007 data.

The hallmark of HIV disease is a profound immunodeficiency resulting from progressive quantitative and qualitative deficiency in the subset of T lymphocytes known as T-helper, or $CD4^+$, cells. Virtually any cell in the body that expresses the CD4 molecule on its cell surface can get infected with the HIV virus, although two major coreceptors, CCR5 and CXCR4, need also to be present to promote efficient HIV entry into the T cell.

Laboratory diagnosis of HIV infection is usually accomplished by detecting HIV antibodies using a highly sensitive enzyme immunoassay (EIA) and a confirmatory Western blot test that detects antibodies to HIV antigens of specific molecular weights. With the exception of patients who may be presenting with very early HIV infection, prior to the development of HIV antibodies, the combination of a positive EIA and confirmatory Western blot is considered the gold standard for the diagnosis of HIV infection.

For HIV-infected patients, measurement of the $CD4^+$ T-cell count and the level of plasma HIV RNA replication (also known as their viral load) are considered as part of routine evaluation and monitoring. The $CD4^+$ T-cell count provides information about the present immunological status of the patient, with the viral load predicting the likely future immunological health of the patient. More specifically, CD4 counts will help prognosticate which complications an infected individual is at greatest risk of developing, along with guiding the use of available prophylactic medications to help prevent infections. The viral load is also used to assess a patient's adherence to and the effectiveness of a given antiretroviral regimen. The goal of therapy is to maximally suppress the measurable plasma HIV to below the lower limit of detection of the viral load assay.

A complete discussion of the clinical manifestations of HIV infection is beyond the scope of this chapter, but severe and disabling conditions associated with HIV become more common as the patient's CD4 count declines as the illness progresses. The key elements in treating symptomatic complications of HIV disease are simultaneously achieving control of HIV replication through the use of combination antiretroviral therapy and implementing therapies directed at curing or mitigating the disabling HIV-associated conditions.

The remainder of this chapter will describe and discuss specific conditions that may create disability in persons infected with HIV.

PERIPHERAL NEUROPATHIES

It is estimated that nearly one third of people with HIV/AIDS experience some degree of peripheral nerve damage. Peripheral neuropathy is the most common neurological complication in these patients. For patients with HIV/AIDS, peripheral neuropathy can be caused by the virus itself, by medications used in the treatment of HIV/AIDS, or as a result of opportunistic infections. The symptoms of peripheral neuropathy that patients usually experience include uncomfortable sensations that are often described as burning, stiffness, prickling, tingling, or numbness. Patients often note a loss of feeling in the toes and soles of the feet. Sometimes the nerves in the fingers, hands, and wrists are also affected. This pattern of symptoms is referred to as a "stocking-glove" distribution, which is characteristic of peripheral neuropathy. Although relatively uncommon, symptoms may progress above the ankles or wrists; this indicates more severe nerve damage.

Distal Sensory Polyneuropathy

The most common form of peripheral neuropathy in this patient population is distal sensory polyneuropathy (DSP) (Cornblath & McArthur, 1988). There are two forms of DSP in HIV patients: one which is associated with the HIV disease itself and the other which is an antiretroviral-induced toxic neuropathy.

DSP, like most peripheral neuropathies, typically causes symptoms of painful or uncomfortable paresthesias. Symptoms may include allodynia, a painful response to a stimulus which is not typically painful, pins and needles sensation, burning discomfort, and/or numbness, which usually begins in the feet and progresses proximally into the legs. DSP has been found to be more common in the late stages of HIV disease when the disease is advanced and generalized wasting and cachexia may be present. The clinical presentation of antiretroviral-induced neuropathy is similar to that associated with DSP, directly related to HIV infection. The exact mechanism of DSP is not known; however, when associated with antiretroviral treatment, the underlying mechanism is thought to be related to mitochondrial toxicity caused by these agents. Among the pharmacological treatments, nucleoside analogues such as abacavir, didanosine, lamivudine, and stavudine are most commonly associated with this neuropathy. Loss of sensation may result, placing the affected individual at risk for injury to the skin of the affected area and related soft tissue or bone infections. In addition, loss of sensation places the affected individual at increased risk for falls and related injuries.

With regard to treatment, the practitioner should search for nutritional or metabolic deficiencies as these may contribute to the development of neuropathy. Treatment is primarily symptomatic and may include various medications to dampen the intensity of the uncomfortable sensations. These include medications such as tricyclic antidepressants, anticonvulsants, and other typical and atypical pain medications. Experimentally, pathogenesis-based approaches have shown promising results, such as highly active antiretroviral therapy (HAART) (Dwyer,

Mayer, & Lee, 1992). Recombinant human nerve growth factor has also been used experimentally with significant improvement in patients' pain (Engsig et al., 2009).

Necrotizing Vasculitis–Associated Neuropathy

Necrotizing vasculitis has been described in patients with HIV (Garstang, 2002). This condition is an immunologically induced process causing an inflammatory reaction and necrosis in the vasa nervorum, the blood vessels that nourish the peripheral nerves. The resulting clinical syndromes may include a distal symmetrical neuropathy or a mononeuritis multiplex, which results from damage to multiple individual nerves. Distal neuropathy, the most common clinical manifestation of vasculitic neuropathy, is usually painful and associated with weight loss and myalgia. CD4 counts are usually below 600/ml. This type of neuropathy is relatively rare and affects 0.1–0.3% of patients with AIDS. The clinical course can be monophasic; however, patients often have relapses. In many patients, there is an overlap with the presence of hepatitis B or C and cryoglobulinemia may be present as well. An evaluation for opportunistic infections associated with vasculitis such as cytomegalovirus (CMV), *Mycobacterium tuberculosis*, fungi, and parasites should be performed. The diagnosis of necrotizing vasculitic neuropathy is made by nerve and muscle biopsies, which reveal inflammatory cell infiltrates and necrosis of blood vessels. The therapy presents a particular problem as most immunosuppressive or cytotoxic agents regularly used to treat vasculitis are contraindicated in HIV, though corticosteroids, IV γ-globulin, and plasmapheresis have been used successfully in combination with antiretroviral treatment (Gonzalez-Duarte, Robinson-Papp, & Simpson, 2008).

MUSCLE DISORDERS

Severe muscle wasting from repeated infections, malignancy, malabsorption, and nutritional deficiency often accounts for weakness and disability seen in patients with HIV/AIDS. Such wasting is characterized by loss of lean body muscle mass and is associated with weakness. Although weakness may be associated with nervous system involvement from infections or immunologically mediated neuropathies in these patients, the possibility of a primary skeletal muscle disease should not be overlooked as several skeletal muscle disorders causing weakness have been identified in HIV-infected patients.

Myopathy

In a review of almost 5,000 HIV-infected patients, myopathy was present in 0.2% (Griffiths, 2004). The affected patients typically present with myalgias, muscle tenderness, and symmetric proximal muscle weakness with a predilection for the lower extremities. Patients may rarely encounter myopathy as the presenting manifestation of HIV infection, or it may occur in the setting of already established AIDS. Unlike neuropathy, the development of myopathy does not correlate with the degree of immunosuppression or the level of CD4+ T cells in the circulation.

HIV-associated myopathies include polymyositis and dermatomyositis, zidovudine (AZT) myopathy, rhabdomyolysis, nemaline rod myopathy, HIV wasting syndrome, myopathy associated with local neoplasm, and myopathy associated with local infection. Opportunistic muscle infections are encountered in untreated patients, whereas treated patients are more likely to develop inflammatory myopathies or drug-induced muscle involvement.

In early HIV infection, polymyositis and dermatomyositis or nemaline rod myopathy may occur. Polymyositis and dermatomyositis are immune mediated and are similar in presentation to patients who do not have HIV. Symptoms are usually generalized and include progressive muscle weakness that develops gradually and tends to affect proximal muscles such as those in the hips, thighs, shoulders, upper arms, and the neck. Nemaline rod myopathy is characterized by slowly progressive weakness and muscle wasting which may be autoimmune in nature (Haas et al., 2004). Later in the disease process, AZT-related myopathy may occur (Hall et al., 2008). Under this condition, patients present with proximal muscle weakness, myalgias of the calves and thighs, and easy fatigability. In the later stages of HIV disease, myopathy may be caused by a local infection or from neoplasm, such as lymphoma or Kaposi's sarcoma. In the setting of an infection, affected muscles become painful and swollen; fever and fatigue may be present as well.

Treatment of HIV-related myopathy is based on its etiology. Polymyositis and dermatomyositis are treated with corticosteroids. Patients who are unresponsive to steroids are often treated with an alternative immunosuppressant, such as azathioprine, cyclosporine, or methotrexate. Intravenous immunoglobulin treatments may help some people who are also unresponsive to other immunosuppressants. Patients with nemaline rod myopathy also respond to corticosteroid treatment (Horberg et al., 2008). In AZT myopathy, the offending medication is discontinued and alternative medications are substituted. Muscle enzymes and muscle strength usually return to normal within a few months after AZT is discontinued.

HIV-Associated Neuromuscular Wasting Syndrome

This syndrome includes neuromuscular clinical manifestations, such as progressive myopathy and a rapidly progressing sensorimotor polyneuropathy. In HIV-associated neuromuscular wasting syndrome (HANWS), patients present with progressive weakness, weight loss, and metabolic abnormalities such as elevated serum lactate and liver function tests. Neurological manifestations vary, as there is a spectrum of pathologies. Many patients exhibit features of demyelination clinically, which is caused by loss of myelin that surrounds the axons that normally increases the speed of nerve condition. However, the majority of patients have primarily axonal pathology, caused by direct involvement of the nerve. The axonal form of this syndrome has a worse prognosis than the demyelinating form. When elevated serum lactate develops in the setting of therapy with nucleoside reverse transcriptase inhibitors, there is a high likelihood that HANWS will develop. Systemic symptoms may include nausea, vomiting, abdominal distention, weight loss, and hepatomegaly (abnormal increase in the size of the liver), which are associated with a rapidly ascending motor weakness that develops over days to weeks. This syndrome may mimic Guillain-Barre syndrome, and it can result in respiratory failure and death (Griffiths, 2004).

The pathogenesis of HANWS in HIV-infected patients is likely to be multifactorial, and may result from a combination of mitochondrial and immunological mechanisms caused by HIV disease; though HAART therapy may contribute as well. Although a majority of patients present with axonal alterations, intravenous immunoglobulin or plasmapheresis could be considered as possible treatment options with the prevalence of demyelination. The treatment of HANWS is controversial, and important, because it is a potentially fatal syndrome. It is therefore important to interrupt HAART therapy in such cases. The reintroduction of HAART then becomes quite challenging; other treatment options should be considered.

SPINAL CORD DISEASES

Vacuolar Myelopathy

Vacuolar myelopathy is the myelopathy most commonly associated with HIV; it is a slowly progressive painless spastic paraparesis, with sensory ataxia and neurogenic bladder and bowel. Histopathologically, vacuolar myelopathy is characterized by prominent vacuolar changes in the ascending and descending tracts of the spinal cord, with a particular affinity

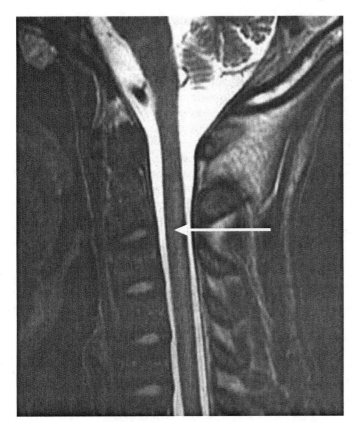

FIGURE 2.1 Sagittal T2-weighted MRI scan of the cervical spinal cord in a patient with vacuolar myelopathy. There is increased signal in the spinal cord noted by arrow. (Photo courtesy of Rona Woldenberg, MD.)

for the thoracic region (Figure 2.1). This type of myelopathy is only clinically symptomatic in about 5–10% of AIDS patients. Most patients who develop this disease die within 6 months of developing related symptoms. This typically occurs during the later stages of HIV infection, when other neurological problems may be present as well, including peripheral neuropathies, dementia, and opportunistic central nervous system and peripheral nervous system infections or malignancies. Vacuolar myelopathy is not typically fatal but rather a cause of significant disability (Jose, Saravu, Jimmy, & Shastry, 2007).

There is no specific treatment that has been proven to be effective for vacuolar myelopathy. Treatments are symptomatic and aimed at relief of typical symptoms of myelopathy including spasticity, neurogenic bladder and bowel, and improving function with multidisciplinary rehabilitation.

Infectious Myelitis

Infectious myelitis in patients with HIV may result from a variety of different etiologies. The involvement of the spinal cord in patients with HIV can be caused either by HIV itself or other opportunistic infections. These infections may be bacterial, viral, or fungal in nature.

Varicella zoster is one of the viruses associated with HIV in many cases. Varicella zoster myeloradiculitis in patients with HIV sometimes involves related encephalitis as well. Varicella myelitis usually involves the posterior horns of the spinal cord because the infection spreads from the dorsal root ganglia through the posterior roots. Patients often note burning pain and hypersensitive skin, which is then followed by the characteristic rash. The blistering rash follows a dermatomal pattern, which appears as a band-like pattern on the skin. The lesions will eventually crust over and heal later. The duration of a typical outbreak usually takes 3–4 weeks for full resolution. Motor weakness may accompany the typical sensory symptoms. Treatment includes pain medications as well as antiviral agents and oral corticosteroids.

Bacterial infections causing myelitis tend to be rare in HIV patients; the most common such pathogen is *M. tuberculosis*. Tuberculosis (TB) is the most common opportunistic infection worldwide affecting HIV-infected persons and is the most common cause of death in patients with AIDS. Involvement of the spine by TB is known as Pott's disease. The signs and symptoms of Pott's disease include back pain, fever, night sweats, weight loss, and focal neurological deficits determined by the level of spinal involvement and paraspinal masses. In adults, the lumbar region is the most commonly involved. Treatment includes long-term multidrug antituberculous therapy. Surgery may occasionally be indicated to prevent progressive neurological decline or spinal deformity. Overall, the prognosis for recovery is excellent with a recovery rate of more than 90% with appropriate treatment (Kalichman, Heckman, Kochman, Sikkema, & Bergholte, 2000).

HTLV-I Myelopathy

Human T-cell lymphotropic virus type I (HTLV-1) is a virus commonly found in the Caribbean and is transmitted through sexual, parenteral, and maternal routes. Risk factors for infection with this virus include intravenous drug use, promiscuous sexual activity, and the presence of HIV disease. HTLV-1 myelopathy is found in a small percentage of patients infected with the virus and causes pyramidal, spinocerebellar, and spinothalamic tract injury. The clinical manifestations of HTLV-1 myelopathy include a slowly progressive spastic paraparesis, segmental sensory abnormalities, urinary dysfunction, and back pain. HTLV-1 is diagnosed based on clinical suspicion and is confirmed with laboratory testing demonstrating HTLV-1 antibodies in the serum and cerebrospinal fluid (CSF). Magnetic resonance imaging of the spinal cord may show abnormalities in the periventricular white matter tracts. There is no long-term disease-altering treatment available for this disease, and potential treatments including corticosteroids, cyclophosphamide, AZT, and vitamin C have been ineffective. Plasmapheresis has also been tried with minimal success (Kalichman et al., 2000). The mainstay of treatment, as with vacuolar myelopathy, involves the symptomatic treatment of associated conditions, prevention of secondary complications such as falls, pressure ulcers, and urinary tract infections, and the rehabilitation interventions to maximize function and preserve independence for as long as possible.

BRAIN DISORDERS

Progressive Multifocal Leukoencephalopathy

Progressive multifocal leukoencephalopathy (PML) is a fatal viral disease characterized by progressive inflammation of the white matter of the brain at multiple locations. This disease typically occurs in patients who are immunocompromised, most commonly in patients with HIV or AIDS. PML is caused by a virus called the John Cunningham (JC) virus. Antibodies to the JC virus are actually found in a large percentage of the general population. In healthy individuals though, the virus typically remains latent and harmless. JC virus produces disease only when one's immune system is severely compromised. Research has shown that the effect of HIV on brain tissue enables viral activation in the brain, which results in the clinically detrimental effects. The symptoms and signs of PML result from the loss of white matter in many areas of the brain (Figure 2.2). PML is a demyelinating disease, which results in a slowing of nerve conduction. Patients experience symptoms that include weakness or paralysis, dysarthria, impaired vision, and cognitive dysfunction. Patients affected with PML typically deteriorate very rapidly; the average survival of HIV patients with PML is about 6 months. There is no known cure for PML; however, patients have been able to survive longer when treated with HAART (Power, Boisse, Rourke, & Gill, 2009). Other antiviral medications have also been studied as possible treatment options; however, more research is required in this area.

CMV Encephalitis

CMV belongs to the family of herpes viruses. CMV infection is endemic; the majority of adults with HIV have evidence of previous CMV infection when blood work for antibodies is performed. CMV encephalitis is a disease typically diagnosed based on clinical suspicion in HIV-infected patients who have a history of infection with CMV disease. These patients present with a clinically progressive encephalopathy, and imaging studies often reveal the evidence of ventriculitis. The diagnosis is then confirmed with polymerase chain reaction (PCR) testing and CSF cultures revealing presence of the virus. CSF-PCR is the diagnostic test of choice.

CMV encephalitis, when associated with HIV infection, can vary in the way in which it presents clinically. Patients who have ventriculoencephalitis suffer an acute onset and rapid deterioration characterized by confusion and lethargy. The cranial nerves may also be affected causing focal neurological deficits. Other medical problems that may be associated with CMV encephalitis include myelitis, retinitis, esophagitis, neuropathy, and adrenal insufficiency.

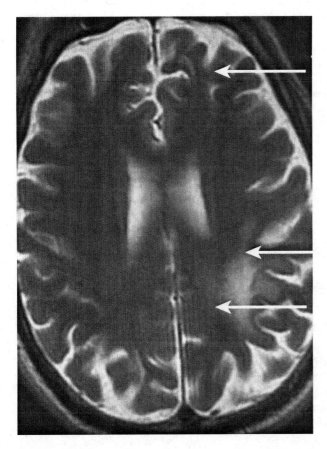

FIGURE 2.2 Axial T2-weighted image of the brain in an HIV-infected patient with progressive multifocal leukoencephalopathy who presented with behavioral changes as his initial manifestation of HIV infection. Arrows indicate multiple areas of abnormal signal change within the brain. (Photo courtesy of Rona Woldenberg, MD.)

If CMV encephalitis is not treated, it typically progresses to death in a period of days to weeks. The treatment consists of ganciclovir, foscarnet, or cidofovir. Patients are usually treated with induction doses initially and then continued on maintenance doses of medication (Robinson-Papp & Simpson, 2009).

Dementia

HIV-associated dementia produces a wide spectrum of disabilities that range from reduced work efficiency and quality of life to complete dependence for self-care. The HIV virus enters the central nervous system very early in the disease process. HIV-associated dementia is thought to arise from an HIV-induced defect in immune cellular signaling that produces neuronal damage in the brain (Said & Lacroix, 2005).

The clinical syndrome known as the AIDS dementia complex (ADC) is one of the most common and clinically important central nervous system complications of late HIV infection. ADC includes behavioral changes, cognitive dysfunction, or brain-related motor impairment, that is not directly attributable to a specific etiologic agent such as PML or CMV. It is quite common for patients with HIV to have deficits in cognition, including in areas such as memory, concentration, problem solving, and mood. These symptoms may be present in different stages of severity. Because ADC is a diagnosis of exclusion, it is important to consider multiple etiologic possibilities, including the possibility of cognitive impairment caused by medications. For example, Efavirenz has been associated with multiple CNS side effects, including impaired concentration (Simpson & Bender, 1988).

Prior to the advent of treatment with HAART, dementia was associated with a high mortality and was seen in many patients before their death. The incidence of dementia in HIV has declined with HAART treatment; however, the prevalence has remained the same, as persons with HIV live longer. Treatment with HAART has even been found to reverse some of the neurological deficits caused by HIV. HAART also delays the onset of dementia in HIV, though it does not seem to prevent the onset of cognitive impairment.

The treatment of HIV-associated dementia is with HAART combined with an aggressive treatment of related psychiatric disorders that may be present. For example, patients who present with depression along with dementia should be evaluated for the need for antidepressant medications. The commonly used antidepressants in patients with HIV include citalopram, escitalopram, fluoxetine, paroxetine, and sertraline. The treatment of concomitant depression not only results in improvement of mood but also better adherence to the patient's antiretroviral medication regimen (Simpson, Citak, Godfrey, Godbold, & Wolfe, 1993).

Psychological Conditions

The introduction of HAART changed the lives of patients with HIV dramatically. Before HAART treatment was available, patients with HIV suffered from extremely poor health characterized by a downward spiral of negative medical events, which dramatically affected life span, as well as quality of life. Patients often became very depressed as they began to lose their jobs and sources of income because of the severity of their illness. With the introduction of HAART, the life expectancy for patients with HIV has been prolonged, and their overall health has improved, which has obvious psychological benefits. Occasionally, the disease is less likely to result in disability. However, the importance of psychologists and mental health professionals remains critical in patients with HIV. Patients with HIV often experience social and psychological distress and require mental health intervention to address these important issues. Patients may suffer from various psychological conditions, including depression, anxiety, panic attacks, and adjustment disorders. The stigma associated with HIV infection alone is a psychological burden to those individuals with HIV and

AIDS. These patients, as a result, often have higher rates of suicide when compared with the general population. In one study that evaluated the psychological status of HIV patients in New York City, significantly more persons with HIV disease exhibited suicidal behavior as compared with patients with an unknown HIV serostatus (Wu, Zhao, Tang, Zhang-Nunes, & McArthur, 2007). Psychological support is therefore critical in HIV patients, and families and friends should be included as part of the support system. It is important for mental health providers to allow the patients to share their feelings and experiences in order to help them remain optimistic and maintain hope throughout the course of the disease. The different services that should ideally be available for these patients include crisis intervention, individual psychotherapy, family interventions and support, support groups, and treatment for those with substance abuse. Those who counsel these patients should have a good understanding of the different psychosocial aspects involved with HIV and the social aspects involved with HIV-associated disability.

REFERENCES

Bradley, W. G., & Verma, A. (1996). Painful vasculitic neuropathy in HIV-1 infection: Relief of pain with prednisone therapy. *Neurology, 47,* 1446–1451.

CDC. (2009). *HIV/AIDS Surveillance Report 2007.* Vol. 19. Atlanta: United States Department of Health and Human Services, CDC. http://www.cdc.gov/hiv/topics/surveillance/resources/reports/2007report/default.htm

Cornblath, D. R., & McArthur, J. C. (1988). Predominantly sensory neuropathy in patients with AIDS and AIDS-related complex. *Neurology, 38,* 794–796.

Dwyer, B. A., Mayer, R. F., & Lee S. C. (1992). Progressive nemaline (rod) myopathy as a presentation of human immunodeficiency virus infection. *Archives of Neurology, 49,* 440.

Engsig, F. N., Hansen, A. B., Omland, L. H., Kronborg, G., Gerstoft, J., Laursen, A. L., et al. (2009). Incidence, clinical presentation and outcome of progressive multifocal leukoencephalopathy in HIV-infected patients during the highly active antiretroviral therapy era: A nationwide cohort study. *Journal of Infectious Diseases, 199,* 77–83.

Garstang, S. V. (2002). Infections of the spine and spinal cord. In S. Kirshblum, D. I. Campagnolo, & J. A. DeLisa (Eds.), *Spinal cord medicine* (pp. 498–512). Philadelphia: Lippincott, Williams and Wilkins.

Gonzalez-Duarte, A., Robinson-Papp, J., & Simpson, D. M. (2008). Diagnosis and management of HIV-associated neuropathy. *Neurologic Clinics, 26,* 821–832.

Griffiths, P. (2004). Cytomegalovirus infection of the central nervous system. *Herpes, 11,* 95A–104A.

Haas, D. W., Ribaudo, H. J., Kim, R. B., Tierney, C., Wilkinson, G. R., Gulick, R. M., et al. (2004). Pharmacogenetics of efavirenz and central nervous system side effects: An Adult AIDS Clinical Trials Group Study. *AIDS, 18,* 2391–2400.

Hall, H. I., Ruiguang, S., Rhodes, P., Prejean, J., An, Q., Lee, L. M., et al. (2008). Estimation of HIV incidence in the United States. *JAMA, 300,* 520–529.

Horberg, M. A., Silverberg, M. J., Hurley, L. B., Towner, W. J., Klein, D. B., Bersoff-Matcha, S., et al. (2008). Effects of depression and selective serotonin reuptake inhibitor use on adherence to highly active antiretroviral therapy and on clinical outcomes in HIV-infected patients. *Journal of Acquired Immune Deficiency Syndrome, 47,* 384–390.

Jose, J., Saravu, K., Jimmy, B., & Shastry, B. A. (2007). Distal sensory polyneuropathy in human immunodeficiency virus patients and nucleoside analogue antiretroviral agents. *Annals of Indian Academy of Neurology, 10,* 81–87.

Kalichman, S. C., Heckman, T., Kochman, A., Sikkema, K., & Bergholte, J. (2000). Depression and thoughts of suicide among middle-aged and older persons living with HIV-AIDS. *Psychiatric Services, 51,* 903–907.

Power, C., Boisse, L., Rourke, S., & Gill, M. J. (2009). NeuoAIDS: An evolving epidemic. *Canadian Journal of Neurological Sciences, 36,* 285–295.

Robinson-Papp, J., & Simpson, D. M. (2009). Neuromuscular diseases associated with HIV-1 infection. *Muscle & Nerve, 40,* 1043–1053.

Said, G., & Lacroix, C. (2005). Primary and secondary vasculitic neuropathy. *Journal of Neurology, 252,* 633–641.

Simpson, D. M., & Bender, A. N. (1988). Human immunodeficiency virus-associated myopathy: Analysis of 11 patients. *Annals of Neurology, 24,* 79–84.

Simpson, D. M., Citak, K. A., Godfrey, E., Godbold, J., Wolfe, D. E. (1993). Myopathies associated with human immunodeficiency virus and zidovudine: Can their effects be distinguished? *Neurology, 43,* 971–976.

Wu, Y.-C., Zhao, Y.-B., Tang, M.-G., Zhang-Nunes, S. X., & McArthur, J. C. (2007). AIDS dementia complex in China. *Journal of Clinical Neuroscience, 14,* 8–11.

3

Alzheimer's Disease

Barry Reisberg, MD, Emile H. Franssen, MD,
Liduïn E. M. Souren, RN, MSN, Sunnie Kenowsky, DVM,
Imran A. Jamil, MD, Salman Anwar, MD, and Stefanie Auer, PhD

Evidence suggests that approximately 10–15% of community-residing persons in the United States, aged 65 and older, may be afflicted with Alzheimer's disease (AD) or closely related dementing illnesses of late life (Evans et al., 1989; Katzman, 1986). Presently, it is estimated that in the United States more than 5 million persons aged 65 and older and approximately 200,000 persons younger than 65 years have AD (Executive Summary, Alzheimer's Association, 2009). At the other end of the demographic spectrum, half of persons older than 85 years in the United States are believed to have AD. More specifically, in the United States, dementia, secondary to AD, in entirety or in part in the great majority of cases, affects about 30% of community-residing persons between 85 and 89 years of age and about 50% of those in the community between 90 and 94 years of age. For community-residing U.S. persons 95 years or older, nearly 75% are found to have dementia (Graves et al., 1996; Montine & Larson, 2009). Worldwide, it has been estimated that more than 24 million persons have AD (Ferri et al., 2005). The prevalence of AD approximately doubles every 5 years after the age of 65 in developed nations and every 7 years in developing nations (Larson & Langa, 2008; Lobo et al., 2000).

In the United States, AD is the fourth leading cause of death in the elderly, after heart disease, cancer, and stroke. AD is the single major cause of institutionalization of aged people in the United States and in many other industrialized nations in the world. Studies have indicated that a large majority of approximately 1.5 million residents in nursing homes in the United States manifest a dementia syndrome generally associated with AD (Chandler & Chandler, 1988; Rovner, Kafonek, Filipp, Lucas, & Folstein, 1986). In addition, the institutional or "semi-institutional" burden of AD, depending upon the precise definition of institutionalization, is truly much greater. Approximately 1 million persons in the United States reside in assisted living facilities, which are "depicted as residential settings for cognitively intact older people with functional limitations" (Kaplan, 2005). In a study of 22 such facilities in Maryland, approximately two thirds of these persons have been found to have dementia, and the great majority of these persons with dementia were found to have AD (Rosenblatt et al., 2004). These statistics may be applicable to the broader U.S. assisted living population. The dimensions of the institutional burden associated with AD are even more striking when it is noted that well under 1 million persons are in U.S. hospitals at any particular time.

Pre-AD conditions add further to the true burden of the disease. For example, approximately 15% of persons aged 65 and older in the United States have mild cognitive impairment (MCI)

(Executive Summary, Alzheimer's Association, 2009). This condition, which is a precursor of overt AD, is associated with a decrease in performance in complex occupational and social tasks (also referred to as executive activities), as well as a generalized decrement in cognitive performance and an increased susceptibility to delirium (Gauthier et al., 2006). MCI is also associated with a decrease in balance and coordination (Franssen, Souren, Torossian, & Reisberg, 1999). These MCI-related disabilities likely have considerable economic, social, and medical consequences, the dimensions of which are largely uncharted. In addition, a pre-MCI condition, termed subjective cognitive impairment (SCI), is now increasingly recognized as an early antecedent of eventual AD. Very subtle cognitive and functional changes appear to occur in this SCI stage of eventual AD, which have unknown consequences, apart from heralding an eventual decline to MCI and, ultimately, the dementia of AD (Reisberg, Shulman, Torossian, Leng, & Zhu, 2010). However, it is clear that large proportions of older persons take a variety of medications, nutriceuticals, vitamins, and other substances in an effort to mitigate their perceived symptoms, and the economic costs associated with this self-prescribing are very considerable (Reisberg, Franssen, Souren, Kenowsky, & Auer, 1998; Reisberg & Shulman, 2009).

The course of AD has been described in increasing detail over the past several years. The cognitive, functional, and behavioral concomitants at each stage of the illness can presently be described in detail (see Figure 3.1). The clinically observable symptomatology of AD dramatically changes in form from the earliest manifest deficits to the most severe stage; therefore, recognition and differentiation of the stages of this illness is imperative for proper diagnosis, prognosis, management, and treatment. Progressive cognitive changes that occur are manifest in concentration, recent memory, past memory, orientation, functioning and self-care, language, praxis ability, and calculation, among other areas (Reisberg, London, Ferris, et al., 1983; Reisberg, Schneck, Ferris, Schwartz, & de Leon, 1983). Characteristic behavioral symptoms are also a frequent component of AD (Finkel, 1996; Finkel & Burns, 2000; Kumar, Koss, Metzler, Moore, & Friedland, 1988; Lyketsos et al., 2000; Reisberg, Franssen, Sclan, Kluger, & Ferris, 1989; Rubin, Morris, Storandt, & Berg, 1987). These behavioral symptoms peak in occurrence at various points in the course of AD and subsequently recede in magnitude and frequency with the progression of the disease. A comprehensive view of the nature and progression of these cognitive, functional, and behavioral changes is critical for the optimization of residual capacity and the identification and management of excess disability in these patients.

An outline of global cognitive, functional, and behavioral changes in normal aging and progressive AD is provided in the Global Deterioration Scale (GDS) (Reisberg, Ferris, de Leon, & Crook, 1982), outlined in Table 3.1 and described in greater detail in the following sections.

GLOBAL DESCRIPTION OF NORMAL BRAIN AGING AND AD

Seven major, clinically distinguishable, global stages from normality to most severe AD have been described (Reisberg et al., 1982; Reisberg, Sclan, Franssen, et al., 2008). These stages and their implications are as follows:

Stage I: No Cognitive Impairment—Diagnosis: Normal
No objective or subjective evidence of cognitive decrement is seen. A significant proportion, although possibly only a minority, of persons more than age 65, fall within this category (Blazer, Hays, Fillenbaum, & Gold, 1997; Brucki & Nitrini, 2008; Gagnon et al., 1994; Jonker, Geerlings, & Schmand, 2000; Reinikainen et al., 1990; Tobiansky, Blizard, Livingston, & Mann, 1995; Wang et al., 2000). The prognosis is excellent for continued adequate cognitive functioning (Geerlings, Jonker, Bouter, Ader, & Schmand, 1999; Kluger, Ferris, Golomb, Mittelman, & Reisberg, 1999; Reisberg, Shulman, Torossian, et al., 2010).

Stage 2: Subjective Cognitive Decline Only—Diagnosis: SCI

Many persons older than 65 years have subjective complaints of cognitive decrement such as a subjective perception of forgetting names of people they know well or of forgetting where they placed particular objects such as keys or jewelry. These subjective complaints may be elicited by comparing the person's perceived abilities with perceptions of their performance 5–10 years previously.

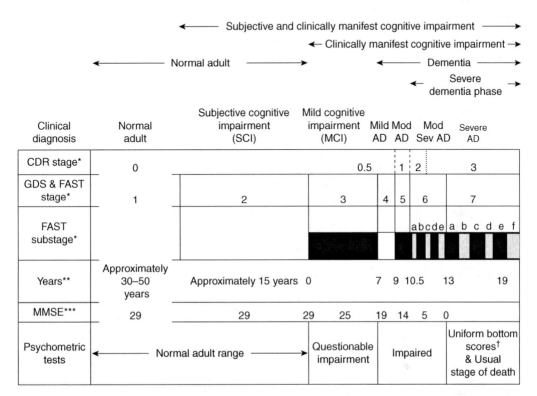

FIGURE 3.1   Typical time course of normal brain aging, mild cognitive impairment associated with Alzheimer's disease, and the dementia of Alzheimer's disease. AD - Alzheimer's disease; CDR - Clinical Dementia Rating (Hughes, Berg, Danziger, Coben, & Martin, 1982; Morris, 1993); FAST - Functional Assessment Staging (Reisberg, 1988; Sclan & Reisberg, 1992); GDS - Global Deterioration Scale (Reisberg et al., 1982; Reisberg et al., 1988); MMSE - Mini-Mental State Examination (Folstein, Folstein, & McHugh, 1975); Mod AD - Moderate Alzheimer's disease; Mod Sev AD - Moderately severe Alzheimer's disease. *Stage range comparisons shown between the CDR and GDS/FAST stages are based upon published functioning and self-care descriptors. **Numerical values represent time in years. For GDS and FAST stage 1, the temporal values are subsequent to the onset of adult life. For GDS and FAST stage 2, the temporal value is prior to onset of mild cognitive impairment symptoms. For GDS and FAST stage 3 and above, the values are subsequent to the onset of mild cognitive impairment symptoms. In all cases, the temporal values refer to the evolution of Alzheimer's disease pathology. All temporal estimates are based upon the GDS and FAST scales and were initially published based upon clinical observations in Reisberg (1986). These estimates have been supported by subsequent clinical and pathological cross-sectional and longitudinal investigations (e.g., Bobinski et al., 1995; Bobinski et al., 1997; Kluger et al., 1999; Prichep et al., 2006; Reisberg & Gauthier, 2008; Reisberg et al., 1996; Reisberg et al., 2010; Wegiel et al., 2008). The spacing in the figure is approximately proportional to the temporal duration of the respective stages and substages, with the exception of GDS and FAST stage 1, for which the broken lines signify abbreviated temporal duration spacing for this normal adult condition which lasts approximately 30–50 years. ***MMSE scores are approximate mean values from prior published studies. †For typical adult psychometric tests. Copyright © 2007, 2009 Barry Reisberg, MD. All rights reserved.

TABLE 3.1   *Global Deterioration Scale (GDS) for Age-Associated Cognitive Decline and Alzheimer's Disease (AD)*

GDS Stage	Clinical Characteristics	Diagnosis
1	No subjective complaints of memory deficit No memory deficit evident on clinical interview	Normal
2	Subjective complaints of memory deficit, most frequently in following areas: (a) forgetting where one has placed familiar objects (b) forgetting names one formerly knew well No objective evidence of memory deficit on clinical interview No objective deficit in employment or social situations Appropriate concern with respect to symptomatology	Subjective cognitive impairment
3	Earliest subtle deficits Manifestations in more than one of the following areas: (a) person may have gotten lost when traveling to an unfamiliar location (b) coworkers become aware of person's relatively poor performance (c) word and/or name-finding deficit become evident to intimates (d) person may read a passage or book and retain relatively little material (e) person may demonstrate decreased facility remembering names upon introduction to new people (f) person may have lost or misplaced an object of value (g) concentration deficit may be evident on clinical testing Objective evidence of memory deficit obtained only with an intensive interview Decreased performance in demanding employment and social settings Denial begins to become manifest in person Mild to moderate anxiety frequently accompanies symptoms	Mild cognitive impairment
4	Clear-cut deficit on careful clinical interview Deficit manifest in following areas: (a) decreased knowledge of current and recent events (b) may exhibit some deficit in memory of one's personal history (c) concentration deficit elicited on serial subtractions (d) decreased ability to travel, handle finances, etc. Frequently no deficit in following areas: (a) orientation to time and place (b) recognition of familiar persons and faces (c) ability to travel to familiar locations Inability to perform complex tasks Denial is dominant defense mechanism Flattening of affect and withdrawal from challenging situations occur	Mild AD

Continued

TABLE 3.1 *Continued*

GDS Stage	Clinical Characteristics	Diagnosis
5	Patient can no longer survive without some assistance	Moderate AD
	Patient is unable during interview to recall a major relevant aspect of their current life, e.g.:	
	(a) their address or telephone number of many years	
	(b) the names of close members of their family (such as grandchildren)	
	(c) the name of the high school or college from which they graduated	
	Frequently some disorientation to time (date, day of the week, season, etc.) or to place	
	An educated person may have difficulty counting back from 20 by 2s	
	Persons at this stage retain knowledge of many major facts regarding themselves and others	
	They invariably know their own names and generally know their spouse's and children's names	
	They require no assistance with toileting or eating, but may have difficulty choosing the proper clothing to wear	
6	May occasionally forget the name of the spouse upon whom they are entirely dependent for survival	Moderately severe AD
	Will be largely unaware of all recent events and experiences in their lives	
	Retain some knowledge of their surroundings; the year, the season, etc.	
	May have difficulty counting by 1s from 10, both backward and sometimes forward	
	Will require some assistance with activities of daily living:	
	(a) may become incontinent	
	(b) will require travel assistance but occasionally will be able to travel to familiar locations	
	Diurnal rhythm frequently disturbed	
	Almost always recall their own name	
	Frequently continue to be able to distinguish familiar from unfamiliar persons in their environment	
	Personality and emotional changes occur. These are quite variable and include:	
	(a) delusional behavior, e.g., patients may accuse their spouse of being an imposter; may talk to imaginary figures in the environment, or to their own reflection in the mirror	
	(b) obsessive symptoms, e.g., person may continually repeat simple cleaning activities	
	(c) anxiety symptoms, agitation, and even previously nonexistent violent behavior may occur	
	(d) cognitive abulia, e.g., loss of willpower because an individual cannot carry a thought long enough to determine a purposeful course of action	

Continued

TABLE 3.1   *Continued*

GDS Stage	Clinical Characteristics	Diagnosis
7	All verbal abilities are lost over the course of this stage	Severe AD
	Early in this stage words and phrases are spoken but speech is very circumscribed	
	Later there is no speech at all—only babbling	
	Incontinent of urine and feces; requires assistance bathing, dressing, toileting, and feeding	
	Basic psychomotor skills (e.g., ability to walk) are lost with the progression of this stage	
	The brain appears to no longer be able to tell the body what to do	
	Generalized and cortical neurological signs and symptoms are frequently present	

Apart from the occurrence of complaints of cognitive impairment with, what appears to be seemingly "normal aging," these complaints may also occur with other, frequently more serious common conditions in the elderly, notably, MCI, dementia and depression. Persons with comparatively benign complaints associated with this stage can usually recall the names of two or more primary school teachers, classmates, or friends and are oriented to the time of day, date, day of week, month, season, and year (although, of course, occasional minor errors may occur). They also display normal recall when queried about recent events and normal concentration and calculation abilities, for example, when asked to perform serial subtractions of sevens from one hundred. The terminology "subjective cognitive impairment" has been suggested for this condition (Reisberg, Prichep, Mosconi, et al., 2008). The American Psychiatric Association's *Diagnostic and Statistical Manual of Mental Disorders, 4th Edition,* refers to this condition under the more inclusive category of "age-related cognitive decline" (American Psychiatric Association, 1994). Clinical interview reveals no objective evidence of memory deficit, and there are no deficits in employment or social situations. However, physiological studies have shown clear, significant decrements in persons with these symptoms in comparison with age-matched subjects free of subjective complaints. For example, a recent study found an 18% decrement in cerebral metabolism in a particular brain region, the parahippocampal gyrus, as well as significant metabolic decrements in some other brain regions, in older persons with SCI in comparison with age-matched subjects who were healthy and free of SCI (Mosconi et al., 2008). Significant increases in urinary cortisol levels have also been reported in SCI subjects in comparison with age-matched control subjects (Wolf, Dziobek, McHugh, et al., 2005).

Current data from prospective longitudinal study indicates that these subjective impairments are in most cases a harbinger of subsequently manifest cognitive impairments after an average of about 7.5 years (Prichep et al., 2006; Reisberg & Gauthier, 2008). The total duration of this stage has been estimated to be an average of about 15 years prior to the onset of more overtly manifest impairments such as those associated with MCI (Reisberg, 1986; Reisberg & Gauthier, 2008). Although medications, nutriceuticals, and nostrums are frequently taken for these perceived deficits, largely in order to prevent further decline, there is no convincing evidence of their efficacy in treating the symptoms of this stage at the present time.

Stage 3: Mild Cognitive Decline—Diagnosis: MCI

This now widely recognized condition was first described, and subsequently named, in association with the GDS (Reisberg et al., 1988; Reisberg, Ferris, Kluger, et al., 2008). Various subsequent definitions of MCI have been proposed (e.g., Petersen et al., 1999; Petersen et al., 2001); however, current consensus definitions are consistent with the original GDS descriptions of the MCI entity (Gauthier et al., 2006; Winblad et al., 2004). MCI is a condition in which subtle deficits in cognition and cognition-associated functioning occur. Subtle evidence of objective decrement in complex occupational or social tasks may become evident in various ways. For example, the person may become confused or hopelessly lost when traveling to an unfamiliar location; relatively poorer performance may be noted by coworkers in a demanding occupation; persons may display overt word- and name-finding deficits; concentration deficits may be evident to family members and upon clinical testing; relatively little material may be retained after reading a passage from a book or newspaper; and/or an overt tendency to forget what has just been said and to repeat oneself may be manifest. A teacher who had routinely recalled the names of all of the students in his class by the end of a semester now may have difficulty recalling the names of any students. This same teacher may, for the first time, begin to miss important appointments. Similarly, a professional who had previously completed hundreds, perhaps thousands, of reports in the course of her lifetime now, for the first time, may be unable to accurately complete a single report. The person may lose or misplace objects of value. Mild to moderate anxiety is frequently observed and is an appropriate reaction to the awareness of impairment.

The prognosis associated with these subtle but objectively identifiable symptoms varies. In some cases, these symptoms are the result of brain insults, such as small strokes, which may not be evident from the clinical history, neurological examination, or neuroimaging findings. In other cases, symptoms are due to subtle and perhaps not clearly identifiable psychiatric, medical, and neurological disorders of diverse etiology. These symptoms are benign in many of the subjects who report them. However, in most cases, where other conditions have been ruled out in terms of etiology, these symptoms do represent the earliest symptoms of subsequently manifest AD. The mean true duration of this stage as a precursor of subsequently manifest mild AD has been estimated to be approximately 7 years (Reisberg, 1986). A review of 19 longitudinal studies found that the "overall conversion rate" (of MCI subjects per annum) was 10%, with large differences between studies (Bruscoli & Lovestone, 2004). They noted that self-selected clinic attendees had the highest conversion rates. In a rigorous 4-year prospective study of otherwise healthy subjects, fulfilling the exclusionary criteria for probable AD at baseline (except for the presence of dementia), MCI subjects declined at a rate of 17.8% per year to dementia, a rate quite similar to the 14.3% per annum change which would be anticipated from a stage which lasts approximately 7 years (Kluger, Ferris, Golomb, Mittelman, & Reisberg, 1999).

However, subjects commonly present with these symptoms well into this stage, and mild AD frequently becomes manifest after a much briefer period (Bowen et al., 1997; Daly et al., 2000; Devanand, Folz, Gorlyn, Moesller, & Stern, 1997; Flicker, Ferris, & Reisberg, 1991; Morris et al., 2001; Petersen et al., 1999; Tierney et al., 1996). Presently, no pharmacological agents have been approved for preventing further decline or in treating cognitive impairments in MCI.

Stage 4: Moderate Cognitive Decline—Diagnosis: Mild AD

Clinical interview at this stage reveals clearly manifest deficits in various areas, such as concentration, recent and past memory, orientation, calculation, and functional capacity. Concentration deficit may be of sufficient magnitude that patients may have difficulty subtracting serial 4s from 40. Recent memory may be affected to the degree that some major events of the previous week are not recalled, and there may be superficial or scanty knowledge of current events and activities. Detailed questioning may reveal that the spouse's knowledge of the patient's past is superior to the patient's own recall of his or her personal history, and the patient may confuse the chronology of past life events. The patient may mistake the date by 10 days or more but generally knows the year and the season. The patient may manifest decreased ability to handle such routine activities as shopping or managing personal and household finances.

Psychiatric features that may be prominent in this stage include decreased interest in personal and social activities, accompanied by a flattening of affect and emotional withdrawal. These behavioral changes are related to the person's decreased cognitive abilities rather than to depressed mood. However, they are frequently mistaken for depression. True depressive symptoms may also be noted but are generally mild, requiring no specific treatment. In cases where depressive symptoms are of sufficient severity to warrant treatment, a low dose of an antidepressant is frequently effective in reducing affective symptoms. At this stage patients are still capable of independent community survival if assistance is provided with complex but essential activities such as bill paying and managing the patient's bank account. Denial is the dominant defense mechanism protecting the patient from the devastating consequences of awareness of dementing illness.

The diagnosis of probable AD can be arrived at with confidence in this stage. It is possible to follow patients through the course of this stage, whose mean duration has been estimated to be approximately 2 years (Reisberg, 1986; Reisberg, Ferris, Franssen, et al., 1996). The cholinesterase inhibitors (donepezil, rivastigmine, and galantamine) have been approved for treating the symptoms of AD in this stage and appear to slow cognitive decline.

Stage 5: Moderately Severe Cognitive Decline—Diagnosis: Moderate AD

Cognitive and functional deficits are of sufficient magnitude that patients can no longer survive without assistance.

Patients at this stage can no longer recall major relevant aspects of their lives. They may not recall the name of the current president, their correct current address or telephone number, or the names of schools they attended. Patients at this stage frequently do not recall the current year and may be unsure of the weather or season. Concentration and calculation deficits are generally of sufficient magnitude as to create difficulty in subtracting serial 4s from 40 and possibly even serial 2s from 20. Patients at this stage retain knowledge of many major facts regarding themselves and others and generally require no assistance with toileting or eating, but they may have difficulty choosing the appropriate clothing to wear for the season or the occasion and may begin to forget to bathe regularly unless reminded.

Psychiatric symptoms in this stage of moderate AD are in many ways similar, although generally more overt, than those noted in mild AD. The patient's denial and flattening of affect tend to be more evident. True depressive symptoms, with mild to moderate mood dysphoria, may occur. Anger and other more overt behavioral symptoms of AD, such as anxieties, paranoia, and sleep disturbances, are frequently evident. Paranoid and delusional ideation peak in occurrence at this stage, with almost 75% of patients exhibiting one or more delusions. Such delusions as people stealing the patient's belongings or money, that one's house is not one's home, or that one's spouse is an impostor, are common. Aggressivity may include verbal outbursts, physical threats and violence, or general agitation. Depending on the nature and magnitude of the psychiatric symptomatology, treatment with an antidepressant or an antipsychotic medication may be indicated. When the latter is used, the dictum for the treatment of psychosis in the elderly applies: "Start low and go slow."

Patients who are living alone in the community at this stage require at least part-time assistance for continued community survival. When additional community assistance, such as day care or home health aides, is not feasible or available, institutionalization or a more protective environment such as an assisted-living facility may be required. Patients who are residing with a spouse frequently resist additional assistance at this stage as an invasion of their privacy and home. The duration of this stage is approximately a year and a half (Reisberg, 1986; Reisberg, Ferris, Franssen, et al., 1996). The cholinesterase inhibitor medications have been approved for the treatment of AD symptoms at this stage. Another class of pharmacological treatment, which has been shown to be efficacious in slowing the course of AD in this stage, is glutamatergic antagonist treatment. Memantine, the first and only medication in this more recently developed class of agents, is believed to reduce the glutamate-induced excitotoxicity caused by presynaptic neuronal injury. Memantine reversibly blocks glutamate transmission postsynaptically at the N-methyl-D-aspartate receptor. A pivotal study has indicated that memantine slowed the progression of AD in this stage and the subsequent stage by about 50% in terms of cognitive and functional outcomes (Reisberg, Doody, Stöffler, et al., 2003). A subsequent study has indicated that the effects of memantine remain robust and may even be enhanced, when memantine is given in combination with the cholinesterase inhibitor, donepezil (Tariot et al., 2004).

Stage 6: Severe Cognitive Decline—Diagnosis: Moderately Severe AD

Cognitive and functional deficits are of sufficient magnitude as to require assistance with basic activities of daily living.

Recent and remote memories are increasingly affected. Patients at this stage frequently have no idea of the date and may occasionally forget the name of the spouse upon whom they are dependent for survival but usually continue to be able to distinguish familiar from unfamiliar persons in their environments. Patients know their own names but frequently do not know their correct address, although they may be able to recall some important aspects of their domicile, such as the street or town. Patients have generally forgotten the schools they attended but recall some aspect of their early lives, such as their birthplace, their former occupation, or one or both of their parents' names. Concentration and calculation deficits are of such magnitude that patients with moderately severe AD frequently have difficulty counting backward from 10 by ones and may even begin to count forward during this task.

Agitation and even violence frequently occur in this stage. Language ability declines progressively so that by the end of this stage speaking is impaired in obvious ways. At this point in the late sixth stage, stuttering and word repetition are common; patients who learned a second language in adulthood sometimes revert, to a varying degree, to their childhood language; other patients may use neologisms, or nonsense words, interspersed to a varying degree in the course of their speech.

In this stage, emotional and behavioral problems generally become most manifest and disturbing, with 90% of patients exhibiting one or more behavioral symptoms (Reisberg, Franssen, Sclan, et al., 1989). A fear of being left alone or abandoned is frequently exhibited. Agitation, anger, sleep disturbances, physical violence, and negativity are examples of symptoms that commonly require treatment at this point in the illness. Low doses of so-called atypical antipsychotics may be useful for many patients. Side effects can be avoided if the medication is titrated upward with intervals of weeks between dosage adjustments. Present efficacy data on the treatment of these symptoms are most compelling for the atypical antipsychotic risperidone (Brodaty et al., 2003; De Deyn et al., 1999; De Deyn et al., 2005; Katz et al., 1999).

However, the dosage of antipsychotic medications given by clinicians and the titration schedules used by clinicians are frequently much higher and many times more rapid than those which are recommended. For example, for risperidone, the recommendation for treatment is as follows:

> In terms of pharmacological treatment of behavioral and psychological symptoms of dementia (BPSD) symptomatology, the clinical adage "start low, go slow" applies. For risperidone treatment, this rule translates into an optimal starting dose of 0.25 mg daily. Although clinical circumstances dictate the schedule of dosage titration, an optimal clinical response is not achieved for many weeks on any particular dosage of medication. Also, extrapyramidal side effects may not peak until a patient has been on a particular dosage of medication for as long as 6 months (Stephen & Williamson, 1984). Therefore, ideally, the clinician should endeavor to leave a patient on a particular dosage of medication for many weeks before further dosage

adjustments. The exigencies of particular situations, of course, will frequently not permit this time luxury in dose adjustments, and clinicians will frequently need to make rapid dosage adjustments. However, the clinician should also be prepared to adjust medication dosage downward as well as upward in response to particular patient needs and the emergence of side effects. After some months of treatment, a steady-state dosage of approximately 0.25–1 mg of risperidone daily is frequently effective in controlling BPSD symptoms. (Reisberg & Saeed, 2004)

In clinical trials of atypical antipsychotic medications in the treatment of BPSD in AD patients, dosages considerably greater than these recommended amounts titrated over a much more rapid time interval have been used. For example, in the study of Katz et al. (1999), dementia patients with BPSD were randomly assigned to treatment with placebo or 0.5, 1.0, or 2 mg/day of risperidone for 12 weeks. The mean age of the patients was 83 years, and 96% of the patients had moderately severe or severe AD as evidenced by Functional Assessment Staging (FAST) (Reisberg, 1988) scores of ≥6a and Mini-Mental State Examination (MMSE) (Folstein, Folstein & McHugh, 1975) mean scores of 6.6. When a meta-analysis was used to review the results of this and similar studies, an increased mortality associated with atypical antipsychotic medication used in dementia patients was found (Schneider, Dagerman, & Insel, 2005). This finding of Schneider et al. (2005) resulted in the U.S. Food and Drug Administration "black boxing" with a warning of "Increased Mortality in Elderly Patients with Dementia-Related Psychosis" antipsychotic medications used for the treatment of BPSD. This warning states in part that: "Analyses of 17 placebo-controlled trials (modal duration of 10 weeks), largely in patients taking atypical antipsychotic drugs, revealed a risk of death in drug-treated patients of ... 1.6 to 1.7 times the risk in placebo-treated patients" (PDR Network, 2009, p. 2683). The warning also notes that the increased mortality is due to varied causes, of which most were related to cardiovascular (heart failure or sudden death) or infectious (such as pneumonia) factors. The Schneider et al., (2005) study and subsequent studies (eg., Wang et al., 2005) have also found an increased mortality associated with the treatment of BPSD (psychosis) in dementia patients with so-called "typical" antipsychotic medications (e.g., haloperidol). In general, the risk of mortality has been found to be greater for "typical" than so-called "atypical" (e.g., risperidone) antipsychotic medications, although one major study found no difference between the two classes of antipsychotic medication in terms of mortality (Kales et al., 2007).

Unfortunately, even more recently published studies of antipsychotic medications in dementia such as the CATIE-AD Study Group report (Schneider et al., 2006) continue to begin with higher dosages of medication than those suggested by Reisberg and Saeed (2004). For example, the Schneider et al. (2006) published study (which was embarked upon in April, 2001) used a starting dose of risperidone of 0.5 mg.

In summary, with respect to the treatment of BPSD symptoms in dementia patients (primarily persons with AD), current consenses have concluded that treatment with antipsychotic medications, approached judiciously, continues to be a necessary option. In the words of a 2008 consensus "there is insufficient evidence to suggest that psychotropics other than antipsychotics represent an overall effective and safe, let alone better, treatment choice for psychosis or agitation in dementia" (Jeste et al., 2008).

In the moderately severe AD stage, the magnitude of cognitive and functional decline, combined with disturbed behavior and affect, make caregiving especially burdensome to spouses or other family members. They literally must devote their lives to helping patients who often can no longer even recall their name, much less appreciate in all the ways which may be desired, the kindness and care being provided. The caregivers' burden may be alleviated, for example, through regular participation in a dementia caregivers' support group, utilization of day care and respite centers for patients, or utilization of home health aides, either part-time or full-time. Clinical experience suggests that if behavioral disturbances are not successfully managed, they become the primary reason for institutionalization, and successful management of the disturbances can postpone this need. The mean duration of this stage is approximately two and a half years (Reisberg, 1986; Reisberg, Ferris, Franssen, et al., 1996). Memantine has been approved for treatment of AD in this stage and does appear to be useful in slowing the progression of cognitive and functional decline (Reisberg, Doody, Stöffler, et al., 2003; Tariot, et al., 2004; Winblad & Poritis, 1999). In 2006, donepezil became the first and still the only cholinesterase inhibitor approved for treating symptoms in this stage.

Stage 7: Very Severe Cognitive Decline—Diagnosis: Severe AD

A succession of functional losses in this stage results in the need for continuous assistance in all aspects of daily living. Verbal abilities are severely limited early in this stage, to approximately a half-dozen different intelligible words during the course of an average day, frequently interspersed with unintelligible babbling. Eventually, only a single word remains: commonly "yes," "no," or "OK." Subsequently, the ability to speak even this final single word is largely lost, although the patient may utter seemingly forgotten words and phrases in response to various circumstances for years after meaningful, volitional speech is lost. It is important to recognize that although the patient may no longer be capable of speaking, thinking capacity remains. Test measures originally developed for infants are able to demonstrate continuing thinking capacities of the patient (Auer, Sclan, Yaffee, & Reisberg, 1994). Although agitation can be a problem for some patients at this stage, psychotropic medication can generally be reduced as this stage progresses and ultimately discontinued.

Memantine has been approved for treating the symptoms (cognitive and functional) of AD patients in this stage. However, only one published memantine study has included these patients. That study (Winblad & Poritis, 1999) did investigate memantine's efficacy in institutionalized, primarily nursing home-residing patients. However, very few of the patients in the Winblad and Poritis study were in this final, severe AD stage. Therefore, there is very little current information regarding the role of memantine in this final stage of the disease.

Donepezil is the only cholinesterase inhibitor approved for the treatment of AD at this stage. The pivotal trial of Winblad et al. (2006) included 61 randomized and treated patients with a FAST stage of 7a or greater (25% of the study population). Hence, fully a quarter of the subjects in this pivotal trial had little or no remaining speech. In addition, 23 randomized and treated subjects were losing the ability to ambulate independently (FAST stage 7c). Hence, the most robust pivotal trial data for any medication in the treatment of persons in this final stage of AD at the present time is that available for donepezil treatment. However, even this trial had a requirement of a minimum MMSE score of 1 at entry. Since most stage-7 subjects, even in the early part of stage 7, have MMSE scores of zero (bottom), even this study of Winblad et al., (2006) included relatively cognitively less impaired final stage AD subjects (Reisberg, 2007).

Nursing homes or similar care facilities may be better equipped than spouses for the management of patients in this stage. If family members maintain the patient at home, round-the-clock health care assistance may be necessary to manage incontinence and basic activities of daily living such as bathing and feeding. Human contact continues to make a great difference in the quality of life of a patient, whether in the home or in an institution. A loving voice, attention, and gentle touch are important for the patient's emotional and physical well-being. As described subsequently, movement and physical activity are particularly important.

AD patients who survive until some point in the severe stage generally die from pneumonia, traumatic or decubital ulceration, or a less specific failure in the central regulation of vital functions. Although approximately half of all patients who reach this stage are dead within 2–3 years, patients may potentially survive for 7 years or longer in this final stage.

FUNCTIONAL CHANGES IN AD

Understanding the progression of AD from the standpoint of change and deterioration in functional abilities is of great importance to both clinicians and families. In terms of a primary diagnosis, as well as differential diagnosis, it is useful to determine whether the nature of the dementia is consistent with uncomplicated senile dementia of the Alzheimer type, because dementing processes associated with other causes frequently proceed differently from AD in terms of functional progression. Knowledge of the functional progression of AD can assist in this differential diagnostic process and, additionally, in identifying possible remediable complications of the illness. Furthermore, even the most severe AD patients can be assessed in terms of a functional level when all traditional mental status and psychometric assessment measures produce uniform bottom (zero) scores (Reisberg, Franssen, Bobinski, et al., 1996; Reisberg, Wegiel, Franssen, et al., 2006b). Functional assessment is presently capable of producing a detailed, meaningful map of the entire course of AD and, from the standpoint of physical rehabilitation, is extremely important in describing the AD patient's level of incapacity and areas of residual capacity.

Requirements for the management of AD fall into two categories: those relating to the patient and those relating to the primary caregiver. It is essential for the benefit of both that management advice be appropriate to each stage of the illness.

Functional Description of AD

A practical diagnostic and assessment tool, the FAST of AD (Reisberg, 1988; Sclan & Reisberg, 1992) permits identification of the stages of characteristic decline in functional activities in AD and their estimated duration (outlined in Table 3.2). Because of their utility, these FAST stages of AD are mandated for usage for certain purposes by the Center for Medicare Services in the United States, as well as in certain international jurisdictions (Health Care Financing Administration, 1998). These stages of functional deterioration in AD correspond optimally with the GDS stages described above. Table 3.2 indicates the approximate corresponding mean MMSE scores for each of the FAST stages and substages (Folstein et al., 1975). Research has indicated strong relationships between progressive functional deterioration assessed on the FAST and progressive cognitive deterioration in AD (e.g., Pearson correlation coefficients of ~0.8 or greater between MMSE and FAST scores have been reported [Reisberg et al., 1984; Sclan & Reisberg, 1992]). Therefore, the relationships shown between FAST and MMSE scores are approximations of likely findings in individual patients, although there is variability. Functionally, the late stages of AD can be subdivided into stages 6a–e and stages 7a–f. Consequently, a total of 16 functioning stages can be recognized, that describe in detail the characteristic changes which occur with the progression of AD. In uncomplicated dementia of the Alzheimer's type, progression through each of the functional stages described below occurs in a generally ordinal (sequential) pattern (Sclan & Reisberg, 1992).

Stage 1: No Objective or Subjective Functional Decrement
The aged subject's objective and subjective functional abilities in occupational, social, and other settings remain intact, compared with prior performance. The prognosis is excellent for continued adequate cognitive functioning.

Stage 2: Subjective Functional Decrement but No Objective Evidence of Decreased Performance in Complex Occupational or Social Activities
The most common age-related functional complaints are forgetting names and locations of objects or decreased ability to recall appointments. Subjective decrements are generally not noted by acquaintances or coworkers, and complex occupational and social functioning is not compromised.

When affective disorders, anxiety states, or other remediable conditions have been excluded, the elderly person with these symptoms can be reassured with respect to the relatively benign prognosis for persons with these subjective symptoms.

TABLE 3.2 *Functional Assessment Stages (FAST) and Time Course of Functional Loss in Normal Aging and Alzheimer's Disease (AD)*

FAST Stage	Clinical Characteristics	Clinical Diagnosis	Estimated Duration in AD[a]	Mean MMSE[b]
1	No decrement	Normal adult		29–30
2	Subjective deficit in word finding or recalling location of objects	Subjective cognitive impairment	15 years	29
3	Deficits noted in demanding employment settings	Mild cognitive impairment	7 years	24–27
4	Requires assistance in complex tasks, e.g., handling finances, planning dinner party	Mild AD	2 years	19–20
5	Requires assistance in choosing proper attire	Moderate AD	18 months	15
6a	Requires assistance in dressing	Moderately severe AD	5 months	9
b	Requires assistance in bathing properly		5 months	8
c	Requires assistance with mechanics of toileting (such as flushing, wiping)		5 months	5
d	Urinary incontinence		4 months	3
e	Fecal incontinence		10 months	1
7a	Speech ability limited to about a half-dozen words	Severe AD	12 months	0
b	Intelligible vocabulary limited to a single word		18 months	0
c	Ambulatory ability lost		12 months	0
d	Ability to sit up lost		12 months	0
e	Ability to smile lost		18 months	0
f	Ability to hold head up lost		12 months or longer	0

[a]In subjects without other complicating illnesses who survive and progress to the subsequent deterioration stage.
[b]MMSE = Mini-Mental State Examination score (Folstein et al., 1975). Estimates based in part on published data summarized in Reisberg, Ferris, de Leon, et al. (1989) and obtained in Reisberg, Ferris, Torossian, et al. (1992).

Source: Adapted from Reisberg, B. (1986). Dementia: A systematic approach to identifying reversible causes. *Geriatrics*, *41*(4), 30–46. Copyright © 1984 by Barry Reisberg, MD.

Stage 3: Objective Functional Decrement of Sufficient Severity to Interfere With Complex Occupational and Social Tasks

This is the stage at which persons may begin to forget important appointments, seemingly for the first time in their lives. Functional decrements may become manifest in complex psychomotor tasks, such as ability to travel to new locations. Persons at this stage have no difficulty with routine tasks such as shopping, handling finances, or traveling to familiar locations, but they may stop participating in demanding occupational and social settings. These symptoms, although subtle clinically, can considerably alter lifestyle. When psychiatric, neurological, and medical concomitants apart from AD have been excluded, the clinician may advise withdrawal from complex, anxiety-provoking situations. Because patients at this stage can still perform all basic activities of daily living satisfactorily, withdrawing from demanding activities may result in complete symptom amelioration for a period of years.

Stage 4: Deficient Performance in the Complex Tasks of Daily Life

Aspects of decreased functioning from former levels are apparent. At this stage, shopping for adequate or appropriate food and other items is noticeably impaired. The person may return with incorrect items or inappropriate amounts of a certain item. The individual may have difficulty preparing meals for family dinners and may display similar deficits in the ability to manage complex occupational and social tasks. Family members may note that the patient no longer is able to balance the checkbook, no longer remembers to pay bills properly, and may make significant financial errors. Persons who are still able to travel independently to and from work may not recall names of clients or details of their employment duties. Because choosing clothing, dressing, bathing, and traveling to familiar locations can be adequately performed at this stage, persons may still function independently in the community, although supervision is often useful.

Maximizing the patient's functioning at this stage is the goal of the family and health care professionals. Financial supervision and structured or supervised travel should be arranged. Identification bracelets, ID cards, or clothing labels with a name, address, and telephone number may be useful for unusually stressful situations where anxiety or other factors further impair the person's capacities.

Stage 5: Incipient Deficit in Performance in Basic Tasks of Daily Life

At this stage, persons with AD can no longer satisfactorily function independently in the community. The person not only requires assistance in managing financial affairs and marketing but also begins to require help in choosing the appropriate clothing for the season and the occasion. The person may wear obviously incongruous clothing combinations or wear the same clothing day after day unless supervision is provided.

At this stage, some patients develop anxieties and fears about bathing. Another functional deficit that frequently becomes manifest at this stage is difficulty in driving an automobile. The patient may slow down or speed up the vehicle inappropriately or may go through a stop sign or traffic light. Occasionally, the person may have a collision with another vehicle for the first time in many years. The person with moderate AD may be sufficiently alarmed by these deficits to voluntarily discontinue driving. Sometimes, however, intervention and coercion are necessary from family members or even from the patient's physician or licensing authorities. A useful strategy for the physician is to arrange for an automobile driving retest.

It is important that functional abilities be maximized. Persons at this stage are still capable of putting on their clothing with minimal guidance once it has been selected for them. They are also capable of bathing and washing themselves, even though they may have to be cajoled into performing these activities. A supportive environment that provides adequate stimulation, in addition to adequate protection, is desirable. It is important that the person continue to engage in and practice skills in which they remain capable.

Stage 6: Decreased Ability to Dress, Bathe, and Toilet Independently

Throughout the course of stage 6, which lasts for approximately two and a half years and encompasses five substages, increasing deficits in dressing and bathing occur. In addition to not being able to choose the proper clothing, early stage-6 patients develop difficulties in putting on their clothing properly (stage 6a). Other dressing difficulties include putting on street clothing over night clothing, putting clothing on backward or inside out, and putting on multiple and inappropriate layers of clothing. The patient may also have difficulty zippering or buttoning their clothing or tying their shoelaces. More overt dressing difficulties develop as this stage progresses and the patient requires increasing assistance in dressing.

A bathing difficulty that becomes apparent at this stage is a decreased ability to adjust the temperature of shower or bath water (substage 6b). Subsequently, taking a bath or shower without assistance becomes increasingly problematic, ultimately with difficulty getting into and out of the bath and washing properly. Fear of bathing may develop, combined with resistance to bathing. This fear of bathing sometimes precedes actual difficulties in handling the mechanics of bathing.

Later in the course of this stage, patients begin to have difficulties with the mechanics of toileting: initially, they may forget to flush the toilet, dispose of toilet tissue improperly, and clean themselves inadequately (stage 6c).

Subsequently, urinary incontinence begins (stage 6d), followed by fecal incontinence (stage 6e), both of which appear to be the result of decreased cognitive capacity to respond appropriately to urinary or fecal urgency. Assisting the patient to use the toilet often helps to forestall and remediate incontinence. Anxieties regarding toileting are frequently noted in stage 6c prior to the actual development of incontinence. Patients may go to the toilet repeatedly even in the absence of a true need for elimination.

Motor capacity deficits also become notable during stage 6. Walking becomes more halting and steps generally become smaller and slower, but the ability to ambulate is still maintained. Because orientation in space is affected, patients may approach a chair and sit down with greater difficulty. Patients may also require assistance in walking up and down a staircase.

Full-time home health care is frequently useful at this time, and it may be appropriate or necessary to discuss nursing home placement with the caregiver and family members. Management strategies and supportive techniques must be developed to assist the patient in bathing, dressing, and toileting, as well as in minimizing the emotional stress of the caregiver.

Stage 7: Loss of Speech and Locomotion

This final stage of AD is marked by decreased vocabulary and speech abilities. Speech becomes increasingly limited from a vocabulary of a half-dozen different intelligible, purposeful, and meaningful words (stage 7a) to at most a single distinguishable purposeful word that may be uttered repeatedly (stage 7b). Eventually, speech becomes limited to babbling, unintelligible utterances, and occasional, intelligible, random utterances.

Prior to the loss of ambulatory ability, patients may exhibit a twisted gait, take progressively smaller and slower steps, or lean forward, backward, or sideways while walking. Eventually, the ability to walk unassisted is lost with the progression of AD (stage 7c). It should be noted that after the loss of speech ability, the ability to walk is invariably lost. However, AD patients, for various reasons, especially excess disability, are susceptible to the loss of ambulation from the beginning of the final 7th AD stage, as well as subsequently.

Approximately a year after ambulatory ability is lost, the ability to sit up without assistance (such as lateral chair rests) is also lost (stage 7d). Subsequently, the abilities to smile (stage 7e) and to hold up the head independently (stage 7f) are also lost. At this point, babbling and grasping may still be observed, and patients can still move their eyes, although familiar persons or objects are apparently no longer recognized. Approximately 3–4 years after the onset of stage 7, generally after the loss of ambulatory ability, many patients die. However, some patients survive in this stage for 7 years or longer. Pneumonia, which is often associated with aspiration, is a frequent cause of death.

Full-time assistance at home or in an institution is a necessity at this stage, and as AD patients are increasingly well cared for, it is likely that more will survive to these final substages of the illness.

FEEDING CONCOMITANTS OF AD

Progressive changes in the ability to prepare meals and in feeding skills have been observed in AD patients and enumerated in accordance with the corresponding GDS and FAST stages (Reisberg et al., 1990). These "Feeding Concomitants of Alzheimer's Disease" are outlined in Table 3.3. The progression of these disturbances in meal preparation and self-feeding,

TABLE 3.3   *Feeding Concomitants of Alzheimer's Disease (AD)*

Stage[a]	Clinical Characteristics
1–2	No objective or subjective decrement in the ability to adequately prepare meals, order food and beverages in a restaurant setting, or in table etiquette
4	Decreased facility in preparing and/or serving relatively complex meals, and/or decreased facility in ordering food and beverages in restaurant setting
5	Decreased ability in preparing simple foods or beverages (e.g., coffee or tea); may occasionally make mistakes in eating food (e.g., improper use of seasoning or condiments)
6	(a) Occasional difficulty with proper manipulation or choice of eating utensils
	(b) Meat and similar foods must be cut up for the patient
	(c) No longer trusted to use a knife; may also eat foods that would have formerly been refused
	(d) No longer trusted to properly use a knife and decreased ability to use a fork, but can still properly use a spoon; may also display occasional misrecognition of dietary substances (pica)
	(e) Capable of going to the refrigerator or cupboard but has difficulty discerning and choosing food, may have difficulty chewing hard food
7	(a) Capable of picking up spoon or fork; will occasionally drop food or misutilize silverware (e.g., may attempt to drink soup or other liquids with a fork); capable of reaching for a cup when desirous of fluid
	(b) Must be assisted in actual feeding; generally, patients are not permitted to handle a knife or fork; may not be able to properly lift a cup
	(c) Can reach for and pick up food with hands; cannot properly pick up a fork or a spoon but can grasp a spoon or other utensil; must be spoon-fed, but can chew
	(d) Cannot distinguish foods from nondietary substances; will reach out for objects, including food

[a]Stages have been enumerated to be optimally concordant with the corresponding Global Deterioration Scale (GDS) and Functional Assessment Staging (FAST) stages in Alzheimer's disease.

Source: Reisberg, B., Pattschull-Furlan, A., Franssen, E., Sclan, S. G., Kluger, A., Dingcong, L., et al. (1990). Cognition related functional, praxis and feeding changes in CNS aging and Alzheimer's disease and their developmental analogies. In K. Beyreuther & G. Schettler (Eds.), *Molecular mechanisms of aging* (pp. 18–40). Berlin: Springer-Verlag. Copyright © 1988 by Barry Reisberg, MD.

as with the progression of deterioration in cognitive and functional abilities, appears to be characteristic of AD.

BALANCE AND COORDINATION

Although it is clear from the preceding description of functional losses in AD that balance and coordination are eventually lost with the progression of the illness process, these aspects are actually very early changes, coincident with the advent of MCI and mild AD. For example, a detailed study indicated that tandem walking, foot-tapping speed, hand pronation and supination speed, and finger-to-thumb apposition speed all decreased significantly in MCI subjects in comparison with normal elderly controls (Franssen et al., 1999). Additional decrements were noted in mild AD subjects.

Another study has demonstrated that complex motor and fine motor measures can be just as robust markers of MCI and mild AD as a cognitive psychometric battery (Kluger et al., 1997). These observations of motor and equilibrium changes in MCI and AD are consistent with neuropathological observations of robust clinicopathological correlations with cerebellar atrophy in AD (Wegiel et al., 1999).

RIGIDITY AND CONTRACTURES

In the latter stages of AD, rigidity becomes increasingly manifest (Franssen, Kluger, Torossian, & Reisberg, 1993; Franssen, Reisberg, Kluger, Sinaiko, & Boja, 1991). Initially, this rigidity is of a paratonic type, for example, elicited in response to an irregular motion of an extremity, such as an irregular movement of an elbow. Later, the rigidity becomes increasingly evident. Figure 3.2 depicts the emergence of paratonic rigidity in AD. Although infrequently manifest in patients with mild AD (i.e., GDS stage 4), approximately 50% of patients with moderate AD (GDS stage 5), 75% of patients with moderately severe AD (GDS stage 6), and virtually all patients with severe AD (GDS stage 7) manifest at least a mildly detectable form of paratonic rigidity. Figure 3.3 illustrates the methodology for the elicitation of this paratonic rigidity by the clinician.

One probable result of this increasing rigidity is the development of contractures (Figure 3.4). Contractures are irreversible deformities of joints, limiting range of motion. In a study by Souren, Franssen, & Reisberg (1995), a contracture was defined as a limitation of 50% or more of the passive range of motion of a joint, secondary to permanent muscle shortening, ankylosis, or both. Souren et al. found that contractures meeting this definition were present in 10% of moderately severe AD patients with incipient incontinence (i.e., AD patients at FAST stages 6d and 6e). In severe AD, contractures are very common. Forty percent of incipient averbal AD patients (FAST stages 7a and 7b) manifested contractures and 50% of incipient nonambulatory AD patients (FAST stage 7c) manifested these deformities. By late stage 7, that is, in immobile patients (FAST stages 7d–f), 95% of AD patients manifested these deformities. Furthermore, at all stages, when contractures occurred, they generally were present in more than one extremity. Specifically, the great majority of patients with contractures (69%) had contractures involving all four extremities. All but one of the 39 patients found to have contractures (97%) had at least two limbs affected. By limiting mobility, contractures predispose patients to further morbidity, such as decubital ulcerations. One third of the patients with contractures in the study of Souren et al. (1995) had decubital ulcerations, either noted by direct patient observation or in the patient's medical record.

There is evidence based upon patient observations that contractures may be prevented until very late in the course of AD by maintenance of patient activities, stretching, other movements, and, especially, specific range of motion exercises of all joints including the hands and fingers.

DIFFERENTIAL DIAGNOSTIC IMPLICATIONS OF THE CHARACTERISTIC FUNCTIONAL COURSE OF AD

Cognitive and functional deficits in patients with AD characteristically follow the progression outlined in the preceding sections. However, other disorders frequently associated with the presence of dementia do not necessarily follow this characteristic pattern. It has been observed that the characteristic pattern of functional loss in AD is useful in differential diagnosis (Reisberg, 1986; Reisberg, Ferris, & Franssen, 1985). Common functional presentations of non-AD dementing disorders are outlined in Table 3.4. For example, normal-pressure hydrocephalus (NPH) commonly presents with gait disturbance as the earliest symptom, antedating any overt cognitive disturbance. In NPH, this ambulatory disturbance is commonly followed by urinary incontinence. Only subsequently, after the advent of ambulatory disturbance and urinary incontinence in NPH, may cognitive disturbances become manifest. As summarized in Table 3.2, the sequence of functional loss in AD is very different. In AD, overt cognitive disturbance precedes urinary incontinence, which in turn precedes ambulatory loss.

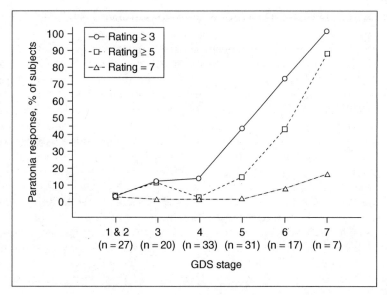

FIGURE 3.2 Percentage of subjects with increased paratonic rigidity in normal aging and Alzheimer's disease of progressively increasing severity. The graph depicts the percentage of subjects showing paratonia as a function of the Global Deterioration Scale (GDS) stage, using three different ratings of activity. Paratonic rigidity, defined as stiffening of a limb in response to contact with the examiner's hand and an involuntary resistance to passive changes in position and posture, was graded according to the amount of passive force necessary to elicit it. A rating of 1 denotes an absence of paratonic rigidity, whereas a rating of 7 indicates that minimal passive force is required for elicitation of the sequence. Further detail regarding the scoring procedure can be found in Franssen, E. (1993). Neurologic signs in aging and dementia. In A. Burns (Ed.), *Aging and Dementia: A Methodological Approach* (pp. 144–174). London: Edward Arnold. *Source:* Data and figure are from Franssen, E. H., Reisberg, B., Kluger, A., Sinaiko, E., & Boja, C. (1991). Cognition independent neurologic symptoms in normal aging and probable Alzheimer's disease. *Archives of Neurology, 48,* 148–154.

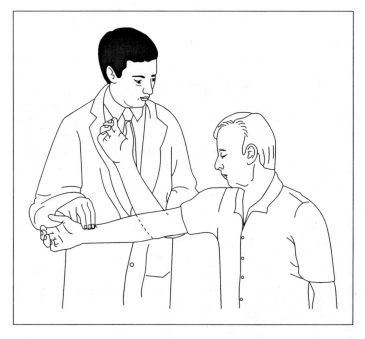

FIGURE 3.3 In the final stages of Alzheimer's disease, patients manifest increasing rigidity. Rigidity is evident to the examiner in the Global Deterioration Scale (GDS) stage 7 patient upon passive range of motion of major joints such as the elbow. Copyright © 1999 Barry Reisberg, MD.

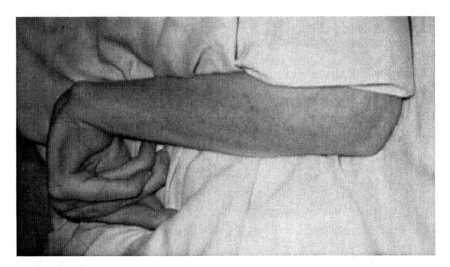

FIGURE 3.4   A stage 7 Alzheimer's disease patient with contractures of the left hand and fingers. Copyright © 1997 Liduïn Souren, RN, MSN.

Creutzfeldt-Jacob disease is a rare form of rapidly progressive dementia that presents with ambulatory disturbance as the earliest symptom in approximately one third of cases. In AD, the ambulatory disturbance is a much later event. The two conditions also may be distinguished temporally. The course of AD extends over many years, as outlined in Table 3.2, and is frequently much slower than the relatively rapid course of the acute and subacute forms of Creutzfeldt-Jacob disease.

Multi-infarct dementia, or dementia associated with an overt, large infarction, may produce speech disturbance as the only symptom. Alternatively, the infarction may produce urinary incontinence as the major overt manifestation. Commonly, ambulatory loss may be the major sequela of a stroke. Clearly, the evolution of functional losses in AD follows a very different and much more stereotyped pattern (as outlined in Table 3.2). As shown in Table 3.4, the evolution of functional disturbance in dementia associated with multiple infarctions may follow a very different course from that which is characteristic of AD.

Depression is a psychiatric disturbance associated with mood dysphoria and other symptoms. Among these other symptoms are negativity and subjective complaints of cognitive impairment. Occasionally, the depression produces a dementia-like syndrome that is potentially reversible when the underlying mood disturbance is treated. This potentially reversible dementia syndrome of depression, formerly called pseudodementia, does not necessarily follow the functional course outlined in Table 3.2. For example, as outlined in Table 3.4, depression may be accompanied by a refusal to dress and bathe as a result of the patient's negativity. However, the patient may be able to point to exactly the clothes he or she wishes to wear. In AD, the loss of ability to pick out clothing properly precedes the loss of ability to put on one's clothing properly.

As outlined in Table 3.4, dementia associated with hyponatremia or other electrolyte disturbances, CNS metastases, and other conditions all may follow a course markedly at variance with the course of AD as outlined in the FAST.

In a patient with AD, a variety of coexisting conditions may result in functional disturbances that may occur prematurely or nonordinally (i.e., out of sequence) in terms of the FAST predictions. Examples of conditions that may be associated with premature (i.e., nonordinal) functional losses in an AD patient are outlined in Table 3.5. For example, if an AD patient is at GDS stage 5 and FAST stage 5 and develops urinary incontinence, this incontinence may,

TABLE 3.4 *Examples of the Order of Functional Loss in Non-Alzheimer Disorders Associated With Progressive or Gradual Onset of Dementia and Characteristic FAST Order of Functional Loss in AD*

	Functional Loss in Non-Alzheimer Disorders			FAST AD Distinctions	
Disorder	*Pathology or Presumed Etiology*	*Example of the Order of Functional Loss in Non-AD Disorder[a]*	*Equivalent FAST Stage*	*Order of Functional Loss in AD per FAST*	*FAST Stages in AD*
Normal-pressure hydrocephalus	Dilated cerebral ventricles	1. Gait disturbance	7c	1. Loss of ability to perform complex tasks	4
		2. Urinary incontinence	6d	2. Urinary incontinence	6d
		3. Loss of ability to perform complex tasks	4	3. Ambulatory (gait) disturbance	7c
Creutzfeldt-Jakob disease	Prion	1. Gait disturbance	7c	1. Loss of ability to perform complex tasks	4
		2. Loss of ability to perform complex tasks	4	2. Gait (ambulatory) disturbance	7c
Multi-infarct dementia	Multiple cerebral infarctions	1. Loss of speech	7a–7b	1. Loss of ability to perform complex tasks	4
		2. Loss of urinary continence	6d	2. Loss of ability to pick out clothing properly	5
		3. Loss of ability to put on clothing	6a	3. Loss of ability to put on clothing without assistance	6a
		4. Loss of ability to bathe without assistance	6b	4. Loss of ability to bathe without assistance	6b
		5. Loss of ambulatory capacity	7c	5. Loss of urinary continence	6d
		6. Loss of ability to perform complex tasks	4	6. Loss of fecal continence	6e
		7. Loss of ability to pick out clothing	5	7. Loss of speech	7a–7b
		8. Fecal incontinence	6e	8. Loss of ambulatory capacity	7c
Dementia syndrome of depression ("pseudodementia")	Affective disorder associated with neurotransmitter imbalance	1. Loss of ability to perform complex tasks	4	1. Loss of ability to perform complex tasks	4
		2. Refusal to put on clothing (associated with negativity)	6a	2. Inability to pick out clothing properly	5

Continued

TABLE 3.4 *Continued*

| | | Functional Loss in Non-Alzheimer Disorders | | FAST AD Distinctions | | |
Disorder	Pathology or Presumed Etiology	Example of the Order of Functional Loss in Non-AD Disorder[a]	Equivalent FAST Stage	Order of Functional Loss in AD per FAST	FAST Stages in AD
		3. Refusal to bathe (associated with negativity)	6b	3. Inability to put on clothing without assistance.	6a
		4. Loss of ability to pick out clothing properly	5	4. Inability to bathe without assistance	6b
Dementia associated with hyponatremia	Electrolyte disturbance	1. Loss of ability to perform complex tasks	4	1. Loss of ability to perform complex tasks	4
		2. Loss of ability to pick out clothing properly	5	2. Loss of ability to pick out clothing properly	5
		3. Loss of ability to dress, bathe and toilet independently	6a–6c	3. Loss of ability to dress, bathe, and toilet independently	6a–6c
		4. Loss of ambulation capacity	7c	4. Loss of urinary and fecal continence	6d–6e
		5. Loss of urinary and fecal continence	6d–6e	5. Loss of speech	7a–7b
		6. Loss of speech	7a–7b	6. Loss of ambulatory capacity	7c
Dementia associated with diffuse CNS metastasis	Neoplastic diffuse cerebral trauma	1. Loss of ability to perform complex tasks	4	1. Loss of ability to perform complex tasks	4
		2. Loss of ability to dress, bathe, and toilet independently	6a–6c	2. Loss of ability to dress, bathe, and toilet independently	6a–6c
		3. Loss of ambulation capacity	7c	3. Loss of urinary and fecal continence	6d–6e
		4. Loss of urinary and fecal continence	6d–6e	4. Loss of speech	7a–7b
		5. Loss of speech	7a–7b	5. Loss of ambulatory capacity	7c

[a]The sequences of functional loss shown are typical for normal-pressure hydrocephalus and Creutzfeldt-Jakob disease; the sequence for multi-infarct dementia is one of various common presentations; the sequences in the dementia syndrome of depression, dementia associated with hyponatremia, and dementia associated with diffuse CNS metastasis are previously observed examples of the presentation of these dementias. It should be noted that in some of the non-AD disorders, particularly multi-infarct dementia, the "sequence" described may appear abruptly, rather than over an extended time interval. FAST = Functional Assessment Staging.

Source: Reisberg, B., Pattschull-Furlan, A., Franssen, E., Sclan, S. G., Kluger, A., Dingcong, L., et al. (1990). Cognition related functional, praxis and feeding changes in CNS aging and Alzheimer's disease and their developmental analogies. In K. Beyreuther & G. Schettler (Eds.), *Molecular mechanisms of aging* (pp. 18–40). Berlin: Springer-Verlag.

TABLE 3.5   *Differential Diagnostic Considerations in Cases of Deviations From FAST*

Stage	FAST Characteristics	Differential Diagnostic Considerations (Particularly if FAST Stage Occurs Prematurely in the Evolution of Dementia)
1	No functional decrement, either subjectively or objectively, manifest	
2	Complains of forgetting location of objects; subjective work difficulties	Anxiety neurosis, depression
3	Decreased functioning in demanding employment settings evident to co-workers, difficulty in traveling to new locations	Depression, subtle manifestations of medical pathology
4	Decreased ability to perform complex tasks such as planning dinner for guests, handling finances, and marketing	Depression, psychosis, focal cerebral process (e.g., Gerstmann's syndrome)
5	Requires assistance in choosing proper clothing, may require coaxing to bathe properly	Depression
6	(a) Difficulty putting on clothing properly	(a) Arthritis, sensory deficit, stroke, depression
	(b) Requires assistance in bathing, may develop fear of bathing	(b) Arthritis, sensory deficit, stroke, depression
	(c) Inability to handle mechanics of toileting	(c) Arthritis, sensory deficit, stroke, depression
	(d) Urinary incontinence	(d) Urinary tract infection, other causes of urinary incontinence
	(e) Fecal incontinence	(e) Infection, malabsorption syndrome, other causes of fecal incontinence
7	(a) Ability to speak limited to one to five words	(a) Stroke, other dementing disorder (e.g., diffuse space-occupying lesions)
	(b) Intelligible vocabulary lost	(b) Stroke, other dementing disorder (e.g., diffuse space-occupying lesions)
	(c) Ambulatory ability lost	(c) Parkinsonism, neuroleptic-induced or other secondary extrapyramidal syndrome, Creutzfeldt-Jakob disease, normal-pressure hydrocephalus, hyponatremic dementia, stroke, hip fracture, arthritis, overmedication
	(d) Ability to sit up independently lost	(d) Arthritis, contractures
	(e) Ability to smile lost	(e) Stroke
	(f) Ability to hold up head lost	(f) Head trauma, metabolic abnormality, other medical abnormality, overmedication, encephalitis, other causes

FAST = Functional Assessment Staging.
Source: Reisberg, B. (1986). Dementia: A systematic approach to identifying reversible causes. *Geriatrics, 41*(4), 30–46. Copyright © 1984 by Barry Reisberg, MD.

at this early point in AD, be a remediable complication, perhaps secondary to a urinary tract infection.

Similarly, if a patient with AD at GDS stage 5 and FAST stage 5 develops loss of independent ambulation, this may be the result of a stroke or possibly of a variety of potentially treatable conditions common in the elderly, such as medication-induced parkinsonian symptoms, arthritis, fracture, and so on. Table 3.5 provides an extensive list of causes of premature functional losses in an AD patient, many of which are potentially remediable.

The relationship between the FAST and the GDS, or the FAST and the MMSE, is also useful in the identification of excess functional disability that may be remediable. Specifically, if an

AD patient is notably more impaired functionally, in comparison with the magnitude of the cognitive impairment (e.g., a GDS stage 5 patient who is at stage 6d on the FAST), this is an indication of the likely presence of excess functional disability. For example, the patient may have coexisting arthritis and AD. As a result of the combination of arthritis and dementia, in addition to not being able to handle finances and to pick out clothing without assistance (deficits that occur only because of the patient's AD), the patient may be unable to dress, bathe, and toilet without assistance, the latter resulting in occasional urinary incontinence. The arthritis may or may not be remediable. Similarly, the excess functional disability may or may not be remediable. Interestingly, when excess functional disability occurs in AD patients, it tends to occur "along the lines of the FAST." It appears that AD predisposes to functional losses outlined on the FAST. When an insult occurs, the closer the AD patient is to the inevitable point of loss of a functional ability on the FAST, the more predisposed the AD patient is to the premature loss of that capacity on the FAST. Not only illnesses but also psychological stressors may produce these premature losses. For example, if an AD patient at GDS stage 6 and FAST stage 6c is moved to an unfamiliar environment, the patient may develop urinary and fecal incontinence that remits when the patient is returned to familiar surroundings. Subsequently, these capacities will, tragically, be lost with the advance of AD.

Knowledge of the FAST progression of AD, in conjunction with the global concomitants, feeding concomitants, and other aspects, also provides invaluable information on the potential for treatment of disability, even in AD that is uncomplicated by the presence of additional pathology. For example, strategies for forestalling incontinence can be contemplated in FAST stage 6c. In FAST stage 6d or 6e, treatment of incontinence requires different strategies, such as frequent toileting. With the advance of deficits in FAST stage 7, strategies and goals for the management of incontinence need to be modified.

Other symptoms in AD, notably symptoms associated with the behavioral syndrome as outlined in Table 3.6, also require treatment. These symptoms are commonly treated with neuroleptics or other psychotropic medications. It should be noted that treatment of these symptoms may also be related to the treatment of functional disabilities. For example, it has been observed that AD patients with excess functional disability in relation to the magnitude of their cognitive disturbances may frequently have particularly marked behavioral disturbances. Conversely, marked behavioral disturbances may be associated with excess functional disability. This excess functional disability may be remediated in part by successful treatment of the behavioral symptoms.

OVERALL MANAGEMENT SCIENCE

As shown in Table 3.7, a very interesting and important aspect of the functional progression of AD is that the order of losses on the FAST is a precise reversal of the order of acquisition of the same functions in normal human development (Reisberg, 1986; Reisberg, Ferris, & Franssen, 1986). Subsequent work has indicated that AD also reverses normal development in terms of other functional parameters such as feeding abilities and figure drawings (Reisberg et al., 1990), as well as cognitively (Auer et al., 1994; Ouvrier, Goldsmith, Ouvrier, & Williams, 1993; Sclan, Foster, Reisberg, Franssen, & Welkowitz, 1990; Shimada et al., 2003).

For example, the MMSE is a well known and widely used cognitive assessment developed for the assessment of dementia patients (Folstein et al., 1975). The MMSE score has shown approximately as robust a relationship to the mental age of children, as it has shown to any noncognitive measure of dementia pathology. Initially, in a study of Australian children, a 0.83 Pearson correlation of the MMSE score to the mental age of children was found (Ouvrier et al., 1993). A subsequent study, in Spanish children, found a 0.76 Pearson correlation between childhood mental ages and MMSE scores, and a 0.80 correlation between MMSE scores and children's chronological ages (Rubial-Álvarez et al., 2007).

Conversely, a study was conducted in AD patients of a cognitive assessment measure specifically developed for infants and small children, the Ordinal Scales of Psychological

TABLE 3.6   *Behavioral and Psychological Pathological Symptomatology in Alzheimer's Disease*

Paranoid and delusional ideation
  The "people are stealing things" delusion
  The "house is not one's home" delusion
  The "spouse (or other caregiver) is an imposter" delusion
  The "abandonment" delusion
  The "infidelity" delusion
  Other suspicions, paranoid ideation, or delusions

Hallucinations
  Visual hallucinations
  Auditory hallucinations

Activity disturbances
  Wandering
  Purposeless activity (cognitive abulia)
  Inappropriate activities

Aggressivity
  Verbal outbursts
  Physical outbursts
  Other agitation

Diurnal rhythm disturbance
  Day/night disturbance

Affective disturbance
  Tearfulness
  Other depressive manifestations

Anxieties and phobias
  Anxiety regarding upcoming events (Godot's syndrome)
  Other anxieties
  Fear of being left alone
  Other phobias

Source: Reisberg, B., Borenstein, J., Franssen, E., Shulman, E., Steinberg, G., and Ferris, S. H. (1986). Potentially remediable behavioral symptomatology in Alzheimer's disease. *Hospital and Community Psychiatry, 37,* 1199–1201. Also adapted from "Behavioral Pathology in Alzheimer's Disease (BEHAVE-AD)." Copyright © 1986 by Barry Reisberg, MD. All rights reserved. Published in: Reisberg, B., Borenstein, J., Salob, S. P., Ferris, S. H., Franssen, E., and Georgotas, A. (1987). Behavioral symptoms in Alzheimer's disease: Phenomenology and treatment. *Journal of Clinical Psychiatry, 48*(5, Suppl.), 9–15.

Development (OSPD) assessment (Uzgiris & Hunt, 1975). This OSPD test was slightly modi-fied for use in severe dementia patients. The resulting modified-OSPD measurement of cog-nition (the M-OSPD) showed approximately the same relationship to the FAST stage in stage 6 and stage 7 AD patients (a 0.8 correlation) as is seen between the FAST functional stage and MMSE cognitive assessment in somewhat less severe AD patients who are testable with the MMSE (Auer et al., 1994; Reisberg, Ferris, Torossian, Kluger, & Monteiro, 1992).

Similarly, a widely used intelligence test measure for children, the Binet scale, has been applied to AD patients in FAST stages 5, 6, and 7. A Spearman correlation of −0.85, between the Binet test measure basic age value and the FAST stage, was found (Shimada et al., 2003). This is at least as robust as the relationship between the MMSE and the FAST assessment in dementia patients in the corresponding FAST range (Reisberg et al., 1992).

Table 3.7 illustrates that the FAST stages of AD can be expressed in terms of developmen-tal ages (DAs). Remarkably, so-called developmental infantile reflexes appear to be equally good markers of the emergence of the stage of severe AD, corresponding to a DA of infancy, as the same reflexes are in marking the emergence from infancy in normal development (Franssen, Souren, Torossian, & Reisberg, 1997) (see Figure 3.5). Similar to the findings

Alzheimer's Degeneration
Approximate Total Duration: 20 Years

TABLE 3.7 Functional Landmarks in Normal Human Development and Alzheimer's Disease (AD)

Approximate Age	Approximate Duration in Development	Acquired Abilities	Lost Abilities	Alzheimer Stage	Approximate Duration in AD	Developmental Age of AD
Adolescence	13–19 years	Hold a job	Hold a job	3—Incipient	7 years	19–13 years: Adolescence
Late childhood	8–12 years	Handle simple finances	Handle simple finances	4—Mild	2 years	12–8 years: Late childhood
Middle childhood	5–7 years	Select proper clothing	Select proper clothing	5—Moderate	1.5 years	7–5 years: Middle childhood
Early childhood	5 years	Put on clothes unaided	Put on clothes unaided	6a—Moderately severe	2.5 years	5–2 years: Early childhood
	4 years	Shower unaided	Shower unaided	b		
	4 years	Toilet unaided	Toilet unaided	c		
	3–4.5 years	Control urine	Control urine	d		
	2–3 years	Control bowels	Control bowels	e		
Infancy	15 months	Speak 5–6 words	Speak 5–6 words	7a—Severe	7 years or longer	15 months to birth: Infancy
	1 year	Speak 1 word	Speak 1 word	b		
	1 year	Walk	Walk	c		
	6–10 months	Sit up	Sit up	d		
	2–4 months	Smile	Smile	e		
	1–3 months	Hold up head	Hold up head	f		

Normal Development
Approximate Total Duration: 20 Years

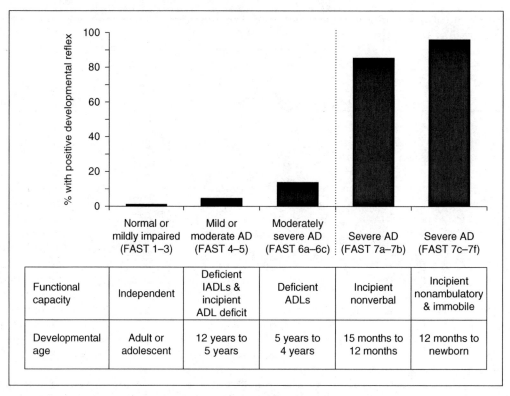

	Normal or mildly impaired (FAST 1–3)	Mild or moderate AD (FAST 4–5)	Moderately severe AD (FAST 6a–6c)	Severe AD (FAST 7a–7b)	Severe AD (FAST 7c–7f)
Functional capacity	Independent	Deficient IADLs & incipient ADL deficit	Deficient ADLs	Incipient nonverbal	Incipient nonambulatory & immobile
Developmental age	Adult or adolescent	12 years to 5 years	5 years to 4 years	15 months to 12 months	12 months to newborn

FIGURE 3.5 Neurologic retrogenesis. Percentages of patients with one or more of the following developmental reflexes (also known as primitive reflexes or frontal release signs) are shown: the tactile sucking reflex, the palmar grasp (hand grasp) reflex, the plantar grasp (foot grasp) reflex, and the plantar extensor (Babinski) reflex. All reflexes were elicited according to standard procedures and were assessed as being present when they were prominent and persistent, defined by a rating of ≥5 on the scale of Franssen (Franssen, 2003; Franssen et al., 1991, 1993). For the three reflexes which were assessed bilaterally, specifically, the palmar grasp reflex, the plantar grasp reflex, and the plantar extensor reflex, a positive response on either side was assessed as positive. Subject samples were as follows: Deficient ADLs (FAST stages 6a to 6c), n = 113; Incipient nonverbal (FAST stages 7a to 7b), n = 29; Incipient non-ambulatory and immobile (FAST stages 7c to 7f), n = 32. IADLs are instrumental (complex) activities of daily life; ADLs are basic activities of daily life. *Source:* Data and figure are adapted from Franssen, E. H., Souren, L. E. M., Torossian, C. L., & Reisberg, B. (1997). Utility of developmental reflexes in the differential diagnosis and prognosis of incontinence in Alzheimer's disease. *Journal of Geriatric Psychiatry and Neurology, 10,* 22–28.

with neurological reflexes, a leading investigator in neurometabolism, Michael Phelps, has reported remarkable similarities between the pattern of brain metabolic activity in the late-stage AD patient and that in the normal infant brain (Phelps, 2000). These findings, obtained using positron emission tomography (PET) techniques, are very different from the metabolic patterns observed in the normal adult brain.

Neuroanatomic brain changes in AD have also been observed to mirror in various ways, the brain changes in normal human development. In early studies of the neuropathology of AD, Brun and Gustafson (1976) noted that "maximal cortical degeneration occurred in the medial temporal (limbic) area and in the lateral hemisphere" and that other brain regions were notably spared. These brain regions, which were observed to be relatively free of AD-related pathology, were observed to be "mainly the anterior cingulate gyrus and the calcarine and cortical motor areas (primary projection areas)." The investigators concluded that, "the pattern described may be related to ontogenic [developmental] features" (Brun & Gustafson, 1976). Subsequently, McGeer et al. (1990), noting the patterns of neuronal loss described by Brun and Englund (1981), and their own PET studies of neurometabolic changes in AD, concluded that the AD neurodegenerative process appears to relate to the pattern and process of brain myelination in normal development (McGeer et al., 1990). They observed that the areas of the brain, which are the last to be myelinated in normal development (and which are therefore the most thinly myelinated) (Flechsig, 1920), appear to be the areas that are the most vulnerable to the pathology of AD in terms of neuronal losses and decrements in cerebral metabolism (reviewed in Reisberg, Franssen, Hasan, et al., 1999). The pattern of neurofibrillary pathology in AD has also been related to the developmental pattern of myelinization of the brain in reverse (Braak & Braak, 1991, 1996). Raz (1999) has provided a numerical value for these anatomic relationships between myelinization in normal human development and myelin loss in the AD pathological process as seen with neuroimaging. He noted that, "The gradient of vulnerability seems to follow the rules of last (....ontogenetically) in—first out... the later a region completes its myelination, the greater age-related difference in volume it exhibits, $r = .60$, $p < 0.05$" (Raz, 1999). This process by which the degenerative changes in AD, and to some extent other dementias, reverse the order of acquisition of capacities and processes in normal development has been termed retrogenesis (Reisberg, Franssen, Hasan, et al., 1999). The process of myelin loss, which is associated with the retrogenic process occurring in AD, has been termed "arboreal entropy" (Reisberg et al., 2002). "Just as the bark of a tree protects it from... injury and, to some extent, the thicker the bark, the greater the protection, the myelin protects the axon and its neuron. Hence, to some extent, ... the thicker the myelin, [and the earlier in development the neuron is myelinated] the greater the protection" (Reisberg et al., 2002).

Interestingly, the retrogenesis process can explain many of the other symptoms and findings in AD, such as the nature of patient behavioral disturbances (Reisberg, Auer, Monteiro, Franssen, & Kenowsky, 1998), and the kind of symptoms that are progressively and invariably lost, such as speaking and walking, in comparison with the kind of symptoms that are more variable, such as the behavioral disturbances (Reisberg, Franssen, Souren, Auer, & Kenowsky, 1998). Most importantly, the retrogenic process provides a rapid appreciation of the general care and management needs of the AD patient at each stage of the disease (Reisberg, Kenowsky, Franssen, Auer, & Souren, 1999) (Table 3.8).

An understanding of the retrogenic process in AD also provides the basis for a detailed management science (Reisberg et al., 2002). This science includes care axioms, care postulates, and care caveats. The care axioms apply to all human beings and to AD patients at all stages (Table 3.9). The postulates are testable hypotheses of AD patient care based on the DA retrogenesis model (Table 3.10). Finally, the caveats are based on acknowledged differences between AD patients and their DA peers (Table 3.11). The combination of these care axioms, postulates, and caveats forms the nascent science of AD management.

RELATIONSHIP BETWEEN AD'S CLINICAL COURSE AND MANAGEMENT AND ITS OBSERVED PATHOLOGICAL AND BIOMOLECULAR FEATURES

The classical observed pathology accompanying the dementia of AD, as viewed upon microscopic examination of the brain, is extracellular plaques containing a substance called amyloid and intraneuronal neurofibrillary tangles. The amyloid plaques are primarily composed of a protein called β-amyloid. The intracellular neurofibrillary tangles are derived from neuronal microtubules. These microtubules are the "tubes" that are used to transport nutrients and other essential substances through the axonal fibers. The axons can be very long, and the axons degenerate in the absence of this essential neurotubular transport.

As noted earlier, the amyloid protein in the amyloid plaques is mainly composed of β-amyloid protein. This β-amyloid protein, like all proteins, is made up of amino acids. There

TABLE 3.8 *Stages of Aging and Alzheimer's Disease (AD) and Corresponding Developmental Ages (DAs): Care Needs and Care Recommendations*

GDS Stage	Diagnosis	Developmental Age (DA)	Care Needs	Care Recommendations
1	Normal	Adult	None	None
2	Subjective cognitive impairment	Aged adult	None	Reassurance with respect to relatively benign prognosis
3	Mild cognitive impairment	Adolescence	None	"Tactical" withdrawal from situations that have become, by virtue of their complexity, anxiety provoking
4	Mild AD	Late childhood	Independent survival still attainable	Assistance towards goal of maximum independence with financial supervision; structured or supervised travel; identification bracelets and labels may be useful
5	Moderate AD	Middle childhood	Patient can no longer survive in the community without assistance; needs supervision with respect to travel and social behavior	Part-time home health care assistance can be very useful in assisting the patient's caregiver. Driving becomes hazardous and should be discontinued at some point over the course of this stage. Family may require guidance in handling patient's emotional outbursts
6	Moderately severe AD	Early childhood	Patient requires assistance with basic activities of daily life. Early in this stage, assistance with dressing and bathing is required. Subsequently, assistance with continence becomes necessary as well	Full-time home health care assistance is frequently very useful in assisting the patient's caregiver. Strategies for assistance with bathing, toileting, and in the management of incontinence should be discussed with the family. Emotional stress in the caregiver should be minimized with supportive techniques
7	Severe AD	Infancy	Early in this stage assistance with feeding as well as dressing, bathing, and toileting is required. Subsequently, assistance with ambulation and	Full-time assistance in the community home residence or institutional setting is a necessity. Strategies for maintaining locomotion should be

Continued

TABLE 3.8   *Continued*

GDS Stage	Diagnosis	Developmental Age (DA)	Care Needs	Care Recommendations
			purposeful movement becomes necessary. Prevention of aspiration, contractures, and decubiti is a major issue in care	explored. The need for psychopharmacological intervention for behavioral disturbances decreases. Soft food or liquid diet is generally tolerated. Patients must be fed and instructed and encouraged to maintain chewing and basic eating skills

are generally 40–42 amino acids in the β-amyloid protein. This β-amyloid protein is itself derived from a much larger protein, the amyloid protein precursor (APP) protein, which is 365–770 amino acids long. The APP protein is known as a transmembrane protein, because it crosses the cell membrane of the neuron. Part of the APP is outside the neuronal cell membrane, part is inside the neuronal cell membrane, and part of this protein is inside the cell, in the cytosol, the neuronal cell substance. The APP protein is normally cleaved by an enzyme known as α-secretase, which cleaves the APP outside the cell membrane. When α-secretase cleavage occurs, there is no amyloid β (Aβ) produced. Alternatively, the APP is cleaved by another enzyme, the β-secretase enzyme, which is, like the α-secretase, located outside the cell membrane. β-Secretase cleavage is followed by cleavage within the cell membrane by an enzyme known as γ-secretase. The result of this β- and γ-secretase cleavage is the Aβ protein, which is in the plaques in AD. Both aging and AD are associated with increased Aβ protein in the brain (Näslund et al., 2000; Seubert et al., 1992).

TABLE 3.9   *Alzheimer's Disease (AD) Care Axioms*

Axiom I	All human beings avoid trauma and humiliation
Axiom II	All human beings seek a sense of accomplishment
Axiom III	All human beings seek a sense of dignity and self-worth
Axiom IV	All human beings are social organisms
Axiom V	All human beings seek praise and acceptance
Axiom VI	All human beings have the capacity to learn
Axiom VII	All human beings require love
Axiom VIII	All human beings have the capacity for happiness if basic needs are fulfilled
Axiom IX	All human beings have the need for physical movement
Axiom X	All human beings have the capacity to remember
Axiom XI	All human beings have the capacity to think
Axiom XII	All human beings seek to influence their environment
Axiom XIII	All human beings have a sense of "taste," i.e., likes and dislikes

TABLE 3.10 *Alzheimer's Disease (AD) Care Postulates*

Postulate I	The magnitude of care and supervision required by an AD patient, at a developmental age (DA), is mirrored by the amount of care and supervision required by a child or infant at the corresponding DA
Postulate II	The kinds of activities enjoyed by an AD patient, at a particular DA, are mirrored by the kinds of activities enjoyed by children at a corresponding DA
Postulate III	The capacity of an AD patient to perform in an area of residual expertise is dependent on the patient's DA
Postulate IV	Previous experiences may determine the kinds of activities enjoyed by an AD patient
Postulate V	The emotional level of the AD patient is dependent on the DA
Postulate VI	Life experiences appropriate to the DA become most relevant for AD patients at any particular stage
Postulate VII	Socialization of the AD patient is dependent on the DA
Postulate VIII	Diversity in children's and infants' activities and interests is mirrored in diversity in AD patient's interests and activities at a corresponding DA
Postulate IX	The emotional changes that occur in AD at a DA are mirrored by the emotional changes observed in children at a corresponding DA
Postulate X	Care settings appropriate to AD patients at a DA are mirrored by care settings appropriate to children at the corresponding DA
Postulate XI	Vulnerability (emotional, physical, and cognitive) of the AD patient at a DA is mirrored by the vulnerability of children at the corresponding DA
Postulate XII	The need of an AD patient for physical movement is mirrored by the corresponding DA
Postulate XIII	Just as one judges development in an infant or child by what the infant or child can do and has achieved, not by what the infant or child cannot do, the AD patient at any particular DA should be assessed in terms of his or her residual skills and accomplishments, what they have learned and relearned, not by what they cannot do
Postulate XIV	The developmental analogy is sufficiently strong to trigger DA-appropriate childhood memories, beliefs, and anxieties in the AD patient
Postulate XV	The language changes of the AD patient are mirrored by the DA

DA = Developmental ages. Copyright © 2002, 2004 by Barry Reisberg, MD. All rights reserved.

TABLE 3.11 *Alzheimer's Disease (AD) Care Caveats*

Caveat I	Development in infants and children is accompanied by increasing expectations, whereas AD at all stages is accompanied by progressively diminished expectations
Caveat II	AD patients experience developmentally analogous brain changes; however, they do not undergo developmentally analogous physical changes
Caveat III	AD patients can, to some extent, draw upon previously mastered skills, whereas infants and children may not have access to these skills
Caveat IV	AD patients can, to some extent, draw upon previously mastered knowledge, whereas infants and children may not have access to this knowledge
Caveat V	AD patients are older than their DA peers, and old age predisposes to various physical disabilities that influence the life and experience of an AD patient
Caveat VI	AD patients appear to be more prone to rigidity than their DA peers
Caveat VII	AD patients can potentially concentrate on a task longer than infants or children at a corresponding DA
Caveat VIII	AD patients appear to be less fascinated by the world and less inquisitive than infants and children at a corresponding DA

DA = Developmental ages. Copyright © 2002, 2004 by Barry Reisberg, MD. All rights reserved.

The neurofibrillary tangles in AD, seen inside the neuron, are composed of paired helical filaments (Kidd, 1963). The major constituent of these paired helical filaments is a protein known as "tau" (Kondo et al., 1988; Wischik, Novak, Edwards, et al., 1988; Wischik, Novak, Thøgersen, et al., 1988). Tau is believed to be a scaffolding molecule, which maintains the structural integrity of the microtubules in the neurons.

The relationship between the clinically observed "plaques and tangles" of AD (including the more recently discovered biomolecular constituents of the plaques and tangles) and the observed behavioral course of AD, described in the preceding sections of this chapter, can presently be elucidated.

As described in the prior sections, remarkably similar patterns between the neurometabolic activity of a late-stage AD patient and those of the infant brain have been noted (Phelps, 2000). In 2002, Reisberg et al., hypothesized that these patterns could be explained if "the most metabolically active regions of the brain in AD … are the regions which are the most vulnerable in AD" (Reisberg et al., 2002). In 2005, it was found by Buckner et al. that, in fact, the pattern of deposition of amyloid plaques in the brain of AD patients appeared to occur in the regions of the brain that are the most active during the resting, so-called, default state, when the brain is not focused upon any particular activity (Buckner et al., 2005). Hence, there appears to be a direct relationship between the metabolic activity of the brain and a major form of microscopically evident AD pathology, the amyloid plaques, containing β-amyloid.

In 1980, Ferris and associates reported, using the then new PET scanning techniques, that there is a continuous decrease in metabolism in many brain regions, with the advance of the behaviorally evident AD process (Ferris et al., 1980). These findings have been replicated and supported in numerous subsequent studies. This process of continuing neurometabolic loss in AD has been termed "neurometabolic entropy" (Reisberg, Wegiel, Franssen, et al., 2006a). The continuing neurometabolic entropy, affecting first, the most metabolically active brain regions, appears to provide an explanation for the observed neurometabolic retrogenesis seen in AD.

Recent studies have provided an understanding of the mechanisms underlying these metabolic changes in AD. The insulin receptor and the insulin-like growth factor (IGF) receptor signaling pathway play a major role in controlling maximum lifespan and age-associated diseases in all species of multicellular organisms that have been studied, including yeast, worms, flies, and mammals (Puglielli, 2008). Interestingly, a decrease in IGF-1 blood levels occurs with normal aging in a retrogenic-like pattern. Specifically, there is a continuing increase in IGF-1 blood levels from infancy to about 15 years of age and this is followed by a continuing decrease in levels of IGF-1 in the blood, reaching an infant and early childhood level by about age 80–85 (Laboratory Corporation of America, accessed 2003; Reisberg, Wegiel, Franssen, et al., 2006a). These circulating blood changes in IGF-1 levels may be related to currently observed changes in the IGF-1 insulin receptor in aging and AD. A decreased number of neurons are now being reported to express the IGF-1 receptor in AD (Moloney et al., 2010). Also, Moloney et al. are reporting that the IGF-1 receptor is aberrantly distributed in AD, particularly in neurons affected by neurofibrillary tangles, in that it is concentrated intracellularly rather than at the neuronal cell membrane. Related to this, Moloney et al. are reporting decreased insulin receptor substrate levels in AD neurons, and these decrements are localized with the neurofibrillary tangles. Interestingly, in terms of the other major microscopically observed pathology in AD, the β-amyloid, formed in part by γ-secretase cleavage, the same enzyme, γ-secretase, is also being related to the IGF-1 receptor. Specifically, γ-secretase has now been reported to be involved in the proteolysis (breakdown) of the IGF-1 receptor (McElroy, Powell, & McCarthy, 2007).

In addition to direct relationships between the IGF-1 receptor and AD pathology, the insulin receptor is also being directly related to AD pathology. Soluble, Aβ (Townsend, Mehta, & Selkoe, 2007), as well as Aβ oligomers (Zhao, DeFelice, Fernandez, et al., 2008) have been shown to impair insulin receptor function.

The net result of these changes in the IGF-1 receptor and in insulin receptor signaling is that the neurons which degenerate in AD may be more resistant to these signals (Moloney et al., 2010). This resistance is being widely observed, and AD is now frequently referred to as type 3 diabetes (Hoyer, 1998; Steen et al., 2005). As with many changes in biology, the arrows, in terms of etiopathogenesis of metabolic deficits in the brain in AD, appear to point in both directions. The decrease in oxidative metabolism, which occurs in the brain in AD, has been observed to be associated with amyloid accumulation in several studies (Pluta, 2002; Popa-Wagner, Schröder, Walker, & Kessler, 1998; Sinigaglia-Coimbra, Cavalheiro, & Coimbra, 2002).

To fully understand the nature of the pathology in AD, together with associated pathogenic mechanisms, and their relationship to the clinical manifestations of AD, an additional principle must be recognized and addressed. This is that there is a homeostatic, regenerative, developmental, physiological response to the progressive pathology of AD. This regenerative physiological response in AD has many elements, which notably include: (1) there is a reactivation of the cell cycle enzymes in terminally differentiated neurons in AD (reviewed in Reisberg et al., 2002); (2) there is an activation of neurogenesis (new neuron production) in a region of the hippocampus (the dentate gyrus) in AD; (3) the activation of the β-secretase enzyme appears to be associated with a myelin regeneration effect; (4) the activation of γ-secretase may also be associated with a regenerative effect; (5) the production of Aβ may be associated with injury repair in the brain; and (6) the reduction in IGF-1 signaling appears to delay age-associated protein-related toxicity (e.g., from toxic soluble and oligomeric forms of Aβ).

For example, to the extent that the function of the β-secretase enzyme is known, apart from its role in the generation of amyloid β, it plays an important role in cleavage associated with the production of myelin (Glabe, 2006; Willem et al., 2006). Interestingly, IGF-1 also plays a role in myelin production, causing the oligodendrocytes, the myelin producing brain cells, to produce more myelin (Carson, Behringer, Brinster, & McMorris, 1993; Flores et al., 2008). β-Secretase knock-out mice show decreased myelin production and decreased IGF-1 signaling (Hu et al., 2006). Therefore, the β-secretase response in AD appears to be a homeostatic compensation for the decrease IGF-1 activity with aging and AD. Nevertheless, as described above, there are continuing IGF-1 signaling abnormalities in AD, and these can account for the observed myelin arboreal atrophy and myelin retrogenesis seen in AD.

Activation of γ-secretase also appears to be a developmental response to the pathology in AD, in addition to its role in the production of β-amyloid and in the protein breakdown of the IGF-1 receptor. For example, notch, an element of the γ-secretase complex, is involved in signaling, which is "crucial for long-term memory" (Costa, Drew, & Silva, 2005). Also, "the notch pathway has been shown to regulate neurite growth and adult neurogenesis" (Breunig, Silbereis, Vaccarino, Sestan, & Rakic, 2007; Costa et al., 2005).

Aβ itself appears to be involved in brain injury repair. Brody et al. (2008) have shown that there is an increase in Aβ in the brain interstitial fluid in the 72-hour period after a brain trauma associated with coma, in the persons who show signs of recovering from a coma. However, this increase in Aβ in the brain interstitial fluid is not seen in the persons with poor signs of coma recovery.

Additionally, the reduced insulin and IGF-1 signaling in AD appears to be, in part, a physiological homeostatic response to toxic proteins produced by the AD process. For example, a recent study showed that reduction in IGF signaling in an Alzheimer mouse model decreased behavioral impairment, neuroinflammation, and neuronal loss (Cohen et al., 2009).

Hence, there is a complex homeostatic, physiological response to the behavioral and biomolecular changes associated with AD. This response can presently provide a good understanding of the nature of the changes seen in AD, including the retrogenic physiological process and the consequent management needs in AD.

CONCLUSIONS

AD is a very common condition in elderly persons, marked by a characteristic cognitive and functional course of disability. Knowledge of this characteristic course is essential for the identification and treatment of excess functional disability and for many other aspects of patient management and care. Proper management and care can alleviate, indeed, even eliminate suffering in the patient and reduce burden in the caregivers of AD victims.

ACKNOWLEDGMENT

This work was supported in part by U.S. Department of Health and Human Services (DHHS) grants AG03051, AG08051, AG09127, and AG11505 from the National Institute on Aging of the U.S. National Institutes of Health; by grants 90AZ2791, 90AM2552, and 90AR2160 from the U.S. DHHS Administration on Aging; by grant NCRRM01 RR00096 from the General Clinical Research Center Program and by Clinical and Translational Science Institute grant 1UL1RR029893 from the National Center for Research Resources of the U.S. National Institutes of Health; by the Fisher Center for Alzheimer's Disease Research Foundation; by a grant from Mr. William Silberstein; by the Leonard Litwin Fund for Alzheimer's Disease Research; by the Woodbourne Foundation; and by the Hagedorn Fund.

REFERENCES

American Psychiatric Associations (1994). *Diagnostic and Statistical Manual of Mental Disorders (Fourth Edition)*. Washington, D.C.: American Psychiatric Association.

Auer, S. R., Sclan, S. G., Yaffee, R. A., & Reisberg, B. (1994). The neglected half of Alzheimer's disease: Cognitive and functional concomitants of severe dementia. *Journal of the America Geriatrics Society, 42*, 1266–1272.

Blazer, D. G., Hays, J. C., Fillenbaum, G. G., & Gold, D. T. (1997). Memory complaint as a predictor of cognitive decline: A comparison of African American and White elders. *Journal of Aging and Health, 9*, 171–184.

Bobinski, M., Wegiel, J., Wisniewski, H. M., Tarnawski, M., Reisberg, B., Mlodzik, B., et al. (1995). Atrophy of hippocampal formation subdivisions correlates with stage and duration of Alzheimer disease. *Dementia, 6*, 205–210.

Bobinski, M., Wegiel, J., Tarnawski, M., Bobinski, M., Reisberg, B., de Leon, M. J., et al. (1997). Relationships between regional neuronal loss and neurofibrillary changes in the hippocampal formation and duration and severity of Alzheimer disease. *Journal of Neuropathology and Experimental Neurology, 56*, 414–420.

Bowen, J., Teri, L., Kukull, W., McCormick, W., McCurry, S. M., & Larson, E. B. (1997). Progression to dementia in patients with isolated memory loss. *Lancet, 349*, 763–765.

Braak, H., & Braak, E. (1991). Neuropathological stageing of Alzheimer-related changes. *Acta Neuropathologica, 82*, 239–259.

Braak, H., & Braak, E. (1996). Development of Alzheimer-related neurofibrillary changes in the neocortex inversely recapitulates cortical myelogenesis. *Acta Neuropathologica, 92*, 197–201.

Breunig, J. J., Silbereis, J., Vaccarino, F. M., Sestan, N., & Rakic, P. (2007). Notch regulates cell fate and dendrite morphology of newborn neurons in the postnatal dentate gyrus. *Proceedings of the National Academy of Sciences of the United States of America, 104*, 20558–20563.

Brodaty, H., Ames, D., Snowdon, J., Woodward, M., Kirwan, J., Clarnette, R., et al. (2003). A randomized placebo-controlled trial of risperidone for the treatment of aggression, agitation, and psychosis of dementia. *Journal of Clinical Psychiatry, 64*, 134–143.

Brody, D. L., Magnoni, S., Schwetye, K. E., Spinner, M. L., Esparza, T. J., Stocchetti, N., et al. (2008). Amyloid-beta dynamics correlate with neurological status in the injured human brain. *Science, 321*, 1221–1224.

Brucki, S. M. D., & Nitrini, R. (2008). Subjective memory impairment in a rural population with low education in the Amazon rainforest: An exploratory study. *International Psychogeriatrics, 21,* 164–171.

Brun, A., & Englund, E. (1981). Regional pattern of degeneration in Alzheimer's disease: Neuronal loss and histopathological grading. *Histopathology, 5,* 549–564.

Brun, A., & Gustafson, L. (1976). Distribution of cerebral degeneration in Alzheimer's disease. *Archiv für Psychiatrie und Nervenkrankheiten, 223,* 15–33.

Bruscoli, M., & Lovestone, S. (2004). Is MCI really just early dementia? A systematic review of conversion studies. *International Psychogeriatrics, 16,* 129–140.

Buckner, R. L., Snyder, A. Z., Shannon, B. J., LaRossa, G., Sachs, R., Fotenos, A. F., et al. (2005). Molecular, structural, and functional characterization of Alzheimer's disease: Evidence for a relationship between default activity, amyloid, and memory. *The Journal of Neuroscience, 25,* 7709–7717.

Carson, M. J., Behringer, R. R., Brinster, R. L., & McMorris, F. A. (1993). Insulin-like growth factor I increases brain growth and central nervous system myelination in transgenic mice. *Neuron, 10,* 729–740.

Chandler, J. D., & Chandler, J. E. (1988). The prevalence of neuropsychiatric disorder in a nursing home population. *Journal of Geriatric Psychiatry and Neurology, 1,* 71–76.

Cohen, E., Paulsson, J. F., Blinder, P., Burstyn-Cohen, T., Du, D., Estepa, G., et al. (2009). Reduced IGF-1 signaling delays age-associated proteotoxicity in mice. *Cell, 139,* 1157–1169.

Costa, R. M., Drew, C., & Silva, A. J. (2005). Notch to remember. *Trends in Neurosciences, 28,* 429–435.

Crook, T., Bartus, R. T., Ferris, S. H., Whitehouse, P., Cohen, G. D., & Gershon, S. (1986). Age-associated memory impairment: Proposed diagnostic criteria and measures of clinical change-report of a NIMH work group. *Developmental Neuropsychology, 2,* 261–276.

Daly, E., Zaitchik, D., Copeland, M., Schmahmann, J., Gunther, J., & Albert, M. (2000). Predicting conversion to Alzheimer disease using standardized clinical information. *Neurology, 57,* 675–680.

De Deyn, P. P., Katz, I. R., Brodaty, H., Lyons, B., Greenspan, A., & Burns, A. (2005). Management of agitation, aggression, and psychosis associated with dementia: A pooled analysis including three randomized, placebo-controlled double-blind trials in nursing home residents treated with risperidone. *Clinical Neurology and Neurosurgery, 107,* 497–508.

De Deyn, P. P., Rabheru, K., Rasmussen, A., Bocksberger, J. P., Dautzenberg, P. L., Eriksson, S., et al. (1999). A randomized trial of risperidone, placebo, and haloperidol for behavioral symptoms of dementia. *Neurology, 53,* 946–955.

Devanand, D. P., Folz, M., Gorlyn, M., Moesller, J. R., & Stern, Y. (1997). Questionable dementia: Clinical course and predictors of outcome. *Journal of the American Geriatrics Society, 45,* 321–328.

Evans, D. A., Funkenstein, H., Albert, M. S., Soherr, P. A., Cook, N. R., Chown, M. J., et al. (1989). Prevalence of Alzheimer's disease in a community population of older persons. *Journal of the American Medical Association, 262,* 2551–2556.

Executive Summary, Alzheimer's Association (2009). *2009 Alzheimer's Disease Facts and Figures.* Chicago, IL: Alzheimer's Association.

Feldman, H., Gauthier, S., Hecker, J., Vellas, B., Subbiah, P. W. E., & the Donepezil MSAD Study Investigators Group (2001). A 24-week, randomized, double-blind study of donepezil in moderate to severe Alzheimer's disease. *Neurology, 57,* 613–620.

Ferri, C. P., Prince, M., Brayne, C., Brodaty, H., Fratiglioni, L., Ganguli, M., et al. (2005). Global prevalence of dementia: A Delphi consensus study. *Lancet, 366,* 2112–2117.

Ferris, S. H., de Leon, M. J., Wolf, A. P., Farkas, T., Christman, D. R., Reisberg, B., et al. (1980). Positron emission tomography in the study of aging and senile dementia. *Neurobiology of Aging, 1,* 127–131.

Finkel, S. I. (Ed.) (1996). Behavioral and psychological signs and symptoms of dementia: Implications for research and treatment. *International Psychogeriatrics, 8* (Suppl. 3), 552 pp.

Finkel, S., & Burns, A. (Eds.) (2000). Behavioural and psychological symptoms of dementia (BPSD): A clinical and research update. *International Psychogeriatrics, 12* (Suppl. 1), 424 pp.

Flechsig, P. (1920). *Anatomie des menschlichen Gehirns und Rückenmarks auf myelogenetischer Grundlage.* Thieme, Leipzig.

Flicker, C., Ferris, S. H., & Reisberg, B. (1991). Mild cognitive impairment in the elderly: Predictors of dementia. *Neurology, 41,* 1006–1009.

Flores, A. I., Narayanan, S. P., Morse, E. N., Shick, H. E., Yin, X., Kidd, G., et al. (2008). Constitutively active Akt induces enhanced myelination in the CNS. *The Journal of Neuroscience, 28,* 7174–7183.

Folstein, M. F., Folstein, S. E., & McHugh, P. R. (1975). Mini-mental state: A practical method for grading the cognitive state of patients for the clinician. *Journal of Psychiatry Research, 12,* 189–198.

Franssen, E. (2003). Neurologic signs in aging and dementia. In A. Burns (Ed.), *Aging and dementia: A methodological approach* (pp. 144–174). London: Edward Arnold.

Franssen, E. H., Kluger, A., Torossian, C. L., & Reisberg, B. (1993). The neurologic syndrome of severe Alzheimer's disease: Relationship to functional decline. *Archives of Neurology, 50*, 1029–1039.

Franssen, E. H., Reisberg, B., Kluger, A., Sinaiko, E., & Boja, C. (1991) Cognition independent neurologic symptoms in normal aging and probable Alzheimer's disease. *Archives of Neurology, 48*, 148–154.

Franssen, E. H., Souren, L. E. M., Torossian, C. L. & Reisberg, B. (1999). Equilibrium and limb coordination in mild cognitive impairment and mild Alzheimer's disease. *Journal of the American Geriatrics Society, 47*, 463–499.

Franssen, E. H., Souren, L. E. M., Torossian, C. L., & Reisberg, B. (1997). Utility of developmental reflexes in the differential diagnosis and prognosis of incontinence in Alzheimer's disease. *Journal of Geriatric Psychiatry and Neurology, 10*, 22–28.

Gagnon, M., Dartigues, J. F., Mazaux, J. M., Dequae, L., Letenneur, L., Giroire, J. M., et al. (1994). Self-reported memory complaints and memory performance in elderly French community residents: Results of the PAQUID Research Program. *Neuroepidemiology, 13*, 145–154.

Gauthier, S., Reisberg, B., Zaudig, M., Petersen, R. C., Ritchie, K., Broich, K., et al. on behalf of the participants of the IPA Expert Conference on MCI. (2006). Mild Cognitive Impairment. *Lancet, 367*, 1262–1270.

Geerlings, M. I., Jonker, C., Bouter, L. M., Ader, H. J., & Schmand, B. (1999). Association between memory complaints and incident Alzheimer's disease in elderly people with normal baseline cognition. *American Journal of Psychiatry, 156*, 531–537.

Glabe C. (2006). Biomedicine. Avoiding collateral damage in Alzheimer's disease treatment. *Science, 314*, 602–603.

Graves, A. B., Larson, E. B., Edland, S. D., Bowen, J. D., McCormick, W. C., McCurry, S. M., et al. (1996). Prevalence of dementia and its subtypes in the Japanese American population of King County, Washington State: The Kame Project. *American Journal of Epidemiology, 144*, 760–771.

Health Care Financing Administration (HCFA). (1998). Hospice-determining terminal status in non-cancer diagnoses-dementia. *The Medicare News Brief/Empire Medical Services*, (MNB-98–7), 45–47.

Hoyer, S. (1998). Is sporadic Alzheimer disease the brain type of non-insulin dependent diabetes mellitus? A challenging hypothesis. *Journal of Neural Transmission, 105*, 415–422.

Hughes, C. P., Berg, L., Danziger, W. L., Coben, L. A., & Martin, R. L. (1982). A new clinical scale for the staging of dementia. *British Journal of Psychiatry, 140*, 566–572.

Hu, X., Hicks, C. W., He, W., Wong, P., Macklin, W. B., Trapp, B. D., et al. (2006). Bace1 modulates myelination in the central and peripheral nervous system. *Nature Neuroscience, 9*, 1520–1525.

Jeste, D. V., Blazer, D., Casey, D., Meeks, T., Salzman, C., Schneider, L., et al. (2008). ACNP White Paper: Update on use of antipsychotic drugs in elderly persons with dementia. *Neuropsychopharmacology, 33*, 957–970.

Jonker, C., Geerlings, M. I., & Schmand, B. (2000). Are memory complaints predictive for dementia? A review of clinical and population-based studies. *International Journal of Geriatric Psychiatry, 15*, 983–991.

Kales, H. C., Valenstein, M., Kim, H. M., McCarthy, J. F., Ganoczy, D., Cunningham, F., et al. (2007). Mortality risk in patients with dementia treated with antipsychotics versus other psychiatric medications. *The American Journal of Psychiatry, 164*, 1568–1576.

Kaplan, A. (2005). High rates of dementia, psychiatric disorders found in assisted living facilities. *Psychiatric Times, 22*, 1 & 5–6.

Katz, I. R., Jeste, D., Mintzer, J. E., Clyde, C., Napolitano, J., & Brecher, M. (1999). Comparison of resperidone and placebo for psychosis and behavioral disturbances associated with dementia: A randomized, double-blind trial. *Journal of Clinical Psychiatry, 60*, 107–115.

Katzman, R. (1986). Alzheimer's disease. *New England Journal of Medicine, 314*, 964–973.

Kidd, M. (1963). Paired helical filaments in electron microscopy of Alzheimer's disease. *Nature, 197*, 192–193.

Kluger, A., Ferris, S. H., Golomb, J., Mittelman, M. S., & Reisberg, B. (1999). Neuropsychological prediction of decline to dementia in nondemented elderly. *Journal of Geriatric Psychiatry and Neurology, 12*, 168–179.

Kluger, A., Gianutsos, J. G., Golomb, J., Ferris, S. H., George, A. E., Franssen, E., et al. (1997). Patterns of motor impairment in normal aging, mild cognitive decline and early Alzheimer's disease. *Journal of Gerontology: Psychological Sciences, 52B*, P28–P39.

Kondo, J., Honda, T., Mori, H., Hamada, Y., Miura, R., Ogawara, M., et al. (1988). The carboxyl third of tau is tightly bound to paired helical filaments. *Neuron, 1,* 827–834.

Kumar, A., Koss, E., Metzler, D., Moore, A., & Friedland, R. (1988). Behavioral symptomatology in dementia of the Alzheimer's type. *Alzheimer Disease and Associated Disorders, 2,* 363–365.

Laboratory Corporation of America. Holdings and Lexi-Comp Inc. (2003). Retrieved 2003, from http://www.labcorp.com/datasets/labcorp/html/chapter/mono/sr003600.htm

Larson, E. B., & Langa, K. M. (2008). The rising tide of dementia worldwide. *Lancet, 372,* 430–432.

Lobo, A., Launer, L. J., Fratiglioni, L., Andersen, K., Di Carlo, A., Breteler, M. M., et al. (2000). Prevalence of dementia and major subtypes in Europe: A collaborative study of population-based cohorts. Neurologic Diseases in the Elderly Research Group. *Neurology, 54,* S4–S9.

Lyketsos, C. G., Steinberg, M., Tschanz, J. T., Norton, M. C., Steffens, D. C., & Breitner, J. C. (2000). Mental and behavioral disturbances in dementia: Findings from the Cache County Study on Memory in Aging. *American Journal of Psychiatry, 157,* 708–714.

McGeer, P. L., McGeer, E. G., Akiyama, H., Itagaki, S., Harrop, R., & Peppard, R. (1990). Neuronal degeneration and memory loss in Alzheimer's disease and aging. *Experimental Brain Research,* (Suppl. 21), 411–426.

McElroy, B., Powell, J. C., & McCarthy, J. V. (2007). The insulin-like growth factor 1 (IGF-1) receptor is a substrate for gamma-secretase-mediated intramembrane proteolysis. *Biochemical and Biophysical Research Communications, 358,* 1136–1141.

Moloney, A. M., Griffin, R. J., Timmons, S., O'Connor, R., Ravid, R., & O'Neill, C. (2010). Defects in IGF-1 receptor, insulin receptor and IRS-1/2 in Alzheimer's disease indicate possible resistance to IGF-1 and insulin signaling. *Neurobiology of Aging, 31,* 224–243.

Montine, T. J., & Larson, E. B. (2009). Late-life dementias: Does this unyielding global challenge require a broader view? *Journal of the American Medical Association, 302,* 2593–2594.

Morris, J. C. (1993). The Clinical Dementia Rating (CDR): Current version and scoring rules. *Neurology, 43,* 2412–2414.

Morris, J. C., Storandt, M., Miller, P., McKeel, D. W., Price, J. L., Rubin, E. H., et al. (2001). Mild cognitive impairment represents early-stage Alzheimer disease. *Neurology, 58,* 397–405.

Mosconi, L., De Santi, S., Brys, M., Tsui, W. H., Pirraglia, E., Glodzik-Sobanska, L., et al. (2008). Hypometabolism and altered cerebrospinal fluid markers in normal apolipoprotein E E4 carriers with subjective memory complaints. *Biological Psychiatry, 63,* 609–618.

Näslund, J., Haroutunian, V., Mohs, R., Davis, K. L., Davies, P., Greengard, P., et al. (2000). Correlation between elevated levels of amyloid ß-peptide in the brain and cognitive decline. *The Journal of the American Medical Association, 283,* 1571–1577.

Ouvrier, R. A., Goldsmith, R. F., Ourvrier, S., & Williams, I. C. (1993). The value of the mini-mental state examination in childhood: A preliminary study. *Journal of Child Neurology, 8,* 145–148.

PDR Network (2009). *Physicians' Desk Reference.* Montvale, New Jersey: PDR Network, p. 2683.

Petersen, R. C., Smith, G. E., Waring, S. C., Ivnik, R. J., Tangalos, E. G., & Kokmen, E. (1999). Mild cognitive impairment: Clinical characterization and outcome. *Archives of Neurology, 56,* 303–308.

Petersen, R. C., Stevens, J. C., Ganguli, M., Tangalos, E. G., Cummings, J. L., & DeKosky, S. T. (2001). Practice parameter: Early detection of dementia: Mild cognitive impairment (an evidence-based review). Report of the Quality Standards Subcommittee of the American Academy of Neurology. *Neurology, 56,* 1133–1142.

Phelps, M. E. (2000). Positron emission tomography provides molecular imaging of biological processes. *Proceedings of the National Academy of Sciences of the United States of America, 97,* 9226–9233.

Pluta, R. (2002). Astroglial expression of the beta-amyloid in ischemia-reperfusion brain injury. *Annals of the New York Academy of Sciences, 977,* 102–108.

Popa-Wagner, A., Schröder, E., Walker, L. C., & Kessler, C. (1998). ß-Amyloid precursor protein and ss-amyloid peptide immunoreactivity in the rat brain after middle cerebral artery occlusion: Effect of age. *Stroke, 29,* 2196–2202.

Prichep, L. S., John, E. R., Ferris, S. H., Rausch, L., Fang, Z., Cancro, R., et al. (2006). Prediction of longitudinal cognitive decline in normal elderly using electrophysiological imaging. *Neurobiology of Aging, 27,* 471–481.

Puglielli, L. (2008). Aging of the brain, neurotrophin signaling, and Alzheimer's disease: Is IGF1-R the common culprit? *Neurobiology of Aging, 29,* 795–811.

Raz, N. (1999). Aging of the brain and its impact on cognitive performance: Integration of structural and functional findings. In F. I. M. Craik & T. A. Salthouse (Eds.), *Handbook of aging and cognition.* Mahwah, NJ: Erlbaum.

Reinikainen, K. J., Koivisto, K., Mykkänen, L., Hanninen, T., Laakso, M., Pyorala, K., et al. (1990). Age-associated memory impairment in aged population: An epidemiological study. *Neurology, 40,* 177.

Reisberg, B. (1986). Dementia: A systematic approach to identifying reversible causes. *Geriatrics, 41*(4), 30–46.

Reisberg, B. (1988). Functional assessment staging (FAST). *Psychopharmacology Bulletin, 24,* 653–659.

Reisberg, B. (2007). Global measures: Utility in defining and measuring treatment response in dementia. *International Psychogeriatrics, 19,* 421–456.

Reisberg, B., Auer, S. R., Monteiro, I., Franssen, E., & Kenowsky, S. (1998). A rational psychological approach to the treatment of behavioral disturbances and symptomatology in Alzheimer's disease based upon recognition of the developmental age. *International Academy for Biomedical and Drug Research, 13,* 102–109.

Reisberg, B., Borenstein, J., Franssen, E., Shulman, E., Steinberg, G., & Ferris, S. H. (1986). Remediable behavioral symptomatology in Alzheimer's disease. *Hospital and Community Psychiatry, 37,* 1199–1201.

Reisberg, B., Borenstein, J., Salob, S. P., Ferris, S. H., Franssen, E., & Georgotas, A. (1987). Behavioral symptoms in Alzheimer's disease: Phenomenology and treatment. *Journal of Clinical Psychiatry, 48*(5, Suppl.), 9–15.

Reisberg, B., Doody, R., Stöffler, A., Schmitt, F., Ferris, S., & Möbius, H.-J., for the Memantine Study Group. (2003). Memantine in moderate-to-severe Alzheimer's disease. *New England Journal of Medicine, 348,* 1333–1341.

Reisberg, B., Ferris, S. H., Anand, R., de Leon, M. J., Schneck, M. K., Buttinger, C., et al. (1984). Functional staging of dementia of the Alzheimer's type. *Annals of the New York Academy of Sciences, 435,* 481–483.

Reisberg, B., Ferris, S. H., de Leon, M. J., & Crook, T. (1982). The global deterioration scale for assessment of primary degenerative dementia. *American Journal of Psychiatry, 139,* 1136–1139.

Reisberg, B., Ferris, S. H., de Leon, M. J., Kluger, A., Franssen, E., Borenstein, J. et al. (1989). The stage specific temporal course of Alzheimer's disease: Functional and behavioral concomitants based upon cross-sectional and longitudinal observation. In K. Iqbal, H. M. Wisniewski, & B. Winblad (Eds.), *Alzheimer's Disease and Related Disorders: Progress in Clinical and Biological Research* (Vol. 317, pp. 23–41). New York: Alan R. Liss.

Reisberg, B., Ferris, S. H., de Leon, M. J., Sinaiko, E., Franssen, E., Kluger, A., et al. (1988). Stage-specific behavioral, cognitive, and in vivo changes in community residing subjects with age-associated memory impairment and primary degenerative dementia of the Alzheimer type. *Drug Development Research, 15,* 101–114.

Reisberg, B., Ferris, S. H., & Franssen, E. (1985). An ordinal functional assessment tool for Alzheimer's-type dementia. *Hospital and Community Psychiatry, 36,* 593–595.

Reisberg, B., Ferris, S. H., & Franssen, E. (1986). Functional degenerative stages in dementia of the Alzheimer's type appear to reverse normal human development. In C. Shagass, R. Josiassen, W. H. Bridger, K. Weiss, D. Stoff & G. M. Simpson (Eds.), *Biological Psychiatry,* 1985 (Vol. 7, pp. 1319–1321) New York: Elsevier Science Publishing Co.

Reisberg, B., Ferris, S. H., Franssen, E. H., Kluger, A., & Borenstein, J. (1986). Age-associated memory impairment: The clinical syndrome. *Developmental Neuropsychology, 2,* 401–412.

Reisberg, B., Ferris, S. H., Franssen, E., Shulman, E., Monteiro, I., Sclan, S. G., et al. (1996). Mortality and temporal course of probable Alzheimer's disease: A five-year prospective study. *International Psychogeriatrics, 8,* 291–311.

Reisberg, B., Ferris, S. H., Kluger, A., Franssen, E., Wegiel, J., & de Leon, M. J. (2008). Mild cognitive impairment (MCI): A historical perspective. *International Psychogeriatrics, 20,* 18–31.

Reisberg, B., Ferris, S. H., Oo, T., & Franssen, E. (2003). Staging: Relevance for trial design in vascular burden of the brain. *International Psychogeriatrics, 15* (Suppl. 1), 231–239.

Reisberg, B., Ferris, S. H., Torossian, C., Kluger, A., & Monteiro, I. (1992). Pharmacologic treatment of Alzheimer's disease: A methodologic critique based upon current knowledge of symptomatology and relevance for drug trials. *International Psychogeriatrics, 4*(Suppl. 1), 9–42.

Reisberg, B., Franssen, E., Bobinski, M., Auer, S., Monteiro, I., Boksay, I., et al. (1996). Overview of methodologic issues for pharmacologic trials in mild, moderate, and severe Alzheimer's disease. *International Psychogeriatrics, 8,* 159–193.

Reisberg, B., Franssen, E. H., Hasan, S. M., Monteiro, I., Boksay, I., Souren, L. E. M., et al. (1999). Retrogenesis: Clinical, physiologic and pathologic mechanisms in brain aging, Alzheimer's and other dementing processes. *European Archives of Psychiatry and Clinical Neuroscience, 249*(Suppl. 3), 28–36.

Reisberg, B., Franssen, E., Sclan, S. G., Kluger, A., & Ferris, S. H. (1989). Stage specific incidence of potentially remediable behavioral symptoms in aging and Alzheimer's disease: A study of 120 patients using the BEHAVE-AD. *Bulletin of Clinical Neuroscience, 54,* 95–112.

Reisberg, B., Franssen, E. H., Souren, L. E. M., Auer, S. R., Akram, I., & Kenowsky, S. (2002). Evidence and mechanisms of retrogenesis in Alzheimer's and other dementias: Management and treatment import. *American Journal of Alzheimer's Disease, 17,* 202–212.

Reisberg, B., Franssen, E. H., Souren, L. E. M., Auer, S., & Kenowsky, S. (1998). Progression of Alzheimer's disease: Variability and consistency: Ontogenic models, their applicability and relevance. *Journal of Neural Transmission, 54* (Suppl.), 9–20.

Reisberg, B., Franssen, E., Souren, L., Kenowsky, S., & Auer, S. (1998). Severity scales. In A. Wimo, B. Jönsson, G. Karlsson, & B. Winblad (Eds.) *Health Economics of Dementia* (pp. 327–357). Chichester: John Wiley and Sons.

Reisberg, B., & Gauthier, S. (2008). Current evidence for subjective cognitive impairment (SCI) as the pre-mild cognitive impairment (MCI) stage of subsequently manifest Alzheimer's disease. *International Psychogeriatrics, 20,* 1–16.

Reisberg, B., Kenowsky, S., Franssen, E. H., Auer, S. R., & Souren, L. E. M. (1999). President's Report: Towards a science of Alzheimer's disease management: A model based upon current knowledge of retrogenesis. *International Psychogeriatrics, 11,* 7–23.

Reisberg, B., London, E., Ferris, S. H., Borenstein, J., Scheier, L., & de Leon, M. J. (1983). The Brief Cognitive Rating Scale: Language, motoric, and mood concomitants in primary degenerative dementia. *Psychopharmacology Bulletin, 19,* 702–708.

Reisberg, B., Pattschull-Furlan, A., Franssen, E., Sclan, S. G., Kluger, A., Dingcong, L., et al. (1990). Cognition related functional, praxis and feeding changes in CNS aging and Alzheimer's disease and their developmental analogies. In K. Beyreuther & G. Schettler (Eds.), *Molecular mechanisms of aging* (pp. 18–40). Berlin: Springer-Verlag.

Reisberg, B., Prichep, L., Mosconi, L., John, E. R., Glodzik-Sobanska, L., Boksay, I., et al. (2008). The pre-mild cognitive impairment, subjective cognitive impairment stage of Alzheimer's disease. *Alzheimer's & Dementia, 4*(Suppl. 1), S98–S108.

Reisberg, B., & Saeed, M. U. (2004). Alzheimer's disease. In J. Sadovoy, L. F. Jarvik, G. T. Grossberg, & B. S. Meyers (Eds.), *Comprehensive Textbook of Geriatric Psychiatry,* Third Edition (pp. 449–509). New York: W.W. Norton.

Reisberg, B., Schneck, M. K., Ferris, S. H., Schwartz, G. E., & de Leon, M. J. (1983). The brief cognitive rating scale (BCRS): Findings in primary degenerative dementia (PDD). *Psychopharmacology Bulletin, 19,* 47–50.

Reisberg, B., Sclan, S., Franssen, E., de Leon, M. J., Kluger, A., Torossian, C., et al. (2008). The GDS Staging System: Global Deterioration Scale (GDS), Brief Cognitive Rating Scale (BCRS), Functional Assessment Staging (FAST). In A. J. Rush, Jr., M. B. First, & D. Blacker (Eds.), *Handbook of Psychiatric Measures, Second Edition* (pp. 431–435). Washington, D.C.: American Psychiatric Publishing.

Reisberg. B., & Shulman, M. B. (2009). Commentary on "A Roadmap for the Prevention of Dementia II: Leon Thal Symposium 2008." Subjective cognitive impairment as an antecedent of Alzheimer's dementia: Policy import. *Alzheimer's & Dementia, 5,* 154–156.

Reisberg, B., Shulman, M. B., Torossian, C., Leng, L., & Zhu, W. (2010). Outcome over seven years of healthy adults with and without subjective cognitive impairment. *Alzheimer's & Dementia, 6,* 11–24.

Reisberg, B., Wegiel, J., Franssen, E., Auer, S., Shimada, M., Meguro, K., et al. (2006a). Behavioral and neuropathophysiologic course of Alzheimer's disease (AD): A synthesis based on retrogenesis, arboreal and neurometabolic entropy and possible etiopathogenic events. In: K. Iqbal, B. Winblad, & J. Avila (Eds.), *Alzheimer's Disease: New Advances* (pp. 219–222). Bologna, Italy: Medimond International Proceedings.

Reisberg, B., Wegiel, J., Franssen, E., Kadiyala, S., Auer, S., Souren, L., et al. (2006b). Clinical features of severe dementia: staging. In A. Burns & B. Winblad (Eds.), *Severe Dementia* (pp. 83–115). London: John Wiley & Sons.

Rosenblatt, A., Samus, Q. M., Steele, C. D., Baker, A. S., Harper, M. G., Brandt, J., et al. (2004). The Maryland Assisted Living Study: Prevalence, recognition, and treatment of dementia and other psychiatric disorders in the assisted living population of central Maryland. *Journal of the American Geriatrics Society, 52,* 1618–1625.

Rovner, B. W., Kafonek, S., Filipp, L., Lucas, M. J., & Folstein, M. F. (1986). Prevalence of mental illness in a community nursing home. *American Journal of Psychiatry, 143,* 1446–1449.

Rubial-Álvarez, S., Machado, M.-C., Sintas, E., de Sola, S., Böhm, P., & Peña-Casanova, J. (2007). A preliminary study of the mini-mental state examination in a Spanish child population. *Journal of Child Neurology, 22,* 1269–1273.

Rubin, E., Morris, J., Storandt, M., & Berg, L. (1987). Behavioral changes in patients with mild senile dementia of the Alzheimer's type. *Psychiatry Research, 21,* 55–61.

Schneider, L. S., Dagerman, K. S., & Insel P. (2005). Risk of death with atypical antipsychotic drug treatment for dementia: Meta-analysis of randomized placebo-controlled trials. *Journal of the American Medical Association, 294,* 1934–1943.

Schneider, L. S., Tariot, P. N., Dagerman, K. S., Davis, S. M., Hsiao, J. K., Ismail, M. S., et al. for the CATIE-AD Study Group. (2006). Effectiveness of atypical antipsychotic drugs in patients with Alzheimer's disease. *The New England Journal of Medicine, 355,* 1525–1538.

Sclan, S. G., Foster, J. R., Reisberg, B., Franssen, E., & Welkowitz, J. (1990). Application of Piagetian measures of cognition in severe Alzheimer's disease. *Psychiatric Journal of the University of Ottawa, 15,* 221–226.

Sclan, S. G., & Reisberg, B. (1992). Functional assessment staging (FAST) in Alzheimer's disease: Reliability, validity and ordinality. *International Psychogeriatrics, 4,* 55–69.

Seubert, P., Vigo-Pelfrey, C., Esch, F., Lee, M., Dovey, H., Davis, D., et al. (1992). Isolation and quantification of soluble Alzheimer's beta-peptide from biological fluids. *Nature, 359,* 325–327.

Shimada, M., Hayat, J., Meguro, K., Oo, T., Jafri, S., Yamadori, A., et al. (2003). Correlation between functional assessment staging and the 'Basic Age' by the Binet scale supports the retrogenesis model of Alzheimer's disease: A preliminary study. *Psychogeriatrics, 3,* 82–87.

Sinigaglia-Coimbra, R., Cavalheiro, E. A., & Coimbra, C.G. (2002). Postischemic hyperthermia induces Alzheimer-like pathology in the rat brain. *Acta Neuropathologica (Berlin), 103,* 444–452.

Souren, L. E. M., Franssen, E. M., & Reisberg, B. (1995). Contractures and loss of function in patients with Alzheimer's disease. *Journal of the American Geriatrics Society, 43,* 650–655.

Steen, E., Terry, B. M., Rivera, E. J., Cannon, J. L., Neely, T. R., Tavares, R., et al. (2005). Impaired insulin and insulin-like growth factor expression and signaling mechanisms in Alzheimer's disease–Is this type 3 diabetes? *Journal of Alzheimer's Disease, 7,* 63–80.

Stephen, P. J., & Williamson, J. (1984). Drug-induced parkinsonism in the elderly. *Lancet, 2,* 1082–1083.

Tariot, P. N., Farlow, M., Grossberg, G. T., Graham, S. M., McDonald, S., & Gergel, I., for the Memantine Study Group (2004). Memantine treatment in patients with moderate to severe Alzheimer Disease already receiving Donepezil. *Journal of the American Medical Association, 3,* 317–324.

Tierney, M. C., Szalai, J. P., Snow, W. G., Fisher, R. H., Nores, A., Nadon, G., et al. (1996). Prediction of probable Alzheimer's disease in memory-impaired patients: A prospective longitudinal study. *Neurology, 46,* 661–665.

Tobiansky, R., Blizard, R., Livingston, G., & Mann, A. (1995). The Gospel Oak Study stage IV: The clinical relevance of subjective memory impairment in older people. *Psychological Medicine, 25,* 779–786.

Townsend, M., Mehta, T., & Selkoe, D. J., (2007). Soluble Abeta inhibits specific signal transduction cascades common to the insulin receptor pathway. *Journal of Biological Chemistry, 282*(46), 33305–33312.

Uzgiris, I., & Hunt, J. Mc V. (1975). *Assessment in Infancy: Ordinal Scales of Psychological Development.* Urbana: University of Illinois.

Wang, P.-N., Wang, S.-J., Fuh, J-L., Teng, E. L., Liu, C. Y., Lin, C. H., et al. (2000). Subjective memory complaint in relation to cognitive performance and depression: A longitudinal study of a rural Chinese population. *Journal of the American Geriatrics Society, 48,* 295–299.

Wang, P. S., Schneeweiss, S., Avorn, J., Fischer, M. A., Mogun, H., Solomon, D. H., et al. (2005). Risk of death in elderly users of conventional vs. atypical antipsychotic medications. *The New England Journal of Medicine, 353,* 2335–2341.

Wegiel, J., Dowjat, K., Kaczmarski, W., Kuchna, I., Nowicki, K., Frackowiak, J., et al. (2008). The role of overexpressed DYRK1A protein in the early onset of neurofibrillary degeneration in Down syndrome. *Acta Neuropathologica, 116,* 391–407.

Wegiel, J., Wisniewski, H. M., Dziewiatkowski, J., Badmajew, E., Tarnawski, M., Reisberg, B., et al. (1999). Cerebellar atrophy in Alzheimer's disease—clinicopathological correlations. *Brain Research, 819,* 41–50.

Willem, M., Garratt, A. N., Novak, B., Citron, M., Kaufmann, S., Rittger, A., et al. (2006). Control of peripheral nerve myelination by the beta-secretase BACE1. *Science, 314,* 664–666.

Winblad, B., Kilander, L., Eriksson, S., Minthon, L., Båtsman, S., Wetterholm, A.-L., et al. for the Severe Alzheimer's Disease Study Group. (2006). Donepezil in patients with severe Alzheimer's disease: Double-blind, parallel-group, placebo-controlled study. *Lancet, 367,*1057–1065.

Winblad, B., Palmer, K., Kivipelto, M., Jelic, V., Fratiglioni, L., Wahlund, L. O., et al. (2004). Mild cognitive impairment—beyond controversies, towards a consensus: Report of the International Working Group on Mild Cognitive Impairment. *Journal of Internal Medicine, 256,* 240–246.

Winblad, B., & Poritis, N. (1999). Memantine in severe dementia: Results of the M-BEST Study (Benefit and efficacy in severely demented patients during treatment with memantine). *International Journal of Geriatric Psychiatry, 14,* 135–146.

Wischik, C. M., Novak, M., Edwards, P. C., Klug, A., Tichelaar, W., & Crowther, R. A. (1988). Structural characterization of the core of the paired helical filament of Alzheimer disease. *Proceedings of the National Academy of Sciences of the United States of America, 85,* 4884–4888.

Wischik, C. M., Novak, M., Thøgersen, H. C., Edwards, P. C., Runswick, M. J., Jakes, R., et al. (1988). Isolation of a fragment of tau derived from the core of the paired helical filament of Alzheimer disease. *Proceedings of the National Academy of Sciences of the United States of America, 85,* 4506–4510.

Wolf, O. T., Dziobek, I., McHugh, P., Sweat, V., de Leon, M. J., Javier, E., et al. (2005). Subjective memory complaints in aging are associated with elevated cortisol levels. *Neurobiology of Aging, 26,* 1357–1363.

Zhao, W. Q., De Felice, F. G., Fernandez, S., Chen, H., Lambert, M. P., Quon M. J., et al. (2008). Amyloid beta oligomers induce impairment of neuronal insulin receptors. *Federation of American Societies for Experimental Biology Journal, 22*(1), 246–260.

4

Traumatic Brain Injury

Brian Im, MD, Mary Hibbard, PhD, ABPP (RP), Ilana Grunwald, PhD,
Patrick T. Swift, PhD, and Negin Salimi, DO

OVERVIEW

In this chapter, medical aspects of traumatic brain injury (TBI) will be reviewed with attention paid to its epidemiology, etiology, mechanisms of injury, measurement of injury severity, and potential complications. The role of an interdisciplinary treatment team in addressing the unique cognitive and behavioral rehabilitation needs of individuals with varying severity of TBI in both the acute inpatient rehabilitation setting and in the community will be discussed.

INTRODUCTION

A TBI often results in devastating and lifelong challenges that can impact a person's physical, cognitive, and psychological functioning. These challenges reveal the importance of understanding TBI and its impact on both persons who have experienced the injury and their family/friends. Although post-TBI physical impairments undoubtedly can hinder functional independence, the behavioral, cognitive, emotional, psychosocial, and personality changes associated with TBI frequently lead to even greater functional dependency. Although not all TBIs result in dysfunction in all of these domains, it is also not uncommon for some or all of these domains to be affected. As typical of many disabilities, the more functional domains that are impacted by the TBI, the more challenging the recovery course would be. When the cultural, social, and personality backgrounds of each individual are also considered, it is easy to see how all individuals with a TBI require a unique approach to their acute care management and their postacute rehabilitation efforts to optimize recovery.

Although there has been improved education in medical schools, professional training programs in rehabilitation interventions, and the public, regarding the unique cluster of challenges that emerge postbrain injury, more than superficial knowledge about the challenges faced by individuals following TBI and appropriate and targeted interventions have been slow to develop. Increased awareness on the part of clinical assessment teams will allow for appropriate referral of patients for either inpatient or outpatient rehabilitation services.

EPIDEMIOLOGY OF TBI

TBIs occur worldwide resulting in many deaths (i.e., mortality) as well as in significant disability and dysfunction (i.e., morbidity) within a subset of every nation's population. In 1996, one estimate attributed at least 10 million deaths or hospitalizations to TBIs worldwide, with an estimated 57 million people living who have been hospitalized with one or more TBIs. Undoubtedly, there are many more people who were never diagnosed or who never sought treatment after a TBI (Langlois et al., 2006), indicating that these figures underestimate the true burden of this condition.

Long-term outcomes after a TBI differ across nations significantly. In general, mortality secondary to TBI is greater in low- and middle-income countries, whereas disability rates after TBI are less in these countries when compared with high-income countries (De Silva et al., 2009). One probable reason for these findings is that high-income nations have developed better detection and acute care interventions for severe TBI resulting in more individuals surviving with significant disabilities.

In the United States, the Centers for Disease Control and Prevention (CDC) reported from 1995 to 2001 that an average of approximately 50,000 deaths, 235,000 hospitalizations, and 1,111,000 emergency department visits occurred as a result of TBIs annually. High incidences of TBI in both the young and the elderly formed two peak age groups, with the highest risk of TBI occurring among 0- to 4-year-olds and 15- to 19-year-olds. However, later studies with modified age ranges revealed that the young adult and middle-aged population were equally at elevated risk of TBI. A significantly higher risk of severe TBI resulting in hospitalizations and mortality was identified in those older than 65 years. Men were one-and-a-half to two times as likely to experience a TBI than women, except in the elderly where the gender ratio is fairly even (Langlois et al., 2006).

Findings across select nations suggest that certain subgroups of individuals are at elevated risk of TBI. For example, multiple studies from Australia, New Zealand, and the United States reveal more than half of prisoners surveyed had sustained a TBI in their past (Schofield et al., 2006).

Available CDC data probably underestimates the full impact of TBI as many mild injuries remain undiagnosed (Powell, Ferraro, Dikmen, Temkin, & Bell, 2008), many people who experience a TBI do not seek treatment despite experiencing problems related to their injury, and many injuries are treated outside of a traditional hospital system such as in private clinics and/or doctors' offices (Langlois et al., 2006). Mild TBIs, even among individuals seen in emergency departments, often remain undetected, especially if the deficits are subtle enough not to interfere with basic functioning. This is particularly the case when an individual has experienced other life-threatening body trauma, which shifts the focus of acute care interventions to these injuries. Injuries resulting in a TBI may also go unreported in the work place if there is motivation by either the worker or employer not to report an injury.

Sports-related TBIs are notoriously underreported and underdiagnosed. This may be a result of numerous factors including a lack of understanding and recognition of concussions, a lack of proper personnel available with the understanding and training to fully evaluate the impact of a potential concussion, pressure among players and staff to minimize the severity of sports injuries, and/or an existing false belief that there are no long-term consequences from a concussion. The CDC estimates that 1.6–3.8 million sports-related concussions occur in the United States each year with many of these athletes never seeking medical treatment beyond that given by a sideline medical specialist (Langlois et al., 2006). A large percentage of these injuries do not result in a loss of consciousness further hindering detection (Guskiewicz, Weaver, Padua, & Garrett, 2000). Yet, even for those without loss of consciousness, a concussion can result in significant cognitive decline (Collins et al., 1999). Football is estimated to account for the majority of these injuries with a significant number occurring among high school athletes (McCrea, Hammeke, Olsen, Leo, & Guskiewicz, 2004). It is important to note that sports-related concussions are not limited to men and football; high incidences of concussions occur in other sports, even those not usually associated with high-impact collisions, for both men and women. The existing fallacy that there were no long-term consequences from a concussion is now being challenged by multiple studies showing that individuals can have residual cognitive deficits on neuropsychological testing for a significant period of time postconcussion, even when the patient reports being symptom free (Broglio, Macciocchi, & Ferrara, 2007; Fazio, Lovell, Pardini, & Collins, 2007). Furthermore, individuals who have experienced one concussion are at a greater risk of having a second concussion (Guskiewicz et al., 2003).

Substance abuse often plays an indirect role in the onset of a TBI. By far the most widely used substance is alcohol, with more than 50% of patients who experience a TBI found to have elevated blood-alcohol levels at the time of injury (Kolakowsky-Hayner et al., 1999; Levy et al., 2004).

Another large source of underreporting in current databases is due to lack of integration of data on individuals in the military who sustain TBIs. Although there is some controversy as to the exact number of military personnel who sustain a TBI due to potential misdiagnosing of posttraumatic stress disorder (PTSD) as TBI (Hoge, Goldberg, & Castro, 2009), it is undeniable that TBI is a significant source of disability among injured soldiers and the signature injury of the Afghanistan/Iraq wars. Better protective equipment and improved acute care interventions in the field have increased the probability of survival from blast injuries in combat. Therefore, it is not unreasonable to expect that the number of nonfatal TBIs among soldiers will only continue to increase (Okie, 2005).

In much the same way that a prior concussion increases the risk of a subsequent concussion, a prior TBI of any severity also places an individual at increased risk of a repeat TBI. This risk rises further with each subsequent TBI (Annegers, Grabow, Kurland, & Laws, 1980). Most TBI surveillance systems do not include these repeat TBIs in their data. When these varied sources of undetected TBI are combined with the known prevalence of TBI, it is clear that the incidence of TBI is much higher than reported in any one source.

COST OF TBI

The burden on the United States due to TBI is significant. The care and medical costs of a person with a severe TBI can easily surpass 1 million dollars over a lifetime. In a study on the public health implications of TBI, approximately 3.17 million Americans were determined to be living with long-term disability related to TBI (Zaloshnja, Miller, Langlois, & Selassie, 2008). The cost to caretakers, both financially and emotionally, can be significant. Family members of individuals who suffer a TBI often need to leave their jobs or reduce their responsibilities at work in order to take care of their injured relative. Given that there are probably a significant number of TBIs that go undetected and even a seemingly mild TBI can lead to permanent disabilities, which limit a person's functional independence and/or capacity to maintain employment, this is undoubtedly a low estimate of the actual proportion of the population that is affected socioeconomically (Langlois, Rutland-Brown, & Wald, 2006). Consequently, the 60 billion dollars calculated to be the financial toll from medical expenses and lost productivity due to TBI in this country in the year 2000 (Finkelstein, Corso, & Miller, 2006) is likely underestimated.

CAUSES OF TBI

According to the CDC, falls are the leading cause of TBI, followed closely by motor vehicle accidents, struck by/against events (where either intentional or unintentional contact is made between one person and another person/object or where a person is caught between two people/objects), and assaults (Langlois, Rutland-Brown, & Thomas, 2004). Other researchers feel that motor vehicle accidents may be the leading cause of TBI, especially if all forms of transportation, and not just automobiles, are considered (Silver, McAllister, & Yudofsky, 2005).

When the causes of injury are examined with respect to specific subsets of the general population, there are differences as compared with the population as a whole. In young children and the elderly, falls are the leading cause of TBI. In adolescents and young adults, motor vehicle accidents followed by violence, assault, and suicide attempts are the most common causes (Cuccurullo, 2004). Sports- and bicycle-related injuries are also a leading cause of TBI, especially mild TBI, in children, teenagers, and young adults. Firearm use is the leading cause of death related to TBI with a large percentage of these events being suicidal in nature (Langlois et al., 2004). In the 1990s, firearm use replaced motor vehicle accidents as the leading cause of mortality due to TBI, most likely as a result of better motor vehicle safety measures (Sosin, Sniezek, & Waxweiler, 1995). As previously mentioned, blast injuries are a leading cause of TBI among soldiers involved in combat (Okie, 2005). Understanding the causes of TBIs within specific subsets of the population is crucial for developing focused and effective prevention programming.

MECHANISMS OF TBI

Mechanisms of TBI are typically described by either the timing of the injury in relationship to the inciting TBI event (primary vs. secondary injuries) or the characteristics of the traumatic event itself (open vs. closed injuries, blunt vs. sharp trauma, and penetrating vs. nonpenetrating injuries). Each mechanism is described below:

Primary injuries occur at the moment of impact directly due to the actual trauma. These injuries include contusions or bruises of the brain itself, lacerations or tears in the lining of the brain, diffuse axonal injury (DAI), rupture of blood vessels leading to hemorrhages, and cranial nerve injuries.

Secondary injuries occur as a consequence of the primary injury and can develop anywhere from hours to days after the initial injury. The mechanisms of secondary injuries include compression of brain structures, hypoxia (lack of oxygen to the brain), cerebral edema or swelling, and metabolic cellular damage. Causes of these injuries include intracranial hypertension, hypotension, intracranial or intraventricular hemorrhage or fluid collection, vasospasm (spasm of cerebral blood vessels), infection, electrolyte and metabolic disturbances, hyperthermia (elevated body temperature), anemia, endocrine disturbances, and seizures.

Closed injuries are those injuries where the skull and lining of the brain are left intact. Open injuries are those injuries where the intracranial vault is exposed to the outside environment. These injuries expose the patient to a higher risk of infection.

Nonpenetrating injuries are caused by a trauma that does not break skin or enter the body. Penetrating injuries are those which do enter the body. In those penetrating injuries caused by a projectile such as a bullet, the velocity of the projectile directly influences the extent of brain damage that occurs. The velocity of the projectile is important to consider because the size of the fluid wave, which is dependent on how fast the projectile was traveling as it entered the brain, usually causes more widespread damage to the brain than the actual path of the projectile itself.

Blunt force trauma refers to impact against a relatively flat object or surface. Blunt trauma does not necessarily imply a closed head injury since blunt forces can cause skull fractures and soft tissue injury as well. Sharp force trauma is caused by an object with an edge or point and usually implies a penetrating injury.

Blast injuries such as those experienced by many military personnel do not necessarily fit completely into any of the above categories since blast injuries typically result from acceleration–deceleration type forces on the brain as well as a unique mechanism of injury by which blast waves enter the brain itself causing neuronal damage (Courtney & Courtney, 2009).

The mechanism of injury does not necessarily indicate the severity of the TBI or its clinical presentation. Counterintuitively, open skull, sharp force, and penetrating injuries may lead to less brain damage than closed skull, blunt force, or nonpenetrating traumas if the skull fracture is nondisplaced and/or the penetration is minor. Fracturing the skull may actually lead to a dissipation of forces lessening the movement of the brain and its impact against the skull.

POST-TBI: PRIMARY SEQUELAE

Trauma to the brain can result in significant pathology. Typically, individuals identified as having experienced a TBI are seen in an emergency room and, along with a clinical examination, undergo immediate neuroradiological assessment, usually with a noncontrast head computed tomography (CT) scan. Those with identified brain pathology on CT scans are typically admitted to a trauma or neurological/neurosurgical unit for close observation and needed interventions. Common pathology associated with TBI is discussed in this section.

Brain contusions, or bruises of the brain, occur due to impact of the brain against the bony ridges of the skull and are detected on head CT and magnetic resonance imaging (MRI) as areas of localized hemorrhages and/or different attenuation as compared to the rest of the brain. Two types of injury leading to contusions are coup and contrecoup injuries: coup injuries refer to damage caused by the initial impact of the brain against the skull; contrecoup injuries occur at the opposite side of the brain as a result of the brain rebounding against the skull. These contusions manifest in a wide variety of neurological and behavioral dysfunction depending on the area of the brain impacted. The most common area affected in TBI is the lower frontotemporal region of the brain due to the bony anatomy at the base of the skull.

DAI results in shearing forces on the brain from acceleration–deceleration and rotational forces that are often associated with high-velocity impact, such as those occurring in a motor vehicle accident and/or blast injury. These shearing forces disrupt nerve cells in the brain, especially where the more freely moving portion meets the more fixed portion of the brain. DAI is a common underlying reason for the abrupt onset of neurological deficits in a significant proportion of patients with TBI. Patients can present with variable severity of cognitive deficits, from those detectable only under stressful situations to altered levels of consciousness, depending on the severity of injury. CT and MRI of the brain may reveal microhemorrhages in select areas of the brain (i.e., the corpus callosum, central white matter, and midbrain) but many times there are no discernible findings on imaging. As a result, the diagnosis of TBI is often based on clinical examination and subjective complaints of new onset neurological symptoms, especially in those with mild injuries.

Intracranial hemorrhages or hematomas are caused by bleeding underneath the skull from ruptured blood vessels. They are most commonly described by the layer of the brain within which the bleeding occurs. The brain is lined by three layers of tissue: the dura mater, pia mater, and arachnoid mater.

Epidural hematomas are collections of blood between the skull and the outermost layer of the brain called the dura mater. This type of hematoma grows rapidly in size and can lead to death within a matter of hours if untreated. The presence of a lucid interval, where the patient appears to recover from the initial trauma for a short period of time soon after the event, often confuses the clinical presentation. In these situations, the patient's level of arousal rapidly declines after this brief lucid time interval.

Subdural hematomas are collections of blood between the dura and pia mater layers of the brain. These bleeds are usually slower growing, and if they grow slow enough, they can increase for weeks or even months before obvious clinical symptoms of dysfunction are noted.

Subarachnoid hematomas occur between the pia mater and the arachnoid membrane, the closest lining surrounding the brain. They often develop as a result of blood vessel abnormalities (i.e., rupture of an arteriovenous malformation or saccular aneurysm) but also occur as a result of trauma. The classic presentation is that of the patient describing "the worst headache of my life" followed by a sudden loss of consciousness.

Intracerebral or intraventricular hematomas are collections of blood within the brain or ventricles of the brain itself. As with the other hemorrhagic injuries, the patient can develop subsequent neurological deficits and can present with symptoms of increasing headaches, visual changes, nausea, vomiting, dizziness, confusion, weakness, difficulties with balance, and ultimately loss of consciousness and death. Although intracranial hemorrhages can lead to ischemia due to decreased blood supply to parts of the brain, pressure on the brain as the hematoma grows is usually the more life-threatening and devastating cause of neurological decline. In cases of ischemia, where there is cell death, treatment is aimed at reducing the extent of surrounding swelling and inflammation in an attempt to preserve nerve function.

Skull fractures themselves do not usually cause neurological deficits, but the potential complications associated with certain fractures can be significant. Depressed skull fractures are associated with worse neurological deficits and outcomes as opposed to nondepressed fractures, and any open injury will increase the risk of infection as mentioned earlier. With temporal bone fractures there is an increased risk of epidural hematomas due to the vascularity of the area. Basilar skull fractures can damage the facial, acoustic (i.e., hearing), and vestibular (i.e., balance) nerves.

Cranial nerve damage can occur following more severe TBIs. The type of injury, such as compressive versus direct insult to the nerve, will also affect the nature of the deficit, the most appropriate treatment, and the prognosis for recovery. The most common cranial nerve injury after a TBI is to the olfactory nerve (cranial nerve I) leading to anosmia (i.e., a loss of the sense of smell and possible alterations in taste) (Marion, 1999). A lack of awareness of this deficit can potentially lead to significant safety risks such as if the patient fails to detect smoke or a gas leak in the home. Depending on the nerve injured, cranial nerve damage can result in other deficits such as monocular blindness, diplopia, visual field deficits, blurring, blind spots, paralysis of the eyes, ptosis of the eyelid, abnormal dilation of the pupil, numbness of the face, decreased salivation, corneal drying, paralysis of the face, hypersensitivity to sound, ringing in the ears, hearing loss, positional vertigo, autonomic system dysfunction, tongue dysfunction, swallowing and speech difficulties, and shoulder muscle dysfunction.

CLASSIFICATION OF TBI

According to the CDC, a diagnosis of a TBI must involve a known traumatic impact to the head which has resulted in disruption of brain functioning. Often, especially in milder TBIs, there is lack of documented physical evidence of the injury on either exam and/or CT and MRI since microscopic damage after TBI is often not visible on standard neuroradiological assessment tools. In such cases, more advanced neuroradiological imaging such as positron emission tomography, single photon emission computed tomography, and diffusion tensor imaging scans may be of greater help in identifying neuronal damage secondary to trauma. However, the clinical history, neurological exam, and neuropsychological testing remain important diagnostic assessment tools.

Traumatic brain injuries are categorized along a continuum of severity: severe, moderate, and mild injury. Approximately 15% of TBIs are classified as moderate to severe whereas the remainder of TBIs (approximately 85%) are classified as mild in nature (Cuccurullo, 2004). Guidelines for classification typically consider factors such as the presence or absence of consciousness, the duration of the posttraumatic amnesia (PTA) state, and the initial level of function postinjury. In general, the more severe the TBI, the more likely the patient is to have a longer recovery course and permanent functional deficits. However, the prognosis for any given individual after a TBI depends on multiple factors including, but not limited to, age, occupation, education, medical and surgical history, severity of injury, location of injury, medical complications of injury, and recovery course to date.

ALTERED LEVELS OF CONSCIOUSNESS

Consciousness, defined as the state of being alert, aware, and responsive to one's environment, is a function of the ascending reticular activating system. In the early phase of recovery after a TBI, a more severely injured patient typically presents with an altered level of consciousness. Altered states of consciousness are usually divided into coma, vegetative state, and minimally conscious state, with coma representing the least responsive state. Once beyond the minimally conscious state, patients usually evolve through some combination of confused, agitated, and amnestic states before behaviors become appropriate. The duration of altered consciousness after an injury is indicative of the level of TBI severity. Some patients never progress beyond the lower levels of consciousness and ultimately require long-term care and/or placement. Each level of altered consciousness requires differing acute and long-term rehabilitation interventions. Significant research has been done and continues to investigate these altered levels of consciousness and possible interventions, including medications and devices (such as surgical implants), to facilitate recovery from lowered levels of consciousness.

Coma

Coma is a state of unconsciousness from which the patient cannot be aroused; the eyes remain continuously closed, there is no spontaneous purposeful movement or communication, there is no ability to localize noxious stimuli, and there is no evidence of a sleep–wake cycle on electroencephalography (EEG).

Vegetative State

The transition to vegetative state is apparent when the patient exhibits spontaneous or stimulus-induced arousal through eye opening, but there is no evidence of purposeful behavior or verbal or gestural communication. The defining characteristic of a vegetative state is intermittent wakefulness with the presence of a sleep–wake cycle on EEG. The Multi-Society Task Force on Persistent Vegetative State (1994) devised the terms persistent and permanent vegetative state:

- The persistent vegetative state is defined as a vegetative state that is present for more than one month after a brain injury.
- The permanent vegetative state is defined as a vegetative state lasting for more than 3 months after a non-TBI or a vegetative state lasting more than a year following a TBI.

The different timelines suggest that the usual period of most rapid recovery is longer following a TBI than in a non-TBI.

Minimally Conscious State

The detection of visual tracking is indicative of the transition out of the vegetative state into the minimally conscious state. The Aspen workgroup (Giacino et al., 2002) described the minimally conscious state as a state in which there is evidence of minimal, but definite, awareness to self or the environment. The patient is able to demonstrate inconsistent yet reproducible behaviors, such as simple command-following, intelligible verbalization, gestural responses, or object manipulation. The Aspen workgroup proposed that the patient has progressed beyond the minimally conscious state when there is demonstration of consistent command-following, functional object use, and functional interactive communication.

ASSESSMENT TOOLS TO CLASSIFY TBI

Several standardized assessment measures are commonly used to assess the severity of TBI and to track patients' progress and recovery. Several of these measures are described below:

The Glasgow Coma Scale (GCS) is traditionally used by early response, emergency, and trauma teams to rapidly determine the level of responsiveness of a patient (Table 4.1).

TABLE 4.1   *Glasgow Coma Scale*

Score	Best Motor Response	Best Verbal Response	Eye Opening
1	None	None	None
2	Decerebrate posturing (extension) to pain	Mutters unintelligible sounds	Opens eyes to pain
3	Decorticate posturing (flexion) to pain	Utters inappropriate words	Opens eyes to loud voice (verbal commands)
4	Withdraws limb from painful stimuli	Able to converse—confused	Opens eyes spontaneously
5	Localizes pain/pushes away noxious stimuli	Able to converse—alert and oriented	
6	Obeys verbal commands		

Source: Adapted from Teasdale, G., & Jennett, B. (1974). Assessment of coma and impaired consciousness. A practical scale. *Lancet, 2*, 81–84.

Although multiple factors should be considered when trying to classify the severity of a TBI, many times the GCS is used alone to make a simplified determination of severity. The GCS quickly assesses the depth of impaired consciousness across three categories: eye opening, verbal response, and motor response. Each category is scored and totaled together to obtain a composite score between 3 and 15 with higher scores suggesting a greater level of responsiveness. Scores of 3–8 are considered an indicator of a severe TBI, 9–12 of a moderate TBI, and 13–15 of a mild TBI. Of the three items in the GCS, the motor response is the best acute predictor of long-term outcome. The best GCS score within the first 24 hours of recovery has been described as the best predictor of recovery (Jennett, 1979).

The Galveston Orientation and Attention Test (GOAT) is a standardized tool used to evaluate the duration of PTA. PTA is a state of acute confusion marked by difficulty with perception, thinking, and concentration that occurs during the early stages of recovery post-TBI. Patients often cannot form new memories (anterograde amnesia) or recall memories that were made just prior to the injury (retrograde amnesia). The duration of PTA is a common predictor of long-term outcome, with longer duration of PTA an indication of a poorer prognosis. The GOAT includes evaluation of a person's orientation, ability to recall the events prior to and after the injury, and ability to describe the circumstances of the hospitalization. Scores can range from 0 to 100, with a score of 75 or higher for 2 consecutive days indicative that the patient is no longer in a state of PTA (Levin, O'Donnell, & Grossman, 1979).

The JFK Coma Recovery Scale Revised (CRS-R) is a measure used to determine when a patient enters into, and progresses beyond, the minimally conscious state. The scale consists of six subscales that investigate the auditory, visual, motor, oromotor, communicative, and arousal functions of a patient with an altered level of consciousness. Evidence of purposeful activity with testing at any time indicates a patient has entered into the minimally conscious state (Giacino, Kezmarsky, DeLuca, & Cicerone, 1991).

The Rancho Los Amigos Levels of Cognitive Function Scale is an instrument used to categorize a patient's level of postinjury cognitive function and characterize behavioral and cognitive patterns typically seen during acute brain injury recovery (Kay, & Lezzak, 1990). The original eight stages are described in Table 4.2 with a revised version of this measure subsequently developed to further differentiate areas of higher functioning. The lowest level is described as no response and the highest level describes a patient who exhibits purposeful/appropriate behavior. This scale has proven helpful in treatment planning and in helping the inpatient rehabilitation team focus on, and understand, a patient's strengths and weaknesses.

TABLE 4.2 *Rancho Los Amigos Levels of Cognitive Function Scale*

Level	Behaviors Exhibited
I	No response
II	Generalized response to stimulation
III	Localized response to stimulation
IV	Confused and agitated behavior
V	Confused with inappropriate behavior (nonagitated)
VI	Confused but appropriate behavior
VII	Automatic and appropriate behavior
VIII	Purposeful and appropriate behavior

Source: Adapted from Hagen, C., Malkmus, D., & Durham, P. Levels of cognitive functions. In: *Rehabilitation of the head-injured adult: Comprehensive physical management.* Downey, CA: Professional Staff Association, Rancho Los Amigos Hospital, 1979.

EARLY-ONSET COMPLICATIONS OF TBI

Medical complications occur fairly often during the acute phase of recovery after a TBI and can be life threatening if not addressed in a timely fashion. The most common early-onset medical complications include:

Increases in intracranial pressure (ICP) due to cerebral edema or intracranial fluid collection or bleeding can cause compression of brain structures, reduce cerebral blood perfusion leading to cerebral ischemia, or cause brain herniations (brain pushing through the skull). Physicians can detect elevated ICPs by finding papilledema (swelling at the rear of the eye) on exam, evidence of brain compression on head CT scans, or elevated pressures with a lumbar puncture or ICP monitoring device. Clinically, a reduction in the patient's level of consciousness may occur with an elevated ICP ultimately resulting in death if untreated. Establishing an airway for breathing, or a mechanical ventilation, and restoring adequate blood flow to the brain are the first steps in medical management with intracranial surgery often necessary. In cases where neurosurgical intervention is not needed immediately, declines in cognitive or neurological functioning on repeat screening or evidence of worsening findings on serial head CT imaging may still occur. These findings are suggestive of delayed neurological compromise, and intracranial surgery may ultimately be needed to limit secondary brain injury (Braddom, 2007).

Posttraumatic hydrocephalus (PTH) is caused by blockage of normal cerebrospinal fluid (CSF) flow, overproduction of CSF, or insufficient absorption of CSF back into the body. If PTH is left untreated, there is an increased risk of morbidity and mortality (Mazzini et al., 2003). Symptoms associated with PTH consist of incontinence, ataxia, gait disturbances, and dementia. The first symptoms of PTH can also be intermittent headache, vomiting, confusion, and/or drowsiness. CT imaging of the brain is helpful in determining whether PTH is present and to what extent. A surgically inserted ventricular drain may be indicated in some cases for treatment of hydrocephalus. In more severe cases, a ventricular shunt emptying somewhere else in the body (usually into the abdominal cavity) may be permanently placed.

Posttraumatic agitation, described as a subtype of delirium, is marked by restlessness, impulsivity, aggression, emotional lability, disinhibition, and confusion. Posttraumatic agitation has been reported in more than 50% of patients with TBI during early recovery in the acute care setting (Cuccurullo, 2004). The first line of treatment is nonpharmacological, with the focus being on reducing environmental stimulation and providing calm and reassuring cues. The protection of the patient from harming themselves or others is paramount and can be facilitated using nonpharmacological means such as de-escalation techniques, close monitoring, safety devices, and nonthreatening barriers. Assessing for and addressing potential medical issues such as pain, urinary issues, constipation, and infection are important since they can trigger or exacerbate agitation. When conservative interventions fail and/or the safety of the patient or others is jeopardized, there is a role for pharmacological intervention. The most commonly used agents are mood stabilizers, antipsychotic medications, β-blockers, and anxiolytic (antianxiety) medications. Neurostimulants have also been utilized to decrease agitation based on the principle that improving cognitive function may help the patient behave more appropriately. However, these medications should be used judiciously as these same medications may increase agitation or promote delirium in some patients. Certain classes of medications used for agitation management in other situations, such as benzodiazepines or anticholinergic medications, are avoided as much as possible in the TBI population due to their sedating and cognitively impairing effects.

ONGOING COMPLICATIONS OF TBI

TBIs can be complicated by a wide variety of chronic physical, cognitive, and emotional sequelae, which are discussed below. They often require lifelong medical and rehabilitation management.

Hypertension, estimated to develop in 11–25% of patients following a TBI, often resolves spontaneously with time (Cuccurullo, 2004). Earlier generation β-blockers such as propranolol are commonly mentioned to treat hypertension in TBI patients because they provide additional cardiovascular benefits and can help decrease anxiety and restlessness.

Headaches occur commonly after a TBI, both in patients with and without evidence of intracranial bleeding. Typically, these headaches will improve with time if it is a result of the TBI and not related to any other pathology or condition. However, a small proportion of TBI patients continue to have chronic headaches, especially under situations of stress or intense cognitive activity. Treatment includes addressing any other causes for the headache besides TBI, minimizing stress, avoiding other triggers if possible, and using analgesic medications.

Sleep disturbances are often seen in patients after a TBI. Early on, patients usually present with decreased sleep, poor quality sleep, and/or altered sleep–wake cycles. These problems usually improve during the course of recovery. Measures taken to facilitate these improvements include fostering better sleep hygiene, decreasing stimuli during desired sleep hours, addressing any pain or medical issues that may be a source of irritation, and using medications that promote sleep. Although all sleep-promoting medications have a sedating effect by their very nature, those with longer lasting effects and those known to cause more cognitive inhibition such as benzodiazepines and anticholinergics are typically avoided. Long-term sleep disturbances may still exist and often shift to excessive sleepiness. In these cases, addressing any psychiatric disturbances such as depression is important. Furthermore, neurostimulant medications, psychological counseling, better sleep hygiene, and attempts to engage patients regularly in social interactions, activities, and hobbies may be beneficial.

Dysautonomia, also called autonomic dysfunction syndrome, can occur after a TBI as a result of damage to sections of the brain involved in regulating the autonomic system. Clinical symptoms may include fever, hypertension, rapid heartbeat, increased respiratory rate, agitation, sweating, pupillary dilatation, and extensor posturing. Treatment involves addressing both the symptoms as well as any underlying medical triggers for the dysautonomic episode. As a result, multiple classes of medications are used to treat dysautonomia.

Posttraumatic seizures can develop after a TBI. Seizures occurring in the first 24 hours after a TBI are classified as immediate; those in the first week are called early seizures and those after that time period are late seizures (Temkin, Dikmen, & Winn, 1991). The American Association of Physical Medicine and Rehabilitation and the American Association of Neurological Surgeons recommend all TBI patients with postresuscitation GCS scores of less than 12 receive a course of antiseizure medication (phenytoin is often the drug of choice) for 1 week. If the patient has an immediate or early-onset seizure, there is no substantial evidence that ongoing antiepileptic medication is necessary. However, a seizure in the late period may necessitate ongoing antiepileptic medications. Attention must be paid to the use of antiepileptic medications as certain medications such as Dilantin may impair cognitive recovery (Timble, 1987).

Deep venous thrombosis (DVT) is a common complication after a TBI and is associated with immobility, fractures, and soft tissue damage during the early stages of TBI recovery. Although DVTs can be painful and cause swelling, the more serious concern associated with having a DVT is that it increases the risk of developing a pulmonary embolus, a blood clot that travels to the lung vasculature and can be fatal. The most commonly used diagnostic tool for DVT detection is a Doppler ultrasound. Due to the serious health risk posed by pulmonary emboli, DVT prevention is important. Preventative measures include early ambulation or the use of anticoagulation medications and sequential compression devices in nonambulatory patients.

Malnutrition can occur after a TBI as patients may be less responsive, confused and agitated, or have impaired swallow function. In addition, energy demands after a TBI are estimated to be approximately twice that of a noninjured individual. Appetite stimulant medications may be used in cases where the patient has an intact swallow but inadequate nutritional intake. If the patient is at risk for aspiration due to swallowing dysfunction, a softer consistency or thickened diet may be necessary. If the patient has severe enough swallow dysfunction or decreased overall function to the point where they are unable to engage in oral intake, a nasogastric tube or gastrostomy tube can be placed to provide access for nutritional support.

Bowel-related issues such as delayed gastric emptying, constipation, nausea, and gastroesophageal reflux are commonly encountered problems in the TBI patient with impaired mobility and more severe deficits. Stool softeners, laxatives, and motility agents are often used to try to keep the patient's bowel movements regular. Antiemetic agents and proton pump inhibitors are used to decrease symptoms of nausea and reflux. Attempts are usually made to avoid anticholinergic and antihistamine medications as they can impair cognition.

Urological dysfunction after a TBI can result in both overactivity and retention of urine. Bladder overactivity can lead to incontinent episodes as the bladder contracts uncontrollably. These patients benefit from a timed voiding program and the use of medications to increase the bladder capacity or decrease bladder contractility. Urinary retention can also develop after a TBI due to bladder hyporeflexia, where the bladder fails to contract normally, or bladder sphincter dyssynergia, where the bladder contracts against a closed urethral sphincter. These patients often require intermittent catheterizations to empty the bladder and the use of medications to relax the sphincter muscle and facilitate voiding. Urodynamic studies may be beneficial in determining the mechanism of dysfunction.

Spasticity, or an involuntary velocity-dependent increase in muscle resistance to passive range of motion, can occur in any patient with a brain injury (Cuccurullo, 2004). Evaluating and managing spasticity is important to avoid such complications as pain, skin breakdown, functional compromise, and joint contractures. Noninvasive treatments include removing noxious stimuli, repositioning and stretching the affected extremity, pressure or vibration mechanisms, and in more severe cases of spasticity, splinting, or serial casting the affected extremity in a stretched position. Options for the management of spasticity cases that are resistant to noninvasive treatments include oral antispasticity medications (often with limited efficacy), nerve blocks, neuromuscular blocks, intrathecal baclofen pumps, and surgical interventions.

Pressure ulcers in the TBI population most commonly occur in those patients with altered levels of consciousness due to their decreased spontaneous repositioning. Pressure ulcers develop as a result of prolonged pressure or friction over bony surfaces of the body, such as the sacrum, heels, and hips, leading to tissue ischemia. Moisture on the skin can decrease skin integrity making incontinent patients more at risk for pressure ulcer formation. Keys to prevention are diligent skin care and minimization of prolonged pressure on one area of the body. Repositioning every 2 hours is a common practice adopted in the nursing care for these patients since pressure ulcer formation has been seen after 1–4 hours of sustained pressure on research studies (Gefen, 2008). When a significant skin breakdown does occur, local infection and osteomyelitis (bone infection) must be considered. These infections can lead to extensive tissue damage and even become life threatening if not treated promptly. Treatment involves addressing any infectious issues, either locally or systemically as needed. For clean wounds, local wound care and proper nutrition to prevent infection and promote healing are important.

Endocrine dysfunction can occur as a result of damage to select structures within the brain. Overt and subtle hormonal abnormalities can increase fatigue or exacerbate behavioral and cognitive impairments. Treatment entails management of symptoms and sequelae and/or hormone replacement, if necessary. Abnormalities may resolve spontaneously with time as well.

Heterotopic ossification (HO) is the formation of bone in soft tissue or muscle. The risk factors for the formation of HO include prolonged coma and/or immobility, spasticity, edema, trauma, and pressure ulcers. The joints commonly involved are the hips, elbows, shoulders, and knees. HO can cause a low-grade fever as well as pain, decreased range of motion, swelling, redness, and warmth at the involved joint. Range of motion exercises, medications, and radiation treatment have been used to prevent the formation and slow the growth of HO. Surgical resection of calcified soft tissue or muscle is usually reserved for more severe cases of HO, and it is often best to wait until new bone formation has stopped before undergoing resection (Braddom, 2007).

Balance and coordination deficits may develop after a TBI due to injury to the vestibular system or the cerebellum. Injury to cranial nerve VIII, also known as the vestibulocochlear nerve, can result in hearing loss as well as vertigo. Treatment involves physical therapy for balance, vestibular therapy, medications to decrease dizziness and nausea, and patient education. Symptoms of dizziness and lightheadedness can also be seen in patients who are beginning to mobilize after a prolonged period of decreased mobility. This is often due to orthostatic hypotension which is a significant decrease in blood pressure upon sitting or standing from a prone or supine position. Pressure support devices such as abdominal binders and stockings, avoidance of rapid changes in position, and physical therapy to try to acclimate the patient to changes in positioning are used to minimize the pressure change. In severe cases of orthostasis resistant to nonpharmacological treatment, medications can be used to sustain a normal blood pressure.

Cognitive and behavioral dysfunction after a TBI can range from severe debilitating impairments to milder subtle deficits only noticeable under situations of increased stress or fatigue. Cognitive issues can include decreased attention, reduced processing speed, memory and learning difficulties, and executive functioning difficulties in planning/organization and flexible problem solving. Behavioral problems can include disinhibition, personality alterations, outbursts of profanity, poor hygiene practices, hypersexuality (increased libido), and hyposexuality. Decreased awareness of deficits and behavioral disturbances often hinder progress in therapy. Inpatient and outpatient management of these challenges require interventions by rehabilitation professionals experienced and knowledgeable regarding TBI. Both cognitive and behavioral issues can be confusing, distressing, and/or difficult for a patient's family to manage. Family education and support by the treating team in both the inpatient and outpatient settings can serve to minimize family distress. Further discussion regarding these issues including interventions and treatment will be addressed in later sections of this chapter.

Emotional lability, depression, and PTSD are common after TBI and can hinder progress and recovery from the injury. Treatment includes counseling, supportive therapy, and medication management. In patients with significant cognitive impairments, effective counseling may not be feasible. In these cases, a greater focus on medication management is indicated. Some patients develop inappropriate laughter or crying after their TBI (pathological laughter and crying). Treatment usually consists of selective serotonin reuptake inhibitor medications but other antidepressant and mood stabilizing medications have been used as well.

Medications to facilitate cognitive recovery or manage behavioral issues are commonly used in the management of TBI throughout the course of recovery. Although there are few, if any, conclusive studies supporting the use of these medications in TBI management, there is significant evidence indicating that many of these medications can be beneficial (Warden et al., 2006). As such, a discussion between the treating team and the patient and/or family should occur when considering these medications. Furthermore, there may be some ethical concerns to consider when patients are unable to make decisions regarding medication use for themselves, especially with the use of medications that can alter mood or sexual behavior.

TBI patients are often more sensitive to the effects of medications possibly as a result of the dysfunction and susceptibility to further insult within the brain itself. Consequently, they are more sensitive to the side effects of these medications since side effects are simply the effects of a medication that are not desired at that moment. For this reason, nonpharmacological management options should always be considered before initiating medications as many issues may be more effectively and safely addressed without the initiation of medications at all, unless there is an immediate danger to the patient or others. When medications are indicated or needed, care should be taken to avoid unnecessary medications, doses should be titrated up slowly to monitor for side effects, and medications with side effects that may impede cognitive recovery or exacerbate behavioral problems such as sedatives or anticholinergics should be avoided. Although there are usually better tolerated medications for most issues associated with TBI, at times it is necessary to use medications that may have significant detrimental effects on cognition or behavior when there are more pressing medical issues. In these cases, the risks and benefits of the medication must be considered, and vigilance must be maintained to discontinue the medication as soon as it is appropriate to do so.

TBI REHABILITATION: A TEAM APPROACH

TBI-focused rehabilitation services are delivered by a team of specially trained professionals with specific knowledge of interventions for TBI-related issues. An interdisciplinary team approach facilitates communication among team members and allows for rapid sharing of goals for treatment that are tailored to each patient's unique rehabilitation needs. This communication among all team members is vital for an effective rehabilitation program. The rehabilitation team consists of different health care professionals under the leadership of a physician in addition to the patient and their family and friends. The roles of the specific team members in both inpatient and outpatient settings are outlined below. However, there is significant overlap among team members in regards to interventions and treatment goals.

The TBI rehabilitation physician specializes in rehabilitation medicine for individuals with cognitive and physical deficits due to a brain injury. The physician is responsible for the overall coordination of care and continuous, often lifelong, medical and medication management of the patient.

Neurorehabilitation psychologists address alterations in brain functioning that impact the patient's thinking processes, behavior, and emotions after a brain injury. The neuropsychologist will deliver psychological as well as neurocognitive interventions in both inpatient and outpatient settings to maximize the patient's awareness, adjustment to injury, and overall cognitive functioning.

Rehabilitation nurses and nurse's aides address a patient's needs in relation to safety, self-care, medication administration, proper nutrition, dressing, bowel and bladder functions, and mobility.

Physical therapists evaluate and intervene to enhance a patient's independence with mobility tasks including ambulation and transfers. This often involves treating weakness and ROM restriction issues. They also often address cognitive barriers to safe mobility.

Occupational therapists evaluate and intervene to decrease difficulties identified in the performance of basic activities of daily living (ADLs) such as feeding, dressing, bathing, and personal grooming. Occupational therapists may also address sensory, perceptual, and cognitive deficits that can interfere with the completion of higher level ADL such as preparing meals, managing household chores, managing child care responsibilities, and handling finances.

Speech–language pathology therapists evaluate the communication and cognitive abilities of a patient after a TBI. Most speech–language pathology therapists will also evaluate a patient's swallow function and provide treatment to improve swallow safety as needed.

Recreational/art therapists identify areas of leisure and social interest for patients and design social and leisure programs to increase their independence, while providing a healthy outlet for expression. Often, with input from other team members, therapeutic activities are selected to increase awareness of cognitive and behavioral challenges which can impact social functioning.

Vocational counselors assist a patient with transition back into the workforce or school once the patient is deemed safe and ready for return to these activities by the rehabilitation team. If necessary, the vocational counselor may assist the patient to find alternative employment options if acquired physical or cognitive deficits prohibit return to a prior profession or occupation.

Social workers/case managers work as part of both inpatient and outpatient teams. On the inpatient unit, they offer supportive counseling to patients and families, address financial and insurance issues related to the inpatient stay, and assist with plans regarding post-hospital care. In the outpatient setting, they serve as liaisons between the rehabilitation program, insurance carriers, disability offices, and other community resources.

Patients and their families are key members of the rehabilitation team as well. (For the purposes required here, family refers to any person who is involved in the support or care of the patient, whether related to the patient or not.) Family members provide direct care and emotional support as well as insight into each patient's unique social history and behaviors. Although it is not always possible to engage the patient actively, especially early in the recovery course after a TBI, when the patient and family are invested in the rehabilitation program, the effectiveness of a treatment program improves greatly.

INPATIENT TBI REHABILITATION

Once an individual with moderate to severe TBI-related functional, cognitive, and behavioral problems has achieved medical stability in an acute care hospital setting, the patient is typically transferred to an inpatient TBI rehabilitation program. These TBI rehabilitation units can be embedded within a larger medical center or within a free-standing rehabilitation facility. Usually, acute inpatient TBI rehabilitation is the most appropriate setting for initial rehabilitation management. To be eligible for acute inpatient rehabilitation, as opposed to subacute inpatient rehabilitation, patients must be able to engage in and benefit from 3 hours of physical and occupational therapy daily versus less daily therapy at subacute rehabilitation centers. In addition, to be eligible for inpatient rehabilitation at all, most insurers require the patient to have residual physical impairments that would benefit from continued physical rehabilitation. These conditions for coverage do not recognize that cognitive and behavioral dysfunction alone can result in functional limitations as significant as those caused by physical impairments. They also tend to ignore the benefits that acute inpatient TBI rehabilitation offers in addressing the medical complications of TBI early on. Furthermore, most families (assuming the patient has a social support system at all), home care agencies, and subacute rehabilitation facilities are not equipped to manage the significant agitation and behavioral problems that may be present early on after a TBI.

In TBI inpatient rehabilitation units, the patient's functional, cognitive, and neurobehavioral impairments are addressed by the team. Communication among the different team members, family, and patient is emphasized since this approach has been shown to yield the most effective treatment after a TBI (Kosmidis, 2007). The Rancho Levels of Cognitive Functioning Scale (Rancho), described earlier in this chapter (see Table 4.2), is often used by the interdisciplinary inpatient rehabilitation team to facilitate rapid identification of the patient's level of postinjury cognitive and neurobehavioral functioning (Leon-Carrion, 2006) and implement treatment programming appropriate to that level of functioning.

Through the course of their stay, the team establishes a plan that the patients and families can eventually carry out on their own to manage the patient's medical, cognitive, and emotional issues after discharge from the unit. At the point of admission to inpatient rehabilitation, each member of the rehabilitation team completes an initial assessment of each patient's medical issues and physical and cognitive functioning to develop a plan of treatment. Collectively, the team determines each patient's functional level, motivation, and ability to engage in treatment. They then implement the treatment plan with the goal of maximizing the patient's medical stability, participation in therapy, safety awareness, and functional independence. As patients progress through their rehabilitation stay, team members discuss their progress within their programs on a regular basis and try to address any problematic issues that develop. Goals are adjusted as needed. Findings from these evaluations are shared with family members and patients if appropriate. Although each patient presents with a unique combination of challenges, some generalizations can be made, and these approaches are described below in relation to the differing Rancho levels.

Rancho Level I–III Programming

For patients admitted to acute inpatient rehabilitation in a coma or with Rancho levels of II–III, enhancing arousal and responsiveness become the primary goals of rehabilitation interventions. In combination with medications prescribed by the physician, the team will initiate a stimulation program to enhance the patient's level of arousal. The JFK CRS-R is frequently used on inpatient TBI units to help guide programmatic interventions for patients at these levels (Giacino et al., 2002). Using the CRS-R, the team plans interventions utilizing all sensory modalities. In addition, the rehabilitation team will emphasize prevention of contractures and skin breakdown. Families are instructed on how best to communicate with their loved one and how to avoid overstimulating the patient. The amount and variety of stimulation provided increases as the patient improves.

Rancho IV–V Programming

For patients with a Rancho IV–V level, the primary target of rehabilitation interventions is the treatment of inappropriate behaviors. During this phase of recovery, individuals typically present with psychomotor restlessness, agitation, and aggressive behaviors such as kicking and hitting. The overarching goal in treatment is to maintain patient safety while at the same time facilitate the ability to self-regulate behavior. Scales such as the Agitated Behavior Scale may be used to assess the degree of behavioral dysregulation and track the efficacy of rehabilitation treatment efforts (Bogner, 2000; Corrigan, 1989). The use of behavior modification strategies and environmental modifications, such as limiting the number of visitors a patient receives, have proven beneficial in reducing agitation in TBI patients (Herbel, Schermerhorn, & Howard, 1990). Often in this phase, pharmacological agents are prescribed by the physician in order to manage confusion, psychomotor restlessness, and/or aggression.

Rancho V–VI Programming

Patients with a Rancho V–VI level may present with improved orientation but significant cognitive impairments and confusion which can limit their safety awareness and ability to complete ADLs. At this phase, in TBI recovery, the Galveston Orientation and Amnesia Test is frequently used to determine when a patient is demonstrating consistent orientation to place and time. Cognitive impairments may include reduced orientation to place and time, attention, information processing speed, memory, language skills, visuospatial skills, and abstract reasoning. These problems can be further exacerbated by emerging symptoms of depression and anxiety in the patient. Family members may feel relief that their loved one has survived a brain injury, but increased confusion or sadness when the cognitive and behavioral impairments become more apparent. This makes ongoing supportive services for families important. Education of the family and patient now progresses to detailed discussions of cognitive and behavioral changes after a TBI. Based typically on a brief neuropsychological assessment, treatment planning by the team is directed at maximizing cognitive strengths while trying to compensate for cognitive weaknesses using compensatory strategies. A memory book involving a calendar and a to-do list is typically implemented to address memory, orientation, and planning deficits. The physician may prescribe medications to try to facilitate cognitive recovery and address depression and anxiety issues as well.

Rancho VII–VIII Programming

Patients with a Rancho VII–VIII level may be able to follow a structured schedule and perform routine self-care tasks with minimal supervision. These patients continue to benefit from inpatient rehabilitation to increase their awareness of how residual moderate-to-mild cognitive impairments will impact functioning in the community. Their time in therapy allows for practicing of compensatory techniques needed for community living. The interdisciplinary goals also focus on having patients become involved in completion of more complex cognitive and linguistic tasks, while maximizing their physical mobility and independence in ADLs. At this phase of TBI recovery, the risk of depression and anxiety increases due to increasing self-awareness of deficits (Hibbard, Uysal, Kepler, Bogdany, & Silver, 1998; Malec, Testa, Rush, Brown, & Moessner, 2007). As with patients in the Rancho V–VI level, the physician considers medications to treat these issues as well as facilitate cognitive recovery. The neuropsychologist closely monitors the patient and family's ongoing emotional adjustment.

Once a patient remains medically stable and has progressed to a level of functional independence (i.e., able to perform most ADLs independently, live relatively independently and safely in the community, and has an adequate support network to return to the community), the patient is ready for discharge back to the community. Careful patient and family education about discharge plans and needed follow-up appointments is important as the patient may still have problems with organizational skills. If patients are not completely independent or safe on their own, the team may still plan for a discharge to home if appropriate family supervision and follow-up outpatient services can be arranged. In these cases, family education is crucial as the patient may have poor awareness into their deficits and limited compliance with instructions regarding maintaining safe function. If the patient does not reach independence in a timely manner and is unsuitable for return home with family support but remains medically stable, placement in a subacute rehabilitation facility is an option with most TBI patients best suited for TBI specific subacute rehabilitation facilities. Regardless of the discharge plan, families are provided with recommendations on how to best care for the patient going forward, with emphasis placed on the importance of a structured daily routine, maintaining safety, and appropriate environmental accommodations.

OUTPATIENT TBI REHABILITATION

Although moderate to severe TBI patients with significant residual functional, cognitive, and behavioral deficits may return home with substantial family support and continue their rehabilitation as an outpatient, patients with mild TBI or those with significant recovery of cognitive functioning after their TBI represent by far the greater proportion of the patients seen for TBI rehabilitation in the outpatient setting. Approximately 5–15% of individuals with documented mild TBIs remain symptomatic for their entire lives (Alexander, 1995; Cassidy et al., 2004; Iverson, 2005), with many of these individuals eventually seen by outpatient TBI services. Mild TBI has been called the "invisible injury" since the majority of individuals present without noticeable physical deficits or obvious cognitive and behavioral issues at first glance. However, upon closer examination, they often have difficulty across cognitive, behavioral, and emotional domains of functioning. Ongoing physical deficits, especially balance impairments, may also be seen. Indeed, individuals with mild TBI typically present with a growing concern about how their newly acquired cognitive and behavioral changes post-TBI are impacting their former roles and their current safety in the community. Often these individuals are able to function independently in the community with minimal support from family or friends, but unable to resume the former threads of their life as related to work and relationships. Sometimes, cognitive and physical symptoms only emerge after the person with a mild TBI has attempted to return to these former life activities and roles. In many cases, it takes rejection or failure with these former relationships and roles for the patient to seek treatment.

However, even after experiencing rejection or failure, the individual may fail to connect these new difficulties with a prior mild TBI. The variable nature of mild TBI symptoms and the time postinjury when these symptoms become problematic may result in the person never seeking treatment or seeking inappropriate treatment. Those who are able to function marginally in society may be labeled as lazy or malingering. For these reasons, the CDC has prepared an online tool kit to educate the professional community about mild TBI, improve diagnosis of mild TBI symptoms, minimize the risk of misdiagnosis, and help physicians educate patients about mild TBI and its potential long-term sequelae.

Most patients with TBI seeking outpatient rehabilitation services present with a wide array of physical (i.e., increased fatigue, decreased motor dexterity and speed, loss of the sense of smell, dizziness, visual disturbances), cognitive (i.e., reduced attention capacity, disturbances in memory and executive functioning), and emotional problems (i.e., depression, anxiety, impulsivity, restlessness, aggression, emotional lability, decreased initiation, altered libido). A focused outpatient program is typically implemented to improve the patient's overall function and quality of life while attempting to maintain maximal involvement in work/school and family roles each step of the way. However, oftentimes, a delay in return to work or school is needed so that the patient is cognitively and emotionally ready to resume these roles. Treatment duration is usually weekly sessions for 6 months to a year. The goal is for patients to incorporate compensation strategies into their lives at the same time as they are trying to improve their cognitive skills. After completing their initial treatment course, it is not unusual for an individual to return briefly for further counseling in response to a significant life change such as the birth of a child, loss of a job, new responsibilities at work, or relationship changes.

During the outpatient treatment course, sessions are scheduled with the patient and family members together at times to address interpersonal issues. These may include issues related to adjusting to new family roles, changes in relationship, including sexual interactions between the patient and significant other, and concerns over the family's involvement in the patient's life (whether it is too much or too little). At other times, group sessions may be planned with other patients to address issues with social interactions and group dynamics.

As in inpatient settings, the initial treatment plan evolves out of discipline-specific assessments and team decisions regarding the appropriate approach and interventions for each patient.

Neuropsychologists initiate an in-depth neuropsychological evaluation to identify the cognitive and behavioral strengths and weaknesses of each patient. The neuropsychological evaluation includes a review of medical records, comprehensive clinical interviews with the patient and significant others, and administration of a wide array of neuropsychological tests to assess attention and concentration (simple, complex, divided, and sustained), short- and long-term memory (for both visual and verbal material), language and verbal fluency abilities, information processing, and executive functioning (planning, sequencing, organization, and abstraction). Mood, personality characteristics, and behavioral issues are evaluated as well. Test performance is interpreted within the context of each patient's prior level of functioning, which is influenced by education, occupation, and age at the time of injury. In select cases, such as for those patients showing a history of pre-TBI superior intellectual abilities, exhibiting more subtle deficits, or attempting to return to academic pursuits or a high-level job, an additional focused assessment is indicated. The results of the neuropsychological evaluation are shared with the patient, appropriate family, and treatment team. Recommendations for psychology interventions based on these findings typically include cognitive remediation, individual psychotherapy, family therapy, and/or group therapy.

Cognitive remediation is aimed at identifying cognitive issues and trying to address them through retraining exercises and compensation strategies. Overall goals of cognitive remediation include increasing awareness of strengths and weaknesses, improving attention and concentration, learning to use compensatory strategies to minimize the functional impact of deficits, improving basic problem-solving skills, and enhancing social pragmatics (i.e., giving and receiving feedback, improving social skills). Cognitive therapy can be rendered simultaneously by several disciplines including neuropsychologists, occupational therapists, speech therapists, and/or vocational rehabilitation counselors with each discipline emphasizing a different aspect of retraining to increase a patient's functional, behavioral, and emotional well being. Through communication and teamwork, cognitive remediation by the rehabilitation team can be much more effective than by one discipline alone. Without focused cognitive interventions, the patient with a mild-to-moderate TBI may repeatedly reexperience failures in everyday functioning. Repeated failures in valued aspects of daily functioning, such as at work and in relationships, can lead to a downward spiral in both cognitive and emotional functioning, and often results in increased depression, anxiety, or emotional dyscontrol. Medications to facilitate cognitive recovery such as neurostimulants and antianxiety, antidepressant, or mood stabilizing medications may have a role in outpatient management as an adjunct to these nonpharmacological therapies. These medications are overseen by the treating physician.

Social workers, case managers, vocational counselors, and rehabilitation counselors all can be very helpful in facilitating patients' transition back into life roles at home, work, school, and even with leisure activities. In the most effective programs, these members of the treatment team work closely with the therapists to optimize the appropriate services, supportive counseling, and education for their patients and families.

Psychotherapy is a vital component of treatment for those with mild-to-moderate TBI. The neuropsychologist traditionally addresses these issues with both the patient and the family. Many patients struggle with disparities between "how they functioned before the injury" and "how they are functioning postinjury." This discrepancy is a major focus of therapeutic treatment and patients are helped with dealing with loss, adjusting to permanent alterations in self, and managing depression and anxiety. Individuals with mild TBI may be unaware of subtle changes in their cognitive functioning and/or behavior. Education, direct feedback, and feedback from others are often utilized to help increase their awareness. Behavioral changes are commonly experienced after a mild TBI. Patients are taught behavioral management techniques to minimize dyscontrol episodes.

Although physical therapy often has a reduced role, if having a role at all, in outpatient TBI management, there may still be residual physical impairments that need ongoing treatment. Furthermore, balance issues can recur or remain for an extended period of time after a brain injury, and outpatient physical and vestibular therapy can be beneficial for this reason.

Individuals who have survived a catastrophic accident as the cause of their TBI, such as returning military servicemen and servicewomen, may present with additional challenges after their TBI such as PTSD. Erbes et al. (2007) found that 12% of returning soldiers from the Afghanistan and Iraq conflicts met criteria for PTSD, whereas Hibbard et al. (1998) reported that PTSD can be observed in approximately 17% of nonmilitary individuals after a TBI. Common symptoms of PTSD, such as increased irritability, trouble sleeping, and not resuming "normal" activities, are very similar to symptoms typical of mild TBI and can significantly impede recovery after a TBI if unrecognized and not addressed. Counseling and therapy are essential to help patients identify and cope with symptoms of PTSD.

Medical management of TBI in the outpatient setting, regardless of its severity, may be lifelong. At any point after injury, appropriate medical monitoring and interventions may be necessary to address ongoing complications of TBI (discussed in an earlier section of this chapter). In addition to nonpharmacological management, medications are often necessary both in outpatient rehabilitation and after rehabilitation services have ended.

Other therapy disciplines may be involved during outpatient rehabilitation upon referral by the physician. Referrals are based on the presenting physical and functional complaints of the patient. Physical therapists may become involved with the patient who presents with issues of decreased mobility, weakness, and poor balance after a TBI. Many specialized PT programs will also provide vestibular therapy to address complaints of post-TBI dizziness. Vision or eye movement dysfunction can occur after a mild TBI as well. In these situations, the physician may refer the patient to a neuro-ophthalmologist and/or a neuro-optometrist who specializes in the treatment of TBI-related vision disorders.

CONCLUSION

Traumatic brain injuries can be devastating and have widespread and far-reaching effects. A TBI can affect multiple facets of a person's life, including his/her behavior, emotions, cognitive function, personality, physical appearance, and physical function. This can lead to functional failures and medical complications in the acute and long-term phases of TBI recovery, and may result in long-standing and permanent disability. Treatment often necessitates addressing multiple problems over many years even after a mild TBI. The impact of a TBI often extends even further changing family dynamics, altering social interactions, and placing a financial burden on the family and society. For these reasons, it is important to address the needs of those with a TBI and the family members who support them from the initial point of injury onwards. This approach requires increased awareness regarding TBI within the medical community, society as a whole, the patient's family, and, often most challengingly, the TBI patient.

Treatment following a TBI often consists of a combination of medical management of issues that arise through the life span post-TBI, as well as specialized TBI rehabilitation interventions designed to optimize functional recovery. The goal of most treatment programs is to maintain medical stability while providing therapy and treatment to maximize functional ability and independence at each stage of recovery. Although it is unclear to what extent the brain actually heals versus creates new pathways to try to restore function, there is no doubt that early and intensive clinical interventions are important for recovery and safety.

As with most other medical conditions, the best treatment for TBI is to prevent its occurrence. Prevention of TBI is especially important given that many of these injuries are avoidable. Increasing the use of helmets and better safety equipment in sports, developing better substance and alcohol abuse prevention programs, observing proper safety practices in motor vehicles such as avoiding reckless driving and wearing seatbelts, removing tripping hazards and installing safety equipment in the homes of the elderly, implementing ideas to decrease TBI risk in children, such as including softer playground surfaces and providing education programs for both parents and children, and even simply paying closer attention to traffic laws when crossing the street are all simple yet effective ways to decrease the incidence of TBIs.

REFERENCES

Alexander, M. P. (1995). Mild traumatic brain injury: Pathophysiology, natural history, and clinical management. *Neurology, 45,* 1253–1260.

Annegers, J. F., Grabow, J. D., Kurland, L. T., & Laws, E. R. (1980). The incidence, causes, and secular trends of head trauma in Olmsted County, Minnesota, 1935–1974. *Neurology, 30,* 912–919.

Bogner, J. (2000). *The agitated behavior scale. The center for outcome measurement in brain injury.* Retrieved July 9, 2009, from http://www.tbims.org/combi/abs

Braddom, R. L. (2007). Physical medicine and rehabilitation. Philadelphia, PA: W.B. Saunders Company.

Broglio, S. P., Macciocchi, S. N., & Ferrara, M. S. (2007). Neurocognitive performance of concussed athletes when symptom free. *Journal of Athletic Training, 42,* 504–508.

Cassidy, J. D., Carroll, L. J., Peloso, P. M., Borg, J., von Holst, H., Holm, L., et al. (2004). Incidence, risk factors and prevention of mild traumatic brain injury: Results of the WHO collaborating centre task force on mild traumatic brain injury. *Journal of Rehabilitation Medicine, 43,* 28–60.

Collins, M. W., Grindel, S. H., Lovell, M. R., Dede, D. E., Moser, D. J., Phalin, B. R., et al. (1999). Relationship between concussion and neuropsychological performance in college football players. *Journal of American Medical Association, 282,* 964–970.

Corrigan, J. D. (1989). Development of a scale for assessment of agitation following traumatic brain injury. *Journal of Clinical and Experimental Neurospychology, 11,* 261–277.

Courtney, A. C., & Courtney, M. W. (2009). A thoracic mechanism of mild traumatic brain injury due to blast pressure waves. *Mount Sinai Journal of Medicine: A Journal of Translational and Personalized Medicine, 76,* 111–118.

Cuccurullo, S. J. (2004). *Physical medicine and rehabilitation board review.* New York: Demos Publishing.

De Silva, M. J., Roberts, I., Perel, P., Edwards, P., Kenward, M. G., Fernandes, J., et al. (2009). Patient outcome after traumatic brain injury in high-, middle- and low-income countries: Analysis of data on 8927 patients in 46 countries. *International Journal of Epidemiology, 38,* 452–458.

Erbes, C., Westermeyer, J., Engdahl, B., & Johnsen, E. (2007). Post-traumatic stress disorder and service utilization in a sample of service members from Iraq and Afghanistan. *Military Medicine, 172,* 359–363.

Fazio, V. C., Lovell, M. R., Pardini, J. E., & Collins, M. W. (2007). The relation between post concussion symptoms and neurocognitive performance in concussed athletes. *NeuroRehabilitation, 22,* 207–216.

Finkelstein, E. A., Corso, P. S., & Miller, T. R. (2006). *The incidence and economic burden of injuries in the United States.* New York: Oxford University Press.

Giacino, J. T., Ashwal, S., Childs, N., Cranford, R., Jennett, B., Katz, D. I., et al. (2002). The minimally conscious state. Definition and diagnostic criteria. *Neurology, 58,* 349–353.

Giacino, J. T., Kezmarsky, M. A., DeLuca, J., & Cicerone, K. D. (1991). Monitoring rate of recovery to predict outcome in minimally responsive patients. *Archives of Physical Medicine and Rehabilitation, 72,* 897–901.

Guskiewicz, K. M., McCrea, M., Marshall, S. W., Cantu, R. C., Randolph, C., Barr, W., et al. (2003). Cumulative effects associated with recurrent concussion in collegiate football players: The NCAA concussion study. *JAMA, 290,* 2549–2555.

Guskiewicz, K. M., Weaver, N. L., Padua, D. A., & Garrett, W. E. (2000). Epidemiology of concussion in collegiate and high school football players. *American Journal of Sports Medicine, 28,* 643–650.

Herbel, K., Schermerhorn, L., & Howard, J. (1990). Management of agitated head-injured patients: A survey of current techniques. *Rehabilitation Nursing, 15,* 66–69.

Hibbard, M. R., Uysal, S., Kepler, K., Bogdany, J., & Silver, J. (1998). Axis I psychopathology in individuals with traumatic brain injury. *Journal of Head Trauma Rehabilitation, 13,* 24–39.

Hoge, C. W., Goldberg, H. M., & Castro, C. A. (2009). Care of war veterans with mild traumatic brain injury—flawed perspectives. *New England Journal of Medicine, 360,* 1588–1591.

Kay, T., & Lezak, M. (1990). *Nature of head injury. Traumatic brain injury and vocational rehabilitation.* Menomonie, WI: University of Wisconsin-Stout Research and Training Center.

Kolakowsky-Hayner, S. A., Gourley, E. V., III., Kreutzer, J. S., Marwitz, J. H., Cifu, D. X., & Mckinley, W. O. (1999). Pre-injury substance abuse among persons with brain injury and persons with spinal cord injury. *Brain Injury, 13,* 571–581.

Kosmidis, M. H. (2007). Review of interdisciplinary approach to the treatment of traumatic brain injury. *Journal of the International Neuropsychological Society, 13,* 557–558.

Langlois, J. A., Rutland-Brown, W., & Thomas, K. E. (2004). *Traumatic brain injury in the United States: Emergency department visits, hospitalizations, and deaths.* Atlanta, GA: Centers for Disease Control and Prevention, National Center for Injury Prevention and Control.

Langlois, J. A., Rutland-Brown, W., & Wald, M. M. (2006). The epidemiology and impact of traumatic brain injury: A brief overview. *The Journal of Head Trauma Rehabilitation, 21,* 375–378.

Leon-Carrion, J. (2006). Methods and tools for the assessment of outcome after brain injury rehabilitation. In J. Leon-Carrion, K. V. Wild, & G. Zitney (Eds.), *Brain injury treatment: Theories and practices.* Philadelphia, PA: Taylor & Francis.

Levin, H. S., O'Donnell, V. M., & Grossman, R. G. (1979). The Galveston orientation and amnesia test. A practical scale to assess cognition after head injury. *The Journal of Nervous and Mental Disease, 167,* 675–684.

Levy, D. T., Mallonee, S., Miller, T. R., Smith, G. S., Spicer, R. S., Romano, E. O., et al. (2004). Alcohol involvement in burn, submersion, spinal cord, and brain injuries. *Medical Science Monitor, 10,* 17–24.

Malec, J. F., Testa, J. A., Rush, B. K., Brown, A. W., & Moessner, A. M. (2007). Self-assessment of impairment, impaired self-awareness, and depression after traumatic brain injury. *Journal of Head Trauma Rehabilitation, 22,* 156–166.

Marion, D. W. (1999). *Traumatic brain injury.* New York: Thieme Publishing Group.

Mazzini, L., Campini, R., Angelino, E., Rognone, F., Pastore, I., & Oliveri, G. (2003). Posttraumatic hydrocephalus: A clinical, neuroradiologic, and neuropsychologic assessment of long-term outcome. *Archives of Physical Medicine and Rehabilitation, 84,* 1637–1641.

McCrea, M., Hammeke, T., Olsen, G., Leo, P., & Guskiewicz, K. (2004). Unreported concussion in high school football players: Implications for prevention. *Clinical Journal of Sport Medicine, 14,* 13–17.

Schofield, P. W., Butler, T. G., Hollis, S. J., Smith, N. E., Lee, S. J., & Kelso, W. M. (2006). Traumatic brain injury among Australian prisoners: Rates, recurrence and sequelae. *Brain Injury, 20,* 499–506.

Silver, J. M., McAllister, T. W., & Yudofsky, S. C. (2005). *Textbook of traumatic brain injury.* Arlington, VA: American Psychiatric Publishing, Inc.

Temkin, N. R., Dikmen, S. S., & Winn, H. R. (1991). Management of head injury. posttraumatic seizures. *Neurosurgery Clinics of North America, 2,* 425–435.

The Multi-Society Task Force on PVS. (1994). Medical aspects of the persistent vegetative state. *New England Journal of Medicine, 330,* 1499–1508.

Timble, M. R. (1987). Anticonvulsant drug and cognitive function: A review of literature. *Epilepsia, 28,* S37–S45.

Warden, D. L., Gordon, B., McAllister, T. W., Silver, J. M., Barth, J. T., Bruns, J., et al. (2006). Guidelines for the pharmacologic treatment of neurobehavioral sequelae of traumatic brain injury. *Journal of Neurotrauma, 23,* 1468–1501.

Zaloshnja E., Miller T., Langlois J. A, & Selassie, A. W. (2008). Prevalence of long-term disability from traumatic brain injury in the civilian population of the United States, 2005. *Journal of Head Trauma Rehabilitation, 23,* 394–400.

Additional Readings

Asikainen, I., Kaste, M., & Sarna, S. (1999). Early and late posttraumatic seizures in traumatic brain injury rehabilitation patients: Brain injury factors causing late seizures and influence of seizures on long-term outcome. *Epilepsia, 40,* 584–589.

Baguley, I. J. (2008). Autonomic complications following central nervous system injury. *Seminars in Neurology, 28,* 716–725.

Baguley, I. J., Heriseanu, R. E., Cameron, I. D., Nott, M. T., & Slewa-Younan, S. (2008). A critical review of the pathophysiology of dysautonomia following traumatic brain injury. *Neurocritical Care, 8,* 293–300.

Baguley, I. J., Heriseanu, R. E., Gurka, J. A., Nordenbo, A., & Cameron, I. D. (2007). Gabapentin in the management of dysautonomia following severe traumatic brain injury: A case series. *Journal of Neurology, Neurosurgery, and Psychiatry, 78,* 539–541.

Baguley, I. J., Nott, M. T., Slewa-Younan, S., Heriseanu, R. E., & Perkes, I. E. (2009). Diagnosing dysautonomia after acute traumatic brain injury: Evidence for overresponsiveness to afferent stimuli. *Archives of Physical Medicine and Rehabilitation, 90,* 580–586.

Barnfield, T. V., & Leathem, J. M. (1998). Incidence and outcomes of traumatic brain injury and substance abuse in a New Zealand prison population. *Brain Injury, 12,* 455–466.

Brown, C. V., Weng, J., Oh, D., Salim, A., Kasotakis, G., Demetriades, D., et al. (2004). Does routine serial computed tomography of the head influence management of traumatic brain injury? A prospective evaluation. *Journal of Trauma, 57,* 939–943.

Centers for Disease Control and Prevention. (1999). *Facts about concussion and brain injury.* Atlanta, GA: CDC.

Centers for Disease Control and Prevention. (2003). *Report to Congress on mild traumatic brain injury in the United States: Steps to prevent a serious public health problem.* Atlanta, GA: National Center for Injury Prevention and Control, CDC.

Christensen, A., & Caetano, C. (1999). Cognitive neurorehabilitation. In D. T. Stuss, G. Winocur, & I. H. Robertson (Eds.), *Neuropsychological rehabilitation in the interdisciplinary team: The postacute stage.* New York: Cambridge University Press.

Englander, J., Bushnik, T., Duong, T. T., Cifu, D. X., Zafonte, R., Wright, J., et al. (2003). Analyzing risk factors for late posttraumatic seizures: A prospective, multicenter investigation. *Archives of Physical Medicine and Rehabilitation, 84,* 365–367.

Fiser, S. M., Johnson, S. B., & Fortune, J. B. (1998). Resource utilization in traumatic brain injury: The role of magnetic resonance imaging. *The American Surgeon, 64,* 1088–1093.

Frey, L. C. (2003). Epidemiology of posttraumatic epilepsy: A critical review. *Epilepsia, 44,* 11–17.

Fugate, L. P., Spacek, B. A., Kresty, L. A., Levy, C., Johnson, J., & Mysiw, W. (1997). Measurement and treatment of agitation following traumatic brain injury-II. A survey of the brain injury special interest group of the American Academy of Physical Medicine and Rehabilitation. *Archives of Physical Medicine and Rehabilitation, 78,* 924–928.

Gefen, A. (2008). How much time does it take to get a pressure ulcer? Integrated evidence from human, animal, and in vitro studies. *Ostomy Wound Management, 54,* 26–28, 30–35.

Graham, D. P., & Cardon, A. L. (2008). An update on substance use and treatment following traumatic brain injury. *Annals of New York Academy of Sciences, 1141,* 148–162.

Hoge, C. W., McGurk, D., Thomas, J. L., Cox, A. L., Engel, C. C., & Castro, C. A. (2008). Mild traumatic brain injury in U.S. soldiers returning from Iraq. *New England Journal of Medicine, 358,* 453–463.

Iverson, G. L. (2005). Outcome from mild traumatic brain injury. *Current Opinions in Psychiatry, 18,* 301–317.

Ivins, B. J., Schwab, K. A., Warden, D., Harvey, L. T., Hoilien, M. A., Powell, C. O., et al. (2003). Traumatic brain injury in the U.S. army paratroopers: Prevalence and character. *Journal of Trauma Injury, Infection and Critical Care, 55,* 617–621.

Jagoda, A. S., Bazarian, J. J., Bruns, J. J., Cantrill, S. V., Gean, A. D., Howard, P. K., et al. (2009). Clinical policy: Neuroimaging and decision making in adult mild traumatic brain injury in the acute setting. *Journal of Emergency Nursing, 35,* e5–e40.

Jennett, B. (1979). Defining brain damage after head injury. *Journal of Royal College of Physicians of London, 4,* 197–200.

Kaups, K. L., Davis, J. W., & Parks, S. N. (2004). Routinely repeated computed tomography after blunt head trauma: Does it benefit patients? *Journal of Trauma, 56,* 475–480.

Manolakaki, D., Velmahos, G. C., Spaniolas, K., de Moya, M., & Alam, H. B. (2009). Early magnetic resonance imaging is unnecessary in patients with traumatic brain injury. *Journal of Trauma, 66,* 1008–1012.

Meythaler, J. M., Peduzzi, J. D., Eleftheriou, E., & Novack, T. A. (2001). Current concepts: Diffuse axonal injury-associated traumatic brain injury. *Archives of Physical Medicine and Rehabilitation, 82,* 1461–1471.

Murray, C. J. L., & Lopez, A. D. (1996). *Global health statistics: A compendium of incidence, prevalence, and mortality estimates for over 200 conditions.* Cambridge, MA: Harvard University Press on behalf of the World Health Organization and the World Bank.

Nampiaparampil, D. E. (2008). Prevalence of chronic pain after traumatic brain injury: A systematic review. *Journal of American Medical Association, 300,* 711–719.

National Institute of Neurological Disorders and Stroke. (2002). *Traumatic brain injury: Hope through research.* No. 02. Bethesda, MD: NIH.

Okie, S. (2005). Traumatic brain injury in the war zone. *New England Journal of Medicine, 352,* 2043–2047.

Owens, B. D., Kragh, J. F., Jr., Wenke, J. C., Macatis, J., Wade, C. E., & Holcomb, J. B. (2008). Combat wounds in operation Iraqi freedom and operation enduring freedom. *Journal of Trauma, 64,* 295–299.

Powell, J. M., Ferraro, J. V., Dikmen, S. S., Temkin, N. R., & Bell, K. R. (2008). Accuracy of mild traumatic brain injury diagnosis. *Archives of Physical Medicine and Rehabilitation, 89*, 1550–1555.

Roberts, I., Yates, D., Sandercock, P., Farrell, B., Wasserberg, J., Lomas, G., et al. (2004). Effect of intravenous corticosteroids on death within 14 days in 10008 adults with clinically significant head injury (MRC CRASH trial): Randomised placebo-controlled trial. *Lancet, 364*, 1321–1328.

Rossitch, E. Jr., & Bullard, D. E. (1988). The autonomic dysfunction syndrome: Aetiology and treatment. *British Journal of Neurosurgery, 2*, 471–478.

Slaughter, B., Fann, J. R., & Ehde, D. (2003). Traumatic brain injury in a county jail population: Prevalence, neuropsychological functioning and psychiatric disorders. *Brain Injury, 17*, 731–741.

Sosin, D. M., Sniezek, J. E., & Thurman, D. J. (1996). Incidence of mild and moderate brain injury in the United States, 1991. *Brain Injury, 10*, 47–54.

Sosin, D. M., Sniezek, J. E., & Waxweiler, R. J. (1995). Trends in death associated with traumatic brain injury, 1979 through 1992. Success and failure. *Journal of American Medical Association, 273*, 1778–1780.

Tagliaferri, F., Compagnone, C., Korsic, M., Servadei, F., & Kraus, J. (2006). A systematic review of brain injury epidemiology in Europe. *Acta Neurochirurgica, 148*, 255–268.

Teasdate, G., & Jennett, B. (1974). Assessment of coma and impaired consciousness. A practical scale. *Lancet, 2*, 81–84.

Temkin, N. R. (2009). Preventing and treating posttraumatic seizures: The human experience. *Epilepsia, 50*, 10–13.

Temkin, N. R., Haglund, M. M., & Winn, H. R. (1995). Causes, prevention, and treatment of post-traumatic epilepsy. *New Horizons, 3*, 518–522.

Thurman, D. J., Alverson, C., Dunn, K. A., Guerrero, J., & Sniezek, J. E. (1999). Traumatic brain injury in the United States: A public health perspective. *Journal of Head Trauma Rehabilitation, 14*, 602–615.

Wang, M. C., Linnau, K. F., Tirschwell, D. L., & Hollingworth, W. (2006). Utility of repeat head computed tomography after blunt head trauma: A systematic review. *Journal of Trauma, 61*, 226–233.

Williams, G., Morris, M. E., Schache, A., & McCrory, P. R. (2009). Incidence of gait abnormalities after traumatic brain injury. *Archives of Physical Medicine and Rehabilitation, 90*, 587–593.

5

Rehabilitation in Burns

*Alan W. Young, DO, W. Scott Dewey, PT, CHT, OCS,
and Steven E. Wolf, MD*

The skin is the body's largest organ. It functions as a physical protective barrier, a reservoir of immune activity, regulator of homeostasis through thermoregulation and fluid balance, and the foundation of our appearance, one of the primary determinants of how we are evaluated by society. A major burn is possibly the most traumatic injury a person can sustain. Not only does it have the potential to cause terrible pain but also it can have a global impact physically, spiritually, psychologically, and emotionally. No other injury so directly affects, probably the most important aspect our self-esteem, our appearance. Even a minor burn can leave scars that are physically and emotionally difficult. It can be disastrous for a family emotionally and economically. A problem of this complex is best addressed in a specialty center where a multidisciplinary approach can be brought to bear to optimize outcome.

Data from the American Burn Association study in 2007 show an incidence of 500,000 burns per year, with 40,000 hospitalizations, 25,000 to specialty burn treatment centers, and approximately 4,000 deaths per year. Only 10% of admissions had more than 30% total body surface area (TBSA) involved; 70% of those injured are men and 31% are uninsured. In addition, military casualties are often seen with additional injuries including multiple orthopedic trauma, soft tissue injuries from fragmentation weapons, amputations, traumatic brain injury, and spinal cord injuries that have to be addressed concurrently. At times, the treatment required for one aspect of the constellation of injuries is not beneficial for another. Here, the multidisciplinary team approach can be important in determining the hierarchy of patient treatment requirements.

CAUSATIVE AGENTS

Eighty-six percent of all burns are thermal, which are caused by an application of either heat or cold (Miller et al., 2008). Heat will create a zone of coagulation with actual tissue destruction and a zone of stasis with decreased blood flow. This area may improve or deteriorate depending on treatment. Cold injury occurs as a result of actual freezing and an area of ischemia caused by decreased blood flow. Severity is determined by duration and intensity of the exposure. It is not possible to determine the depth of the injury until rewarming takes place.

Four percent of burns are electrical, but these in particular have unique consequences that must be addressed in rehabilitation in addition to the loss of skin. The severity of the burn can be initially deceiving; superficially, there may be little apparent injury. The electrical current, however, follows the path of least resistance traveling along nerves, vessels, and muscle, which can all be damaged along its route. Electrical energy generates heat that accumulates in tissue and is explosively released resulting in much more severe damage at the exit wound compared with the entrance. In addition, current flows in all the tissue linearly, and therefore, more current will flow in a given area in those regions with small cross-sectional areas, such as the fingers or wrist, generating more damage. Oftentimes, the amount of injury to the tissues is not manifest for 4–5 days; therefore, we recommend waiting for at least this amount of time before determination of the most appropriate technique for closure of any open wounds or determination of level of amputation, if indicated. According to Hanumadass, Voora, Kagan, and Matsuda (1986), creatine kinase is a sensitive indicator of total muscle damage. Below 2,500 V there is little risk of amputation or skin grafting and above that level there is a greater likelihood for major amputation (Block et al., 1995). Specific complications related to electrocution injuries include cardiopulmonary arrest, cognitive impairment, long bone fractures, neuropathies, and in longer term the early formation of cataracts and hearing loss.

Chemical burns comprise 3% of all burns and can have acid, alkali, or vesicant etiologies. The amount and concentration of a substance, its toxicity, the mechanism, and the duration of exposure will determine the extent of the injury. Acids will result in coagulative necrosis, which is typically limited to the skin, but alkalis will cause liquefaction necrosis, which may extend into deeper tissues. Treatment is aimed at irrigation of the chemical away from the wound. Chemical neutralization should be avoided as this will cause an endothermic reaction resulting in further burn. The final severity is typically underestimated initially because some chemicals such as white phosphorus continue to burn despite topical treatment and must be physically removed to stop damage.

Neel (1991) noted that radiation causes injury based upon duration, location, and intensity of exposure. Damage occurs to DNA and RNA cross-linkages and many virulent free radicals are produced. Once exposure reaches the critical level of 400 rads, only 50% of cells will survive; 800 rads of acute exposure is 100% lethal. The most common example of radiation exposure is sunburn. Fortunately, other examples are rare.

CLASSIFICATION

Burns are described by depth, and outcomes are related to the degree of dermal damage. Partial thickness burns involve the epidermis (first degree) and the upper layers of the dermis (second degree). For epidermal burns, there is erythema but no blistering. An example is sunburn. Second degree burns involve the dermis, but enough is left to affect spontaneous local healing. These are characterized into superficial and deep. Superficial burns are localized to the papillary dermis, have blistering and intense pain but are wet in appearance, and should heal in 7–10 days (Figure 5.1). Deep partial-thickness burns are dry, but live dermal elements remain (Figure 5.2). These will heal if treated conservatively over 2–3 weeks but can result in severe hypertrophic scarring. Full thickness burns (third degree) have complete damage to all layers of the skin and is seen as pale and insensate secondary to loss of vascular and neural structures (Figure 5.3).

The extent of the burn, referred to as the TBSA, can be estimated using the rule of nines. This apportions 9% of the body surface to the head and each arm, 18% to each leg, the anterior chest, the posterior chest, and 1% to the perineum. The Lund and Browder method is used to estimate TBSA in children as it takes into account relative changes that occur in body proportions as they mature (Miller, Finley, Waltman, & Lincks, 1991).

Minor burns involve less than 15% TBSA (10% in children) or 2% full thickness. The Committee on Trauma (1999) stated that major burns involve more than 25% TBSA (20% in children) or 10% full thickness or involve the face, eyes, ears, or perineum; involve inhalational injury; or is an electrical injury. All major burns require hospitalization, ideally in a specialty burn unit.

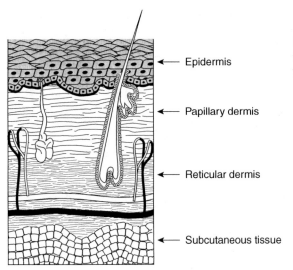

FIGURE 5.1 Superficial burns just involve the upper layers of the epidermis. *Source:* Used with permission from Richard, R. L., 2009.

Epidermis

Papillary dermis

Reticular dermis

Subcutaneous tissue

PATIENT MANAGEMENT

Patient management begins the same as all resuscitation from acute injury with an assessment of airway, breathing, and circulation and identification of all injuries. Once assessed, an estimate of the TBSA and depth of injury is performed. One of the primary problems is management of fluid homeostasis (fluid balance in the body); patients often require massive volumes to maintain homeostasis that is associated with dramatically increased capillary permeability. This allows tremendous fluid shifts to occur that can cause vascular collapse, a catastrophic loss of blood pressure due to fluid that is supposed to be in the blood vessels being lost to the inter- and intra-vascular spaces, particularly in the first 24–48 hours. This is countered by intravenous infusion of fluid using a protocol such as the Parkland formula

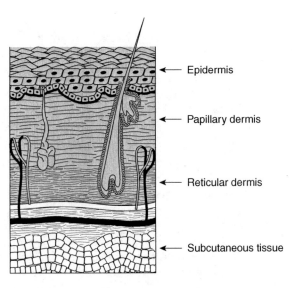

FIGURE 5.2 Partial thickness burns may be superficial or deep. They extend from below the dermis to the reticular dermis. *Source:* Used with permission from Richard, R. L., 2009.

Epidermis

Papillary dermis

Reticular dermis

Subcutaneous tissue

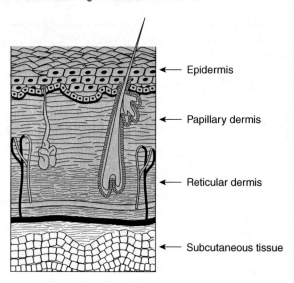

Epidermis

Papillary dermis

Reticular dermis

Subcutaneous tissue

FIGURE 5.3 Full thickness burns extend through the reticular dermis into the subcutaneous tissue. *Source:* Used with permission from Richard, R. L., 2009.

(4 ml/kg/%TBSA burn) in which one half is administered in the first 8 hours with the rest infused over the next 16 hours (Baxter, 1968). Evidence of inhalation of smoke with airway damage is evaluated by bronchoscopy as soon as possible. A nasogastric tube is placed, tetanus toxoid is administered, and gastric bleeding prophylaxis is begun with H2 blockers. The patient is evaluated for compartment syndrome, an elevation of pressure within the extremities caused by fluid shifts into the intravascular spaces. If the pressure is too high or is elevated for a long period of time, the nerves and muscles may be injured or die due to loss of blood flow into the area. A charotomy, an incision through the skin, is performed if indicated to relieve the pressure. The areas are cleaned and topical antimicrobials are placed. IV antibiotics are only given for specific infections and not for prophylaxis.

Risk of mortality is estimated by adding the patient's age with TBSA burned (Baux index, 1961). Index numbers approaching 100 and higher are less likely to be associated with successful outcome. However, survivors among those with high numbers are frequent and increasing each year. One reason is adoption of the practice of excision and grafting of as much burned skin as soon as possible after the injury. Numerous clinical techniques are used to maximize donor area to relatively rapidly close the wound and thus reestablish the function of the skin as a barrier to infection. Wound care proceeds on a daily basis with the use of topical agents to limit wound colonization with microorganisms. Wounds are no longer washed by immersion but mechanical cleansing takes place with flow-by techniques. After epidermal closure, topical emollients are applied to healed areas. The skin is wrapped in a nonadherent dressing as a base and other dressing to absorb drainage and apply pressure as required.

SKIN COVERAGE

The ultimate method to close wounds is either by secondary intention (spontaneous closure) or grafting with the patient's own skin from uninjured areas. For those with large areas of injury, spontaneous closure is not tenable and grafting will be required. These grafts are taken from areas called donor sites as split thickness skin grafts. These are layers of skin that can include all the dermal elements or just the top epidermis that are laid down over the excised burn to close the area. The donor site will then heal spontaneously from the elements that are left. Oftentimes, these grafts are meshed to increase the amount of surface that can be covered; 2:1 to 4:1 are typical ratios (Ong, Samuel, & Song, 2006). The greater the mesh area, the longer it takes for complete closure of the interstices to occur and the worse the potential is for scar to form with contraction and loss of function because of the lack of dermis. Some areas such as the face and hand require sheet grafts or even full thickness skin grafts (Moncrief, Switzer, & Rose, 1964). The latter severely limits the amount of tissue available for grafting but should prevent contracture from occurring.

In a large burn, the amount of donor skin available may be limited, so this may require the use of temporary skin substitutes. Even though they are not permanent, they will decrease fluid loss and provide protection from infection, decrease pain, and aid thermal regulation. Agents used include allograft skin from cadavers, which works well when need exceeds what is available from the donor. Xenograft skin from another species can also be used temporarily. Historically, in the developed world, this is from pigs, and in Brazil, the frog has been used.

Much work has been done to develop synthetic dressings. They can be unilaminate or bilaminate; the most popular of which is a bilaminate dressing called Biobrane (Barret et al., 2000). It is a bilayer of flexible nylon with a collagen cover. This can be applied to open wounds, both partial and full thickness, which adheres to the wound and closes it temporarily. Integra is another product used for this purpose; however, it incorporates into the wound to form a neodermis. The outer layer can be removed once vascularization takes place and then autograft skin is applied. Branski et al. (2007) reviewed the purported advantage of decreased scarring because of the formation of neodermis, but this has never been clearly demonstrated in patients.

Another interesting method of skin closure is by cultured epidermal autografts. A 2.5 cm^2 piece of nonburned skin is sent to a laboratory whereby the keratinocytes are separated and grown in culture dishes to radically expand the available cells for autografting. From this meters of skin can be rapidly grown. Because the patient is the donor there is no risk of rejection. Unfortunately, the skin consists of only the top few layers of cells, which are fragile. Because of this, it is very difficult to discern clinically those areas with successful grafting, and even once grafted, the skin can be easily injured by shear force. In addition, it has difficulty adhering to irregularly shaped surfaces and is frightfully expensive. Barret, Wolf, Desai, and Herndon (2000) showed that only 25% was durable coverage of areas grafted with cultured epithelial autografts. Nevertheless, it can be useful when no other donor source exists.

REHABILITATION

Rehabilitation of burned patients is a complex process that begins at the time of admission and continues throughout the inpatient and outpatient stays culminating in community reintegration. Richard et al., (2008) proposed that it is not a linear progression but moves through a spectrum of treatments with the ultimate goal of enhanced function. There are times that one aspect of therapy may negatively impact another portion of the treatment plan, that is, passive range of motion (PROM) of an axilla may cause tearing of the scarred skin. This then may delay overall wound closure but is necessary to prevent contractures. Fresh skin grafts should not be mobilized for 3–5 days to prevent shear, but this allows surrounding tissue to become tight. Communication among all members of the team, doctors, nurses, and therapists, is a prerequisite for successful treatment. In many burn centers, rounds occur daily with representatives from all disciplines so that decisions regarding that day's priorities and goals can be discussed and implemented based on the patient's condition at the time.

The ultimate goal of the treatment of burn survivors is to preserve function. The greatest impediment in achieving this goal is scar formation (Bombaro et al., 2003), although immobilization and amputation may be complicating factors as well. Scars will grow and contract as they mature over the course of 1–1.5 years after injury. Contracting scars are particularly damaging over joints as these are the areas that can shorten on the skeletal frame. The scar of interest may only be partially over the joint with dysfunction, when it is really the whole scar

TABLE 5.1 *Typical Scar Contractures Involving Joints*

- Boutonnière deformity of the proximal interphalangeal joint
- Extension contracture of the metacarpophalangeal joint
- Abduction contracture of the thumb
- Wrist flexion contracture
- Antecubital flexion contracture
- Anterior and posterior axillary contractures
- Neck flexion contracture
- Lip ectropion
- Microstomia
- Eyelid ectropion
- Hip adduction contracture
- Popliteal flexion contracture
- Toe extension and flexion contractures

that is shortening. An example is antecubital flexion contracture from a scar starting at the hand extending to the trunk. It is the entire scar causing the deformity and not just that over the elbow. Therefore, treatment should be directed at the entire scar. Typical scar contractures involving joints are listed in Table 5.1.

Hypertrophic scars can be cosmetically and psychologically devastating even without effects on mechanical limitation. In addition, these patients are often critically ill and require bed rest for their treatments, and thus, they undergo muscle atrophy. Hypermetabolism also universally develops, which is associated with lean mass catabolism, further contributing to weakness that retards rehabilitative efforts.

POSITIONING

One of the simplest means to prevent contracture in general, regardless of region, is to place the joint of interest in extension and abduction, the reason being that the natural pull of contracting scar is to flexion and adduction. It can help prevent edema and skin breakdown and assist with later mobilization of the joint. For example, maintaining the head and neck in extension can help prevent flexion of the chin onto the chest. One caveat to this general notion is the hand, where the metacarpophalangeal joint of the fingers is best placed in flexion to place the tendons at maximum length as healing of the skin occurs. Positioning measures are generally the first step in burn rehabilitation as skin grafts and burns must remain immobile to initiate healing.

SPLINTS

Splinting is an art and a science. Each burn is unique and will have different requirements as it goes from initial injury to initial autografting to contracting scar. Splint type, location and placement require a dynamic assessment as the patient progresses through the intensive care unit, ward, and outpatient clinic. Splint types are classified as static, static-progressive (Figure 5.4), and dynamic. Serial casting is also commonly used during burn rehabilitation. Splints can be used to provide optimal positioning for protection or scar elongation. Many custom splints have been identified for all areas of the body (Richard, Chapman, Dougherty,

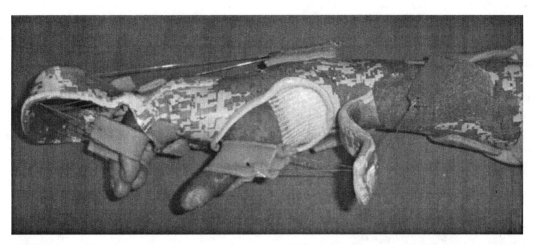

FIGURE 5.4   The splint pictured is a static-progressive PIP extension and thumb radial abduction splint. The indication was development of PIP joint flexion contractures and a thumb adduction contracture status post deep palmar burn. Dynamic and static-progressive splints are typically utilized if adequate ROM is not obtained with static splinting.

Franzen, & Serghiou, 2005). Guidelines proposed by Richard et al. (2009) for hand splinting are based on burn depth, location, and the rehabilitation phase the patient is in. The number of specific hand splints for particular conditions such as boutonnière deformity and distal interphalangeal flexion contracture also exist.

Use of splinting is customized to the patient in an effort to prevent contractures from forming or to correct deformity in others. Contracture correction devices are typically fabricated during the scar maturation phase of wound healing. Use of splints must be tempered by the need for active range of motion to ensure the best outcomes. The best splint for a particular joint or potential contracture is currently based on experience rather than prospective data, for the most part. This has been noted by the burn community, and efforts are currently underway to remedy this shortcoming. The ultimate goal of rehabilitation is to elongate the immature scar tissue prior to maturation to prevent burn scar contracture and subsequent joint contracture. Once the scar matures and is no longer malleable, fixed contractures will generally have to be corrected surgically.

THERAPEUTIC EXERCISE

Though positioning and splinting are important, they must be balanced with motion. Even if immobilized in an appropriate position, a joint or limb will lose motion and become functionally impaired. Active and passive range-of-motion of all joints and skin surfaces are vital. During the acute grafting period, these activities must often be held in order to allow for safe skin graft adherence; however, at the earliest possible time, motion should be initiated. This generally begins 3 days after grafting in an effort to maintain function and improve scar control. When motion is allowed, efforts are generally focused on ambulation and PROM during the acute healing phase (Figure 5.5). The progression to ambulation often begins with sitting and tilting on a tilt-table until regaining proper balance is achieved. Thereafter, ambulation distance is lengthened as appropriate. In particular, it is paramount to regain loading of the spine and large muscle groups to combat the adverse effects of prolonged bed rest on lean body mass. These activities are beneficial to joint mobility, preservation of muscle mass, cardiopulmonary and GI function, wound healing and psychological well being. After this is accomplished, strength of extremity muscle groups can be targeted in an effort to improve function and decrease contractures.

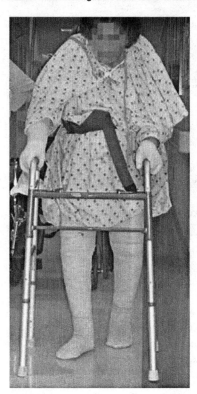

FIGURE 5.5   Patient with a severe burn beginning the process of ambulation. Note the bandages compressing the healing wounds and the use of adaptive equipment.

SCAR MANAGEMENT

When burn wounds heal, hypertrophic scars can form (Spurr & Shakespeare, 1990). This is characterized by raised erythematous (red) borders with significant deviations from normal texture. Estimates in its occurrence range from 4% to 75% of burn scars. There is no clear understanding as to why there is such variability in formation of hypertropic scars. For many years, the standard and only treatment to prevent the formation was the application of pressure directly to the scar. This was accomplished by custom-made compression garments designed to apply 25 mm Hg of circumferential pressure to the surface of the scar for the duration of the scar maturation phase over 1–1.5 years. The garments stretch with use, but it should be replaced approximately every 3 months. These are ideally worn for at least 23 hours a day and are removed only for bathing and skin care.

Problems occur with this treatment. For instance, the face is very difficult to cover with uniform pressure using fabric masks; hence, molded acrylic masks were developed. The garments themselves are very warm and the masks even more so. Patient compliance can be an issue. However, even with good compliance, hypertrophic scar formation is still common. In fact, some studies claim that this type of therapy is not effective for this purpose (Chang et al., 1995). Silastic gel sheets are now commonly used either alone or under pressure garments or incorporated into garments and masks. The mechanism explaining why silicone is effective is unclear. Injection of scars with steroids has been practiced for many years and recent trials have added various substances to intralesional injection of steroids (Koc, Arca, Surucu, & Kurumlu 2008). But to date, no studies have shown a clear benefit of this treatment over no therapy. Scars tend to improve to some degree over time; therefore, controlled studies with no treatment are clearly necessary to discern benefit.

A treatment that appears to offer much promise is the application of 585 nm pulse dye laser, which has been shown clinically to improve color and reduce size of hypertrophic scar without recurrence (Davison et al., 2009). However, definitive evidence to support this practice is still forthcoming.

PAIN MANAGEMENT

Pain with burn care and rehabilitation is a severe problem. In those with open wounds, the causes for pain are obvious, but for those with closed wounds, the reasons may not be so apparent. However, pain is a subjective entity, and those who are burned or are convalescing from burns and have complaints of pain must be treated appropriately.

There are three etiologies of pain that must be addressed: background, breakthrough, and procedural. Background pain is the pain that is caused by the direct injury of the burn to the skin, muscle, and nerves, which can last for weeks, and is associated with inflammation and release of noxious mediators. It is best treated with long-acting agents such as methadone or morphine, because the stimulus is always present, sometimes lasting for months in the most severe cases. Recent evidence suggests that the addition of medications that address the neuropathic components of pain can significantly decrease the requirement for narcotic analgesia that will also result in decreasing the sedation associated with opioid use. Cuignet, Pirson, Soudon, and Zizi (2007) demonstrated gabapentin as an example of this class of mediation.

Procedural pain has a distinct onset and termination that is oftentimes associated with wound care or rehabilitation efforts at mobilization and exercise that acutely activates pain receptors. These occurrences including the duration which is often short can be anticipated; therefore, it is best managed with short-acting agents of sufficient strength to deal with the stimulus appropriately. This typically includes morphine and hydromorphone. The use of fentanyl is avoided because the dosing is likely to be repeated, and the lipophilic characteristics of fentanyl and its metabolites make it long acting in this circumstance, and not short acting.

Breakthrough pain is more ill-defined, and may not have a specific etiology. It is characterized by the complaint of pain in the absence of painful intervention in those whose background pain has presumably been addressed. If it occurs frequently, it is a sign that background pain is not being sufficiently addressed and consideration should be given for increasing the dose of background pain medications. Intermittent episodes of breakthrough pain should be treated with a medium-acting narcotic such as hydrocodone, morphine, oxycodone, or tramadol.

Pain becomes more chronic as the patient progresses into convalescence. Other causes should be identified and treated appropriately. Persistent inflammation, muscle tightness, and nerve regeneration should be treated with agents specific to those problems. Anxiety can be interpreted as pain but is not appropriately addressed by narcotics. The usual clinical picture is that of a patient who is well into recovery with tapering doses of narcotics with increasing function. Since opioids become less effective in these situations, alternative techniques such as acupuncture, transcranial electrical stimulation, and virtual reality may be considered as they show promise as nontraditional means to improve symptomatology (Sharar et al., 2007).

Pruritus, a sense of itching, is common with healing and should be addressed as an important component of a thorough pain management program. It was initially thought to be because of histamine release with treatment concentrated on the use of histamine blockers such as diphenhydramine. However, the cause of pruritus is more complex and likely involves other neurotransmitters such as bradykinins, vanilloids, and various proteinases (Goutos, Dziewulski, & Richardson, 2009). Therefore, treatment options have expanded to include topical tricyclics, gabapentin, and the use of lasers. There is, however, a paucity of evidence-based research (Bell & Gabriel, 2009) to direct treatment options (Demling & DeSanti, 2001; Mendham, 2004).

PSYCHOLOGICAL PROBLEMS

The burn survivor is immediately faced with a severe change to their personal sense of identity and well being. A bad haircut in today's society can be a source of embarrassment with its emphasis on youth and beauty; those with visible burns suffer worse. Many burn survivors cannot bring themselves to look into a mirror for months. There is a significant change in their roles in the family and community. They may suffer financial stress and sometimes experience survivor guilt. Posttraumatic stress disorder (PTSD) has been shown to occur in approximately 25% of all burn survivors (van Loey, van Son, van der Heijden, & Ellis, 2008). Dyster-Aas, Willebrand, Wikehult, Gerdin, and Ekselius (2008) found that preexisting psychiatric disorders are frequently exacerbated during the rehab phase. Adjustment disorder is common, though not universal, and should be monitored throughout the recovery process.

Treatment begins with reassurance and education that often includes peer support for both patients and families. Adjustment disorder requires a multidisciplinary approach and psychiatric and psychological support, antidepressants, and anxiolytics all have their place. PTSD is specifically addressed with counseling and with a pharmacological approach that may include antidepressants imipramine or fluoxetine (Tcheung et al., 2005) or the atypical antipsychotics olanzapine, rispiridone, and quetiapine (Kozaric-Kovacic & Pivac, 2007). Other agents with some effectiveness include prazocin (Raskind et al., 2003) and propranolol (McGhee et al., 2009). Eye movement desensitization and reprocessing, an approach to psychotherapy that involves the use of external stimulation—such as eye movement—to treat the emotional distress that sometimes is the result of trauma, has been shown to be effective and was developed by Shapiro and Maxfield (2002). The treatment of PTSD is currently a very active field of research, and we expect that standardization of treatment for this condition will be available in the near future.

NEUROPATHY

Kowalske, Holavanahalli, and Helm (2001) reported peripheral neuropathy will occur in 15–20% of patients with TBSA of 20% or more, with a much higher incidence in electrical burns. Strength frequently recovers, but paresthesias may persist. It may present as a mononeuropathy, multiple mononeuropathies, or generalized neuropathy involving sensory and motor components. The etiology of such presentations is often not clear; however, these frequently resolve with time. Paresthesias tend to respond well to medication for neuropathic pain such as amitripryline, gabapentin, and pregabalin. Early recognition of a neuropathy is important so that appropriate splinting and/or exercise can be implemented to prevent subsequent soft tissue or joint contracture and maintain function.

HETEROTOPIC OSSIFICATION

Heterotopic ossification (HO), the deposition of ectopic bone around joints and tendons, is a problem shared by those with spinal cord injury, traumatic brain injury, and burns. It is not clear what the common pathway between these various mechanisms of injuries is that drives this process, although for burns some investigators have shown it to be associated with prolonged time to burn wound closure (Klein et al., 2007). The incidence is usually reported as 2–3%, but a recent evaluation of military personnel with burns puts the incidence at 11% (unpublished personal data). The most common location is the elbow (> 90%), oftentimes with bilateral involvement with less frequent involvement of the hip, shoulder, knee, and wrist (Hunt, Arnoldo, Kowalske, Helm, & Purdue, 2006). Interestingly, HO is detected in joints not directly impacted by the burn itself. (Haran, Bhuta, & Lee, 2004)

If the ossification bridges the joint, it diminishes the motion of the affected limb causing severe impairment of function. Traditionally, surgical resection of HO was postponed for more than 1 year after onset to ensure the bone mass was no longer actively growing, decreasing the risk of recurrence. However, some suggest that earlier (6 months to a year after injury) resection accompanied by prophylactic treatment with antiinflammatory drugs and/or etidronate may be effective in preventing recurrence, although adequate studies examining this have not yet been reported. While investigators have shown that early excision of HO can be done safely, it was noted to redevelop in over 10% of patients (Tsionos, Leclercq, & Rochet, 2004). Recurrence is uncommon if resection occurs after burn scar maturation. Bisphosphonate therapy has also been successful in sporadic cases, but when subjected to the rigors of clinical trial or meta-analysis (Shafer, Bay, Caruso, & Foster, 2008) benefit was not seen. No prospective trials or consensus has been reached on the issue at this time.

RECOVERY

Recovery may be a very long-term process; active rehabilitation and reconstructive procedures may continue for several years. Psychological recovery may also be prolonged; however, the majority of patients tend to do well. Brych et al. (2001) found that 90% of patients admitted to a burn unit return to work within 2 years, and children generally maintain school status and go on to live productive lives (Blakeney et al., 1998). Holavanahalli, Helm, Gorman, and Kowalske (2007) found that this remains true even in the population of large percentage TBSA burns with deep partial or full thickness hand burns. Barriers preventing return to normal activities and function are initially pain, wound healing, and physical limitations, but as time progresses, psychosocial issues predominate. These include fear of leaving home, fear of the workplace, nightmares/flashbacks, concern over appearance, and depression.

SUMMARY

Severe burns are a complex problem. Even minor injuries may have significant functional impact depending upon location. Burns are best managed by setting a multidisciplinary program that addresses the numerous surgical, medical, functional, psychological, and social problems that may occur. The solutions may begin in the operating room and ICU and can last years through the outpatient clinic, therapy gym, councilor's office, peer groups, reconstructive surgeon's visits, workplace and home as survivors work to resume their lives.

REFERENCES

Barret, J. P., Dziewulski, P., Ramzy, P. I., Wolf, S. E., Desai, M. H., & Herndon, D. N. (2000). Biobrane versus 1% silver sulfadiazine in second-degree pediatric burns. *Plastic and Reconstructive Surgery, 105,* 62–65.

Barret, J. P., Wolf, S. E., Desai, M. H., & Herndon, D. N. (2000). Cost-efficacy of cultured epidermal autografts in massive pediatric burns. *Annals of Surgery, 231,* 869–876.

Baux, S. (1961). *Contribution a l'etude du traitement local des bruleres thermigues etendues.* Paris: These.

Baxter, C. R. (1968). Physiological response to crystalloid resuscitation of severe burns. *Annals of New York Academy of Science, 150,* 874–883.

Bell, P. L., & Gabriel, V. (2009). Evidence based review for the treatment of post-burn pruritus. *Journal of Burn Care & Research, 30,* 55–61.

Blakeney, P., Meyer, W., Jr., Robert, R., Desai, M., Wolf, S., & Herndon, D. (1998). Long-term psychosocial adaptation of children who survive burns involving 80% or greater total body surface area. *The Journal of Trauma, 44,* 625–634.

Block, T. A., Aarsvold, J. N., Matthews, K. L., Mintzer, R. A., River, L. P., Capelli-Schellpfeffer, M., et al. (1995). The 1995 Lindberg award. Nonthermally mediated muscle injury and necrosis in electrical trauma. *The Journal of Burn Care & Rehabilitation, 16,* 581–588.

Bombaro, K. M., Engrav, L. H., Carrougher, G. J., Wiechman, S. A., Faucher, L., Costa, B. A., et al. (2003). What is the prevalence of hypertrophic scarring following burns? *Burns, 29*, 299–302.

Branski, L. K., Herndon, D. N., Pereira, C. T., Mlcak, R. P., Celis, M. M., Lee, J. O., et al. (2007). Longitudinal assessment of integra in primary burn management: A randomized pediatric clinical trial. *Critical Care Medicine, 35*, 2615–2623.

Brych, S. B., Engrav, L. H., Rivara, F. P., Ptacek, J. T., Lezotte, D. C., Esselman, P. C., et al. (2001). Time off work and return to work rates after burns: Systematic review of the literature and a large two-center series. *The Journal of Burn Care & Rehabilitation, 22*, 401–405.

Chang, P., Laubenthal, K. N., Lewis, R. W., Rosenquist, M.D., Lindley-Smith, P., Kealey, G. P., et al. (1995). Prospective, randomized study of the efficacy of pressure garment therapy in patients with burns. *The Journal of Burn Care & Rehabilitation, 16*, 473–475.

Committee on Trauma ACoS. (1999). *Resources for optimal care of the injured patient.* Chicago: American College of Surgeons.

Cuignet O., Pirson, J., Soudon, O., & Zizi, M. (2007). Effects of gabapentin on morphine consumption and pain in severely burned patients. *Burns, 33*, 81–86.

Davison, S. P., Dayan, J. H., Clemens, M. W., Sonni, S., Wang, A., & Crane, A. (2009). Efficacy of intralesional 5-fluorouracil and triamcinolone in the treatment of keloids. *Aesthetic Surgery Journal, 29*, 40–46.

Demling, R. H., & DeSanti, L. (2001). Topical doxepin significantly decreases itching and erythema in the healed burn wound. *Wounds, 13*, 210–215.

Dyster-Aas, J., Willebrand, M., Wikehult, B., Gerdin, B., & Ekselius, L. (2008). Major depression and posttraumatic stress disorder symptoms following severe burn injury in relation to lifetime psychiatric morbidity. *The Journal of Trauma, 64*, 1349–1356.

Goutos, I., Dziewulski, P., & Richardson, P. M. (2009). Pruritus in burns: Review article. *Journal of Burn Care & Research, 30*, 221–228.

Hanumadass, M. L., Voora, S. B., Kagan, R. J., & Matsuda, T. (1986). Acute electrical burns: A 10-year clinical experience. *Burns, 12*, 427–431.

Haran, M., Bhuta, T., & Lee, B. (2004). Pharmacological interventions for treating acute heterotopic ossification. *Cochrane Database of Systematic Reviews*, (4):CD003321.

Holavanahalli, R. K., Helm, P., Gorman, A. R., & Kowalske, K. (2007). Outcomes after deep full-thickness hand burns. *Archives of Physical Medicine and Rehabilitation, 88*: S30–S35.

Hunt, J. L., Arnoldo, B. D., Kowalske, K., Helm, P., & Purdue, G. F. (2006). Heterotopic ossification revisited: A 21-year surgical experience. *Journal of Burn Care & Research, 27*, 535–540.

Klein, M. B., Logsetty, S., Costa, B., Deters, L., Rue, T. C., Carrougher, G. J., et al. (2007). Extended time to wound closure is associated with increased risk of heterotopic ossification of the elbow. *Journal of Burn Care & Research, 28*, 447–450.

Koc, E., Arca, E., Surucu, B., & Kurumlu, Z. (2008). An open, randomized, controlled, comparative study of the combined effect of intralesional triamcinolone acetonide and onion extract gel and intralesional triamcinolone acetonide alone in the treatment of hypertrophic scars and keloids. *Dermatologic Surgery, 34*, 1507–1514.

Kowalske, K., Holavanahalli, R., & Helm, P. (2001). Neuropathy after burn injury. *The Journal of Burn Care & Rehabilitation, 22*, 353–357; discussion 352.

Kozaric-Kovacic, D., & Pivac, N. (2007). Quetiapine treatment in an open trial in combat-related post-traumatic stress disorder with psychotic features. *The International Journal of Neuropsychopharmacology, 10*, 253–261.

McGhee, L. L., Maani, C. V., Garza, T. H., Desocio, P. A., Gaylord, K. M., & Black, I. H. (2009). The effect of propranolol on posttraumatic stress disorder in burned service members. *Journal of Burn Care & Research, 30*, 92–97.

Mendham, J. E. (2004). Gabapentin for the treatment of itching produced by burns and wound healing in children: A pilot study. *Burns, 30*, 851–853.

Miller, S. F., Bessey, P., Lentz, C. W., Jeng, J. C., Schurr, M., Browning, S., et al. (2008). National burn repository 2007 report: A synopsis. *Journal of Burn Care & Research, 29*, 862–870.

Miller, S. F., Finley, R. K., Waltman, M., & Lincks, J. (1991). Burn size estimate reliability: A study. *The Journal of Burn Care & Rehabilitation, 12*, 546–559.

Moncrief, J. A., Switzer, W. E., & Rose, L. R. (1964). Primary excision and grafting in the treatment of third-degree burns of the dorsum of the hand. *Plastics and Reconstructive Surgery, 33*, 305–316.

Neel, J. V. (1991). Update on the genetic effects of ionizing radiation. *Journal of the American Medical Association, 266*, 698–701.

Ong, Y. S., Samuel M., & Song, C. (2006). Meta-analysis of early excision of burns. *Burns, 32*, 145–150.

Raskind, M. A., Peskind, E. R., Kanter, E. D., Petrie, E. C., Radant, A., Thompson, C. E., et al. (2003). Reduction of nightmares and other PTSD symptoms in combat veterans by prazosin: A placebo-controlled study. *The American Journal of Psychiatry, 160,* 371–373.

Richard, R. L., Hedman, T. L., Quick, C. D., Barillo, D. J., Cancio, L. C., Renz, E. M., et al. (2008). A clarion to recommit and reaffirm burn rehabilitation. *Journal of Burn Care & Research, 29,* 425–432.

Richard, R., Baryza, M. J., Carr, J. A., Dewey, W. S., Dougherty, M. E., Forbes-Duchart, L., et al. (2009). Burn rehabilitation and research: Proceedings of a consensus summit. *Journal of Burn Care & Research, 30,* 543–573.

Richard, R., Chapman, T., Dougherty, M., Franzen, B., & Serghiou, M. (2005). *An atlas and compendium of burn splints.* San Antonio, TX: Reg Richard, Inc.

Shafer, D. M., Bay, C., Caruso, D. M., & Foster, K. N. (2008). The use of eidronate disodium in the prevention of heterotopic ossification in burn patients. *Burns, 34,* 355–360.

Shapiro, F., & Maxfield, L. (2002). Eye movement desensitization and reprocessing (EMDR): Information processing in the treatment of trauma. *Journal of Clinical Psychology, 58,* 933–946.

Sharar, S. R., Carrougher, G. J., Nakamura, D., Hoffman, H. G., Blough, D. K., & Patterson, D. R. (2007). Factors influencing the efficacy of virtual reality distraction analgesia during postburn physical therapy: Preliminary results from 3 ongoing studies. *Archives of Physical Medicine and Rehabilitation, 88*: S43–S49.

Spurr, E. D., & Shakespeare, P. G. (1990). Incidence of hypertrophic scarring in burn-injured children. *Burns, 16,* 179–181.

Tcheung, W. J., Rhonda R., Rosenberg, L., Rosenberg, M., Villarreal, C., Thomas, C., et al. (2005). Early treatment of acute stress disorder in children with major burn injury. *Pediatric Critical Care Medicine, 6,* 676–681.

Tsionos, I., Leclercq, C., & Rochet, J. M. (2004). Heterotopic ossification of the elbow in patients with burns. Results after early excision. *The Journal of Bone Joint Surgery, 86,* 396–403.

van Loey, N. E. E., van Son, M. J., van der Heijden, P. G., & Ellis, I. M. (2008). PTSD in persons with burns: An explorative study examining relationships with attributed responsibility, negative and positive emotional states. *Burns, 34,* 1082–1089.

6

The Role of Rehabilitation in Cancer Patients

Reema Batra, MD, and Parul Jajoo, DO, FAAPMR

INTRODUCTION

No word is feared by people more than the word "cancer." It is a disease that does not discriminate between young and old, rich and poor, healthy and sick. Unfortunately, in many cases, it is silent, until it is often too late. It is these characteristics that differentiate cancer from other illnesses.

Cancer is an umbrella term for a group of diseases that are caused by the uncontrolled growth and spread of abnormal cells. The proliferation of cells is unchecked, creating an imbalance between the cancer cells and healthy cells. It is the intractability of the cancer cells that eventually leads to the demise of the individual. The causes of most cancers are still relatively unknown, but we do understand that it can be due to both external and internal factors. External factors include radiation exposure, cigarette smoke, and infectious organisms, whereas internal factors include inherited mutations and abnormalities of the immune system. It is certain that the development of most cancers requires multiple steps that may take over many years.

One in eight deaths is attributed to cancer (American Cancer Society, 2008) around the world. In developed countries, cancer is the second leading cause of death, whereas in poorer countries it is the third leading cause of death. As more people are living longer and adapting lifestyle behaviors such as smoking and high-fat diets, the rates of cancer are increasing and there is an overwhelming growth of health care systems in both developed and developing countries.

In the United States, cancer is the second most common cause of death followed by heart disease. It accounts for about one in four deaths. In 2009, about 560,000 Americans were expected to die from cancer, about 1,500 per day. Lung cancer remains the leading cause of death from cancer in both males and females. The most common cancers in men and women are prostate and breast cancer, respectively (American Cancer Society, 2008).

Because of these staggering numbers, financial support both from public and private funding has poured into research for cancer treatment, as well as prevention and screening strategies. It is this dedication to research that has changed the landscape of cancer treatment, in many cases making it a chronic disease rather than a death sentence. Five-year survival rates have increased significantly from 1996 to 2004, 66%, up from 50% in 1975–1977 (American Cancer Society, 2008). These statistics vary depending on cancer type, stage, and patient variability; however, the numbers do tell us that more people are living longer with modern cancer treatment than ever before.

Treatment of cancer is specific to site and stage, but general principles are applied to all cancer types. Treatments can generally include surgery, radiation, and chemotherapy, utilizing a multidisciplinary approach that most often achieves optimal results for the patient. From the time of diagnosis to the start of treatment, most patients have encountered a surgeon, radiation oncologist, and medical oncologist. A treatment plan has likely been developed, and the patient is ready to embark on a journey that will likely be physically and emotionally draining.

The therapeutic modalities that are used in cancer management have, no doubt, significantly changed the way we see cancer as a population. Although many of our patients survive many years after the initial diagnosis, the actual treatment process can compromise patients' normal functioning. Because of this potentially drastic side effect of the treatment, rehabilitation specialists are vital to the multidisciplinary approach to the cancer patient.

The origin of cancer rehabilitation can be traced back to the National Cancer Act in 1971 (Goreczny, 1995), which directed funding toward this aspect of cancer treatment. This eventually led to the National Cancer Rehabilitation Conference in 1972, sponsored by the National Cancer Institute. Four objectives were developed at this conference to improve rehabilitative support to cancer patients: psychosocial support, optimal physical functioning, vocational counseling, and optimal social functioning (Dudas & Carlson, 1988). With the increasing complexity of cancer treatment and the prolongation of survival of these patients, the issues of functionality for the patient have become an integral part of the therapeutic planning. Multiple definitions have been proposed for cancer rehabilitation. One such example is given by Mayer and O'Connor (1989), who proposed that cancer rehabilitation is a process that assists patients in optimizing functionality in their individual environments. In general, rehabilitation in cancer patients uses the same general principles as rehabilitation in, for example, stroke, traumatic brain disease, and heart disease. As cancer increasingly becomes a chronic long-term illness with an unpredictable course, rehabilitation in these patients becomes a more unique process.

The more modern approach to rehabilitation in cancer patients addresses the scope and course of the disease as well as the diversity of problems that may arise at unpredictable times. Dietz (1981) described four phases in the rehabilitation process: prevention, restoration, support, and palliation. Preventive strategies focus on the patient's physical functioning prior to the initiation of treatment. Restorative strategies are used to bring patients back to their original level of functioning after the treatment. An example of this would be range-of-motion exercise in postmastectomy patients. Rehabilitation for supportive measures, such as the use of a prosthetic device in a patient who has had a limb amputation for sarcoma, is performed to help patients adapt to permanent disabilities. If a patient reaches a phase in which the goal is palliation, there may be increasing disability as the disease progresses. These goals include, but are not limited to, pain control, psychological support, and prevention of contractures and bed sores secondary to inactivity.

It has been seen in the past that the utilization of rehabilitation in cancer patients has been suboptimal. In 1978, Lehmann et al. were one of the first to describe the problems encountered by cancer patients, which required rehabilitative services. They screened more than 800 patients with all types of cancers, including hematological malignancies, and found that more than 50% of patients had issues related to physical medicine, many of which could be treated with rehabilitation. Another observation was that more than 50% of patients who were experiencing physical problems also had psychological problems. It was concluded that this population of patients would benefit from an intervention by a rehabilitation team.

Although there have been many studies that have concluded that cancer patients can benefit from rehabilitation, there is still an underutilization of the rehabilitative services. This may be due to a lack of awareness of services by the clinical staff and an underrecognized eligibility of patients. This can be improved by education of the clinical staff with a capacity of referring patients to the rehabilitation service. Clinicians should be trained to assess outcomes such as side effects from the treatment and the disease itself, performance status and the ability to perform activities of daily living, and psychosocial needs. It is important to also assess the patient's quality of life, and this can be done using well-established scales developed by the Eastern Cooperative Oncology Group and European Organisation for Research and Treatment of Cancer.

BREAST CANCER

In the United States, breast cancer is ranked as the most common cancer and the second leading cause of cancer death in women (Jemal et al., 2008). It is also the leading cause of cancer death in women between the ages of 45 and 55. Many risk factors, including age, female gender, and personal and family history of breast cancer, have been associated with breast cancer (Jemal et al., 2008). In the United States, breast cancer affects women of all racial groups, but the incidence is highest in Whites, about 133/100,000 women (American Cancer Society, 2008). Although the rate is lower in Black women (118/100,000), the incidence is much higher at younger ages and the mortality is higher than in White women. This is likely due to the cancers being more aggressive in Black women and diagnosis at a late stage. Other risk factors include, but are not limited to, younger age at onset of menarche, older age at onset of menopause, nulliparity, and older age at first birth.

Treatment options for breast cancer vary widely depending on the stage of the disease and tumor characteristics. Treatment modalities used are surgery, radiation therapy, chemotherapy, and hormonal therapy. In recent years, there have been many advancements in breast cancer therapy, resulting in improvements in survival rates.

Surgery is usually the first step in the treatment of breast cancer, unless patients have very large tumors, in which case they are offered neoadjuvant therapy, or if they have metastatic disease, wherein they are started on systemic chemotherapy. The type of surgery that is performed for a patient is usually a decision made by the breast surgeon, oftentimes in consultation with the medical oncologist and radiation specialist. The most common surgeries are breast conservation therapy (BCT) and mastectomy.

With BCT, the breast tumor is removed along with a small amount of normal tissue from the breast. This is then followed by radiation therapy to the area. The combination of BCT and radiation therapy has been compared with mastectomy alone, and the results showed that the procedures were similar with regard to patient survival (Fisher, et al., 2002). During the procedure, the surgeon usually removes sentinel lymph nodes to ensure that the cancer cells have not spread to the axilla. If cancer is present in the sentinel nodes, the patient will subsequently have all the axillary nodes removed. The complications that patients can experience after BCT and radiation treatment include infection, fluid collection at the incision site, rib fracture, shortness of breath, and secondary cancers. Cosmetic outcomes after BCT are usually good to excellent after surgery using modern surgical techniques. Some of the factors that may influence the cosmetic outcome include the amount of breast tissue removed, patient variability such as breast size, and timing of adjuvant chemotherapy and radiation.

Although there has been a shift toward BCT, mastectomies are still performed in the United States. This procedure is usually performed if the size of the tumor is too large or if the location of the tumor makes a lumpectomy difficult. Many times, the patient herself may opt for a mastectomy, even if a lumpectomy is feasible. There are two types of mastectomies: the modified radical mastectomy (MRM) and the simple mastectomy. MRM is removal of the tumor from the breast, the normal breast tissue surrounding the tumor, some of the chest wall tissue underlying the breast, and the nodes in the axillae. Oftentimes, an axillary lymph node dissection is performed, especially if there is concern for spread of the cancer. A simple mastectomy is the entire removal of the breast tissue without the axillary nodes. A sentinel node biopsy is performed during the procedure, and if the results are positive for metastatic cancer, the patient is brought back for an axillary lymph node dissection. A smaller percentage of women undergo skin-sparing mastectomies. This technique involves the removal of the nipple and areola, but the skin is maintained and the patient has immediate reconstruction of the breast after the breast tissue is removed.

Many women opt for breast reconstruction after a mastectomy. This can be done immediately after the mastectomy or at a later time, that is, after treatment is completed. There are now many options for reconstruction, and women should consult with a plastic surgeon prior to the initial surgery to discuss which option is best for them.

Although mastectomies are relatively safe procedures, complications can occur. The more common ones are postoperative bleeding and/or hematomas, seromas, wound infection, and lymphedema. Depending on the stage of the cancer, the characteristics of the tumor found, and the type of surgery performed initially, chemotherapy and radiation may be used to decrease the chance of recurrence. Radiation is definitely performed if the patient has BCT, ensuring that cancer cells that may have been left behind in the normal breast tissue are eradicated and local control of the tumor is optimized. Radiation can also be used after mastectomy; it is usually recommended in patients who have a tumor larger than 5 cm or if there are more than four lymph nodes positive with cancer. The possible long-term complications of radiation therapy are listed above, but the benefits far outweigh the small risks. Chemotherapy and hormonal therapy are also possible treatments for breast cancer. Again, the choice and duration of treatment depends largely on the tumor characteristics, such as hormone receptor positivity and the human epidermal growth factor receptor 2, or Her2neu status. It also depends on the stage of the tumor at diagnosis. The side effects of common chemotherapy medications are discussed elsewhere in the chapter.

Patients with primary or recurrent breast cancer can have shoulder and arm pain as well as lymphedema. The pain that is experienced includes phantom breast pain, neuroma pain, or neuralgia. Pain can extend to the neck, axilla, or chest wall. There is often a loss of shoulder function that occurs postmastectomy, lumpectomy, axillary lymph node dissection, or reconstruction. Exercise in cancer patients has numerous benefits that include decreased fatigue, increase of lean body mass, improved cardiovascular function, and decrease of depression.

Rehabilitation exercises for breast cancer are often prescribed with consideration of the type of surgery that was performed. If patients have a radical mastectomy or axillary lymph node dissection they are discharged from the hospital within a day. It is necessary to instruct the patient on how to incorporate shoulder range-of-motion activities with a home exercise program. This can include wall walking exercises to improve flexibility in the shoulder. The patient has to stand about two feet from a wall, raise her arm to shoulder level and climb her fingers up the wall, hold for a few seconds, and descend back to shoulder level with stretching in between. Shoulder roll exercises can also be implemented, which include standing with arms at the side of the body, moving shoulders forward and shrugging them up, and moving them backward; the patient can repeat it five times in a slow circular action. Isometric exercises can be started by using elastic bands that are differentiated by color, depending on the resistance they provide. The patient can gradually advance to isotonic exercises, which strengthens the muscle by moving the joint. Postsurgical shoulder mobilization should be gradual with consideration of the number of days postoperation. The shoulder can be subject to internal and external rotations as much as the patient can tolerate starting the first postoperative day. At postoperative day 3, the patient can flex and abduct the shoulder up to 45°, and at postoperative day 6, the patient can flex the shoulder 90° and abduct it up to 45° (Braddom, 2006). One week after surgery, the shoulder can be ranged to tolerance.

Axillary web syndrome can be seen after axillary node dissection. It is a cord-like visual tissue within the axilla that can develop months or years postoperation. These palpable cords can extend all the way below the elbow. This can occur with a sudden increase in activity after a period of decreased range of motion. Treatment plans for axillary web syndrome should include heat, manipulation, and gradual range of motion.

LYMPHEDEMA

Lymphedema is the blockage of lymph vessels that causes increased fluid retention in the tissues. Lymphedema can occur in more than 20% of patients postmastectomy secondary to breast cancer (O'Sullivan & Schmitz, 2006). The role of the lymphatic system is to transport fluid, including protein, large molecules, and fat. It reacts to cells that the body recognizes as foreign, such as the cancer cell, and produces white blood cells. Lymph nodes are a part of the immune system through which most of the lymph fluid enters the venous system.

Lymphedema occurs when the lymph load exceeds the transportation capacity of the lymph system. A dilation of lymph vessels occurs causing valve incompetence. This fluid is filled with protein and can attract bacteria resulting in infection. These infections can cause thrombosis and clotting of the lymph vessels. Lymphedema is classified as primary and secondary. Primary lymphedema is due to a hereditary condition where the node or vessel is malformed. This can be due to a degenerative or inflammatory process (Casley-Smith, Morgan, & Piller, 1993). In primary lymphedema, females are more affected than males and this occurs soon after birth. Secondary lymphedema is more common than primary, and it is due to a blockage of the lymph system that can occur after surgery or cancer treatment, such as radiation. Filariasis, caused by a worm larva that can live in the lymph vessels, is a cause of secondary lymphedema in underdeveloped nations.

In the initial diagnosis of lymphedema, one can find several features such as swelling with or without pitting that is painful at times and relieved with elevation, an increase in skin folds, asymmetry of the limb, and change in skin texture. Skin lesions, such as ulcerations, fungi, rashes, or trauma, can occur (O'Sullivan & Schmitz, 2006). Other causes of swelling that may not be due to lymphedema are trauma, cellulitis, malignancy, complex regional pain syndrome, and deep vein thrombosis.

Medical treatments of lymphedema can include controversial means such as pneumatic compression pumps that show some benefit but can increase proximal edema. Diuretics can be used to decrease fluid retention but it only works in the early stages. Benzopyrone is yet to be approved by the FDA as a treatment for lymphedema but is used in some countries and can cause liver toxicity (Casley-Smith et al., 1993).

Lymphedema can be treated with physical therapy. The advantage of this treatment is a more conservative approach to decrease edema that can increase range of motion and cosmesis. Treatment of lymphedema can be accomplished with a two-stage program known as complete decongestive therapy. The first phase includes manual lymph drainage, bandaging, compression garments in the daytime, and exercise. Compression garments should use from 30 to 50 mm Hg (Delisa, Gans, & Bocknek, 1998). The second phase is a self-managed and modified version of the first phase.

In metastatic disease, the goals for rehabilitation professionals should include attaining tolerable pain relief, allowing the patient to self-care and perform activities of daily living, maintaining energy levels allowed for a safe environment that will ensure the patient will not fall, and maintaining bone stability.

HEAD AND NECK CANCER

Head and neck cancer is not as common as some other types of cancers, but the treatment of this disease requires a prudent multidisciplinary approach, and oftentimes the patient is referred for rehabilitation because of the effects of surgery and radiation. The annual incidence of this cancer is about 47,000 in the United States, and it has declined over the last 30 years (Jemal et al., 2008; Sikora, Toniolo, & DeLacure, 2004). The cancer is more frequently seen in men, but women with risk factors are susceptible to the disease.

There are many causes of head and neck cancer, but the two strongest associations are tobacco and alcohol (Spitz, 1994), and the risk is higher in people who combine smoking and drinking. Other risk factors include viral associations, in particular, human papillomavirus (HPV), radiation exposure, occupational exposure, and genetic susceptibility.

Head and neck cancer is a general term for a variety of subtypes of cancers that are classified according to the origin of the tumor. Head and neck cancer is usually classified into five categories: oral cavity, pharynx, larynx, nasal cavity and paranasal sinuses, and salivary glands. The treatment of head and neck cancer can become quite complicated as this is largely due to a number of subtypes, the anatomical complexity of the head and neck region, and the need to maintain quality of life and ensure organ preservation. After treatment of the cancer, many patients find themselves working on their quality of lives, undergoing rehabilitation and restoration of speech and/or swallowing.

The modalities most often used in the treatment of head and neck cancer are surgery, radiation, and systemic chemotherapy. Approximately one third of the patients present in early-stage disease, and, in general, either surgery or radiation can cure a patient. The choice between the two modalities depends largely on the patient's comorbidities, functional outcomes, and accessibility. In some cases, a patient may receive adjuvant radiation, for example, if there are positive margins at surgery, bone erosion, or positive lymph nodes. These patients may also benefit by the addition of chemotherapy in the adjuvant setting if they have an adequate performance status that will allow them to tolerate the treatment regimen.

When the cancer is more advanced, but not yet metastatic, the treatment is not as straightforward. Many patients are not resectable at this stage; however, by using chemotherapy and/or radiation in the neoadjuvant setting, patients can potentially go for surgery. When a patient is found to have metastatic disease, the only modality that is used is chemotherapy. At this stage, patients are not curable and the goal of treatment is control of the spread of the disease and palliation.

The side effects of the treatment of head and neck cancer largely depend on the modalities used. There are several chemotherapy medications that are used, and their side effects will be discussed elsewhere in the chapter. Radiation therapy can have both acute and long-term sequelae, and these occur largely because of the loss of parenchymal cells. The most common acute side effects are mucositis, odynophagia, dysphagia, hoarseness, xerostomia, dermatitis, and weight loss, and these effects resolve as the cells are replaced. These side effects can vary, and largely depend on the type of tumor being treated and patient-related factors, such as cigarette use and comorbid conditions. It is important to be aware of these potential side effects in these patients and to initiate any preventive measures and/or prompt treatment when they occur, as the symptoms oftentimes are so severe that they can delay treatment and ultimately affect the patient's outcome.

One of the more important preventable measures is encouraging smoking cessation once the patient begins treatment. Other than being a known cause of head and neck cancer, it can make the side effects more pronounced in patients receiving radiation, even after it is completed. Patients who smoke throughout treatment also have a suboptimal outcome, as seen in a clinical trial (Browman et al., 1993). Patients should also be instructed on appropriate skincare to prevent or decrease the dermatitis that radiation can cause. The patient should avoid UV rays, wind exposure, lotions, creams, and fragrances to minimize irritation by chemicals.

Unfortunately, late effects can also occur in these patients after radiation. This is usually the result of injury to the stromal elements or the supportive structures. Some of the more common side effects include permanent xerostomia, osteoradionecrosis of the jaw, radiation-induced fibrosis, chronic pain, airway edema leading to tracheostomy placement, and hypothyroidism.

Surgery is also an integral part of the treatment of head and neck cancer, and if a patient's tumor is resectable, that is often the treatment of choice if the patient is a good surgical candidate. The goals of surgical resection are to cure the patient, but without the compromise of organ function and cosmetic outcome, both of which ultimately affect quality of life. In early-stage cancers, surgery is often utilized as first-line treatment because of the resectability of the tumor and low potential of organ compromise. However, as the tumor becomes more advanced, surgical options become more limited, and, if utilized, it is oftentimes in combination with chemotherapy and/or radiation. There are many surgical options when it comes to head and neck cancer, and the procedure that is selected for the patient largely depends on the location of the tumor. Again, the more advanced cancers are usually treated with chemotherapy, radiation, or a combination of both prior to attempting a surgical resection.

Speech and Swallowing in the Head and Neck Cancer Patient

There are three phases of swallowing numbered according to the route the bolus travels in as it reaches the stomach (Delisa et al., 1998). The first is the oral phase that includes the preparation of the bolus prior to being swallowed. At this time, food is chewed and moistened with saliva that helps break down food and the mouth sequentially opens and closes. At the end of this phase, when the bolus is prepared, the tongue moves up and pushes the bolus of the food into the oropharynx. This begins the second phase of swallowing known as the pharyngeal phase. The bolus is pushed by the tongue, and at the same time, the epiglottis covers the trachea. The food moves from the larynx through the pharyngoesophageal sphincter and into the esophagus beginning the third phase. The bolus goes through the esophagus and into the stomach via the gastroesophageal sphincter.

Head and neck cancer can affect any or all of these stages as well as give a patient speech impairments, shoulder dysfunction, neck weakness, and disfigurement that can lead to depression. If a patient has a glossectomy, there is a risk of aspiration and may need prosthesis for the palate. A laryngectomy or radiation to the area may call for communication aides such as electrolarynx.

Head and neck cancers can affect a patient's ability to swallow. Treatments for dysphagia, which is pain with swallowing, should be implemented with a modification of the diet. One should have a pureed diet and thickened liquids to prevent aspiration. Exercises can be practiced at home including strengthening of the oral musculature to prevent food coming out of the oral cavity. This should include techniques to exercise the tongue such as moving the tongue several times in a horizontal manner, exercising the posterior pharynx by gargling, exercising the larynx by saying "ah" in a deep voice, and exercising the jaw by moving it side by side as described by Braddom (2006). Patients should also learn how to eat with the chin tuck method. This involves sitting up straight and flexing the neck by placing the chin toward the chest when swallowing to prevent aspiration by protecting the airway.

Patients who suffer from head and neck cancer and seek out treatment must be evaluated for nutritional needs. This includes the consideration of a feeding tube if needed. Many of these patients, after radiation treatment, have significantly reduced saliva and must increase their fluid intake and have an appropriate soft diet. The reduction of saliva can damage dental enamel as well; this can be prevented by the use of a special toothpaste that increases saliva production.

Several head and neck cancer patients come out of surgery with partial or total spinal accessory nerve injury (Braddom, 2006). This occurs less often because radical neck dissections are falling out of favor as compared with functional dissections. Functional dissections spare the muscles, nerves, and veins of the neck. If the spinal accessory nerve is somewhat compromised, one must consider some rehabilitation techniques. The patient can suffer from scapular instability that can cause winging and shoulder weakness with decreased range of motion causing frozen shoulder and decreased flexibility of the chest wall. It is important to strengthen the elevators of the scapula, range the shoulder, and use heat, such as ultrasound, on the shoulder.

Radiation can also cause disfigurement such as severe contracture of the neck. Aggressive active and passive range of motion should be implemented during and after the radiation therapy. The patient can be given a home exercise program that includes stretching and self-massage.

Head and neck cancer treatment can cause impaired vocal cords. This can be extremely debilitating for the patients. Patients can be taught other sources of communication such as writing, mouthing their words, or using gestures. A tracheoesophageal puncture can be done; this creates a connection between the trachea and esophagus (Delisa et al., 1998). A valve is placed to allow air to come into the esophagus and close off the trachea. Some patients do not prefer this and choose an electrolarynx. This device senses vibrations; however, the sound can be monotonous and not as similar to the human voice.

MUSCULOSKELETAL CANCERS

The most common tumors seen afflicting the musculoskeletal system are sarcomas. These are rare tumors that can arise from any area of the mesenchymal system—about 10,000 cases are diagnosed per year, contributing to 0.7% of the new cancer diagnoses. However, mesenchymal cells have the capacity to mature into striated muscle, bone, cartilage, soft tissue, and adipose tissue, and the treatment of these cancers oftentimes can leave the patient with a new handicap and/or a suboptimal cosmetic outcome. Therefore, even though these tumors are rare, the rehabilitation needs are high.

The biological behaviors of these tumors are varied, from indolent to aggressive, and this is largely dependent on the specific histology of the tumor cells. The tumors can affect the soft tissues, bones, and peripheral nerves. Because of the wide array of tumors that present under the sarcoma classification and the relative rarity of these tumors itself, there has been a relatively less understanding of the biology of the tumors and their responsiveness to treatment. These have also limited our understanding of the best treatment that can be given for these types of cancers. Multimodality treatment is often used, including surgery, radiation, and chemotherapy; the choice of treatment oftentimes depends on the location of the tumor and the stage. Soft tissue sarcomas can occur at any anatomical site, most commonly the thigh, buttocks, and groin areas (Lawrence et al., 1987). In many cases, surgical resection is utilized, however, leaving patients with a functional deficit that they must learn to live with.

Rehabilitation for musculoskeletal cancers, including sarcomas, begins prior to treatments and surgeries. This gives an opportunity to educate the family and patient about the goals that should be reached to increase strength and endurance and about ambulatory devices and fall precaution.

Cancers of the limb can be treated with limb-sparing surgeries. Immediate postoperative care for these patients includes rest for wound healing to decrease edema and maintain alignment of the limb and joint. Occasionally, muscles are resected and splints and orthotics can be taken into consideration. Along with adaptive equipment to assist in activities of daily living, such as larger-handled utensils for eating or reachers for grabbing garments so patients can dress themselves, immediate passive range of motion is important with the surgeon's permission. If the limb is amputated, it may result in a shorter residual limb secondary to ensuring the tumor margins are eliminated. Thus, edema and wound healing may delay the fitting of an upper or a lower extremity prosthesis. With limb amputations, the health care professional should take into consideration phantom pain, which is pain of the amputated part of the limb, phantom sensation, which is a sensation that the limb is still present, and stump pain, which is pain at the stump site. This can be treated by the physician with various medications.

Cancers of the trunk can result in splinting on the side of surgery. This should be discouraged and early ambulation should be encouraged. In lower extremity cancers, it is important to differentiate between possible infections causing cellulitis versus deep venous thrombosis and lymphedema. All three are possible and have different treatment options. The limb would appear red, swollen, and tender to touch if it is cellulitic and can be treated with antibiotics. If it is a deep vein thrombosis or blood clot, the limb would be swollen and tender to touch with squeezing, requiring treatment with blood thinners. Lymphedema would result in a swollen limb and at times the limb would have decreased range of motion and treatment would include physical therapy.

Sexual dysfunction is a notable side effect of several types of cancers and secondary to treatments, and this is common in musculoskeletal cancers. Chemotherapy can cause a decrease in testosterone production, which decreases the libido, and radiation therapy can cause fibrosis of the mucus epithelium that can decrease lubrication to the vagina. Counseling should be part of the treatment process with both the patient and partner encouraged to show other possible ways of intimacy.

Bone Metastases

Metastasis to the bone is a frequent complication in patients with advanced cancer. Breast and prostate cancers are the two most common malignancies to spread to the bone; however, most solid tumors have a propensity to affect the bone when the disease is advanced (Coleman & Rubens, 1987). The incidence of bone metastasis is unknown, but it is thought that about one half of patients who die from metastatic cancer have bone involvement (Mundy, 2002). There are many consequences of the metastasis to the bone, some common ones being severe pain, fractures, spinal cord compression, and hypercalcemia.

Bone lesions are usually classified as osteolytic or osteoblastic. Osteolytic bone lesions result from the destruction of bone, whereas osteoblastic lesions result from deposits of new bone. Patients can have one or the other type of lesion, but many patients can have characteristics of both. The common denominator of the two types of processes is that they result from an interruption of normal bone remodeling.

Patients are suspected of having bone metastasis when they present with symptoms resulting due to bone lesion. As a result, the diagnostic tests, rather than a standard test, will usually focus on the patient's symptoms. For example, a patient may experience pain in a certain area that is severe and that can negatively impact the patient's daily activities. These symptoms would prompt the practitioner to evaluate the area with a radiological exam, usually an X-ray. Bone scans are helpful if bone metastases are strongly suspected, but the plain film is negative; this is because they can detect the lesions at earlier stages. The limitation with bone scans is that they can detect osteoblastic lesions better than osteolytic lesions that may go undetected. Other examinations that can be used are MRI and CT scans.

Spinal cord compression is another consequence of bone metastasis, but this will be discussed later in the chapter. Hypercalcemia results from an increased bone resorption and a release of calcium from the bone. This is most commonly seen in patients with breast cancer, who most often present with osteolytic lesions (Guise et al., 1996). This can result in neuropsychiatric abnormalities, gastrointestinal disturbances, renal dysfunction, and cardiac conduction abnormalities.

The treatment of bone metastasis focuses largely on the improvement of the patient's quality of life and activities of daily living. Chemotherapy and/or hormonal therapy can be used if the patient is still a candidate based on performance status and organ function. The goals of palliative treatment in these patients are elimination of pain, preservation of skeletal integrity, and functional maintenance. One method of palliation is radiation therapy, most commonly external beam radiation therapy. This is best used when the lesions are limited to a certain number of sites, rather than diffuse disease. More than 80% of patients who have external beam radiation therapy experience some relief of pain, whereas more than half of the patients have a complete response (Arcangeli et al., 1998). Because of these statistics, several groups advocate the use of radiation for the palliation of pain from bone metastases (Hoskin, Yarnold, Roos, & Bentzen, 2001; National Comprehensive Cancer Network, 2004).

Bisphosphonates are also used for their ability to inhibit osteoclastic activity and can help patients with bone metastases. The use of bisphosphonates is especially important in patients with hypercalcemia, but can also be used in those with bone lesions and no evidence of the metabolic abnormality. They have been demonstrated in clinical trials to decrease the frequency of skeletal events (Theriault et al., 1999), thereby decreasing the frequency of pathological fractures, hypercalcemia, and the need for radiation therapy.

Bony metastatic lesions cause localized pain to the area, which is worse at night and severe at times. It is important to aggressively range the patient. The fall risk must be considered in the patients with long lower extremity bone involvement. Surgery should be considered when lesions are greater than 2.5 cm in diameter and are more than half of the cortical diameter or greater than half of the cross-sectional area (Delisa et al., 1998). If the patient is not a surgical candidate, he/she should be partial to non-weight-bearing. The patient should be encouraged to ambulate using aides such as walkers or crutches, and if there is an unstable spine, a spinal orthotic can be prescribed.

CENTRAL NERVOUS SYSTEM TUMORS

Central nervous system (CNS) tumors arise from various cells within the CNS or they are metastatic from another primary cancer. Because of these differing etiologies, CNS tumors can behave differently, and hence, the treatment and prognosis vary widely. The symptoms of CNS tumors are numerous. They are usually caused by local invasion into the brain by the tumor itself, compression of vital structures, and increased intercranial pressure caused by edema and inflammation.

CNS Metastases

More than half of the brain tumors that are found in adult patients are metastases from other cancers, making this the most common type of intracranial cancers in this age group (Wen & Loeffler, 1999). About 10–30% of adult patients with cancer eventually develop brain metastases (Johnson & Young, 1996) and the most common primary tumors are lung cancer, breast cancer, renal cell cancer, and colorectal cancer, with lung cancer being the most common (Patchell, 1997). The incidence of brain metastasis is increasing, and this is thought to be partially due to longer survival rates of patients and new imaging modalities that detect smaller cancers.

The mechanism of metastasis is primarily due to hematogenous spread (Delattre, Krol, Thaler, & Posner, 1988). Many tumors are found at watershed areas whereas about 80% of the patients have metastases in the cerebral hemispheres, the remaining being in the cerebellum and the brain stem.

Clinically, the symptoms vary depending on the location and the size of the tumor, as well as the surrounding edema associated with it. Because of the variability of the location of the metastases, the signs and symptoms can vary widely from patient to patient. The most common complaint is headache with or without associated nausea and vomiting, but patients can also present with focal neurological abnormalities, seizures, and cognitive dysfunction. Stroke is also a possibility, either due to hemorrhage into the tumor site or invasion or compression of a vessel from a tumor.

The management of brain metastases is usually tailored to the patient's overall prognosis. This is largely dependent on the patient's performance status, age, and extent of the primary tumor. Patients with the best prognosis have a median survival of about 7 months, whereas those with the worst prognosis have a median survival of about 2 months. If a patient has a good overall prognosis, the treatment is tailored to eradicate the brain metastases. Surgical resection is an option if the tumor location is favorable and if there are only a limited number of lesions. Whole brain radiation is also recommended after the surgery to decrease the local recurrence risk. Treatment of patients with a poor prognosis is focused on the control of symptoms and maintenance of quality of life and neurological functioning. Whole brain radiation is the first line of treatment in these patients to achieve a quick relief of symptoms. Systemic chemotherapy can be used, but this is usually after radiation and surgery have not worked and the goal is for palliation only.

The treatment of the brain metastases can cause complications themselves. When patients receive whole brain radiation therapy, they are at risk of both acute and long-term complications. Acute toxicities include cerebral edema, nausea and vomiting, encephalopathy, dermatitis and alopecia, and myelosuppression. Some more chronic problems are brain atrophy, neurocognitive dysfunction, radiation necrosis at the site of the tumor, and neuroendocrine disease. Acute toxicities are usually self-limiting, but chronic side effects can be helped with supportive care with rehabilitative efforts.

Other treatments that are used for brain metastases include supportive measures, such as corticosteroids for the treatment of the vasogenic edema and its associated edema, and anticonvulsants for seizure control.

Primary CNS Tumors

Primary brain tumors arise from different cells in the CNS, thereby creating a diverse group of tumors. It is a relatively uncommon malignancy, with the annual incidence being roughly 7 in every 100,000 people in the United States (Central Brain Tumor Registry of the United States, 2004). In adults, the most common primary brain tumors are gliomas, as they make up more than 80% of these cancers. They arise from the glial cells, and can be further classified as astrocytomas, anaplastic astrocytomas, and gliomas. Some other primary CNS tumors that are seen are meningiomas, pituitary tumors, lymphomas, and oligodendrogliomas. Unfortunately, even though primary CNS tumors are rare, the 5-year survival rate for the malignant types is around 33% (Surveillance, Epidemiology and End Results Program 1975–2001). The treatment for malignant gliomas and the other types of malignant brain tumors utilizes a multimodality approach to maximize the outcome of the patient. This includes, when safe, optimal surgical resection with adjuvant chemotherapy and/or radiation. As noted above, these modalities are associated with side effects, and the utilization of rehabilitative efforts can really influence the patient's quality of life.

Spinal cord metastasis can affect the thoracic spine 70% of the time, lumbar spine 20% of the time, and less likely the cervical spine, which is only 10% of the time. Cord compression can occur in 5% of cancer patients (Delisa et al., 1998). Pain can be located in the spine itself or seen as radicular pain. Deep palpation of the spine can elicit the pain or radicular pain can be seen with electric, shooting type pain that radiates down the extremity. Myelopathy can also develop. It is important to note the patient's ambulatory status and if they are falling often. Symptoms of myelopathy can include imbalance, falls, or near falls. The patient can suffer from motor deficits prior to sensory deficits. Treatments for this can include oral steroids conservatively, or, if necessary, considering the life expectancy, one can refer to a spine surgeon for laminectomy (Delisa et al., 1998).

Brain tumor rehabilitation mimics stroke rehabilitation. Health care providers should consider similar occurrences in patients with brain tumors and strokes. Hydrocephalus is a complication that can occur in both disorders. Three symptoms of hydrocephalus can be seen in patients while in therapy: urinary incontinence, gait imbalance, and dementia. At times, these symptoms are not manifested and hydrocephalus can be diagnosed if a patient is simply not progressing in therapy. Brain tumors close to the third and fourth ventricles can obstruct the flow of cerebral spinal fluid and can cause hydrocephalus. At times, brain tumors can cause new blood vessels to form that can create edema and if severe enough, a full herniation of the brain (Glantz et al., 1996).

A complication that can be seen in both brain tumors and stroke is hemiparesis, which is weakness to one or both sides of the body. It is important to implement aggressive active and passive range of motion to increase function and decrease the chance of contractures of the limb.

Primary or secondary brain tumors can also cause cognitive deficits that differ from traumatic brain injury or stroke in that brain tumor cognitive deficits can be temporary and reversible. After surgery is performed to a certain area and the pressure is relieved, function can be rapidly resolved. It is important to involve speech therapy and neuropsychology for the cognitive deficits the patient may be experiencing. If there are unresectable metastases in several areas, decline can be gradual and downward.

CNS cancers can be rehabilitated according to their life expectancy and clinical course. If a patient has a fair neurological status and functional ability, the rehabilitation course can be aggressive. If the patient is not able to ambulate and is bound to the bed, the course should include prevention of ulcers, passive range of motion, customized adaptive equipment, cognitive exercises, and aggressive pain management.

Peripheral Nervous System and Oncological Issues

Patients with cancer can present with manifestations on the peripheral nervous system (PNS). This can be related to the cancer, such as paraneoplastic syndromes, or it can be related to the treatment, such as chemotherapy-induced peripheral neuropathy. Other factors that may influence the functioning of the PNS are metabolic derangements, poor nutrition, and comorbid conditions. These neurological impairments can cause disabilities in the cancer patient that ultimately affect quality of life.

Brachial plexopathy can occur a month or several years after radiation. Initially, a patient can experience paresthesias and pain, and there can be a decrease in sensation and weakness as well. Pain can be controlled by using the World Health Organization ladder, once controlled exercise and range of motion are implemented. If the patient has weakness in the shoulder, a sling can be used to prevent shoulder subluxation in addition to hand and wrist orthosis (Braddom, 2006).

Paraneoplastic syndromes are a diverse group of syndromes that can affect the nervous system at any point and can damage one or multiple areas. These syndromes are generally unrelated to metastases or treatment of the cancer, and although the mechanism is poorly understood, it is believed that an immunological response against certain tissues is the likely cause (Dalmau, Gultekin, & Posner, 1999). Some syndromes have also been found to be the result of oversecretion of hormones and/or cytokines, generating an abnormal metabolic response (Posner, 1995). The most common paraneoplastic syndromes seen are Lambert-Eaton syndrome, which affects 3% of patients with small-cell lung cancer, and myasthenia gravis, which affects 15% of patients with thymoma. For patients with other tumors, the incidence of these syndromes is much less than 1% (Rudnicki & Dalmau, 2000). Again, these syndromes can affect any part of the nervous system, so diagnosis is usually made with the help of a neurologist who can assess the patient's symptoms and relate it to the corresponding part of the system.

Because most of the syndromes are immune mediated, many of the treatments are centered around immune suppression and treatment of the tumor itself. For example, patients with Lambert-Eaton syndrome and myasthenia gravis are treated with intravenous immunoglobulin, which is an infusion of antibodies, or plasma exchange; both treatments can suppress the immune response and improve neurological status in the short term. If patients do not improve, it may be that the damage is irreversible at the time the treatment is instituted.

Chemotherapy can cause a wide array of neurological side effects either from the direct toxic effects of the medication itself or from the manifestations on the metabolic system. The most common drugs to cause neurotoxicity are the platinum compounds, although many others can also be responsible.

Cisplatin, most commonly used in the treatment of lung cancer and head and neck cancer, is known to cause peripheral neuropathy and ototoxicity. The neuropathy is largely axonal and affects myelinated sensory fibers. The patient usually begins to feel numbness, paresthesias, and sometimes pain; this usually begins distally in the toes and fingers, and ends proximally in the legs and arms. This side effect is dose dependent, as most patients can tolerate doses up to 400 mg/m^2, but this can vary from patient to patient. Once the patient develops the symptoms, there is no treatment. Patients with mild neuropathy can continue treatment, but those with more disabling symptoms will need to have a discussion with their oncologist regarding the risks and benefits of continuing treatment. The discontinuation of treatment generally reverses the condition, although many patients never recover fully.

Carboplatin is a drug similar to cisplatin, but the side effects of neuropathy are generally not seen in standard treatment. However, in very high doses used for hematopoietic stem cell transplant, patients can experience a severe neuropathy. Oxaliplatin, another platinum compound used in the treatment of colorectal cancer, is associated with two neurotoxicities: an acute neurosensory complex, which can occur during the first few infusions of the drug, and a cumulative sensory neuropathy, which is associated with a distal loss of sensation. Many preventive efforts for the oxaliplatin-induced neuropathy are available, including stopping and reintroducing the medication, prolonging the infusion time, and administering various pharmacological agents such as calcium and magnesium infusions, glutathione, and glutamine.

Other chemotherapeutic drugs that can cause neurological side effects are the vinca alkaloids, the most common being vincristine. This antineoplastic agent is widely used, and its dose-limiting toxicity is an axonal neuropathy. Patients generally have symptoms that are synonymous with diabetic neuropathy. Taxanes are antimicrotubule agents that can also cause peripheral neuropathy, usually affecting the sensory fibers. The manifestations usually involve burning paresthesias of the hands and feet. Paclitaxel, a compound from the taxane family, can also cause a motor neuropathy affecting the proximal muscles. Docetaxel can also cause motor and sensory neuropathies, but these side effects are usually much less than with paclitaxel.

CANCER FATIGUE

Fatigue is a common problem seen in cancer patients. This can be associated with many causes, including the side effect of the treatment, anemia, pain, emotional distress, and nutritional deficiencies. Fatigue is important in the determination of the patient's quality of life, both for the patient and their family members. Despite this finding, cancer fatigue is not routinely assessed by health care practitioners. Screening is now recommended at all cancer-related visits, as it has been shown to play a large role in determining the patient's quality of life (Dy et al., 2008).

Cancer Pain

Cancer patients experience pain that is often left untreated. Pain can be secondary to the tumor itself or bony metastases. This can be due to nociceptive pain and/or neuropathic pain (Robb, Williams, Duviver, & Newham, 2006).

Pain in spinal cord injury secondary to metastases to the spinal cord can be due to nociceptive pain and/or neuropathic pain. Nociceptive pain can be due to sprains, fractures, or other injuries. Symptoms for nociceptive pain include a localized, constant aching or throbbing pain. Nociceptive pain can also be due to instability of the spine, muscle spasms, and pain secondary to overuse. The nociceptive pain can be treated with nonsteroidal anti-inflammatory medication and muscle spasms treated with antispasmodics. In neuropathic pain, trauma and neural alterations of the pain pathways can occur. The pain is described as nerve root entrapment and is described as lancinating, burning, or stabbing that can occur in a pattern of the nerve. Root avulsion can occur, creating a burning sensation to an area that is denervated. This can occur often with metastasis to the spine. Pain below the level of injury can be called central dysesthesia. This pain is constant and has been described as a burning sensation with numbness and tingling. This is often treated with neuropathic pain medication and possibly epidural steroid injections. When discussing treatment options, one should consider the type of pain the patient is experiencing and the appropriate long-term goal.

Pain can also be due to neuropathic pain that is secondary to chemotherapy. Postsurgical pain can occur secondary to organ removal from cancer itself. It is important to know the type of pain being treated secondary to the cancer to develop a proper treatment plan. The goal to treat the patients with this pain should be to improve their function and create a sense of independence so they can deal with their illness in a positive manner. It is important to control their pain when it is acute and severe, and if it is inadequately controlled, patients are more likely to develop chronic pain. The pain should be controlled after surgery and during chemotherapy and radiation. A balance of interventional, pharmacological, behavioral, and rehabilitation therapy should be maintained.

Oral medications can be considered first, which can be prescribed by using the World Health Organization guidelines. This was developed specifically for pain secondary to cancer. If a patient has bone metastasis, the best treatment is a nonsteroidal anti-inflammatory agent. This is the first suggested medication to use with the WHO pain ladder. This step also includes adjuvant medication, such as antiepileptics, for neuropathic pain that can be caused by chemotherapy or plexopathies secondary to radiation therapy. The second step includes a mild opioid, if the first step did not adequately control the patient's pain. The third step can be a strong opioid, if necessary. Prior to this, one can use interventional therapies to help with oral medications (World Health Organization, 1990), for example, epidural injections or continuous catheters, including neurolytic agents (phenol or alcohol) to help with thoracic pain secondary to thoracotomy or transforaminal injections into the lower thoracic foramen to help with thoracic pain (Burton, Fanciullo, Beasley, & Fisch, 2007).

Celiac plexus blocks can be used for most of the organs in the abdomen, excluding the liver. A block of the plexus can stop nociception from the visceral organs, and eventually reduce or stop pain to the area. If a patient is on chronic narcotics, has adverse side effects to the medication, and has a life expectancy of more than 3 months, an intrathecal pump can be inserted to deliver medications such as morphine.

SUMMARY

As cancer treatments become more advanced and patients start to live longer, rehabilitation issues become more apparent as patients begin to ease back into their daily lives and activities. It is imperative that practitioners who encounter a cancer patient make assessments on their functional outcomes during and after cancer treatment. Although many survivors will eventually seek the help to integrate back into the community, patients with poor prognoses can benefit from rehabilitative services to improve on the quality of life and palliation from the cancer effects. Our goal as practitioners is ultimately to make the experience from the cancer diagnosis more positive and less ridden with side effects and poor functioning. An early intervention from the rehabilitation team can make all the difference.

REFERENCES

American Cancer Society. (2008). *Cancer Facts and Figures 2008.* Atlanta: American Cancer Society. Retrieved from http://www.cancer.org

Arcangeli, G., Giovinazzo, G., Saracino, B., D'Angelo, L., Giannarelli, D., & Micheli, A. (1998). Radiation therapy in the management of symptomatic bone metastases: The effect of total dose and histology on pain relief and response duration. *International Journal of Radiation Oncology Biology Physics, 42,* 1119–1126.

Braddom, R. L. (2006). *Physical medicine and rehabilitation.* St. Louis, MO: Elsevier Health Sciences.

Browman, G. P., Wong, G., Hodson, I., Sathya, J., Russell, R., McAlpine, L., et al. (1993). Influence of cigarette smoking on the efficacy of radiation therapy in head and neck cancer. *New England Journal of Medicine, 328,* 159–163.

Burton, A. W., Fanciullo, G. J., Beasley, R. D., & Fisch, M. J. (2007). Chronic pain in the cancer survivor: A new frontier. *Pain Medicine, 8,* 189–198.

Casley-Smith, J. R., Morgan, R. G., Piller, N. B. (1993). Treatment of lymphedema of the arms and legs with 5,6-benzo-[alpha]-pyrone. *New England Journal of Medicine, 329,* 1158–1163.

Central Brain Tumor Registry of the United States. (2004). *CBTRUS Statistical Report.* Hinsdale, IL.

Coleman, R. E., & Rubens, R. D. (1987). The clinical course of bone metastases from breast cancer. *British Journal of Cancer, 55,* 61–66.

Dalmau, J., Gultekin, H. S., & Posner, J. B. (1999). Paraneoplastic neurologic syndromes: Pathogenesis and pathophysiology. *Brain Pathology, 9,* 275–284.

Delattre, J. Y., Krol, G., Thaler, H. T., & Posner, J. B. (1988). Distribution of brain metastases. *Archives of Neurology, 45,* 741–744.

Delisa, J. A., Gans, B. M., & Bockenek, W. L. (1998). *Rehabilitation medicine: Principles and practice.* Philadelphia, PA: Lippincott Williams & Wilkins.

Dietz, J. H. (1981). *Rehabilitation oncology.* Somerset, NJ: John Wiley & Sons.

Dudas, S., & Carlson, C. E. (1988). Cancer rehabilitation. *Oncology Nursing Forum, 15,* 183–188.

Dy, S. M., Lorenz, K. A., Naeim, A., Sanati, H., Walling, A., & Asch, S. M. (2008). Evidence-based recommendations for cancer fatigue, anorexia, depression, and dyspnea. *Journal of Clinical Oncology, 26,* 3886–3895.

Fisher, B., Anderson, S., Bryant, J., Margolese, R. G., Deutsch M., Fisher, E. R., et al. (2002). Twenty-year follow-up of a randomized trial comparing total mastectomy, lumpectomy, and lumpectomy plus irradiation for the treatment of breast cancer. *New England Journal of Medicine, 347,* 1233–1241.

Glantz, M. J., Cole, B. F., Friedberg, M. H., Lathi, E., Choy, H., Furie, K., et al. (1996). A randomized, blinded, placebo-controlled trial of divalproex sodium prophylaxis in adults with newly diagnosed brain tumors. *Neurology, 46,* 985–991.

Goreczny, A. J. (1995). *Handbook of health and rehabilitation psychology.* New York: Springer.

Guise, T. A., Yin, J. J., Taylor, S. D., Kumagai, Y., Dallas, M., & Boyce, B. F., et al. (1996). Evidence for a causal role of parathyroid hormone-related protein in the pathogenesis of human breast cancer-mediated osteolysis. *The Journal of Clinical Investigation, 98,* 1544–1549.

Hoskin, P. J., Yarnold, J. R., Roos, D. R., & Bentzen, S. (2001). Radiotherapy for bone metastases. *Clinical Oncology (R Coll Radiol), 13,* 88–90.

Jemal, A., Siegel, R., Ward, E., Hao, Y., Xu, J., Murray, T., et al. (2008). Cancer Statistics, 2008. *CA: A Cancer Journal for Clinicians, 58,* 71–96.

Johnson, J. D., & Young, B. (1996). Demographics of brain metastasis. *Neurosurgery Clinics of North America, 7,* 337–344.

Lawrence, W. Jr., Donegan, W. L., Natarajan, N., Mettlin, C., Beart, R., & Winchester, D. (1987). Adult soft tissue sarcomas. A pattern of care survey of the American College of Surgeons. *Annals of Surgery, 205,* 349–359.

Lehmann, J. F., DeLisa, J. A., Warren, C. G., deLateur, B. J., Bryant P. L., & Nicholson C. G. (1978). Cancer rehabilitation: Assessment of need, development, and evaluation of a model of care. *Archives of Physical Medicine and Rehabilitation, 59,* 410–419.

Mayer, D., & O'Connor L. (1989). Rehabilitation of persons with cancer: An ONS position statement. *Oncology Nursing Forum, 16,* 433.

Mundy, G. R. (2002). Metastasis to bone: Causes, consequences, and therapeutic opportunities. *Nature Reviews Cancer, 2,* 584–593.

National Comprehensive Cancer Network. (2004). *Practice guidelines in oncology: Cancer pain.* Retrieved June 2009 from www.nccn.org

O'Sullivan, S. B., & Schmitz, T. J. (2006). *Physical Rehabilitation.* Philadelphia, PA: F.A. Davis.

Patchell, R. (1997). Brain metastases. *Handbook of Neurology, 25,* 135–149.

Posner, J. B. (1995). *Neurologic complications of cancer.* Philadelphia, PA: F.A. Davis.

Robb, K. A., Williams, J. E., Duvivier, V., & Newham, D. J. (2006). A pain management program for chronic cancer-treatment-related pain. *Journal of Pain, 7,* 82–90.

Rudnicki, S. A., & Dalmau, J. (2000). Paraneoplastic syndromes of the spinal cord, nerve, and muscle. *Muscle Nerve, 23,* 1800–1818.

Sikora, A. G., Toniolo, P., & DeLacure, M. D. (2004). The changing demographics of head and neck squamous cell carcinoma in the United States. *Laryngoscope, 114,* 1915–1923.

Spitz, M. R. (1994). Epidemiology and risk factors for head and neck cancer. *Seminars in Oncology 1994, 21,* 281–288.

Surveillance, Epidemiology and End Results Program. (1975–2001). National Cancer Institute. Retrieved June 2009 from http://seer.cancer.gov/csr/1975–2001

Theriault, R. L., Lipton, A., Hortobagyi, G. N., Leff, R., Glück, S., Stewart, J. F., et al. (1999). Pamidronate reduces skeletal morbidity in women with advanced breast cancer and lytic bone lesions: A randomized, placebo-controlled trial. Protocol 18 Aredia Breast Cancer Study Group. *Journal of Clinical Oncology, 17,* 846–854.

Wen, P. Y., & Loeffler, J. S. (1999). Management of brain metastases. *Oncology (Huntingt), 13,* 941–954, 957–961, discussion 961–962, 9.

World Health Organization (1990). *Cancer Pain Relief and Palliative Care.* Geneva, Switzerland.

7

Cardiovascular Disorders

Ana Mola, MA, RN, ANP-BC, Jonathan H. Whiteson, MD,
and Mariano J. Rey, MD, FACC

Cardiovascular disorders constituted the major health epidemic of the 20th century and it will continue to be so in the 21st century also unless effective measures are taken to control or eliminate this epidemic. In the United States and in most other industrialized countries, nearly two thirds of all deaths are now caused by cardiovascular diseases (CVDs)—killing one person every minute. In countries of the developing world, CVDs presently account for a quarter of all deaths, and this fraction will increase with increasing economic development and urbanization. It is estimated that CVD will be the major killer in the world by the year 2025. As the deaths from infectious diseases decrease, the unhealthy lifestyles of Western society will spread across the globe and will result in a greater relative mortality from cardiovascular disorders. Moreover, by the year 2050, about 70% of the world's population will be urbanized and the prevalence of these disorders will increase not only in relative but also in absolute terms.

CVDs also represent the most common cause of disability in the United States. The American Heart Association (AHA), in 2006, estimated that there were 80 million people in the United States who had one or more forms of CVD. In the same year, there were an additionally estimated 73 million Americans afflicted with at least one cardiovascular risk factor for CVD. Both the presence of the diseases and its determinant factors often result in physical impairments and limitations of activities of daily life. Also, every year in the United States, about 1 million Americans survive an acute major cardiac event or undergo a cardiac intervention. About 500,000 Americans suffer heart attacks, another 250,000 have coronary artery bypass graft (CABG) surgery, and 250,000 more undergo coronary artery angioplasty (percutaneous transluminal coronary angioplasty [PTCA]) nowadays, with the vast majority of individuals also having an intracoronary stent placement. Every year, a significant percentage of this million having either a cardiac event or a cardiac procedure will develop either physical or psychological disabilities or both.

In the United States, at present, there are about 6 million Americans who have symptoms of CVD—which can be major causes of disability by themselves. In the last decade, congestive heart failure (CHF), a condition with many symptoms, shortness of breath being the most common, became the most common diagnosis upon discharge from U.S. hospitals. The ever-growing prevalence of chronic atrial fibrillation, and its main symptom of palpitations, is on the rise as the average age of the American population increases and a greater number of individuals live beyond the age of 80 years. Such is the magnitude of the continuing cardiac disease epidemic that it is rare to find an American family that is not affected by its mortality and morbidity. Cardiovascular disorders still constitute the major health challenge to all providers of rehabilitative, physical, psychological, and vocational services. Therefore, it is imperative for all health care professionals to acquire a comprehensive understanding of the cardiovascular system and its diseases.

It is imperative that the health care professionals who work with patients with CVDs and disabilities should become aware of the general definitions used in rehabilitative medicine. In 1980, the World Health Organization (WHO) developed a general definition of disability: the International Classification of Impairments, Disabilities and Handicaps (ICIDH), which has become the leading classification system for defining and understanding the term "disability." The ICIDH was formally reassessed in the late 1990s, and the review process eventually led in 2002 to the establishment of the International Classification of Functioning, Disability and Health (ICF). According to the ICIDH, "impairment" refers to the physical status of a person; disability means the restriction of activities because of the impairment; and "handicap" expresses the limitation in terms of the fulfillment of a social role. In other words, impairment refers to a body organ or part having a functional or structural abnormality; "disability" means the effect of the impairment on the performance of the individual; and a handicap is the overall consequence of the impairment or of the disability on the whole person as a member of a society. This classification places less emphasis on the individual deficiencies of a person. Thus, a "continuum of health status" is recognized that stresses the environmental factors (including the physical, social, and political environments) that may facilitate or restrict a person's potential to participate in daily life. The ICF never accepts either a medical model or a social model alone as being valid as a definition of "disability"—which is always best appreciated as a complex system that evaluates the individual within the structure of society in a "biopsychosocial model." CVDs and their resulting disabilities are best understood and addressed by this biopsychosocial model and it is the interactive dysfunction of its dynamic components that results in the development of the diseases and the initial failure of their prevention (World Health Organization, 2002).

CARDIOVASCULAR DISORDERS

Cardiovascular disorders are those that affect the heart and the vascular system. By structural and functional criteria (or by anatomy and physiology), the heart has five components: the coronary arteries, the pericardium, the myocardium, the endocardium, and the electrical conduction system.

The Coronary Arteries

The coronary arteries are deemed to be the most important blood vessels in the body because they supply blood to the heart itself. Without normal coronary blood flow, the heart cannot carry out its function of supplying blood to the rest of the body. There are two coronary arteries: the left coronary artery and the right coronary artery. The left coronary vessel, after a short main segment, bifurcates. One of the branches is the left anterior descending coronary artery, which brings blood to the septum (the muscle between the two ventricles) and to the anterior wall of the left ventricle; the other branch is the circumflex coronary artery and is the vessel that supplies blood to the right ventricle and to the inferior wall of the left ventricle. The right coronary artery does not bifurcate and supplies blood mainly to the right ventricle. Although there are minor variations in the coronary artery network, the blood supply system is fairly similar in humans. The main variation is that in any one individual, the blood supply to the posterior wall of the left ventricle can originate from either the left circumflex artery or the right coronary artery, or from both (Figure 7.1).

Cardiovascular disorders resulting from primary disease of the coronary arteries is the single leading cause of death in the United States today. The cause of this coronary heart

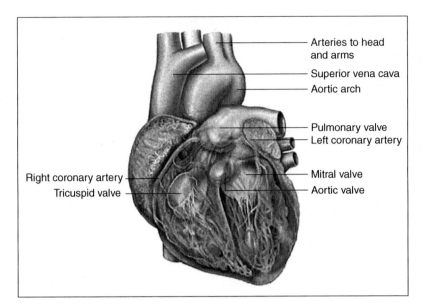

Arteries to head and arms
Superior vena cava
Aortic arch
Pulmonary valve
Left coronary artery
Mitral valve
Aortic valve
Right coronary artery
Tricuspid valve

FIGURE 7.1 Interior structures of the heart. Image located at www.ynhh.org/cardiac2/heart/

disease (CHD) can be best described as a "biopsychosocial failure"—as has already been mentioned. It is this complex constellation of biological, psychological, and social factors that has resulted in the epidemic of CHD. The risk factors for coronary atherosclerosis are elevated blood cholesterol, high blood pressure, cigarette smoking, diabetes, obesity, and a sedentary but stressful life style. Recently, depression has been determined to be a separate and independent risk factor. These risk factors, alone or in multiple combinations, create the initial lesion of CHD, the atherosclerotic plaque, or atheroma. Researchers have learned that the progression of atherosclerosis is a lifelong process, beginning early in life as a fatty streak in the coronary arteries and progressing to an occlusive fibrous atherosclerotic plaque. The inflammatory pathological process is one in which the endothelium, the single-cell lining of the inner surface of the coronary arteries, becomes structurally or functionally damaged. The risk factors directly or indirectly release inflammatory cytokines and other toxic enzymes that result in endothelial dysfunction. Once this endothelial barrier is altered, there is deposition of fats, calcium, and amorphous debris inside the arterial wall, which results in the development of plaques.

Eventually, the atherosclerotic plaques create rigid arterial walls and lead to progressive narrowing of the arteries, which is termed as "coronary stenosis." Once the coronary vessel has a 70% stenosis of the coronary artery lumen, there is reduced blood flow that may still meet the metabolic needs of the heart while that individual is in a state of rest. However, during exercise, such a narrowing can no longer allow an increase in blood flow to meet the heart tissue's increased metabolic and oxygen needs that occur with activity. Such an imbalance between oxygen demand and supply, which results in the metabolic derangement of heart cells, is called myocardial ischemia. Therefore, this type of coronary artery disease (CAD) is also known as ischemic heart disease.

Moreover, the atherosclerotic plaque is an unstable structure that can easily become damaged. At the site of an ulcerated or fissured plaque, there is a tendency to form a clot, or thrombus, and to have arterial spasm. Alone or in combination, thrombus and spasm lead to more severe stenosis and at times to, a total or, 100% occlusion of the artery. This complete cessation of all blood flow to the segment of heart muscle supplied by that artery results in the death of that muscle segment or to a heart attack or myocardial infarction (MI). An understanding of the clinical presentations of CHD must be based on this understanding of atheroma pathophysiology.

Factors that help establish the risk of this inflammatory atherosclerotic process are circulating inflammatory biomarkers that have been identified in the blood of patients with ischemic heart disease. One of the most studied inflammatory biomarkers is the high-sensitivity C-reactive protein (hs-CRP). Numerous clinical studies have shown that measuring systemic CRP levels with a highly sensitive assay provides a significant clinical prognostic value across clinical evaluations ranging from risk screening in apparently healthy people to stable and unstable angina. Studies have demonstrated that people with higher hs-CRP levels are on average at a higher risk of adverse cardiovascular events. Supportive of this concept have been recent publications, which demonstrate that apparently healthy people who have low levels (<130 mg/dl) of low-density lipoprotein (LDL) cholesterol but had elevated levels (>2 mg/L) of hs-CRP levels—who were treated with statin, a cholesterol-lowering agent—had a significant relative risk reduction (as high as 44% in one study) in the composite end points of the following: unstable angina, need of coronary revascularization, and a confirmed death from cardiovascular causes. However, controversy remains as to whether hs-CRP plays a causative role in plaque formation and growth and in acute coronary artery atherosclerosis syndromes or whether it is a mere predictive biomarker of the presence of CAD and its clinical complications.

Ischemic chest pain, or angina pectoris, is the only cardiac symptom in the relatively fortunate group of cardiac patients who have stable atheromas that result in coronary narrowing more than 70% but in less than a total occlusion. Angina pectoris is described as a visceral pain because it is usually felt deeply, rather than superficially, in the chest. The angina sufferer describes the discomfort as squeezing, pressing, or crushing or as heaviness or a dull ache. Angina is usually felt in the mid-chest or the sternal area. It often radiates to the left arm or the jaw. It is brought on by physical exertion or by mental stress. It is relieved by the cessation of the activity that caused it. Angina usually lasts less than 5 minutes. Patients with this typical pattern are said to have the clinical syndrome of stable angina. It is estimated that at any given time there are about 5 million Americans with stable angina pectoris. Angina that occurs at rest, without obvious provocation, or with less effort than usual, is unstable angina. This syndrome is usually a manifestation of an unstable atheroma, which has a superimposed thrombus and spasm that has caused further acute stenosis of the coronary artery. When such unstable angina is severe in intensity or sustained in duration, it is termed preinfarction angina. It may be an indication that a 100% coronary artery occlusion is taking place. If there is total blood flow cessation for 30 minutes or more, the usual consequence is death to the segment of heart muscle supplied by the occluded artery. This muscle death is an MI, popularly known as a heart attack. The main presenting symptom of an acute MI is angina that is much more severe in intensity and that lasts for a much longer time than the typical episode of stable angina syndrome. The pain often occurs in the context of generalized symptoms such as weakness, sweating, and anxiety.

Women may be more likely to present with atypical or subtler symptoms during an acute coronary event. Although women probably experience chest pain as an acute coronary symptom as often as men, they may complain less of chest pain and be more likely than men to report neck, jaw, or back pain alone. Therefore, it can be more difficult to diagnose an MI in women than in men. Women's symptoms are not as predictable as those of men and they may appear approximately a month before the acute event occurs. In about two thirds of the cases, the initial presentation of ischemic heart disease in women may be an acute MI or a sudden cardiac death. A National Institutes of Health-sponsored research study of 515 women diagnosed with acute MI on hospitalization at five different medical centers revealed that prodromal symptoms had occurred frequently 4–6 months before the event. Ninety-five percent of the women reported experiencing various warning signals approximately a month before the acute event. In some of the cases, the women reported ignoring their own symptoms; in others, they sought medical assistance only to have their symptoms minimized, misdiagnosed, or ignored. The most common acute symptoms were as follows: shortness of breath, weakness, and fatigue. Notably, less than one-third reported having chest pain or discomfort immediately prior to their heart attack and nearly one-half reported no chest pain during any phase of the event.

During an evolving MI, many persons have a sense of impending doom and they feel they are going to die. Contrary to popular misinformation, MIs are seldom a result of physical activity. They nearly always strike at rest and often during the early morning hours, shortly after awakening. The timing of the event reflects its pathophysiology. MIs are not a consequence of myocardial demand of exercise outstripping a compromised blood supply but are caused by the sudden thrombus formation on an unstable atheroma, which then totally occludes the atherosclerotic coronary artery. In 2004, the National Center for Health Statistics reported 1,565,000 hospitalizations for primary or secondary diagnosis of an acute coronary syndrome (ACS), 669,000 for unstable angina, and 896,000 for MIs. The American College of Cardiology (ACC) and the AHA have national guidelines for the clinical care of various cardiac diagnoses and the most recent guidelines have been updated in 2007 to incorporate results from major clinical trails in the past 5–10 years. A greater emphasis has been placed on the earlier access to medical evaluation of ACSs that include unstable angina, non-ST elevation myocardial infarction (NSTEMI), and ST elevation myocardial infarction (STEMI).

Faster community EMS response time and facilitated emergency department triage of ACS have occurred over the last two decades because of the more definite detection of sensitive cardiac biomarkers of necrosis such as troponins and of emerging cardiac imaging diagnostics such as cardiac magnetic resonance and coronary computed tomographic angiography. Clinical trials have further defined the best practices of initial medical or surgical interventions in patients presenting with ACS. The guidelines recommend that upon hospital discharge, patients who have been diagnosed with ACS should be prescribed the following medication regimen: aspirin (unless contraindicated), clopidogrel (PLAVIX), β-blockers, angiotensin-converting enzyme inhibitors (ACEI) or angiotensin-receptor blockers if intolerant of the ACEI, and statins. Over the last decade, aggressive treatment of hospitalized MI patients with acute thrombolytic (clot-dissolving) therapy and with β-receptor blockers has drastically reduced both the in-hospital death rate and the 1-year death rate to less than 10% for treated patients. Unfortunately, about 60% of all deaths from an acute infarction occur within 1 hour after the onset of symptoms—thus, one-half of all individuals die before they reach the hospital and before they can receive the benefits of these new therapies. Yearly, approximately 500,000 Americans have MIs, and in spite of all these recent advances, these acute MIs still account for 25% of all deaths in the United States every year.

Sudden cardiac death is best defined as an unexpected demise with a lack of warning symptoms or prodrome. About 80% of victims of sudden death have CHD. Sudden death is usually the result of a lethal ventricular rhythm disturbance that has its origin in the unstable electrical milieu of heart muscle cells that are affected by ischemia or that are adjacent to an area of scar caused by a prior MI. Some persons are fortunate to have the benefit of prompt cardiopulmonary resuscitation within a few minutes of being stricken. They are said to be sudden-death survivors. Their long-term prognosis is poor, with a chance of about 50% of a subsequent fatal event within a year or two. It is estimated that there are about 300,000 sudden cardiac deaths in the United States yearly. They account for about 50% of all the deaths from CVD. Two recent developments may help decrease the frequency of sudden electrical cardiac death. One is the creation of small defibrillators (about the size of the better known pacemakers) that can be permanently implanted within the chest wall of survivors of sudden death (or of those deemed susceptible to such a tragic event). These devices can deliver a resuscitative electric shock to the heart whenever a potentially lethal arrhythmia occurs. The other development is the more extensive availability of external defibrillators in public places such as airports and train and bus stations, so that victims of severe arrhythmias can be quickly brought back to stable rhythms and to life itself.

The concept of silent myocardial ischemia, although no longer relatively new, is still not shared by the general population and by many health care workers. It is based on the observation that the cardiac muscle can be ischemic (or even infarcted) without any symptoms. Such silent ischemia has been detected by electrocardiogram changes in 24-hour ambulatory recordings by Holter monitors and described in the findings of the Framingham study and other investigations that show that as many as 25% of all MIs can be silent. Such individuals with silent ischemia and infarction can have as their first presentation a sudden cardiac death. They can also present with an ischemic cardiomyopathy, a heart that has suffered small multiple silent infarctions and has become boggy and dilated. Their symptoms will be those of CHF. Silent myocardial ischemia is a major component of the total ischemic burden for patients with CAD. It is estimated that approximately 2–3 million persons with stable CAD have evidence of silent ischemia. Approximately 40% of patients with ischemic heart disease have acute episodes of myocardial ischemia during their lifetime and 75% of these episodes cause no symptoms and are considered "silent." The management of silent ischemia should be directed to reduce or eliminate myocardial ischemia by risk factor modification, aggressive medical therapy and, if deemed needed, myocardial revascularization.

Every year in the United States, approximately 1 million men in the total male population older than 30 years manifest symptomatic CHD for the first time. About 40% present with angina pectoris, another 40% with an acute MI, and another 10% have sudden death as their first, last, and the only symptom. In the remaining 10%, the first symptoms are those of heart failure, palpitations, or syncope, the sudden loss of consciousness. One should not adopt the common misconception that CHD afflicts only men. Coronary atherosclerosis and its clinical syndromes affect just as many women as men. Although the prevalence of CVD is not higher among women (33.9%) when compared with the total population (34.2%), more women than men die of CVD (53.2% of CVD deaths). The percentage of deaths caused by CVD was highest for White (39.8%) and African American (39.6%) women followed by Asian (35.8%), Hispanic or Latino (32%), and Native American (24.5%) women. CAD was the cause of half of all CVD deaths among women, and stroke was responsible for 20%. One in four women have some form of CVD and almost 6 million have a history of MI, angina pectoris, or both. Out of these, approximately 3 million have a history of MI and these women are at higher risk than men for CHF. In 2001, 33,023 women died of CHF (62.5% of deaths from CHF). On average, however, women experience their clinical CHD 10 years later than men do. For example, women in their 60s have an incidence of coronary syndromes similar to that of men in their 50s. This is because of the loss of the protective effect of the female hormones, mainly estrogens, whose production is greatly decreased at the onset of menopause.

Oral postmenopausal hormone therapy appears to a have positive effect on lipid panels (with the exception of triglycerides), but its effect on inflammatory markers shows considerable variability from study to study. Oral postmenopausal hormone therapy lowers LDL cholesterol levels, increases high-density lipoprotein (HDL) cholesterol, and lowers lipoprotein (a) levels—all changes shown to reduce CHD risks. Triglyceride levels increase (more so with unopposed estrogen therapy compared with estrogen/progestin combination therapy) and is associated with greater LDL particle numbers and smaller particles that are atherogenic. Lipid and lipoprotein changes are less pronounced with transdermal preparations. CRP tends to increase with oral hormone therapy, whereas transdermal preparations seem to have no effect. Tumor necrosis factor-α levels, cell adhesion molecules, and monocyte chemoattractant protein 1, which all implicated in the progression of CHD, tend to decrease with hormone therapy. However, hormone therapy also has both potentially procoagulant and fibrinolytic effects that tend to mitigate endothelium dysfunction. Hormone-induced changes seem to vary based on age and clinical characteristics of the women receiving therapy as well on the dose and route of administration (Rossouw et al., 2008)

Current guidelines from the AHA for the prevention of CVD in women have classified postmenopausal hormone therapy as a Class III intervention—a form of therapy that should not be used for the purpose of primary or secondary prevention of CVD (Mosca et al., 2007).

These guidelines are based on the revolutionary study of the Women's Health Initiative (WHI) in 2002 when results demonstrated that combined estrogen and progestin therapy increased the risk of CHD, stroke, pulmonary embolism, and breast cancer. This study of 16,608 women with a mean age of 63 years was terminated 3.3 years early because the risks were deemed to outweigh any potential benefits. The European Society of Cardiology, the American College of Obstetrics and Gynecology (ACOG), and the North American Menopause Society (NAMS) similarly concluded that hormone therapy cannot be recommended for the purpose of CVD preventions (ACOG Committee on Gynecologic Practice, 2008; Stramba-Badiale et al., 2006; Utian et al., 2008). The current iterations of recommendations make a clear distinction between hormone prescribing for younger compared with older women. NAMS suggests that hormone therapy for symptom control does not seem to increase the risk of CHD among younger women (aged 50–59 years) and highlights to emerging evidence that initiation of hormone therapy in early post-menopause may reduce the risk of CHD (Rossouw et al., 2007). A more recent reanalysis of the WHI explored whether the timing of the start of hormone therapy might influence its effect on CVD in 24,317 women aged 50–79 years. The researchers found an increased risk for stroke in all women, regardless of age. However, hormone therapy may be safe, or even beneficial, in terms of reduced CHD risk if taken in the early postmenopausal years. A summary of WHI with estrogen-only results demonstrated that estrogen therapy alone is neutral for heart disease. The effect of hormone replacement therapy may depend on the age and the stage of atherosclerosis in the vessel. As an example, in younger women with a healthy vessel, estrogen may be beneficial but not in older women with an abnormal vessel (Grodstein, Clarkson, & Manson, 2003).

Function and Disability

The major determinant of impaired function and disability in CHD is angina. Coronary artery atherosclerosis is not a stable condition. For a myriad of reasons, the tonicity of the muscles in the vessel wall varies during any given time interval and so does the severity of coronary artery stenosis. Thus, an individual patient's angina pattern may have minor weekly, and even daily, variations in severity, frequency, and the level of exertion needed to provoke it. Nonetheless, the typical patient with a typical stable angina syndrome usually has a predictable functional impairment. That is, a similar number of blocks walked on a level surface or on an incline, a similar number of flights of stairs climbed, and a similar weight that he lifted or carried will reproducibly, time after time, result in the same intensity and duration of angina pectoris. The functional impairment and disability can be best determined based on a careful history, which is unique for each individual. On the basis of this unique individual history, medical therapy can be instituted, referral to surgical intervention can be made, and rehabilitation protocols can be carried out. The estimated functional capacity and subsequent disability of an individual with angina can be confirmed by exercise stress testing. Exercise tests, whether performed on a treadmill or on a bicycle, approximate the exertion of normal activities of daily living. The goal of all stress testing is to increase the work of the heart and its muscle oxygen demand by increasing the exerciser's heart rate and systolic blood pressure. The age-adjusted target heart rate is roughly the number 220 minus the patient's age. For example, the exercise target heart rate of a 40-year-old is 180 beats per minute and that of a 60-year-old is 160 beats per minute. The systolic blood pressure should rise about 60 mm from the rest level to the peak exercise level, and the diastolic blood pressure should drop slightly or remain unchanged. The increasing heart rates and blood pressures are achieved by increasing the workload. On a treadmill, workload is increased by a progressively faster speed and higher incline, and on a bicycle, by gradual greater pedal resistance.

The most widely used treadmill protocol for establishing functional capacity, as well as diagnosis and prognosis, is the Bruce protocol. For patients who are undergoing evaluation before or after a program of cardiac rehabilitation and for individuals in whom gas-exchange metabolic evaluation is also being performed, at the New York University Medical Langone Medical Center Joan and Joel Smilow Cardiopulmonary Rehabilitation and Prevention

Center, the Bensen protocol is used to evaluate the rehabilitation status of the patients. This is a gentler protocol of 2-minute stages in which energy expenditure increases in each stage by only 25% over the prior stage. By comparison, the Bruce protocol elicits more demanding increases of 50% in work with each successive stage. Heart-imaging techniques with exercise, such as with thallium or the newer technetium myocardial perfusion agents, nuclear ventriculograms, and echocardiography, have independent values in establishing diagnosis and prognosis and give insightful understanding of the anatomical and physiological basis for an individual's exercise tolerance and functional capacity. Whenever possible, as determined by the information gained by a medical history, a physical exam, and an exercise stress test, the functional capacity of the individual with heart disease should be described according to the classification system of the New York Heart Association (NYHA). This system establishes four functional classes, which are as follows: Class IV, symptomatic at rest (no effort); Class III, symptomatic with minimal effort; Class II, symptomatic with moderate effort; and Class I, asymptomatic at any effort level. This traditional functional classification is useful because it provides a common language and point of reference for all health care professionals.

Treatment and Prognosis

The definite and ultimate treatment of CAD is the radical correction of the biopsychosocial failure that is at its root. Primary prevention (i.e., before any clinical event has taken place) of CHD should be the main mission of all health care professionals and can be accomplished by the reduction or elimination of all of the risk factors for atherosclerosis. An elevated serum cholesterol level is considered by some investigators to be the primary culprit in atherosclerosis. Some families have an autosomal dominant genetic condition called familial hypercholesterolemia. Patients who are homozygous for the gene have serum cholesterol levels as high as 1,000 mg/dl and have severe coronary and peripheral atherosclerosis during childhood and adolescence. Heterozygous individuals have a serum cholesterol level that ranges from 300 to 500 mg/dl. They also have premature and severe atherosclerosis. Homozygous individuals are only about one in a million and heterozygous only about 2 in a million of the U.S. population, however. Thus, the atherosclerosis epidemic is not the result of an unalterable genetic disorder but is the consequence of an atherogenic lifestyle that can be altered. It has been recently shown that chronic mental and emotional stress can elevate cholesterol. Numerous epidemiological and population studies, human trials of dietary intervention, and experimental animal investigations have shown the high causative correlation between an elevated serum cholesterol and atherosclerosis.

Cholesterol can be lowered below the recommended 200 mg/dl by weight loss and by reducing the consumption of animal fats that contain cholesterol and of saturated fats in general. It is now well documented that one of the lipoproteins that carries cholesterol in the blood, high-density lipoprotein (HDL), has an opposite and protective effect by scooping up circulating cholesterol and bringing it to the liver for degradation. HDL cholesterol can be raised by frequent exercise and by the judicious moderate daily drinking of alcoholic beverages. Hypertension can be lowered by weight loss, exercise, and a diet low in salt. When these natural measures are not successful, or while they are being undertaken, aggressive control of the elevated blood pressure with medication is indicated. Few are the individuals who cannot attain blood pressure control by a combination of interventions.

Most adult-onset diabetic patients have their metabolic disease because of obesity. Weight reduction significantly lowers serum glucose levels in these patients even to normal levels. It is still controversial whether obesity by itself is an independent risk factor. There can be no argument, however, that obesity has a causative relation with all of the atherosclerotic risk factors except for smoking. The smoking of cigarettes doubles the risk of CHD. Beyond being a causative factor for atherosclerosis, it may constitute an additional separate risk for MI. The reduction of risk for infarction may be an astounding 50% within only 1 year after complete smoking cessation. Multiple studies have shown that exercise, through many mechanisms, results in reduced atherosclerosis and in a lower risk of clinical events if atherosclerosis is already present. CHD, however, is usually first treated with medications. The medical therapy of stable angina pectoris is based on an understanding of its pathophysiological basis: ischemia from an increased metabolic demand that cannot be met by a fixed supply.

Pharmaceutical intervention has as its goal the reduction or prevention of that ischemia through two main pharmacological means: an increased supply of blood to the heart muscle and a decreased demand of the heart muscle for that blood. These desired effects are accomplished by the three principal classes of cardiac pharmaceutical agents: nitrates, β-receptor blockers, and calcium channel blockers. Nitrates are vasodilators. They exert their beneficial effects by dilating coronary arteries directly, thus increasing blood flow to the heart muscle. They also dilate peripheral veins, resulting in the peripheral pooling of blood, with a subsequent reduction in blood return to the heart, less stress on the heart wall, and finally a decreased need for oxygen. β-Receptor blockers reduce oxygen demand by lowering the heart rate (or chronotropy) and are termed negative chronotropic agents. Calcium channel blockers combine the effects of nitrates and β-blockers. Most of the available calcium channel blocker agents have both vasodilatory and chronotropic effects. Most patients with a stable angina pectoris syndrome can have their angina controlled and their functional impairment and disability eradicated with the use of one of these agents alone or with some combination or all three. Unless a contraindication exists, patients with CHD and also perhaps asymptomatic individuals with atherosclerosis risk factors should take low-dose prophylactic daily aspirin.

Patients with unstable angina pectoris require immediate hospitalization as they are at risk for an acute infarction. The treatment is based on its pathophysiology basis: an unstable atherosclerotic plaque that creates a substrate for new thrombus and artery spasm, which in turn may result in total vessel occlusion and heart muscle death. Treatment with intravenous heparin is directed at the inhibition of further thrombus formation. The treatment with intravenous nitrates aims to reduce and prevent arterial spasm. Patients with an acute MI should receive immediate intravenous thrombolytic therapy with either streptokinase or tissue plasminogen activator. The prompt breaking up of the occluding thrombus results in a restoration of blood flow. If this is done within the first hour or two after the onset of symptoms, there is considerable myocardial salvage. The earlier these agents are administered, the greater is the rescue of heart muscle and the patient's chance of survival. The nonmedical therapy of CHD is PTCA and CABG. About an equal number of these procedures are now performed in the United States yearly. Several randomized studies comparing the efficacy of each treatment are currently under way and preliminary reports indicate no clear superiority of one treatment modality over the other. In PTCA, a balloon-tipped catheter is introduced through a peripheral artery and then manipulated around the aortic arch and inserted into the coronary artery that has the occluding atheroma. The balloon inflation causes an increase of the overall vessel diameter and increased blood flow by the process of atheroma fracture and compression and by stretching of the vessel wall. The initial success rate is now more than 90%, but restenosis occurs at a rate of about 25% within 1 year of the procedure. The recent development of stents, cylindrical rigid metal devices that are placed within a coronary artery at the site of an angioplasty, has decreased the frequency of post-PTCA restenosis.

Percutaneous coronary artery intervention (PCI) developed about 30 years ago, improves the quality of life by relieving angina in patients with stable CAD and can be life saving in patients with extensive ischemia and ACSs. The safety of the PCI procedures has been enhanced significantly by the use of adjunctive pharmacotherapy, most importantly antithrombotic and antiplatelet agents (Brar & Stone, 2009). PCI is best used in patients to relieve angina symptoms, to reduce medication requirements in patients with stable ischemic syndromes, and to prevent MI in patients with ACSs: unstable angina, NSTEMI, and STEMI. A recent meta-analysis of 17 randomized trials (Schomig et al., 2008), including the Clinical Outcomes Utilizing Revascularization and Aggressive Drug Evaluation (COURAGE) trial, with a total of 7,513 patients with stable angina treated with PCI or medical therapy demonstrated that a 20% reduction in the odds ratio (OR) of all cause of death with PCI compared with medical treatment alone. In the nuclear substudy of COURAGE, 314 patients underwent myocardial perfusion scanning before and after PCI. The PCI group had a greater reduction in ischemia when compared with the medical therapy alone (33–19%). Overall, in the COURAGE trial, the aggregate data suggest that among the patients with small areas of ischemia and mild symptoms, intensive medical therapy is a viable first option, with PCI reserved for those in whom medical therapy alone is inadequate or in whom symptoms progress. In the COURAGE trial, many quality of life measures were superior in the PCI group for 3 years with the greatest benefits noted in patients with the most severe symptoms at baseline. In patients with moderate to severe ischemia or significant symptoms, an initial PCI strategy likely will lead more rapidly to an improved symptomatic state, reduce medication requirement and rehospitalization, improve quality of life, and possibly increase event-free survival (Brar & Stone, 2009).

PCI of more complex disease has become a more standard practice and has resulted in recent declines in the rates of surgical revascularization. Several recent randomized trials have defined the role of PCI in the management of complex CAD. For example, the SYNTAX trial compared PCI using a drug-eluting stent (DES) with CABG among patients with triple-vessel disease or unprotected left main artery disease. Patients were randomly assigned to PCI or CABG and at 12 months there were no significant differences in the rates of death or MI between the two groups. However, the incidence of stroke was significantly higher in the CABG arm whereas the repeat revascularization need was greater in the PCI arm. Moreover, in patients with unprotected left main artery disease, events were similar in the CABG and PCI groups (Serruys et al., 2009). Results similar to the SYNTAX trial were reported from the CARDIA trial in which 510 patients with diabetes mellitus and multivessel disease were randomly assigned to DES, bare metal stents (BMS), or CABG. The composite rate of death, MI, or stroke at 1 year did not significantly differ between the groups, although there were more revascularization events and fewer strokes with PCI. The results of the SYNTAX and CARDIA trials suggest that patients with complex CAD can undergo PCI without an increase in the rates of death or MI. DESs have continued to evolve since the late 1990s. Pooled analyses have noted a small incremental risk in late stent thrombosis with DES compared with BMS, although the rates of death or MI are comparable with the two types of stents. The marked reduction in restenosis with DES likely offsets the excess risk of late stent thrombosis by decreasing the need for revascularization, including CABG and reducing the occurrence of ACSs after restenosis (Mauri et al., 2007). Another novel stent under investigation is the bioabsorbable stent that fully degrades in approximately 3–4 years. These stents may have theoretical advantages over traditional stents in that they may permit the vessel to normally remodel, minimize the frequency of late stent thrombosis, allow the vessel to respond normally to endothelial factors, and permit noninvasive stent assessments such as with multi-detector CT scanning (Brar & Stone, 2009).

In CABG, saphenous veins from the legs (or an internal mammary artery from inside the chest wall) are used as conduits to restore blood flow by bypassing the site of the atherosclerotic plaque. CABG is performed at present with an operative mortality approaching only 2%. More than 90% of operated patients achieve total or significant symptom relief. Progressive atherosclerotic occlusion of the vein grafts, through the same process that affected the native coronary arteries, is likely to occur within 10 years of surgery if the treated individuals do not change their lifestyles to reduce the risk factors for atherosclerosis. Both procedures are indicated in patients with stable angina pectoris who cannot obtain symptom relief with medical therapy. Emergency PTCA should also be performed when medical treatment alone does not appear to arrest ongoing cardiac muscle damage in unstable angina or in acute MI. Bypass surgery is indicated, regardless of symptoms, in patients who are found, by coronary angiography, to have a significant disease of the main left coronary artery segment or to have severe triple-vessel disease, especially if they have impaired left ventricular function. Several studies have shown improved survival with surgical (compared with medical) therapy in these patient subgroups with more extensive CHD. Newer alternative revascularization techniques include removal of the coronary atheroma by mechanical excision (coronary atherectomy) or by ablation using laser energy (laser angioplasty). Both procedures are considered experimental, but they hold great promise because both may supplant the major surgical procedure of CABG and solve the problem of restenosis in coronary angioplasty. Perhaps the most recent significant development in the management of CHD is the evidence that coronary atherosclerosis is reversible. It has now been convincingly shown by coronary angiography studies that coronary atherosclerosis can be reversed by lowering cholesterol with lipid-lowering agents or with changes in lifestyle.

The major determinants of prognosis in CHD are the extent and severity of the coronary atherosclerosis and of the ventricular dysfunction. CAD can be best diagnosed and evaluated by exercise stress tests and by cardiac catheterization with coronary angiography. Echocardiography and nuclear ventriculography can assess the ventricular function. The lower the left ventricular ejection fraction (the percentage of blood in the left ventricle ejected with each heart beat, normal being 50% or higher), the worse the prognosis. Even though the atherosclerotic epidemic still rages, there has been a significant decline in the age-adjusted mortality from all CVDs over the past 20 years. The death rate from MI alone declined by about 30% during the 1980s. This reduction in mortality is partly accounted for by the creation of hospital coronary care units, development of sophisticated diagnostic tools, and advances in medical and surgical therapies. Most of the reduction is the result of changes in lifestyle.

Psychological and Vocational Implications

There is an undisputed relationship between CHD and psychological disorders. Psychological disorders are definite contributors to atherosclerosis and the clinical syndromes of CAD. In turn, the diagnosis and treatment of CHD may create or worsen psychological disorders. The mechanisms whereby psychological disorders cause or accelerate coronary atherosclerosis have not been well defined. Psychosocial stresses result in increased sympathetic nervous system activity, however, with a greater release of circulating catecholamines (epinephrine and norepinephrine). These, in turn, lead to elevated heart rates, elevated systemic blood pressures, and elevated cholesterol levels, and also perhaps to enhanced platelet aggregation and thrombus formation. High catecholamine levels also lower the triggering threshold for ventricular arrhythmias. Recent primate experiments appear to indicate that atherosclerotic vessels may respond with vasoconstriction when the experimental subjects are exposed to several psychosocial stresses. Moreover, far too many individuals in our society respond to mental or emotional stress by resorting to the immediate oral gratification of smoking or overeating. Poor dietary habits, with the wrong quality and quantity of foods, lead indirectly through obesity—and directly through elevated cholesterol, sugar, and salt intake—to a worse atherosclerosis risk profile. More specifically, several studies have shown that emotional or mental stress precedes the clinical manifestations of CHD. There seems to be a positive correlation between an exacerbation of anxiety or depression just before the onset of the symptoms of stable and unstable angina, and prior to the occurrence of both fatal and nonfatal MI and sudden electrical death. Psychiatric patients with previously diagnosed depression have been shown to have a much greater mortality from CHD than the general population. Social isolation, both of individuals and of large populations, seems to result in higher rates of sudden death.

Depression is highly prevalent after acute cardiac events, with 20–45% of patients having significant depression after acute MI. Over a hundred studies have given evidence that depression has a prevalence from 25–35% in populations with CVD and is independently predictive of adverse outcomes among patients with existing cardiac disease. In addition, depression precedes CVD in multiple studies, including a first MI and cardiac death (Rumsfeld & Ho, 2005). It has been noted that CABG surgery patients may have substantial perioperative depression, and graded inverse relationship has been found between the severity of perioperative depressive symptoms and improvement in physical functional status one year after surgery. Depressive symptoms were a stronger predictor of the lack of functional improvement than were variables such as previous MI, diabetes, and ventricular ejection fraction. The relationship is more pronounced in women than in men. This finding may explain why women may derive less functional benefit from CABG surgery and suggests the importance of considering depression as an existing factor among women undergoing cardiac surgery (Mallik et al., 2005).

There are important gender differences between depression and the age of onset and symptom presentation of CVD (Eastwood & Doering, 2005). After a MI, younger women (60 years or younger) had a depression risk that was 3.1 times higher than that of men older than 60 years. When compared with men, CAD risk in women is more strongly increased by traditional factors (diabetes, hypertension, hypercholesterolemia, and obesity) as well as by socioeconomic and psychosocial factors. Current evidence suggest that depression causes a greater increase in CAD incidence in women, and that female CAD patients experience higher levels of depression than men (Moller-Leimkuhler, 2008). Depression rates double in the presence of diabetes and depressed diabetic women have a more rapid development of CAD than nondepressed diabetic women (Clouse et al., 2003). Patients who are depressed are significantly less likely to adhere to prescribed medications, follow lifestyle recommendations (exercise prescription and smoking cessation), and practice self-management (e.g., monitor weight and salt diet restriction in heart failure). Patients who are depressed may not adhere to a cardiac plan of the best practices of aspirin, β-blockers, statins, and ACEI. Hence, depression serves as a barrier to the delivery of optimal cardiac care. Further studies are needed to prove that treating depression can improve cardiovascular mortality and morbidity. Some patients treated with selective serotonin reuptake inhibitors (SSRIs) have had significantly lower overall and cardiovascular mortality. Observational data also suggest that SSRIs may be associated with a reduction in MI (Berkman et al., 2003).

Over the past 30 years perhaps the most studied relationship between the mind and the heart has been Type A behavior. Excessive drive, competitiveness, an exaggerated sense of time urgency, and free-floating hostility characterize this behavior. The earlier data seemed to support the thesis that such behavior was a significant independent risk factor for CHD. Then, over the past decade, several major studies found no correlation. One investigation even suggested that Type A behavior may confer a survival advantage by reducing the death rate in survivors of MI. Recently, a consensus seems to be developing that the subset of patients with Type A behavior who show cynical hostility and suppressed anger may be the only ones at risk for coronary disease. The conflicting findings may be a consequence of the differing methods (self-administered questionnaires, structure, interviews, videotaped observation of subjects) used in defining the behavior and evaluating the individuals who display it. The issue remains controversial.

CHD leads to psychological distress and the development of psychiatric symptoms. Denial, a useful defense mechanism in some circumstances, may be injurious when it leads to self-destructive behavior such as a delay in getting to the hospital after the first symptoms of a MI. Denial is an acute adaptive and beneficial reaction during hospitalization, but when chronic it can be maladaptive and is detrimental because it may lead to noncompliance with prescribed medical therapy or risk factor modification. Anxiety, as both an appropriate response and as an inappropriate one when excessive, is seen during most diagnostic cardiac procedures from the most innocuous, such as echocardiography, to the most tedious and dangerous, such as electrophysiology testing. An additional interface of psychological disorders and CHD occurs with the presentation of primary psychiatric disorders as cardiac disease when no cardiac disease exists. Such cardiac presentations are most commonly seen in patients who carry psychiatric diagnoses of hypochondriasis, chronic depression, and chronic anxiety. It is of interest that whereas in the United States anxiety disorders have a prevalence of about 10% in the population, a higher percentage of patients with anxiety disorders consult cardiologists. Specifically, patients with panic attacks are frequent visitors to emergency rooms and the offices of cardiologists. These patients can have many of the symptoms of an acute MI: chest pain, palpitations, shortness of breath, dizziness, nausea, sweating, and a sense of impending doom. Many of them are treated erroneously, as if they had CHD. Indeed, as many as a third of all patients with chest pain syndromes referred for diagnostic coronary angiography who are found to have normal coronary arteries have a panic attack syndrome.

CHD has significant vocational implications. CHD causes more economic loss in the United States than any other disease or disorder. Millions of Americans are unemployed or underemployed because of the effects of CHD. The vocational counselor should consider, however, the magnitude of the problem in the context of the fact that the energy requirements of work have decreased in industrialized countries in this century. This is a result of the mechanization, automation, and computerization of labor. In 1950, 65% of all work was considered heavy labor, while in 1990 only 5% was deemed heavy. Therefore, through creative vocational counseling, if the economy and the job market allow, many now unemployed cardiac patients could rejoin the work force. The vocational counselor should take into account the individual's cardiac diagnosis; his or her functional capacity as determined by a careful history, personal observation, and the results of the exercise stress test; and an occupational history that incorporates physical, mental, emotional, and environmental job requirements. Whenever possible, the functional status should be expressed as an NYHA class. Both the exercise tolerance on the stress test and the energy costs of work or other physical activities should be expressed in metabolic equivalents (METs). One MET is defined as the amount of oxygen consumed by an awake individual at rest. It is equivalent to 3.5 cc of oxygen per kilogram of body weight per minute. Stages of exercise and many vocational and recreational activities have been traditionally classified in terms of how many METs or multiples of the resting oxygen consumption are required by the activity. By the use of this method, results of the exercise stress test can be translated, though not precisely, to the level of exertion at work that the individual may safely perform. Rates of return to work after a cardiac event or procedure have a range of 35–95%.

Factors associated with a lower reemployment are severity of the cardiac condition; older age of the patient, social class or educational level; coexisting psychological conditions; and family environment that is either not supportive or too protective. After a MI, men return to work at a rate of about 75%. Women have a lower rate of reemployment. Surprisingly, the rate for patients after coronary bypass surgery is lower at about 60%. This is paradoxical because 100% of patients have reduced myocardial function after an infarction and 90% have improved myocardial blood flow after the bypass surgery. Formal rehabilitation programs with a multidisciplinary approach that incorporates supervised exercise, education, and nutritional and psychological counseling are increasingly proving to be beneficial in many aspects. They provide an excellent environment for the effective modification of atherosclerotic risk factors, improve psychological status, and increase rates of return to work. Moreover, several recent meta-analytic studies (in which data from similar randomized controlled studies are pooled and analyzed) indicate a secondary-prevention (the avoidance of a subsequent cardiac event) benefit of increased survival and decreased cardiovascular complications.

The Pericardium

The pericardium is the sac that contains the heart. It helps to fix the heart inside the thorax, protecting it from excessive movement. It prevents direct contact with other organs in the chest, reducing friction during constant cardiac motion. It is thought to slow the spread of infection to the heart from other organs such as the lungs. The lack of a pericardium is quite compatible with life, however, and if removed, there are usually no clinical consequences.

Disease Description
The most common pericardial disease is pericarditis, or inflammation of the pericardium. This can be caused by infections with tuberculosis, bacteria, or viruses. Other causes are trauma, metabolic or autoimmune diseases, and adverse reactions to medications. Pericarditis can result in the accumulation of fluid within the two layers that make up the pericardium, termed pericardial effusion. When severe, it may result in cardiac tamponade—a choking of

the heart that prevents its proper filling and emptying and may result in death. Tumors in the pericardium, either by adjacent spread or by metastasis from a distant site, can also cause pericardial effusion. Some patients, months after the acute episode of pericarditis, especially those with tuberculous pericarditis, may develop chrome constrictive pericarditis. As the inflamed pericardium heals, it scars, contracts, and constricts the heart, resulting in a condition similar to cardiac tamponade. The pericardium can be best visualized and pericardial diseases diagnosed and evaluated, with echocardiography.

Function and Disability
Functional impairment and disability are usually not considerations in individuals with acute pericarditis because it is a short limited process without sequelae. The most common symptom in the individual with acute pericarditis is chest pain, quite similar to that of angina pectoris. However, it is usually the so-called pleuritic kind because, just as with inflammations of the pleura (the lining of the lungs), the pain comes about at rest, is of a sharp quality, and is worsened by motion, breathing, or coughing. Cardiac tamponade's main symptoms are similar to those of CHF. Chronic constrictive pericarditis presents with symptoms similar to tamponade, but its time course is more insidious. The patient may be ill for months, even years and may appear emaciated, as if suffering from terminal cancer. Functional impairment and disability in chronic constrictive pericarditis are similar to those of myocardial failure. With the notable exception that in chronic pericarditis, the complete elimination of the functional impairment or disability may be possible by surgical excision of the constricting pericardium.

Treatment and Prognosis
The treatment of acute pericarditis is the direct treatment of the underlying disease causing the inflammation or infection. The threatening fluid of pericardial effusion or cardiac tamponade can be removed by inserting a small needle in the pericardial space. This procedure is called pericardiocentesis. A persistent or recurrent pericardial effusion of physiological import can be eradicated by the definitive curative procedure of surgical resection of the pericardium. This is also the treatment for chronic constrictive pericarditis. Great care must be taken that a patient with constrictive pericarditis not be medically managed as if ventricular failure was present. Such treatment may cause fluid depletion and dehydration and further decrease cardiac output, which will worsen symptoms and even lead to death. Prognosis for patients with pericarditis is excellent; it depends on the nature of the condition causing the pericardial inflammation. Proper management of the acute condition, prompt recognition and drainage of pericardial fluid, and correct diagnosis and management of chronic constrictive pericarditis should result in a normal life span.

Psychological and Vocational Implications
The psychological and vocational implications of pericardial disease are not well studied or described. This is mainly because pericardial disorders are neither common nor chronic. The most usual psychological manifestation is the anxiety provoked by the pain of pericarditis because it is confused by the patients, their families, and even by health care professionals, with the ischemic pain of angina or an acute MI. This situation is particularly devastating because the majority of patients with viral or traumatic pericarditis are young people. Patients with chronic constrictive pericarditis often suffer from clinical chronic depression. Their vocational evaluation should include both physiological and psychological factors.

The Myocardium

The myocardium is the heart muscle itself. It is divided into the left and the right ventricles. The left ventricle receives oxygenated blood from the lungs via the left atrium, and then pumps that blood to the body via the aorta and its branches. The right ventricle receives deoxygenated blood from the body via the right atrium, and then delivers that blood to the lungs for reoxygenation via the pulmonary artery.

Disease Description

Diseases of the myocardium are termed cardiomyopathy. There are three anatomical and physiological categories of cardiomyopathy, which are as follows: dilated (an enlarged heart with a thin or normal-thickness muscle wall), hypertrophy (a normal-size or only slightly enlarged heart with a thick muscle wall), and restrictive (a normal-size heart with a thick or normal muscle wall of increased rigidity). The cardiomyopathies are best diagnosed and evaluated with echocardiography. In the United States, dilated cardiomyopathies are usually caused by alcoholism, diabetes, and, principally, by CHD (ischemic cardiomyopathy). Another cause of dilated cardiomyopathy is inflammation of the myocardium, or myocarditis. This is most frequently caused by a viral infection and unfortunately occurs in young individuals. Some cardiomyopathies that were previously deemed idiopathic, or of unknown cause, are probably viral in origin. Hypertrophic cardiomyopathies are most often the result of chronic untreated or improperly treated elevated blood pressure, or hypertension. These myopathies, secondary to pressure overloads, usually result in a symmetrical or concentric type of hypertrophy. A different type, asymmetric hypertrophy, which includes idiopathic hypertrophic subaortic stenosis (IHSS), has an unknown etiology, is often familial, and is associated with sudden death in young people. Restrictive cardiomyopathies are the least common in the United States. They are caused by the infiltration or deposition of extraneous material in the heart muscle. In the case of patients with metabolic diseases or multiple blood transfusions, iron is an example of such extraneous material, as is amyloid in the case of those with chronic infections.

Function and Disability

The major determinant of impaired function and disability in myocardial disease is the degree of myocardial dysfunction. All of the cardiomyopathies, by definition, entail myocardial dysfunction. In dilated cardiomyopathies there is impaired ventricular contraction, or systole. In the hypertrophic and restrictive cardiomyopathies the initial dysfunction is in ventricular relaxation, or diastole. In their advanced stages, the latter two myopathies may also exhibit systolic dysfunction and cardiac dilation and may progressively begin to resemble both anatomically and physiologically, a dilated cardiomyopathy. All of the cardiomyopathies may create a decreased cardiac blood output state that is insufficient to meet the metabolic needs of the peripheral tissues. This altered physiological state is called CHF. CHF is usually the pathophysiological endpoint of most CVDs because eventually the myocardium is affected. Therefore, whether the initial disorder originated in the coronary arteries or in the cardiac valves, or whether it was the result of a systemic condition such as diabetes or hypertension, it is myocardial failure that produces the symptoms that determine functional capacity and disability.

The decreased blood flow in CHF signals the kidneys to retain fluid. When the excess fluid accumulates in the lungs, it causes the most common symptom of heart failure: difficult breathing or dyspnea. In the beginning stages of heart failure, when there is only mild impairment, dyspnea occurs only with significant exertion. As the condition becomes more severe and the ventricular function deteriorates, dyspnea may occur with minimal effort and even at rest. When dyspnea occurs while the patient is lying down, it is termed orthopnea; when it suddenly wakens a patient, it is called paroxysmal nocturnal dyspnea. The excess fluid may also cause abdominal distension, or ascites. It may cause the liver to be enlarged, a condition called hepatomegaly. The fluid deposition in the legs, which usually begins about the ankle area, is termed edema. The symptoms of weakness, fatigue, and lethargy indicate even more severe heart failure and reflect a greatly decreased cardiac blood output.

Functional impairment and disability are best assessed by a careful interview, with special attention given to the patient's daily activities. Treadmill exercise stress testing can be useful in determining factional capacity in patients with cardiomyopathies and are of greatest help in those with dilated cardiomyopathies. They are not particularly useful in patients with restrictive cardiomyopathies because often their primary disease is the major contributor to their functional impairment and disability. Moreover, it must be specifically emphasized that patients with IHSS should not (as a rule with occasional exceptions) undergo exercise stress testing. In the natural history of their disease, these individuals can have syncope and sudden death with exercise. To exercise them on purpose is a risk. This is particularly true if their ventricular obstruction to blood flow is physiologically significant. For the assessment of functional capacity in the patient with a dilated cardiomyopathy, a gentler exercise is recommended. Before the test, it should be absolutely determined by interview and careful physical examination that the individual does not have active or decompensated CHF. Particularly useful and informative in these patients are exercise tests that use imaging of ventricular function such as nuclear ventriculograms or echocardiograms. The patient's ventricular function, including global ejection fraction and segmental wall motion, at rest and with exercise, can be easily, objectively, and safely determined with both the techniques. Individuals whose ventricular function worsens with exercise are evidently more functionally limited and more likely to be disabled.

It is of great interest that a low left ventricular ejection fraction at rest, without question the best predictor of prognosis in any cardiovascular disorder, may not be predictive of functional capacity. Some patients with ejection fractions below 30% can have a normal exercise tolerance, whereas some patients with normal ejection fractions of more than 50% can have a markedly reduced exercise tolerance. This seeming paradox is accounted for by the differing peripheral adaptation in different individuals. Those with a higher exercise tolerance and greater functional capacity are more physically fit individuals because of their more efficient skeletal musculature and greater oxygen extraction capability.

Treatment and Prognosis

In the medical management of the patient with myocardial failure it is important to consider first the elimination of any conditions that might have helped to precipitate the failure. Such conditions may be internal stresses (e.g., anemia, fevers, infection, rhythm disturbances, and thyroid disorders) or they may be environmental stresses (e.g., high altitudes or excessive heat or cold). After such contributing factors are eradicated, therapy is aimed at creating the optimal hemodynamic milieu for myocardial function. This milieu can be best created by positively intervening in three components of myocardial mechanics and of CHF pathophysiology. This is accomplished by increasing inotropy, or myocardial contractility; by decreasing preload, or diastolic ventricular volume; and by decreasing afterload, or the stress or tension of the heart muscle wall during the ejection of blood. By improving one of the three, the two others are also improved.

Specific treatment includes nitrates to directly decrease preload, diuretics to eliminate excess fluid and indirectly reduce preload, digitalis to directly increase inotropy, and afterload reducing agents such as direct vasodilators or ACEI. Most patients are also advised to restrict their salt intake because excessive dietary salt will cause fluid retention. There is no definite cure for myocardial failure other than complete cardiac transplantation. Patients referred for cardiac transplantation are those who prove refractory to the best possible combination of medical therapy and are in the NYHA Class IV functional status. Without transplantation, some of these individuals may have as high as a 90% 1-year mortality. This mortality is to be compared with the survival rates of transplantation, which are currently about 85% in 1-year and about 70% in 3 years.

The prognosis of patients with cardiomyopathies depends on the kind of cardiomyopathy and the degree of myocardial dysfunction and CHF present. Patients with a dilated cardiomyopathy have the worst average prognosis of all cardiomyopathies. Within that group, the individuals with the ischemic cardiomyopathy fare the worst. As a general rule, the worse the ventricular function, as assessed by resting left ventricular ejection fraction, the worse the prognosis, and the greater the likelihood of death from end-stage CHF, cardiovascular collapse, and shock.

Psychological and Vocational Implications

The psychological and vocational implications of pericardial disease are not well studied or described. This is mainly because pericardial disorders are neither common nor chronic. The most usual psychological manifestation is the anxiety provoked by the pain of pericarditis because it is confused by the patients, their families, and even by health care professionals, with the ischemic pain of angina or of an acute MI. This situation is particularly devastating because the majority of patients with viral or traumatic pericarditis are young people. Patients with chronic constrictive pericarditis often suffer from clinical chronic depression. Their vocational evaluation should include both physiological and psychological factors.

The Endocardium

The endocardium (its inner lining surface that is in contact with systemic blood) disorders are mainly those of the following four cardiac valves: the aortic, the mitral, the pulmonic, and the tricuspid. While rare diseases may primarily involve the endocardial lining and only secondarily the valves, these are quite uncommon in the United States.

Disease Description

The principal etiologic factor of endocardial and valvular heart disease, in the developed as well as the developing countries of the world, has been rheumatic fever, a result of the body's immune response against a streptococcal infection. Rheumatic fever can result in both valvular insufficiency (or "leaky" valves) and valvular stenosis (or "tight" valves). With the introduction and widespread use of penicillin and other antibiotics to treat streptococcal infections, the incidence of rheumatic heart disease, and of valvular disease in general, has progressively and significantly decreased over the past half-century in economically developed nations. This decrease, at the same time that coronary atherosclerosis is on the increase, has limited endocardial and valvular diseases to fewer than 10% of all cases of CVD in these countries, while its prevalence remains high in underdeveloped areas of the world.

Mitral stenosis, with very few exceptions, is always secondary to rheumatic heart disease. About 70% of patients with mitral stenosis are women. Even though the left ventricle is usually normal in mitral stenosis, symptoms similar to those of CHF, such as dyspnea and orthopnea, begin in these patients when they are in their 40s or 50s. The elevated pressures in the left atrium and the pulmonary vasculature that must be generated to force the blood through the stenotic mitral valve cause these symptoms. Complications of mitral stenosis such as arrhythmias can lead to symptoms of palpitations. Mitral regurgitation is caused in 50% of cases by rheumatic fever. Pure rheumatic mitral regurgitation is more common in men than in women. Infective endocarditis, which preferentially attacks valves previously damaged by rheumatic disease, also leads to mitral regurgitation. Causative are also a variety of conditions that affect the supporting structures of the valve. There can be dilation or calcification of the mitral annulus, the ring-like orifice between the left atrium and the ventricle that the valve occupies. Also, there can be fibrosis of the papillary muscles, which through the net-like chordae tendineae attach the valve leaflets to the left ventricle. A unique disease entity of the mitral valve is the mitral valve prolapse syndrome. In this condition, the leaflets of the mitral valve prolapse into the left atrium during valve closure. Echocardiographic studies have suggested that the incidence of this condition may be about 5% in the female population. Aortic stenosis may be caused by rheumatic fever, by degenerative calcification of the cusps, or by a congenital condition called bicuspid aortic valve. Bicuspid aortic valve is abnormal because it has two instead of three cusps. This abnormality, the most common congenital cardiac abnormality, occurs in about 2% of the population. In only a small portion of that group does this congenital condition result in clinical disease. As opposed to stenosis of the mitral valve, where mainly women are affected, about 80% of adult patients with isolated aortic stenosis are men.

Aortic regurgitation is mainly rheumatic in origin, especially when found in combination with mitral valve disease. Nearly 80% of patients with pure aortic regurgitation are men. Women are the majority of those who have concomitant mitral disease. A bicuspid aortic valve can also become insufficient. An increasing incidence of aortic regurgitation is caused by infective endocarditis. Diseases that result in the dilation of the aorta itself may also dilate the aortic valve annulus and lead to secondary aortic insufficiency. Disorders of the valves of the right side of the heart are far less common than those of the valves of the left side of the heart. Tricuspid stenosis is very uncommon and is usually secondary to rheumatic heart disease and found in association with disease of the other valves. Tricuspid insufficiency is more common than stenosis and results directly from infective endocarditis in users of intravenous drugs or indirectly from right ventricular enlargement and accompanying tricuspid annular dilation. Of all valvular disorders, those of the pulmonic valve are the rarest. The most common pulmonic valve disorder is insufficiency, secondary to pulmonary hypertension.

Function and Disability
The major determinant of impaired function and disability in endocardial disease is the severity of the valvular stenosis or insufficiency and the degree of secondary myocardial dysfunction. Valvular insufficiency and valvular stenosis both interfere with normal cardiac blood flow. Valvular insufficiency leads to a volume overload and eventual dilation of the cardiac chambers. Aortic and pulmonic stenosis may cause a pressure overload, and ventricular hypertrophy and atrial dilation. These overloads, if severe and left untreated, will invariably lead to CHF. The time for the onset of symptoms is related to the severity of the valvular lesion and also to the age and physical fitness of the individual patient. Individuals with valvular disease may have the following symptoms: chest pain that has some of the features of angina pectoris, palpitations from both atrial and ventricular arrhythmias, and dyspnea most often when mitral regurgitation is present. In addition to the symptoms of CHF, patients with aortic stenosis can also have chest pain indistinguishable from angina pectoris and can also have sudden death as their only clinical presentation. Disease classification by NYHA criteria is similar to that of the patient with CHD or with a cardiomyopathy. If an appropriate functional history cannot be obtained, exercise stress testing is a good objective indicator of function in these patients. It should be noted, however, that exercise testing is relatively contraindicated in patients with mild to moderate mitral stenosis and aortic stenosis and absolutely contraindicated when the stenoses are severe. With exercise testing, those with stenotic valvular disease may develop acute pulmonary edema and those with aortic stenosis may also have syncope.

Treatment and Prognosis
Treatment is the surgical replacement of the diseased valve with either a porcine (pig) valve or a metal valve prosthesis. The use of porcine valves is rapidly falling into disfavor because it is becoming evident that they may become dysfunctional within 10 years after implantation. Replacement with a metal prosthesis results in the need for lifelong anticoagulation. Regurgitant valves can at times be surgically repaired, rather than replaced, in what essentially can be considered plastic surgery of the heart.

The treatment of patients with mitral valve prolapse is mainly reassurance that they have a good prognosis. Medical treatment with β-blockers may be necessary to treat symptoms of palpitations from their benign yet symptomatic arrhythmias. A mitral valve prolapse patient with significant mitral regurgitation, like all other patients with valvular disease or with prosthetic valves, should have antibiotic prophylaxis before dental work or surgery to prevent acquiring endocarditis from a potential bacteremia (the introduction of bacteria into the blood) that may happen with such procedures. The prognosis of patients with valvular disease is excellent as long as replacement, repair, or valvuloplasty is performed before there is damage to the ventricles, the atria, or the pulmonary vasculature. Once the chronic volume or pressure overloads have irreversibly damaged these structures, the surgical mortality is markedly increased, from about 1% in uncomplicated cases to more than 15% in those with failing ventricles. These unfortunate individuals have a decreased lifespan even if the surgery is successful and the prosthetic valve has perfect function. Severely dysfunctional cardiac valves, if not repaired or replaced, usually will lead to death within 5 years.

During the last decade, there has been an increase in valve surgery through minimal access valve surgery (MAVS). Reported benefits include better cosmetics and reduced surgical trauma, blood loss, incidence of atrial fibrillation, pain, and hospital stay, and a more rapid return to functional activity. Current best available evidence from randomized clinical trials (Grade A, Level 1b) does not show any significant quantitative differences between MAVS and conventional valve surgery for the following: perioperative mortality, stroke, renal failure, or respiratory failure (Bakir et al., 2006).

Psychological and Vocational Implications

In many respects, the psychological and vocational implications of endocardial and valvular heart disease are the same as those of the dilated cardiomyopathies, especially when secondary ventricular dysfunction exists. Unique psychological situations in the valvular diseases arise because many of the patients with rheumatic valvular disease are young women of child-bearing age. Often, some patients who are childless must make a decision as to whether to become pregnant even though pregnancy may worsen their cardiac condition and lead to risk of death. At times, the stress-laden decision is not whether to become pregnant but whether to terminate an advanced wanted pregnancy. Psychological intervention and support is needed before, during, and particularly after the time of decision making. Patients with mitral valve prolapse present a difficult challenge to the psychologist. These individuals, with cardiac symptoms but with a good prognosis, are often disabled for psychological, and not physiological, reasons. A team approach, with the cardiologist, psychologist, and other caregivers working together, is often more effective than an uncoordinated approach that often confuses the patient and results in further distress.

Unique vocational implications exist with patients with valvular heart disease because this is the only group of CVDs in which women constitute a majority. Patients with mitral valve prolapse and rheumatic mitral valve disease are often young women who have to care for a family and work outside the home in the context of their mitral disease. Surgical valve replacement often occurs in older women in their late 50s or early 60s who are near retirement age. Many do not return to work after the surgery. Many live alone because they have survived their husbands, who have already died from their own CHD. The rehabilitative and vocational challenges are great in this group of patients.

The Electrical Conduction System

The cardiac conduction system, made of specialized fibers, has two functions. The main cardiac pacemaker, the sinus, or sinoatrial node, generates the rhythmic electrical impulse that is the basis of life. The other parts of the system include the atrioventricular node (the backup or auxiliary pacemaker), the bundle of His, the bundle branches, and the Purkinje fibers. They all ensure the sequential and uniform propagation of the electrical current so that the cardiac cycle of ventricular systole and diastole is an organized and effective activity. As the population ages, atrial fibrillation will become more prevalent. The Framingham Heart Study showed that the lifetime risk of developing atrial fibrillation at age 40 and older is approximately one in four. The prevalence of atrial fibrillation is increasing, with predictions that the number of individuals suffering from atrial fibrillation will increase from the approximately 2.5 million at present to roughly 5.6 million over the next decades.

Disease Description

Disorders of the electrical system can result in bradycardia (slow rates of less than 60 beats per minute), tachycardia (fast rates at more than 100 beats per minute), or arrhythmias or dysrhythmias (irregular rhythms). Arrhythmias of a slow rate are bradyarrhythmias and those of a fast rate are tachyarrhythmias. Dysrhythmias can be further classified as those with an abnormal current originating from the atria or supraventricular arrhythmias, and those with an abnormal origin in the ventricles or ventricular arrhythmias. Supraventricular arrhythmias are paroxysmal atrial tachycardia (PAT), atrial flutter, atrial fibrillation, and multifocal atrial tachycardia (MAT). Although the atrial rates vary, the ventricular rate in these arrhythmias, even if untreated is generally relatively slow, about 1 SO beats per minute, because the impulses are slowed or blocked at the level of the AV node and the His bundle. MAT occurs mostly in patients with pulmonary disease. PAT can occur in normal persons without heart disease and is most commonly precipitated by anxiety or by the ingestion of irritants such as alcohol and caffeine. Atrial flutter and fibrillation occur in patients with atria that are enlarged either because of ventricular dysfunction, or mitral or tricuspid valvular disease. An overly active thyroid gland, or hyperthyroidism, may cause atrial fibrillation.

Ventricular arrhythmias are of two types: ventricular tachycardia and ventricular fibrillation. Ventricular tachycardia and fibrillation usually occur in patients with a dilated cardiomyopathy or a prior MI. They are rare, but do occur, in people with normal ventricles.

A rare congenital anomaly of the conduction system occurs in the presence of an accessory pathway, an extra bundle with conduction properties akin to those of the conduction system. Such a bundle allows the electrical activity from the atria to the ventricles to bypass the AV node and the bundle of His. Patients with these abnormalities, called pre-excitation syndromes, are usually young, are prone to episodes of PAT, and can have very fast ventricular rates with atrial fibrillation. There are two types of pre-excitation syndromes, which are: Wolff–Parkinson–White syndrome and Lown–Ganong–Levine syndrome.

Cardiac electrical block is said to occur when either of the two cardiac pacemakers cannot generate a normal electrical impulse or when a normal impulse is not conducted correctly through the conduction system. Fibrosis of the conduction system, which is part of the aging process, is a cause of electrical blocks in the elderly. Most blocks, however, like most arrhythmias, are the result of CHD.

Function and Disability

The functional impairments and disabilities that result from the cardiac arrhythmias fall into two major categories. One is the physiological disability from the ineffective ventricular contractions and decreased cardiac output that is secondary to a chronic arrhythmia that is too slow, too fast, or too disorganized. (Atrial fibrillation is the prototype and its symptoms place the functional considerations of this arrhythmia with those of CHF.) The other is the psychological disability secondary to an arrhythmia that is not chronic but acute. Such an arrhythmia is unpredictable. It arrives suddenly and without any warning. Ventricular tachycardia is the prototype. The individual may have no physiological functional limitation or disability with the activities of daily life yet may refrain from work because of fear of precipitating the arrhythmia with activity. Patients with supraventricular arrhythmias have palpitation as their most common symptom. PAT and atrial flutter are acute and not chronic arrhythmias and therefore have no functional or disability implications when they are not present. Those with atrial flutter or fibrillation may develop syncope or symptoms of CHF, especially if they have the arrhythmias in the context of impaired ventricular function. Those with coexisting CAD may develop angina pectoris because the fast heart rates of the arrhythmia create metabolic demands that cannot be met by the compromised blood supply through the obstructed coronary arteries. Patients whose heart rate in atrial fibrillation is controlled at rest can still have exertional dyspnea, as in this condition the heart rate may rapidly increase with little exertion. The chaotic atrial electrical activity of atrial fibrillation creates a combination of turbulence and stasis of blood in the atria. This can lead to the complication of thrombus formation in the atria. These thrombi can dislodge and be carried by the circulation to other parts of the body. Such a traveling thrombus, or embolus, may cause obstruction of blood flow to the eyes, leading to blindness, or to the kidneys, causing renal failure. When carried to the brain, it may result in cerebral infarction, or stroke.

If ventricular tachycardia is of a short duration (a few seconds), the patient may experience palpitation. If of a longer duration (a few minutes), syncope may occur. If sustained beyond a few minutes, degeneration to ventricular fibrillation is likely and sudden death may ensue. Individuals with the accessory pathway syndromes will experience palpitation when PAT is their acute arrhythmia. In them, atrial fibrillation, if of prolonged duration and of a very fast ventricular rate, may degenerate into ventricular fibrillation and lead to sudden cardiac death. The health care professional should not be deceived into complacency because the patient looks young, healthy, and vigorous. Atrial fibrillation in a patient with a pre-excitation syndrome is dire. Severe bradycardia or high degrees of block, resulting in heart rates of less than 30 beats per minute, can cause fatigue and dizziness because of the decreased cardiac output and the resultant diminished cerebral perfusion. When the effective rate is even slower or when the bradycardia is sudden in onset, syncope may occur.

Treatment and Prognosis
The treatment of supraventricular arrhythmias involves their prevention, quick termination, or the prompt and effective control of their fast rate. Avoiding stressful situations and the ingestion of alcohol or stimulants such as caffeine and antihistamines can prevent supraventricular arrhythmias. If the initiation of the arrhythmia is not preventable, then it may be terminated, or its fast rate controlled, by medications that slow electrical conduction through the AV node such as digitalis, β-blockers, and calcium channel blockers. Individuals whose atrial fibrillation is chronic or recurrent (paroxysmal atrial fibrillation) need to take such medications for life to control their heart rates. Most of them will also require lifelong anticoagulation with warfarin (Coumadin) to prevent thrombus formation and embolization. If medication fails to abolish the arrhythmia, or if the patient is severely ill because of angina pectoris, of severe CHF, or in shock, then prompt electrical cardioversion to normal sinus rhythm is indicated.

The treatment of sustained ventricular tachycardia and of ventricular fibrillation should be prompt electrical cardioversion to a normal rhythm. Only younger individuals with normal ventricular function can tolerate sustained ventricular tachycardia. Ventricular fibrillation is not compatible with life. Antiarrhythmic agents to prevent these ventricular arrhythmias should be prescribed only by expert cardiologists who have evaluated the arrhythmia with invasive electrophysiological studies. It is no longer acceptable to treat such patients empirically, as these agents have been found to have a high pro-arrhythmic potential. In up to 25% of cases they can precipitate the very arrhythmia they are supposed to prevent or even make it worse. Patients with ventricular arrhythmias who do not respond to medical therapy may require surgical ablation of the myocardial focus from which the arrhythmia originates. Some, with recurrent episodes of ventricular fibrillation, may require the chronic implantation of an antiarrhythmic device, similar to a pacemaker, called an implantable automatic defibrillator, to deliver an electrical shock whenever ventricular fibrillation occurs. The ultimate treatment of ventricular arrhythmias, however, lies in the prevention of CHD, which is present in about 80% of patients with malignant ventricular arrhythmias and sudden electrical death.

The treatment of patients with the pre-excitation syndromes is similar to that of those with supraventricular arrhythmias. However, great caution is needed when giving antiarrhythmic agents to these patients because a paradoxical effect may result, that is, the arrhythmia may be made worse and faster rates may obtain if agents that would normally control the arrhythmia or slow down its rate are administered. In patients where arrhythmia is refractory to medical therapy or those who have the lethal trial fibrillation with a very rapid ventricular rate, ablation of the accessory pathway, possible nowadays by different techniques, is recommended. Cardiac electrical blocks and symptomatic bradycardia are treated with the implantation of permanent pacemakers that substitute for the heart's own pacemakers and conduction system. In recent years, technology has led to the development of ever more sophisticated and smaller pacing devices that nearly duplicate the heart's electrophysiological mechanisms and allow for nearly normal ventricular hemodynamics.

The prognosis for patients with supraventricular arrhythmia under appropriate medical care is excellent. Their mortality depends on the physiological cause of the arrhythmia rather than on the arrhythmia itself. For example, those with normal hearts or with hyperthyroidism have a much better prognosis than do those whose arrhythmias are complications of structural heart disease, such as mitral stenosis or myocardial dysfunction.

The prognosis for the patient who is a survivor of sudden death and who has recurrent episodes of ventricular fibrillation or ventricular tachycardia is dismal. This is particularly the case for those with a dilated cardiomyopathy and a left ventricular ejection fraction of less than 20%. This poor prognosis has been ameliorated by the practice of medical therapy guided by electrophysiological testing, by the newer surgical techniques, and by the use of the implantable defibrillators.

The prognosis in patients with pre-excitation syndrome is excellent because they usually have otherwise normal hearts. If the correct diagnosis is made and expert prompt treatment is rendered the few times it is needed, these individuals will have a normal lifespan. The prognosis of patients requiring pacemakers is excellent if the ventricular function is normal.

Psychological and Vocational Implications

The psychological implications of cardiac arrhythmias are significant. Not only is the psychologist confronted with the psychological consequences of the arrhythmias, but perhaps more importantly, psychological disorders may trigger lethal arrhythmias. As mentioned, a chronic depression or anxiety syndrome that may develop over time after repeated episodes of their sudden and unexpected tachyarrhythmia may disable patients with paroxysmal atrial fibrillation (PAT), recurrent ventricular tachycardia, and ventricular fibrillation. They may progressively and drastically curtail their range of activities as they associate the onset of their arrhythmias with particular events, places, or times. Phobias and a repertoire of superstitious behaviors may develop in many of these individuals. Intensive yet nonthreatening psychological interventions are often necessary. Particularly difficult is the control and prevention of the psychological precipitants of the arrhythmias. It is well documented that about 1% of all patients with malignant ventricular arrhythmias have no demonstrable structural heart disease, and the only causative factor for their arrhythmia is psychological. An even greater percentage of patients with known heart disease have their potentially lethal arrhythmias triggered by psychological factors. A few medical centers have laboratories and testing protocols that elicit and identify specific thoughts, ideas, or mental images that trigger the arrhythmias in a particular individual. The judicious use of antiarrhythmic agents, in combination with β-blockers and directed and focused psychological intervention, has proved quite successful in preventing or reducing the frequency of arrhythmias in such patients. The vocational implications of cardiac arrhythmias are also significant. The vocational counselor must undertake a careful evaluation of the work situation, with special attention given to any environmental, emotional, or mental stress that may precipitate or aggravate the arrhythmia.

DISEASES OF THE VASCULAR SYSTEM

The vascular system, also known as the peripheral vascular system, is responsible for the circulation of blood from the heart to the rest of the body and back again to the heart. Its components are the aorta, the arteries, the arterioles, the capillaries, and the veins. In this chapter, only diseases of the aorta will be considered. Diseases of specific vessels and of the smaller vasculature are covered in other chapters of this book.

The Aorta

The aorta is the largest artery in the body. It receives the blood from the heart and then, through its branches, delivers that blood to the rest of the body. Because of its large size and its unique function as the receiving conduit for blood directly from the left ventricle, the walls of the aorta experience greater tension and stress than do other blood vessels. Therein lies the anatomical and physiological substrate for its diseases.

Disease Description

Arteriosclerosis develops in the aorta just as it does in the coronary arteries. Such is the extent of the process that nearly all adults in the United States are believed to have some measure of aortic arteriosclerosis. Even children and adolescents have been shown to have aortic fatty streaks, the earliest lesion of aortic arteriosclerosis. The vast majority of patients with clinical aortic disease are hypertensive men who smoke cigarettes. There are three main diseases of the aorta: aneurysms, dissections, and obstructive disease. Diseases of the aorta and its branches are best evaluated by angiography. The new technique of transesophageal echocardiography is particularly useful for the evaluation of diseases of the thoracic aorta.

An aortic aneurysm is an abnormal dilation of the aorta that is susceptible to acute rupture. Aneurysms can be found in the thoracic aorta (in both its ascending and descending segments) and also in the abdominal aorta. Ascending aortic aneurysms are the ones that are least likely to be caused by arteriosclerosis. Before our age of antibiotics and organized prevention of sexually transmitted diseases, ascending aortic aneurysms were mainly caused by syphilis. At present, the most common cause of ascending aneurysms is damage of the middle layer of the aortic wall, the media. This condition is termed cystic medial necrosis and is of unknown etiology. Aneurysms of the descending thoracic aorta and of the abdominal aorta are nearly all caused by arteriosclerosis. Many patients who have thoracic aneurysms also have abdominal aneurysms, and about 10% of those with abdominal aneurysms have more than one.

Aortic dissections can occur anywhere in the aorta. A dissection takes place when the innermost of the three layers of the wall of the aorta, the intima, breaks and allows blood to flow into the wall of the aorta itself. The pressure of the blood separates the layers of the aorta. Hypertension plays a significant role in aortic dissections regardless of their location. Surgeons categorize dissections into three types: Type I dissection involves the entire aorta, from its ascending portion, around the arch, and into the abdominal aorta; Type II dissection is limited to the ascending aorta; and Type III dissection is limited to the descending aorta. Aortic obstructive disease, like coronary artery obstructive disease, impedes the adequate flow of blood. Obstruction in the aorta is the most frequently noted in its terminal portion, usually at its bifurcation into the iliac and femoral arteries, the vessels that supply the lower extremities.

Function and Disability

Most patients with aortic aneurysms and dissections are free of functional impairments and disability because they are asymptomatic until the moment of the acute event. Aortic aneurysms are most often found on routine abdominal physical exam or by x-rays. Symptoms, when they do exist, may be only those of a lower back pain syndrome. Some patients may actually have been misdiagnosed as having lumbar vertebral disease.

Obstructive aortic disease does cause disability and chronic functional impairment. The most common symptom is claudication. This is pain of one or both legs, usually in the muscles of the calves, with walking. Patients may be able to walk only a few feet before disabling pain impedes further walking. They may also have pain of the thighs and buttocks with walking and at rest. They often have impotence. The functional capacity of patients with claudication and the degree of their vascular stenosis can be evaluated by Doppler ultrasound of the legs.

This is performed before and after treadmill walking, using special test protocols different from those used for the evaluation of the impairment in CHD.

Treatment and Prognosis

The treatment of aortic aneurysms, of dissections, and of severe obstructive disease is always surgical. The acute rupture of an aortic aneurysm is nearly always a fatal event. When an abdominal aneurysm has a diameter of less that 6 cm, the probability of rupture is about 15% over a 10-year period, but if the aneurismal diameter is 6 cm or greater, there is a 50% probability of rupture in a shorter time span. The operative mortality of elective abdominal aneurysm resection is less than 10%. Resection of aneurysms of the ascending aorta or of the aortic arch carries a greater operative mortality. There is about 20% mortality in the surgical treatment of aortic dissections.

The surgical treatment of obstructive disease of the main branches of the aorta to the lower extremities is aortic–femoral bypass grafting, using synthetic conduits to restore circulation to the legs. Excellent results are achieved with little mortality and morbidity, and claudication is abolished or decreased in about 90% of patients. As in coronary disease, an alternative treatment is percutaneous balloon angioplasty most recently with the additional placement of vascular metal stents. This procedure is particularly feasible in the dilation of discrete lesions of the iliac arteries.

The prognosis of patients with any type of arteriosclerotic disease of the aorta and its branches can be best determined in the context of their coexisting coronary artery arteriosclerosis. It is the extent and severity of the coronary disease that is the major determinant of both the operative mortality and the long-term survival of patients who undergo successful aortic or peripheral vascular surgery.

Psychological and Vocational Implications

There are usually no psychological implications in aortic disorders before the acute events of aortic aneurysm rupture and of aortic dissection because the patterns are usually asymptomatic up to that time. Most of these patients had denied the potential consequences of their smoking or of their uncontrolled hypertension. The acute event has perhaps no match in all of medicine as a truly terrifying experience. Most survivors of the event, and the subsequent surgery, experience a reversal of their present psychological mind-set, become acutely aware of their mortality, and may develop chronic depression and even excessive anxiety and an over-vigilant state. Such individuals can benefit from psychological intervention. A group of patients with a similar problem are those who are informed of the presence of an abdominal aortic aneurysm that is still too small to undergo surgical resection. They may spend months or even years in watchful waiting before surgery is finally indicated. Psychological implications in patients with obstructive aortic disease usually focus on their loss of self-esteem because of their inability to walk and work and principally because of impotence.

There are important vocational implications in aortic diseases. The patients who have had surgical repair of an aortic aneurysm or dissection have an even lower rate of return to work than do those who have had coronary bypass surgery. This may be due to the advanced age of these patients, most of whom are in their 60s and 70s. It may also be because the surgical procedure that was performed on them is perceived as, and is in fact, more complex than coronary bypass surgery. Patients with occlusive disease have specific vocational considerations because they are unable to perform most work activity that entails walking or prolonged standing. They may be employed in jobs that require the performance of work only with the arms, and only while sitting and with infrequent walking for short distances.

CARDIAC REHABILITATION

Cardiac rehabilitation is designed to decrease the physiological and psychological effects of cardiac disease, to reduce the risk for sudden death and of reinfarction, to control cardiac symptoms, to stabilize or reverse the atherosclerotic process, and enhance vocational status of patients. A goal of cardiac rehabilitation is also to help reduce cardiovascular risk factors by lipid control, weight loss, stress management, and increased physical activity. Specifically, a comprehensive transdisciplinary program should improve a patient's exercise performance, promote lifestyle changes, and increase psychosocial well being. Cardiac rehabilitation and secondary prevention programs are recognized as integral to the comprehensive care of patients with CVD and as such are recommended as useful and effective (Class I) by the AHA, ACC, American Association of Cardiovascular and Pulmonary Rehabilitation, and the Agency for Health Care Policy and Research. All conclude that cardiac rehabilitation programs (CRP) should offer a multifaceted and transdisciplinary approach to the overall cardiovascular risk reduction and that programs consisting of exercise training alone are not considered cardiac rehabilitation.

Patients should be formally evaluated at the time they are enrolled in a CRP and should have a comprehensive medical history and physical examination, a review of relevant test results and treatments, and risk stratification. In order to individualize the patient's program, each clinician should design an individualized program of secondary prevention. Appropriate strategies can include nutrition counseling, weight management, blood pressure, lipid and diabetic management, tobacco use cessation, physical activity counseling, targeted physical prescription, medication adherence, and detection and management of depression (Zellwenger et al., 2004). Inherent in the patient's involvement in the CRP is the understanding that successful risk factor modification and the maintenance of a physically active lifestyle is a lifelong process.

An admission to a CRP should include a psychosocial evaluation that encompasses an identification of depression, anxiety, anger or hostility, social isolation, family distress, sexual dysfunction, and any substance abuse, using standard interview and measurement techniques. Individual or group education and counseling are warranted with referral to appropriate specialists as needed. In a study of over 500 consecutive coronary patients enrolled in cardiac rehabilitation compared with control patients not completing rehabilitation, depressive symptoms were assessed by questionnaire and mortality was evaluated at a mean follow-up of 40 months. Depressed patients had a greater than fourfold mortality than nondepressed patients (22% vs. 5%) and depressed patients who completed rehabilitation had a 73% lower mortality (8% vs. 30%) (Milani & Lavie, 2007). Importantly, a reduction in depressive symptoms and the associated decrease in mortality were related to improvement in fitness. Hence, only a mild improvement in the levels of fitness was needed to produce the benefit on depressive symptoms and its associated decrease in mortality.

In terms of the safety and clinical efficacy of cardiac rehabilitation, a meta-analysis of 48 randomized clinical trials (with a total of nearly 9,000 patients out of which only 20% were women) demonstrated that exercised-based cardiac rehabilitation had significant reductions in both all-cause mortality (OR: 0.80; 95% confidence interval (CI): 0.68–0.93) and cardiac specific mortality (OR: 0.74; 95% CI: 0.61–0.96) after a median follow-up of 15 months, in both the genders. In these studies, reductions in all cause mortality ranged from 15–28% and reduction in cardiac mortality from 26–31%. Also, enrollment and participation in community-based CRPs that provide both exercise and secondary prevention education is associated with reduced mortality and fewer recurrent MIs (Witt et al., 2004).

A national study of Medicare beneficiaries to assess referral patterns for cardiac rehabilitation was conducted after individuals were hospitalized for acute MI or CABG surgery. A total of 267,427 beneficiaries who were aged 65 years and above and who survived at least 30 days after hospital discharge were enrolled in the study. Overall, cardiac rehabilitation was used in only 13.9% of patients hospitalized for acute MI and in 31% of patients who underwent CABG. Older patients, women (44% of cohort), non-Whites (8.2% of cohort) and patients with comorbidities (including CHF, previous stroke, diabetes mellitus, or cancer) were significantly less likely to receive cardiac rehabilitation. CABG during index hospitalization, higher median household income, higher level of education, and shorter distance to the nearest cardiac rehabilitation facility were important indicators of higher cardiac rehabilitation utilization (Suaya, Stason, Ades, Norman, & Shepherd, 2009).

A more recent study assessed the effects of CRP on survival in a large cohort of older coronary patients. Randomized controlled trials have shown that rehabilitation improves survival, but in these trials the participants have been predominantly middle age, low, or moderate risk, White men. This study consisted of a population of 601,099 U.S. Medicare beneficiaries who were hospitalized for coronary conditions or cardiac revascularization procedures. One- to five-year mortalities were examined in CRP users and nonusers using Medicare claims and the following three analytic techniques: propensity-based matching, regression modeling, and instrumental variables. The first method used 70,040 match pairs and the other two used the entire cohort. Only 36% of the CRP users were women, compared to the fact that women were 50% of the nonusers. After extensive analyses to control for potential confounding variables, mortalities were 21–34% lower in CRP users than in CRP nonusers in this socio-economically and clinically diverse, older population (Suaya et al., 2009).

A study of 234 women (99 African Americans and 135 Whites) were surveyed 1 month post discharge from the hospital after a PCI, CABG, or MI without revascularization and completed a 6-month follow-up survey. The findings revealed that the overall rate of referral to outpatient cardiac rehabilitation for women was only 19% and it was significantly lower for African American women compared with White women (12% vs. 24%). Only 15% of the referred women went on to enroll in the programs with fewer African American women enrolling compared with the White women (9% vs. 19%). Controlling for age, education, angina class, and comorbidities, women with annual income < $20,000 were 66% less likely to be referred to cardiac rehabilitation and 60% less likely to enroll when compared with women with incomes > $20,000. Diversity in the population of individuals referred and enrolled in cardiac rehabilitation programs and diversity of the professional caregivers of cardiac rehabilitations remains a challenge that must be addressed (Allen, Scott, Stewart, & Rohm-Young, 2004).

SUMMARY

The challenge of cardiovascular disorders will continue to grow as long as their prevention is not given emphasis and priority. If present trends continue, the diagnostic and therapeutic advances of the past decades may reduce cardiovascular mortality without a reduction in the prevalence of CVD and its attendant functional limitation and disability. The need of individuals with CVD for medical, psychological, rehabilitative, and vocational services may be greater than ever.

REFERENCES

ACOG Committee on Gynecologic Practice. (2008). ACOG Committee Opinion 420. November 2008: hormone therapy and heart disease. *Obstetrics & Gynecology, 112,* 1189–1192.

Allen, J. K., Scott, L. B., Stewart, K. J., Rohm-Young, D. (2004). Disparities in women's referral to and enrollment in outpatient cardiac rehabilitation. *Journal of General Internal Medicine, 19,* 747–753.

Bakir, I., Casselman, F. P., Wellens, F., Jeanmart, H., De Geest, R., Degrieck, I., et al. (2006). Minimally invasive versus standard approach aortic valve replacement: A study in 506 patients. *The Annals of Thoracic Surgery, 81,* 1599–1604.

Berkman, L. F., Blumenthal, J., Burg, M., Carney, R. M., Catellier, D., Cowan, M. J., et al. (2003). Enhancing recovery in coronary heart disease patients' investigators (ENRICHD). Effects of treating depression and low perceived social support on clinical events after myocardial infarction: The enhancing recovery in coronary heart disease patients (ENRICHD) randomized trial. *Journal of American Medical Association, 289,* 3106–3116.

Brar, S., & Stone, G. (2009). Advances in percutaneous coronary intervention. *Current Cardiology Reports, 11,* 245–251.

Clouse, R. E., Lustman, P. J., Freedland, K. E., Griffith, L. S., McGill, J. B., & Carney, R. M. (2003). Depression and coronary heart disease in women with diabetes. *Psychosomatic Medicine, 65,* 376–383.

Eastwood, J. A. & Doering, L. V. (2005). Gender differences in coronary artery disease. *Journal of Cardiovascular Nursing, 20*, 340–351.

Grodstein, F., Clarkson, T. B., & Manson, J. E. (2003). Understanding the divergent data on postmenopausal hormone therapy. *New England Journal of Medicine, 348*, 645–650.

Mallik, S., Krumholz, H. M., Lin, Z., Kasl, S. V., Mattera, J. A., Roumanis, S. A., et al. (2005). Patients with depressive symptoms have lower health status benefits after coronary artery bypass surgery. *Circulation, 111*, 271–277.

Mauri, L., Hsieh, W. H., Massacre, J. M., Ho, K. K., D'Agostino, R., & Cutlip, D. E. (2007). Stent thrombosis in randomized clinical trials of drug eluding stents. *New England Journal of Medicine, 356*, 1020–1029.

Milani, R., & Lavie, C. J. (2007). Impact of cardiac rehabilitation on depression and its associated mortality. *American Journal of Medicine, 120*, 799–806.

Moller-Leimkuhler, A. (2008). Women with coronary artery disease and depression: A neglected risk group. *The World Journal of Biological Psychiatry, 9*, 92–101.

Mosca, L., Banka, C. L., Benjamin, E. J., Berra, K., Bushnell, C., Dolor, R. J., et al. (2007). Evidence-based guidelines for cardiovascular disease prevention in women: 2007 update. *Circulation, 115*, 1481–1501.

Rossouw, J. E., Cushman, M., Greenland, P., Lloyd-Jones, D. M., Bray, P., Kooperberg, C., et al. (2008). Inflammatory, lipid, thrombotic, and genetic markers of coronary heart disease risk in the Women's Health Initiative Trials of Hormone Therapy. *Archives of Internal Medicine, 168*, 2245–2253.

Rossouw, J. E., Prentice, R. L., Manson, J. E., Wu, L., Barad, D., Barnabei, V. M., et al. (2007). Postmenopausal hormone therapy and risk of cardiovascular disease by age and years since menopause. *Journal of American Medical Association, 297*, 1465–1477.

Rumsfeld, J., & Ho, M. (2005). Depression and cardiovascular disease: A call for recognition. *Circulation, 111*, 250–253.

Schomig, A., Mehilli, J., de Waha, A., Seyfarth, M., Pache, J., & Kastrati, A. (2008). A meta-analysis of 17 randomized trials of a percutaneous coronary intervention-based strategy in patients with stable coronary artery disease. *Journal of American College of Cardiology, 52*, 894–904.

Serruys, P. W., Morice, M. C., Kappertein, A. P., Colombo, A., Holmes, D. R., Mack, M. J., et al. (2009). Percutaneous coronary intervention versus coronary-artery bypass grafting for severe artery disease. *New England Journal of Medicine, 360*, 961–972.

Stramba-Badiale, M., Fox, K. M., Priori, S. G., Collins, P., Daly, C., Graham, I., et al. (2006). Cardiovascular disease in women: a statement from the policy conference of the European Society of Cardiology. *European Heart Journal, 27*, 994–1005.

Suaya, J., Stason, W., Ades, P., Norman, S., & Shepard, S. (2009). Cardiac rehabilitation and survival in older coronary patients. *Journal of the American College of Cardiology, 54*, 25–33.

Utian, W. H., Archer, D. F., Bachman, G. A., Gallagher, C., Grodstein, F., Heiman, J. R., et al. (2008). North American Menopause Society. Estrogen and progestogen use in postmenopausal women. July 2008 position statement of the North American Menopause Society. *Menopause, 15*, 584–602.

Wilson, P. (2004). Prediction of coronary heart disease events: The contribution of lifestyle factors. *Cardiology Round, 8*, 2–12.

Witt, B. J., Jacobsen, S. J., Weston, S. A., Killian, B. S., Meverden, R., Allison, T., et al. (2004). Cardiac rehabilitation after myocardial infarction in the community. *Journal of American College of Cardiology, 44*, 988–996.

World Health Organization. (2002). *Toward a Common Language for Functioning, Disability and Health*. ICF: Geneva.

Zellwenger, M. J., Osterwalder, R. H., Langewitz, W., & Pfisterer, M. E. (2004). Coronary artery disease and depression. *European Heart Journal, 25*, 3–9.

8

Chronic Pain Syndromes

Christopher G. Gharibo, MD, and M. Fahad Khan, MD, MHS

Chronic pain syndromes are composed of a multifactorial relationship between biologically based neurological triggers and pathways; psychologically mediated moods, emotions, and behaviors; and socially developed responses, interactions, and consequences. The complex interplay between all of these factors is part of what can devastate a patient's quality of life, as well as make the diagnosis, treatment, and ongoing management of chronic pain syndromes by health care professionals exceedingly difficult and ultimately result in psychological and physical disability.

Chronic pain differs from acute pain in many key tenets. In acute pain, there is a gradual abatement in the normal signals triggered from a noxious stimulus as the cause of the perceived stimulus heals and ceases to exist as a triggering mechanism. In chronic pain, the imprinted signals and perceived pain may persist for several weeks, months, or even years after the original injury has healed. In addition, the acute pain pathway is triggered by the presence of an immediate noxious stimulus, whereas the chronic pain pathway may be activated in the absence of an immediate physical trigger (i.e., prior traumatic injury or infection) or in some cases by the absence of any physiological or pathological trigger (i.e., psychogenic).

PREVALENCE AND IMPACT

It is clear that the development of a chronic pain syndrome can contribute to significant morbidity in an affected individual, and when the effects are examined across a population, it is also easy to surmise that chronic pain syndromes can have significant psychosocial and medical consequences, if not identified and dealt with appropriately. Various researchers have suggested that approximately 20–30% of the U.S. population (Bonica, 1990) and nearly 35% of the Canadian population (Toth, Lander, & Wiebe, 2009) suffer from a chronically painful condition, and the amount of medical resources that is spent annually in the diagnosis and treatment of these conditions coupled with the cost of lost productivity due to inability to work is a number that reaches the hundreds of billions of dollars (Gill & Frymoyer, 1997).

Although chronic pain syndromes can affect a significant portion of a population, their prevalence and impact is not equal across gender lines, age, and/or socioeconomic status (Wenig, Schmidt, Kohlmann, & Schweikert, 2009). In addition, coexisting psychopathology (i.e., major depressive disorder, anxiety, attention deficit disorder) is another major component of this cohort, which not only predisposes individuals to developing a chronic pain syndrome but may also exacerbate the symptoms of a newly acquired syndrome.

The complexity of the various syndromes that will be discussed in this chapter has made it difficult to address chronic pain syndromes within the traditional medical model of care. Thus, the fact that these conditions require a multidisciplinary approach and a thorough understanding and commitment to addressing their respective biological, psychological, and social aspects is no surprise and has been convincingly proved as effective in numerous studies.

PATHOPHYSIOLOGY OF CHRONIC PAIN

Although an extensive discussion of physiology of acute pain and pathophysiology of chronic pain is beyond the scope of this chapter, an understanding of what exactly is occurring neurologically is necessary. Chronic pain is more than just "low back pain." Why is chronic pain spontaneous? Why does it exist longer than expected after an injury? Why is it physically and emotionally disabling? How does it reduce a person's quality of life? To begin to address these questions we need to discuss how this pain is initiated.

To understand the progression of acute pain to chronic pain pathophysiology, we need to understand that the process of neurological change in the peripheral and central nervous system is a continuum that starts with the basic mechanisms of nociception and eventually includes the structural and chemical changes in the peripheral and central nervous system that are ultimately responsible for the more complex mechanisms of chronic pain. The process of neurological peripheral and central sensitization starts from "time zero" with the initiation of peripheral tissue injury and is imprinted in the chronic pain population rather than initiated but reversed in the rest of the population.

The International Association for Study of Pain categorizes pain into two distinct classes, which may present together in the same patient: nociceptive and neuropathic pain includes acute, subacute, and inflammatory pain. Nociceptive pain results from noxious stimuli and inflammation and is largely considered protective, adaptive, and "normal."

Neuropathic pain often implies chronic pain and has peripheral and central nervous system components. Chronic pain often is mixed nociceptive and neuropathic (e.g., failed back surgery syndrome and osteoarthritis) or primarily neuropathic and is associated with imprinted neuroanatomical (e.g., neuroplastic rewiring, sodium channel, and α-receptor upregulation) and chemical changes (e.g., glutamate and aspartate release) in the peripheral and central nervous systems that results in abnormal processing.

Such changes often result in clinical symptoms and signs of spontaneous and paresthetic pain that is associated with dysesthesias (unpleasant sensations evoked by various stimuli), allodynia (pain evoked by a normally nonpainful stimulus), and hyperalgesia (disproportionate pain due to a stimulus considered to be already painful).

Peripheral "nociceptors" are free nerve endings that exist throughout the body and respond to potential tissue-damaging stimuli (Bonica, 1990). In the chronic pain patient, often in the absence of a noxious stimulus, long-term lowering of peripheral nociceptor activation threshold or aberrant spontaneous firing by a peripheral neuroma maintains the sensitizing reaction of the central nervous system to sensory input. The peripheral signals are transmitted by myelinated A-δ and A-β fibers, as well as unmyelinated C fibers, which can respond to a variety of chemical, mechanical, and thermal stimuli in the periphery.

The first-order nociceptive afferents terminate in the various Rexed lamina of the dorsal horn. For example, the unmyelinated C fibers terminate primarily in the Rexed lamina 1 and the myelinated pain fibers terminate in lamina 1, 3, 4, and 5. The second-order neurons that project from the dorsal horn to the thalamus and cortex, some of which are known as wide dynamic range (WDR) neurons, expand to receive a wider range of impulses. In essence, WDR neurons are activated by both noxious and non-noxious stimuli and are thought to be responsible for central mechanisms of allodynia. These second-order neurons project to the higher centers primarily via the spinothalamic tracts and project to the medial and posterior nuclei of the thalamus, which in turn projects to the sensory cortex (Raj, 1996).

The Gate Control Theory of Pain published by Wall and Melzack introduced the concept of spinal pain modulation. The pain modulation concept has since been broadened to encompass the pain-processing parts of the peripheral and central nervous systems, including the descending pathways that are all thought to be responsible for the elements of chronic pain pathophysiology and individual differences of pain perception (Figure 8.1).

The descending cerebrospinal pathways can be inhibitory or excitatory. These tracts involve connections from periaqueductal gray in the midbrain to the nucleus raphe magnus, reticular formation, and lower dorsal horn centers that receive the primary afferents. These pathways are modulated primarily by noradrenergic and serotonergic neurotransmitters, which help explain why certain antidepressants are effective treatments for chronic pain. Antidepressants can also address the patient's coexisting anxiety and depression, which are inextricably linked to the chronic pain population.

Immediately following an injurious stimulus, the barrage of stimuli that are generated in the primary afferents in the periphery travel toward the second-order neurons and higher centers in the central nervous system. This process induces peripheral and central sensitization, also known as "windup," where the primary afferents, dorsal horn, and higher centers become progressively hypersensitized to repetitive afferent stimulation. In the chronic pain patient, this is often coupled with diminished descending inhibition on the afferent impulses. The end result is exaggerated afferent impulse activity that reaches the higher centers that are ultimately processed as chronic pain.

In essence, there are neuroanatomic, neuroplastic, and neurochemical changes and associated sensitization in the progression from acute to chronic pain pathophysiology. The

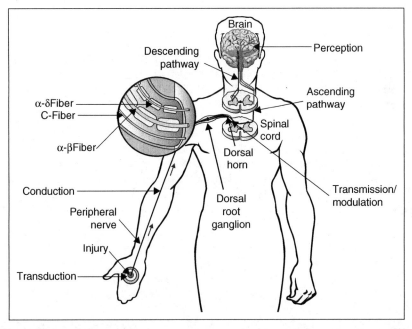

FIGURE 8.1 Physiology of pain perception. *Source*: From Galer, B. S., & Dworkin, R. H. (2000). *A clinical guide to neuropathic pain*. Minneapolis, MN: McGraw-Hill; Irving, G. A., & Wallace, M. S. (1997). *Pain management for the practicing physician*. New York, NY: Churchill Livingstone; Woolf, C. J. (2004). Pain: Moving from symptom control toward mechanism-specific pharmacologic management. *Annals of Internal Medicine, 140*, 441–451.

neurological sensitization process starts immediately upon tissue injury, which typically reverses, resulting in the resolution of the pain. However, when this neurological process does not reverse, chronic pain results. The interactions between the ascending and descending pathways are potent and ultimately play a determinant role in chronic pain development, perception, and modulation.

COMPONENTS OF DISABLING CHRONIC PAIN SYNDROMES

Biopsychosocial Component

In addition to the biological and physiological basis for chronic pain, there are strong correlations with psychological and social factors that contribute to the etiology, onset, and progression of chronic pain syndromes. Major psychological contributors to chronic pain may include problems such as a lack of self-control, poor coping, emotional turmoil, low self-esteem, and negative thinking. Social factors that affect chronic pain syndromes are numerous and, among other factors, include gender, culture, family dynamics, employment issues, socioeconomic status, religion, and income.

The importance of understanding and addressing psychosocial contributors to chronic pain syndromes is underscored by the fact that these nonbiological factors can have both an direct and indirect effect on the patient's mind and body. For instance, patients' persistence of negative thinking may preclude them from allowing themselves to ever believe the notion that treatment modalities will relieve their pain. Furthermore, patients' cultural beliefs may limit them from being able to effectively communicate all aspects of their pain to a practitioner. In light of these factors, it is clear that a multidisciplinary approach to the chronic pain patient, including physicians, nurses, psychologists, social workers, and other allied health care professionals, is crucial in the care of a chronic pain patient.

Neuropathic Component

In addition to the nociceptive components that can contribute to acute pain and eventually lead to chronic pain, more subtle neuropathic pain conditions need to be identified early to direct targeted treatment. Neuropathic components are prevalent in scenarios where direct injury to nerve components is obvious (i.e., mechanical nerve trauma) and in settings where obvious pathology to nerves is less explicit (i.e., chronic low back pain). Commonly, the neuropathic component may manifest as numbness, paresthesias, allodynia, hyperalgesia, motor weakness, anhidrosis, and/or dysautonomia. In addition to chronic pain and the aforementioned symptoms, systemic neuropathies due to conditions such as diabetes or chronic alcoholism may produce bowel and bladder dysfunction, heat and cold intolerance, and sexual dysfunction. Therefore, the importance of identifying the neuropathic components is essential for the effective management of any chronic pain syndrome.

Depression and Anxiety Components

An undiagnosed mental illness, especially a depressive or anxious mood disorder, can interfere with the effective treatment of a chronic pain syndrome. Given the high prevalence of depression, anxiety, and other psychiatric conditions in chronic pain patients, it is important to screen patients for the presence of such conditions and refer them for appropriate treatment (Alschuler, Theisen-Goodvich, Haig, & Geisser, 2008). Mental health issues may manifest themselves as lack of motivation, lack of general physical activity, and/or feelings of hopelessness or worthlessness and are often best elucidated by a mental health care professional such as a pain psychologist or psychiatrist. Without addressing the depressive components of chronic pain, patients will continue not only to experience significant impairment in their ability to participate in treatment modalities, but will also be markedly limited in the performance of their basic activities of daily living.

Quality of Life

Given the high incidence of physical and psychosocial impairment in chronic pain patients, the negative effect on a patient's quality of life can be enormous. Detailed functional and psychological assessments of the chronic pain patient can identify areas to address to improve the patient's quality of life. One aspect of coping with chronic pain that has been shown to have a positive association with quality of life is a patient's willingness to accept his or her pain (Mason, Mathias, & Skevington, 2008). The assessment of improvements in the quality of life of a patient suffering from a chronic pain syndrome over time is a useful outcome measure that can be applied to determine the effectiveness of the overall management of a single patient or to assess the advantages of a specific chronic pain therapy.

HEADACHES

Migraine and chronic headache accounts for a large amount of lost work days and costs billions of dollars annually in health care costs and loss of productivity in the United States. Migraineurs cost American employers about 13 billion dollars per year because of missed work days and impaired work function. Direct medical costs for migraine care are about 1 billion dollars per year (Hu, Markson, Lipton, Stewart, & Berger, 1999).

Migraine is a prevalent episodic chronic disease that affects sufferers during their most productive years. Individuals with severe migraine are typically incapacitated by a throbbing headache, nausea and/or vomiting, and sensitivity to light and/or sound (Levin, 2008). A migraine headache is debilitating due to the fact that it interferes with family obligations and social plans, impairs work responsibilities, produces emotional stress, and challenges a health-related quality of life (Levin, 2008).

As opposed to the vast majority of medical syndromes, the diagnosis and development of a treatment plan for headaches relies almost solely on a patient's historical description of his or her symptomatology. The value of laboratory analysis and radiological testing is not in the confirmation of a primary diagnosis of a headache syndrome, but instead in the value of ruling out a secondary cause of pain related to entities such as increased intracranial pressure or vascular pathology.

It is important to assess the extent of impairment and disability in headache sufferers. Self-administered questionnaires that are reliable, validated, and short can be clinically helpful. A number of these have been developed to quantify disability such as the Subjective Symptom Assessment Profile, the Headache Disability Inventory, and the Migraine Disability Assessment Questionnaire.

Migraine and chronic daily headache are serious afflictions with a need to be recognized as serious chronic pain syndromes that can result in disabling problems. Although there are numerous pharmacological, interventional, and behavioral modalities aimed at treating headache syndromes, there is a need for further research into the etiologies, innovative therapies, and economic benefit (Kernick, 2005) that can result in improved management of these chronic pain syndromes.

LOW BACK AND LEG PAIN

Low back pain is one of the most common experiences of humankind. Although studies reveal that back pain affects 60–80% of the adult population in the United States, it is probably experienced by nearly everyone at some point in their life. The point prevalence of low back pain is estimated to be approximately 30%. The diagnosis and treatment of refractory chronic low back pain represents one of the greatest challenges to medicine.

The Quebec Task Force on Spinal Disorders found that more than 90% of low back pain episodes improve spontaneously within 3 weeks of onset. The Task Force recommended against diagnostic tests, including imaging studies, for low back pain within the first 4–6 weeks. In 1994, the Agency for Health Care Policy and Research published guidelines for the treatment of acute low back pain (Bigos et al., 1994). The consensus was that more than 90% of acute low back pain patients recover spontaneously within 1 month regardless of treatment.

Surveys conducted in the United States reveal that low back pain accounts for approximately 15 million office visits annually with total associated health care–related and productivity losses exceeding $100 billion annually. Because of the limitations of currently available medical therapies for low back pain and other conditions, up to 40% of the population resorts to alternative therapeutic modalities (Bigos et al., 1994; Derby, Bogduk, Anat, & Schwarzer, 1993). The portion that continues with conventional medical treatment will often undergo progressively more invasive and expensive therapeutic modalities that may end in one or more surgeries in an attempt to obtain pain relief.

Low back pain is a leading cause of disability in people younger than 45 years and accounts for roughly 40% of all disability claims. The cost of medical treatments, days off from work, and worker's compensation payments result in an annual cost to society of tens of billions of dollars.

The vast majority of low back pain is acute and muscular in origin, although other etiologies should be considered. The differential diagnosis of low back pain is vast, as noted in Table 8.1, which includes visceral and nonmusculoskeletal processes as well. However, the vast majority of low back pain is caused by biomechanical processes that develop with years of poor posture and age-related degenerative changes. The spine and its attached elements degenerate simultaneously, resulting in pain that may originate from multiple sources.

The most common examples include muscle sprains and strains, osteoarthritis of the lumbosacral spine, and other anatomical abnormalities such as herniated nucleus pulposus, degenerative disc disease, and spinal stenosis. The structures that can be major contributors to low back pain are muscles, intervertebral disks, zygapophysial joints, the posterior longitudinal ligament, nerve roots, dura, and ligamentum flavum. Extraspinal sciatica is extremely rare, occurring in 1 in 1,000 patients.

TABLE 8.1 *Some of the Causes of Low Back Pain*

Muscle sprain/strain

Herniated nucleus pulposus

Degenerative disc disease

Annular fissure/tear

Zygapophysial joint arthropathy

Spinal central canal or foraminal stenosis

Osteoarthritis of the hip

Spondylolisthesis

Ankylosing spondylitis

Epidural abscess/hematoma

Discitis

Osteomyelitis

Primary or metastatic cancer

Referred: Abdominal aortic aneurysm, pancreatitis, renal colic, etc.

Other

The typical low back pain patient often suffers from more than one musculoskeletal diagnosis and presents with multiple pain generators. A thorough history and physical examination with particular attention to the musculoskeletal and nervous systems is essential while ruling out more serious conditions such as low back pain of cancer, infection, or vascular etiology. Although commonly performed, the use of magnetic resonance imaging (MRI) and computed tomography (CT) of the lumbar spine has been criticized for their sensitivity, causing the physician to focus on anatomic abnormalities that are unrelated to the patient's pain. The results of MRI or CT scan of the lumbar spine and electromyography (EMG) are not diagnostic and are mainly useful to corroborate clinical suspicions identified during the history and physical examination.

One common pain generator of low back pain is a lumbosacral radiculopathy (spinal nerve root pathology) caused by degeneration of or injury to an intervertebral disc in the spinal column. Disc disease is accompanied by the triggering of an inflammatory cascade, whose chemical mediators in turn exert a noxious effect on the nearby spinal nerves (Mchaourab & Knight, 2009). As these spinal nerves, which exit the spinal cord in the lower back and link the back and the lower extremities to the central nervous system, are irritated, they can transmit inflammatory pain that travels from the lower back to the legs. This is typically manifested in patients' describing pain that starts in their back and characteristically "shoots" down one or both of their legs toward their feet.

Another prevalent cause of low back pain is related to spinal arthropathy and the accompanying inflammation of a key joint of the spinal column known as the zygapophysial or facet joint. The facet joints of the spine run from the cervical region all the way down to the lumbosacral area and are in almost constant motion and play a significant role in allowing twisting, bending, and rotation of the human body. Over time facet joints, similar to any other joint in the body, can become arthritic, destabilize, or lose their cartilage, which causes the bony components of the joint to enlarge and hypertrophy (Czervionke & Fenton, 2008). These changes are accompanied once again by inflammation, which can be a significant pain generator.

Routine clinical evaluations of low back pain patients fail to provide a specific diagnosis in up to 85% of cases (Bigos et al., 1994). Diagnostic spinal injections can provide additional information, which in conjunction with the history, physical examination, and results of imaging studies, may aid in identifying the most probable anatomic basis for the pain. Subsequently, a precisely directed therapeutic spinal injection can provide significant relief with minimal risk to the patient when compared with surgery. The challenge presented to the physician is to identify the major pain generator(s) and to decide which to treat first, while avoiding the structures that appear abnormal on the MRI but do not contribute to the patient's symptoms.

Although some references recommend bed rest for the treatment of low back pain, it has been shown to impede recovery. Prolonged inactivity and deconditioning propagate the conditions underlying the low back pain, making recovery more difficult. Currently, maintenance of the patient's activity and work status, participation in a physical rehabilitation program, and pain management have become the cornerstones of treating low back pain patients.

Because of the dire statistics on persistent low back pain, a patient with low back pain that has persisted beyond a 4-week period should be referred to a specialist. This level of care is necessary to provide the patient with sufficient pain control to allow physical therapy and reverse the physical deconditioning that insidiously develops. For example, Katz (2006) has published that "80 percent of workers who report an episode of low back pain return to work within one month; more than 90% return by 3 months, less than 25% return to work within one year and less than 5 percent never return." Essentially, the longer an individual remains out of work due to low back pain, the lesser the likelihood of them returning back to work.

Low back pain affects costs related to work loss, disability, and worker's compensation. According to published data, there are approximately 150 million work days lost as a result of low back pain every year, and low back pain has been reported to be responsible for 40%

of absences from work, the second leading source of work absences after the common cold (Shaw, Linton, & Pransky, 2006).

Furthermore, back pain is the most common cause for filing worker's compensation claims and the most common cause of work-related disability in people younger than 45 years. Economically, the average cost of a worker's compensation claim for low back pain was $8,300, more than twice the average cost of $4,075 for other compensable claims.

Katz also noted that the 5% of patients who have low back pain and do not return to work by 3 months account for 75% of health care costs incurred by those with low back pain (Katz, 2006). These costs include medications, outpatient visits, physical therapy, peripheral and spinal injections, emergency department visits, hospitalizations, and surgery. As the volume of low back pain–related health care utilization increases without evidence of corresponding clinical improvement, more scientifically validated therapies are demanded by insurers, employers, and other stakeholders.

COMPLEX REGIONAL PAIN SYNDROME

Complex regional pain syndrome (CRPS) is predominantly a neuropathic pain syndrome that develops because of an overreactive peripheral and central nervous system. It often involves the distal extremities, although it has been described in other parts of the body including the head, neck, back, shoulders, and even the viscera. What used to be referred to as "reflex sympathetic dystrophy" and "causalgia" have been reclassified by the International Association for the Study of Pain as "CRPS Type I" and "CRPS Type II," respectively. The syndromes are similar in that they are both characterized by a spectrum of sensory, motor, autonomic, trophic, and dystrophic changes. The differentiating factor between them is the evidence of obvious nerve damage in CRPS Type II that is lacking in CRPS Type I.

Although the pain and characteristic symptoms of CRPS are usually localized over an initial injured location, it is not uncommon for the symptoms to spread to both adjacent and remote unaffected areas. Typically, the most bothersome symptoms for patients can be "electrical" shooting and "burning" pains, but additional complaints may include allodynia, dysesthesia, hyperalgesia, tremors, swelling, hyperhidrosis, edema, color and temperature changes of the skin, inability to use muscles secondary to pain, and painful range of motion leading to atrophy and motion-limiting contractures.

When making the diagnosis of CRPS, it is important to note that the pain and above symptoms need not be confined to the territory of a single peripheral nerve nor does the pain need to be proportionate to the proposed injury from which they presumably arose. In addition, to make the diagnosis of CRPS, the symptoms cannot be attributable to another pathology or condition.

Early recognition and referral of the CRPS patient to a multidisciplinary pain treatment clinic is essential so that the diagnosis can be made and appropriate therapy initiated. A delay in diagnosis and treatment can be a source of devastating impairment as it can result in irreversible physical, neurological, and psychological damage. Common therapies include rehabilitation, pharmacological treatment (i.e., antidepressants, antiinflammatories, bisphosphonates, neuropathic medications, and opioids), psychological counseling, and interventional approaches including diagnostic and therapeutic central and peripheral neural blockade, as well as peripheral nerve or dorsal column stimulation.

PELVIC PAIN

Chronic pelvic pain has been defined as pain causing functional disability that has lasted for at least 6 months and is otherwise not solely attributable to pathologies such as malignancy, inflammatory bowel disease, prostatitis, pelvic inflammatory disease, endometriosis, or dysmenorrhea. It is an ailment that negatively affects a significant number of men and women across the world. In some family practice cohorts, it has been estimated that upward of 20–25% of women suffer from this chronic pain syndrome, a number that rivals that of migraine headaches, back pain, and asthma (Grace & Zondervan, 2004). Although the overall prevalence of the condition is likely much less than that, chronic pelvic pain is a problem that leads to increasing morbidity, health care utilization, and economic impact every year. The appropriate diagnosis and subsequent treatment of pelvic pain can help prevent the deleterious consequences this syndrome can have on patient's personal and occupational well-being.

To date, the etiologies of chronic pelvic pain have yet to be thoroughly elucidated. According to published results, more than 60% of chronic pelvic pain sufferers stated that the cause of their pain had no single identifiable causative factor (Latthe, Latthe, Say, Gülmezoglu, & Khan, 2006). Several immunohistochemically based hypotheses have led to the identification of specific upregulated molecules in human tissues of chronic pelvic pain sufferers. Transient receptor potential vanilloid type-1 has been shown to inhabit a greater percentage of biopsied endometriotic lesions in women with chronic pelvic pain in comparison with their unaffected cohorts (Poli-Neto et al., 2009). In addition, it has been proven that vascular endothelial growth factor manifests a significantly higher expression in association with subsequent immature vascularization in chronic pelvic pain patients (Kiuchi et al., 2009). These exciting new discoveries have not only expanded on previous hypotheses relating the etiology of chronic pelvic pain to vascular and neuropathic causes, but have also laid the groundwork for potential drug therapies that will target the cause of this syndrome, as opposed to the symptomatic treatment that is the current mainstay of treatment.

Despite the myriad of modalities that have been commonly prescribed by physicians for the treatment of chronic pelvic pain, there is no consensus regarding the choice of treatment because of a lack of scientifically proven data regarding various interventions. The spectrum of therapeutic options ranges from the noninvasive to surgery, as depicted in Table 8.2.

A recent Cochrane Library review outlined the documented efficacy and ineffectiveness of several commonly used treatment regimens for chronic pelvic pain (Stones, Cheong, & Howard, 2005). On the basis of data garnered from several randomized controlled trials, the review supported the use of ultrasound scanning in conjunction with reassurance and counseling, the prescription of progesterone or goserelin (a synthetic hormonal analog) for pelvic congestion, and the utilization of a multidisciplinary approach to assessment and treatment as proven effective treatment modalities. Although adhesiolysis, laparoscopic uterine nerve

TABLE 8.2 *Interventions Aimed at Relief of Chronic Pelvic Pain*

Noninvasive	Pharmacological	Surgical
Exercise	NSAIDs	Laparoscopy
Diet modification	Oral contraceptives	Adhesiolysis
Acupuncture	Progesterone	Ventral suspension
Cognitive behavioral therapy	Danazol	Presacral neurectomy
Psychotherapy	GnRH analogs	Laparoscopic uterine nerve ablation
Biofeedback	Intrauterine contraceptive devices	Ovarian vein ligation
Meditation	Antidepressants	Hysterectomy/oophorectomy
Hypnosis	Anticonvulsants	Ovarian drilling
	Analgesics	Endometrial ablation

Note. NSAID = nonsteroidal antiinflammatory drug. *Source:* From Stones, W., Cheong, Y. C., & Howard, F. M. (2005). Interventions for treating chronic pelvic pain in women. *Cochrane Database of Systematic Reviews.* Art. No.: CD000387. DOI: 10.1002/14651858. CD000387.

ablation, extracorporeal shock wave therapy, and the prescription of selective serotonin reuptake inhibitor antidepressants have yet to show a statistically significant benefit in the chronic pelvic pain population in appropriately powered and replicated randomized controlled trials, positive outcomes using these modalities have been described in the literature and thus continue to be used as part of treatment regimens.

With the significant burden that chronic pelvic pain places on both individuals and our society as a whole, further research in the field elucidating the etiology and best practices in diagnosis is needed. In addition, as this chronic pain syndrome continues to cause significant disability and economic hardship related to its multifaceted treatment options, outcomes-based research focusing on the efficacy of both expensive and affordable invasive and noninvasive therapies is warranted.

MULTIDISCIPLINARY PAIN TREATMENT

Over the years, a multidisciplinary approach to the treatment of chronic pain has been proven to be superior to single-discipline treatments such as medication management or rehabilitation alone. As evaluation methods and treatment modalities have evolved, the development of multidisciplinary pain centers has led to the consolidation of a patient's overall chronic pain management. The growth of multidisciplinary centers has also allowed for more effective management of chronic pain patients by not only identifying and alleviating physical and emotional pain, but also implementing effective strategies to help cope with chronic pain. To provide a comprehensive slate of services, a multidisciplinary approach often includes physicians (i.e., anesthesiologists, neurologists, physiatrists, surgeons, radiologists, and psychiatrists), physical therapists, occupational therapists, nurses, psychologists, and providers of complementary medicine.

In addition to its multipronged therapeutic approach to the chronic pain condition, the success of a multidisciplinary approach is rooted in the effective sharing of information and data between members of the multidisciplinary team. Communication and knowledge sharing among team members can help to elucidate the true etiology of a patient's pain and in turn better direct specific therapeutic interventions.

Physiatric Approach

The physiatric approach to chronic pain syndromes emphasizes the performance of a comprehensive musculoskeletal and appropriate neuromuscular history and examination with an emphasis on both structure and function as it applies to diagnosing chronic pain problems and developing rehabilitation programs. The approach includes assessments of static and dynamic flexibility, strength, coordination, and agility of peripheral joint, spinal, and soft tissue in patients with pain conditions. The physiatric approaches discussed elsewhere in the textbook are integrated and utilized concomitantly with the pharmacological, interventional, and sometimes surgical treatments that a patient may also be prescribed to achieve functional restoration by treating multiple problems multidimensionally.

Neurological Approach

The neurological approach entails a detailed neurological history and physical and neurological examination that includes an assessment of mental status, cranial nerves, motor function, sensory function, reflexes, cerebellar function, and gait. Obtaining and interpreting neuroimaging of the brain and/or spine, as well as radiographs of bony structures and joints will not only aid in the diagnosis of a chronic pain pathology but will also help direct appropriate therapy.

Psychiatric Approach

The full psychiatric evaluation of a chronic pain patient to elucidate psychiatric and pain comorbidities can be helpful in the management of chronic pain syndromes. Unrecognized conditions such as substance abuse, mood, anxiety, somatoform, factitious, and personality disorders can hinder the treatment of chronic pain if not simultaneously and appropriately addressed. In addition to counseling patients regarding the potential effects of pain and psychotropic medications on mental status, this arm of the multidisciplinary pain treatment program can be effective at tackling psychosocial contributors to chronic pain pathologies by referring patients for psychological or psychiatric treatments, as well as by teaching patients coping and stress-relieving strategies.

Psychological Approach

Cognitive behavioral therapy (CBT) is a treatment strategy that is commonly used as part of a comprehensive approach to managing chronic pain syndromes. Through CBT, a patient is able to reconceptualize beliefs that pain is uncontrollable and unavoidable into beliefs that it is manageable and does not have to control his or her life. The success of CBT lies in its ability to distract a patient from his or her pain, which will reduce autonomic activity and in turn provide an enhanced sense of self-control. Four commonly used techniques of this approach are explained in the following sections.

Guided Imagery
This technique has the patient focus on a multisensory imaginary scene. Typically, the image is elicited from the patient, and the therapist guides the patient through the image, substituting sensations such as warmth or numbness for pain.

Progressive Muscular Relaxation
By being taught to alternately tense and relax individual muscle groups throughout the body, the patient is able to learn the difference between feelings of tension and relaxation.

Biofeedback
Through the use of modalities such as EMG or nerve stimulation, a chronic pain patient can learn relaxation techniques and the ability to self-regulate physiological pain processes.

Hypnosis
This technique teaches relaxation strategies and enables the patient to experience an analgesic reinterpretation of the pain, experiencing numbness, for example, instead of pain.

CONCLUSION

In sum, it is important to note that successful chronic pain management is best achieved via a coordinated multimodal, multidisciplinary approach. The complex and sometimes cryptic nature of chronic pain syndromes often lend themselves to being best approached in both diagnosis and treatment by providers and modalities from differing specialty backgrounds. In addition, recent literature has shown outcomes supporting the fact that a multidisciplinary approach to chronic pain may actually result in a reduction in overall health care costs (Cunningham, Rome, Kerkvliet, & Townsend, 2009). This fact is important to keep in mind, as the prevalence of and costs associated with chronic pain syndromes are continuing to rise as mentioned throughout this chapter. Therefore, a successful and efficient approach to chronic pain involves a number of different practitioners specializing in multiple disciplines, concurrently applying various interventions in a coordinated, multidisciplinary fashion.

REFERENCES

Alschuler, K. N., Theisen-Goodvich, M. E., Haig, A. J., & Geisser, M. E. (2008). A comparison of the relationship between depression, perceived disability, and physical performance in persons with chronic pain. *European Journal of Pain, 12*, 757–764.

Bigos, S., Bowyer, O., Braen, G., Brown, K., Deyo, R., Haldeman, S., et al. (1994). *Acute low back problems in adults* (Clinical Practice Guidelines No. 14. AHCPR Publication No. 95–0642). Rockville, MD: Agency for Health Care Policy and Research, Public Health Service, U.S. Department of Health and Human Services.

Bonica, J. J. (1990). Anatomic and physical basis of nociceptive and pain. In J. J. Bonica (Ed.), *The management of pain* (2nd ed., pp. 28–94). Philadelphia: Lea & Febiger.

Cunningham, J., Rome, J., Kerkvliet, J., & Townsend, C. (2009). Reduction in medication costs for patients with chronic nonmalignant pain completing a pain rehabilitation program: A prospective analysis of admission, discharge, and 6-month follow-up medication costs. *Pain Medicine, 10*, 787–796.

Czervionke, L., & Fenton, D. (2008). Fat-saturated MR Imaging in the detection of inflammatory facet arthropathy (facet synovitis) in the lumbar spine. *Pain Medicine, 9*, 400–406.

Derby, R. D., Bogduk, N., Anat, D., & Schwarzer, A. (1993). Precision percutaneous blocking procedures for localizing spinal pain. *Pain Digest, 3*, 89–100.

Gill, K., & Frymoyer, J. W. (1997). Management of treatment failures after decompressive surgery. In J. W. Frymoyer (Ed.), *The adult spine: Principles and practice* (2nd ed., 2111–2133). Philadelphia: Lippincott-Raven.

Grace, V. M., & Zondervan, K. T. (2004). Chronic pelvic pain in New Zealand: Prevalence, pain severity, diagnoses and use of the health services. *Australia and New Zealand Journal of Public Health, 28*, 369–375.

Hu, H., Markson, L. E., Lipton, R. B., Stewart, W. F., & Berger, M. L. (1999). Burden of migraine in the United States—Disability and economic costs. *Archives of Internal Medicine, 1*, 813–818.

Katz, J. N. (2006). Lumbar disc disorders and low-back pain: Socioeconomic factors and consequences. *The Journal of Bone Joint Surgery, 88-A*(Suppl.), 21–24.

Kernick, D. (2005). An introduction to the basic principles of health economics for those involved in the development and delivery of headache care. *Cephalalgia, 25*, 709–714.

Kiuchi, H., Tsujimura, A., Takao, T., Yamamoto, K., Nakayama, J., Miyagawa, Y., et al. (2009). Increased vascular endothelial growth factor expression in patients with bladder pain syndrome/interstitial cystitis: Its association with pain severity and glomerulations. *BJU International, 104*, 826–831.

Latthe, P., Latthe, M., Say, L., Gülmezoglu, M., & Khan, K. S. (2006). WHO systematic review of prevalence of chronic pelvic pain: A neglected reproductive health morbidity. *BMC Public Health, 6*, 177.

Levin, M. (2008). The international classification of headache disorders and classification and diagnosis of migraine. In M. Levin (Ed.), *Comprehensive review of headache medicine* (pp. 59–72). New York: Oxford University Press.

Mason, V. L., Mathias, B., & Skevington, S. M. (2008). Accepting low back pain: Is it related to a good quality of life? *Clinical Journal of Pain, 24*, 22–29.

Mchaourab, A., & Knight, K. (2009). Management of axial back pain: A critical view. *Techniques in Regional Anesthesia and Pain Management, 13*, 65–66.

Poli-Neto, O. B., Filho, A. A., Rosa e Silva, J. C., Barbosa, Hde F., Candido Dos Reis, F. J., & Nogueira, A. A. (2009). Increased capsaicin receptor TRPV1 in the peritoneum of women with chronic pelvic pain. *Clinical Journal of Pain, 25*, 218–222.

Raj, P. P. (1996). Pain mechanisms. In P. P. Raj, *Pain medicine: A comprehensive review* (pp. 12–23). St. Louis, MO: Mosby.

Shaw, W., Linton, S., & Pransky, G. (2006). Reducing sickness absence from work due to low back pain: How well do intervention strategies match modifiable risk factors? *Journal of Occupational Rehabilitation, 16*, 591–605.

Stones, W., Cheong, Y. C., & Howard, F. M. (2005). Interventions for treating chronic pelvic pain in women. *Cochrane Database of Systematic Reviews.* Art. No.: CD000387. DOI: 10.1002/14651858. CD000387.

Toth, C., Lander, J., & Wiebe, S. (2009). The prevalence and impact of chronic pain with neuropathic pain symptoms in the general population. *Pain Medicine, 10*, 918–929.

Wenig, C. M., Schmidt, C. O., Kohlmann, T., & Schweikert, B. (2009). Costs of back pain in Germany. *European Journal of Pain, 13*, 280–286.

9

Diabetes Mellitus

David G. Marrero, PhD

INTRODUCTION

Diabetes mellitus is one of the major public health threats in the United States today. There are currently 24 million Americans estimated to have diabetes (American Diabetes Association [ADA], 2004; Centers for Disease Control and Prevention [CDC], 2004; Harris et al., 1998; Mokdad et al., 2001; National Diabetes Fact Sheet, 2003). Moreover, there are more than 65 million Americans with evidence of "prediabetes," a term that has come to represent two less severe disorders of glucose metabolism that precede the clinical diagnosis of type 2 diabetes (National Diabetes Fact Sheet, 2003; HHS, 2002).

Many of these individuals will go on to develop diabetes. As a result, diabetes is now viewed as an "epidemic" by the CDC. Diabetes accounts for more than 220,000 deaths and costs the United States almost $174 billion annually. Individuals with diabetes are significantly more likely than their nondiabetic peers to develop macrovascular (large blood vessel) disease, as well as the microvascular problems of retinopathy, neuropathy, and nephropathy. Such multiple morbidity problems can lead to various forms of functional limitation and disability.

Diabetes is most accurately viewed as a family of diseases characterized by the body's inability to effectively metabolize glucose. This inability is due to defects in insulin secretion and/or insulin action. The result is chronic hyperglycemia (i.e., elevated blood glucose). The chronicity and degree of elevated glucose is associated with many of the long-term diabetes-related health problems (Eastman, 1995; Klein & Klein, 1995).

Classification of Prediabetes and Diabetes

Prediabetes is the term used to describe two less severe disorders of glucose metabolism that precede the clinical diagnosis of type 2 diabetes. The first is the presence of impaired fasting glucose (IFG) defined as a fasting plasma glucose (FPG) of 100–125 mg/dl. The second is the presence of impaired glucose tolerance defined by a plasma glucose level of 140–199 mg/dl, 2 hours after a 75-g oral glucose meal (Knowler Barrett-Connor, et al., 2002; Tuomilehto, Lindstrom, et al., 2001).

The National Diabetes Data Group (1979) and the World Health Organization (WHO, 1980) made similar recommendations for a system of classification and nomenclature of diabetes. The result of their work was a general agreement on five types of diabetes: insulin-dependent diabetes mellitus (IDDM), noninsulin-dependent diabetes mellitus (NIDDM), gestational diabetes mellitus (GDM), malnutrition-related diabetes mellitus, and other types. Each is characterized by fasting hyperglycemia or elevated glucose concentrations during an oral glucose tolerance test (OGTT) in which the individual ingests 75 g of glucose and then has glucose level measured at the fasting state and 1 and 2 hours post-ingestion. The 1979 NDDG classification further included the category of impaired glucose tolerance (IGT), marked by an OGTT (i.e., glucose levels in response to a 75-g glucose meal) response above normal but below the diabetes diagnostic criteria. (For historical purposes, the terms type I and type II replaced "juvenile-onset" and "adult-onset," respectively. One problem with the age-based descriptors is that the elderly may be diagnosed with type I diabetes and increasingly, the young with type 2, hence the elimination of terms referring to age.)

The classification of diabetes further evolved in 1997. The terms IDDM and NIDDM were eliminated and replaced with the terms type 1 and type 2, respectively (The Expert Committee on the Diagnosis and Classification of Diabetes Mellitus, [ECDCDM], 1997). Arabic numbers (1 and 2) are used instead of roman numerals to avoid confusing II with 11. The new terms are used according to etiology: type 1 for diabetes resulting from β-cell destruction typically mediated by the immune system, and type 2 for diabetes resulting from defects in insulin resistance and/or insulin secretion (ECDCDM, 2003). The classification terms IGT and GDM have been retained.

Diagnostic Criteria

In addition to a new nomenclature, the diagnostic criteria for diabetes have also been modified. A diagnosis of diabetes can be based upon any of three criteria (ECDCDM, 1997): (1) a plasma glucose value ~200 mg/dl at any time plus the presence of classic symptoms, such as polyuria (i.e., excessive urination) or polydipsia (i.e., excessive thirst); (2) FPG ~126 mg/dl; or (3) elevated plasma glucose in response to an OGTT performed according to WHO guidelines ~200 mg/dl at the 2-hour time period. Confirmation on a subsequent day of any of these three criteria is strongly recommended. In clinical practice, however, diagnostic confirmation on a subsequent day is rare if the person presents with values significantly above the minimum values.

Prevalence and Incidence of Prediabetes and Diabetes

Prediabetes
Current estimates suggest that more than 64 million persons have prediabetes. When defined by IFG, the annual incidence is between 0.3% and 0.6% (Nichols, Hiller, & Brown, 2008). When the more definitive IGT test is utilized, annual incident increases to 5.1% (de Vegt et al., 2001). When both factors are present, the annual incidence increases to 5.8%. For persons with prediabetes, between 5% and 15% will convert to diagnosed diabetes annually (Mokdad et al., 2001; ADA, 2004).

Diabetes
It is estimated that 24 million Americans or approximately 8% of the U.S. population have diabetes (CDC, 2008). The number of persons with diabetes (and the corresponding prevalence rate) has increased steadily over the past several decades with a steady 5% annual increase since 1990 (Cowie et al., 2009). This is due in part to decreased mortality in persons with diabetes, better and more widespread screening efforts, and corresponding increases in associated risk factors such as obesity and sedentary lifestyle behavior (Kenny, Aubert, & Geiss, 1995).

Approximately 186,000 individuals aged 19 years and 300,000–500,000 persons of all ages have type 1 diabetes in the United States. Consequently, type 1 diabetes accounts for a very small percentage of all cases of diabetes. Although studies vary in their estimates, it is generally accepted that 1.7 per 1,000 individuals have type 1 diabetes, making this one of the most prevalent chronic diseases of childhood. Incidence estimates in the United States suggest a rate of 30,000 new cases per year (Cowie et al., 2009; LaPorte, Matsushima, & Fang, 1995).

Type 2 is clearly the most pervasive form of diabetes in the United States, with an estimated 17.9 million diagnosed cases and an additional 5.7 estimated to have diabetes but not yet diagnosed (National Diabetes Statistics, 2007). Considering persons of all ages, type 2 constitutes 90% or more of all cases of diabetes. In 2007, type 2 had a prevalence rate of about 7% for persons between ages 18 and 44 but climbed to 23% for those 65 and older. The average annual incidence rate for all ages is approximately 625,000 cases, or more than one new case of type 2 diabetes diagnosed every 60 seconds (CDC, 2008; Kenny, Aubert, & Geiss, 1995). A recent study by Narayan, Boyle, Thompson, Sorensen, and Williamson (2003) used data from the National Health Interview Survey (1984–2000) to estimate age-, sex-, and race-/ethnicity-specific lifetime risk of diabetes in the cohort born in 2000 in the United States. These data were used to estimate residual lifetime risk of diabetes, duration with diabetes, and life-years and quality-adjusted life-years lost from diabetes. The estimated lifetime risk of developing diabetes for individuals born in 2000 was 32.8% for men and 38.5% for women. Women have higher residual lifetime risks at all ages. The highest estimated lifetime risk for diabetes is among Hispanics (men 45.4% and women 52.5%) (Narayan et al., 2003).

GDM occurs in approximately 4% of all U.S. pregnancies (Cousins, 1995). Testing for GDM between weeks 24 and 28 of gestation is therefore an important part of obstetric care for women who are at increased risk, for example, above normal body weight, or have a family history of diabetes (ECDCDM, 1997). Identification of GDM is important to reduce the associated fetal morbidities and mortality complications.

Risk Factors for the Development of Diabetes

In general, the stress-diathesis model of illness applies to the development of both types of diabetes—a genetic predisposition interacts with one or more environmental factors, conferring the expression of diabetes. Many factors thought to increase the risk of diabetes have been studied, including demographic, genetic, environmental lifestyle, and physiological. Risk factors are very different for type 1 and type 2, reflecting the differences in etiology between the two forms of the disease. Type 1 is viewed as an autoimmune disease caused by a pathogen that results in the destruction of β cells responsible for the production of insulin. Type 2 is understood as a problem in insulin action (decreased insulin sensitivity) and/or insulin secretion (in a relative, rather than absolute, manner). Whether intervening to reduce a given risk factor would prevent or delay the onset of diabetes is unknown. However, diabetes prevention trials are currently underway for both type 1 and type 2.

Type 1 Risk Factors
SEX, AGE, RACE/ETHNICITY. Men and women have similar incidence rates, indicating gender is not a risk factor for type 1 diabetes. The odds of developing type 1 are greatest at the age of puberty (age 10–14, depending on gender). This increased risk period is thought to be due in part to hormonal changes or growth activity (Dorman, McCarthy, O'Leary, & Koehler, 1995). Whites are generally more susceptible to type 1, with the countries of Finland and Sweden having the highest prevalence of the disease (Dorman et al., 1995). LaPorte et al. (1995) examined racial differences in type 1 incidence across several studies and found a significantly higher rate in Whites compared to either African Americans, Hispanics, or Asians.

GENETIC. Only 20% of new cases of type 1 diabetes are linked to a family history of the disease. The risk of diabetes before age 30 for those with siblings, parents, and offspring with type 1 is 1–15% compared with <1% for those without a family history of the disease (Dorman et al., 1995). The concordance rate for identical twins is 25–50% compared with 10% for a sibling of a person with diabetes (ADA, 1996). The identical twin concordance rates reflect the importance of environmental factors.

ENVIRONMENTAL/LIFESTYLE. There is a seasonal tendency toward greater type 1 diagnosis during winter months. Since flu strains are more common in winter, this lends evidence to a viral agent or other pathogen as a potential, associated contributing factor. Coxsackie B viruses (B2, B3, B4, and B5) and cytomegalovirus have been implicated in type 1 onset, but their potential contribution is not well understood (Dorman et al., 1995).

Nutrition may play a part in the onset of type 1 diabetes, for example, consumption of cow milk. The putative mechanism is a link between bovine serum albumin (BSA) antibodies and diabetes. (BSA may trigger an autoimmune response involving the β cells of the pancreas.) Scott, Norris, and Kolb (1996) examined animal and human dietary evidence and suggest that there are at least three type 1 diabetogenic foods—wheat, soy, and cow milk. More research is needed to better understand the potential contribution of nutritional factors in the onset of type 1 diabetes.

PHYSIOLOGICAL. Compared with people without diabetes, individuals with type 1 are much more likely to exhibit islet cell cytoplasmic antibodies, antibodies to insulin, and/or antibodies to the enzyme glutamic acid decarboxylase (Dorman et al., 1995). It is not known whether these antibodies are directly or indirectly involved in the pathophysiology of type 1.

Type 2 Risk Factors
SEX, AGE, RACE/ETHNICITY. Although some studies suggest a greater prevalence of type 2 in women than in men (ADA, 1996), such observations can be attributable to other risk factors rather than gender, per se. When variables such as obesity and greater utilization of health care services are considered (both more common in women), the female:male ratio approaches 1 (Pareschi & Tomasi, 1989). Regarding age, the onset of type 2 is rare before age 30. After 30, age is directly and strongly related to the development of type 2 in most populations (Rewers & Hamman, 1995). Reaven and Reaven (1985) suggest that much of the association can be attributed to age-related variables such as obesity and physical inactivity (discussed in the "Environmental/lifestyle" factors below).

Prevalence rates of type 2 vary markedly depending on race and ethnic group. The highest rates are found in the American Pima Indians (50%), compared with the near zero prevalence rate in traditional societies such as the Mapuche Indians in Chile (Rewers & Hamman, 1995). United States data indicate that African Americans and Hispanics have rates nearly twice that of non-Hispanic Whites (ADA, 1996).

GENETIC. There is an 11% chance of developing type 2 diabetes by age 70 with no family history of the disease (ADA, 1996). This increases to 45% if both parents have type 2 diabetes. In reviewing studies assessing both monozygotic (MZ) and dizygotic (DZ) twin data, Rewers and Hamman (1995) noted at least a doubling of the concordance rate for MZ versus DZ twin pairs. The MZ concordance rates ranged from 34% to 80% in these reports, with the mean rate substantially lower than 100%. Thus, environmental factors are important in the onset of type 2 diabetes.

Racial admixture data also reflect the (indirect) influence of genetic predisposition toward type 2. The percentage of Native American admixture across different groups (e.g., Pima Indians 100%, Barrio Mexican Indians 46%, and mid-income Mexican Americans 27%) is strongly related to the prevalence rate of type 2 in each group (ADA, 1996). Potential group differences in environmental/lifestyle factors may also play a role in developing the disease.

More than 50 studies have investigated candidate genes for type 2 diabetes (Rewers & Hamman, 1995). Given the methodological challenges involved in this kind of research, how type 2 diabetes is inherited remains unclear. Overall, the data indicate polygenic influences rather than a single major locus influence.

ENVIRONMENTAL/LIFESTYLE. The question of whether specific dietary components (e.g., high sugar, high fat, and low fiber) are diabetogenic has generated much research. Interpretation of such studies is difficult due to methodological concerns. Perhaps the biggest concern is that few dietary components appear to promote diabetes independent of obesity. An exception is a prospective study by Marshall and Hamman (1988) who reported a sevenfold increased risk for a 40 g/day higher fat intake controlling for obesity and other factors. Overall, however, the available longitudinal (prospective) data do not support the hypothesis that dietary composition, per se, promotes the onset of type 2 diabetes (e.g., Bennett, Knowler, Baird, Butler, & Reid, 1984).

Physical inactivity may be a risk factor for type 2 diabetes. Research using a prospective epidemiological design has found that increased caloric expenditure is significantly related to a decreased risk of type 2 diabetes (Helmrich, Ragland, Leung, & Paffenbarger, 1991; Manson et al., 1992). Acute exercise enhances insulin sensitivity, but insulin sensitivity benefits diminish or disappear after only 3 days of inactivity (Schneider, Amorosa, Khachadurian, & Ruderman, 1984). Such evidence suggests adopting a lifestyle of physical activity (e.g., every 2–3 days) for both preventing and controlling type 2 diabetes.

Epidemiological evidence also suggests a strong link between obesity and the risk of developing diabetes. Figure 9.1 shows data combined from two studies, the Nurses Health Study (Carey et al., 1997) and the U.S. Health Professionals Study (Chan, Rimm, Colditz, Stampfer, & Willett, 1994). Both are longitudinal studies that look at the effect of lifestyle on chronic illness. In the male health professional study, men with a body mass index (BMI) more than 35 had a 42.1 times greater age-adjusted risk than men with a BMI less than 23 for developing diabetes. A similar trend was observed in female nurses, with the risk increasing to a staggering 93.2 of developing diabetes with a BMI of greater than 35 kg/m². Moreover, the longer a person

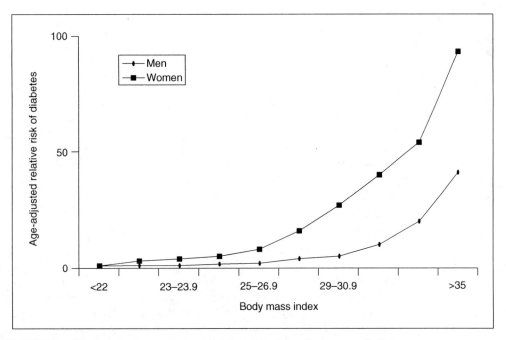

FIGURE 9.1. The link between obesity and the risk of developing type 2 diabetes.

remains obese, the higher the risk of developing type 2 diabetes. In one study, people who have been at a BMI of greater than 30 for more than 10 years have over twice the risk of type 2 diabetes compared with those who have been obese for less than 5 years (Chan et al., 1994).

However, it is important to note that most overweight individuals do not develop diabetes, and conversely, nonobese persons are diagnosed with type 2.

The distribution of a person's adipose (fat) tissue has been repeatedly shown to predict the presence of diabetes. A common index of body fat distribution is the waist-to-hip ratio (WHR), obtained by dividing the circumference of the waist by the circumference of the hip. WHR is a significant predictor of type 2 diabetes (Vague, DeCastro, & Vague, 1986). Intra-abdominal fat assessed by computed tomography scans has also been shown to predict the onset of type 2 (Bergstrom et al., 1990).

PHYSIOLOGICAL. Between 1% and 5% of persons with impaired glucose tolerance develop type 2 each year (ADA, 1996; Meigs, Muller, Nathan, Blake, & Andres, 2003). Thus, while the majority of patients with IGT either remains so or reverts to normal glucose tolerance, elevated blood or plasma glucose is a risk factor for diabetes. Insulin levels have been studied since impairment of insulin secretion/utilization is considered a primary metabolic abnormality in these patients. Both reduced insulin secretion (Kadowaki et al., 1984) and hyperinsulinemia (Haffner & Stem, 1989) have been found to predict diabetes development.

FUNCTIONAL PRESENTATION OF DIABETES

Type 1: At Onset

The onset of symptoms for a person with type 1 diabetes is acute. Classic symptoms include polyuria (frequent urination), polydipsia (frequent drinking), polyphagia (frequent eating), and weight loss. Since the β cells in the pancreas are no longer producing insulin, the body is unable to transfer glucose from the bloodstream into the organs, muscles, and so on. Although there is plenty of fuel (glucose) available in the blood, it cannot reach the target tissues without insulin. The result is often referred to as "starving in the midst of plenty."

Unable to effectively utilize and store food intake, the individual is caught in a vicious cycle. The sensation of hunger promotes polyphagia. Because of polyphagia and lack of insulin, the high concentration of glucose circulates through the kidneys. At or above concentrations of 160–180 mg/dl (the renal threshold), the overload of glucose is excreted in the urine (glycosuria). The body's drive to eliminate excessive glucose promotes polyuria. In turn, the person experiences dehydration, which promotes polydipsia. Caloric loss via glycosuria can be substantial and promote weight loss. In addition, since circulating glucose cannot be used as energy, the body begins to break down fat stores (lipolysis) as an energy source, further promoting weight loss. Lipolysis causes an increase in the blood level of free fatty acids and ketone bodies. Depending on the severity of symptoms, a person may reach a state of diabetic ketoacidosis (DKA), which reflects a dangerously high level of acid in the bloodstream. Although DKA is preventable and treatable, coma and possibly death may result if diagnosis and treatment are delayed.

Type 2: At Onset

The onset of symptoms for a person with type 2 diabetes is much more insidious. This explains in part the large number of undiagnosed cases in the United States. Since increasing age is associated with type 2 diabetes, many individuals perceive the slow onset of symptoms such as loss of energy, getting up at night to urinate, vision difficulties, and so on, as signs of aging. Individuals with type 2 diabetes rarely experience DKA as they do not suffer from absolute insulin deficiency. Given the insidious development of type 2 diabetes, the discrepancy for some patients between meeting the diagnostic criteria for diabetes and actual diagnosis can be years.

Type 1 and 2: Acute Complications

There are several acute complications associated with the disease. Individuals with poorly controlled type 1 diabetes are at risk for DKA, a very serious (but preventable and correctable) metabolic problem. Hospital discharge records note DKA on 3–4% of all diabetes admissions (ADA, 1996). Hypoglycemic episodes are fairly common in persons with type 1 (also called "insulin reactions"), but individuals with type 2 taking insulin or oral medication may also experience hypoglycemia. Two acute, though rather rare, metabolic conditions associated with type 2 are hyperosmolar hyperglycemic nonketotic syndrome and lactic acidosis. In addition, people with diabetes are at greater risk for various forms of infections.

Prediabetes, Type 1 and 2: Long-Term Complications

Microvascular Complications
There are a number of morbidities associated with diabetes that typically take years to develop and may be evidenced during the prediabetes phase (The Diabetes Prevention Program Research Group, 2007). Patients with diabetes are very susceptible to microvascular disease, which can result in damage to the eye (retinopathy), kidney (nephropathy), and nerve functioning (neuropathy). Compared with nondiabetics, individuals with diabetes are 25 times more likely to become blind, 17 times more likely to develop renal disease, and 20 times more likely to develop gangrene (Davidson, 1986). It is believed that chronically elevated glucose levels (duration of diabetes interacting with degree of hyperglycemia) are primarily responsible for these problems (The Diabetes Control and Complications Trial Research Control Group [DCCT Research Group], 1993).

Regarding retinopathy, diabetes is a leading cause of new cases of blindness in adults (12% of all new cases) (ADA, 1996). New research shows that approximately 8% of persons with IGT have evidence of retinopathy (The Diabetes Prevention Program Research Group, 2007). Klein and Klein (1995) reported 97% of insulin-taking and 80% of noninsulin-taking persons who have had diabetes for 15 or more years suffer some form of retinopathy. Bernbaum and Albert (1996) note that many diabetes patients with proliferative retinopathy are not referred for vision-related rehabilitation services by their ophthalmologist or diabetes care provider. There is a strong need to improve referrals to such services.

Nephropathy and renal disease are a common complication of diabetes. Diabetic nephropathy is defined as protein in the urine at a concentration > 30 mg/dl. Approximately 10–21% of persons with diabetes have nephropathy. Progression of nephropathy can lead to end-stage renal disease (ESRD). Diabetes is the primary cause of ESRD and is responsible for approximately one third of new cases. Individuals with type 2 diabetes constitute the majority of new ESRD cases that are related to diabetes. From 1982 to 1991, the percentage of ESRD cases attributable to diabetes increased from 23% to 36%. In a parallel fashion, the mortality for diabetes-related renal disease doubled between 1979 and 1990. ESRD usually develops after some extended diabetes duration, often more than 25 years, and requires dialysis or a kidney transplant for survival (ADA, 1996).

The general definition of neuropathy refers to nerve damage, and there are many forms of diabetic neuropathy. Approximately 60–70% of individuals with type 1 and type 2 diabetes suffer from subclinical or clinical neuropathy (Eastman, 1995). The various neuropathic conditions can have pervasive effects throughout the body. The most common form is peripheral sensory neuropathy, affecting the hands, feet, and legs. Fifty-four percent of individuals with type 1 and 45% of those with type 2 have this form. Carpal tunnel syndrome affects one third of persons with diabetes. Impotence, delayed gastric emptying, and bladder and bowel dysfunction are examples of autonomic neuropathy. Increased risk of silent myocardial infarction and sudden death in patients with diabetes are due in part to autonomic neuropathy (ADA, 1996).

Macrovascular Complications

Persons with prediabetes and type 2 diabetes are at increased risk for large blood vessel disease, the leading cause of mortality in this population. Individuals with diabetes are 2–12 times more likely to suffer from cardiovascular disease (CVD) and 2–4 times more likely to die from heart disease compared with those without diabetes (ADA, 1996). Peripheral arterial disease (PAD) affects about 10% of all patients with diabetes, but the rate is much higher with a disease duration > 20 years. Peripheral vascular disease (PVD)/PAD interferes with blood and oxygen flow to the lower extremities. PVD/PAD in concert with peripheral sensory neuropathy can lead to foot ulcerations, gangrene, and amputation. Approximately half of all nontraumatic amputations in the United States occur in patients with diabetes (ADA, 1996; Palumbo & Melton, 1995). In addition, stroke is 2–4 times more common, making cerebrovascular disease another significant morbidity associated with diabetes.

Mortality

Persons with prediabetes have a 150% increase in their 5-year risk for CVD-related mortality and a 50–60% increase in total mortality (Barr et al., 2007; Morrish, Wang, Stevens, Fuller, & Keen, 2001). Portuese and Orchard's (1995) review indicates that more than 15% of persons diagnosed with type 1 in childhood will be dead by the age of 40, reflecting a mortality some 20 times that seen in the general population. Improved therapeutic modalities, however, have improved these statistics (Dahlquist & Kallen, 2005; Orchard et al., 2004). Mortality in type 2 individuals is also elevated compared with the general U.S. population but to a lesser degree. When type 2 onset occurs in middle age, these persons are observed to lose about 5–10 years of life expectancy. The onset of type 2 in people ≥ 70 years of age has negligible effects on life expectancy (Geiss, Herman, & Smith, 1995).

Economic Costs of Prediabetes and Diabetes

Prediabetes

Prediabetes is associated with statistically higher rates of ambulatory visits for hypertension; endocrine, metabolic, and renal complications and general medical conditions. It is also associated with a slight, but not statistically significant, increase in visit rates for neurological symptoms, PVD, and CVD. Extending these findings to the 57 million adults with prediabetes in 2007 suggests that national annual medical costs of prediabetes exceed $25 billion. Prediabetes is also associated with excessive use of ambulatory services for comorbidities known to be related to diabetes (Zhang et al., 2009).

Diabetes

Given the extensive morbidity and mortality problems related to diabetes, estimates of the direct and indirect costs attributable to the disease in 2007 totaled more than $174 billion with $116 billion attributed to medical expenditures with $27 billion for diabetes care, $58 billion for chronic diabetes-related complications, and $31 billion for excess general medical costs. Indirect costs resulting from increased absenteeism, reduced productivity, disease-related unemployment disability, and loss of productive capacity because of early mortality totaled $58 billion. This is an increase of $42 billion since 2002. This 32% increase means the dollar amount has raised $8 billion more each year. The 2007 per capita annual costs of health care for people with diabetes is $11,744 a year and of which $6,649 (57%) is attributed to diabetes. One out of every five health care dollars is spent caring for someone diagnosed with diabetes, while one in ten health care dollars is attributed to diabetes. Since the prevalence of type 2 diabetes is significantly greater than the prevalence of type 1, type 2 diabetes is responsible for most of the economic burden of diabetes (ADA, 2008).

Gestational Diabetes

There are an estimated 180,000 GDM pregnancies resulting in delivery each year. Because of complications in both birthing and neonatal factors associated with GDM, there is an additional average increase of $3,305 per pregnancy plus $209 in the newborn's first year of life. As a result of these statistics, GDM increased national medical costs by $636 million in 2007 to $596 million for maternal costs and $40 million for neonatal costs (Chen et al., 2009).

Reducing or Preventing the Incidence of Diabetes

Randomized controlled trials have shown that modest lifestyle changes can prevent or delay the onset of diabetes in adults who have impaired glucose tolerance (IGT), a form of prediabetes that is defined by a plasma glucose level of 140–199 mg/dl, 2 hours after a 75-g oral glucose meal. The Diabetes Prevention Program (DPP) found that the development of diabetes could be reduced by 58% over 3 years when overweight or obese adults with IGT were offered an intensive lifestyle intervention involving modest weight loss and regular physical activity (Knowler et al., 2002). Unfortunately, the DPP lifestyle intervention remains unavailable in most settings, because the study's recruitment and intervention strategies have been challenging to implement in the "real world" (Glasgow et al., 2003).

Treatment of Prediabetes and Diabetes

Prediabetes

There are currently two approaches to the treatment of prediabetes (Padwal, Majumdar, Johnson, Varney, & McAlister, 2005). First is the use of selected pharmacological agents that are used for the treatment of diabetes. In controlled research studies, the use of Acarbose was associated with a 27% reduction in risk for diabetes in persons with IGT (Chiasson et al., 2003). In the DPP study, metformin was associated with a 31% reduction in risk. The use of thiazolidinediones has also been shown to reduce risk for diabetes in persons with IGT (Durbin, 2004). In all of these cases, it is important to note that all of the medications that have been used for prevention research are not FDA approved for the indication of prediabetes.

The second treatment approach is the use of personalized lifestyle interventions. Three major research studies have demonstrated that lifestyle interventions that promote modest weight loss and increased physical activity can significantly delay or possibly prevent the onset of type 2 diabetes in persons with prediabetes. The first was the Da Qing study, which screened more than 110,000 men and women for IGT in 33 health centers in China. The investigators identified 577 persons (mean age 45 and mean BMI 25.8 kg/m^2) with IGT and randomized them by clinic to receive either standard care (i.e., the control condition) or one of three interventions: diet only, exercise only, or a combined diet and exercise intervention. After 6 years of observation, the Da Qing study showed a 31% reduction in risk of developing diabetes for the diet intervention, a 46% reduction for the exercise intervention, and a 41% reduction for the combined diet and exercise intervention. This was the first study that clearly demonstrated that implementing a personalized lifestyle intervention was both feasible and effective for the prevention of type 2 diabetes (Pan et al., 1997).

The next major clinical trial of lifestyle as a prevention modality for type 2 diabetes was the Finish Diabetes Prevention (FDP) study. The FDP recruited and randomized 522 adults aged 40–65 with IGT to receive either a control or a lifestyle intervention. Subjects assigned to the control condition received written and oral general information about a weight loss diet and benefits of exercise provided at baseline and annually. Subjects assigned to the intervention condition were provided detailed, individualized instructions on achieving study goals: weight loss of at least 5% of their body weight at entry into the study and moderate exercise for at least 30 minutes per day. At the end of 4 years, subjects in the intervention condition showed a 58% reduction in risk of developing diabetes compared with controls.

The largest and most rigorous prevention trial to date is the DPP. The DPP recruited 3,234 subjects aged 25–75 with IGT. Subjects were randomized into one of three conditions: an intensive lifestyle intervention, a medication intervention, or a medication placebo control condition. Subjects in the lifestyle intervention were encouraged to lose at least 7% of their initial body weight and to maintain this weight loss throughout the trial.

At the end of 3 years, trial data warranted an early termination of the study. Subjects in the lifestyle condition had a 58% reduction in risk of developing diabetes, and subjects in the medication arm had a 31% reduction when compared with control subjects. In addition, the interventions were effective regardless of race or age (Knowler et al., 2002)

Since the DPP, at least four trials have been conducted that reinforce the ability of lifestyle modification to significantly reduce the risk of developing diabetes in persons with prediabetes (Gilles et al., 2007). Collectively, if results of the primary prevention trials that assessed lifestyle interventions are pooled, they average a 51% reduction in risk, as noted below in Figure 9.2.

Treatment of Diabetes

Although diabetes is a medical problem, effective management relies heavily on the patient to perform the appropriate self-care behaviors. Given the complexity and chronicity of diabetes self-management coupled with the lack of an effective health care model for managing diabetes (Etzwiler, 1997), most patients with diabetes do not achieve proper glycemic control.

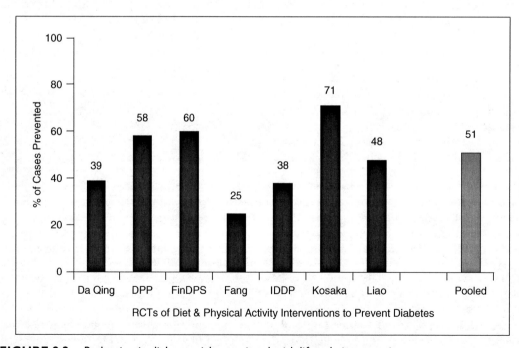

FIGURE 9.2. Reduction in diabetes risk associated with lifestyle interventions.

Treatment Goals

For prediabetes, the primary treatment is reducing body weight by at least 7% of baseline or by the selective use of medications. Type 1 and 2 diabetes are characteristically different in terms of age at onset (and hence developmental challenges), level of obesity, lipid abnormalities, and other factors. Consequently, the focus of treatment is not identical for both forms of the disease.

The primary goals of treatment for type 1 diabetes are to (1) establish and maintain medical and psychological well-being; (2) avoid severe and frequent episodes of hypoglycemia, symptomatic hyperglycemia, and DKA; and (3) promote proper growth and development in children and adolescents (ADA, 1994a). A secondary goal is to provide the individual family with the resources required to achieve optimal glycemic control in order to prevent/delay the diabetes-related micro- and macrovascular complications. The primary goals are viewed as very reasonable; the secondary goal requires much more effort and resources to achieve, however, they also provide greater benefits.

Primary treatment goals for patients with type 2 diabetes are to (1) promote normal metabolism (glucose and lipid) and (2) prevent or minimize micro- and macrovascular complications (ADA, 1994b). Since the majority of patients with type 2 diabetes are obese, normalizing lipid levels, blood pressure, and body weight are important for managing potential macrovascular complications.

Treatment Components

There are four basic components to the treatment of diabetes: medication (insulin, oral hypoglycemic agents), nutrition therapy, exercise, and self-monitoring of blood glucose (SMBG). Each component must be individualized for the patient. Medication, food intake, and exercise must be carefully balanced so the person maintains desirable glucose levels and avoids hypo- and hyperglycemia. SMBG is used as feedback to determine which aspects of the treatment regimen need adjustment.

Medication

For type 1 diabetes, all patients must take exogenous insulin to survive as they have an absolute or near-absolute deficiency in endogenous insulin production. The optimal goal of insulin administration is to mimic normal insulin secretion. However, this requires multiple daily injections (≥ 3/day) or use of an insulin infusion pump. Many type 1 patients do not want such an intensive regimen and opt for a twice-daily regimen, mixing both short-term and long-term insulins in each injection. In general, a twice-daily regimen yields poorer glycemic control compared to an MDI or pump approach (ADA, 1994a). The diabetes health care team and the patient must work together to determine an insulin administration plan that is acceptable to both parties while achieving the best possible glycemic control.

Medications for patients with type 2 include oral agents and insulin. Some type 2 patients are able to control their blood glucose with diet and exercise and do not need medication. However, this is a small minority. When diet alone is not successful, oral agents and possibly insulin are typically introduced in a stepped care approach.

Medical Nutrition Therapy

Regarding type 1 diabetes, current guidelines for macro nutrient intake suggest calories be distributed as follows: protein—10–20%; fat—< 10% from saturated fat, $\leq 10\%$ from polyunsaturated fat; this leaves the remaining 60–70% to come from carbohydrate and monounsaturated fat (ADA, 1998b). These guidelines are much more flexible than those used in the past. Consequently, terms such as "Medical Nutrition Therapy" (MNT) or "meal planning" are used to better convey the current approach of determining proper caloric intake according to a set of nutrition-related goals. The primary aim of MNT is to promote proper glucose metabolism. Additional MNT goals for type 1 include healthy lipid levels, distribution of calories and types of foods to promote normal growth and development in children and adolescents, and prevention/treatment of hypoglycemic episodes (ADA, 1998b). All of these goals are developed with the individual while considering the person's health status, eating habits, cultural food preferences, and exercise habits.

MNT goals for persons with type 2 diabetes emphasize problems commonly seen in this population, for example, obesity, hypertension, and elevated lipid levels. Thus, in addition to normalizing glucose levels, primary goals for type 2 include modifying the quantity and quality of food intake to reduce weight, blood pressure, and blood lipids.

Exercise

Exercise is recommended for individuals with diabetes. The potential benefits may include (1) decreased risk of CVD via reducing obesity, blood pressure, and elevated lipid levels, and by increasing HDL levels; (2) increased insulin sensitivity which may enhance glycemic control and decrease dosage of antidiabetic medication; (3) improvements in mood and self-esteem; (4) enhancing quality of life and activities of daily living (ADLs) by improving muscle strength and joint flexibility; and (5) promoting weight reduction and maintenance of weight loss (ADA, 1994a, 1994b).

Potential risks associated with exercise for patients with diabetes are also numerous. These may include (1) cardiovascular effects such as arrhythmias due to ischemic heart disease, significant increases in blood pressure, and orthostatic hypotension following exercise; (2) microvascular problems such as retinal hemorrhage and increased proteinuria in patients with such preexisting problems; (3) metabolic decompensation such as promoting hyperglycemia due to too little insulin when exercise is started, or hypoglycemia if too much insulin is present; and (4) musculoskeletal and related problems such as aggravating preexisting joint disease, and orthopedic injury and foot ulcers related to neuropathy (ADA, 1994a,b). The benefit:risk ratio can be maximized by careful planning (with appropriate diabetes care providers) and tailoring physical activities to the person.

Self-Monitoring of Blood Glucose

SMBG provides feedback regarding the effects of recent behavior (medication use, food intake, exercise) on blood glucose control. When used appropriately (i.e., accurate measurement and results properly used to modify regimen behavior), SMBG can be a powerful tool in optimizing glycemic control (The DCCT Research Group, 1993). However, SMBG performance and/or its results to guide eating or insulin adjustments are used by a minority of type 1 patients seen in an outpatient clinic setting (Fekete, Guare, Marrero, & Orr, 1997). Thus, SMBG is best viewed as a self-management tool, and there is no reason to believe it will enhance glycemic control unless it is used properly.

PSYCHOLOGICAL AND VOCATIONAL IMPLICATIONS

There are a number of psychological/behavioral and vocational issues relevant to diabetes. This section addresses adherence, stress, depression, eating disorders, insulin manipulation for weight control, sexual dysfunction, and adjustment to disability. These topics are representative of the psychosocial concerns in the diabetes literature and should not be construed as exhaustive.

Adherence

Given the multiple health behaviors involved in the self-management of diabetes, adherence should not be viewed as a unitary construct. Research has shown that an individual may adhere well to one behavior (e.g., SMBG) but not another (e.g., meal plan) (Johnson, 1994). Consequently, attempts to measure diabetes adherence behavior should be domain specific.

Issues with adherence are also more commonplace with pediatric patients, notably adolescents (Sussman-Stillman, Hyson, Anderson, & Collins, 1997).

Partial or inconsistent adherence to one's diabetes treatment regimen is common (Kovacs, Goldston, Obrosky, & Iyengar, 1992). Patients often report greatest difficulty following the meal plan component (Ary, Toobert, Wilson, & Glasgow, 1986). Research also indicates that an average of 16% (range 0–50%) of the foods consumed by patients in a typical week would promote hyperglycemia (Fekete et al., 1997). The least difficult aspect of the regimen involves taking medication. However, though most patients take their medication, many do not wait the appropriate amount of time between insulin administration and eating (Hains, Berlin, Davies, Parton, Alemzadeh, 2006; Johnson, 1994).

Stress

Psychological stress has been thought to promote hyperglycemia and thus worsen glycemic control. Two mechanisms have been proposed to account for this hypothesis. Stress may indirectly affect blood glucose by interfering with one's behavior, for example, eating, exercise, and so on, which in turn promotes hyperglycemia. Another possibility is that glucose metabolism may be directly compromised by the neuroendocrine effects associated with stress, for example, increased catecholamine and/or cortisol levels.

Overall, the evidence that stress promotes metabolic decompensation in persons with diabetes is equivocal. The hypothesis that stress interferes with adherence to the type 1 regimen and consequently raises blood glucose has received mixed support (Hanson, Henggeler, & Burghen, 1987; Schafer, Glasgow, McCaul, & Dreher, 1983). Correlational studies have found that increased levels of stressful life events or daily hassles is significantly related to poorer glycemic control in persons with type 1 (Cox, Taylor, Nowacek, Holley-Wilcox, & Pohl, 1984) and type 2 diabetes (Aikens & Mayes, 1997). Conversely, lack of stress-induced hyperglycemia has been reported in laboratory research manipulating acute stressors in type 1 (Kemmer et al., 1986) and type 2 diabetes (Bruce, Chisholm, Storlien, Kraegen, & Smythe, 1992). Stabler, Morris, Litton, Feinglos, and Surwit (1986) reported a greater blood glucose elevation in response to a competitive video task in Type A behavior versus Type B behavior children with diabetes. Thus, the need to account for individual differences in response to stress is important.

Depression

Individuals with diabetes have to cope with the demands of managing an incurable disease, possibly putting them at risk for certain psychological problems. Depression has received the most attention in the area of diabetes. The finding that depression is more common in individuals with diabetes than healthy persons is well established. Garvard, Lustman, and Clouse (1993) conducted a systematic review of the depression and diabetes prevalence literature (20 studies). They concluded that approximately 15–20% of persons with type 1 or 2 diabetes experience major depression at some point during their life, a rate several times that of the general population. However, it is unclear whether persons with diabetes are more likely to experience depression compared to persons with other chronic medical conditions. Thus, the question remains if the increased risk is due to having a chronic disease or diabetes, per se.

Griffith and Lustman (1997) note the limited data addressing gender and suggest that depression in diabetes seems to follow the 2:1 female-to-male ratio seen in the general population. Given the recurring nature of depressive episodes and their significant impact on the person, diagnosing and treating depression in patients with diabetes should be an integral part of diabetes care. This is especially true for women.

Eating Disorders

There is substantial pressure on women in our society to be thin. Successful management of diabetes requires close attention to food intake. It has been hypothesized that young women with diabetes are at increased risk of eating disorders, especially bulimia nervosa. Initial research using self-report measures of eating-disordered behavior seems to support this hypothesis; however, two problems exist with self-report measures (Wing, Nowalk, Marcus, Koeske, & Finegold, 1986). One, while such measures are informative, they cannot be used to make a diagnosis of eating disorders. Two, persons with diabetes often endorse items that are appropriate for diabetes management, resulting in an artificially inflated score, for example, "I pay close attention to the food I eat."

Recent research using a structured interview format and appropriate comparison subjects indicates that the prevalence of eating disorders is relatively low in women with diabetes and comparable to that of their nondiabetic peers (Peveler, Boller, Fairburn, & Dunger, 1992). However, subclinical eating-disordered behavior is a substantial problem. For example, scores on the Bulimia test-revised (BULIT) were a significant and independent predictor of glycemic control in adolescents and young adult females with diabetes (Guare et al., 1997a).

Insulin Manipulation for Weight Control

Adolescent females with diabetes are significantly more dissatisfied with their weight/body shape than their male counterparts, and such attitude differences diverge even more so as adolescence progresses (Guare & Orr, 1995). Individuals with type 1 diabetes can reduce/omit their insulin dose which will promote loss of calories via glycosuria. Recent research indicates that type 1 females aged 14–24 both decrease and skip their insulin dose specifically for weight control purposes significantly more often than type 1 males (Guare et al., 1997b). Screening for weight dissatisfaction and possible insulin manipulation should be considered in type 1 females in this age category.

Sexual Dysfunction

Erectile dysfunction or impotence is reported by 50% of men with diabetes (Waxman, 1980). Both physiological and psychological factors may contribute to this problem. Women with type 2 (but not type 1) diabetes also report greater disturbance in sexual functioning compared to healthy women without diabetes in areas of sexual desire, orgasmic capacity, and lubrication (Schreiner-Engel, Schiavi, Vietorisz, & Smith, 1987). However, research addressing sexual dysfunction in women with diabetes is relatively new and has produced mixed results. It is also not clear if diabetes has an organic contribution to sexual problems in women as it does in men. Future sexual dysfunction research should stress the importance of assessing psychological and physiological factors and emphasize the study of women.

Disability and Employment

The following is based on a review of disability and diabetes by Songer (1995). Between 20 and 50% of persons with diabetes report some form of disability, rates substantially higher than the general population. Activity limitations as well as restricted-activity days are reported 2–3 times as often by patients with diabetes. Increasing age and minority group status are associated with greater impairment in activity and/or work. Reported activity limitations affect persons with type 2 (50.2%) more so than type 1 (42.3%), and is especially high for type 2 individuals taking insulin (63.5%). Long-term complications are a primary cause of disability.

Individuals with type 1 who are also disabled have higher rates of unemployment (49%) compared to nondisabled persons (12%). The same pattern holds true for absenteeism, 13.8 versus 3.0/days per year. The average number of physician visits per year is double that for disabled persons with diabetes compared to those without disability. ADLs are more likely to be limited by persons with diabetes (type 1—8.8%, type 2—4.9%) than by those without (2.3%).

SUMMARY/FUTURE DIRECTIONS

Diabetes is a serious medical disorder that places significant demands on the person and health care system. However, substantial progress has been made in the field of primary prevention and the care of diabetes. Strong evidence illustrates that type 2 diabetes can be significantly delayed or even prevented by modest lifestyle changes in persons with increased risk. Pharmaceutical companies have developed new antidiabetic medications (both oral and insulin) whose effects on long-term glycemic control are promising but as yet undetermined. Nonpharmacological efforts such as behavioral weight loss and interventions for overweight patients with type 2 diabetes have demonstrated improved glucose metabolism (Williams, Kelley, Mullen, & Wing, 1998). In addition, the ongoing development of minimally-invasive and noninvasive blood glucose meters for daily patient use will hopefully improve diabetes self-care behavior. Perhaps most importantly, intensive management of type 1 diabetes significantly reduces the risk of diabetes-related sequelae. Whether the health care system will support and patients choose an intensive treatment approach to reduce long-term complications and disability remains to be seen.

REFERENCES

Aikens, E., & Mayes, R. (1997). Elevated glycosylated albumin in NIDDM is a function of recent everyday environmental stress. *Diabetes Care, 20,* 1111–1113.

American Diabetes Association. (1994a). *Medical management of insulin dependent (type II) diabetes* (2nd ed.). New York: American Diabetes Association.

American Diabetes Association. (1994b). *Medical management of non-insulin dependent (type II) diabetes* (3rd ed.). New York: American Diabetes Association.

American Diabetes Association. (2008). Economic costs of diabetes in the U.S. in 2007. *Diabetes Care, 31,* 596–615.

American Diabetes Association. (1996). *Diabetes vital statistics.* New York: American Diabetes Association.

American Diabetes Association. (1998a). Economic consequences of diabetes mellitus in the U.S. in 1997. *Diabetes Care, 21,* 296–309.

American Diabetes Association. (1998b). Nutritional recommendations and principles for people with diabetes mellitus. *Diabetes Care, 21,* S32–S35.

American Diabetes Association. *National Diabetes Fact Sheet.* Retrieved May 2, 2004, from http://www. diabetes.org/diabetes-statistics/national-diabetes-fact-sheet.jsp

Ary, D. V., Toobert, D., Wilson, W., & Glasgow, R. E. (1986). Patient perspective on factors related to nonadherence to diabetes regimen. *Diabetes Care, 9,* 168–172.

Barr, E. L., Zimmet, P. Z., Welborn, T. A., Jolley, D., Magliano, D. J., Dunstan D.W., et al. (2007). Risk of cardiovascular and all-cause mortality in individuals with diabetes mellitus, impaired fasting glucose, and impaired glucose tolerance: The Australian Diabetes, Obesity, and Lifestyle Study (AusDiab). *Circulation, 116,* 151–157.

Bennett, P. H., Knowler, W. C., Baird, H. R, Butler, D. J., & Reid, I. M. (1984). Diet and development of non-insulin-dependent diabetes mellitus: An epidemiological perspective. In G. Pozza, P. Micossi, A. L. Catapano, & R. Pauletti (Eds.), *Diet, diabetes and atherosclerosis* (pp. 109–119). New York: Raven Press.

Bergstrom, R. W., Newell-Morris, L. L., Leonetti, D. L., Shuman, W. P., Wahl, W. P., & Fujimoto, W. Y. (1990). The association of elevated C-peptide level and increased intraabdominal, fat distribution with development of NIDDM in Japanese-American men. *Diabetes, 39,* 104–111.

Bernbaum, M., & Albert, S. G. (1996). Referring patients with diabetes and vision loss for rehabilitation: Who is responsible? *Diabetes Care, 19,* 175–177.

Bruce, D. G., Chisholm, D. J., Storlien, L. H., Kraegen, E. W., & Smythe, G. A. (1992). The effects of sympathetic nervous system activation and psychological stress on glucose metabolism and blood pressure in subjects with type II non-insulin dependent diabetes mellitus. *Diabetologia, 35,* 835–843.

Carey, V. J., Walters, E. E., Colditz, G. A., Solomon, C. G., Willet, W. C., Rosner, B. A., et al. (1997). Body fat distribution and risk of non-insulin-dependent diabetes mellitus in women: the Nurses' Health Study. *American Journal of Epidemiology, 145,* 614–619.

CDC. (2008). State-specific incidence of diabetes among adults—Participating states, 1995–1997 and 2005–2007. *MMWR, 57,* 1169–1173.

Centers for Disease Control and Prevention (2008). State-specific prevalence of obesity among adults—United States, 2007. *Morbidity and Mortality Weekly Report, 57,* 765–768.

Chan, J. M., Rimm, E. B., Colditz, G. A., Stampfer, M. J., & Willett, W. C. (1994). Obesity, fat distribution, and weight gain as risk factors for clinical diabetes in men. *Diabetes Care, 17,* 961–969.

Chen, Y., Quick, W. W., Yang, W., Zhang, Y., Baldwin, A., Moran, J., et al. (2009). Cost of gestational diabetes in the United States in 2007. *Popular Health Management, 12,* 165–174.

Chiasson, J., Josse, R., Gomis, R., Hanefeld, M., Karasik, A., & Laakso, M. (2003). Acarbose for prevention of type 2 diabetes mellitus: The STOP-NIDDM randomised trial. *The Lancet, 359,* 2072–2077, 2003.

Cousins, L. (1995). Obstetric complications. *Diabetes mellitus and pregnancy: Principles and practice* (2nd ed.). New York: Churchill Livingstone.

Cowie, C. C., Rust, K. F., Ford, E. S., Eberhardt, M. S., Byrd-Holt, D. D., Li, C., et al. (2009). Full accounting of diabetes and pre-diabetes in the U.S. population in 1988–1994 and 2005. *Diabetes Care, 32,* 287–294.

Cox, D. J., Taylor, A. G., Nowacek, G., Holley-Wilcox, P., & Pohl, S. (1984). The relationship between psychological stress and insulin-dependent diabetic blood glucose control: preliminary investigations. *Health Psychology, 3,* 63–75.

Dahlquist, G., & Kallen, B. (2005) Mortality in childhood—Onset type 1 Diabetes. A population-based study. *Diabetes Care, 28,* 2384–2387.

Davidson, M. B. (1986). *Diabetes mellitus: Diagnosis and treatment.* New York: Wiley.

de Vegt, F., Dekker, J. M., Jager, A., Hienkens, E., Kostense, P. J., Stehouwer, C. D., et al. (2001). Relation of impaired fasting and postload glucose with incident type 2 diabetes in a Dutch population: The Hoorn Study. *Journal of the American Medical Association, 285,* 2109–2113.

Dorman, J. S., McCarthy, B. J., O'Leary, L. A., & Koehler, A. (1995). *Risk factors for insulin dependent diabetes. Diabetes in America* (2nd ed.). Bethesda, MD: NIH publication No. 95–1468.

Durbin, R. J. (2004). Thiazolidinedione therapy in the prevention /delay of type 2 diabetes in patients with impaired glucose tolerance and insulin resistance. *Diabetes, Obesity, & Metabolism, 6,* 280–285.

Eastman, R. C. (1995). *Neuropathy in diabetes. Diabetes in America* (2nd ed.). Bethesda, MD: NIH publication No. 95–146.

Etzwiler, D. D. (1997). Chronic care: A need in search of a system. *The Diabetes Educator, 23,* 569–573.

Fekete, D., Guare, G., Marrero, D., & Orr, D. (1997). Self-management of "Off-Diet" food intake by adolescents and young adults with insulin-dependent diabetes mellitus. *Diabetes, 46,* 265A.

Garvard, J. A., Lustman, P. J., & Clouse, R. E. (1993). Prevalence of depression in adults with diabetes: An epidemiological evaluation. *Diabetes Care, 16,* 1167–1178.

Geiss, L. S., Herman, W. H., & Smith, P. I. (1995). Mortality in non-insulin dependent diabetes. *Diabetes in America* (2nd ed.). Bethesda, MD: NIH publication No. 95–1468.

Gilles, C. L., Abrams, K. R., Lambert, P, C., Cooper, N. J., Sutton, A. J., Hsu, R. T., et al. (2007). Pharmacological and lifestyle interventions to prevent or delay type 2 diabetes in people with impaired glucose tolerance: systematic review and meta-analysis. *British Medical Journal, 334,* 299.

Griffith, L. S., & Lustman, P. J. (1997). Depression in women with diabetes. *Diabetes Spectrum, 10,* 216–223.

Guare, J. C., Marrero, D., Orr, D., Kakos-Kraft, S., Fineberg, N., & Friedenberg, G. (1997a). Predictors of diabetic control in male and female adolescents and young adults with IDDM. *Diabetes, 46,* 266A.

Guare, J. C., Marrero, D., Orr, D., Kakos-Kraft, S., Fineberg, N., Friedenberg, G. (1997b). Bulimia symptomatology and insulin manipulation in males and females with 100M. *Diabetes, 46,* 265A.

Guare, J. C., Orr, D. P. (1995). Changes in weight-related attitudes over a 2-year period in male and female adolescents with IODM. *Diabetes, 44,* 97A.

Haffner, S. M., & Stern, M. P. (1989). Hyperinsulinemia is associated with 8-year incidence of NIDDM in Mexican Americans. *Diabetes, 38*(Suppl. 1), 92A.

Hains, A. A., Berlin, K. S., Davies, W. H., Parton, E. A., & Alemzadeh, R. (2006). Attributions of adolescents with type 1 diabetes in social situations. *Diabetes Care, 29,* 818–822.

Hanson, C. L., Henggeler, S. W., & Burghen, G. A. (1987). Model of associations between psychosocial variable and health-outcome measures of adolescents with IODM. *Diabetes Care, 10,* 752–758.

Harris, M. I., Flegal, K. M., Cowie, C. C., Eberhardt, M. S., Goldstein, D. E., Little, R. R., et al. (1998). Prevalence of diabetes, impaired fasting glucose, and impaired glucose tolerance in U.S. adults. The Third National Health and Nutrition Examination Survey, 1988–1994. *Diabetes Care, 21,* 518–524.

Helmrich, S. P., Ragland, D. R., Leung, R. W., & Paffenbarger, R. S. (1991). Physical activity and reduced occurrence of non-insulin-dependent diabetes mellitus. *New England Journal of Medicine, 325,* 147–152.

HHS. (2002). *ADA warn Americans of "pre-diabetes," encourage people to take healthy steps to reduce risks.* U.S. Department of Health and Human Services; HHS Press Release March 27, 2002. Retrieved March 2, 2009 from http://www.hhs.gov/news/press/2002pres/20020327.html.

Johnson, S. B. (1994). Methodological issues in diabetes research: Measuring adherence. *Diabetes Care, 15,* 1658–1667.

Kadowaki, T., Miyake, Y., Hayura, R., Akanuma, Y., Kajinuma, H., Kuznya, N., et al. (1984). Risk factors for worsening to diabetes in subjects with impaired glucose tolerance. *Diabetologia, 26,* 44–49.

Kemmer, F. W., Bisping, R., Steingruber, H. J., Baar, H., Hardtmann, F., Schlaghecke, R., et al. (1986). Psychological stress and metabolic control in patients with type I diabetes. *New England Journal of Medicine, 314,* 1078–1084.

Kenny, S. J., Aubert, R. E., & Geiss, L. S. (1995). Prevalence and incidence of non-insulin-dependent diabetes. In: *Diabetes in America,* 2nd ed., National Diabetes Data Group. National Institute of Diabetes and Digestive and Kidney Diseases. Bethesda, MD: National Institutes of Health, Publication no. 95-1468, pp. 47–67.

Klein, R., & Klein, B. E. K. (1995). Vision disorders in diabetes. *Diabetes in America* (2nd ed.). Bethesda, MD: NIH publication No. 95–1468.

Kovacs, M., Goldston, D., Obrosky, D. S., & Iyengar, S. (1992). Prevalence and predictors of pervasive non-compliance with the medical treatment among youths with insulin dependent diabetes mellitus. *Journal of the American Academy of Child and Adolescent Psychiatry, 31,* 1112–1119.

LaPorte, R. E., Matsushima, M., & Fang, Y. (1995). *Diabetes in America* (2nd ed.). Bethesda, MD: NIH publication No. 95–1468.

Manson, I. E., Nathan, D. M., Krowleski, A. S., Stampfer, M. J., Coldlitz, G. A., Willett, W. C., et al. (1992). A prospective study of exercise and incidence of diabetes among U.S. male physicians. *Journal of the American Medical Association, 268,* 63–67.

Marshall, J. A., & Hamman, R. F. (1988). Low carbohydrate, high fat diet, and the incidence of non-insulin-dependent diabetes mellitus. *Diabetes, 37,* 115A.

Meigs, J. B., Muller, D. C., Nathan, D. M., Blake, D. R., & Andres, R. (2003). The natural history of progression from normal glucose tolerance to type 2 diabetes in the Baltimore Longitudinal Study of Aging. *Diabetes, 52,* 1475–1484.

Mokdad, A. H., Bowman, B. A., Ford, E. S., Vinicor, F., Marks, J. S., & Koplan, J. P. (2001). The continuing epidemics of obesity and diabetes in the United States. *Journal of the American Medical Association, 286,* 1195–1200.

Morrish, N. J., Wang, S. L., Stevens, L. K., Fuller, J. H., & Keen, H. (2001). Mortality and causes of death in the WHO multinational study of vascular disease in diabetes. *Diabetologia, 44,* S14–S21.

Narayan, V., Boyle, J. P., Thompson, T. J., Sorensen, S. W., & Williamson, D. F. (2003). Lifetime risk for diabetes mellitus in the United States. *Journal of the American Medical Association, 290,* 1884–1890.

National Diabetes Clearing House. NIDDK. *National Diabetes Statistics, 2007.* Available from http://diabetes.niddk.nih.gov/index.htm.

National Diabetes Data Group. (1979). Classification and diagnosis of diabetes mellitus and other categories of glucose intolerance. *Diabetes, 28,* 1039–1057.

National Diabetes Fact Sheet. (2003). American Diabetes Association. Retrieved May 2, 2004, from http://www.diabetes.org/diabetes-statistics/national-diabetes-fact-sheet.jsp.

National Diabetes Fact Sheet. (2003). *General information and national estimates on diabetes in the United States, 2003.* Department of Health and Human Services, Centers for Disease Control and Prevention. Retrieved May 5, 2004 from http://www.cdc.gov/diabetes/pubs/pdf/ndfs_2003.pdf.

National Institutes of Health. (2007). *Diabetes statistics.* (NIH Publication No. 96–3926). Bethesda, MD: Author.

Padwal, R., Majumdar, S. R., Johnson, J. A., Varney, J., & McAlister, F. A. (2005). A systematic review of drug therapy to delay or prevent type 2 diabetes. *Diabetes Care, 28,* 736–744.

Palumbo, P. I., & Melton, L. J. III (1995). *Diabetes in America* (2nd ed.). Bethesda, MD: NIH publication No. 95–1468.

Pan, X. R., Li, G. W., Hu, Y. H., Wang, J. X., Yang, W. Y., An, Z. X., et al. (1997). Effects of diet and exercise in preventing NIDDM in people with impaired glucose tolerance. The Da Qing IGT and Diabetes Study. *Diabetes Care, 20,* 537–544.

Pareschi, P. L., & Tomasi, F. (1989). Epidemiology of diabetes mellitus. In M. Morsiani (Ed.), *Epidemiology and screening of diabetes* (pp. 77–113). Boca Raton, FL: CRC Press.

Peveler, R. C., Boller, I., Fairburn, C. G., & Dunger, D. (1992). Eating disorders in adolescents with IDDM. *Diabetes Care, 15,* 1356–1368.

Portuese, E., & Orchard, T. (1995). Mortality in insulin-dependent diabetes. *Diabetes in America* (2nd ed.). Bethesda, MD: NIH publication No. 95–1468.

Reaven, G. M., & Reaven, E. P. (1985). Age, glucose intolerance, and non-insulin dependent diabetes mellitus. *Journal of the American Geriatrics Society, 33,* 286–290.

Rewers, M., & Hamman, R. F. (1995). Risk factors for non-insulin-dependent diabetes. *Diabetes in America* (2nd ed.). Bethesda, MD: NIH publication No. 95–1468.

Schafer, L. C., Glasgow, R. E., McCaul, K. D., & Dreher, M. (1983). Adherence to IDDM regimens: Relationship to psychological variables and metabolic control. *Diabetes Care, 6,* 493–498.

Schneider, S. N., Amorosa, L. F., Khachadurian, A. K., & Ruderman, N. B. (1984). Studies on the mechanism of improved glucose control during regular exercise in type II (non-insulin dependent) diabetes. *Diabetologia, 26,* 355–360.

Schreiner-Engel, P., Schiavi, R. C., Vietorisz, D., & Smith, H. (1987). The differential impact of diabetes type on female sexuality. *Journal of Psychosomatic Research, 31,* 23–33.

Scott, F. W., Norris, I. M., & Kolb, H. (1996). Milk and type I diabetes: Examining the evidence and broadening the focus. *Diabetes Care, 19,* 379–383.

Songer, T. I. (1995). *Diabetes in America* (2nd ed.). Bethesda, MD: NIH publication No. 95–1468.

Stabler, B., Morris, M. A., Litton, J., Feinglos, M. N., & Surwit, R. S. (1986). Differential glycemic distress in type A and type B individuals with IDDM. *Diabetes Care, 9,* 550–552.

Sussman-Stillman, A., Hyson, D. M., Anderson, F. S., & Collins, W. A. (1997). Adolescent psychosocial development and adherence to treatment for insulin-dependent diabetes mellitus. In J. A. McNamara, & C. A. Trotman (Eds.), *Creating the compliant patient* (pp. 73–101). Ann Arbor, MI: University of Michigan Center for Human Growth and Development.

The Diabetes Control and Complications Trial Research Control Group. (1993). The effect of intensive treatment of diabetes on the development and progression of long-term complications in insulin dependent diabetes mellitus. *The New England Journal of Medicine, 329,* 977–986.

The Diabetes Prevention Program Research Group. (2007). The prevalence of retinopathy in impaired glucose tolerance and recent-onset diabetes in the Diabetes Prevention Program. *Diabetic Medicine, 24,* 137–144.

The Expert Committee on the Diagnosis and Classification of Diabetes Mellitus. (1997). Report of the expert committee on the diagnosis and classification of diabetes mellitus. *Diabetes Care, 20,* 1183–1197.

The Expert Committee on the Diagnosis and Classification of Diabetes Mellitus. (2003). Follow-up report on the diagnosis of diabetes mellitus. *Diabetes Care, 26,* 3160–3167.

Vague, P., DeCastro, J. V., & Vague, J. (1986). The role of adipose tissue distribution in the pathogenesis of type II diabetes. In M. Serarano-Rios & P. J. Lefebvre (Eds.), *Diabetes 1985* (pp. 524–528). New York: Elsevier Science Publishers.

Waxman, S. G. (1980). Pathophysiology of nerve condition: Relation to diabetic neuropathy. *Annals of Internal Medicine, 92,* 297–201.

Williams, K. V., Kelley, D. E., Mullen, M. L., & Wing, R. R. (1998). The effect of short periods of caloric restriction on weight loss and glycemic control in type 2 diabetes. *Diabetes Care, 21,* 2–8.

Wing, R. R, Nowalk, M. P., Marcus, M. D., Koeske, R, & Finegold, D. (1986). Subclinical eating disorders and glycemic control in adolescents with type I diabetes. *Diabetes Care, 9,* 162–167.

World Health Organization. (1980). Report of the expert committee on diabetes. *WHO Technical Report Series, 646,* Geneva, Switzerland.

Zhang, Y., Dall, T. M., Chen, Y., Baldwin, A., Yang, W., Mann, S., et al. (2009). Medical cost associated with pre-diabetes. *Population Health Management, 12,* 157–163.

10

Epilepsy

Robert T. Fraser, MD, PhD, CRC, John W. Miller, MD, PhD,
and Erica K. Johnson, PhD, CRC

Epilepsy is one of the most common chronic neurological disorders. The term epilepsy derives from the Greek word for "to be seized." A seizure involves a disruption of the normal activity of the brain through neuronal instability. Neurons become unstable and fire in an abnormally rapid manner, and this excessive electrical discharge is a seizure.

Seizures differ in their presentation, depending on the location of the discharge focus within the brain. For some individuals, the focus of the electrical discharging can be in the motor cortex and simply involve some muscle twitching in a hand (simple partial seizure), whereas for others, it involves most of the brain and results in a severe generalized tonic–clonic (formerly called grand mal) seizure. These seizures involve the whole body in convulsions and result in loss of consciousness.

Causes of epilepsy include traumatic brain injury (TBI), birth trauma, anoxia, brain tumors, infectious diseases (e.g., meningitis), parasitic infections, stroke, and abnormalities of the brain's blood vessels. The general incidence of epilepsy is between 1% and 4% varying with age groups. In the Rochester studies (Hauser, Annegers, & Kurland, 1993), the cumulative risk for having epilepsy by the age of 80 was 4%, with the lifetime risk for a single unprovoked seizure being 9%. Risk factors include alcohol abuse, hypertension, lower socioeconomic status, and depressive illness (Hauser, 1997). As underscored by Lowenstein (2009), the relative risk (RR) for developing epilepsy from TBI is 29-fold compared with the general population, exceeded only by brain tumor (RR = 40) and subarachnoid hemorrhage (RR = 34). Annegers, Hauser, Coan, and Rocca (1998) indicate that at 30 years follow-up, the cumulative incidence of epilepsy was 2.1% for mild TBI, 4.2% for moderate TBI, and 16.7% for severe TBI. It should be underscored that epilepsy involves the occurrence of two or more seizures; the occurrence of one seizure is insufficient to make a diagnosis of epilepsy (Devinsky, 2002).

SEIZURE CLASSIFICATION

Seizures are classified by assessing clinical symptoms, supplemented by wake and sleep electroencephalograms (EEGs) and sometimes by more sophisticated procedures such as 24-hour EEG-video monitoring. Seizures are generally categorized as generalized seizures, which begin in both cerebral hemispheres; and partial seizures, which begin in a specific part of the cerebral hemisphere. Partial seizures are further divided into simple partial seizures, in which consciousness is maintained; complex-partial seizures, which involve more than one symptom and in which consciousness is impaired; and secondarily generalized tonic–clonic seizures, where the seizure spreads to both cerebral hemispheres. The classification proposed by the International League Against Epilepsy (ILAE) Commission on Classification and Terminology was published in 1981 and is provided in Table 10.1. This table provides the reader with a basic overview of the different types of seizure conditions in the generalized and partial categorizations. This classification schema is currently undergoing revision by the ILAE.

Generalized Seizures

Generalized seizures begin in both cerebral hemispheres and involve wide areas of the brain, including the cerebral cortex, thalamus, and brainstem, and are subcategorized into a number of specific types. The most common form of generalized seizure is the generalized tonic–clonic seizure. This type of seizure involves two stages: the tonic stage, in which the body becomes rigid for a period of seconds, and the clonic stage, in which the person experiences a series of rhythmic jerking movements. The entire seizure generally lasts about 1–3 minutes (Devinsky, 2002). It is this type of seizure that is best known by the general public. If the seizure lasts more than 10 minutes or if the individual has multiple seizures in this time without regaining consciousness, it is *status epilepticus*. This is an emergency situation and requires immediate medical intervention. During the tonic–clonic seizure, it is best to discourage a crowd from gathering and to refrain from putting anything into the person's mouth. It is helpful to turn the person on one side and put a soft article of clothing under the head.

The other commonly known type of generalized seizure is the absence seizure (traditionally known as petit mal seizure). It consists of a brief disruption of consciousness (most often less than 20 seconds) and autonomic symptoms such as pupil dilation and mild rhythmic movements of the eyelids. Although some simple absence seizures involve blank stares, most are

TABLE 10.1   *An Abbreviated Classification of Epileptic Seizures*

Generalized Seizures of Nonfocal Origin Tonic–Clonic
Tonic
Clonic
Absence
Atonic/akinetic
Myoclonic

Partial (Focal) Seizures
Simple partial seizures with elementary symptomatology (consciousness is not impaired)
With motor symptoms (including Jacksonism, versive, and postural)
With sensory symptoms (including visual, somatosensory, auditory, olfactory, gustatory, and vertiginous)
With autonomic symptoms
With psychic symptoms (including dysphasia, dysmnesic, hallucinatory, and affective changes)
Compound (i.e., mixed) forms
Complex-partial seizures with complex symptomatology (consciousness is impaired)
Simple partial seizures followed by loss of consciousness
With impairment of consciousness at the outset
With automatisms
Partial seizures evolving to secondarily generalized seizures

Unclassified Seizures

From the International League Against Epilepsy Classification and Terminology Commission. "Revised Terminology and Concepts for Organization of the Epilepsies: Report of the Commission on Classification and Terminology." www.ilae-epilepsy.org

accompanied by the eye blinking (Devinsky, 2002). Absence seizures are distinguished by the generalized spike-and-wave tracings on the EEG. Most patients with this type of epilepsy begin having such seizures before age 14. Although they involve less than 5% of epilepsy cases (Penry, 1986), it is important to intervene medically, because not only can seizures affect a child's learning and influence his or her behavior, but they can also be associated with generalized tonic–clonic seizures. More severe generalized seizures can also occur as the child approaches adolescence.

Many adults who report that they have "petit mal" seizures actually have complex-partial seizures. Absence seizures are relatively uncommon in adults. On a vocational outreach grant at our center, between 25% and 30% of adults entering the study described their seizures as petit mal, which was not correct in most cases (Fraser & Clemmons, 1989). If patients do not know their seizure type, they may also be on an inappropriate medication.

Other types of seizures include atonic seizures, or brief drop attacks, which are more common in children younger than 5 years, and generalized myoclonic jerks in adults, which are brief shock-like contractions affecting the entire body or part of the body.

Partial Seizures

Partial seizures, as described in Table 10.1, can be divided into three categories: simple partial seizures with elementary symptoms; complex-partial seizures with diverse symptoms; and partial seizures evolving into secondarily generalized seizures.

Simple partial seizures may be motor, sensory, or autonomic or they may involve some combination of symptoms without impaired consciousness. Many individuals can function quite well with simple partial seizures that have a duration of only a few seconds.

Complex-partial seizures, however, present a significant problem. First, consciousness is impaired. These seizures may or may not have an associated aura, or warning, which can involve a strange odor, aphasia, dizziness, nausea, headache, unusual stomach sensations, or a déjà vu experience. Common motor activity during the seizures includes repetitive movements, fumbling with hands or clothing, lip smacking, and wandering. Complex-partial seizures without motor components are less common.

Approximately 60% of those with epilepsy have seizures in the partial seizure category (Pedley & Hauser, 1988). If the initial seizures are partial, the diagnosis of epilepsy may not be recognized until a generalized tonic–clonic seizure occurs. Because of the impaired consciousness and strange characteristics of complex-partial seizures (clutching clothing, lip smacking, etc.), clients with complex-partial seizures are sometimes misdiagnosed with a psychiatric condition. This seizure type is often not appropriately identified in unsophisticated assessments. Accurate diagnosis is critical to appropriate medication treatment.

It should be noted that a subgroup of people initially diagnosed with chronic epilepsy is later determined to have psychogenic nonepileptic seizures (PNES, or "pseudoseizures") with behavior during the event that mimics seizure activity. These events have an emotional cause, rather than being actual epileptic seizures. Kloster (1993) estimated this subgroup as between 10% and 20% of those initially diagnosed with syncope, hyperventilation, panic attacks, conversion disorders, dissociative events, and the like. More recent estimates have been that 20% of those being assessed at epilepsy center inpatient units have nonepileptic seizures (Devinsky, 2002); at the University of Washington Center, this incidence is 28%. Diagnosis can sometimes be clarified by recording serum prolactin levels, which would be dramatically elevated 20–30 minutes after generalized tonic–clonic seizures (Betts, 1997). However, the surest way of diagnosing nonepileptic seizures is by capturing a typical event on a EEG-video monitoring study. About 5% of those with established seizures studied in epilepsy monitoring units also have nonepileptic seizures (Betts, 1997). Martin et al. (1997) used a Minnesota Multiphasic Personality Inventory-2 (MMPI-2) stepwise discrimination function to successfully classify 81% of patients with and without epileptic seizures.

CLASSIFICATION OF THE EPILEPSIES

In addition to classifying seizures, which are events that the patient is experiencing, it is also possible to classify the patient's underlying condition, that is, the epilepsy. Epilepsy may be classified according to the underlying cause. Symptomatic (secondary) epilepsy has a known cause, for example, a tumor, prior stroke, or TBI. With cryptogenic epilepsy, the underlying cause is unknown. In idiopathic (primary) epilepsy, the epilepsy has a presumed genetic cause.

Epilepsy can also be classified according to the seizure type. If the seizures are partial or secondarily generalized, the condition is called localization-related epilepsy. If the seizures all begin from both sides of the brain, the condition is generalized epilepsy.

TREATMENT AND PROGNOSIS

Following their first recognized seizure, most individuals receive an initial inpatient or outpatient evaluation. The physician may begin a medical treatment program or refer the individual to a general neurologist. If seizure control is not secured within 3 months, a neurological referral is recommended (National Association of Epilepsy Centers, 1990). Membership in the American Epilepsy Society (AES) is an indication of the physician's commitment to epilepsy treatment.

Neurological consultation includes a history and a physical examination, metabolic studies, and other evaluations, including routine EEG testing and neuroimaging. The awake and sleep EEGs look for abnormalities that may occur even in the absence of actual seizures (interictal spikes or sharp waves), which can confirm a seizure diagnosis and help to classify the epilepsy type. A normal EEG can be seen in some patients with epilepsy, even when two EEGs are obtained (~ 25% of cases). Neuroimaging cannot confirm a diagnosis of epilepsy; rather, its purpose is to find the cause. Magnetic resonance imaging (MRI) of the head is generally superior to computed tomography (CT), also known as a CAT scan, because it is better able to detect small lesions or cerebral cortex abnormalities; however, in an acute situation, if MRI is not available or there are other technical difficulties, a CT scan may be used (International League Against Epilepsy, 1997). Single photon emission CT and positive emission tomography are not used in the initial evaluation of seizures and are only used when patients are evaluated for possible neurosurgical treatment for uncontrolled epilepsy. Multichannel magnetoencephalography is a newer technique for measuring magnetic fields of the brain; it is sometimes used as part of the evaluation for epilepsy neurosurgery, but is largely a research method at the present time.

If seizure control is not achieved by the general neurologist within 9 months, a referral to a tertiary- or fourth-level epilepsy center should be made (National Association of Epilepsy Centers, 1990). These centers have neurologists and allied health teams that specialize in epilepsy (viz., epileptologists), and they address such areas as pharmacological problems, possible PNES, the potential for epilepsy surgery, and the need for complementary psychological or psychiatric expertise. It is important to acknowledge that antiepileptic medications are selectively effective for one or more different types of seizures (Wannamaker, Booker, Dreifuss, & Willmore, 1984). The neurologist matches the appropriate drug to the specific seizure type. Table 10.2 presents an overview of the primary and secondary drugs that are most commonly used for various seizure categories.

To achieve optimal daily-life functioning for a patient (most effective treatment and fewer side effects), the normal course of treatment is the maximum tolerable dosage of one medication. A dosage should be established that maintains an appropriate concentration within the bloodstream throughout the day. Therapeutic ranges and toxicity levels have been established for the major recommended drugs. Table 10.3 shows pharmacological data on the major antiepileptic drugs.

TABLE 10.2   *Epilepsy Types and Indicated Antiepileptic Drugs*

Localization-Related Epilepsy (Simple Partial, Complex-Partial, and Secondarily Generalized Tonic–Clonic Seizures)

Primary drugs	Secondary drugs
Lamotrigine (Lamictal)	Gabapentin (Neurontin)
Carbamazepine (Tegretol, Carbatrol)	Valproate (Depakote, Depakene)
Oxcarbazepine (Trileptal)	Phenobarbital (Luminil)
Levetiracetam (Keppra)	Primidone (Mysoline)
Phenytoin (Dilantin)	Felbamate (Felbatol)
Topiramate (Topamax)	Tiagabine (Gabatril)
Zonisamide (Zonegran)	Methsuximide (Celontin)
	Lacosamide (Vimpat)

Generalized Epilepsies (Myoclonic, Absence Generalized Tonic–Clonic Seizures)

Primary drugs	Secondary drugs
Valproate (Depakote, Depakene)	Felbamate (Felbatol)
Lamotrigine (Lamictal)	Clonazepam (Klonopin)
Zonisamide (Zonegran)	Acetazolamide (Diamox)
Topiramate (Topamax)	Ethosuximide (Zarontin)
Levetiracetam (Keppra)	Methsuximide (Celontin)

Source: Karceski, S., Morrell, M., & Carpenter, D. (2001). The expert consensus guideline series. Treatment of epilepsy. *Epilepsy & Behavior, 2*(Suppl.), A1–A50; Deray, M., Resnick, T., & Alvarez, L. (2004). *Complete pocket reference for the treatment of epilepsy.* Miami, FL: CPR Educational Services, LLC.

Maintenance of an appropriate level of the medication in the bloodstream requires that patients consistently take the correct dose. It is extremely common that individuals with cognitive issues, such as memory, do not take their medication consistently. Excessive concentrations of medication (e.g., patient tries to "catch up") can result in dose-related adverse effects (toxicity), such as double vision, lethargy, impaired mental attention, coordination difficulties, weight change, and other significant medical complications. Laboratory monitoring of medication levels for some antiepileptic medications is sometimes useful for reducing the risk of adverse effects and optimizing seizure control. However, many drug side effects may occur even with serum antiepileptic levels in the so-called therapeutic range.

Since the early 1990s, many new antiepileptic medications (viz., gabapentin, oxcarbazepine, felbamate, lamotrigine, tiagabine, topiramate, levetiracetam, pregabalin, lacosamide, and rufinamide) have been licensed. All were initially tested as "add on" or adjunctive drugs.

TABLE 10.3   *Common Anticonvulsant Properties*

Drug	Therapeutic Range (µg/mL)	Half-life (Hours)
Carbamazepine	4–12	12–17
Lamotrigine	4–20	11–61
Levetiracetam	5–40	6–8
Phenytoin	10–20	7–42
Topiramate	4–10	19–23
Valproate	50–130	9–12
Zonisamide	15–40	60

Half-life may vary depending on age, hepatic or renal function, and interaction with other medications. Time to steady state is approximately 5 times the half-life. *Source:* Deray, M., Resnick, T., & Alvarez, L. (2004). *Complete pocket reference for the treatment of epilepsy.* Miami, FL: CPR Educational Services, LLC.

Most have shown effectiveness against complex-partial and secondarily generalized seizures initially, but over time a majority has shown effectiveness as monotherapy, that is, given without other antiepileptic medications. Some have also proven useful for generalized epilepsies. These newer medications (the "third generation" of anticonvulsants) are not necessarily more effective or always better tolerated than older drugs, but they provide welcome alternatives, which can often lead to better seizure control or fewer adverse effects for individual patients. Brodie and Kwan (2002) indicate that 47% of patients respond to the first antiepileptic medication, 13% are seizure-free on the second, and only 1% respond to the third monotherapy choice. The best prognosis for seizure control is response to the first anticonvulsant. Only 3% were controlled with two simultaneous anticonvulsants and none were controlled with three.

In a staged approach to epilepsy management, Brodie and Kwan (2002, p. 86) emphasize the following:

1. Appropriateness for seizure type, tolerability, and long-term safety are most important in choosing the first antiepileptic.
2. If the first drug is poorly tolerated at low dosages or fails to improve seizure control at adequate doses, an alternative should be substituted.
3. If a well-tolerated drug does not completely abolish seizures, combination therapy may sometimes be tried.
4. Work-up for epilepsy surgery should be considered after failure of two well-tolerated regimens.

There are a number of considerations outside of epilepsy surgery, which may not be an option for some patients. The ketogenic diet is an option for children who do not respond to antiepileptic medications because some long-term studies indicate > 50% seizure reduction for 40–50% of the children treated (Gaillard, Shields, Stafstrom, & Vining, 1997). The vagal nerve stimulator is implanted in the chest wall and stimulates the left vagus nerve at an established cycle and at seizure onset if the patient is able to activate it by passing a magnet over it. Approximately 38% of those using the stimulator achieve > 50% seizure reduction, but extremely few patients become seizure-free (Fisher & Handforth, 1999). Obviously, these individuals have very challenging seizure conditions.

A review of seizure-relapse studies would suggest that patients treated with medication generally achieve a 65–80% seizure-free status (Hauser & Hesdorffer, 1990). Annegers (1988) indicates that 10 years and 20 years after epilepsy diagnosis, 65% and 76% of patients, respectively, are seen in seizure remission. Although the probability of achieving remission after 10 years exceeds 60%, the probability of achieving remission during the next 10 years for those patients not having seizure control at 5 years from diagnosis was only 33%. The most important prognostic indicator for the eventual control of seizures is the duration of seizure occurrences. Other factors include seizure cause, seizure type, and age of onset (Annegers, 1988). After 1–6 years of seizure freedom, 69% of children and 61% of adults remain seizure-free when medications are tapered and stopped (Camfield & Camfield, 2008), with children deserving the opportunity to discontinue medication at 1–2 years and adults at 4 years.

For patients with medically intractable seizures, surgical intervention can be a consideration for up to 25% of patients with localization-related epilepsy, primarily those with partial complex seizures (Hauser & Hesdorffer, 1990). A series of diagnostic studies, including neuropsychological testing and continuous EEG-video monitoring are conducted, in addition to utilization of the previously mentioned neuroimaging techniques, to determine the site of seizure origination, and to determine if it can be safely removed. If surface EEG and neuroimaging techniques fail to definitely locate the seizure focus, then invasive recording with subdural or depth electrodes may be used (Hauser & Hesdorffer, 1990). Neuropsychological data are reviewed carefully, especially with regard to memory and language functions. There are different approaches to the surgeries (Schaul, 1987), including a standard temporal lobectomy and tailoring the tissue resection to the individual patient's seizure focus. Most centers report that 50–80% of those undergoing surgery can become seizure-free (Engel, Wieser, & Spencer, 1997). Available evidence from chiefly nonrandomized observational studies indicate that for appropriately selected patients with drug-resistant temporal lobe surgery, the surgery and medical treatment combination is four times more successful than medical treatment alone to achieve seizure freedom (Schmidt & Stavem, 2009).

In general, seizure-free status is a key variable in predicting psychosocial adjustment and improved vocational functioning (Fraser, 2006), although it can take more than several years to establish the vocational benefit of the surgical intervention (Chin et al., 2007; Jones, Berven, Ramirez, Woodward, & Hermann, 2002).

To some degree, surgical outcome is not completely clear because of different means of establishing outcome across surgical centers. In Schaul's review, it is estimated that there may be up to 120,000 surgical candidates within the United States who could profit from this type of surgery. For those with successful, seizure-free outcomes, medications are sometimes tapered off after 6–12 months.

Neuropsychological Assessment

At the Epilepsy Center of Michigan, over a 5-year period, Rodin, Shapiro, and Lennox (1977) found that only 23% of their medical referrals had epilepsy; among the remainder, brain impairment was the largest presenting difficulty across other psychosocial adjustment issues. In establishing functional abilities, this can be an important area to assess, particularly at epilepsy centers serving those with more severe seizure conditions. Approximately 40% of those applying to the University of Washington's Regional Epilepsy Center Vocational Services indicated on their program application form that they had had a head injury. Additional research has shown that if individuals have more than 75 lifetime generalized tonic–clonic seizures or have an incidence of *status epilepticus* involving extended continuous seizure activity, their neuropsychological performance decreases markedly (Dodrill, 1986).

It is reasonable to assume that those seeking vocational rehabilitation services would have diverse patterns of cognitive impairment that present more barriers to employment than would be common among a mainstream general or medical population. Research by Hermann et al. (2006, 2008), Oyegbile et al. (2004), and Rausch, Le, and Langfitt (1997) indicate that common cognitive concerns for individuals with epilepsy include attention, speed of mental processing, memory, and learning, executive function, and cognitive flexibility. A neuropsychologist can be helpful in providing an analysis of individual brain–behavior relationships relative to specific deficits and also in identifying assets on which the vocational rehabilitation program can be established—assets often being the most important variables in rehabilitation planning. The neuropsychological evaluation moves beyond basic intellectual and psychological assessment to look at more subtle aspects of problem solving, processing speed, sensory-perceptual abilities, memory capacities, motoric capacities, language skills, visual/spatial abilities, and self-regulating activity (Loring, Hermann, & Cohen, 2009).

Commonly used neuropsychological batteries include the Halstead Reitan Neuropsychological Battery (Reitan & Wolfson, 1985) and the Luria-Nebraska Neuropsychological Battery (Goldin, Hammeke, & Parisch, 1980). Dodrill (1978) has established a comprehensive battery of 16 discriminative measures more sensitive to brain impairment and epilepsy. This battery includes Halstead's Neuropsychological Battery for Adults, the Aphasia Screening Test, the Trail Making test, the Logical Memory and Visual Reproduction parts of the Wechsler Memory Scale, Form I, the Sensory-Perceptual Examination, the Stroop Test, and the Seashore Tonal Memory Test. In recent years, other neuropsychological batteries have been adapted incorporating some of the original with newer instruments, to include measures of "malingering." Neuropsychological testing is important both pre- and postsurgery for epilepsy, particularly to assess the surgical impact on memory and language functioning. The testing can also be helpful in clarifying epileptic foci.

It is important to emphasize that among studies conducted at the University of Washington (Fraser, Clemmons, Dodrill, Trejo, & Freelove, 1986) with clients actively engaged in vocational rehabilitation services, aspects of cognitive impairment consistently discriminated between those who were able to go to work and maintain a job for 1 year and those who could not secure a job through our program (i.e., they tried to secure work through the program but were unsuccessful). Specific predictive impairments were visual/spatial problem solving and motor deficits. Most of these clients had job experience that was characterized as unskilled or semiskilled work, and the brain impairments were affecting their employability. Clients with cognitive impairments affecting job stability typically require longer training or coached work experience relative to organizational and speed of functioning to secure and maintain competitive job placement. They also benefit from learning compensatory strategies to cope with their difficulties. For clients with a long history of generalized tonic–clonic seizures, neuropsychological test results can be facilitative relative to rehabilitation planning.

Psychosocial Assessment

Measures traditionally used in the clinical environments are useful in the assessment of the psychosocial functioning of clients with epilepsy. These measures include MMPI-2, the Personality Assessment Inventory (PAI), the Millon Clinical Multiaxial Inventory III, the Beck Depression Inventory-II, the Symptom Checklist-90-Revised, computerized psychiatric diagnostic interviews (Diagnostic Interview Schedule), and structured clinical interviews (the Mini-International Neuropsychiatric Interview, Structured Clinical Interview for *DSM-IV-TR* [SCID II]).

For purposes of clinical interview, the reader might review the next section on psychosocial adjustment to identify risk factors to maladjustment that deserve attention in the interview. Specifically, depression and anxiety are frequently underdiagnosed and undertreated in both pediatric and adult populations (Barry, 2004; Jackson & Turkington, 2005), yet these two disorders are two of the strongest predictors of quality of life, above clinical seizure features such as seizure frequency and severity (Johnson, Jones, Seidenberg, & Hermann, 2004; Strine et al., 2005). The lifetime-to-date rate of Diagnostic and Statistical Manual of Mental Disorders (DSM) defined major depression for people with epilepsy as ~ 30% across published studies (Hermann, Seidenberg, & Bell, 2000) compared with the general population lifetime-to-date estimate of 16% (Johnson et al., 2004; Kessler et al., 2003). Point-prevalence estimates of diagnosed depression and anxiety vary in studies examining samples from the general population of people with epilepsy (~ 13% with depression; Fuller-Thomson & Brennenstuhl, 2009) versus samples with typically more complicated epilepsy from tertiary care clinics (~ 30% with depression and 52% with anxiety disorders; Johnson et al., 2004; Jones et al., 2005). Rates of suicide are higher in adults with epilepsy than in those of the general population, independent of psychiatric comorbidity (Bell & Sander, 2009; Pompili, Girardi, Ruberto, & Tatarelli, 2005). Gilliam (2004) in his review notes a suicide rate in excess of 11%, and this morbidity issue is substantiated in meta-analytic studies (Pompili et al., 2005; Pompili, Girardi, & Tatarelli, 2006). These areas should be consistently addressed in the psychological assessment of adults with epilepsy.

One noteworthy measure for the purposes of psychosocial assessment of a client with epilepsy is the Washington Psychosocial Seizure Inventory (WPSI). This inventory, developed by Dodrill, Batzel, Queisser, and Temkin (1980), is helpful in identifying specific areas of concern to the client (Chang & Gehlert, 2003). This empirically derived measure has 132 items, which clients can typically complete in ~ 20–30 minutes.

Psychosocial concerns are identified across eight scales: family background, emotional, interpersonal, vocational, financial, adjustment to seizures, medicine and medical management, and overall psychosocial functioning. Other quality-of-life instruments have also been developed more recently (e.g., Liverpool Quality of Life Battery, QOLIE-89 item, QOLIE-10 item) and are used to assess psychosocial status, but also as outcome measures related to medication changes or epilepsy surgery.

PSYCHOLOGICAL AND VOCATIONAL IMPLICATIONS

Incidence of Psychosocial Maladjustment

In discussing the psychological and social adjustment issues of those with epilepsy, it is helpful to review findings using the WPSI. Trostle (1988) found that most studies using the WPSI identified 50% of respondents as having moderate to severe problems on a majority of the WPSI scales. Trostle further indicated that 50–60% of those sent for evaluation at a special epilepsy center indicate severe levels of maladjustment, in comparison with 19% in a general sample from Rochester, Minnesota (Trostle, Hauser, & Sharbrough, 1986). Overall, it would appear that those clients referred for evaluation by private physicians have fewer adjustment difficulties than clients referred from a medical center specializing in epilepsy treatment. The former may have less involved seizure conditions and lesser neuropsychological impairment, and may be at lower psychosocial risk.

In conclusion, the WPSI and other quality-of-life instruments (particularly the longer QOLIE-89) can be helpful in initial rehabilitation planning efforts. If there appear to be more significant psychiatric concerns, a referral for a more comprehensive psychological or neuropsychiatric evaluation can be more assistive in problem solving and goal setting.

Factors Influencing Psychosocial Adjustment

A number of factors have been established as relating to psychosocial adjustment for people with epilepsy. Hermann (1988) has synthesized the work of previous investigators in suggesting that four general forces affect adjustment among clients with epilepsy: biological, psychosocial, medication, and demographic factors. In Table 10.4, this multietiological model is presented with some additional factors identified by Fraser and Clemmons (1989). These factors cover most of those identified in the research literature as influencing the community adjustment of those with the disability. In the neurological category, items such as early age of onset, additional disabilities, associated neuropsychological impairment, and type of seizure activity have been found to be important variables. Under the psychosocial category, a number of variables are identified, including perceived stigma and limitations, adjustment to seizures, vocational status, financial status, parental fears, limited socialization and recreation, divisive or dysfunctional parenting styles, and poor relationships with parents, siblings, and intrusive grandparents.

Other more immediate issues, such as considerable life event changes, availability of social support, and perceived locus of control or self-efficacy, seem to affect adjustment. Basic demographic issues such as age, sex, education, and intelligence should also be reviewed. Some older clients adapt well to the seizure condition because of positive prior life experiences and an integrated self-concept. For other individuals, despite their age, the onset of a seizure condition can be unsettling. Young males tend to have more difficulties in adjusting than do females. It is of interest that the vocational interests and academic orientation of young males with more severe, early-onset seizures appear to be affected, compared with a norm group (Fraser, Trejo, Temkin, Clemmons, & Dodrill, 1985), but this is not true for young females. Special education tracking seems to relate to psychosocial maladjustment—this may be a masking variable for neuropsychological impairment (Goldin, Perry, Margolin, Stotsky, & Foster, 1967). In the medication category, the number of medications an individual takes and the appropriateness of medication levels can also affect community adjustment.

TABLE 10.4 *Multietiological Predictor Variables*

Neurological		Psychosocial
Age at outset	Perceived stigma	Parental fears
Duration of epilepsy	Perceived limitations	Divisive/dysfunctional parenting styles
Seizure type	Adjustment to seizures	
Neuropsychological impairment	Vocational adjustment	Limited recreation
Laterality of lesion	Financial status	Poor relationships with siblings, parents, grandparents
Presence/absence of multiple seizure types	Special education tracking	
Etiology	Locus of control	Social support
		Life event changes
Medications	Demographics	
Monotherapy vs. polytherapy	Age	
Presence of barbiturate medications	Gender	
Serum levels of medication	Education	
	IQ	

Note: Reprinted with modifications with permission from the Epilepsy Foundation of America as found in Hermann, B. P. (1988). Interrictal psychotherapy in patients with epilepsy. In W. A. Hauser (Ed.), *Current trends in epilepsy: A self-study course for physicians (Unit 1)*. Landover, MD: Epilepsy Foundation of America.

As emphasized by Hermann (1988), this type of model simply increases the reader's awareness of the range of factors that can influence a client's mental health. When emotional difficulties occur, depression and anxiety appear to be among the most frequent. There is also a significant rate of sexual dysfunction, particularly among males, with a propensity toward those having complex-partial or temporal lobe seizures (Hermann, 1988).

Work at the University of Washington Regional Epilepsy Center has demonstrated that early vocational rehabilitation program dropouts can be discriminated from those who have successfully become employed based on a number of specific items from the WPSI (Fraser, Trejo, Clemmons, & Freelove, 1987). These items identified increased depression and anxiety, financial difficulties, and lack of adjustment to one's seizure condition as being more prominent among program dropouts. New 12-hour interventions were tested at our center as precursors to vocational programming to stabilize dropouts (Fraser et al., 1990), but they were insufficient to render a difference. Other psychosocial adjustment concerns relate to epilepsy surgery—although a seizure-free status is highly correlated with adjustment, some seizure-free patients then experience a "burden of normality" (Wilson, Bladin, & Saling, 2001). For example, it can take several years for epilepsy surgery patients to achieve substantive vocational gains. It would appear that careful psychosocial/vocational goal planning and intervention should begin before the actual surgical intervention.

Self-Management Advances

Since 1997, the Centers for Disease Control and Prevention has promoted a public health agenda related to epilepsy. These efforts culminated in The Living Well With Epilepsy II conference of 2003, where priority recommendations were developed to address the behavioral and social health concerns of individuals with epilepsy. Specific emphasis was placed on the formulation and evaluation of epilepsy management models that emphasize self-management and self-determination in clinical and community care.

Broadly, self-management programs refer to chronic disease patient education programs that involve the patient as an active participant in treatment. The central premise behind such programs is that day-to-day management of chronic illness rests in the hands of the patient, as opposed to medical providers, and wellness management skills are a necessary teaching focus to mitigate disability and improve health outcomes (Furler et al., 2008; Lorig & Holman, 2003; Lorig, Ritter, Laurent, & Plant, 2006). Self-management for the person with epilepsy refers to the adaptive health behaviors and activities that an individual can perform to promote seizure control and enhance well-being (Austin & de Boer, 1997; DiIorio, Escoffery, McCarty, et al., 2009; DiIorio, Escoffery, Yeager, et al., 2009).

Most of the literature relating to epilepsy self-management has focused on psychosocial life adaptation. For example, Hausman et al. (1996) discussed an individualized assessment across diverse life areas such as cognitive abilities, cultural values, emotional status, family dynamics, financial concerns, general lifestyle, other health problems, personality characteristics, preconceived attitudes and beliefs, and available support systems to identify concerns and formulate a targeted educational plan and intervention. Consistent follow-up was also discussed.

Pramuka, Hendrickson, Zinski, and Van Cott (2007) conducted a 6-week psychosocial intervention study involving 2-hour classes to address one's medical care, taking charge of self-advocacy, managing stress, goal setting, managing relationships, and taking charge of one's future. Limited positive findings in relation to the Quality of Life in Epilepsy-89 role limitations-emotional score were reported, but the study was also noted to include a medical sample with more severe disability than what is seen in community-based samples.

In relation *specifically* to epilepsy self-management, the Cochrane review (Shaw et al., 2007) indicates that only the Sepulveda Epilepsy Program (SEP) and the Modular Services Package for Epilepsy (MOSES), a European program, met the criteria for a self-management program intervention within a randomized control context (Shaw et al., 2007). The SEP program involved 16 sessions over 2 days and had significant effects at 4 months in relation to misconceptions about the disability, overall extent of misinformation, and alleviating fears about medical concerns. Although not reaching statistical significance, there was a decided trend toward reducing seizure frequency and improved medical compliance. The nine-session MOSES program resulted in significant improvements in epilepsy knowledge, information-seeking activity, coping with epilepsy, and adherence to medication regimen. Both of these programs involved face-to-face group involvement.

Finally, in an effort to address the important role of behavior theory as well as practical issues such as patient needs and transportation barriers, DiIorio, Escoffery, Yeager, et al. (2009) developed an Internet-based intervention, WebEase. The program was based on the transtheoretical model of behavior change (Prochaska & DiClemente, 1982; Prochaska, Velicer, DiClemente, & Fava, 1988), social cognitive theory (Bandura, 1997), and motivational interviewing (Miller & Rollnick, 2002) to specifically address three behavioral areas: medication, stress, and sleep management. Significant results were seen in epilepsy self-management, sleep quality, self-efficacy, and social support.

A key limitation to the intervention literature, and one that may explain in part the inconsistent findings, is the lack of specific needs assessment/needs identification with consumers having epilepsy. Focus group data from the University of Washington Managing Epilepsy Well Needs Assessment Project indicates that in terms of group leadership, consumers prefer that the group be lead by a professional as well as lay trainer who also has epilepsy. In terms of format, consumers prefer a group meeting format that meets face to face weekly for 1–2 hours at a time, for no longer than 6 weeks consecutively. Focus group participants (two groups, n = 20) stated that topics of interest included understanding epilepsy and life hygiene; optimizing one's epilepsy care; stress and sadness management; employment; low-cost community recreation opportunities; and socializing well with a seizure disorder. Larger sample survey work is underway to confirm these findings. In conclusion, self-management interventions appear to hold promise in their ability to improve patient social and emotional functioning, health adherence, and quality of life. The importance of involving consumers in the identification of self-management needs should be underscored, as inconsistencies in intervention findings may relate to the structure, leadership, and content preferences of participants in contrast to professional opinion.

VOCATIONAL IMPLICATIONS

In epilepsy rehabilitation it is very important to maintain an individualized approach to vocational evaluation and goal planning. Issues tend to arise around the seizure condition itself, associated disabilities, medication concerns, and seizure disclosure. Each of these salient issue categories is reviewed in the following section.

CLARIFICATION OF SEIZURE STATUS

It is important that the counselor has a clear understanding of the client's seizure status. If a seizure status remains unclear, it is important that the client be referred to a major epilepsy center (to which one can be directed by the National Epilepsy Foundation, www.epilepsy-foundation.org) so that more sophisticated assessment and/or 24-hour EEG-video monitoring can be conducted. Some individuals will have nonepileptic seizures, which are emotionally rooted and require a different course of treatment. Recent advances in treatment of these seizures involve close interdisciplinary work and cognitive-behavioral individual and time-limited group intervention (Schöndienst, 2003). Some may have both real seizures, involving electrical discharges within the brain, and nonepileptic seizures. In each case, the counselor must understand the following.

1. The specific type of seizure the client currently has, with a clear description of what occurs during a seizure. Of particular importance is establishing whether there is a loss of consciousness.
2. What type of seizure control has the client achieved? If the seizures are not controlled, it is important to understand whether there is any pattern to their occurrence. Many individuals will have seizures only early in the morning, while sleeping, or when taking a break from the day's work activities. For some clients, certain precipitants seem to trigger the seizures. These can include fatigue, having flu or other illness, flickering lights or screens, certain levels of stress in the work environment (which certainly vary for each client), and other events or health-related issues.
3. Does the client have a specific warning or aura (actually the initial part of the seizure) before the occurrence of a full seizure? A warning can be a feeling of lightheadedness, an uneasy sick feeling, other strange sensations, or déjà vu experiences. A consistent aura is helpful in that it allows an individual to take safety precautions (e.g., sitting down, lying down, or otherwise removing oneself to a safe area before the seizure is in full progress).
4. What is involved in the recovery period? Some individuals can go directly back to work, others will require a brief nap, and some will have to take a sick day and spend the better part of the day recovering.
5. Has the client ever been otherwise injured as a result of a seizure? If not, this is very comforting for the employer.
6. Does the client have any other disabilities? In a recent study at our center (Fraser, Clemmons, Andrechak, Dodrill, & Temkin, 1991)—a tertiary center—89% of the clients served had one or more additional disabilities. It is particularly important to note whether there has been an additional head injury that precipitated the seizures or whether a head injury came about as a result of seizure activity (e.g., due to a

fall). The additional or associated disabilities will often require specific assessment (e.g., neuropsychological).

7. What type of medication is the client taking, is it appropriate, and is he or she complying with the recommended medication and dosages? Might the client with a clear focus and intractable seizures be a surgical candidate? Is the medication evaluation recent?

If the psychologist can answer the above questions, he or she is in a better situation to serve the client more appropriately. For example, recently at our center, as a result of a misunderstanding on the part of a counselor about a seizure type (which he believed to be a minor partial type), an individual was placed in a loading dock position in which he fell during a seizure, breaking his nose and sustaining a significant number of facial contusions and lacerations. In fact, he had had relatively frequent generalized tonic-clonic seizures that resulted in loss of consciousness and falling. In consideration of the heavy physical work he had been assigned and the potential for falling from the dock, the job assignment was inappropriate. It is a good standing policy to confirm the seizure description with a family member or significant other. As discussed earlier, many clients do not understand their seizure type and may provide inaccurate information. Many of them have never even witnessed a seizure and do not understand what occurs. A report (Bryant-Comstock, Hogan, Shumaker, & Tennis, 1997) indicates that a client's own perception of seizure severity, using the Liverpool Seizure Severity Scale, may be a better discriminator of employability than other seizure variables (e.g., seizure frequency).

ADDITIONAL DISABILITIES

As discussed earlier, a majority of clients with epilepsy coming for vocational rehabilitation services will have an additional disability. This is most commonly some type of neuropsychological impairment that has to be clarified. For example, vocational rehabilitation staff who miss detailed information about head injuries and other brain-related difficulties may result in mismatching individuals in the job placement process. An example would be an individual who had significant memory deficits and was placed in a locksmith job-training program, requiring him to remember a large number of different key molds. Clarification of some of these issues earlier would redirect the placement effort or the effort would have begun with more compensatory strategies being used. As discussed previously, clients who drop out of our rehabilitation program tend to do so because of emotional difficulties such as depression, anxiety, and financial fears. Individuals who are placed through the program but lose jobs after they are hired tend to do so because of cognitive or neuropsychological deficits.

To clarify these issues, a neuropsychological, or more specifically, an epilepsy battery that includes Halstead-Reitan and other specialized measures is used to identify brain impairment issues. An MMPI-II or PAI is also standardly used. Although neuropsychological issues and emotional concerns are more common, additional physical disabilities, mental retardation, cerebral palsy, and other medical concerns will be found in a subgroup of referrals. In review of some of these concerns, it becomes apparent that a number of clients will learn better in actual on-the-job training programs versus formal academic vocational/technical school training. Given specific cognitive deficits, it can be much easier to learn and retain the work tasks and requirements by training on the job site. This will be a counseling issue with clients who seek college training.

MEDICATION ISSUES

The area of medication management deserves significant attention. A number of clients are simply on the wrong medication when they come for vocational rehabilitation or are receiving too many medications, which results in poorly managed seizures and negative side effects.

Common side effects can include double vision, blurred vision, balance difficulties, lethargy, behavioral changes, gingival growth, nausea, weight gain, and liver enzyme elevations. As discussed earlier, if a client is not achieving good seizure control and has not been evaluated at an epilepsy center or by a neurological group that specializes in epilepsy, it can be appropriate to make a referral for current medication evaluation. A number of clients referred to our center may still be receiving Dilantin and phenobarbital, prescribed by a general practitioner to manage their seizures, which is often inappropriate. These instances occur more frequently in rural areas.

It is also common that clients do not take their medication as prescribed and do not understand that it can take days (depending upon their medication) to achieve a steady state of the anticonvulsant within their bloodstream. Consequently, a number of them take medication infrequently or in larger doses that result in toxicity and other side effects. They must be cautioned that it is necessary to take their medication consistently. This situation can be improved by taking the medication at a specific time or by using a pill counter or a medication box that has an alarm to remind patients when to take the medications.

DISCLOSURE OF SEIZURE STATUS

Disclosure of a seizure condition is a very individual consideration. For most people, we recommend that seizures be clearly discussed if they could affect work performance, preferably at the end of the interview, after they have had the opportunity to discuss their work-related background and skills. Consequently, they generally do not mention epilepsy on the application, but they have the interviewer note it at the time of their actual meeting with the employer. There can be a number of different approaches to disclosing. Because they do not lose consciousness, only have a seizure while sleeping, or have some other mitigating circumstance, some do not really have to discuss the issue with an employer or coworker. They may prefer to tell an employer or coworker that they have a seizure condition after they have been on the job some time and have established credibility as a worker. Under the Americans with Disabilities Act, which was implemented in 1992, and amended in 2008, reasonable accommodation for many private-sector employers could involve minor modifications to the worksite (layer of padding on a concrete floor or reassignment of work tasks [e.g., having a coworker do some minimal driving that is required on the job if the client lacks a driver's license because of epilepsy]). Although people with epilepsy (whether controlled with medication) are now well covered under the 2008 amendments to the Americans with Disabilities Act, litigation under the Equal Employment Opportunity Commission is slow. It is better to try to negotiate an accommodation with the employer.

In general, most studies show that the attendance and performance records for people with epilepsy are equal to or better than those of the general working population (McLellan, 1987). Risch (1968) demonstrated that time lost as a result of seizures was ~ 1 hour for every 1,000 hours worked by individuals with active seizure conditions. A study by Sands (1961) indicated that over a 13-year period in the state of New York, there were more accidents in the workplace caused by sneezing or coughing on the job than accidents related to seizures. Hiring people with epilepsy does not increase industrial insurance. In addition, second injury funds in most states protect an employer from bearing responsibility for total disability if the client has a seizure on the job that results in inability to work again. Working around machinery is generally not a problem of any significant measure in today's society. Most machinery has plastic guards and other safety features. Even equipment such as farm tractors have been modified with toggle switches to kill the engine when an individual experiences seizure activity while driving. For some individuals with active seizure conditions, however, working around heights may not be a reasonable idea, and in some cases working around boiling or molten materials can also present certain concerns. In these cases, however, safety harnesses or flame-resistant/retardant clothing materials may still enable an individual to perform the job. On issues of accommodation, the Job Accommodation Network in West Virginia (www.jan.wvu.edu) or university departments and their vocational rehabilitation, occupational therapy, or assistive technology units can be contacted for accommodation or ideas specific to individual seizure-related concerns. The Epilepsy Foundation in Washington, D.C., is developing new online website employment resources with some local Epilepsy Foundation affiliates having employment programs (www.epilepsyfoundation.org). The AES has a new resource site for physicians and employers on Epilepsy and Employment within the Practice Tools link (www.aesnet.org).

CONCLUSIONS

This chapter reviews medical, psychosocial, and vocational implications of epilepsy as a disability. With greater understanding of third-generation anticonvulsants' benefits, people with epilepsy should be more employable. It is hoped that, by attention to a number of the concerns presented in this chapter, many human service professionals can be successful in working with the client having a seizure condition. In our experience, with good medical and psychosocial/vocational assessment and targeted intervention, the seizure condition itself and associated disabilities can be worked with and around, resulting in a successful job match and better general community adjustment.

REFERENCES

Annegers, J. F. (1988). The natural history and prognosis of patients with seizures and epilepsy. In W. A. Hauser (Ed.), *Current trends in epilepsy: A self-study course for physicians (Unit 1)*. Landover, MD: Epilepsy Foundation of America.

Annegers, J., Hauser, W., Coan, S., & Rocca, W. (1998). A population-based study of seizures after traumatic brain injuries. *New England Journal of Medicine, 338*, 20–24.

Austin, J., & de Boer, H. (1997). Disruption in social functioning and services facilitating adjustment for the child and adult with epilepsy. In J. Engel & T. Pedley, (Eds.), *Epilepsy: A comprehensive textbook* (pp. 2191–2201). Philadelphia: Lippincott-Raven.

Bandura, A. (1997). *Self-efficacy: The exercise of control*. New York: W. H. Freeman & Co.

Barry, J. J. (2004, December). *The link between mood disorders and epilepsy—why is it important to diagnose and treat?* Paper presented at the Annual Meeting of the American Epilepsy Society, New Orleans, LA.

Bell, G. S., & Sander, J. W. (2009). Suicide and epilepsy. *Current Opinion in Neurology, 22*, 174–178.

Betts, T. (1997). Psychiatric aspects of nonepileptic seizures. In J. Engel & T. A. Pedley (Eds.), *Epilepsy* (pp. 2101–2116). Philadelphia: Lippincott-Raven.

Brodie, M. J., & Kwan, P. (2002). Staged approach to epilepsy management. *Neurology, 58*(Suppl. 5), 52–58.

Bryant-Comstock, I., Hogan, P., Shumaker, S., & Tennis, P. (1997). Relation of seizure severity to employment status and education [Abstract]. *Epilepsia, 38*(Suppl.), 135.

Camfield, P., & Camfield, C. (2008). When is it safe to discontinue AED treatment? *Epilepsia, 49*(Suppl. 69), 1528–1167.

Chang, C. H., & Gehlert, S. (2003). The Washington Psychosocial Seizure Inventory (WPSI): Psychometric evaluation and future applications. *Seizure, 12*, 261–267.

Chin, P. S., Berg, A. T., Spencer, S. S., Sperling, M. R., Haut, S. R., Langfitt, J. T., et al. (2007). Employment outcomes following resective epilepsy surgery. *Epilepsia, 48*, 2253–2257.

Deray, M., Resnick, T., & Alvarez, L. (2004). *Complete pocket reference for the treatment of epilepsy*. Miami, FL: CPR Educational Services, LLC.

Devinsky, O. (2002). *Epilepsy: Patient and family guide* (2nd ed.). Philadelphia: F. A. Davis.

DiIorio, C., Escoffery, C., McCarty, F., Yeager, K. A., Henry, T. R., Koganti, A., et al. (2009). Evaluation of WebEase: An epilepsy self-management Web site. *Health Education Research, 24*, 185–197.

DiIorio, C., Escoffery, C., Yeager, K. A., McCarty, F., Henry, T. R., Koganti, A., et al. (2009). WebEase: Development of a web-based epilepsy self-management intervention. *Preventing Chronic Disease: Public Health Research, Practice, and Policy, 6*, 1–7.

Dodrill, C. B. (1978). A neuropsychological battery for epilepsy. *Epilepsia, 19*, 611–623.

Dodrill, C. B. (1986). Correlates of tonic-clonic seizures with intellectual, neuropsychological, emotional, and social functions in patients with epilepsy. *Epilepsia, 27,* 399–411.

Dodrill, C. B., Batzel, L. W., Queisser, H. R., & Temkin, N. R. (1980). An objective method for the assessment of psychological and social problems among epileptics. *Epilepsia, 21,* 123–135.

Engel, J., Wieser, H. G., & Spencer, D. (1997). Overview: Surgical therapy. In J. Engel & T. A. Pedley (Eds.), *Epilepsy* (pp. 1673–1676). Philadelphia: Lippincott-Raven.

Fraser, R. T. (2006). Psychosocial and vocational outcomes: A perspective on patient rehabilitation. In J. W. R. Miller & D. C. Silvergeld (Eds.), *Controversies in epilepsy surgery* (pp. 735–742). New York: Marcel Dekker.

Fraser, R. T., & Clemmons, D. C. (1989). Vocational and psychosocial interventions for youth with seizure disorders. In B. Hermann & N. I. Siedenberg (Eds.), *Childhood epilepsies: Neuropsychological, psychosocial, and intervention aspects* (pp. 201–220). Chichester, England: John Wiley & Sons.

Fraser, R. T., Clemmons, D. C., Andrechak, N., Dodrill, C. B., & Temkin, N. (1991, December). *Prevocational intervention in epilepsy rehabilitation: Outcome and pre/postintervention employability correlates.* Paper presented at the American Epilepsy Society meeting, Seattle, WA.

Fraser, R. T., Clemmons, D. C., Dodrill, C. B., Trejo, W., & Freelove, C. (1986). The difficult to employ in epilepsy rehabilitation: Predictors of response to an intensive intervention. *Eplepsia, 27,* 220–224.

Fraser, R. T., Clemmons, D. C., Prince, S., Dodrill, C. B., Nelson, H., & Lucas, L. (1990, November). *Preliminary report of an intensive intervention in epilepsy rehabilitation.* Paper presented at the American Epilepsy Society annual meeting, San Diego, CA.

Fraser, R. T., Trejo, W., Clemmons, D. C., & Freelove, C. (1987, November). *Psychosocial adjustment of early dropouts compared to competitive placements.* Paper presented at the annual meeting of the American Epilepsy Society, San Francisco.

Fraser, R. T., Trejo, W., Temkin, N. R., Clemmons, D. C., & Dodrill, C. B. (1985). Assessing the vocational interests of those with epilepsy. *Rehabilitation Psychology, 30,* 29–33.

Fuller-Thomson, E., & Brennenstuhl, S. (2009). The association between depression and epilepsy in a nationally representative sample. *Epilepsia, 50,* 1051–1167.

Furler, J., Walker, C., Blackberry, I., Dunning, T., Sulaiman, N., Dunbar, J., et al. (2008). The emotional context of self-management in chronic illness: A qualitative study of the role of health professional support in the self-management of type 2 diabetes. *BMC Health Services Research, 8,* 214–232.

Gaillard, W., Shields, W. D., Stafstrom, C., & Vining, E. P. G. (1997). Ketogenic diet: What is the evidence that it works clinically and how to study it mechanically [Abstract]. *Epilepsia, 38*(Suppl.), 2.

Gilliam, F. G. (2004, December). *Understanding serious adverse outcomes of epilepsy.* Paper presented at the Annual Meeting of the American Epilepsy Society, New Orleans, LA.

Goldin, C. J., Hammeke, T. A., & Parisch, A. D. (1980). *The Luria-Nebraska neuropsychological battery: Manual.* Los Angeles: Western Psychological Services.

Goldin, C. J., Perry, S. L., Margolin, R. F., Stotsky, B. A., & Foster, J. C. (1967). *Rehabilitation of the young epileptic.* Lexington, MA: D.C. Heath.

Hauser, W. A. (1997). Incidence and prevalence. In J. Engel & T. A. Pedley (Eds.), *Epilepsy* (pp. 47–58). Philadelphia: Lippincott-Raven.

Hauser, W. A., Annegers, J. F., & Kurland, I. T. (1993). The incidence of epilepsy and unprovoked seizures in Rochester, Minnesota. 1935–1984. *Epilepsia, 34,* 453–468.

Hauser, W. A., & Hesdorffer, D. C. (1990). *Epilepsy: Frequency, causes, and consequences.* New York: Demos.

Hausman, S. V., Luckstein, R. R., Zwygart, A. M., Cicora, K. M., Schroeder, V. M., & Weinhold, O. (1996). Epilepsy education: A nursing perspective. *Mayo Clinic Proceedings, 71,* 1114–1117.

Hermann, B. P. (1988). Interrictal psychotherapy in patients with epilepsy. In W. A. Hauser (Ed.), *Current trends in epilepsy: A self-study course for physicians (Unit 1).* Landover, MD: Epilepsy Foundation of America.

Hermann, B. P., Jones, J. E., Sheth, R., Koehn, M., Becker, T., Fine, J., et al. (2008). Growing up with epilepsy: A two-year investigation of cognitive development in children with new onset epilepsy. *Epilepsia, 49,* 1847–1858.

Hermann, B. P., Seidenberg, M., & Bell, B. (2000). Psychiatric co-morbidity in chronic epilepsy: Identification, consequences, and treatment of major depression. *Epilepsia, 41*(Suppl. 2), S31–S41.

Hermann, B. P., Seidenberg, M., Dow, C., Jones, J., Rutecki, P., Bhattacharya, A., et al. (2006). Cognitive prognosis in chronic temporal lobe epilepsy. *Annals of Neurology, 60,* 80–87.

International League Against Epilepsy (Neuroimaging Commission) (1997). Recommendations for neuroimaging of patients with epilepsy. *Epilepsia, 38*(Suppl. 10), 1–2.

Jackson, M. J., & Turkington, D. (2005). Depression and anxiety in epilepsy. *Journal of Neurology, Neurosurgery, and Psychiatry, 76*(Suppl. 1), i45–i47.

Johnson, E. K., Jones, J. E., Seidenberg, M., & Hermann, B. P. (2004). The relative impact of anxiety, depression, and clinical seizure features on health-related quality of life in epilepsy. *Epilepsia, 45,* 544–550.

Jones, J. E., Berven, N. L., Ramirez, L., Woodward, A., & Hermann, B. P. (2002). Long-term psychosocial outcomes of anterior lobectomy. *Epilepsia, 43,* 896–903.

Jones, J. E., Hermann, B. P., Barry, J. J., Gilliam, F., Kanner, A. M., & Meador, K. J. (2005). Clinical assessment of Axis I psychiatric morbidity in chronic epilepsy: A multicenter investigation. *Journal of Neuropsychiatry and Clinical Neurosciences, 17,* 172–179.

Karceski, S., Morrell, M., & Carpenter, D. (2001). The expert consensus guideline series. Treatment of epilepsy. *Epilepsy & Behavior, 2*(Suppl.), A1–A50.

Kessler, R. C., Berglund, P., Demler, O., Jin, R., Koretz, D., Merikangas, K. R., et al. (2003). The epidemiology of major depressive disorder: Results from the National Comorbidity Survey Replication (NCS-R). *Journal of the American Medical Association, 289,* 3095–3105.

Kloster, R. (1993). Pseudo-epileptic versus epileptic seizures: A comparison. In L. Gram, S. Johannessen, P. Osterman, & M. Sillanpas (Eds.), *Pseudoepileptic seizures* (pp. 3–16). Petersfield, UK: Wrightson Biomedical.

Lorig, K. R., & Holman, H. R. (2003). Self-management education: History, definition, outcomes, and mechanisms. *Annals of Behavioral Medicine, 26,* 1–7.

Lorig, K. R., Ritter, P. L., Laurent, D. D., & Plant, K. (2006). Internet-based chronic disease self-management: A randomized trial. *Medical Care, 44,* 964–971.

Loring, D. W., Hermann, B. P., & Cohen, M. J. (2009). Neuropsychological advocacy and epilepsy. *Clinical Neuropsychology, 11,* 1–12.

Lowenstein, D. H. (2009). Epilepsy after head injury: An overview. *Epilepsia, 50*(Suppl. 2), 4–9.

Martin, R., Snyder, P., Gilliam, F., Roth, D., Fraught, E., & Kuzniecky, R. (1997). Classification accuracy of the MMPI-2 in the identification of patients with frontal lobe epilepsy and non-epileptic seizures [Abstract]. *Epilepsia, 38*(Suppl.), 159.

McLellan, D. L. (1987). Epilepsy and employment. *Journal of Social and Occupational Medicine, 3,* 94–99.

Miller, L., & Rollnick, S. (2002). *Motivational interviewing* (2nd ed.). New York: Guilford Press.

National Association of Epilepsy Centers (1990). Recommended guidelines for diagnosis and treatment in specialized epilepsy centers. *Epilepsia, 32*(Suppl. 1), 1–12.

Oyegbile, T. O., Dow, C., Jones, J., Bell, B., Rutecki, P., Sheth, R., et al. (2004). The nature and course of neuropsychological morbidity in chronic temporal lobe epilepsy. *Neurology, 62,* 1736–1742.

Pedley, T. A., & Hauser, W. A. (1988). Classification and differential diagnosis of seizures and of epilepsy. In W. A. Hauser (Ed.), *Current trends in epilepsy: A self-study course for physicians (Unit 1).* Landover, MD: Epilepsy Foundation America.

Penry, J. K. (Ed.) (1986). Epilepsy: *Diagnosis, management, and quality of life.* New York: Raven Press.

Pompili, M., Girardi, P., Ruberto, A., & Tatarelli, R. (2005). Suicide in the epilepsies: A meta-analytic investigation of 29 cohorts. *Epilepsy & Behavior, 7,* 305–310.

Pompili, M., Girardi, P., & Tatarelli, R. (2006). Death from suicide versus mortality from epilepsy in the epilepsies: A meta-analysis. *Epilepsy & Behavior, 9,* 641–648.

Pramuka, M., Hendrickson, R., Zinski, A., & Van Cott, A. (2007). A psychosocial self-management program for epilepsy: A randomized pilot study in adults. *Epilepsy & Behavior, 11,* 533–545.

Prochaska, J. O., & DiClemente, C. C. (1982). Transtheoretical therapy: Toward a more integrative model of change. *Psychotherapy: Theory, Research, and Practice, 19,* 276–288.

Prochaska, J. O., Velicer, W. F., DiClemente, C. C., & Fava, J. (1988). Measuring the process of change: Application to the cessation of smoking. *Journal of Consulting and Clinical Psychology, 56,* 520–528.

Rausch, R., Le, M. T., & Langfitt, J. L. (1997). Neuropsychological evaluation: Adults. In J. Engel & T. A. Pedley (Eds.), *Epilepsy.* Philadelphia: Lippincott-Raven.

Reitan, R. M., & Wolfson, D. (1985). *The Halstead-Reitan test battery: Theory and clinical interpretations.* Tucson, AZ: Neuropsychology Press.

Risch, F. (1968). We lost every game…but. *Rehabilitation Record, 9,* 16–18.

Rodin, E. A., Shapiro, H. L., & Lennox, K. (1977). Epilepsy and life performance. *Rehabilitation Literature, 38,* 34–38.

Sands, H. (1961). Report of a study undertaken for the committee on neurological disorders in industry. *Epilepsy News, 7,* 1.

Schaul, N. (1987). Epilepsy surgery. *New York Journal of Epilepsy, 5,* 14–15.

Schmidt, D., & Stavem, K. (2009). Long-term seizure outcome of surgery versus no surgery for drug-resistant partial epilepsy: A review of controlled studies. *Epilepsia, 50,* 1301–1309.

Schöndienst, M. (2001). Management of dissociative disorders in a comprehensive care setting. In M. Pfäfflin, R. T. Fraser, R. Thorbecke, V. Specht, & R. Wolfe (Eds.), *Comprehensive care for people with epilepsy* (pp. 67–76). London: John Libbey.

Shaw, F., Stokes, T., Camosso-Stefinovic, J., *Baker,* R., Baker, G. A., Jacoby, A. (2007). Self-management education for adults with epilepsy. *Cochrane Database of Systematic Reviews, 2,* 1–14.

Strine, T. W., Kobau, R., Chapman, D. P., Thurman, D. J., Price, P., & Balluz, L. S. (2005). Psychological distress, comorbidities, and health behaviors among U.S. adults with seizures: Results from the 2002 National Health Interview Survey. *Epilepsia, 46,* 1133–1139.

Trostle, J. A. (1988). Social aspects of epilepsy. In W. A. Hauser (Ed.), *Current trends in epilepsy: A self-study course for physicians (Unit 1).* Landover, MD: Epilepsy Foundation of America.

Trostle, J. A., Hauser, W. A., & Sharbrough, F. (1986). Self-regulation of medical regimens among adults with epilepsy in Rochester. *Epilepsia, 27,* 640.

Wannamaker, B. B., Booker, H. E., Dreifuss, F. E., & Willmore, L. J. (1984). *The comprehensive clinical management of the epilepsies.* Landover, MD: Epilepsy Foundation of America.

Wilder, B. J. (1997). Vagal nerve stimulation. In J. Engel & T. A. Pedley (Eds.), *Epilepsy* (pp. 1353–1358). Philadelphia: Lippincott-Raven.

Wilson, S. J., Bladin, P. F., & Saling, M. (2001). The "burden of normality": concepts of adjustment after surgery for seizures. *Journal of Neurology, Neurosurgery, and Psychiatry, 70,* 649–656.

11

Speech, Language, Hearing, and Swallowing Disorders

Nancy Eng, PhD, CCC-SLP, and
Patricia Kerman Lerner, MA, CCC, Fellow, ASHA

INTRODUCTION

Communication is a basic human behavior that has an impact on all aspects of the human experience, including the ability to establish and maintain relationships, to participate in educational programs and recreational activities, to pursue and retain employment, and to achieve full independence. The ability to communicate is a unique behavior influenced by an interaction among biological, psychological, and environmental factors. Adequate speech, language, and hearing systems working in an integrated manner allow for the effective exchange of information among humans.

Speech and language disorders have a direct impact on communication and can also affect the related areas of feeding and swallowing because of the shared use of the neuromuscular speech mechanism. Problems can range from very mild to severe degrees of impairment. Problems can be developmental in nature or acquired by way of disease or trauma. It is conservatively estimated that more than 38 million individuals in the United States have some form of communication impairment (Benson and Marano, 1995). Common causes of speech and language disorders include hearing loss, developmental disabilities, cognitive impairment, brain injury, sensory impairment, and congenital anomalies. In many cases, however, the cause is unknown.

Speech is the verbal means of communication. It is achieved by planning, coordinating, and executing a series of neuromuscular movements to produce the sounds (or phonemes) specific to a particular language. A phoneme is a meaningful speech sound. Each language has a unique set of phonemes and a unique set of rules that allow for combinations of sounds specific to that language. Speech disorders refer to those that interfere with speech production (also referred to as articulation), fluency of speech production, and/or vocal qualities of speech production. Because the oromotor system serves two functions (speech production and nutrition), problems with swallowing and feeding must also be considered in some cases. Regardless of the nature or severity of the speech disorder, the speaker's ability to use language may or may not be affected. For example, speakers who stutter do not necessarily have accompanying language impairments.

Language is a code used to express ideas about the world (Lahey, 1998). It is a socially shared code that is rule-governed; that is, all users of the code (a particular language) agree to follow the rules of the language so as to assure comprehension. For example, English speakers add "ed" onto verbs to indicate past events. Although the symbols are limited in number, languages have rules that allow for the combination of these symbols to create words, phrases, and sentences. For example, English speakers will agree that "splig" or "dsinm" is not a real word, but "splig" could be a real word whereas not "dsinm". Language disorders refer to interference in the ability to use the symbol system in communication. That is, language disorders can affect language comprehension and language expression, including the ability to read and write. Again, regardless of the nature or severity of the language impairment itself, the speaker's ability to produce speech may or may not be affected. For example, speakers with dementia may have excellent articulation skills but fail to understand what is spoken to them and fail to adequately express themselves.

In the sections to follow, speech and language disorders will be discussed in terms of how these can affect individuals across the lifespan. In some cases, the problems identified in childhood may resolve with time, whereas in other cases, these persist into adulthood, having a significant impact on vocational choices and social relationships.

LANGUAGE DEVELOPMENT AND LANGUAGE DISORDERS

The acquisition of language is accomplished effortlessly by almost all children exposed to different languages. Most children demonstrate comprehension of words by 9 months and utter the first words by their first birthdays. The period between birth and 24 months involves a tremendous amount of growth and development. A summary of major language milestones is presented in Table 11.1, which is based on observations of typically developing children who are exposed to English (Lust, 2006).

TABLE 11.1 *Summary of Major Language Milestones*

Age	Ability
Birth–2 months	Distinguishes between speech and nonspeech stimuli Able to distinguish between two different languages Reflexive crying, vegetative sounds (burp, grunt, sigh) Sounds of pleasure and discomfort Some cooing
2–4 months	Detects stress in syllables such as ba-da vs. ba-da Comfort sounds during social exchanges Distinguishes between native and nonnative language
4–6 months	Prefers speech to nonspeech sounds Begins to make association with sounds and mouth Vocal play—experimenting with sounds Plays with yelling, squealing Continues to distinguish between native and nonnative language
6–8 months	Preference for speech from the native language Babbling begins now Remembers words from songs and stories
8–10 months	Distinctive intonation patterns in babbling; vocalization with sound play Begins to search for familiar objects as they are named
10–12 months	Longer and more variability in babbling strings of sounds First words at around 12 months May understand as many as 50 words
12–18 months	Vocabulary expansion Longer words are reduced to one or two syllables
18–24 months	Child is using language-specific word order rules By 2 years, child may understand as many as 1000 words

Source: Lust, B. (2006). *Child language: Acquisition and growth*. Cambridge, MA: Cambridge University Press. Reprinted with permission of Cambridge University Press.

Atypical Development (Language)

Some children will need assistance in language learning. Why some children fail to acquire what appears to be natural to most children remains an enigma to parents, educators, and health care providers alike. Approximately 6% of the school-age population is estimated to present with some form of language delay (Tomblin et al., 1997). Whereas most of these concerns are resolved with time, the long-term impact that language impairment can have on academic achievement, acquisition of literacy skills along with achievement of vocational goals, and socialization cannot be ignored. These children can exhibit difficulties learning to speak and/or understand what is being said to them in conversations and in stories. For example, they may speak in shorter, less mature sentences as compared with age-matched peers, or else they may need multiple repetitions of utterances for comprehension. Because of the developmental lag in language acquisition, these children may have problems in both academic performance and peer relationships.

Specific Language Impairment

The term specific language impairment (SLI) is used to describe children who demonstrate difficulty in acquiring language but are otherwise typically developing in all other areas of development. It is estimated that the disorder affects between 1.5% and 7% of children (Leonard, 1998) with boys at twice the risk of SLI compared with girls (Tomblin, 1996). These children do not exhibit any neurological, sensory, emotional, or cognitive impairments. SLI is synonymous with the terms language impaired, language disorders, language delayed, and language disabled. Children with SLI exhibit a range of speech and language problems and often have difficulty understanding and/or producing complex sentences so that productions are limited to simple sentence structures.

Many late talkers ultimately master language as well as their typically developing peers, whereas some simply fail at the task. Distinguishing between these clinically different groups is the challenge for speech-language pathologists (SLPs). Early and accurate diagnosis for late talkers and subsequently securing early intervention for children at risk for SLI is vital to reducing the risk of later academic and other related problems such as social, emotional, and behavioral difficulties. In fact, many children who struggle academically may be struggling with the language associated with content areas in school. Approximately 80% of prison inmates are described as functionally illiterate, where more than two thirds of prisoners have notable reading comprehension problems (Moody et al., 2000).

Some children with SLI may show weakness in auditory processing. They may not hear subtle differences between sounds in words in the absence of any hearing loss. For many listening to spoken information, understanding it, remembering it, and then recalling it is difficult. The problems are not the result of cognitive or linguistic deficits. Although it is perfectly logical to assume a causative relationship between the auditory processing and the central nervous system (CNS), in many cases, the CNS is intact (Bellis, 1996).

Management Considerations

As with any other diagnostic group, evaluation of children suspected with SLI requires a thorough and careful consideration. Commercially available tests are used in school systems and hospital settings for the purposes of identification. Protocols are available for therapy services that address the academic and social problems that often accompany SLI. Whereas some tests target specific areas of language development, others cover a wider range of skills. Regardless of the test instrument used, a thorough assessment should include evaluation of syntactic skills (comprehension and use of a range of age-appropriate sentence forms), semantic skills (including vocabulary skills, word knowledge, and word retrieval skills), pragmatic skills (ability to use language for different functions such as making requests, expressing feelings, and gaining clarification in socially appropriate and acceptable ways), and metalinguistic abilities (i.e., looking at how well a child is able to think about and manipulate language).

Therapy approaches are designed to address the language deficits identified through formal testing in conjunction with parental input and teacher observations. Interventions target specific areas of language deficits as identified through formal testing procedures. Consistent and notable gains have been reported when intervention services are provided by qualified SLPs (Fey, Cleave, Long, & Huges, 1993). In some cases, children presenting with expressive language delays are more responsive to therapy as compared with those with a mixed receptive and expressive language disorder (Law, Garrett, & Nye, 2003). In some cases, speech/ language therapy continues to be offered beyond the school-age years. Although adults with SLI do not necessarily experience differences with respect to the quality of life (Records, Tomblin, & Freese, 1992), continuous use of compensatory strategies can be viewed as taxing on a daily basis (Gopnik, 1990).

Dyslexia

Dyslexia refers to a learning disability that is associated with problems in reading and spelling. Individuals with dyslexia have difficulty learning to read despite the availability of educational opportunity. Despite public perception, the problems of dyslexia are more complex than visual processing where readers reverse and transpose letters in words and words in phrases. In addition, these individuals have adequate vision and do not demonstrate cognitive impairments. In fact, a number of famous actors including Tom Cruise, Danny Glover, Whoopi Goldberg, and Keanu Reeves have all been reported to have had the reading disability!

Deficits in the processing of linguistic units (in print) are at the root of dyslexia, and hence referred to as a specific reading disability. Common symptoms include difficulty recognizing letters and words in print and poor reading comprehension. In addition, decoding (or pronouncing unfamiliar words) and encoding (or spelling unfamiliar words) problems may occur. Phonological processing problems are also present—this involves the ability to attend to the sounds that make up words in the language. Being able to rhyme, identify initial and final sounds of words, and so on are just some of the skills associated with phonological processing. Without well-developed phonological processing skills, learning how to pronounce and to spell words is compromised. Reading, specifically word identification, involves assigning sounds to printed letters, blending those sounds into meaningful words of the language, and, finally, activating the appropriate meaning for the particular string of sounds. For typical readers, this process is fast and seamless, but for those with phonological processing problems, this process works slowly and deliberately, thus disrupting reading fluency and ultimately interfering with reading comprehension.

Management Considerations

A thorough assessment of the four modalities of language (listening comprehension, verbal expression, reading, and writing) is essential in identifying the specific deficits that impede an individual's reading and writing abilities. It should also be noted that there is a high correlation with attention deficit hyperactivity disorder (ADHD) so that it is important to ask the relevant questions regarding attention behaviors.

One of the best predictors of reading competence is a child's phonological processing ability. Several commercially available tests can be used to evaluate phonological processing skills, and most of these include tasks that tap alphabet knowledge and the ability to manipulate sounds in words (say the word stop but don't say the /t/ sound), recall sequence of sounds and lists of words, repeat sentences, and identify rhyming words and rapid automatic naming. By 3 or 4 years of age, many children are able to perform standardized tasks that tap phonological processing skills.

Following identification of reading problems, initiation of intervention is critical in alleviating their impact. Strategies designed to increase phonemic awareness have been proven to be effective. Activities including manipulating sounds in syllables, sound blending, creating rhyming words, and segmenting words into syllables are ways of improving skills necessary for reading success and spelling confidence. Other skills including recognizing the letters of the alphabet, relating sounds to printed letters, and orthographic knowledge (knowing that "ph" is equivalent to "f") are critical in understanding sound–spelling relationships and ultimately lead to encoding and decoding skills. Programs such as Lindamood Bell Learning Processes (Alexander, Anderson, Heilman, Voeller, & Torgensen, 1991), Wilson Reading System (Wilson, 1998), and the Orton-Gillingham Method (Ritchey & Goeke, 2006) are used with individuals identified to be either at risk for reading disabilities or to have confirmed reading problems. The emphasis of these programs is on helping readers establish sound–symbol relationships for reading and related skills including decoding and encoding.

Autism and Autism Spectrum Disorders

Autism spectrum disorders (ASDs) have received wide media exposure in an effort to heighten awareness of this devastating childhood disorder. The term encompasses disabilities related to a range of social and communication disorders that are typically observed in early childhood, usually by 2 years of age. Children and adults who are diagnosed with ASD have significant problems with social interactions and marked difficulties in both verbal and nonverbal communication. Although cognitive abilities can range from very low functioning levels to much higher levels, such as those observed in Asperger Syndrome, social and communication impairments are common to all individuals with ASD. Verbal fluency can range from nonverbal in lower functioning individuals to relatively fluent productions in higher functioning ones.

The term ASD encompasses several different disorders including classic autism, pervasive developmental disabilities, childhood disintegrative disorder, Rett's Syndrome, and Asperger Syndrome. According to the Centers for Disease Control and Prevention (2007), approximately 1 in 150 births is affected by autism and as many as 1.5 million Americans are said to have some form of the disorder. Rutter and Schopler (1987) estimate that approximately 75% of children with autism are also diagnosed with mental retardation, creating additional diagnostic and treatment challenges. The overlap between the disorders creates challenges in understanding the nature of each of these developmental disabilities and in the differential diagnosis of people in this spectrum.

Parents are usually one of the first to notice behaviors in their children that they consider different from those of other children. Some of these behaviors can be observed in children as young as 18 months of age and include those given in Table 11.2.

TABLE 11.2 *Behaviors Suggestive of ASD*

- Not pointing at objects of interest
- Poor eye contact
- Losing skills that had been acquired (stop using words that were previously used)
- Lack of "pretend" play skills such as pretending to feed a doll
- Prefers to be alone instead of with peers and adults
- Has difficulty transitioning from one activity to another
- Has problems understanding what is being said to them
- Lack of interest in people
- Dislikes being cuddled or hugged
- Preference for sounds over speech
- Repeating actions or gestures over and over again
- Echolalia or repeating words and phrases over and over again
- Confusion in pronoun use, specifically in the use of first and second person pronouns

Management Considerations

Individuals with ASD pose unique challenges in evaluation, given the variability in the communication/language, social, and cognitive domains. Thorough assessments are conducted to identify developmental disabilities, to determine eligibility for support services and current levels of functioning in the cognitive, academic, and emotional domains, and to recognize strengths and weaknesses in development and for the purpose of monitoring progress over time. It is critical to assess across all developmental areas to understand the scope of the disability to determine effective intervention approaches to meet educational, vocational, and behavioral goals. Additionally, input from caregivers, educators, and health care providers is useful for differential diagnosis.

Because behavioral and cognitive factors may interfere with administration of formal testing, clinicians frequently modify these materials for the purposes of gaining a better understanding of underlying issues. For clients whose behavioral and cognitive status may preclude the use of formal testing methods, there is a plethora of questionnaires that are available to clinicians. Some of the more commonly used behavioral checklists for ASD include the Checklist for Autism in Toddlers (CHAT; Baron-Cohen, 1992), Autism Diagnostic Interview-Revised (ADI-R; Lord, Rutter, & Le Couteur, 1994), the Gilliam Autism Rating Scale (GARS; Gilliam, 1995), the Asperger Syndrome Diagnostic Scale (ASDS; Smith-Myles & Southwick, 2001), and the Childhood Autism Rating Scale (CARS; Schopler, Reichler, & Renner, 1988).

Research supports the use of parental reports collected through the use of behavioral checklists (Baird et al., 2000; Baron-Cohen, 1992) citing the accuracy with which parents can judge behaviors as valuable in identifying children who are at risk for ASD and subsequently using this information to secure early assessment and intervention of these children.

There are a number of treatment philosophies with respect to addressing ASD. The three more popular ones are described briefly below. Applied Behavioral Analysis is commonly used to analyze and manage behaviors, both socially appropriate ones and inappropriate ones, such as ritualistic, repetitive, self-injurious, and disruptive behaviors. DeMeyer, Hingtgen, and Jackson (1981) recommended the use of behavioral approaches. They stated that it is the treatment of choice as it allows for expansion of the individual's behavioral repertoire, and if executed properly, allows for interaction with many different therapists, which is ultimately critical in addressing ASD. Floortime, a child-oriented therapeutic play approach is part of developmental, individual-difference, relationship-based therapy. Developed by Stanley Greenspan, it addresses the challenges of autism by using techniques to promote social engagement and emotional reciprocity. In this approach, the therapist follows the lead of the child to gain the latter's attention so as to begin a two-way social exchange. Promoters of this approach assert that Floortime can be incorporated into daily routines, thus providing naturalistic contexts for intervention (Greenspan & Wieder, 1997).

Other approaches include relationship development intervention (RDI), which advocates family-based therapeutic intervention that focuses on what its founder, Steve Gutstein, termed the core deficits of autism. These include deficits in social exchanges, communication, foresight/hindsight, flexibility, and information processing typically observed in ASD. RDI seeks to motivate individuals with ASD to engage in dynamic social exchanges and, in doing so, is believed to address the core deficits of autism (Gutstein, Burgess, & Montfort, 2007).

To date, the various educational treatment approaches for ASD do not have enough evidence with respect to efficacy, though undoubtedly, individuals have had some degree of benefit and improvement following intervention. It is likely that in time, objective and scientific evaluations of technique and progress will be available to shed light on these seemingly promising approaches to ASD.

Developmental Disabilities and Mental Retardation

According to the Developmental Disabilities Act (PL 106–402), a developmental disability is defined as a severe, chronic disability that occurs before the age of 22 and is likely to continue over the life span. A developmental disability results in significant limitations in at least three major life activities (such as language skills, self-help skills, learning, mobility, independent living, and economic self-sufficiency). Those affected will have a need for extended or life-long support services.

Mental retardation is a developmental disability that is observed before the age of 18. It is defined by an individual's intellectual functioning level as measured on standard intelligence tests where results suggest that one's level of functioning is significantly low enough to have an impact on two or more adaptive skill areas. Children with mental retardation have difficulties not only in language and cognitive development but also in gross and fine motor development, acquisition of self-care, and learning. Thus, mental retardation affects a person's language and cognitive abilities and, in turn, that individual's ability to function independently.

The difference between the terms mental retardation and developmental disability is that the former makes reference to IQ scores whereas the latter does not. It is not uncommon for an individual to meet requirements for both categories. There are different causes of mental retardation. Among the more common causes are genetic conditions such as Down Syndrome and Fragile X Syndrome. In addition, problems during or immediately following pregnancy can also lead to mental retardation, such as fetal alcohol syndrome or perinatal asphyxia.

Individuals with mental retardation are described from three distinctive and critical perspectives: intellectual, adaptive, and behavioral (Soenen, van Berckelaer-Onnes, & Scholte, 2009). Individuals with mental retardation exhibit learning styles that reflect their cognitive limitations. Thus, short-term memory and working memory are below average; these individuals are generally much slower in their acquisition of new information. In many cases, attending behaviors are limited, further hindering learning attempts. Bray, Fletcher, and Turner (1997) reported a positive correlation between cognitive impairment and short-term memory deficits so that immediate recall of information is impaired. Individuals with mental retardation require more time to retrieve information as compared with typically developing peers (Merrill, 1990) but once information is established in long-term memory, retention is no worse than that observed in typically developing peers. Memory, motivation, ability to pay attention to relevant information while ignoring the irrelevant, learning rate and ability to generalize new information, and other facets of intellectual functioning must be assessed individually as different patterns of strengths and weaknesses have been reported for this heterogeneous clinical population (Fletcher, Blair, Scott, & Bolger, 2004).

The term adaptive behavior refers to the performance of social and personal activities of daily living; these include self-care skills and interpersonal skills to establish and sustain friendships and to develop coping strategies to deal with problems that are encountered during the course of exchanges with peers. Individuals with mental retardation often have poor language and communication skills, such as speaking out of turn, frequent changes of topic, and inappropriate eye gaze that hinder social exchanges.

Management Considerations

As with any other clinical population, it is important to assess and bring to light the strengths and weaknesses that are unique to the person with mental retardation. Because many of these individuals present with behavioral problems that interfere with administration of conventional tests, adaptations are often used to minimize these distracters. Stagg, Wills, and Howell (1989) cite several reasons for test adaptation including poor attention and motivation, physical limitations (impaired motor skills), and reduced hearing and/or vision. Although altering the way in which testing is administered threatens the validity of the instrument, one of the purposes of formal testing under these circumstances is to unveil true abilities rather than for comparative purposes with nonclinical peers. In some cases, clinicians may choose to test the limits of a client's ability by presenting test items beyond his or her level of functioning.

Attention Deficit (Hyperactivity) Disorder

One of the most common developmental problems that continue from childhood onto adulthood is ADHD. There are three subtypes of ADHD: predominantly hyperactive-impulsive, predominantly inattentive, and a combination of hyperactivity-impulsive and inattentive behaviors. For the most part, symptoms associated with ADHD occur early on in life. The National Institute of Mental Health (2008) identifies the following symptoms as being associated with specific types of ADHD.

Signs of hyperactivity include

- Nonstop talking
- Moving around, touching, and playing with everything in sight
- Trouble sitting still for activities such as mealtimes, story time, and school activities
- Difficulty staying focused on quiet tasks and activities.

Signs of inattention include:
- Easily distracted, forgetful, and frequent switching from one activity to the next
- Difficulty focusing on one activity at a time
- Easily bored by tasks unless these are highly enjoyable
- Difficulty focusing on organization and completion of tasks or learning a new task
- Difficulty in completing assignments, often losing things (e.g., pencils, homework assignments, toys) needed to complete assignments
- Does not seem to listen when spoken to
- Daydreamer, easily confused, and moves very slowly
- Difficulty processing information as quickly as peers
- Difficulty following directions.

Signs of impulsivity include:
- Impatience
- Difficulty waiting for turn in games and so on
- Blurt out inappropriate responses, show emotions without restraint, and act without regard for consequences
- May interrupt conversations or activities of others.

Comorbidity is high in this clinical population. Because of the different learning problems that result from ADHD, many affected children are referred for speech and language assessment and intervention. As a group, these individuals present with a wide range of problems in all aspects of language learning. In addition, assessment of auditory processing skills should be conducted. The language problems are usually not the result of a language delay, rather of impaired language processing. In some cases, the problems go largely undetected until the children enroll in school. Auditory processing deficits, which involve detection, discrimination, and analysis of speech sounds as well as short-term auditory memory, are common in children with ADHD. Many with ADHD are easily distracted in noisy environments and perform better in quiet settings. Reading comprehension is also problematic. Because hearing acuity is not the problem, difficulties relate to what they do with what they hear, not whether they hear well. Their problems in auditory processing can also lead to deficits in other language areas including organization of conversations, ability to follow conversations, difficulties with inferencing, and, in general, difficulties in social situations.

Management Considerations
Typically, a team approach is the best practice because teachers, physicians, and other health care and mental health providers are involved in the care of these individuals. SLPs use a variety of approaches in evaluating those identified as having ADHD. In addition to using

standardized tests to assess different language modalities and different language/speech parameters, classroom observations along with home visits provide information about the quality of peer and adult interactions. Because a language impairment can coexist with ADHD and because the symptoms of ADHD can mimic a language impairment, differential diagnosis aids in designing a treatment program. Initially, other disorders and conditions are ruled out, including underlying medical conditions, hearing and vision problems, anxiety or depression, psychiatric problems (oppositional defiant disorder or conduct disorder), learning disabilities, and any traumatic events that might affect behavior. Language impairment in ADHD has a severe disadvantage on the performance in school because of its impact on working memory and other cognitive functions and places them at risk for academic failure (Cohen et al., 2000).

A range of support services is used to address symptoms associated with ADHD, including medications, psychotherapy, and educational support services such as speech/language therapy. The expertise of different providers is used to direct the planning and execution of treatment approaches so that collaboration will facilitate greater understanding of the individual and ultimately improve outcome.

In some cases, medications (specifically stimulants) are used to treat behaviors associated with ADHD. These work to reduce impulsivity and improve attention. Although medications are not "cures" for ADHD, they are used to control negative behaviors and facilitate positive ones for learning and work-related tasks. Practitioners should be aware of all medications a child is taking and the side effects they may impart. Common side effects of stimulant medications include decreased appetite, anxiety, irritability, difficulties with sleeping, and in some rare cases, tics, which are typically minor in nature and manageable with dose adjustments.

Language Disorders

According to Goodglass, Kaplan, and Barresi (2001, p. 5), "aphasia refers to the disturbance of any or all of the skills, associations and habits of spoken and written language produced by injury to certain brain areas that are specialized for these functions. Disturbances in communication that are due to paralysis or incoordination of the musculature of speech or writing or to impaired vision or hearing are not, of themselves, aphasic." Persons with aphasia can have problems with receptive language (auditory comprehension and reading) and expressive language (verbal expression and writing). Some patients demonstrate sensory impairment as well, affecting hearing and vision. Aphasia can result from focal lesions in the left hemisphere of the brain as well as from more diffuse disease including brain tumors and head injury. Insults including brain tumor, head trauma, and infectious diseases are also causes of aphasia. Right brain damage has also been reported to produce aphasia, specifically with left-handed speakers.

Persons with aphasia can broadly be assigned to one of two groups—fluent versus nonfluent aphasics. Fluent aphasics are those who are able to speak spontaneously without marked hesitations or pauses though their language content is largely meaningless. On the other hand, nonfluent speakers are those whose productions are halting, with a reduced rate of speech.

Nonfluent Aphasia

Nonfluent aphasias include Broca's aphasia, transcortical motor aphasia (TMA), and global aphasia. Damage to Broca's area (frontal lobe) results in nonfluent aphasia, of which Broca's aphasia is the most common form. In these cases, speech is slow and labored so that rate of speech is notably reduced. Articulation is awkward and vocabulary is reduced. Although utterances are brief (in some cases, patients may only use one-word productions), they are meaningful. Comprehension is relatively intact. Verbal output is considered agrammatic in that function words (articles, prepositions, auxiliary verbs, grammatical endings of words, and the like) are omitted, whereas content words (nouns, verbs, adjectives, and adverbs) are better preserved. Speech output is sometimes referred to as telegraphic because of the paucity of function words. Repetition skills are also impaired.

In TMA, patients have limited verbal output except when they are asked to repeat complex words and utterances. On repetition tasks, both articulation skills and grammar are intact. It is the perseveration of repetition skills that distinguishes Broca's aphasia from TMA. Spontaneous production is characterized by errors in the use of grammatical words such as articles, imprecise production of different speech sounds, and perseveration (which refers to uncontrollable repetition of a response even though the stimulus has already been changed). Many patients have difficulty initiating conversational exchanges but are likely able to respond to simple questions. Comprehension is likely fair to excellent.

As the term implies, global aphasia is a severe impairment that is characterized by markedly reduced language comprehension and production. These patients are usually nonverbal and have little, if any, ability to speak (Wepman & Jones, 1961). All aspects of language are so severely impaired that there is no longer a pattern of persevered versus impaired components (Goodglass et al., 2001).

Fluent Aphasia

Fluent aphasias include Wernicke's aphasia, conduction aphasia, and transcortical sensory aphasia (TSA). Damage to Wernicke's area (found in the temporal lobe) results in Wernicke's aphasia, which is the most common of the fluent aphasias. In these cases, language comprehension is impaired and speech, though fluent and without any apparent articulation problems, is meaningless. Because of the fluent but semantically empty productions, the language output of patients with Wernicke's aphasia has often been referred to as "cocktail talk." In many cases, the productions are complex sentence forms. The hallmark feature of language errors is use frequency of verbal paraphasias, which refer to meaning errors in speech. For example, a patient might use the word "coffee" for "tea" where the error was not the intended word but it is semantically linked to the target. Despite apparent verbal fluency, patients with Wernicke's aphasia exhibit poor repetition skills and their productions include use of word substitutions.

Conduction aphasia is a rare form of fluent aphasia and is reported in less than 10% of aphasia cases (Bhatnager & Andy, 1995). Fluent verbal output is observed in these patients, and, interestingly, they make attempts to self-correct. A qualitative difference between language production of patients with conduction aphasia versus Wernicke's aphasia is observed where the former exhibits shorter fluent utterances. Spontaneous productions are more intact than repetition skills. For example, a difficulty in repeating complex words and repeating complex utterances has been reported (Goodglass et al., 2001). Word-finding problems are common. Finally, auditory comprehension is relatively intact for patients with conduction aphasia as compared with those with Wernicke's aphasia.

TSA is an extremely rare form of fluent aphasia that is characterized by intact repetition skills but markedly poor comprehension skills. These patients demonstrate fluent verbal output but have difficulty responding to simple commands. Although these patients are able to repeat complex sentences with good articulation skills, they fail to understand what they are repeating. Other areas of deficit include difficulty naming pictures, that is, these patients are not able to retrieve labels for objects, and on such tasks, they may repeat the words of the examiner. In some cases, output is characterized by use of nonspecific referring terms such as "these," "things," "those," and "the stuff," in place of content words, thus reflecting word retrieval deficits.

Management Considerations

The purpose of assessment is to gain a thorough description of language and cognitive impairment following brain damage. A number of critical skills are targeted during formal testing; these include spontaneous speech production, repetition of words, phrases, and sentences, auditory comprehension skills, and naming ability along with reading and writing skills. Formal assessment of these language modalities is found in a number of commercially available materials including the *Boston diagnostic examination of aphasia* (3rd ed) (Goodglass et al., 2001). Following administration of the examination, areas of language weakness are identified so that results can be used to implement a therapy plan. Severity of impairment is rated on a scale that allows for profiling of speech behaviors and deriving patterns of weaknesses and strengths. Other formal assessments include the Western Aphasia Battery (Kertesz, 1982) and the Communication Activities of Daily Living (Holland, 1980).

Much has been written about the association between initial severity of aphasia and rehabilitation potential where patients with denser (more severe) aphasias will require a longer period of recovery (see Mark, Thomas, & Berndt, 1992; Mazzoni et al., 1992). Initial aphasia severity had been considered a critical variable in ultimate language function where more severely impaired patients are less likely to regain functional skills as compared with mildly affected ones (Pedersen, Jørgensen, Nakayama, Raaschou, & Olsen, 1995). The role and contributions of the right hemisphere following left-hemisphere brain damage have been identified as having a predictive value regarding success in therapy (Richter, Wolfgang, Miltner, & Straube, 2008). Studies have shown that recruitment of the right hemisphere during aphasia therapy positively affects therapy outcomes.

Clinical evidence suggests that recovery is not limited to the immediate period following brain damage but extends well into the postacute phase for some patients with aphasia. For example, Yoko, Tomoyuki, and Masahiro (2000) examined the long-term recovery process of patients with chronic aphasia and reported that progress was still observed after 3 years of uninterrupted speech therapy.

Aside from the site of the brain damage and severity of the aphasia, other factors also directly affect therapy outcomes. These include the patient's age, gender, handedness, and various psychosocial issues such as motivation and emotional adjustment to disability—all of which will have an impact on the process of recovery. The primary goal of therapy is to restore a functional level of communication skills to meet social and emotional needs. Such goals can be addressed either in small group settings or on an individual basis.

Right-Hemisphere Damage

Right-hemisphere damage does not yield any predictable pattern of language impairment. Instead, this hemisphere has been associated with music appreciation, visuoperception skills, and emotions. Documented cases of behavioral problems following right-hemisphere damage suggest higher-level language and cognitive impairments. Deficits include disturbances in attention, initiation of verbal utterances, left-neglect, visual memory, judgment, and the social use of language including understanding and use of humor and body language (Myers, 1997). Paucity in facial expression (e.g., flat affect) while speaking, poor eye contact, failure to use gesture, and a lack of vocal inflection all characterize their interaction style. Right hemisphere-impaired individuals are often labeled "difficult personalities." Problems with social interactions may develop as result of this type of brain damage. These patients may talk endlessly without noticing a change in conversational topic, may fail to recognize a listener's need for clarification (Stierwalt, Clark, & Robin, 2000), or may joke causally about taboo topics, such as sex, without inhibition (Obler & Gjerlow, 1999).

Management Considerations
Higher-level language skills and improved cognition within a communicative context are the primary focus of therapeutic intervention for the person with right-hemisphere impairment. Remediation of attention, recall, and initiation of conversation are three areas frequently addressed. Because of impaired attention, reducing environmental distractions can facilitate communication, as does providing verbal cues that encourage patients to remain on topic. Other organizational devices including calendars, diaries, and clocks are useful in enhancing

organization skills. Repetition of instructions allows for more opportunity to understand and grasp the message. Combined with reduced social awareness, these deficits will invariably affect the quality of peer interactions.

Traumatic Brain Injury

Traumatic brain injury (TBI) is caused by a blow to the head or some type of injury that penetrates the head, causing a disruption in normal brain activity. Unlike strokes, damage to the brain is often diffuse, affecting a variety of perceptual and linguistic behaviors. In fact, thinking (memory and reasoning skills), language (comprehension and expression), perceptual (senses of touch, taste, and smell), and emotional (depression, anxiety, aggression, and personality changes) changes are frequently observed in the patient with TBI. Therefore, language is impaired as part of a complex constellation of memory and cognitive deficits instead of the isolated language impairment noted in aphasia.

Severity of the impairment depends on various factors, including the length of comatose state (if applicable), extent of tissue damage, lack of oxygen to the brain, swelling of the brain, and the buildup of cerebrospinal fluid (Miller, 1984). Because a number of mental changes are observed, the individual may exhibit disorientation and confusion in verbal output, along with anomia (word-finding difficulty). Difficulty integrating, analyzing, and synthesizing information affect the person's abstract reasoning and problem-solving abilities. Subsequent to such impairments, almost all aspects of daily living and communication may be compromised. Functional disability ranges in severity from a comatose state, with little or no response to the environment, to mild brain injury or postconcussive syndrome, which results in subtle manifestation of deficits (Ylvisaker & Szekeres, 1986).

Management Considerations

A number of cognitive and communication problems can be expected following a TBI, although the nature and severity of such will vary from one person to the next. Variables such as the extent of the brain injury, premorbid skills, educational level, and personality traits must be considered. Whereas the effects of brain injury are most serious immediately after the event, residual damage of the TBI is best addressed in therapy. Deficits in cognitive functions, executive functions, and language functions are commonly reported. As a result, these individuals may appear disoriented, inattentive, forgetful, and slow-to-respond. Specifically, the language deficits associated with TBI include word-finding problems (anomia), poor comprehension, inability to stay on topic in conversational exchanges, and poor perception of nuances in language (e.g., these persons may miss the punch line in jokes or misunderstand sarcasm). Speech may be described as dysarthric or apraxic; some may also experience dysphagia (swallowing problems).

During the initial stages of therapy, the SLP may focus on orientation to person, place, and time. If necessary, oromotor exercises may be introduced to address difficulties in speech production and swallowing. Language activities that facilitate comprehension and verbal expression are used to stimulate recovery of lost skills and develop compensatory strategies. Computer-assisted programs for the remediation of language impairments are introduced so that carryover activities can be implemented in the home. These programs have the benefit of portability—that is, individuals can work on therapy activities outside of the home. Evidence-based practice studies have suggested that these approaches have the desired outcomes in terms of meeting intervention goals (Gontkovsky, McDonald, Clark, & Ruwe, 2002). The goal of therapy is to achieve independence in all areas of functioning so as to allow the individual to return to premorbid activities.

It is expected that at least 10% of children with TBI will experience residual memory deficits as compared with problems seen in 30–40% of adult patients (Klonoff & Paris, 1974). The majority of brain-injured victims are younger than 30 years, with concomitant physical disabilities. As a result, treatment must be designed to address the current communication needs and to anticipate the cognitive demands of future educational and vocational endeavors. The direction of treatment is continually modified during the recovery process. Early intervention methods focus on remediation of deficit areas and instructional techniques aimed at restoration of skills. As recovery in function begins to plateau, efforts target implementation and training of compensatory strategies. The culmination of rehabilitation is directed toward carryover of skills and strategies into the everyday life of the client.

SPEECH DEVELOPMENT AND SPEECH DISORDERS

Typically children will follow a developmental course of acquiring the various speech sounds of the language to which they are exposed. Generally speaking, simpler sounds are observed before more complex sounds. By 6 years of age, English-speaking children can be expected to have mastered all of the target sounds of the language.

Atypical Development (Speech)

Whereas most children easily learn to produce the speech sounds of their language, others experience difficulty pronouncing them correctly. There is a predictable development course in speech sound acquisition and up until a certain age, inaccurate productions are acceptable. However, by age 8 most master the speech sounds of English. Some problems such as sensory loss (e.g., hearing), genetic (e.g., Down Syndrome) or neurological (e.g., cerebral palsy [CP]) disorders, developmental disability (e.g., autism), or structural abnormality (e.g., cleft palate) prevent mastery of some sounds. In such cases, intelligibility of speech is compromised.

Articulation Disorders

Articulation problems arise from impaired speech production that results in altered intelligibility. These range from mild to severe and negatively impact how well listeners understand speakers. Problems in articulation are described by the manner in which target sounds are produced. Some target sounds are omitted in production so that the speaker might produce "raf" for "raft" or "ches" for "chest." In other incidences, target sounds are either replaced or substituted. Examples of substitutions include "tat" for "cat" and "wowipop" for "lollipop." In a related example, a target sound may be distorted in production. For example, one may produce "thip" for "sip" or "thoo" for "zoo" where the tongue is thrust forward creating a frontal lisp.

In children, developmental delay is the most likely cause of articulation disorders where the child may have difficulties perceiving the fine details of target sounds and/or producing the features of the target sounds. Articulation problems are also associated with language delay. Other causes of articulation problems in childhood include brain damage, hearing loss, craniofacial anomalies including cleft palate, and dental problems.

Adults can also demonstrate speech disorders due to developmental disorder, sensory loss, structural deficits, or acquired disorder, such as brain damage, that may result in apraxia or dysarthria.

Management Considerations

Evaluation of articulation disorders includes the evaluation of the language status of the patient. Because some disorders may have similar manifestations, differential diagnosis is imperative to establish a precise diagnosis for the purposes of treatment and considerations of prognosis. In the assessment of speech sound production, standard and nonstandard approaches, including the collection of a speech sample followed by an error analysis, and finally assessment of intelligibility of speech in various communication settings, can be used.

Additionally, an examination of the oral cavity and articulators is conducted to determine whether there are structural and/or musculature deficits that contribute to the articulation problem.

Intervention is focused on treatment approaches that will address specific articulation problems. The goal of therapy is to improve speech sound discrimination, if necessary (i.e., if the child has difficulty hearing differences in speech sounds), and to improve sound production by reducing errors and increasing production of target sounds. Tasks are designed to be age appropriate, appealing, and highly motivating so as to provide the child with an opportunity to produce a variety of target sounds. In some cases, goals can be achieved in a relatively short period of time whereas in other cases, therapy may be necessary for longer periods of time.

Apraxia

Apraxia is defined as a disorder in carrying out or learning complex movements that cannot be accounted for by elementary disturbances of strength, coordination, sensation, compensation, or attention (Strub & Black, 1981). Verbal apraxia is characterized by a limited number of consonants and vowels, consistent and inconsistent articulation errors, and a greater number of errors with consonant clusters as compared with single speech sounds. Difficulty in producing fluent, intelligible speech is not due to muscle weakness or paralysis. Movement of the articulators (the tongue, lips, mandible, and velum) is easier in isolation. Sequencing such movements in rapid succession is problematic (Morley, 1965). Additionally, the initiation of these movements can be difficult.

Signs of apraxia in very young children include limited amount of cooing and babbling and late onset of first words. For these children, only a small repertoire of speech sounds is used and a limited number of different consonants are observed. Feeding problems including sensitivity to food tastes and textures have also been reported for this group. In children with apraxia, speech is distinguished from the production of typical peers by the continued immaturity of speech production, difficulty imitating speech sounds, predominance of brief phrases in place of longer utterances where longer utterances result in an increased number of errors, and notable groping behaviors as if they were searching for speech sounds. Some have described the speech sound repertoire of these children as not only being limited in the number of sounds acquired, but more importantly, the system is viewed as deviant (not delayed). The marked inconsistency in speech sound production is a hallmark feature of this disorder (Maassen, 2002).

Unlike peers with functional articulation problems, children with apraxia demonstrate vowel production errors, and general articulation problems persist over a longer period of time (Rosenbek & Wertz, 1972). In addition, features such as speech rhythm, fluency, stress, and intonation are affected in apraxia. In fact, inappropriate use of stress is one feature that is quite salient in calling attention to the speaker. Apraxia of speech in adults, like in children, results from brain damage. No language or cognitive deficits are a part of the apraxia profile though, in some cases, aphasia is a comorbid condition. A number of speech features characterize apraxia including sound substitutions where complex sounds are substituted with simpler ones (Wertz, LaPointe, & Rosenbek, 1984). Speakers with apraxia of speech fail to execute speech production on a volitional basis. Their production is slow, labored, and imprecise with respect to the production of target speech sounds, which disrupts the sequencing of speech sounds. Like in developmental apraxia, production of both consonants and vowels is affected. Such difficulties are evident when patients are asked to repeat words and phrases. LaPointe (1997) described qualitative differences in the production of automatic tasks (e.g., counting and reciting) versus volitional tasks (e.g., word repetition and confrontational naming) where the former is more intelligible. In most cases, speakers are aware of their problems but are unable to control the errors.

Management Considerations

In the management of patients presenting with apraxia of speech, the first goal is to define the problem. Differentiating among functional articulation problems, muscle weakness, sensory loss, and language impairment must be ruled out to arrive at a proper diagnosis. Treatment protocols are designed to address the problem of poor coordination of motor movements.

On many levels, the focus of intervention should be on creating and promoting positive feelings about verbal communication because many clients have the language capacity but are deficient in speech production. In very severe cases, augmentative devices may be used to support communication attempts. In many cases long-term, individualized therapy is necessary, and encouragement and support from family members and peers are vital for success. Treatment programs focus on planning, programming, storing, and retrieving the articulatory gestures necessary for different speech sounds. Approaches include oromotor exercises, visual, and auditory cues for target sounds and other speech sound production exercises and drills.

Dysarthria of Speech

Dysarthria is a neurogenic speech disorder that affects various aspects of speech production. It is caused by brain damage following stroke, head injury, tumors, and neurological disorders such as CP. In children, CP is a nonprogressive disorder that impairs movement and is one of the most common causes of dysarthria. Children with CP demonstrate varying degrees of dysarthria. Rosenbek and Wertz (1972) described speech disruptions as ranging from mild to severe, and they involve aspects of articulation (imprecise production of consonants and vowels), rate of speech production, respiration (which can limit breath support for speech production), laryngeal control (affecting loudness, pitch range, and voice quality where some patients may sound breathy), and feeding (in some cases, patients present with swallowing problems). Weakness in oromotor control can result in drooling.

In adults, dysarthria of speech results from brain damage, which involves paralysis, abnormal muscle tone, and/or incoordination of muscles related to speech production. Dysarthria can also affect respiration, phonation, resonance, articulation, and prosody (Rosenbek & LaPointe, 1985). This disorder does not have an impact on the patient's ability to use language; that is, it is not a language impairment such as aphasia. Instead, it is the production of speech sounds that is impaired.

Management Considerations

The therapy program for persons with dysarthria focuses on increasing effective communication through improving speech intelligibility. For the mildly involved dysarthric speaker, whose speech is fairly intelligible in certain situations, treatment includes enhancing communication efficiency while maintaining clarity and speech naturalness. For those moderately involved dysarthric speakers who are able to communicate with speech but who are not completely intelligible, the primary goal of treatment is to maximize their speech intelligibility. Traditional behavioral methods have focused on improving the strength and coordination of the speech musculature. New technology, encompassing the use of microcomputers and instrumental biofeedback, has facilitated the modification of acoustic parameters in speech performance. In some instances, however, these methods produce only limited changes in function. Compensatory techniques to enhance speech intelligibility may also be used, along with prosthetic devices, to aid vocal intensity and/or resonance (e.g., palatal lift).

For the severely involved dysarthric speaker who has poor or nonfunctional speech intelligibility, little or no verbal, written, or gestural communication, and severe physical disabilities, treatment may include augmentative/alternative communication (AAC). The selection of an appropriate AAC system is dependent upon the communication needs as well as the physical and cognitive abilities of the person. Systems range from simple objects, letter, or word boards (communication boards) where the user makes selections by pointing to more complex computer-based systems that provide synthesized speech, printed output, and memory (Yorkston, Beukelman, & Bell, 1988). The goals of treatment vary with the severity of the disability and, in some cases such as amyotrophic lateral sclerosis, with the progression of the disorder.

Stuttering

Stuttering is a disorder characterized by involuntary interruption of a smooth flow of speech sounds. Approximately 1% of the adult population is reported to have some form of stuttering; the incidence (or the number of new cases at a given time) rate is 5% (Guitar, 1998). It is widely accepted that many adults have stuttered at some time during their lives but have spontaneously recovered from the disorder. Although the onset of stuttering is usually during childhood, it can also occur in adulthood secondary to a discrete neurological, pharmacological, or psychological event. Stuttering tends to occur in males more than females (three of four stutterers are male), and stuttering tends to run in families.

There is no known "cure" for stuttering though some clients report spontaneous recovery from the disorder, and for others, the disorder remains unresolved and it is maintained well into adulthood.

Whereas all speakers will exhibit some disfluency in speech production, it is the type and frequency of disfluency along with associated secondary behaviors, if any, that determine whether a speaker is perceived as a "stutterer." Various aberrant speech behaviors that are considered stuttering may occur within the word whereas others occur in between words. Within-word disfluencies include part-word repetitions ("re-re-report"), sound prolongations ("w—eek"), and silent blocks where a sound is attempted but no phonation is heard. Between-word disfluencies include whole-word repetitions ("he-he-he is home"), interjections ("he...um...um...um is sick"), and revisions ("I purch...bought a car"). Coupled with the frequency with which these behaviors occur, listeners make judgments about stuttering and fluency along with judgments about the severity of stuttering. Listeners' judgments may negatively affect a speaker's fluency and emotional well-being.

Associated or secondary nonspeech behaviors refer to physical/visible behaviors that accompany disfluent speech. Examples of these include finger-tapping, blinking, moving parts of the body, lip tension, and flaring of the nostrils. Initially, such behaviors were produced by being incidentally paired with the disfluent speech. Because the behaviors served as a distractor for the speaker, they seemed to decrease stuttering because they redirected the speaker's attention when speaking. Over time, the speaker draws an erroneous correlation between a behavior such as finger-tapping and fluency and the speaker begins to use finger-tapping to avoid stuttering. With overuse of such strategies, the novelty of the finger-tapping wears off but the stuttering persists. This results in the speaker incorporating finger-tapping as part of his stuttering behavior.

For the person who stutters, there is a wide range of response to the interruption in the flow of speech. For some speakers, disfluencies are not necessarily troublesome; they do not rely on secondary behaviors or devices to escape or avoid stuttering. Yet for others, the disfluencies may be so severe that speakers feel helpless and out of control. Embarrassment, fear, and shame are commonly reported by this group of speakers (Guitar, 1998). For this group, feelings and attitudes must be taken into consideration in the planning of treatment.

Management Considerations

Current literature divides therapy approaches for stuttering into two basic categories: stuttering modification therapy and fluency-shaping therapy. The former focuses on teaching the client to modify his stuttering behaviors and to reduce the fear associated with speaking and stuttering. The client is taught to confront the stuttering, thereby reducing the avoidance of stuttering. The latter focuses on the establishment of a level of speech fluency followed by therapy activities with the primary goal of integrating fluency into conversational speech (Guitar, 1998). The emphasis is on slow, easy-flowing speech. More recently, fluency-enhancing devices have become available to those who stutter. These small units are worn in the ear canal (much like a hearing aid) and are based on the use of altered auditory feedback as a means of reducing stuttering. Specifically, delayed auditory feedback and frequency-altered feedback can be programmed into each unit to meet the particular needs of a client. Research has shown that these devices can markedly reduce and even eliminate stuttering within a brief period of time. Efficacy studies on these devices are currently being conducted so that the long-term benefits of this therapy can be assessed (Van Borsel, Reunes, & Van den Bergh, 2003).

Voice

Phonation, or voice production, is a complex neuromotor activity that requires coordination of respiration, laryngeal function, and resonance. Disruption of any one of these processes can result in a disordered voice, termed dysphonia. Such conditions may result from pathological, neurological, traumatic, or behavioral conditions. This discussion is confined to those conditions that relate to a medical or neurological etiology.

Vocal fold pathologies disrupt the biomechanics of laryngeal function, thereby causing a phonatory disturbance. Vocal nodules, vocal polyps, contact ulcers, and laryngitis are the most prevalent benign conditions. Vocal fold pathologies are usually characterized by hoarse, breathy, strained, or harsh vocal quality and, at times, low vocal intensity. In addition, neurological or traumatic injury to the CNS or the larynx may result in vocal fold paralysis, resulting in a breathy voice quality, low intensity, or, in more severe cases, a total lack of phonation, which is termed aphonia. Laryngeal tumors, of which approximately 80% are malignant, may also exist (English, 1976). Tumors are often suspected when there is a prolonged period of hoarse vocal quality combined with complaints of pain. Depending on the extent of surgical resection of the tumor, the individual can be rendered dysphonic or even aphonic, that is, with reduced voicing or no voice at all.

A common medical procedure that produces aphonia is tracheostomy. When the upper airway is compromised, an artificial airway, or tracheostomy, is surgically created in the neck below the cricoid cartilage of the larynx. Inhalation and exhalation take place below the larynx, precluding the passage of air through the vocal folds that normally produces voice. Individuals may undergo a tracheostomy for a variety of medical conditions, including chronic obstructive pulmonary disease, laryngeal trauma, or progressive neurological diseases such as amyotrophic lateral sclerosis or myasthenia gravis (Dikeman & Kazandjian, 2003).

Management Considerations

Management of voice disorders requires the coordinated efforts of an SLP and various medical specialists including otolaryngologists. Treatment of noncancerous vocal fold pathologies often includes medical intervention (e.g., surgical resection) along with a period of vocal rest. When vocal abuse or misuse is identified as a cause of the pathology, voice therapy is recommended. The goal is the elimination of vocal abuse behaviors and the promotion of good vocal hygiene. Several techniques used include breathing exercises, relaxation approaches, and digital manipulation/pressure.

In the case of vocal fold paralysis, remediation focuses on improving vocal fold approximation to produce voice. Spontaneous recovery is expected in many cases, usually within 6 months of onset. In cases where recovery has not occurred, surgical interventions for paralysis include silastic tube implantation, thyroplasty, vocal cord augmentation, or vocal cord repositioning to aid vocal cord closure (Colton & Casper, 1990). Voice therapy for this condition is usually used to facilitate maximum gains. More recently, botulinum toxin injections have been used experimentally to facilitate increased vocal fold function in specific phonatory disorders, such as spasmodic dysphonia (Adler, Bansberg, Krein-Jones, & Hertz, 2004).

Treatment for malignant vocal fold pathologies incorporates surgical resection, radiation, and/or chemotherapy, along with voice strengthening or restoration. A total laryngectomy, for example, requires the excision of the entire larynx. The laryngectomy renders the patient aphonic, and respiration takes place via a surgically created airway in the neck called the stoma. Restoration of speech is usually accomplished by the use of an artificial larynx, esophageal speech, or a tracheoesophageal puncture.

For the tracheostomized individual with an intact larynx, voice restoration is the primary goal. Finger occlusion or capping of the tracheostomy tube is often adequate to redirect exhaled air through the vocal folds so that normal phonation is produced. Additionally, the use of prosthetic speaking valves or a two-way tracheostomy valve will facilitate the return of voice.

Prognosis for successful intervention depends on the etiology of the disorder, the severity of the dysphonia, and the regeneration of the vocal physiology. Of course, behavioral factors, including motivation, and willingness to accept a modified but functional voice are also important components.

Dysphagia

The ability to swallow is a basic function essential to our health and well-being, affording us both pleasure and nutrition. Eating and swallowing are intertwined in the daily fabric of life. The act of swallowing encompasses the interaction of complex anatomic, neurological, and physiological systems. Even small alterations in these systems—the timing of events, structures, or physiology involved in swallowing—can have a profound influence on the process and significantly alter a person's quality of life.

Difficulty in swallowing, or dysphagia, affects people throughout the age spectrum with a wide range of developmental, neurological, structural, and medical etiologies. Dysphagia can encompass a person's ability to swallow saliva, liquids, and/or food of all consistencies. A person with dysphagia may swallow unsafely, which causes food or saliva to enter his airway, a process termed aspiration, or a person may have a weak and slow swallowing function resulting in difficulty obtaining adequate food and liquids to ensure proper nutrition. Mastication (chewing) may be impaired and some people may experience drooling. Other people may have difficulty propelling their foods through their mouth or pharynx into the esophagus. These deficits create serious problems in sustaining a healthy and satisfying quality of life. Consequences of dysphagia range from discomfort, for example, throat pain, to coughing and choking or even life-threatening illness. Serious sequelae include aspiration pneumonia, severe weight loss, dehydration, and malnutrition.

Swallowing disorders are found in both the pediatric and adult populations. Problems can arise from various causes, including developmental disabilities, neurological diseases, such as stroke, degenerative diseases, alterations of anatomy and physiology following surgery, TBI, cardiovascular and other systemic diseases, congenital defects, failure to thrive, and damage arising from chemoradiation treatment or surgery for head/neck cancer. It may also arise from mechanical problems of the swallowing mechanism or from gastrointestinal disorders (Murry & Carrau, 2006).

The infant or child with a feeding or swallowing problem presents with specific challenges. The child may demonstrate refusal to eat, have difficulty with the act of eating, or be unable to sustain oral feedings to maintain adequate intake (Pitcher, Crandell, & Goodrich, 2008). He/she may have never experienced age-appropriate feeding and swallowing for daily nutrition and hydration needs. This population includes children who have neurological, structural, or developmental disorders and those who are medically fragile or with complex medical diagnoses including gastroesophageal disorders, developmental delays, various genetic syndromes, sensory integration disorders, and craniofacial anomalies. Children who are on the autism spectrum or fail to thrive often show aberrant feeding issues. If a delay or disruption in the feeding process occurs during the child's early years, the child may demonstrate malnutrition, poor growth, delayed development, poor academic achievement, psychological problems, and loss of general good health and well-being (Arvedson & Brodsky, 2002).

Swallowing Stages

Swallowing is a complex series of coordinated events involving the cerebral cortex, brain stem, 6 different cranial nerves, and 31 facial and oral muscles working together to initiate the swallowing process. Normal swallowing is rapid, safe, and efficient, taking a person less than 2 seconds to move foods or liquids from the mouth, through the pharynx, and into the esophagus (Logemann, 1998). Swallowing occurs in three stages: oral, including oral preparatory and oral transit, pharyngeal, and esophageal. The first stage is voluntary and is controlled by cortical centers located in the brain. The next two stages are involuntary and are coordinated by brain stem centers.

In the oral stage, food and liquids are mixed with saliva and, if solid, chewed to an appropriate size and consistency. Oral transit follows as the material is propelled by the tongue from the front toward the back of the mouth and then into the pharynx. When material is in the pharynx (pharyngeal stage), several processes occur simultaneously to halt respiration, protect the airway, open the upper esophageal sphincter (the top portion of the esophagus), and transport the material being swallowed into the esophagus and stomach. Material must be efficiently transported with good airway protection to prevent the misdirection of material into the airway. This misdirection, termed aspiration, of liquids or foodstuffs into the airway, can lead to asphyxiation, pulmonary inflammation, or infections, including bronchitis and pneumonias, and permanently damage the respiratory system.

The speed of swallowing encompasses both the oral and pharyngeal transit times and is normally 2 seconds or less. The final stage of swallowing, the esophageal stage, transports the swallowed material through the length of the esophagus, the gastroesophageal junction, and into the stomach. The esophageal stage normally can take up to 8–10 seconds. If the oral, pharyngeal, and esophageal stages of swallowing are not competent, it is unlikely that the patient will be able to obtain adequate nutrition by mouth for the maintenance of good health.

Management Considerations
Prior to the initiation of swallow treatment and management, the patient receives an evaluation that delineates the oral, pharyngeal, and upper esophageal swallow function. The evaluation of swallow function often includes a clinical or bedside examination and an instrumental assessment.

CLINICAL "BEDSIDE" EXAMINATION. The clinical, or bedside, examination of swallowing determines clinical signs and symptoms of swallow dysfunction and the anatomical and functional status of the swallowing mechanism. It also includes a medical, feeding, and swallowing history, examination and function of the oral structures, assessment of the effect of therapeutic postures or maneuvers on the swallow, and may offer observations of swallow competence if test swallows are given (Goodrich & Walker, 2008). It can provide indirect evidence of difficulty but it does not define the disordered anatomy or physiology of the oropharynx and upper cervical esophagus or the subsequent swallow impairments. With the adult population, the clinical examination is often viewed as a screening assessment and usually does not contain the necessary information to initiate a treatment and swallow management plan.

In evaluating a pediatric case, a comprehensive clinical assessment may include many of the items previously listed in addition to an in-depth analysis of the feeding history, developmental history, oral sensory–motor, feeding skills, and psychosocial environment, including a caregiver interview (Pitcher et al., 2008). An instrumental assessment may be needed if concerns arise regarding the pharyngeal physiology or risks of aspiration. Depending upon the etiology, an instrumental test may not be necessary, rather only an in-depth clinical assessment will be required to obtain a complete evaluation of the child's feeding and swallowing problems.

INSTRUMENTAL SWALLOW ASSESSMENTS. Several instrumental assessments of swallow function are available to the practitioner. The two most widely used are the videoflouroscopic swallow study (VFSS) also termed as the modified barium study (MBS) and the fiberoptic endoscopic evaluation of swallowing (FEES) with or without sensory testing (FEESST) (Aviv, Kim, & Sacco, 1998).

The VFSS is a comprehensive dynamic assessment of the oral, pharyngeal, and esophageal phases of swallowing using videofluoroscopy when dysphagia is suspected. The patient ingests various food consistencies and liquids that are impregnated with barium. The study is recorded and provides a detailed analysis of function, coordination, and timing of swallowing. It identifies the presence/absence of aspiration—the passage of material into the airway instead of the esophagus. It defines the etiology of aspiration and other swallow deficits (Logemann, 1993). It allows testing and examines the effects of specific treatment procedures (Murry & Carrau, 2006). It aids in devising an appropriate treatment plan and identifies the best method of nutritional intake, for example, oral, nonoral, or a combination.

The FEES involves the passage of a fiberoptic laryngoscope through the nostril into the pharynx to view the pharyngeal swallow during ingestion of various materials. It uses a flexible nasoendoscope and evaluates the larynx and pharynx while giving the patient small amounts of liquids and solids mixed with food dye to swallow (Langmore, Shatz, & Olson, 1998). This study, which is also recorded, does not involve any radiation and is more sensitive than the MBS in detecting structural abnormalities of the pharynx and larynx. However, it does not assess the oral stage of swallowing, the cervical esophagus, or view the actual swallowing process when it is occurring. This limits the examiner's information as to the oral, pharyngeal, and cervical esophageal deficits. It also limits the evaluation for aspiration during swallowing. Furthermore, depending upon the endoscope's positioning, the examiner may not be able to observe additional aspects of the swallow, such as swallow modifications, during the study to obtain improved swallow function.

In recent years, with technology-enhanced diagnostics and physiology-based treatment techniques, health care professionals have discovered that active intervention with the swallowing-impaired individual often aids in a person's return to normal feeding and swallowing (Groher, 1997). Treatment is designed to reestablish or increase oral intake, maintain adequate nutrition and hydration, improve the swallowing safety, and eliminate aspiration. When specific anatomical or physiological deficiencies are present, the therapy plan is usually devised from information obtained from clinical and instrumental assessments. Intervention can include swallow rehabilitation and, if needed, specific medical/surgical techniques.

Remediation involves identifying problems and selecting correct swallowing techniques to address these problems. Through exercises and management strategies, many individuals will eventually show improvement in swallowing function. Treatment can be divided into three types: management of the impaired swallow by changing the type and consistencies of foods and liquids to aid intake and reduce risk of aspiration; compensatory strategies to eliminate the symptoms of the swallowing problem while not necessarily changing the swallow physiology; and specific therapy techniques, designed to change the swallow physiology (Groher & Crary, 2010).

Examples of rehabilitation techniques designed to change the swallow physiology include (1) providing exercise programs to improve muscle range of motion, strength, and muscle coordination (Kays & Robbins, 2006); (2) enhancing sensory input to improve the awareness of food in the mouth or the speed at which the pharyngeal swallow is triggered; (3) taking voluntary control over timing and coordination of specific swallowing movements; and (4) using specific maneuvers, designed to change selected aspects of the pharyngeal swallow.

In the past several years, new treatment regimens have been developed utilizing research in muscle strengthening and neuromuscular stimulation. The Iowa Oral Performance Instrument protocol for oral resistance training developed by Robbins Gangnon, Theis, Kays, and Hind (2005) has shown promising results with functional swallow improvements noted. Sapienza and Wheeler (2006) showed the benefits in respiratory muscle training to improve airway protection and enhance swallow function. Recently, surface neuromuscular electrical stimulation has been used to treat various dysphagia impairments. The intent of the stimulation has been to enhance contraction of muscles of swallowing, especially by increasing the number of motor action potentials supplied to the muscles involved (Leonard & Kendall, 2008). The use of neuromuscular electrical stimulation has recently received a lot of attention and positive claims of excellent results. To date, however, the research on its efficacy has been somewhat contradictory (Blumenfeld, Hahn, Lepage, Leonard, & Belafsky, 2006; Ludlow et al., 2007).

In many cases, the individual is best managed when compensatory and direct treatment techniques are used simultaneously, that is, the patient is given a compensatory technique that enables him to eat by mouth while swallow treatment is initiated. The direct treatment will eventually improve oropharyngeal muscle function and enable the patient to eat without compensatory postures.

If swallowing therapy does not prove effective, there are limited prosthetic and surgical options that may be appropriate for select patients. For example, a palatal lift elevates the soft palate to achieve separation between the oral and nasal cavity, thus preventing regurgitation of food through the nose. In the case of a vocal cord paralysis, vocal fold medialization or augmentation of the vocal folds with an absorbable material, such as collagen or fat, to increase vocal cord closure may decrease the chance of aspiration. Dilatation of the upper cervical esophagus may assist in treating cricopharyngeal dysfunction by stretching the upper cervical esophagus so that foods and liquids can pass through into the stomach.

Some patients are unable to take adequate nutrition by mouth. This may be temporary in patients who are recovering from an acute medical condition, such as a stroke, or long term as with patients who have a neuromuscular degenerative disease and are no longer able to manage oral nutrition (Murry & Carrau, 2006). Short- or long-term nonoral feeding options may need to be considered if the person with a feeding or swallowing impairment is unable to maintain necessary nutrition and hydration for daily life and well-being.

HEARING AND HEARING DISORDERS

Hearing is an integral component of communication. Every year in this country, approximately 12,000 infants are born with a permanent hearing loss and 3 of 1000 infants are born with some type of hearing loss; approximately 17% or 36 million Americans have some type of hearing loss (Kochkin, 2007). Early detection and treatment of these conditions are critical in assuring the acquisition of language and cognitive prerequisites for academic and social success. Universal hearing screenings are now available in many states. These efforts have resulted in the provision of early intervention services to the affected child and support services to the family by promoting their interests and advocating for the needs of the child. In comparison with their hearing peers, the academic performance of children who are deaf or hard of hearing is poor. For example, Traxler (2000) reported that the reading comprehension levels of such 18 year olds is estimated to be at the fourth-grade level.

With increased longevity of the American population, the number of individuals with some type and degree of hearing loss continues to rise (National Institute on Deafness and Other Communication Disorders, Better Hearing Institute, 1999). In fact, hearing loss has been identified as the third most prevalent chronic condition among the older population in the United States (National Institute on Deafness and Other Communication Disorders, Better Hearing Institute, 1999).

Hearing losses are identified according to where the damage is found in the auditory system—in the outer/middle ear and/or the inner ear. Thus, the four types of hearing losses are identified as conductive losses that result from damage to the outer or middle ear and sensorineural losses that involve the inner ear (cochlea) and/or the auditory nerve. Mixed hearing losses have both a conductive and sensorineural component. Central hearing losses refer to damage along the auditory pathway or in the brain itself. The term functional hearing loss is reserved for hearing losses for which there is no organic cause for the impairment. Audiological testing is conducted to determine the type and degree of hearing loss.

Conductive Hearing Loss

When sound is not effectively transmitted because of barriers in the outer or middle ear, the result is a conductive hearing loss. Examples of these barriers include malformation of the outer or middle ear, impacted cerumen (ear wax), presence of a foreign body, and middle ear pathology. Any of these conditions impede sound transmission so that the sound that is perceived by the listener is described as "muffled" and of low volume. Under these conditions, speech sounds are not distorted so that by increasing the volume of the signal, speech is understood.

Abnormalities of the outer ear tend to produce a hearing loss of varying degrees. Outer ear pathologies include malformations of the auricle or absence of the external auditory canal (meatus), which may be a hereditary condition, such as Treacher Collins syndrome, or the result of traumatic injury. Otitis externa (swimmer's ear) results in a conductive hearing loss caused by swelling of the skin lining in the external auditory canal. Tumors (both malignant and benign) and cerumen (ear wax) interfere with sound transmission when they completely obstruct the ear canal and eardrum.

As in the outer ear, any barrier or abnormality of the middle ear system often produces a conductive hearing loss. The most common condition arises from otitis media or middle ear infection. In chronic cases, fluid accumulation in the middle ear not only dampens the sound signal but can rupture the tympanic membrane (eardrum). For children, the critical concern is the fluctuating hearing loss that results from each episode of ear infection and the subsequent impact these losses can have on the development of language and speech skills.

Fusion or absence of the ossicles (three small bones of the middle ear) results in an inability to transmit sound from the middle to the inner ear. Otosclerosis is a progressive structural condition that results in the formation of spongy bone over these bones, causing fixation. Damage to the middle ear can also occur following head trauma or perforation of the eardrum from tumors in the middle ear.

Sensorineural Hearing Loss

Damage to the inner ear (cochlea) or auditory nerve results in sensorineural hearing loss. Unlike a conductive loss where sounds are "not loud enough," a sensorineural loss results in not only reduced loudness but it also affects the ability to hear clearly. For example, with a high-frequency loss, certain sounds become more difficult to hear so that distinguishing among words in running speech is problematic. Consequently, word intelligibility is compromised. Patients with sensorineural hearing losses will complain that speech is unclear, even if the signal is loud enough. Hearing is further challenged in noisy conditions where patients have problems distinguishing the signal (speech) from the noise.

A sensorineural loss can result from a congenital condition or an acquired disorder. Congenital hearing losses result from either genetic factors (35–50% of the cases) or prenatal or perinatal conditions (English, 1976). Prenatal conditions that result in hearing loss include rubella, RH incompatibility, anoxia, viruses, and the use of ototoxic drugs during the birth process. Genetic conditions that may result in hearing loss at birth or later in life (perinatal) include Waardenburg's syndrome, Crouzon's disease, and Pierre Robin syndrome.

Acquired hearing loss can result from a number of different conditions, including viruses, degenerative diseases, tumor, ototoxic drugs, or noise exposure. Viruses causing diseases, including measles, mumps, and meningitis, can result in sensorineural hearing loss. Degenerative changes to the auditory system associated with the aging process result in a progressive sensorineural hearing loss called presbycusis. Lesions of the auditory nerve (e.g., acoustic neuromas) are additional causes of acquired hearing loss. Prolonged and excessive use of well-known drugs, such as aspirin, quinine, and certain antibiotics, may produce temporary or permanent hearing loss as well (Martin, 1986).

People of all ages can develop noise-induced sensorineural hearing losses (NHL). NHL usually results from excessive exposure to loud noises or sounds at work or during leisure time activities. For example, attending rock concerts, hunting/shooting, and mowing the lawn are all examples of environmental sounds that at high enough levels can negatively affect hearing sensitivity. The severity is dependent upon the intensity and duration of the noise exposure. Hearing loss due to noise may be temporary, as with brief exposure to high levels of loud sound, or permanent, if the exposure is repetitive over long periods (Martin, 1986).

Meniere's disease, often seen clinically, is characterized by fluctuating sensorineural hearing loss, accompanied by vertigo, vomiting, tinnitus, and fullness in the affected ear. The site of the lesion is cochlear; however, there is no definitive cause for this disease. In the course of Meniere's disease, either cochlear hearing loss or vestibular symptoms may be present but usually will not co-occur. Meniere's disease occurs at any age but is most prevalent in adults (Paparella, DaCosta, Fox, & Yoon, 1991).

Central Hearing Loss

These are quite rare and are caused by hypoxia hyperbilirubinemia/kernicterus or intraventricular hemorrhage (Haddad, 2004).

Functional Hearing Loss

The term functional hearing loss is frequently used to describe a hearing loss for which there is no organic pathology. A functional loss is also referred to as pseudohypoacusis, nonorganic hearing loss, psychogenic hearing loss, or hysterical deafness. The term malingering has been used to describe individuals who consciously falsify physical or psychological symptoms. The audiological evaluation may not be able to determine if a nonorganic hearing loss is the result of an unconscious or a conscious behavior. Financial gain, compensation, and psychological or emotional factors can contribute to this behavior (Katz, 2001).

Classification of Hearing Loss

Classifying hearing impairments by the degree and type of loss is a convenient method of interpreting audiological results and aids in determining the effect of the hearing handicap on communication. Although inferences can be made from interpreting the test results, the degree of impairment is affected by a variety of other factors, including the type, degree, and configuration of hearing loss, age of onset, cognitive status, educational background, and the individual's personality.

The following classification schema, with physical and functional manifestations along with a rating of hearing handicap, may be helpful to the professional's understanding of the hearing-impaired individual.

Mild hearing loss is associated with a 26–40 dB hearing loss. The individual often has difficulty with faint speech, distant speech, or understanding conversational speech in background noise. This is considered a slight hearing handicap.

Moderate hearing loss is associated with 41–55 dB hearing loss. The individual has difficulty understanding conversational speech, especially in noisy environments, if the distance between the speaker and listener is more than 3 feet. This is considered a mild hearing handicap.

Moderately severe hearing loss is a 56–70 dB hearing loss. The individual requires speech to be loud and may have difficulty understanding speech in most listening situations, unable to hear conversational speech. This is considered a marked hearing handicap.

Severe hearing loss is a 71–90 dB hearing loss. The individual hears loud speech approximately 1 foot from the speaker and is aware of some environmental noises; speech sounds in conversation will not be heard. This is considered a severe hearing handicap.

Profound hearing loss is a greater than 90 dB hearing loss. The individual's understanding of speech is poor; conversational speech is not audible, but some loud sounds may be heard; and the individual is unable to rely on hearing as the only modality in communication situations. This is considered an extreme hearing handicap.

Management Considerations

It is useful to view management for the hearing-impaired population as either medical or surgical intervention, followed by appropriate aural rehabilitation as needed. One or all of these treatment modalities may be required to maximize the individual's functional communication capability. Medical intervention is indicated once a conductive or mixed hearing loss is identified. For example, hearing sensitivity is often improved or restored with antibiotics when a middle ear infection is present. Surgery is frequently the treatment of choice for structural or physiological etiologies. Most sensorineural hearing losses are not amenable to medical or surgical intervention. A life-threatening tumor or disease associated with sensorineural hearing loss, however, can necessitate otologic surgery. Hearing preservation is not the primary concern in this situation.

Following the appropriate medical or surgical intervention, aural rehabilitation may be initiated. Aural rehabilitation includes amplification, speech reading, and auditory training. The aim of aural rehabilitation is to maximize the use of residual hearing for the hearing-impaired individual to function in social, educational, and vocational roles. A secondary purpose is to educate the individual to manage his or her hearing aid, to optimize communication strategies, and to prevent the possibility of further hearing impairment.

Amplification is central to a treatment program of aural rehabilitation. Amplification includes hearing aids that intensify the speech signal to a comfortable listening level for the hearing-disordered person. Hearing aids are frequency specific, allowing for amplification of those frequencies in which hearing loss is present (Hartford, 1988).

In recent years, amplification has been improved with advances in hearing aid components. This has resulted in miniaturization of hearing aids with greater frequency specificity. In addition, technology has allowed for the development of programmable or digital hearing aids. These have the capacity to be programmed to acoustically accommodate different listening environments. In a noisy situation, for instance, the hearing aid wearer can adjust the aid to reduce low-frequency input to reduce background noise (Sammeth, 1990).

In some situations, an individual can use both a traditional hearing aid and an assistive listening device. This device captures sound inches from the source and transmits it directly to the listener's ear without losing the sound intensity of the speech signal and without amplifying unwanted environmental sounds. For example, in a lecture hall, the lecturer wears a microphone inches from his or her mouth. The signal is transmitted through the air, by either infrared or FM waves, directly to the listener's hearing aid, a special FM unit, or a special infrared unit. Other assistive listening devices available include a closed caption decoder for television, flashing smoke detectors, flashing alarm clocks, and vibrator alarm beds.

Cochlear implants, a recent breakthrough, are surgically implanted devices available for children and adults who present with severe to profound hearing losses. The cochlear implant is designed to amplify some of the speech spectrum information in an attempt to enhance functional hearing and communication abilities. A cochlear system includes two surgically implanted parts: one is placed behind the outer ear in the mastoid area and the other is implanted into the cochlea. Finally, an externally worn speech processor and a headset are placed behind the ear (Zwolan, 2002). Sounds are transformed into small electrical currents that stimulate auditory nerves found in the cochlea and produce hearing sensation.

For severely hearing impaired or deaf individuals, sign language may be the primary method of communication. The most commonly used form of sign language in the United States is the American Sign Language (ASL). ASL is the third most commonly used language in the United States. Sign language may be implemented as the sole means of communication or used in conjunction with any combination of previously described management methods. Like any other natural language, ASL has its own grammar and vocabulary.

An important piece of technology designed for this population is the telecommunication device for the deaf (TDD). The TDD allows direct interface with a phone line. The message is typed and either transmitted to a visual display screen or printed out at the receiver's TDD. Many phone companies provide toll-free numbers so that a hearing-impaired person using a TDD can communicate via telephone with a normal hearing person.

Finally, speech reading, traditionally called lip reading, consists of using visual cues for the recognition of speech sounds and incorporates the use of facial expressions, body movements, and gestures. Speech reading alone, however, is ineffective because only one third of English speech sounds are visible. Auditory training, instructing the individual to maximize his residual hearing, in conjunction with speech reading, enables the person to use minimal auditory cues most effectively. The combination of speech reading, auditory training, and amplification offers the hearing-disordered individual an enhanced comprehension of speech (Miller, Groher, Yorkston, & Rees, 1988).

CONCLUSIONS

It is appropriate to conclude this chapter by reiterating the critical role that speech, language, and communication skills play in our daily lives. Whereas many of us, thankfully, will never have first-hand experience with the devastation impairment in these areas can cause, it nonetheless can be all encompassing and can affect the daily routines of those afflicted with such disorders. A fair amount of knowledge has been massed about these disorders and there remain important challenges that are still unmet.

REFERENCES

Adler, C. H., Bansberg, S. F., Krein-Jones, K., & Hentz, J. G. (2004). Safety and efficacy of botulinum toxin type B (Myobloc) in adductor spasmodic dysphonia. *Movement Disorders, 19*, 1075–1079.

Alexander, A., Anderson, H., Heilman, P., Voeller, K., & Torgesen, J. (1991). Phonological awareness training and the remediation of analytic decoding deficits in a group of severe dyslexics. *Annals of Dyslexia, 41*, 193–206.

Arvedson, J. C., & Brodsky, L. (2002). *Pediatric swallowing and feeding.* Albany, NY: Singular.

Aviv, J., Kim, T., & Sacco, R. (1998). FEESST: A new bedside endoscopic of the motor and sensory components of swallowing. *Annals of Otolaryngology and Rhinology, 107*, 189–201.

Baron-Cohen, S. (1992). Out of sight or out of mind: Another look at deception in autism. *Journal of Child Psychology and Psychiatry, 33*, 1141–1155.

Bellis, T. J. (1996). *Assessment and management of central auditory processing disorders in the educational setting: From science to practice.* San Diego, CA: Singular.

Benson, V., & Marano, M. (1995). Current estimates from the National Health Interview Survey, 1993. In *Vital and health statistics* (Series 10, No. 190). Atlanta, GA: National Center for Health Statistics.

Bhatnager, S. C., & Andy, O. J. (1995). *Neuroscience for the study of communication disorders* (1st ed.). Baltimore: Williams and Wilkins.

Blumenfeld, L., Hahn, Y., Lepage, A., Leonard, R., & Belafsky, P. C. (2006). Transcutaneous electrical stimulation verses traditional dysphagia therapy: A nonconcurrent cohort study. *Otolaryngology-Head and Neck Surgery, 135,* 754–757.

Bray, N. W., Fletcher, K. L., & Turner, L. A. (1997). Cognitive competencies and strategy use in individuals with mental retardation. In W. W. Maclean Jr. (Ed.), *Ellis' handbook of mental deficiency, psychological theory, and research* (3rd ed., pp. 197–217). Mahwah, NJ: Erlbaum.

Cohen, N. J., Vallance, D. D., Barwick, M., Im, N., Menna, R., Horodezky, N., et al. (2007). The interface between ADHD and language impairment: An examination of language, achievement, and cognitive processing. *Journal of Child Psychology and Psychiatry, 43,* 353–362.

Colton, R. H., & Casper, J. K. (1990). *Understanding voice problems: A physiological perspective for diagnosis and treatment.* Baltimore: Lippincott Williams and Wilkins.

DeMyer, M. K., Hingtgen, J. N., & Jackson, R. K. (1981). Infantile autism reviewed: A decade of research. *Schizophrenia Bulletin, 7,* 388–450.

Dikeman, K., & Kazandjian, M. (2003). *Communication and swallowing management of tracheostomized and ventilator-dependent adults* (2nd ed.). San Diego, CA: Singular.

English, G. M. (1976). *Otolaryngology.* New York: Harper and Row.

Fey, M. E., Cleave, P. L., Long, S. H., & Huges, D. L. (1993). Two approaches to the facilitation of grammar in children with language impairment: An experimental evaluation. *Journal of Speech and Hearing Research, 36,* 141–157.

Fletcher, K. L., Blair, C., Scott, M. S., & Bolger, K. (2004). Specific patterns of cognitive abilities in young children with mental retardation. *Education and Training in Developmental Disabilities, 39,* 270–278.

Gontkovsky, S. T., McDonald, N. B., Clark, P. G., & Ruwe, W. D. (2002). Current directions in computer-assisted cognitive rehabilitation. *Journal of Rehabilitation, 17,* 195–199.

Goodglass, H., Kaplan, E., & Barresi, B. (2001). *The assessment of aphasia and related disorders.* New York: Lippincott Williams and Wilkins.

Goodrich, S. J., & Walker, A. I. (2008). Clinical swallow evaluation. In R. Leonard & K. Kendall (Eds.), *Dysphagia assessment and treatment planning* (2nd ed.). San Diego: Plural.

Gopnik, A. (1990). Developing the idea of intentionality: Children's theories of mind. *The Canadian Journal of Philosophy, 20,* 89–114.

Greenspan, S. T., & Wieder, S. (1997). An integrated developmental approach to interventions for young children with severe difficulties in relating and communicating. *Zero to Three: National Center for Infants, Toddlers, and Families, 17,* 5–18.

Groher, M. (1997). *Dysphagia: Diagnosis and management* (3rd ed.). Boston: Butterworth-Heinemann.

Groher, M., & Crary, M. (2010). *Dysphagia: Clinical management in adults and children.* Maryland Heights, MO: Mosby Elsevier.

Guitar, B. (1998). *Stuttering: An integrated approach to its nature and treatment.* Baltimore: Lippincott Williams & Wilkins.

Hadad, J., Jr. (2004). Hearing loss. In R. E. Behrman, R. Kliegman, H. B. Jenson (Eds.), *Nelson textbook of pediatrics* (17th ed., pp. 2129–2134). Philadelphia: Saunders.

Hartford, E. R. (1988). Hearing aid selection for adults. In M. Pollack (Ed.), *Amplification for the hearing impaired* (3rd ed., pp. 175–210). Orlando, FL: Statton.

Holland, A. (1980). *CADL communicative abilities in daily living.* Baltimore: University Park Press.

Katz, J. (2001). *Handbook of clinical audiology* (5th ed.). Philadelphia: Lippincott Williams and Wilkins.

Kays, S., & Robbins, J. (2006). Effects of sensorimotor exercise on swallowing outcomes relative to age and age-related disease. *Seminars in Speech and Language, 27,* 245–256.

Kertesz, A. (1982). *The Western Aphasia Battery.* New York: Grune and Stratton.

Klonoff, H., & Paris, R. (1974). Immediate, short-term and residual effects of acute head injury in children: Neuropsychological and neurological correlates. In R. M. Reitan & L. A. Davison (Eds.), *Clinical neuropsychology: Current trends and applications.* Washington, DC: V.H. Winston & Sons.

Kochkin, S. (2007). Marke Trake VII: Obstacles to adult non-user adoption of hearing aids. *The Hearing Journal, 60(4),* 27–43.

Lahey, M. (1998). *Language disorders and language development.* Boston: Macmillian.

Langmore, S. E., Shatz, K., & Olson, N. (1998). Fiberoptic endoscopic examination of swallowing safety: A new procedure. *Dysphagia, 2,* 216.

LaPointe, L. (1997). *Aphasia and related neurogenic language disorders* (2nd ed.). New York: Thieme.

Leonard, L. (1998). *Children with specific language impairment.* Cambridge, MA: MIT Press.

Leonard, R., & Kendall, K. (2008). *Dysphagia assessment and treatment planning—A team approach* (2nd ed.). San Diego, CA: Plural.

Logemann, J. (1998). *Evaluation and treatment of swallowing disorders* (2nd ed.). Austin, TX: Pro-ed.

Lord, C., Rutter, M., & Le Couteur, A. (1994). Autism diagnostic interview-revised: A revised version of a diagnostic interview for caregivers of individuals with possible pervasive developmental disorders. *Journal of Autism and Developmental Disorders, 24,* 659–685.

Ludlow, C. L., Humbert, I., Saxon, J., Poletto, C., Sonies, B., & Crujido, L. (2007). Effects of surface electrical stimulation on hyolaryngeal movements in normal individuals at rest and during swallowing. *Dysphagia, 16,* 165.

Lust, B. (2006). *Child language: Acquisition and growth.* Cambridge, MA: Cambridge University Press.

Maassen, B. (2002). Issues contrasting adult acquired versus developmental apraxia of speech. *Seminars in Speech and Language, 23(4),* 257–266.

Mark, V. W., Thomas, B. E., & Berndt, R. S. (1992). Factors associated with improvements in global aphasia. *Aphasiology, 6,* 121–134.

Martin, F. N. (1986). *Introduction to audiology* (3rd ed.). Englewood Cliffs, NJ: Prentice-Hall.

Mazzoni, M., Vista, M., Pardossi, L., Avila, L., Bianchi, F., & Moretti, P. (1992). Spontaneous evolution of aphasia after ischaemic stroke. *Aphasiology, 6,* 387–396.

Miller, E. (1984). *Recovery and management of neuropsychological impairments.* New York: John Riley.

Miller, R. M., Groher, M., Yorkston, K. M., & Rees, T. S. (1988). Speech, language, swallowing and auditory rehabilitation in rehabilitation medicine. In J. A. DeLisa (Ed.), *Principles and practice* (pp. 118–134). Philadelphia: J.B. Lippincott.

Moody, K. C., Holzer, C. E., Roman, M. J., Paulsen, K. A., Freeman, D. H., Haynes, M., et al. (2000). Prevalence of dyslexia among Texas prison inmates. *Texas Medicine, 96,* 69–75.

Morley, M. (1965). Development and disorder of speech in childhood (2nd ed.). Baltimore: Lippincott Williams and Wilkins.

Murry, T., & Carrau, R. C. (2006). *Clinical management of swallowing disorders* (2nd ed.). San Diego, CA: Plural.

Myers, P. S. (1997). Right hemisphere syndrome. In L. LaPointe (Ed.), *Aphasia and related neurologic language disorders* (2nd ed., pp. 201–225). New York: Thieme.

National Institute on Deafness and Other Communication Disorders, Better Hearing Institute. (1999). Bethesda, MD.

Obler, L. K., & Gjerlow, K. (1999). *Language and the brain.* Cambridge, MA: Cambridge University Press.

Paparella, M., DaCosta, S., Fox, R., & Yoon, T. H. (1991). Meniere's disease and other labyrinthine diseases. In M. M. Paparella, D. A. Shumrick, J. C. Gluckman, & J. L. Meyerhoff (Eds.), *Otolaryngology* (3rd ed., pp. 291–321). New York: W.B. Saunders.

Pedersen, P. M., Jørgensen, H. S., Nakayama, H., Raaschou, H. O., & Olsen, T. S. (1992). Aphasia in acute stroke. Incidence, determinants, and recovery. *Annals of Neurology, 3,* 659–666.

Pitcher, J., Crandall, M., & Goodrich, J. (2008). Pediatric clinical feeding assessment. In R. Leonard & K. Kendall (Eds.), *Dysphagia assessment and treatment planning, a team approach* (2nd ed., pp. 117–133). San Diego, CA: Plural.

Records, N. L., Tomblin, J. B., & Freese, P. R. (1992). Quality of life in adults with histories of specific language impairment. *American Journal of Speech Language Pathology, 1,* 44–53.

Richter, M., Wolfgang, H. R., Miltner, R., & Straube, T. (2008). Association between therapy outcome and right-hemispheric activation in chronic aphasia. *Brain, 131,* 1391–1401.

Ritchey, K. D., & Goeke, J. L. (2006). Orton-Gillingham and Orton-Gillingham based reading instruction: A review of the literature. *The Journal of Special Education, 40,* 171–183.

Robbins, J., Gangnon, R., Theis, S., Kays, S. A., & Hind, J. (2005). The effects of lingual exercise on swallowing in older adults. *Journal of the American Geriatrics Society, 53,* 1483.

Rosenbek, J. C., & LaPointe, L. L. (1985). The dysarthrias: Description, diagnosis, and treatment. In D. F. Johns (Ed.), *Clinical management of neurogenic communicative disorders* (pp. 97–152). Boston: Little Brown and Company.

Rosenbek, J. C., & Wertz, R. T. (1972). A review of 50 cases of developmental apraxia of speech. *Language, Speech and Hearing Services in the Schools, 3,* 23.

Sammeth, C. A. (1990). Current availability of digital and hybrid hearing aids. *Seminars in Hearing, 11,* 91–100.

Sapienza, C., & Wheeler, K. (2006). Respiratory muscle strength training: Functional outcomes versus plasticity. *Seminars in Speech and Language, 5,* 123–131.

Smith-Myles, B., & Southwick, J. (2001). *Asperger syndrome and difficult moments: Practical solutions for tantrums, rage and meltdowns.* Shawnee Mission, KS: Autism Asperger.

Soenen, S., van Berckelaer-Onnes, I. A., & Scholte, E. M. (2009). Patterns of intellectual, adaptive and behavioral functioning in individuals with mild mental retardation. *Research in Developmental Disabilities 30,* 433–444.

Stagg, V., Wills, G. D., & Howell, M. (1989). Psychopathology in early childhood witnesses of family violence. *Topics in Early Childhood Special Education, 9,* 73–87.

Stierwalt, J. A. G., Clark, H. M., & Robin, D. A. (2000). Aphasia and related disorders. In J. B. Tomblin, H. L. Morris, & D. C. Spriesterbach (Eds.), *Diagnosis in speech–language pathology* (2nd ed., pp. 315–336). San Diego, CA: Singular.

Strub, R. L., & Black, F. W. (1981). Organic brain syndromes: An introduction to neurobehavioral disorders. Philadelphia: Davis.

Tomblin, J. B. (1996). *Epidemiology of SLI: The association of speech sound disorder with SLI.* Paper presented at the Child Phonology Conference, Iowa City, IA.

Tomblin, J. B., Records, N. L., Buckwalter, P., Zhang, X., Smith, E., & O'Brien, M. (1997). The prevalence of specific language impairment in kindergarten children. *Journal of Speech Language Hearing Research, 40,* 1245–1260.

Traxler, R. (2000). Education outcomes of hard of hearing and deaf students. *Journal of Deaf Studies and Deaf Education, 5,* 337–348.

Van Borsel, J., Reunes, G., & Van den Bergh, N. (2003). Delayed auditory feedback in the treatment of stuttering: Clients as consumers. *International Journal of Language and Communication Disorders, 38,* 119–129.

Wepman, J., & Jones, L. (1961). *The language modalities test for aphasia.* Chicago: University of Chicago.

Wertz, R. T., LaPointe, L. L., & Rosenbek, J. C. (1984). *Apraxia of speech in adults: The disorder and its management.* New York: Grune and Stratton.

Wilson, B. A. (1998). Matching student needs to instruction: Teaching reading and spelling using the Wilson Reading System. In S. A. Vogel & S. Reder (Eds.), *Learning disabilities, literacy, and adult education* (pp. 213–234). Baltimore: Brookes.

Ylvisaker, M. S., & Szekeres, S. F. (1986). Management of the patient with closed head injury. In R. Chapey (Ed.), *Language intervention strategies in adult aphasia* (pp. 474–490). Baltimore: Lippincott Williams and Wilkins.

Yoko, Y., Tomoyuki, G., & Masahiro, N. (2000). Long-term recovery of language impairment in aphasia with various lesion sites and sizes. *Higher Brain Function Research, 20,* 311–318.

Yorkston, K. M., Beukelman, D., & Bell, K. (1988). *Clinical management of dysarthria speakers.* San Diego, CA: College Hill.

Zwolan, T. A. (2002). Cochlea implants. In J. Katz (Ed.), *Handbook of clinical audiology* (5th ed., pp. 740–768). New York: Lippincott Williams and Wilkins.

12

Hematological Disorders

Bruce G. Raphael, MD

Blood contains a variety of mature differentiated cells that have specialized functions. These include the red blood cells that carry oxygen to the tissues, the white blood cells that help fight infection, and the platelets, which are the blood-clotting cells. The white blood cells are further divided into a variety of cell types. The two most important white blood cell types are granulocytes, which fight bacterial infection, and lymphocytes, which make the antibodies, control the immune reactions, and help with viral infections. New cells are required constantly to replace the old, and hence, there is a need for a stem cell, which is defined as self-renewing progenitor cell that, under appropriate stimulus, divide and mature into various blood cells. The majority of these cells are in a resting state in the bone marrow in humans. The process of division and maturation is a complex operation, and mistakes in the control and programmed cell death lead to abnormal accumulation of the precursor cells at various stages of maturation. Cancers that develop because of abnormal proliferation of the white blood cells in the blood are known as leukemia and in the lymph nodes are called lymphoma. The final stage of maturation of B lymphocytes is a plasma cell that produces immunoglobulins to fight infection and a malignant transformation of one of the plasma cells is multiple myeloma.

LYMPHOMA

Disease Description

Lymphomas are a malignant proliferation of one of the white blood cell types: lymphocytes, which are divided into B lymphocytes and T lymphocytes. B lymphocytes are cells that go through a complicated maturation process in which only a portion of the genetic material that codes for antibody production is activated, so each B cell produces a single antibody against a specific foreign protein. T lymphocytes go through similar maturation, with activation of other portions of genetic material. These cells then specialize in helping (helper cells) or suppressing (suppressor cells) the immune reaction. Once formed, these cells migrate to the lymph nodes, and when exposed to a foreign protein or an infectious agent, those lymphocytes programmed to make the specific antibody against the abnormal antigen will divide, enlarge, and multiply, producing large numbers of cells that ultimately mature into plasma cells in the bone marrow, which produce antibodies to neutralize the invading organism. The T-helper cells will aid this reaction; and when the organism is cleared, T-suppressor cells will inhibit the immune reaction, and the swollen lymph gland will shrink back to the quiescent state (Skarin, 1989).

When one of the maturing and dividing lymphocytes undergoes malignant change and divides uncontrollably, an accumulation of these cells occurs as a tumor, called a lymphoma. The cause of this malignant change is chromosomal breaks or gene mutations that occur during the division and maturation of each individual lymphocyte, which leads to activation of genes involved in proliferation and cell death. The result is either uncontrolled growth (Williams, Butler, Erslev, & Lichtman, 1990) or lack of programmed cell death, both of which leads to an accumulation of clonal malignant cells. Although certain viruses (the Epstein-Barr virus and T-cell lymphotrophic virus) have been implicated in a small number of B- and T-cell lymphomas, respectively, most of these mutations occur as a consequence of mistakes in the complex act of gene replication and division. Five percent of all cancers in the United States are lymphomas, with 70–80% of B-cell origin and the rest derived from T cells (Skarin, 1989). There is a rising incidence of aggressive lymphoma in acquired immune deficiency syndrome (AIDS) patients and in patients on immunosuppressive drugs (i.e., post transplant state). The speculative cause of these lymphomas is excessive immune stimulation of B lymphocytes with chromosomal breaks and poor immune surveillance by the reduced number of T lymphocytes, which are destroyed by the AIDS virus (Raphael & Knowles, 1990).

Pathology

The lymphomas are all classified by the appearance of malignant lymphocytes on the biopsy slides of the tumor. As stated earlier, normal lymphocytes go through various stages of maturation. A lymphoma is an accumulation of malignant lymphocytes that are arrested at one stage of maturation. Clinical behavior of the tumor is often correlated with the level of maturation of the abnormal lymphocyte. Hence, classification of lymphomas is divided into three categories: (a) low; (b) intermediate; and (c) high grade (Rosenberg, 1982). Low-grade lymphomas contain cells that are smaller, slower growing, and often asymptomatic. Intermediate-grade lymphomas have cells that are larger and faster growing. High-grade lymphomas are very fast-growing, immature lymphocytes, which often present in extranodal as well as nodal tissues. In addition, the tumor can present in a nodular (follicular) pattern or diffusely, replacing the architecture of the lymph node. Slower growth is associated with the former pattern, and more aggressive behavior is related to the latter (Rosenberg, 1982) (Table 12.1). Subsequently, the realization based on immunologic staining of cells, molecular studies, and the understanding of genetic translocations and mutation have led to further classifications called the REAL classification in 1994 and the World Health Organization (WHO) classification in 2001 (Chan, 2001). Classification based on cytogenetic abnormalities not shown in Table 12.1 is beyond the scope of this report. However, it is important to note that tumors that look the same but have different genetic mutations have led to the understanding of why some patients are cured whereas others with the same disease do not respond to the same treatment. Hence, this new information is being used to develop new protocols targeting the molecular defects resulting from these changes (Schouten, 2007).

Functional Presentation

Patients present with swollen, growing lymph glands (nodal disease) or tumors in other organs (extranodal disease). Patients can be asymptomatic (A) or have one or more of the B symptoms, which include fever, drenching night sweats, loss of 10% of body weight, and itching. An evaluation is done to determine the extent of disease called staging. This includes a proper physical examination to determine any lymph node group that is enlarged or any abnormal organ enlargement. In addition, computed tomography scans of chest, abdomen, and pelvis are done to determine internal organ and nodal involvement. A bone marrow

TABLE 12.1   *Classifications of Lymphoma*

Low grade
  Malignant lymphoma, small lymphocytic
  Malignant lymphoma, follicular, predominantly small cleaved cell
  Malignant lymphoma, follicular, mixed small and large cell

Intermediate grade
  Malignant lymphoma, follicular, predominantly large cell
  Malignant lymphoma, diffuse, mixed small and large cell
  Malignant lymphoma, diffuse large cell cleaved

High grade
  Diffuse large cell, immunoblastic
  Malignant lymphoma, lymphoblastic
  Malignant lymphoma, small noncleaved cell

biopsy is used to examine whether it is involved by lymphoma. In particular, cerebrospinal fluid is analyzed to determine central nervous system involvement in higher grade lymphomas because of a higher chance of spread with these aggressive tumors. Positive emission tomography scans have recently been added to the evaluation of lymphomas. Radioactive sugar is given intravenously which rapidly accumulates in tumor cells because they use more sugar to fuel their increased metabolic activity compared with normal cells. The amount of radioactivity in the tumor cells can be followed both during and after chemotherapy to determine completeness of response to therapy (Friedberg & Chengazi, 2003). The stage of disease is then determined by the number of lymph nodes involved and presence of disease in other organs (Table 12.2). Prognosis is dependent on the type of lymphoma as well as stage and clinical presentation (Matasar & Zelenetz, 2008). This has led to a prognostic index and risk stratification (Table 12.3).

Treatment

The vast majority of lymphomas present in multiple areas of the body, Stage 3 or 4, as abnormal lymphocytes are free to travel to other areas of the body through the blood. Hence, localized treatment with surgery or radiation is rarely curative (Ruthoven, 1987; Skarin, 1989). Treatment is, therefore, primarily chemotherapy, in which chemicals are used to poison the growing malignant cells. Combinations of drugs have resulted in more remissions and cures, although response rates are influenced by the number of poor prognostic factors as noted in Table 12.3. In addition to chemotherapy and external irradiation to shrink disease, in the last 5 years, biologic agents have been added to treatment regimens. These include manufactured monoclonal antibodies directed at proteins on the cancer cell that attack the tumor

TABLE 12.2   *Staging of Lymphoma*

Stage	Characteristics
I	Involvement of a single lymph node region or single extra modal organ or site
II	Involvement limited to one side of the diaphragm with two or more lymph node regions
III	Involvement of lymph node regions on both sides of the diaphragm
IV	Diffuse or disseminated involvement of one or more extra lymphatic organs

TABLE 12.3 *Prognostic Factors and Risk Stratification*

Prognostic factors
  Age > 60 years
  Advanced stage (III or IV)
  >1 Extranodal sites of involvement

Presence of symptoms
  Serum lactate dehydrogenase level increased

Risk group stratification according to the International Prognostic Index (total number of above-listed features)
  0–1: Low risk
  2: Low intermediate risk
  3: High intermediate risk
  4–5: High risk

cells directly, antibodies that are conjugated with a radioactive substance or toxin allowing preferential targeting of the tumor, and a vaccine produced from the tumor cells that stimulate an immune reaction in the patient against the cancer cell. (Hsu et al., 1997) Low-grade lymphomas can be controlled for many years, with median survival of 7–10 years, but are rarely curable (Skarin, 1989). Recently there has been a large number of newer agents and in particular monoclonal antibodies that are manufactured in large quantities that target the lymphocytes. When these new agents were added to existing chemotherapeutic protocols responses improved and it was hoped that either cure or long-term control of the lymphoma growth would result (Berdeja, 2003). A recent study comparing survival in modern combination chemotherapy and monoclonal antibody treatment with historical controls from the 1980s and 1990s appears to suggest that the complete remission and duration of remission is longer and overall survival is also improved. That said, cures in low-grade lymphomas remain rare (Fisher et al., 2005).

The intermediate lymphomas now have a 50–70% cure rate, depending on stage and prognostic factors, using combinations of multiple chemotherapy agents (Skarin, 1989; Williams et al., 1990). The addition of monoclonal antibodies has also influenced these lymphomas and cure rates increased in all prognostic risk categories by 10–15% (Michallet & Coiffier, 2009). High-grade lymphomas are treated with intensive doses of chemotherapy, leading to 80–90% cures in children and 30–50% cure rate in adults, but individuals who relapse often die within a year (Magrath, 1996).

Lymphomas are very sensitive to chemotherapy, but no drug is specific for only the tumor cell. This leads to the side effects of chemotherapy: normal-growing cells are affected as well as specific organs that are sensitive to the toxic effects of these agents. The disability that patients experience may, in part, be due to the presence of the tumor in a disease site, such as shortness of breath with lung involvement and debilitation from fevers and weight loss. Alternatively they may be related to the side effects of the chemotherapy. These drugs are toxins that poison the tumor cells but also may injure normal cells such as Adriamycin which can damage the heart, or Oncovin, which causes peripheral neuropathy. It should be noted that specialized and expensive treatments may add further barriers to care in lower socio-economic groups. A disparity in survival figures between Whites and Blacks has already been demonstrated in lymphoma treatment (Han et al., 2008).

For patients who do not respond to primary treatment, bone marrow transplantation is increasingly used. High-dose chemotherapy is used to kill the lymphoma that was resistant to conventional treatment. Stem cells harvested from the patient (autologous transplant) or from a tissue-matched relative (allogeneic transplant) are stored before the procedure and given back to rescue the patient from the lethal effects of high-dose chemotherapy on the bone marrow. Other organs are damaged during the intensive therapy, infections are frequent, and immune suppressive drugs are needed in the case of allogeneic transplant to prevent the donor's immune cells from infecting the recipient's cells (graft vs. host). The result is a prolonged, complicated hospital stay with multiple manifestations of organ damage. As patients recover, they typically have been bed ridden, unable to eat due to chemotherapy-induced gastric damage, and debilitated from previous infection. Hence, a lengthy recovery period is the norm, with active rehabilitation by physiotherapy, psychology, and dietary services.

LEUKEMIA

Disease Description

Acute leukemia is characterized by an abnormal proliferation of immature white blood cells. As stated earlier, lymphoma represents an accumulation of lymphocytes arrested at one stage of maturation; leukemia is the accumulation of the earliest white blood cells, called blasts or progenitor cells. These cells normally divide and mature into the normal white cells that help fight infections but eventually die. Hence, stem cells also must self-renew so that they can be called upon again and again to repopulate the constant turn over of bone marrow cells. Hence, the effect of lack of maturation is the presence of large numbers of these young cells in the bone marrow and lack of normal bone marrow cells. Patients then present with signs and symptoms of low red blood cell count (anemia) such as weakness and shortness of breath with activity, decreased white blood cells (granulocytopenia) with infection and fever, and a low platelet count (thrombocytopenia) with bleeding. In addition, infiltration of various organs by these tumor cells can lead to enlargement of liver, spleen, and lymph nodes, as well as to gum hypertrophy and skin nodules.

The incidence of acute leukemia is 9 cases per 100,000 individuals, and the incidence rises with age (DeVita, Hellman, & Rosenberg, 1989). Unlike some other tumors, however, acute leukemia occurs in childhood and is the most common childhood malignancy. There are two main forms of acute leukemia: acute lymphoblastic leukemia (ALL) is a cancer of the earliest stages of lymphocyte maturation, and acute nonlymphoblastic leukemia (ANLL) usually is a malignancy of the progenitor of the granulocyte series called the myeloblast. ALL occurs more often in the young; ANLL is more common with adults. Cytogenetic studies show a variety of chromosomal breaks and mutations associated with different types of leukemia. The proteins encoded by these mutated genes cause dysregulation of division and maturation and hence accumulation of myeloblasts or lymphoblasts (Berman, 1997).

Pathology

Patients' routine blood tests show low levels of all blood cells (pancytopenia) and/or early white cell forms (blasts). Bone marrow analysis shows a hypercellular specimen with almost complete replacement by early white cell forms. Only a few remaining normally maturing blood cells can be found. The cells are analyzed by morphology, staining characteristics, biochemistry, and immunologic typing to differentiate between ANLL and ALL. In addition, cytogenetic and molecular analysis is done to characterize the type of leukemia as well as to indicate prognosis (Frankfurt, Licht, & Tallman, 2007). The realization that response to treatment is affected by the genetic mutations led to the WHO recently classifying myeloid leukemia using genetic, morphologic, and previous exposure to DNA-damaging agents (Vardiman, Harris, & Brunning, 2002) (Table 12.4). Survival with

TABLE 12.4 *Classification of Myeloid Leukemia*

Acute myeloid leukemia with recurrent genetic abnormalities

Acute myeloid leukemia with multilineage dysplasia

Acute myeloid leukemia and myelodysplastic syndromes, therapy related

Acute myeloid leukemia, not otherwise categorized

standard chemotherapy would range from 50% to 60% for good-risk cytogenetics to 10% or less for all the others.

Functional Presentation

Patients with lymphoma present with tumor and related symptoms, but they generally have adequate normal blood cells and can tolerate chemotherapy as outpatients. Patients with acute leukemia usually present as critically ill, with signs and symptoms of lack of normal blood elements. If they present late in the course of the disease, the white blood cell counts are elevated because the leukemic cells have multiplied in the bone marrow and spilled into the blood or there is organ dysfunction due to infiltration by the tumor cells. Hence, patients are admitted immediately and stabilized by correcting the anemia with red blood cell transfusions, treated for any uncontrolled infection resulting from lack of mature white blood cells, subjected to platelet transfusions to control bleeding, and started on chemotherapy to kill the leukemia cells. Although treatment for ANLL differs from treatment for ALL, the principle is the same. Induction therapy involves large doses of chemotherapy to poison the tumor cells (Gale & Foon, 1987; Hoelzer & Gale, 1987). However, these drugs are toxic to all blood cells, resulting in the death of the few remaining normal bone marrow cells and the development of aplasia in the bone marrow. Once chemotherapy stops and the tumor cells die, the normal stem cells in the marrow that are resistant to chemotherapy divide and their progeny cells mature and repopulate the marrow over the next 3 weeks. Until sufficient cells grow to produce the necessary mature, functioning peripheral blood cells, the patient is very sick and must receive antibiotics, fluids, and transfusions on a daily basis. Remissions occur in up to 80% of cases, but relapses are common. Additional consolidation chemotherapy is given after recovery to prevent recurrence (Gale & Foon, 1987; Hoelzer & Gale, 1987) but with variable success depending on the cytogenetic abnormality (King & Rowe, 2007). The repetitive chemotherapy injury further slows recovery, adds days of admissions to the hospital, and results in more disability.

Furthermore, the chemotherapy drugs are toxic to other organs as well as bone marrow. Myopathy (disorders of the muscle) caused by steroids and neurotoxicity from the drug vincristine is common in the treatment of ALL. Heart damage from anthracycline chemotherapy drugs and fluid overload due to multiple intravenous fluids and transfusions are common to all patients. Finally, nausea, mouth sores, and gastric irritation are typical with this type of chemotherapy, making adequate nutritional intake difficult and further adding to the general level of debilitation. In cases of relapse, as well as in some experimental protocols for patients in remission, bone marrow transplantation is offered as a way of using very high doses of chemotherapy to rid the body of any remaining leukemia cells and to prevent any further relapses (Williams et al., 1990). The physical problems secondary to this intensive therapy are multiplied, compared with conventional therapy. Hence, patients with leukemia face months of treatment and weeks of hospitalization with each treatment. The resulting physical, psychological, and financial toll is substantial.

Psychological and Vocational Implications

A further discussion of the relationship of cancer and psychosocial adaptation will be found in chapter 6 of this book. However, several points that are unique to lymphoma and leukemia will be discussed here.

As stated earlier, lymphoma and leukemia affect a wider age range than do most cancers, and the psychosocial implications will vary with age. Younger adults, aged 18–36, with leukemia and lymphoma were surveyed by Daiter, Larson, Weddington, and Ultmann, 1988. As might be expected, patients with less favorable prognoses experienced more stress but also significant personal growth and maturation. In addition, family and friends who provided social support reported not only more stress when dealing with the sicker patient with poor prognosis but also sometimes expressed more prolonged anxiety after treatment was completed than did the patient. Psychological stress has been reported to be lower for leukemia than for breast cancer. Treatment with chemotherapy and radiation to younger patients, with acute leukemia, particularly ALL, may add developmental disability to the list of long-term deficits. There is up to a 30% risk of school-related problems especially in those patients treated for central nervous system involvement (Mulhern, Friedman, & Stone, 1988). Adolescents require different types of support and negotiating treatment is more demanding (Penson et al., 2002).

Older patients have additional concerns about financial matters, how their spouses and children are coping and functioning, and interpersonal relationships at work. Depression, sleep disorder, and anxiety over personal appearance are common. Long-term survivors also have persistent problems; one study reported 73% of patients with Hodgkin's disease having at least one of five problems including decreased energy level, negative body image, depression, employment problems, and marital problems (Fobair et al., 1986). In addition, the rising incidence of leukemia with age and secondary leukemia due to previous chemotherapy results in many difficult decisions concerning therapy and quality of life issues (Sekeres et al., 2004). However, a recent review looking at quality of life parameters 6 months after chemotherapy in older patients in remission from acute myeloid leukemia demonstrated that those patients who remained in remission had a gradual improvement of all parameters (Alibhai et al., 2009). Hence, while the chance of long-term remission in patients older than 60 years is smaller, those who do have a remission can have a relative normal quality of life.

Finally, because bone marrow transplantation has become a common therapy for refractory lymphoma and leukemia, studies of the psychosocial morbidity of these procedures have been completed. Jenkins, Linington, and Whittaker (1991) report a 40% prevalence of depression with impaired function, but most cases were temporary and resolved with resumption of normal activities and return to work. Wolcott, Wellisch, Fawzy, and Landsverk (1986) also reported that 15–20% of bone marrow transplant recipients have a degree of psychological distress that would benefit from intervention. Somerfield, Curbow, Wingard, Baker, & Fogarty, 1996 noted a list of most frequently endorsed fears of transplant patients, which included increased vulnerability to illness, uncertain future, reduced energy, and inability to have children. In addition, heightened concern over somatic symptoms leads to panic attacks that the cancer is returning. In particular, patients with continuing medical problems were more likely to need help. In addition to routine physical therapy, aerobic training has been tested in patients after high-dose chemotherapy and shown to reduce fatigue and enhanced physical performance (Dimeo et al., 1997).

In summary, patients with leukemia and lymphoma require intensive chemotherapy and, in some cases, repeated hospitalizations, which can lead to a host of psychological and vocational difficulties. Remarkably, most patients adapt well, but significant numbers may benefit from at least temporary counseling and rehabilitation services. Two recent studies show that both physical and emotional recovery after bone marrow transplantation is delayed with psychological symptoms persisting longer. Three to five years are required before most patients have fully recovered and interventions such as physical, occupational, and psychological therapies are required to speed this process (Broers, Kaptein, Le Cessie, Fibbe, & Hengeveld, 2000; Syrjala et al., 2004).

DISORDERS OF HEMOSTASIS

Hemostasis is the process by which blood clots in response to injury to the vessels. When a vessel is cut, it may constrict, reducing blood flow and bleeding. Platelets, the blood-clotting cells, then adhere to the open wound and clump together to form a plug. In a highly orchestrated and sequential manner, coagulation factors are activated from an inactive proenzyme form one after another ultimately resulting in the last coagulation factor fibrinogen (Factor I) converting to fibrin. Fibrin strands mesh with platelets, forming a stable clot that will not break down until the vessel repairs itself. Abnormal bleeding may occur when there is a defect in the number or function of the platelets or any of the 13 coagulation factors. Hemophilia A and B are the most common congenital deficiencies of these plasma coagulation proteins. We will discuss them in more detail as prototypes of a chronic bleeding disorder.

Hemophilia

Disease Description
As stated previously, there are 13 coagulation factors. Factor XII is activated first, and then a series of factors are converted to their active form. This cascade of activation will be stopped or slowed if there is a deficiency of any one factor required to convert the next factor. Mutations of the genes responsible for the proper levels of the coagulation proteins result in the decreased production and impairment of clot formation. Factor VIII is the most common congenital deficiency, accounting for 75% of hemophilias. It is a rare disease, however, with an incidence of 1 in 10,000 male births (Williams et al., 1990). A gene on the X chromosome encodes the protein. Hence, males need inherit only one defective gene from the mother to be affected. Females, who have two X chromosomes, are rarely affected.

Hemophilia B, a deficiency of Factor IX, is also an X-linked recessive hemorrhagic disease. It occurs in 1 of 75,000 male births and clinically is indistinguishable from hemophilia A (Williams et al., 1990). The diagnosis of both of these disorders is made by functionally assaying the plasma for the level of either protein compared with normal plasma.

Functional Presentation
The genes controlling production of either Factor VIII or IX may have one of many mutations. This can lead to no production, decreased production, or production of a defective protein. Hence, the patient can present with mild, moderate, or severe hemorrhagic disease, depending on the amount of active protein produced. Activity of the protein is measured in a timed clotting assay and compared with normal plasma. Mothers of hemophilia patients are obligate carriers and have 50% or greater activity. Mild hemophiliacs have 6–25% activity, rarely bleed spontaneously, and usually are discovered after excessive bleeding secondary to trauma or surgery. Moderately affected individuals have 1–5% levels of the active protein and have rare episodes of spontaneous bleeding but can hemorrhage with any trauma. Finally, patients with less than a 1% level have severe disease, with frequent spontaneous hemorrhage from early childhood (Williams et al., 1990). Patients can bleed anywhere, but bleeding into joints (hemarthrosis), soft tissue (such as muscle), urine (hematuria), and the brain are common. Chronic bleeding into joints results in inflammation, scaring, and restriction of movement. Bleeding into the brain or spinal canal can lead to nerve damage with both functional and psychological disabilities.

Treatment and Prognosis
The general principle of treatment of hemophilia is, first, to avoid drugs that can interfere with clotting, particularly aspirin and other nonsteroidal antiinflammatory agents that inhibit platelet function (Williams et al., 1990). Second, early recognition of bleeding

episodes or potential trauma and treatment with replacement Factor VIII or IX is imperative. Concentrates of these factors from normal plasma are commercially available. The number of units of coagulation protein infused depends on the initial level of the factor in the patient's plasma and the level of factor desired. Minor trauma or bleeding may require factor levels of only 20% of normal to stop bleeding, whereas major hemorrhage, especially intracranial, will require larger doses to raise levels of the factor to more than 50% of normal (Kasper & Dietrich, 1985; Williams et al., 1990). If surgery is required, Factors VIII and IX must be raised before the operation. Because Factor VIII is degraded in the plasma, half the dose is gone in 8–12 hours; treatment is given every 12 hours for several days to allow healing and prevent late hemorrhage. Factor IX has a longer half-life, 18–24 hours, and reinfusion can take place less often.

Prognosis improved with the advent of factor concentrate treatment in the 1960s, with fewer severe bleeds, less crippling arthritis from hemarthrosis, and less intracranial bleeding. Complications of multiple transfusions, such as hepatitis and AIDS, have greatly influenced the prognosis. New preparation techniques have eliminated the hepatitis and human immunodeficiency virus (HIV) from Factor VIII concentrates and the risks of infection now is very small. However, many older hemophiliacs, particularly those who were severely affected and hence needed many transfusions, were infected by HIV in the 1980s and ultimately died of AIDS. Since the advent of highly active antiretroviral therapy, the prognosis of patients who were infected has dramatically improved but because healthy but infected adult hemophiliacs are sexually active, the risk of sexually transmitting the AIDS virus is problematic. New patients appear safe from transmission of these viruses because of the new concentrates, but it will be many years before the problem of transfusion-related viral infections in the older patients will disappear.

Psychological and Vocational Implications

The medical advancement of efficient factor replacement led to a great improvement in the psychosocial aspect of caring for hemophilia patients. A study from the Netherlands (Rosendaal et al., 1990) showed that most patients consider their health and quality of life no different from that of the general population. In addition, those who were employed had positions consistent with their education. In the older patient, however, joint damage correlated with increased disability and decrease in successful marriage and having children. Twenty-two percent of patients were unemployed and receiving some disability compensation. Vocational training should stress jobs that limit potentially hazardous situations. Patients who are on effective replacement therapy can compete equally for most jobs. It is clear that programs like home therapy slow the rate of progression of arthropathy, and most young hemophiliacs who are under appropriate medical care can and should be fully employed and leading normal lives.

However, the patients who were infected with the AIDS virus during therapy from 1980 to 1985 will require special psychological help and will experience greater disability. Social counseling for sexual partners is imperative. The impact of this tragic complication should be temporary as future patients are protected by the newer generation of coagulation factor replacement products.

Sickle Cell Disease

Disease Description

Normal red blood cells have a biconcave shape with a pliable cell membrane and cytoplasm in the center filled with a protein called hemoglobin. This protein is a combination of two α-globin chains and two β-globin chains, forming a complex molecule that binds an iron-containing heme molecule in the center, which allows the protein to bind oxygen. Hemoglobin is soluble in the cytoplasm, so the red cell shape can change and thereby squeeze through small vessels to deliver the oxygen to the tissues. Sickle cell disease occurs when both β chains have one amino acid changed from a glutamic acid to valine in the sixth position of a 146-amino acid chain that makes up the β-globin protein molecule (Williams et al., 1990). This substitution of one amino acid for another cause lining up of the hemoglobin molecules producing stacking, forming a tubular insoluble structure, and causing the red cell to assume a nonpliable sickle shape. This process occurs only when the hemoglobin molecule has lost the oxygen molecule at the level of the tissue, and it can be reversed by reoxygenating the hemoglobin in the lungs as the blood returns to the left side of the heart. However, permanent membrane change occurs after several cycles of sickling and unsickling, resulting in an irreversibly sickled cell. The resultant cellular defect leads to the main manifestations of disease, which include (a) premature destruction of the cells, called hemolytic anemia; (b) vascular occlusion of vessels (due to plugging of vessels by sickle cells that cannot pass through the small capillaries) and subsequent tissue infarction; and (c) increased susceptibility to infection.

Sickle cell disease patients are homozygous for the abnormal gene controlling β-chain production. Hence, both parents must be at least heterozygous for the abnormal gene. The frequency of one abnormal gene in the Black population of America is 1 in 12, and the incidence of sickle cell anemia is 1 in 650 in American Blacks (Williams et al., 1990). Milder forms of this disease can be seen with one sickle β-gene and either deletion of the other β-gene (thalassemia) or occurrence of a second type of sickle gene, called sickle C. The latter results from replacement of the glutamic acid by lysine at the sixth position on the β chain (Williams et al., 1990).

Functional Presentation

Patients usually present in the first decade of life with complications of the three main characteristics of sickle cell disorder. As stated earlier, anemia results from hemolysis secondary to irreversible shape change and the quick breakdown of blood cells, with large amounts of hemoglobin being released into the blood, converted into bilirubin, and secreted into the bile. Bile stones develop early, and the clinical picture is that of a patient with anemia, jaundice, and gallstone attacks. Also, the bone marrow expands, producing extra red blood cells to make up for the anemia, causing bone deformity. This hypercellular marrow is susceptible to vitamin deficiency and viral infection, leading to an abrupt decrease in production, a condition called aplastic crisis.

The second set of clinical symptoms results from the plugging of small blood vessels by the nonpliable sickle cells. Infarction of any organ and in particular, bone results in a painful crisis. In addition, strokes and cardiac and pulmonary infarction are major complications of the vascular occlusive disease. Leg ulcers develop for the same reason, heal poorly because of poor tissue perfusion, and can cause physical disability. In a recent study, children with more severe sickle cell disease and more vascular episodes had language processing deficits (Schatz, Puffer, Sanchez, Stancil, & Roberts, 2009). Finally, the spleen, an organ that helps clear certain infectious agents from the blood, shrinks and is nonfunctional as a result of many infarctions in early childhood. The result is a susceptibility to infections, particularly pneumococcal pneumonia. Another infectious complication results from the combination of devitalized bone and a propensity for salmonella to lodge in the diseased gallbladder, leading to seeding of the bone and salmonella osteomyelitis.

Treatment and Prognosis

There is no specific treatment for sickle cell disease; hence, most therapy is supportive in treatment of the complications. Painful crises are treated with fluids, pain medication, and careful search for causes, such as an infection (Charache, 1974). Pain control usually requires narcotics in the acute crisis and doctors have been reluctant to prescribe enough medication because of the manifestation of vaso-occlusive disease, the sociocultural factors in pain assessment, and fears of potential addiction (Wright & Adeosum, 2009). This appears to be worse for the patients with more or longer crisis following a hospital admission. A recent study demonstrated that postdischarge pain control and functional limitation outcomes were worse for the group of 2- to 18-year-old sickle cell patients (Brandow, Brousseau, & Panepinto, 2009) who had more severe crisis. Early recognition of infection, administration of prophylactic antibiotics, and vaccination may forestall or prevent other complications (Scott, 1985). If painful crisis persists or there is infarction of a major organ (brain, lung, or heart), exchange transfusion is performed to remove some of the sickle red cells. Normal red cells are transfused to lower the concentration of sickle hemoglobin to 50% (Charache, 1974). At this level no significant sludging, further thrombosis, or complications will occur. This effect is temporary; however, as the transfused red cells die, new cells with hemoglobin S (Hb S) are produced. In addition, transfusion carries risks of infection, allergy, and sensitization to donor blood. Hence, this mode of treatment is used only for severe cases. New approaches to therapy are centered on the reduction of intracellular Hb S concentration and pharmacologic induction of hemoglobin F (Hb F) as a substitute for Hb S (Bunn, 1997). This has resulted in the use of hydroxyurea, an oral chemotherapeutic agent, which can cause an increase in Hb F and reciprocal decrease in Hb S. The decreased concentration of Hb S then leads to reduced sickling and reduction in symptoms. The exposure to chemotherapy and potential complications has limited its use to patients with more frequent and severe attacks. In this group, however, efficacy and cost effectiveness have been established (Moore, Charache, Terrin, Barton, & Ballas, 2000).

Bone marrow transplantation and possible gene therapy, in which the normal β-globin gene is placed in the patient's stem cell, hold hope for the future, but many technical hurdles still remain. Prognosis has improved with good supportive care, particularly in pediatric mortality although the reduction in the last 20 years is less for older children (Yanni, Grosse, Yang, & Olney, 2009). However, frequent admissions for painful crisis, the complication of sickle cell disease, narcotic use and abuse due to chronic pain, and absence from school and work lead to significant psychological and vocational problems.

Psychological and Vocational Implications
Several authors have documented the psychological impact on a patient with chronic painful disease (Barrett et al., 1988; Damlouji, Kevess-Cohen, Charache, Georgopoulos, & Folstein, 1982). In one study, the findings suggested that a relationship between the chronicity and dependence on the medical care system was the best predictor of psychosocial functioning (Damlouji et al., 1982). Others have shown links between medical complications and psychopathology (Barrett et al., 1988). The psychological impact can include drug addiction, hysterical conversion reaction, and malingering, as well as low self-esteem, dependency, and depression (Barrett et al., 1988).

Adolescents with sickle cell disease must deal with defining their personal identity along with their chronic illness. Delays in sexual maturation and adolescent growth spurt contribute to poor self-image. Physical limitations, particularly in sports, also lead to low self-esteem. Fifteen percent of patients between the ages of 13 and 40 have been reported to be depressed (Kinney & Ware, 1996).

Physical limitations stemming from stroke in childhood, along with decreased IQ (Hariman, Griffith, Hartig, & Keehn, 1991) and medical complications, may contribute to both psychosocial and vocational limitations. The greatest dysfunction was found in areas of employment, finances, sleep habits, and performance of daily activities (Barrett et al., 1988). Hence, the implications of these findings suggest a strong need for vocational rehabilitation services, training in areas of communication and self-esteem (Barrett et al., 1988), medical treatment, and psychological help for depression and drug dependence. The prevalence of this disease in the Black population, who are chronically underserved by the health care system and the difficulty of obtaining affordable insurance as well as maintaining a job with insurance benefits, has necessitated development of a national policy to pay for the costs and develop treatments for these patients (Nietert, Silverstein, & Abboud, 2002).

A national sickle cell disease program with 10 regional centers has been established to provide the comprehensive care required, but many patients and families still have difficulty in obtaining the help they need (Scott, 1985). The centers provide cost-effective day treatment to handle the majority of patient complaints that are neither emergent nor life threatening. As discussed earlier, the physical and psychological damage from repeated painful crisis require continued care as an outpatient and the mission of these centers is also to provide psychological, rehabilitation, and vocational services for the patient and family (Koshy & Dorn, 1996).

REFERENCES

Alibhai, S. M. H., Leach, M., Gupta, V., Tomlinson, G. A., Brandwein, J. M., Saiz, F. S., et al. (2009). Quality of Life beyond 6 months after diagnosis in older adults with acute myeloid leukemia. *Critical Reviews in Oncology-Hematology, 69,* 168–174.

Barrett, D. H., Wisotzek, I. E., Abel, G. G., Rouleau, J. L., Platt, A. F., Pollard, W. E., et al. (1988). Assessment of psychosocial functioning of patients with sickle cell disease. *Southern Medical Journal, 81,* 745–750.

Berdeja, J. G. (2003). Immunotherapy of lymphoma: Update and review of the literature [Review]. *Current Opinion in Oncology, 15,* 363–370.

Broers, S., Kaptein, A. A., Le Cessie, S., Fibbe, W., & Hengeveld, M. W. (2000). Psychological functioning and quality of life following bone marrow transplantation: A 3-year follow-up study. *Journal of Psychosomatic Research, 48,* 11–21.

Berman, E. (1997). Recent advances in the treatment of acute leukemia. *Current Opinion in Hematology, 4,* 256–260.

Brandow, A. M., Brousseau, D. C., & Panepinto, J. A. (2009). Postdischarge pain, functional limitations and impact on caregivers of children with sickle cell disease treated for painful events. *British Journal of Haematology, 144,* 782–788.

Bunn, H. F. (1997). Pathogenesis and treatment of sickle cell disease. *New England Journal of Medicine, 337,* 762–769.

Chan, J. K. C. (2001). The new World Health Organization classification of lymphomas: The past, the present and the future. *Hematological Oncology, 19,* 129–150.

Charache, S. (1974). The treatment of sickle cell anemia. *Archives of Internal Medicine, 133,* 698–705.

Daiter, S., Larson, R. A., Weddington, W. W., & Ultmann, J. E. (1988). Psychosocial symptomatology, personal growth and development among young adult patients following the diagnosis of leukemia or lymphoma. *Journal of Clinical Oncology, 6,* 613–617.

Damlouji, N. F., Kevess-Cohen, R., Charache, S., Georgopoulos, A., & Folstein, M. F. (1982). Social disability and psychiatric morbidity in sickle cell anemia and diabetes patients. *Psychosomatics, 23,* 925–931.

DeVita, V. T., Hellman, S., & Rosenberg, S. A. (Eds.). (1989). *Cancer: Principles and practice of oncology* (3rd ed.). Philadelphia, PA: J. B. Lippincott.

Dimeo, F. C., Tilmann, M. H., Bertz, H., Kanz, L., Mertelsmann, R., & Keul, J. (1997). Aerobic exercise in the rehabilitation of cancer patients after high dose chemotherapy and autologous peripheral stem cell transplantation. *Cancer, 79,* 1717–1722.

Fisher, R., Leblanc, M., Press, O. W., Maloney, D. G., Unger, J. M., & Miller, T. P. (2005). New treatment options have changed the survival of patients with follicular lymphoma. *Journal of Clinical Oncology, 23,* 8447–8452.

Fobair, P., Hoppe, R. T., Bloom, J. R., Cox, R., Varghese, A., & Spiegle, D. (1986). Psychosocial problems among survivors of Hodgkin's Disease. *Journal of Clinical Oncology, 4,* 805–814.

Frankfurt, O., Licht, J. D., & Tallman, M. S. (2007). Molecular characterization of acute myeloid leukemia and its impact on treatment. *Current Opinion in Oncology, 19,* 635–649.

Friedberg, J. W., & Chengazi, V. (2003). PET scans in the staging of lymphoma: Current status. *Oncologist, 8,* 438–447.

Gale, R. P., & Foon, K. A. (1987). Therapy of acute myologenous leukemia. *Seminars in Hematology, 24,* 40–54.

Hariman, L. M. P., Griffith, E. R., Hartig, A. L., & Keehn, M. T. (1991). Functional outcomes of children with sickle-cell disease affected by stroke. *Archives of Physical Medicine and Rehabilitation, 12,* 498–502.

Han, X., Kilfoy, B., Zheng, T., Holford, T. R., Zhu, C., Zhu, Y., et al. (2008). Lymphoma survival patterns by WHO subtype in the United States, 1973–2003. *Cancer Causes & Control, 19,* 841–858.

Hoelzer, D., & Gale, R. P. (1987). Acute lymphoblastic leukemia in adults: Recent progress, future directions. *Seminars in Hematology, 24,* 27–39.

Hsu, F. J., Caspor, C. B., Czerwinski, D., Kwak, L. W., Liles, T. M., Syrengelas, A., et al. (1997). Tumor-specific idiotype vaccines in the treatment of patients with B-cell lymphoma: Long term results of a clinical trial. *Blood, 89,* 3129–3135.

Jenkins, P. L., Linington, A., & Whittaker, J. A. (1991). A retrospective study of psychosocial morbidity in bone marrow transplant recipients. *Psychosomatics, 32,* 65–71.

Kasper, C. K., & Dietrich, S. L. (1985). Comprehensive management of hemophilia. *Clinics in Haematology, 14,* 489–512.

King, M. E., & Rowe, J. M. (2007). Recent developments in acute myelogenous leukemia therapy. *The Oncologist, 12,* 14–21.

Kinney, T. R., & Ware, R. E. (1996). The adolescent with sickle cell anemia. *Hematology-Oncology Clinics of North America, 10,* 1255–1264.

Koshy, M., & Dorn, L. (1996). Continuing care for adult patients with sickle cell disease [Review]. *Hematology-Oncology Clinics of North America, 10,* 1265–1273.

Magrath, I., Adde, M., Shad, A., Venzon, D., Seibel, N., Gootenberg, J., et al. (1996). Adults and children with small non-cleaved-cell lymphoma have a similar excellent outcome when treated with the same chemotheraphy regimen. *Journal of Oncology, 14,* 925–934.

Matasar, M. J., & Zelenetz, A. D. (2008). Overview of lymphoma diagnosis and management. *Radiologic Clinics of North America, 46,* 175–198.

Michallet, A. S., & Coiffier, B. (2009). Recent developments on the treatment of aggressive non-Hodgkin Lymphoma. *Blood Reviews, 23,* 11–23.

Moore, R. D., Charache, S., Terrin, M. L., Barton, F. B., & Ballas, S. K. (2000). Cost-effectiveness of hydroxyurea in sickle cell anemia. Investigators of the Multicenter Study of Hydroxyurea in Sickle Cell Anemia. *American Journal of Hematology, 64,* 26–31.

Mulhern, R. K., Friedman, A. G., & Stone, P. A. (1988). Acute lymphoblastic leukemia: Long-term psychological outcome [Review]. *Biomedicine & Pharmacotherapy, 42,* 243–246.

Nietert, P. J., Silverstein, M. D., & Abboud, M. R. (2002). Sickle cell anaemia: Epidemiology and cost of illness. *Pharmacoeconomics, 20(6),* 357–366.

Penson, R. T., Rauch, P. K., McAfee, S. L., Cashavelly, B. J., Clair-Hayes, K., Dahlin, C., et al. (2002). Between parent and child: Negotiating cancer treatment in adolescents. *Oncologist, 7,* 154–162.

Raphael, B. G., & Knowles, D. M. (1990). Acquired immunodeficiency syndrome-associated non-Hodgkin's lymphoma. *Seminars in Oncology, 17,* 361–366.

Rosenberg, S. A. (Chairman). (1982). National Cancer Institute sponsored study of classifications of non-Hodgkin's lymphomas: Summary and description of a working formulation for clinical usage. *Cancer, 49,* 2112–2135.

Rosendaal, F. R., Smit, C., Varekamp, L., Bröcker-Vriends, A. H., Van Dijck, H., Saurmeijer, T. P., et al. (1990). Modern hemophilia treatment: Medical improvements and quality of life. *Journal of Internal Medicine, 228,* 633–640.

Ruthoven, J. J. (1987). Current approaches to the treatment of advanced-stage non-Hodgkin's lymphoma. *Canadian Medical Association Journal, 136,* 29–36.

Schatz, J., Puffer, E. S., Sanchez, C., Stancil, M., & Roberts, C. W. (2009). Language processing deficits in sickle cell disease in young school-age children. *Developmental Neuropsychology, 34,* 122–136.

Schouten, H. C. (2007) Diagnosis, staging and prognostic factors. *Annals of Oncology,* 18(suppl 1), i22–i28.

Scott, R. B. (1985). Advances in the treatment of sickle cell disease in children. *American Journal of Diseases of Children, 139,* 1219–1222.

Sekeres, M. A., Stone, R. M., Zahrieh, D., Neuberg, D., Morrison, V., De Angelo, D. J., et al. (2004). Decision-making and quality of life in older adults with acute myeloid leukemia or advanced myelodysplastic syndrome. *Leukemia, 18,* 809–816.

Syrjala, K. L., Langer, S. L., Abrams, J. R., Storer, B., Sanders, J. E., Flowers, M. E., et al. (2004). Recovery and long-term function after hematopoietic cell transplantation for leukemia or lymphoma. *JAMA, 291,* 2335–2343.

Skarin, A. T. (1989). Non-Hodgkin's lymphoma. *Archives of Internal Medicine, 34,* 209–242.

Somerfield, M. R., Curbow, B., Wingard, J. R., Baker, F., & Fogarty, L. A. (1996). Coping with the physical and psychosocial sequelae of bone marrow transplantation among long-term survivors. *Journal of Behavioral Medicine, 19,* 163–184.

Vardiman, J. W., Harris, N. L., & Brunning, R. D. (2002). The World Health Organization (WHO) classification of myeloid neoplasms. *Blood, 100,* 2292–2302.

Williams, W. J., Butler, E., Ersley, A. J., & Lichtman, M. A. (Eds.). (1990). *Hematology* (4th ed.). New York: McGraw-Hill.

Wolcott, D. L., Wellisch, D. K., Fawzy, F. I., & Landsverk, J. (1986). Adaptation of adult bone marrow transplant recipient long-term survivors. *Transplantation, 41,* 478–484.

Wright, K., & Adeosum, O. (2009). Barriers to effective pain management in sickle cell disease. *British Journal of Nursing, 18,* 158–161.

Yanni, E., Grosse, S. D., Yang, Q., & Olney, R. S. (2009). Trends in pediatric sickle cell disease-related mortality in the United States 1983–2000. *Journal of Pediatrics, 154,* 541–545.

13

Developmental Disabilities

Richard J. Morris, PhD, and Yvonne P. Morris, PhD

Developmental disability can be traced to the work of Jean Itard, a French physician, and his attempts, beginning in 1799, to educate Victor, the Wild Boy of Aveyron (Itard, 1962). According to Humphrey (1962), Itard believed that Victor's condition could be cured. Itard felt that the reason for Victor's "apparent subnormality" was his lack of typical language experiences and social interactions that form an integral part of the development of a "normal civilized person." He placed Victor under his care for 5 years at the Paris Institution where he worked. Although Victor improved over this period, he did not achieve Itard's initial expectations and predictions of becoming "normal."

Itard's work influenced the writings, research, and treatment practices of a number of early workers in the field of developmental disabilities, notably, Edouard Seguin. Their writings, in turn, led directly to the building of residential schools and facilities in the United States for individuals having intellectual or other developmental disabilities.[1] The first facility was established in Watertown, Massachusetts, in 1848, as part of the Perkins Institution for the Blind (MacMillan, 1982), and the second was built in Syracuse, New York, in 1851, as an independent facility for people with intellectual and other developmental disabilities. Although the primary residents of these facilities were children, adults and adolescents were also placed in these institutions. These persons in the 1850s—as well as those who manifested similar characteristics over almost the next 100 years—were referred to as "feebleminded" or, later, as "mentally defective." In addition to these labels, more specific levels of "feebleminded" and "mentally defective" were given to these persons depending on their level of intellectual functioning. Specifically, "moron" was applied to those people who were in the highest intellectual functioning category of feeblemindedness, followed by "imbeciles" who were in the middle range of intellectual functioning, and "idiots," who were in the lowest intellectual functioning category (Kanner, 1948).

Seguin and others (e.g., Samuel Howe) intended these facilities to be established on an experimental basis as educational institutions rather than as custodial asylums (Morris & Kratochwill, 2008). The hypothesis underlying this form of intervention was that after people with intellectual disability (or other types of developmental disability) received education

---

[1] The term "mental retardation" has been used for decades throughout the United States to describe a group of individuals who have a particular type of developmental disability that is characterized by significant subaverage deficits in adaptive and intellectual functioning, with such deficits occurring prior to 18 years of age. Since this term has often resulted in social stigma of these individuals (e.g., Matson, Terlonge, & Minshawi, 2008), throughout this chapter we will use the term "intellectual disability" to describe persons having this type of developmental disability.

and training to help them to function adequately in society, they would then be returned to their original homes within the community. The hypothesis, however, was not supported by empirical data (Baumeister, 1970). In fact, few persons who entered these institutions ever returned to society, and by the beginning of the 20th century, the state educational schools became the state custodial institutions (Baumeister, 1970; Blatt, 1984; Brown et al., 1986; Kanner, 1964; Morris & Kratochwill, 2008; Wolfensberger, 1972). This custodial emphasis began to change in the late 1960s and early 1970s with positive developments in the deinstitutionalization and normalization movements (e.g., Blatt, 1968, 1984; Blatt & Kaplan, 1966; Nirje, 1969; Wolfensberger, 1969, 1972), legal advocacy for individuals with intellectual disability (e.g., Friedman, 1975; Halderman v. Pennhurst, 1977; New York State Association for Retarded Children v. Rockefeller, 1973; Pennsylvania Association for Retarded Children v. Commonwealth of Pennsylvania, 1971; Wyatt v. Stickney, 1971), and the introduction of behavior modification treatment (e.g., Ayllon & Azrin, 1968; Baer, Wolf, & Risley, 1968; Gardner, 1971; Kazdin, 1975; Lovaas & Bucher, 1974; Morris, 1976; Schaefer & Martin, 1969; Thompson & Grabowski, 1972; Watson, 1973).

DESCRIPTION OF DISABILITY

Developmental disability encompasses a wide range of diagnostic conditions and behaviors (e.g., Blackman, 1983; Wright, 1987) and typically refers to those chronic or lifelong intellectual, behavioral, and/or physical conditions that develop in individuals prior to 18 years of age and require specific forms of agency services and intervention strategies that may occur over an extended duration (Ehlers, Prothero, & Langone, 1982; Scheerenberger, 1987). In addition, social adaptability and competence enter into the specific definition of one of these disabilities, namely, intellectual disability (American Association on Mental Retardation, 1992; Leland, 1991; Luckasson et al., 2002; Matson, Terlonge, & Minshawi, 2008; Scheerenberger, 1987). The major forms of developmental disability are intellectual disability, cerebral palsy, epilepsy, and other types of seizure disorder, as well as pervasive developmental disorders (PDDs), such as autism and Asperger's syndrome. Some of the common characteristics that are often found in persons with developmental disabilities are functional limitations in some or most of the following areas: self-care and self-help skills, receptive and/or expressive language, cognition and learning ability, mobility, self-direction, economic independence, and the ability to live on their own without assistance (American Psychiatric Association, 2000; Cole & Gardner, 1993; Developmental Disabilities Act, 1984; Developmental Disabilities Assistance and Bill of Rights Act, 2000). In addition, these persons are often characterized as scoring in the below average range on individually administered standardized tests of intelligence. This chapter will focus on two broad types of developmental disability: intellectual disability and PDDs.

FUNCTIONAL PRESENTATION

Mental Retardation

In 1959, the American Association of Mental Deficiency—now called the American Association on Intellectual and Developmental Disabilities (AAIDD)—defined mental retardation in terms of a person's level of intellectual ability and level of adaptive behavior. This statement has been revised over the years; the current definition is as follows: "Mental retardation is a disability characterized by significant limitations both in intellectual functioning and in adaptive behavior as expressed in conceptual, social, and practical adaptive skills. This disability originates before age 18" (Luckasson et al., 2002, p. 1).

This definition reflects the multidimensional underpinnings in approaching mental retardation as well as the expanding conceptualization of this condition. The dimensions included are intellectual abilities and adaptive behavior, with intellectual disability being defined as a state of intellectual and adaptive functioning that begins in childhood (Luckasson et al., 2002). Consistent with good testing practice, the evaluation of intellectual and adaptive functioning should be assessed within the context of environmental and personal factors, including culture, race and ethnicity, linguistic diversity, and sensory, motor, and behavioral factors.

Intelligence refers to overall mental ability, including capacity to problem solve and learn. Limitations in *intellectual functioning* are generally assessed through the use of standardized individually administered IQ tests. Scores that are two or more standard deviations below the mean for the specific assessment instruments used—taking into consideration the assessment instrument's standard error of measurement (SEM), as well as the instrument's strengths and limitations—are viewed as falling into the intellectual disability range (Luckasson et al., 2002). As most IQ tests have a mean of 100, a standard deviation of 15, and an SEM of 5, the requisite IQ score for a diagnosis of intellectual disability is generally 70 or lower. With the inclusion of the SEM criterion, the ceiling IQ score for intellectual disability is raised to 75, with IQ being reported as a confidence band (e.g., 65–75) rather than a finite score (Luckasson et al., 2002).

Adaptive behavior is defined by the AAIDD (see, e.g., Luckasson et al., 2002) as the conceptual, social, and practical skills that people use in order to function in their everyday lives. Conceptual skills include communication skills, money and calculation skills, and self-direction. Social skills include interpersonal skills and the ability to understand and follow rules and laws. Practical skills include skills in personal and instrumental activities of daily living (e.g., eating, meal preparation), as well as occupational job-related skills (Luckasson et al., 2002).

Tests of adaptive behavior usually assess these skills by observing the individual in situations where these skills are required, by interviewing those who know the individual well, or through a combination of these procedures. Adaptive behavior is typically assessed by the use of standardized tests of adaptive behavior that have been normed on the general population, including nondisabled and disabled individuals. *Adaptive functioning* limitations in intellectual disability are generally conceptualized as scores on these standardized tests that are two or more standard deviations below the mean for adaptive behavior overall or for at least one of the three types of adaptive functioning: conceptual, social, or practical (Luckasson et al., 2002). One assessment instrument that has been frequently used to assess adaptive behavior in persons who may have an intellectual disability is the *Vineland Adaptive Behavior Scales, Second Edition* (VABS; Sparrow, Cicchetti, & Balla, 2005).

Intellectual disability has traditionally been divided into levels of severity, with these levels linked to level of functioning or to IQ scores. In the early 1900s, Goddard proposed a classification system for intellectual disability based on the Binet-Simon concept of mental age. Individuals having intellectual disability with the lowest mental age level (less than 3 years of age) were identified as *idiots*. *Imbeciles* had a mental age of 3–7 years, and *morons* had a mental age between 7 and 10 years (Mash & Wolfe, 1999). In 1959, Heber developed a classification system based on deficits in measured intelligence and adaptive behavior (personal-social and sensory-motor) (Heber, 1959). This system proved unworkable and in 1961 Heber revised the intellectual disability classification manual (Brison, 1967). Heber (1961) linked retardation in measured intelligence to the following IQ scores on the *Stanford-Binet Intelligence Scale*: borderline (IQ range of 68–83), mild (IQ range of 52–67), moderate (IQ range of 36–51), severe (IQ range of 20–35), and profound (IQ below 20). Slightly higher IQ score ranges were reported for the same categories using the Wechsler intelligence scale: borderline (IQ range of 70–84), mild (IQ range of 55–69), moderate (IQ range of 40–54), severe (IQ range of 25–39), and profound (IQ below 25). A subsequent revision in the categories (Grossman, 1983) reduced the categories to four levels of intellectual disability (i.e., mild, moderate, severe, and profound).

In 1968, the American Psychiatric Association's (APA) *Diagnostic and Statistical Manual of Mental Disorders, Second Edition* (DSM-II; APA, 1968), linked IQ scores to levels of intellectual disability, with borderline mental retardation indicating IQ scores of 68–83, mild mental retardation indicating IQ scores of 52–67, moderate mental retardation indicating IQ scores of 36–51, severe mental retardation indicating IQ scores of 20–35, and profound mental retardation indicating an IQ score under 20. Prior to 1973, the recommended IQ cutoff scores for intellectual disability were 84 or 85. With the publication of the *Manual on Terminology and Classification in Mental Retardation* by the American Association on Mental Deficiency (Grossman, 1973), the cutoff score was revised downward to approximately 70, where it remains today.

In the most recent edition of APA's *Diagnostic and Statistical Manual of Mental Disorders, Fourth Edition*, Text Revision (*DSM-IV-TR*; APA, 2000), mental retardation is "…characterized by significantly subaverage intellectual functioning (an IQ of approximately 70 or below) with onset before age 18 years and concurrent deficits or impairments in adaptive functioning" (p. 39). The areas of concurrent impairment in adaptive functioning include "…at least two of the following skill areas: communication, self-care, home living, social/interpersonal skills, use of community resources, self-direction, functional academic skills, work, leisure, health, and safety … (*DSM-IV-TR*, 2000, p. 41). The *DSM-IV-TR* lists four "degrees of severity of mental retardation": mild mental retardation encompasses an IQ range of 50–55 to approximately 70, moderate retardation encompasses an IQ range of 35–40 to 50–55, severe mental retardation encompasses an IQ range of 20–25 to 35–40, and profound mental retardation encompasses an IQ range below 20 or 25 (APA, 2000, p. 42). Other classification systems that include sections on intellectual disability are the World Health Organization's *International Classification of Diseases: Tenth Revision* (ICD-10, 1992), and United States federal government's *Individuals With Disabilities Improvement Education Act* (IDEIA) (2004).

Beginning in 1992, the American Association on Mental Retardation (AAMR; now the AAIDD) proposed a reconceptualization of the levels of severity of mental retardation based on intensities of support a person required in order to function successfully in society. The AAMR definitions of system levels of needed support are listed in Table 13.1 (AAMR, 1992; Luckasson et al., 2002).

The AAMR's levels of intensities of supports has not been as widely accepted as the traditional system based on IQ scores (Conyers, Martin, Martin, & Yu, 2002), and a number of concerns have been raised about the differences between this system and state and federal statutes pertaining to intellectual disability, which are usually composed of wording similar to the *DSM-IV-TR*'s severity levels and the AAIDD's earlier conceptualization of mental retardation (see, e.g., Gresham, MacMillan, & Siperstein, 1995; Hodapp, 1995; MacMillan,

---

TABLE 13.1 *Definition and Examples of Intensities of Supports*

Intermittent supports on an "as needed basis." Characterized by episodic nature, person not always needing the support(s), or short-term supports needed during life-span transitions (e.g., job loss or acute medical crisis) Intermittent supports may be high or low intensity when provided.

Limited supports. An intensity of supports characterized by consistency overtime, time limited but not of an intermittent nature, may require fewer staff members and cost less than more intense levels of support (e.g., time-limited employment training or transitional supports during the school-to-adult provided period)

Extensive supports. This is characterized by regular involvement (e.g., daily) in at least some environments (such as work or home) and not time limited (e.g., long-term support and long-term home living support)

Pervasive supports. This is characterized by their constancy and high intensity; provided across environments; potentially life-sustaining in nature. Pervasive supports typically involve more staff members and intrusiveness than do extensive or time-limited supports

Note: From American Association of Mental Retardation. *Mental Retardation. Definition, Classification, and Systems of Support* (9th ed.). Washington, DC. American Association of Mental Retardation. Copyright 1992 by the American Association of Mental Retardation. Reprinted with permission.

Gresham, & Siperstein, 1993; Matson, 1995). The AAIDD (Luckasson et al., 2002) acknowledged these concerns and added the caveat that clinicians may classify individuals with intellectual disability using support intensity, IQ range, adaptive behavior limitations, etiology, mental health category, or other classification systems as necessary for the person having intellectual disability to meet statutory requirements to qualify for local, state, and federal services.

Estimates of the prevalence of intellectual disability in the general population in the United States range between 1% and 3% (Boyle et al., 1996; Daily, Ardinger, & Holmes, 2000; Grossman, 1983; Lee et al., 2001; McLaren & Bryson, 1987). Prevalence rates for children and youth in U.S. public schools who receive special education services under the IDEIA category "mental retardation" have dropped significantly over the past 25 years, to approximately 1% of the school population (U.S. Department of Education, 2002). This decline may reflect increased differentiation of these students from other children and youth who have overlapping disabilities (e.g., autism), a reluctance on the part of school administrators to diagnose mild mental retardation, and/or an increased use of nondiagnostic multicategorical classrooms. From a global perspective, in 1994, the World Health Organization estimated a worldwide prevalence of mental retardation to be 3% (WHO, 1992).

An appreciable amount of research has been devoted to determining the causes of intellectual disability, as well as to developing techniques and strategies for intervention and prevention (see, e.g., AAMR, 1992; Aman & Singh, 1991; Bielecki & Swender, 2004; Cole & Gardner, 1993; Coutler, 1991; Curry et al., 1997; Daily et al., 2000; Gullone, King, & Cummins, 1996; Handen, 2007; Luckasson et al., 2002; Matson et al., 2008; Matson, Laud, & Matson, 2004; Pennington, McGrath, & Peterson, 2009a; Peterson & Martens, 1995; Williams, Kirkpatrick-Sanchez, & Crocker, 1994; Zigler & Hodapp, 1986). For example, hundreds of recognized genetically based syndromes associated with intellectual disability are listed online in the database of the *Online Mendelian Inheritance in Man* database, authored and edited by the McKusick-Nathans Institute of Genetic Medicine at the Johns Hopkins University School of Medicine (<www.ncbi.nih.gov/omim>). These genetically based syndromes (e.g., Angelman syndrome) as well as various nongenetically based syndromic disorders (e.g., fetal alcohol syndrome) have been found to be associated with intellectual disability. As a general rule, the more severe the intellectual disability, the more likely it is that the intellectual disability can be attributable to an identifiable medical or physical condition. The three major known causes of intellectual disability are Down syndrome, fetal alcohol syndrome, and fragile X syndrome. However, the etiology of 50% of all cases of intellectual disability is presently unknown. For known cases, prenatal factors (e.g., trisomy 21 Down syndrome, maternal alcohol consumption) are implicated as causal factors more often than are perinatal (e.g., hypoxia, fetal malnutrition, various infections) or postnatal (e.g., head injury, malnutrition, seizure disorder) factors (Handen, 2007; Matson et al., 2008; McLaren & Bryson, 1987). Table 13.2 lists some of the physical conditions associated with intellectual disability (Baraitser & Winter, 1996; Gorlin, Cohen, & Hennekam, 2001; Jones, 1997; Stevenson, Schwartz, & Schroer, 2000). For individuals whose intellectual disability is not accounted for by known conditions, social deprivation, neglect, abuse, and inadequate level of environmental stimulation are often considered to be primary contributing factors to the etiology of intellectual disability (Handen, 2007; Matson et al., 2008).

Pervasive Developmental Disorders

Pervasive developmental disorders (PDD) is an umbrella term created by the APA (1980) for a group of neurodevelopmental disorders characterized by impaired social interaction, deficits in verbal and nonverbal communication, and restrictive and/or stereotyped patterns of behavior, activities and/or interests. This umbrella term is also used by the IDC–10 (WHO, 1992), with these two diagnostic systems having converging definitions and diagnostic criteria for autism and related disorders (Volkmar, State, & Klin, 2009). PDD is a generic label

TABLE 13.2 *Conditions or Events Which Are Often Associated With Intellectual Disability*

Period of Development	Type of Condition or Event	Examples
Pre- and periconceptual	Brain malformation	Encephalocele, hydranencephaly, neural tube defects, agenesis of the corpus callosum
	Chromosomal abnormalities: trisomy	Down's syndrome
	Chromosomal abnormalities: deletions	Prader Willi syndrome, Angelman syndrome, Wolf-Hirschhorn syndrome
	Chromosomal abnormalities: sex chromosome-linked disorders	Fragile X, Rett's syndrome
	Chromosomal abnormalities: autosomal dominant conditions	Tuberous sclerosis, Williams syndrome
	Chromosomal abnormalities: autosomal recessive conditions	Tay-Sachs, Niemann-Pick, Lesch-Nyhan
Prenatal	Teratogens	Chemicals, radiation, maternal substance abuse (alcohol, drugs) Prescription medications (e.g., anticonvulsants, warfann)
	Infection	TORCH viruses: rubella, toxoplasmosis, cytomegalovirus, herpes simplex
	Fetal malnutrition	Mother with high blood pressure or kidney disease
Perinatal	Prematurity	Complications such as poor oxygenation of the brain and intracranial hemorrhage
	Metabolic abnormalities	Hypoglycemia, phenylketonuria
	Trauma	Misapplication of forceps
	Infection	Herpes simplex encephalitis
Postnatal	Infection	Meningitis, encephalitis, general inflammatory disease with high fever
	Trauma; Lack of oxygen	Automobile accidents, child abuse, near drowning, strangulation
	Severe nutritional deficiency	Kwashiorkor, iodine deficiency
	Environmental toxins	Lead, carbon monoxide, household products
	Environmental and social problems	Psychosocial deprivation, parental psychiatric disorders

Adapted from: Blackman, J. A. (Ed.). (1983). *Medical aspects of developmental disabilities in children birth to three*. Iowa City, IA: University of Iowa Press.

(Szatmari, 2000) and incorporates a wide range of impairments that a child is born with or born with the potential of developing (Frith, 1991).

The *DSM-IV-TR* (APA, 2000) includes five specific disorders under the PDD umbrella: autistic disorder (or autism), Asperger's disorder (also referred to as Asperger's syndrome), Rett's disorder (commonly abbreviated as RTT), childhood disintegrative disorder (CDD), and pervasive developmental disorder not otherwise specified (PDDNOS). These five disorders have overlapping diagnostic criteria and are commonly viewed as related disorders. The National Institute of Mental Health discusses these disorders under the general rubric of *autism spectrum disorders* (ASD). There is some confusion in the literature regarding the definition of ASD, with some researchers limiting the term ASD to autism and Asperger's disorder (Lewis, Murdoch, & Woodyatt, 2007; Ritvo, Ritvo, Guthrie, & Ritvo, 2008), whereas others include autism, Asperger's disorder, and PDDNOS (e.g., Fombonne, 2003a; Witwer & Lecavalier, 2008). Significant overlap in the clinical and demographic characteristics, neuropsychological profiles, and comorbidities of individuals diagnosed with these specific PDD diagnoses has been reported. RTT and CDD, which are characterized by a period of normal development followed by severe regression and loss of skills, along with the development of ASD symptoms, are very low-incidence disorders and are not included in most discussions of ASD.

It is increasingly common for ASD to be viewed as a continuum of problems that range from absent to severe in each of the three main symptom areas of social interaction, communication, and behavior (Attwood, 1998; Eisenmajer et al., 1996; Fombonne, 2003a; Schopler, 1996). Some researchers have posited that the continuum extends to typical behaviors, so that it includes milder, nonclinical forms of the behaviors found in the ASD diagnosis. For example, Baron-Cohen and his associates have speculated that the "systematizing" symptoms of ASD are manifestations of "the extreme male brain" (Auyeung et al., 2009; Baron-Cohen, 2002). Similarities in the response patterns to questionnaires and to psychological tests, given by individuals diagnosed with ASD and their family members, have led some researchers to also conclude that there is a "broad autism phenotype" (e.g., Losh et al., 2009).

Estimates of the prevalence of ASD have varied widely, ranging between 30 and 67 per 10,000 individuals (Bertrand et al., 2001; Chakrabarti & Fombonne, 2001, 2005; Croen, Grethner, Hoogstrate, & Selvin, 2002; Fombonne, 2002, 2003b; Fombonne, Simmons, Ford, Meltzer, & Goodman, 2001; Newschaffer, Falb, & Gurney, 2005; Yeargin-Allsopp et al., 2003). Estimates from the U.S. Centers for Disease Control and Prevention Autism and Developmental Disabilities Monitoring Network (2007) resulted in an overall United States ASD prevalence rate of 67 per 10,000, or 1 in 150, with a 4 to 1 ratio of boys to girls. The Autism and Developmental Disabilities Monitoring Network assessed rates at different sites at two points in time, with rates being fairly consistent across time, and varying between survey sites in different states. These prevalence rates are consistent with the findings of other recent surveys of ASD (e.g., Chakrabarti & Fombonne, 2005; Charman, 2002; Fombonne, 2003b; Fombonne et al., 2001; Mahoney et al., 2001; Wing & Potter, 2002). Fombonne (2003b) speculated that older surveys underestimated the true prevalence for ASD, and that the true prevalence rate was likely to be close to 60 per 10,000. He noted that (1) children with milder or high-functioning types of ASD are often missed in surveys; (2) younger children are underrepresented because assessment techniques used in the diagnosis of infants and preschool-aged children are less sensitive than techniques used for older children; (3) older children are underidentified because the newer diagnostic criteria for ASD were not in place when they were diagnosed; and (4) with the increasing availability in the 1990s of developmental disability services for children with ASD, schools and other educational services agencies have become more likely to identify and provide programs for children with ASDs. Williams, Higgins, and Brayne (2006) conducted a meta-analysis of 60 studies that estimated the prevalence of typical autism and of all ASDs. Based on their analyses, 61% of the variation in prevalence estimates of typical autism could be attributed to differences in diagnostic criteria, age of children screened, and/ or study location (or some other unknown variables for which these three study characteristics were acting as a proxy). In a study conducted in California, Croen et al. (2002) found that the prevalence rate for ASD increased over time, whereas the prevalence rate for intellectual disability went down. They speculated that some children who would have been diagnosed with intellectual disability in the past were now being diagnosed with ASD.

A link between prevalence rates for ASD and environmental factors, especially environmental pathogens, has long been suspected. However, no environmentally based causal factors have been identified to date (Newschaffer et al., 2007). Among the most frequently mentioned pathogens is some component of childhood vaccinations, usually the combined measles, mumps, and rubella (MMR) vaccination, or thimerisol, a mercury-based preservative used in some vaccinations (though not the vaccination for MMR) (e.g., Hviid, Stellfeld, Wohlfahrt, & Melbye, 2003; Madsen et al., 2002). Despite the fact a link between vaccinations and ASD has not been found, the belief that vaccinations are a cause of ASD persists (Waterhouse, 2008).

Autism and ASD

More than 65 years ago, Leo Kanner (1943) described a group of 11 children who displayed a similar pattern of specific symptoms that were significantly different from those of other childhood behavior disorders. Kanner called this form of childhood psychopathology "early infantile autism" and noted that among its characteristics were marked withdrawal; dislike of being held; unresponsiveness to people as well as to the environment; manipulation of objects in a rigid, stereotyped manner; lack of appropriate play; failure to acquire normal speech; echolalia and difficulties with pronoun use; anxious insistence on sameness in the environment; excellent rote memories; normal physical appearance; and good cognitive potential.

Currently, autism is characterized by deficits in the following three categories: (a) qualitative impairment in reciprocal social interaction and/or activities; (b) qualitative impairment in verbal and nonverbal communication, as well as in imaginative activity; and (c) restricted and stereotyped patterns of behavior, interests, and/or activities. Each category includes four deficit classes, comprising a total of 12 deficits, or symptoms of impairment. At least 6 of the 12 specified deficits are necessary to diagnose autism, including at least two deficits in reciprocal social interaction and at least one each in difficulty in communication and restricted, repetitive behaviors, interests, or activities. Onset of at least one of these deficits must occur prior to 3 years of age and the disturbance cannot be better accounted for by RTT or CDD (APA, 2000). Impairment in reciprocal social interaction can be demonstrated through difficulty in using nonverbal behaviors to regulate social interaction, failure to develop age-appropriate peer relationships, limited sharing of pleasure, achievements, or interests with others, and a lack of social or emotional reciprocity. Impairment in communication can be manifested by a delay or failure to develop language, difficulty holding conversations, difficulty using unusual or repetitive language, and failure to demonstrate developmentally appropriate play. Having restricted and stereotyped patterns of behavior, interests, and/or activities is exemplified by the person having interests that are narrow, overly intense, and/or unusual; having an unreasonable insistence on sameness and following familiar routines; engaging in repetitive motor movements; and in attachment to unusual objects or preoccupations with parts of objects (Ozonoff, Goodlin-Jones, & Solomon, 2007). Reportedly half of the individuals diagnosed with autism never develop meaningful speech (Tanguay, 2000).

With regard to etiology, Gupta and State (2007) have stated that ASD is a strongly genetic disorder, with an estimated heritability of more than 90%. Pennington, McGrath, and Peterson (2009b) noted the association between ASD and known genetic disorders, including tuberous sclerosis and fragile X syndrome. Most cases of ASD are thought to be the result of a polygenic disorder (Gupta & Slate, 2007; Tsai, 2006). The genetic markers for several of the behavioral features of autism have been identified (Gillberg, 1999; Ritvo, Freeman, Mason-Brothers, Mo, & Ritvo, 1985; Ritvo, Spence, et al., 1985), and studies using data gathered by the Autism Genetic Resource Exchange (2009), a DNA repository and family registry of genotypic and phenotypic information, have identified loci on several genes that are significantly associated with autism.

Neuroimaging studies using magnetic resonance imaging and computed tomography scans, as well as postmortem examinations, have revealed a higher incidence of structural brain defects, particularly in the cerebellum, in individuals diagnosed with autism, as compared with nondiagnosed individuals (e.g., Allen & Courchesne, 2003; Courchesne, 1989; Courchesne et al., 1994; Haas et al., 1996; Rapin & Katzman, 1998). Other studies have reported a pattern of atypical head growth and brain enlargement in children diagnosed with autism. Although these children reportedly had a head circumference that was within normal limits at birth, a significant minority (around 20% of autistic individuals) developed macrocephaly in their first year, with an atypical pattern of brain growth, followed by early cessation of brain growth (Brambilla et al., 2003; Courchesne, Carper, & Akshoomoff, 2003, Dawson et al., 2007; White, O'Reilly, & Frith, 2009). Abnormal patterns of brain function have been noted in individuals diagnosed with ASD, including reduced responsiveness to novel stimuli, lower activation of mirror neurons on certain tasks, increased variability in regional metabolic rates on positron emission tomography scans, and differences in brain substrates, especially in the fusiform gyrus and amygdala (Amaral, Schumann, & Nordahl, 2008; Pennington et al., 2009b). Altered serotonergic function in individuals with autism has also been reported (Anderson, Horne, Chatterjee, & Cohen, 1990; Anderson et al., 2002; Cook et al., 1990; Freeman & Ritvo, 1984; Minderaa et al., 1989), with this finding being considered one of the most robust and well-replicated in the neurobiology of autism (Buitelaar & Willemsen-Swinkels, 2000). However, the significance of this finding is not known, as studies focusing on pharmacological treatment to reduce blood serotonin levels have generally failed to yield behavioral or other improvements (e.g., Duker et al., 1991; Ekman, Miranda-Linne, Gillberg, & Garle, 1989).

It should be noted that many individuals with ASD have comorbid psychiatric diagnoses, including anxiety disorders, attention deficit/hyperactivity disorder, and oppositional defiant disorder (Leyfer et al., 2006, Simonoff et al., 2008). Additional comorbid disorders include intellectual disability, sleep problems (Liu, Hubbard, Faber, & Adams, 2006), and gastrointestinal problems (Tsai, 2006). In general, pharmacological treatment of children with ASD has had limited success, with most drug treatments focusing on the reduction or alleviation of disruptive symptoms and behaviors (Charlop-Christy, Malmberg, Rocha, & Schreibman, 2008, Ozonoff et al., 2007; Tsai, 2006). In this regard, it has been reported that about 70% of children older than 8 years, who have been diagnosed with ASD, receive some form of psychoactive medication in a given year (Oswald & Sonenklar, 2007).

Asperger's Disorder

About the time Kanner (1943) was studying early infantile autism in the United States, Hans Asperger in Austria identified a group of young boys presenting with what he called *autistic psychopathy*. These boys were described as having normal intelligence and language development, with autistic-like behaviors and deficiencies in social and communication skills. However, it was not until Asperger's research was translated from German to English in 1991 that it began to gain attention, with Wing describing children with Asperger's disorder as tending to have "good grammatical speech from early in life, passive, odd, or subtly inappropriate social interaction and poor gross motor coordination on gait and posture" (in Frith, 1991, pp. 115).

In 1994, Asperger's disorder (also known as Asperger's syndrome) was added to the *DSM-IV* (APA, 1994). According to the *DSM-IV-TR* (APA, 2000), Asperger's disorder (AD), like autism, includes severe and sustained impairment in social interaction and restricted, repetitive patterns of interest, behaviors, and activities. The symptom categories for AD are identical to those for autism, with the exception of difficulties in communication. In AD, the development of language abilities is not impaired (e.g., there must be communicative use of single words by age two and use of meaningful phrases or speech by age three), and there should be no clinically significant delay in cognitive development (e.g., there should be no apparent delay in the first years of life, although mild mental retardation may be diagnosed during the school years) or in the development of age appropriate self-help skills, adaptive behavior, and curiosity about the environment. In the *DSM-IV-TR*, a diagnosis of autistic disorder takes precedence over a diagnosis of AD, and autistic disorder must be ruled out before a diagnosis of AD can be made. The mean age for diagnosis of AD is reported to be 8 years (Eisenmajer et al., 1996). It should be noted that the diagnostic criterion of no clinically significant delays in language development does not preclude the presence of unusual qualities in language skills.

Speech and language peculiarities may be present and are most likely to involve difficulties in the areas of pragmatics and prosody (Attwood, 1998; Safran, 2002).

Generally, individuals with AD may move into the personal space of others, fail to recognize body language and other nonverbal communicative gestures, and fail to recognize verbal cues that he or she has behaved in a socially inappropriate fashion (Safran, 2001, 2002). For example, the person with AD may discuss pet topics at length despite cues from the listener that he or she is not interested (Safran, 2002). In this regard, Attwood (1998) has suggested that individuals having AD tend to have one-sided conversations and frequently uses questioning as a social tool. Individuals with AD are usually disinterested in games, sports, and play activities, are indifferent to peer pressure, and lack precision in expressing emotions.

In practice, it may be difficult to differentiate between those individuals diagnosed with AD and those with high-functioning autism (Matson & Wilkins, 2008; Ritvo et al., 2008). Ozonoff, South, and Miller (2000) have suggested that the differences between high-functioning autism and AD are likely to be artifacts, with both groups having similar trajectories when followed over time, and both groups having reportedly similar neuropsychological research findings (Ozonoff et al., 2007; Pennington et al., 2009b).

Pervasive Developmental Disorder, Not Otherwise Specified

PDDNOS does not have specific criteria for a diagnosis. According to the *DSM-VI-TR* (APA, 2000), PDDNOS is considered an appropriate diagnosis "when there is a severe and pervasive impairment in the development of reciprocal social interaction, verbal and nonverbal communication skills, or the development of stereotyped behavior, interests, and activities, but the criteria are not met for a specific Pervasive Developmental Disorder, Schizophrenia, Schizotypal Personality Disorder, or Avoidant Personality Disorder" (p. 84). It is used for children who have difficulties in at least two of the three autism symptom areas, but who do not meet the criteria for a diagnosis of autism or of the other PDDs. It is also used to diagnose individuals whose symptoms developed after 30 months and/or who present with atypical or fewer symptoms necessary for diagnosis (Tanguay, 2000). Tsai (2000) has noted that some children initially given a diagnosis of PDDNOS may develop additional diagnostic features as they mature, and may receive a subsequent diagnosis of autism. Ozonoff et al. (2007) have noted that PDDNOS is a very heterogeneous category and that the diagnosis is often misused, with children having this diagnosis either meeting the criteria for an autism diagnosis or not meeting the criteria for any PDD diagnosis. They therefore recommend a reevaluation of any child that comes into a clinic or agency with a PDDNOS diagnosis.

Rett's Disorder

RTT was named for Austrian physician Adreas Rett, who in 1966 described two severely disabled young girls with stereotypical hand-wringing movements (Hagberg, Aicardi, Dias, & Ramos, 1983). It is a progressive neurodevelopmental disorder characterized by apparently normal prenatal and perinatal development for the first six to 18 months of life, followed by the development of clinical symptoms, including decreased head circumference growth and microcephaly, loss of muscle tone and previously purposeful hand movements, and characteristic hand-wringing stereotypical behaviors. Children with RTT experience cognitive and functional regression (Mount, Hastings, Reilly, Cass, & Charman, 2003). Hagberg (2002) has developed a detailed four-stage system of development of this disorder.

RTT is caused by a genetic mutation of the *MeCP2* gene, which is located on the X chromosome (Amir et al., 1999). The protein encoded by this gene suppresses gene activation in neurons and leads to developmental delays and neurological disorders. A genetic mutation in the *MeCP2* gene can be identified in 80–85% of RTT cases, with unidentified aberrations in the *MeCP2* gene region thought to be responsible for cases in which a genetic mutation is not apparent (Bienvenu et al., 2000). Recent research has suggested that the *MeCP2* gene regulates the expression of brain-derived neurotropic factor (BDNF), which modulates neuronal survival, neurogenesis, and plasticity. Individuals with RTT with BNDF polymorphism are likely to have more severe symptoms of this disorder (Zeev et al., 2009).

Initially, it was thought that RTT occurred exclusively in females; however, it is now known to occur at a much lower frequency in males. The true incidence and prevalence of RTT is not known but is thought to affect one in every 10,000–15,000 live female births. Although male fetuses can have RTT, they are likely to be spontaneously aborted during pregnancy or to die shortly after birth. It is believed that RTT males with an extra X chromosome may survive longer.

Childhood Disintegrative Disorder

Although the diagnostic category, CDD, was first added to the *DSM-IV* in 1994, it has a long history and can be traced back to Theodore Heller's 1908 discussion of "Dementia Infantilis" (Hendry, 2000). Children with this disorder develop a condition similar to autism, with significant loss of skills in communication, social relationships, play, and adaptive behavior, after a period of at least 2 years of apparently normal development. According to the *DSM-IV-TR*, the clinical presentation of CDD includes (a) significant loss, prior to age 10, of previously acquired skills in at least two of the following areas: expressive or receptive language, social skills or adaptive behavior, bowel or bladder control, play, or motor skills; and (b) abnormalities in functioning in at least two of the following areas: qualitative impairment in social interaction, qualitative impairment in communication, and restricted, repetitive and stereotyped patterns of behavior.

CDD is a very rare disorder, and its prevalence is unknown. In his review of past epidemiological surveys of autism and other PDDs, Fombonne (2002) found four surveys that included CDD. Prevalence rates reported in those surveys ranged from 1.1 to 6.4 per 100,000 individuals. Fombonne (2002) calculated a pooled prevalence estimate for CDD, resulting in an estimated prevalence rate of 1.7 per 100,000 individuals. Behaviorally, individuals diagnosed with CDD are similar to those with ASD, and the treatments for the two disorders are similar, although less improvement over time than is expected in individuals with CDD than in individuals with autism (Ozonoff et al., 2007).

TREATMENT AND PROGNOSIS

Historically, treatment programs for individuals with developmental disabilities have been limited, with more severely impaired individuals typically living in institutional settings where they received custodial care (Morris & Kratochwill, 2008). Educational programs may have been provided for higher functioning individuals within institutional settings, and community-based educational programs were likely to be found in private and church-related schools. Individuals functioning in the moderately and mildly intellectually disabled range were likely to be educated in a segregated classroom setting (i.e., classrooms for the trainable and educable), and sheltered workshop activities, both within and outside the custodial institution, may have been available for older youths and adults. Psychotherapy and counseling services for individuals with developmental disabilities were not widely available (see, e.g., Cowen, 1963; Stacey & DeMartino, 1957).

Most contemporary approaches to the treatment of persons with developmental disabilities can be traced to the behavior modification treatment research of the 1960s and early 1970s (see, e.g., Ayllon & Azrin, 1968; Gardner, 1971; Kazdin, 1975; Lovaas, 1977; Lovaas, Berberich, Perloff, & Schaeffer, 1966; Matson & McCartney, 1981; Morris, 1976; Tharp & Wetzel, 1969; Thompson & Grabowski, 1972; Ullmann & Krasner, 1965; Ulrich, Stachnik, & Mabry, 1966). Many contemporary behavioral treatment programs use an applied behavior analysis approach and are based on the assumptions that the antecedents of a behavior, as well as the consequences of a behavior, can be manipulated so that the likelihood a behavior will be repeated is increased. Behavioral treatment programs have been widely used in helping individuals with developmental disabilities develop and strengthen their positive behavior skills, including adaptive behavior and coping skills, functional language skills, and social skills.

Mental Retardation

So much has been written about the relative effectiveness of behavior modification procedures with people who have an intellectual disability that few writers today would question its utility and the role that these procedures have played in assisting people to live more comfortable and humane lives, independent of their level of intellectual disability (see, e.g., Alberto, Heflin, & Andrews, 2002; Brown et al., 1986; Carr, Turnbull, & Horner, 1999; Cole & Gardner, 1993; Handenm, 2007; Matson et al., 2008; Matson, Laud, & Matson, 2004; Pennington et al, 2009a; Wacker & Berg, 1988). Behavior modification procedures have been used successfully to develop and strengthen positive behaviors and to reduce and eliminate problem behaviors.

Reinforcement Procedures

Reinforcement is typically defined as an event that immediately follows a specific behavior that has been designated for change (called the target behavior) and that results in an increase in the frequency of occurrence of that behavior (e.g., Skinner, 1938, 1953). Because reinforcement is defined for our purposes in terms of its effects on the person, something that might be reinforcing to one person may not be reinforcing to another person. It is therefore very important when using reinforcement procedures to make sure that the clinician, teacher, counselor, parent, or other care provider knows what a reinforcer is for the person with whom she or he is working.

There are typically five categories of positive reinforcement: social praise ("Very Good," "That's right," "Fine," "You're terrific," etc.), nonverbal messages (smiling, tickling, hugging, kissing, etc.), edibles (small amounts of the person's favorite foods, snacks, or drinks), objects (pencil, paper, book, coupons, toys, cosmetics, etc.), and activities (playing catch, playing video games or other electronic games, going to the county fair, going to a shopping mall or park, etc.) (Morris, 1985). The positive reinforcers used by the clinician, teacher, counselor, parent, or other care provider should be appropriate for the person's age, and if possible, the clinician or other behavior modifier should avoid the use of edibles or liquids.

Use of edibles and liquids is usually reserved for clients with severe to profound intellectual disability. The most commonly used method for distributing positive reinforcers is through the use of a conditioned reinforcer, called a token, within a token economy program (see, e.g., Ayllon & Azrin, 1968; Kazdin, 1975, 2001; Morris, 1985). A token is an object (such as a metal washer, poker chip, credit card receipt, or check mark on a personalized identity card) that can be earned by the client each time he or she engages in the target behavior and that has a quantitative relationship to the obtainment (i.e., purchasing) of particular positive reinforcers such as those listed earlier.

Positive reinforcement can be applied on a continuous or intermittent basis, but whenever possible, should be applied on an intermittent basis. In addition, reinforcement can be applied when the client performs the target behavior or, in the case of *differential reinforcement of other behavior* (DRO) or *differential reinforcement of incompatible behavior* (DRI), when the client engages, respectively, in a behavior(s) other than the target behavior (DRO) or a behavior(s) that is incompatible with the target behavior (DRI). Another procedure, *shaping*, is used when the clinician or other behavior modifier wants to teach a complex target behavior to the client in successive steps, with each step gradually leading to an approximation of the desired behavior. For example, instead of attempting to teach a severely handicapped client a whole complex behavior pattern, the behavior modifier would break up the behavior into its component parts and teach each component in successive steps that lead eventually to the performance of the complex behavior pattern (Morris, 1985).

Each of these reinforcement procedures has been used successfully with persons with intellectual disability to teach them a variety of target behaviors, such as self-help/self-care skills, social skills, reading, math, writing, job interview skills, job-finding skills, independent living skills, assertiveness, speech and sign language, and vocational/prevocational skills (see, e.g., Cole & Gardner, 1993; Lovaas, 2003; Matson et al., 2004, 2008; Matson & McCartney, 1981; Morris & McReynolds, 1986).

Behavior-Reduction Procedures

Behavior-reduction procedures involve the introduction of a dissatisfying or unpleasant event immediately following a person's performance of the target behavior that results in a decrease in the probability that the target behavior will occur again the next time the same antecedent or situational stimuli are present (Skinner, 1938, 1953). The most commonly used behavior-reduction procedures are extinction, time-out from positive reinforcement, response cost, and overcorrection (Morris, 1985). *Extinction* refers to the removal of the reinforcing consequences that normally follow a particular target behavior (Skinner, 1953). To use this procedure, the clinician, teacher, or other care provider must be able to (a) identify those consequences that are reinforcing or maintaining the client's undesirable behavior, (b) determine whether those consequences will follow the client's behavior each time the behavior is performed, (c) control the occurrence of those consequences, and (d) be consistent in the use of the procedure each time the target behavior is performed (Morris, 1985). If these conditions cannot be met, another behavior-reduction procedure should be used.

Time-out from positive reinforcement involves removing the person from an attractive and positively reinforcing situation (or withdrawing a positive reinforcing activity) for a particular period of time immediately following the client's performance of the undesirable target behavior. The type of time-out setting in which the client is placed is very important and should contain fewer positive aspects than the positive reinforcing area. Three types of time-out procedures have been applied with persons with intellectual disability. "Contingent observation" involves having the client who performs the undesirable target behavior step away from the reinforcing setting (e.g., small group discussion, athletic event, and group vocational activity) for a specified period and watch the other people in the setting perform appropriate behaviors and receive positive reinforcement from the clinician or other behavior modifier. The client then rejoins the group after a specific time has elapsed. A second time-out method is called *exclusion time-out*. In this method, the person is removed from the reinforcing setting for a specific time and placed in a situation that has a lower reinforcement value to the client each time he or she performs the undesirable target behavior. Typically, the client is not removed to another room or environment with this procedure; rather, he or she is placed in an isolated area in the same room with his or her back to the group activity.

A third procedure is *seclusion time-out*, in which the client is removed from the reinforcing situation for a specific period and placed in a supervised isolated area (e.g., vacant room and cubicle) that is separate from the reinforcing setting. The isolated area must be well ventilated, well lighted, and unlocked, and the person must be monitored on a regular basis (Morris, 1985).

Another behavior-reduction procedure is *response cost*. This procedure is typically combined with a token-economy positive reinforcement method and involves placing a cost on a client's performance of a specific undesirable target behavior. Thus, this procedure consists of the removal or withdrawal of a particular quantity of reinforcers (tokens) from the person each time he or she performs the target behavior.

These methods have been used effectively to decrease the frequency or eliminate the occurrence of a wide variety of target behaviors, including physical aggression, verbal aggression, disruptive behaviors, property destruction, stealing, noncompliance, head banging and other self-injurious behavior (SIB), and self-stimulation. However, they should be used only in conjunction with positive reinforcement procedures where the clinician, teacher, counselor, or parent is also teaching the client alternative desirable target behaviors (Morris, 1985). Matson et al. (2008) have commented that a number of writers in the field of intellectual disability have objected to the use of behavior-reduction methods with clients, maintaining that such methods are not necessary. Instead, they are promoting the use of positive behavior support (PBS) in interventions with people having an intellectual disability (see, e.g., Carr et al., 1999). The foundation of this approach is in applied behavior analysis and involves the replacement of undesirable or challenging behaviors with more desirable prosocial behaviors and skills. The assumption underlying PBS is that it reduces the need for behavior-reduction methods like time-out procedures while also promoting positive changes in the person's behavior(s). PBS makes use of "functional behavioral assessment" to determine the frequency, antecedents, and consequences of the person's challenging behavior(s), as well as the situations and settings under which the behavior(s) occurs. Once this assessment is completed, an intervention plan can be implemented that focuses on preventing the undesirable or challenging behavior(s) from occurring and/or providing the person with PBS for engaging in more desirable behaviors. Matson et al. (2008) maintain, however, that no direct comparison outcome studies have been conducted in which PBS procedures and behavior-reduction methods have been compared regarding their relative effectiveness in reducing various types of challenging behaviors (such as aggressive behaviors, SIB, etc.) in people who have an intellectual disability.

Modeling/Imitation Learning Procedures
Behavior change that results from the observation of another person has been typically referred to as *modeling* (Bandura, 1969; Bandura & Walters, 1963). The modeling procedure consists of an individual called the model (e.g., therapist, teacher, parent, and aide) and a person called the observer (e.g., the client). The observer typically observes the model performing the desirable target behavior in a familiar setting, where the model experiences reinforcement for engaging in the behavior. Another approach to modeling follows Skinner's (1938, 1953) position, in which the clinician, teacher, counselor, parent, or other care provider first demonstrates the target behavior and then reinforces the person for successfully imitating the target behavior of the therapist. Modeling or imitation learning often reduces the amount of time that a person needs to learn a particular behavior.

Although modeling and imitation learning have been found effective in teaching persons having an intellectual disability, there are certain preconditions that must be met for it to be helpful. First, the person should be able to attend to the various aspects of the modeling situation. Second, the person should be able to reproduce motorically the modeled behavior. Third, the person should be motivated to perform the target behavior that she or he has observed (Bandura, 1969; Rimm & Masters, 1979). If any of these factors are absent, the clinician should consider using another behavior modification procedure to teach the target behavior. Modeling has been used effectively to teach such behaviors as social skills, speech and related conversational skills, and recreational activities.

Self-Management Procedures
Self-management refers to a group of procedures in which the person becomes the primary agent directing and controlling his or her behavior to lead to preplanned and specific behavior changes and/or consequences (e.g., Goldfried & Merbaum, 1973; Kanfer, 1980; Karoly & Kanfer, 1982; Liaupsin & Scott, 2008; Lloyd, Hallahan, Kauffman, & Keller, 1998). Self-management methods have the following as their common base: (a) the recognition of the contribution of self-statements to behavior change and (b) the view that individuals can regulate their own behavior. A third common base involves the presence of a clinician, teacher, counselor, parent, or other care provider to motivate the person to begin the self-management plan and to teach him or her how, when, and where to use it (Kanfer, 1980).

The essence of a self-management approach involves the following general steps: (a) having the person with an intellectual disability discuss with the clinician, teacher, counselor or parent the negative self-statements that may be preventing the person from working effectively or that may lead him or her to become emotionally upset; (b) developing with the person specific self-statements, rules, or strategies that can be used to assist him or her in performing the appropriate target behavior, educational task, or work activity; and (c) providing the person with positive reinforcement and feedback for his or her use of the self-management procedure (e.g., Meichenbaum & Genest, 1980).

Self-management procedures represent a potentially effective approach for changing the behaviors of individuals with mental retardation (Ferretti, Cavalier, Murphy, & Murphy, 1993). The relative effectiveness of this approach, however, is tied not only to the level of structuring provided by the clinician, teacher, counselor or parent but also to the receptiveness, interest, and motivational level of the client in implementing the procedure. Moreover, if the level of cognitive functioning in the client is low, then this procedure may be contraindicated— although there is research literature to suggest that this procedure can be used effectively with these clients (e.g., Ferretti et al., 1993; Rusch, McKee, Chadsey-Rusch, & Renzaglia, 1988; Shapiro, 1981, 1986). Self-management has been used effectively with teaching such behaviors as on-task activity, exercise skills, chores, and social skills.

Pervasive Developmental Disorders

Although both Kanner (1943) and Asperger originally postulated that autism and Asperger's disorder were organic or genetic in origin, until the mid-1960s, it was commonly assumed that the basis for autism was a pathological parent-infant relationship (see, e.g., Bettelheim, 1950, 1967, 1974; Kanner, 1943, 1948). As a result, the most widely used therapeutic approach was psychoanalytically based treatment. An early alternative approach was associated with the organic theory of autism as proposed by Rimland (1964). After thoroughly reviewing the literature on autism, Rimland concluded that the disorder had a biological basis. His book stimulated a great deal of interest in the biological bases of autism and treatment programs based on his assumption of a neurological or a biochemical dysfunction were developed (see, e.g., Perry & Meiselas, 1988; Schopler, 1965; Schopler & Reichler, 1971). Alternative theories regarding the etiology of autism and its treatment began to appear in the mid-1960s (Harris, 1988).

Most contemporary intervention programs for the treatment of PDDs are based on the use of *behavior modification procedures*, and the behavioral approach is reported to be the major treatment model that has been empirically demonstrated to be effective in treating children with autism (Charlop-Christy et al., 2008, Ozonoff et al., 2007; Pennington, 2009). Many contemporary behavior modification programs focus on a prescribed and structured teaching of objectively defined behaviors, skills, and facts. Focus is initially on student compliance with the teacher/adult, with rewards given for correct responses, with the behavioral program largely directed through oral language (Tanguay, 2000; Odom et al., 2003).

One of the earliest behavioral programs for the treatment of autism was proposed by Lovaas and his associates (e.g., Lovaas, 1977; Lovaas et al., 1966). They used behavior modification techniques to treat many of the behaviors associated with autism, including increasing the frequency of eye contact, developing functional speech and social skills, and reducing self-injurious and stereotypic behaviors. Lovaas and his associates used an approach called discrete trial training (DTT) in which every task given to the child consisted of a request to perform a specific action, followed by a response from the child, and a reaction from the therapist. Lovaas (1987) reported on the results of a treatment study in which preschool children with autism received intensive behavioral treatment (i.e., more than 40 hours per week of intensive one-to-one behavioral intervention), while similar children in a control group received less intensive treatment (i.e., 10 hours per week of behavioral treatment).

Results indicated that 47% of the children in the intensive treatment group, compared with 2% of the children in the control group, achieved normal intellectual functioning and were placed in the regular first-grade education program. These findings were maintained over time (McEachin, Smith, & Lovaas, 1993). More recent comparative reviews of intervention programs for preschool children with autism have concluded that the most successful programs use a structured, functional approach to problem behaviors, focus on teaching attention, imitation, communication, and social and play skills, incorporate strategies to facilitate generalization, have a low student to staff ratio, and have a high level of family involvement, with family members involved in the treatment program (Dawson & Osterling, 1997; National Research Council, 2001).

A review of behavioral treatment programs for individuals with ASD suggests that most studies have focused on the use of behavior modification procedures to develop and strengthen social and communication skills and to reduce or eliminate behavior problems (e.g., tantrums, aggression, SIB, and self-stimulation). Although, as noted earlier, DTT programs for teaching communication and social skills have been found to be effective, problems in generalizing treatment results to other behaviors, other people, and other environments have been noted. In addition, robotic responding to stimulus cues were sometimes reported, and prompt dependency was sometimes a problem (Charlop-Christy et al., 2008). To address these problems, behavioral treatment programs that focused on teaching behaviors in the natural environment using natural contingencies were developed: pivotal response training (e.g., Koegel et al., 1989); incidental teaching (McGee, Krantz, & McClannahan, 1985); milieu training (Kaiser, Yoder, & Keetz, 1992); and modified incidental teaching sessions (Charlop-Christy, Carpenter, Le, LeBlanc, & Kellet, 2002). These programs are reported to have good generalization of treatment effects, and they are described as more likely to be used by parents and others in naturally occurring situations (Charlop-Christy et al., 2008).

Behavioral treatment methods, including modeling and imitation learning, have also been used as methods to teach primary social skills, such as eye contact, attention, and response to the immediate environment, as well as more complex social skills, including play, verbally based social behaviors, and perspective taking (including theory of mind activities). For example, Strain and his associates (e.g., Odom, Hoyson, Jamieson, & Strain, 1985; Odom & Strain, 1984; Strain, Ken, & Ragland, 1979) integrated autistic and nonautistic peers in a naturalistic setting, with the socially competent children acting as peer models in initiating and carrying out social interactions. Laushey and Helfin (2000) created a class-wide buddy system wherein several students were assigned to support the social interaction of peers with autism. Other social skill studies have used adults to model social interactions, used verbal prompts to initiate social interaction patterns, and used self-management and self-reinforcement procedures for developing social interaction (e.g., Koegel & Frea, 1993; Krantz, MacDuff, & McClannahan, 1993).

Behavioral treatment methods have also been used to teach communication skills to children diagnosed with ASD. It has been estimated that approximately 50% of children diagnosed with ASD are nonverbal or have limited verbal skills, and many children with ASD have receptive and/or expressive language deficits (Rimland, 1964). Behavioral programs for teaching language to these children have included both verbal language and sign language training (e.g., Carr, 1979; Carr, Kologinsky, & Leff-Simon, 1987; Fay & Schuler, 1980; Lovaas, 1977). Most such programs focus primarily on the development of functional language, using positive reinforcement and shaping procedures for imitating the clinician's vocalizations. Language enhancement programs, such as natural language programming (NLP), have been developed to teach nonverbal children autism to talk (see, e.g., Koegel, O'Dell, & Koegel, 1987). Koegel et al. (1987) have reported higher rates of imitated verbalization, as well as greater generalization of verbalizations to other settings, with the use of NLP than with the more traditional forms of functional language training.

Behavioral procedures have also been used in augmentative communication programs for nonverbal individuals. For example, the *Picture Exchange Communication System* (PECS;

Bondy & Frost, 1994) uses behavioral methods to teach functional communication skills. Nonverbal individuals are reinforced for exchanging a picture of something they want (such as a glass of water or swinging on a swing) for the actual item or activity. Programs that use visually based communication systems and activity schedules have been found to promote language and decrease inappropriate behavior (Bondy & Frost, 1998, 2002; Charlop-Christy et al., 2002; Matson, Sevin, Box, Francis, & Sevin, 1993; Morrison, Sainato, Benchaaban, & Endo, 2002; Wood, Lasker, Siegel-Causey, Beukelman, & Ball, 1998). When compared with auditory presentation alone, visual strategies, such as picture icons, drawings, objects, and/ or written word, provide a more concrete way of presenting information, support, and/or instruction (Hodgdon, 1996; MacDuff, Krantz, & McClannahan, 1993; Pierce & Schreibman, 1994). Charlop-Christy et al. (2008) have noted that children diagnosed with ASD are more likely to be responsive to visual, as opposed to auditory, cues in their environment.

Charlop-Christy et al. (2008) have also noted that difficulties in the use of positive reinforcement programs with children with ASD may arise because the children may not be motivated to learn the behaviors or skills being taught. In addition, it may be difficult to identify salient reinforcers (or any reinforcers other than food, liquids, and the avoidance of pain). In this regard, they report that some researchers have used internal reinforcers (e.g., opportunities to engage in self-stimulatory behaviors), which are commonly seen as problematic behaviors when teaching new skills (e.g., Charlop, Kurtz, & Casey, 1990).

Programs for treating behavior problems have traditionally used extinction, as well as such positive reinforcement techniques as DRO and DRI (Odom et al., 2003). Many programs for treating problem behaviors incorporate a functional analysis, or "functional behavior assessment" prior to the start of treatment in order to determine the frequency, antecedents, and consequences of variables in the environment that are maintaining the behavior, and so that an appropriate replacement behavior can be identified (e.g., Dunlap & Fox, 1999; Durand & Carr, 1991; Horner & Day, 1991, Keen, Sigafoos, & Woodyatt, 2001). As noted earlier, the use of functional behavior assessment in developing a behavior program is consistent with the use of positive behavioral support (Matson et al., 2008).

Charlop-Christy et al. (2008) have noted that many functional analyses of maladaptive behaviors of children diagnosed with ASD result in the problem behavior falling into one of three groups: attention-motivated behavior, escape-motivated behavior, and sensory reinforcement-motivated behavior (automatic reinforcement). Developing a behavior plan to address these behaviors may be especially difficult as the functions of a behavior may change during a given activity or period of time and some behaviors have multiple or unclear functions (LaBelle & Charlop-Christy, 2003).

Behavioral principles, including charting and reinforcement, have been incorporated into comprehensive curriculums for individuals with autism, such as the Treatment and Education of Autistic and related Communication-Handicapped Children (TEACCH) program developed at the University of North Carolina. This structured teaching program is heavily grounded in controlling the environment and providing routine. It uses visual strategies as part of the program (Schopler, Mesibov, & Hearsey, 1995).

There are many firsthand accounts by individuals diagnosed with autism, Asperger's syndrome, or other ASD, noting difficulties with multichannel receptivity and processing (e.g., Grandin, 1986; Stehli, 1992; Williams, 1992). Treatment procedures addressing hyper- and hyporeactivity to sensory stimulation, as well as problems with distortion of sensory input, have been reported in the literature. Perhaps, the best known and most widely used of these procedures is sensory integration therapy (Ayers, 1972, 1979). This treatment focuses primarily on three senses: tactile (i.e., touch), vestibular (i.e., motion and balance), and proprioception (i.e., joints and ligaments). Although numerous anecdotal reports emphasize the beneficial effects of sensory integration therapy, empirical reviews of its efficacy do not document reliable treatment effects for any specific patient population (see, e.g., Dawson & Wathing, 2000; Reilly, Nelson, & Bundy, 1983; Shaw, 2002; Smith, Mruzek, & Mozingo, 2005). In 2003, Miller argued that the lack of empirical documentation supporting the use of sensory integration therapy was the result of (1) the absence of controlled experimental studies of sensory integration treatments, (2) problems in developing measures to reliably and accurately assess the physiologic and behavioral manifestations of sensory processing impairments, and (3) difficulties in reaching conclusions based on studies that use different subject populations and different treatment protocols. Despite these problems, sensory integrative therapy continues to be popular. Pennington (2009) has speculated that the continued use of this therapy may be due, in part, to the proprietary interest of professional practitioners, namely, occupational therapists.

Specific treatment programs have also been developed to address problems in hypo- and hypersensitivity to auditory and visual stimuli as well as problems with sound discrimination and visual attention. Many auditory interventions, such as Berard's Auditory Integration Training (Berard, 1993) and the Tomatis method, focus on reducing oversensitivity to sound and involve repeated listening to a variety of different sound frequencies coordinated to the person's level of impairment. Recent reviews of auditory integration programs note that there is no clear evidence that these auditory programs address the symptoms of ASDs, nor is there evidence that they cause or reverse autism (see, e.g., American Speech-Language Hearing Association (ASHA), 2004; Dawson & Wathing, 2000; Gravel, 1994). In 1998, the American Academy of Pediatrics issued a statement cautioning against its use of auditory interventions as a treatment for autism.

The most commonly used programs for the treatment of sensitivity to visual stimuli are vision training programs and the use of colored lenses (Irlen lenses) to minimize print distortions when reading. There is no empirical research documenting the efficacy of vision training programs for individuals with ASD or with any other developmental disorder (Pennington, 2009).

PSYCHOLOGICAL AND VOCATIONAL IMPLICATIONS

As a result of the deinstitutionalization and normalization movements that began in the late 1960s and early 1970s, as well as the research advances in behavior modification treatment, many individuals with developmental disabilities are living in group homes, semi-independent apartments/homes, or independent living residences rather than in institutional settings. Although this situation certainly reflects the advances that have taken place over the past 25–30 years in implementing intervention methods that address various social, emotional, academic, and behavior problems found in some people having a developmental disability, certain issues continue to be present in the field, including peoples' living conditions, activity status, and their perceptions of their quality of life and level of productivity (e.g., Migliore & Butterworth, 2008; Salkever, 2000). In addition, issues remain involving the maximization of treatment gains through the generalization of behaviors that have been modified or successfully developed in these individuals. Such generalization involves transferring the acquired behaviors to a variety of settings in the person's natural environments (stimulus generalization) and in the maintenance of the person's treatment gains over time (temporal generalization) (see, e.g., Brown et al., 1986; Cole & Gardner, 1993; Hammel, Lai, & Heller, 2002; Lovaas & Buch, 1992; Luftig & Muthert, 2005; Matson et al., 2008; Smith, Parker, Taubman, & Lovaas, 1992).

These issues have significant implications when assessing the long-term success of both the psychological and vocational aspects of a person's intervention and habilitation plans (see, e.g., Handen, 2007; Luce, Christian, Anderson, Troy, & Larsson, 1992; Matson & Coe, 1992; Matson et al., 2008; Perel, 1992; Wacker & Berg, 1988; Wetzel, 1992). Future research needs to continue to address these areas to further assist people having a developmental disability in moving forward socially, educationally, emotionally, and vocationally in order for them to be able to lead meaningful, fulfilling, and productive adult lives with as much independence and personal satisfaction as possible.

REFERENCES

Alberto, P., Heflin, L. J., & Andrews, D. (2002). Use of the timeout ribbon procedure during community-based instruction. *Behavior Modification, 26*, 297–312.

Allen, G., & Courchesne, E. (2003). Differential effects of developmental cerebellar abnormality on cognitive and motor functions in the cerebellum: An fMRI study of autism. *American Journal of Psychiatry, 160*, 262–274.

Aman, M. G., & Singh, N. N. (1991). Pharmacological intervention. In I. L. Matson & I. A. Mulick (Eds.), *Handbook of mental retardation* (2nd ed., pp. 347–372). New York: Pergamon Press.

Amaral, D. S., Schumann, C. M., & Nordahl, C. W. (2008). Neuroanatomy of autism. *Trends in Neuroscience, 31*, 137–145.

American Academy of Pediatrics. (1998). Policy statement: Auditory integration training and facilitated communication for autism. *Pediatrics, 102*, 431–433.

American Association on Mental Retardation. (1992). *Mental retardation: Definition, classification, and systems of supports* (9th ed.). Washington, DC: Author.

American Psychiatric Association. (1968). *Diagnostic and statistical manual of mental disorders* (2nd ed.). Washington, DC: Author.

American Psychiatric Association. (1980). *Diagnostic and statistical manual of mental disorders* (3rd ed.). Washington, DC: Author.

American Psychiatric Association. (2000). *Diagnostic and statistical manual of mental disorders* (4th ed., Text Revision). Washington, DC: Author.

American Psychological Association. (1994). *Resolution on facilitated communication by the Council of Representatives of the American Psychological Association.* Los Angeles, CA: Author.

American Speech-Language Hearing Association (ASHA). (2004). *Auditory integration training* [Technical Report]. Retrieved from www.asha.org/docs/html/TR2004-00260.

Amir, R. E., Ignatia, B., Van den Veyver, I. B., Wan, M., Tran, C. Q., Francke, U., et al. (1999). Rett syndrome is caused by mutations in X-linked MECP2 encoding methyl-CpG-binding protein 2. *Nature Genetics, 23*, 185–188.

Anderson, G. M., Gutkecht, L., Cohen, D. J., Brailly-Tabard, S., Cohen, J. H. M., Ferrari, P., et al. (2002). Serotonin transporter and promoter variants in autism: Functional effects and relationship to platelet hyperserotonemia. *Molecular Psychiatry, 7*, 831–836.

Anderson, G. M., Horne, W. C., Chatterjee, D., & Cohen, D. J. (1990). The hyperserotonemia of autism. *Annals of the New York Academy of Science, 600*, 331–342.

Attwood, T. (1998). *Asperger's syndrome: A guide for parents and professionals.* London: Jessica Kingsley.

Autism Genetic Resource Exchange. (2009). *Autism speaks.* Retrieved from www.agre.org/index.cfm.

Auyeung, B., Baron-Cohen, S., Ashwin, E., Knickmeyer, R., Taylor, K., & Hackett, G. (2009). Fetal testosterone and autistic traits. *British Journal of Psychiatry, 100*, 1–22.

Ayers, A. J. (1972). *Sensory integration and learning disorders.* Los Angeles: Western Psychological Associates.

Ayers, A. J. (1979). *Sensory integration and the child.* Los Angeles: Western Psychological Associates.

Ayllon, T., & Azrin, N. H. (1968). *The token economy: A motivational system for therapy and rehabilitation.* New York: Appleton-Century-Crofts.

Baer, D. M., Wolf, M., & Risley, T. R. (1968). Some current dimensions of applied behavior analysis. *Journal of Applied Behavior Analysis, 1*, 91–97.

Bandura, A. (1969). *Principles of behavior modification.* New York: Holt.

Bandura, A., & Walters, R. H. (1963). *Social learning and personality development.* New York: Holt.

Baraitser, M., & Winter, R. M. (1996). *Color atlas of congenital malformations.* London: Mosby-Wolfe.

Baron-Cohen, S. (2002). The extreme male brain theory of autism. *Trends in Cognitive Sciences, 6*, 248–254.

Baumeister, A. A. (1970). The American residential institution: Its history and character. In A. A. Baumeister & E. Butterfield (Eds.), *Residential facilities for the mentally retarded* (pp. 1–28). Chicago: Aldine.

Berard, G. (1993). *Hearing equals behavior.* New Canaan, CT: Keats.

Bertrand, J., Mars, A., Boyle, C., Bove, F., Yeargin-Allsopp, M., & Decoufle, P. (2001). Prevalence of autism in a United States population: The Brick Township, New Jersey investigation. *Pediatrics, 108*, 1155–1161.

Bettelheim, B. (1950). *Love is not enough.* Glencoe, IL: Free Press.

Bettelheim, B. (1967). *The empty fortress.* New York: Free Press.

Bettelheim, B. (1974). *A home for the heart.* New York: Knopf.

Bielecki, J., & Swender, S. L. (2004). The assessment of social functioning in individuals with mental retardation: A review. *Behavior Modification, 28,* 694–708.

Bienvenu, T., Carrié, A., de Roux, N., Vinet, M., Jonveaux, P., Couvery, P. V., et al. (2000). MECP2 mutations account for most atypical forms of Rett syndrome. *Human Molecular Genetics, 9,* 1377–1384.

Blackman, J. A. (Ed.). (1983). *Medical aspects of developmental disabilities in children birth to three.* Iowa City, IA: University of Iowa.

Blatt, B. (1968). The dark side of the mirror. *Mental Retardation, 6,* 42–44.

Blatt, B. (1984). Biography in autobiography. In B. Blatt & R. J. Morris (Eds.), *Perspectives in special education: Personal orientations* (pp. 263–307). Glenview, IL: Scott, Foresman.

Blatt, B., & Kaplan, F. (1966). *Christmas in purgatory: A photographic essay on mental retardation.* Boston: Allyn & Bacon.

Bondy, A., & Frost, L. (1998). The picture exchange communication system. *Topics in Language Disorders, 19,* 373–390.

Bondy, A., & Frost, L. (2002). *A picture's worth: PECS and other visual communication strategies in autism.* Bethesda, MD: Woodbine House.

Bondy, A., & Frost. L. (1994). The Delaware autistic program. In S. L. Harris & J. S. Handleman (Eds.), *Preschool education for children with autism* (pp. 37–54). Austin, TX: PRO-ED.

Boyle, C. A., Yeargin-Allsopp, M., Doernberg, N. S., Holmgreen, P., Murphy, C. C., & Schendel, D. E. (1996). Prevalence of selected developmental disabilities in children 3-10 years of age: The Metropolitan Atlanta Developmental Disabilities Surveillance Program, 1991. *MMWR Morbidity and Mortality Weekly Report Surveillance Summaries, 45,* 1–14.

Brambilla, P., Hardan, A., Ucelli di Nemi, S., Perez, J., Soares, J. C., & Barale, F. (2003). Brain anatomy and development in autism: Review of structural MRI studies. *Brain Research Bulletin, 61,* 557–570.

Brison, D. W. (1967). Definition, diagnosis, and classification. In A. A. Baumeister (Ed.), *Mental retardation* (pp. 1–19). Chicago: Aldine.

Brown, L., Shiraga, B., Ford, J. R., Nisbet, J., VanDeventer, P., Sweet, M., et al. (1986). Teaching severely handicapped students to perform meaningful work in nonsheltered vocational environments. In R. J. Morris & B. Blatt (Eds.), *Special education: Research and trends* (pp. 131–189). New York: Pergamon Press.

Buitelaar, J. K., & Willemsen-Swinkels, S. H. N. (2000). Medication treatment in subjects with autsitic spectrum disorders. *European Child & Adolescent Psychiatry, 9,* 85–97.

Carr, E. G. (1979). Teaching autistic children to use sign language: Some research issues. *Journal of Autism and Developmental Disorders, 9,* 345–359.

Carr, E. G., Horner, R. H., Turnbill, A. P., Marquis, J. G., McLaughlin, D. M., McAree, M. L., et al. (1999). *Positive behavior support as an approach for dealing with problem behavior in people with developmental disabilities.* Washington, DC: American Association on Mental Retardation.

Carr, E. G., Kologinsky, E., & Leff-Simon, S. (1987). Acquisition of sign language by autistic children: 3. Generalized descriptive phases. *Journal of Autism and Developmental Disorders, 17,* 217–229.

Carr, E. G., Turnbull, A. P., & Horner, R. H. (1999). *Positive behavior support in people with developmental disabilities: A research synthesis.* Washington, DC: AAMR.

Center for Disease Control and Prevention Autism and Developmental Disabilities Monitoring Network. (2007). Prevalence of autism spectrum disorders. *Center for Disease Control and Prevention Surveillance Summaries, 56*(SS04), 12–18. Retrieved from www.cdc.gov/mmwr/preview/mmwrhtml/SS5601a2.htm

Chakrabarti, S., & Fombonne, E. (2001). Pervasive developmental disorders in preschool children. *Journal of the American Medical Association, 285,* 3093–3099.

Chakrabarti, S., & Fombonne, E. (2005). Pervasive developmental disorders in preschool children: Confirmation of high prevalence. *American Journal of Psychiatry, 162,* 1133–1141.

Charlop, M. H., Kurtz, P. F., & Casey, F. G. (1990). Using aberrant behaviors as reinforcers for autistic children. *Journal of Applied Behavior Analysis, 22,* 275–285.

Charlop-Christy, M. H., Carpenter, M., Le, L., LeBlanc, L. A., & Kellet, K. (2002). Using the picture exchange communication system (PECS) with children with autism: Assessment of PECS acquisition, speech, social-communicative behavior, and problem behavior. *Journal of Applied Behavioral Analysis, 35,* 213–231.

Charlop-Christy, M. H., Malmberg, D. B., Rocha, M. L., & Schreibman, L. (2008). Treating autistic spectrum disorder. In R. J. Morris & T. R. Kratochwill (Eds.), *The practice of child therapy* (3rd ed., pp. 299–335). New York: Lawrence Erlbaum & Associates.

Charman, T. (2002). The prevalence of autism spectrum disorders: Recent evidence and future challenges. *European Child and Adolescent Psychiatry, 11,* 249–256.

Cole, C. L., & Gardner, W. I. (1993). Psychotherapy with developmentally delayed children. In T. R. Kratochwill & R. J. Morris (Eds.), *Handbook of psychotherapy with children and adolescents* (pp. 426–471). Boston: Allyn & Bacon.

Conyers, C., Martin, T. L., Martin, G. L., & Yu, D. (2002). The 1983 AAMR Manual, the 1992 Manual, or the Developmental Disabilities Act: Which do researchers use? *Education and Training in Mental Retardation and developmental Disabilities, 37,* 310–316.

Cook, E. H. J., Leventhal, B. L., Heller, W., Metz, J., Wainwright, M., & Freedman, D. X. (1990). Autistic children and their first-degree relatives: Relationships between serotonin and norepinephrine levels and intelligence. *Journal of Neuropsychiatry and Clinical Neuroscience, 2,* 268–274.

Coulter, D. L. (1991). Theoretical basis of the definition. In R. Luckasson (Ed.), *Classification in mental retardation: Draft-1991.* Washington, DC: American Association on Mental Retardation.

Courchesne, E. (1989). Neuroanatomical systems involved in infantile autism: The implications of cerebellar abnormalities. In G. Dawson (Ed.), *Autism: New perspectives on diagnosis, nature, and treatment* (pp. 119–143). New York: Guilford Press.

Courchesne, E., Carper, R., & Akshoomoff, N. (2003). Evidence of brain overgrowth in the first year of life in autism. *Journal of the American Medical Association, 290,* 337–345.

Courchesne, E., Saitho, O., Yeung-Courchesne, R., Press, G. A., Lincoln, A. J., Haas, R. H. et al. (1994). Abnormality of cerebellar vermian lobules VI and VII in patients with infantile autism: Identification of hypoplastic and hyperplastic subgroups by MR imaging. *American Journal of Roentgenology, 162,* 123–130.

Cowen, E. (1963). Psychotherapy and play techniques with the exceptional child and youth. In W. M. Cruickshank (Ed.), *Psychology of exceptional children and youth* (2nd ed., pp. 526–592). Englewood Cliffs, NJ: Prentice-Hall.

Croen, L. A., Grether, J. K., Hoogstrate, J., & Selvin, S. (2002). The changing prevalence of autism in California. *Journal of Autism and Developmental Disorders, 32,* 207–215.

Curry, C. J., Stevenson, R. E., Aughton, D., Byrne, J., Carey, J. C., Cassidy, S., et al. (1997). Evaluation of mental retardation: Recommendations of a consensus conference. *American Journal of Medical Genetics, 72,* 468–477.

Daily, D. K., Ardinger, H. H., & Holmes, G. E. (2000). Identification and evaluation of mental retardation. *American Family Physician, 61,* 1059–1065.

Dawson, G., & Osterling, J. (1997). Early intervention in autism: Effectiveness and common elements of current approaches. In M. J. Guralnick (Ed.), *The effectiveness of early intervention* (pp. 307–325). Baltimore: Brookes.

Dawson, G., & Wathing, R. (2000). Intervention to facilitate auditory, visual, and motor integration in autism: A review of the evidence. *Journal of Developmental Disabilities, 30,* 415–421.

Dawson, G., Munson, J., Webb, S. J., Abbott, R., Toth, K., & Nalty, T. (2007). Rate of head growth decelerates and symptoms worsen in the second year of life in autism. *Biological Psychiatry, 61,* 458–464.

Developmental Disabilities Act. (1984). Washington, DC: U.S. Government Printing Office.

Developmental Disabilities Assistance and Bill of Rights Act (PL 106-402). (2000). Washington, DC: U.S. Government Printing Office.

Duker, P. C., Welles, K., Seys, D., Rensen, H., Vis, A., & van der Berg, G. (1991). Brief report: Effects of fenfluramine on communicative, stereotypic and inappropriate behaviors of autistic-type mentally handicapped individuals. *Journal of Autism and Developmental Disorders, 21,* 355–363.

Dunlap, G., & Fox, L. (1999). A demonstration of behavioral support for young children with autism. *Journal of Positive Behavior Interventions, 1,* 77–87.

Durand, V. M., & Carr, E. G. (1991). Functional communication training to reduce challenging behavior: Maintenance and application in new settings. *Journal of Applied Behavior Analysis, 25,* 251–264.

Ehlers, W. H., Prothero, J. C., & Langone, J. (1982). *Mental retardation and other developmental disabilities* (3rd ed.). Columbus, OH: Merrill.

Eisenmajer, R., Prior, M., Leekham, S., Wing, L., Gould, J., Welham, M., et al. (1996). Comparison of clinical symptoms in autism and Asperger's disorder. *Journal of the Academy of Child & Adolescent Psychiatry, 35,* 1523–1531.

Ekman, G., Miranda-Linne, F., Gillberg, C., & Garle, M. (1989). Fenfluramine treatment of 20 children with autism. *Journal of Autism and Developmental Disabilities, 19,* 511–532.

Fay, W. H., & Schuler, A. L. (1980). *Emerging language in autistic children.* Baltimore: University Park Press.

Ferretti, R. P., Cavalier, A. R., Murphy, M. J., & Murphy, R. (1993). The self-management of skills by persons with mental retardation. *Research in Developmental Disabilities, 14,* 189–206.

Fombonne, E. (2002). Prevalence of childhood disintegrative disorder. *Autism, 6,* 149–157.

Fombonne, E. (2003a). Editorial. *Journal of the American Medical Association, 289,* 49.

Fombonne, E. (2003b). Epidemiological surveys of autism and other pervasive developmental disorders: An update. *Journal of Autism and Developmental Disorders, 33,* 365–382.

Fombonne, E., Simmons, H., Ford, T., Meltzer, H., & Goodman, R. (2001). Prevalence of pervasive developmental disorders in the British nationwide survey of child mental health. *Journal of the American Academy of Child and Adolescent Psychiatry, 40,* 820–827.

Freeman, B. J., & Ritvo, E. R. (1984). The syndrome of autism: Establishing the diagnosis and principles of management. *Pediatric Analysis, 13,* 284–305.

Friedman, P. (1975). *The rights of the mentally retarded.* New York: Avon.

Frith, U. (1991). Asperger and his syndrome. In U. Frith (Ed.), *Autism and Asperger syndrome* (pp. 1–36). Cambridge, MA: Cambridge University.

Gardner, W. I. (1970). *Behavior modification in mental retardation.* Chicago: Aldine.

Gardner, W. I. (1971). *Behavior modification: Applications in mental retardation.* Chicago: Aldine.

Gillberg, C. (1999). Neurodevelopmental processes and psychological functioning in autism. *Development and Psychopathology, 11,* 567–587.

Goldfried, M. R., & Merbaum, M. A. (1973). A perspective on self-control. In M. R. Goldfried & M. Merbaum (Eds.), *Behavior change through self-control* (pp. 127–143). New York: Holt.

Gorlin, R. J., Cohen, M. M., & Hennekam, R. C. M. (2001). *Syndromes of the head and neck* (4th ed.). Oxford, England: Oxford University Press.

Grandin, T. (1986). *Emergence: Labeled autistic.* Novato, CA: Academic Therapy.

Gravel, J. S. (1994). Auditory integrative training: Placing the burden of proof. *American Journal of Speech and Language Pathology, 3,* 25–29.

Gresham, F. M., MacMillan, D. L., & Siperstein, G. N. (1995). Critical analysis of the 1992 AAMR definition: Implications for school psychology. *School Psychology Review, 10,* 1–19.

Grossman, H. J. (Ed.). (1973). *Manual on terminology and classification in mental retardation.* Washington, DC: American Association on Mental Deficiency.

Grossman, H. J. (Ed.). (1983). *Classification in mental retardation.* Washington, DC: American Association on Mental Deficiency.

Gullone, E., King, N. J., & Cummins, R. A. (1996). Fears of youth with mental retardation: Psychometric evaluation of the Fear Survey Schedule for Children-II (FSSC-II). *Research in Developmental Disabilities, 17,* 269–284.

Gupta, A., & State, M. (2007). Recent advances in the genetics of autism. *Biological Psychiatry, 61,* 429–437.

Haas, R. H., Townsend, J., Courchesne, E., Lincoln, A. J., Schreibman, L., & Yeung Courchesne, R. (1996). Neurologic abnormalities in infantile autism. *Journal of Child Neurology, 11,* 84–92.

Hagberg, B. (2002). Clinical manifestations and stages of Rett syndrome. *Mental Retardation and Developmental Disabilities Research Review, 8,* 61–65.

Hagberg, B., Aicardi, J., Dias, K., & Ramos, O. (1983). A progressive syndrome of autism, dementia, ataxia, and loss of purposeful hand use in girls. Rett's syndrome: Report of 35 cases. *Annals of Neurology, 14,* 471–479.

Halderman v. Pennhurst, 446 F. Supp. 1295 (1977).

Hammel, J., Lai, J.-S., & Heller, T. (2002). The impact of assistive technology and environmental interventions on function and living situation status with people who are ageing with developmental disabilities. *Disability and Rehabilitation, 24,* 93–105.

Handen, B. L. (2007). Intellectual disability (mental retardation). In E. J. Mash & R. A. Barkley (Eds.), *Assessment of childhood disorders* (4th ed., pp. 551–597). New York: Guilford Press.

Harris, S. L. (1988). Autism and schizophrenia: Psychological therapies. In J. L. Matson (Ed.), *Handbook of treatment approaches in childhood psychopathology* (pp. 289–300). New York: Plenum.

Heber, R. F. (1959). A manual on terminology and classification in mental retardation. *American Journal on Mental Deficiency, 64*(Monograph Supp) 1–111.

Heber, R. F. (1961). Modifications in the manual on terminology and classification in mental retardation. *American Journal on Mental Deficiency, 65,* 499–500.

Hendry, C. N. (2000). Childhood disintegrative disorder: Should it be considered a distinct diagnosis? *Clinical Psychology Review, 2,* 77–90.

Hodapp, R. M. (1995). Definitions in mental retardation: Effects on research, practice, and perceptions. *School Psychology Review, 10,* 24–28.

Hodgdon, L. A. (1996). *Visual strategies for improving communication.* Troy, MI: Qirk Roberts.

Horner, R. H., & Day, H. M. (1991). The effects of response efficiency on functionally equivalent competing behaviors. *Journal of Applied Behavior Analysis, 24,* 719–732.

Humphrey, G. (1962). Introduction. In J. M. C. Itard (Ed.), *The wild boy of Aveyron* (G. Humphrey & H. Humphrey, Trans.). New York: Appleton-Century-Crofts.

Hviid, A., Stellfeld, M., Wohlfahrt, J., & Melbye, M. (2003). Association between thimerosal-containing vaccine and autism. *Journal of the American Medical Association, 290,* 1763–1766.

Individuals with Disabilities Education Improvement Act. (2004). Public Law 108-446. 118 Stat. 2647.

Itard, J. M. C. (1962). *The wild boy of Aveyron* (G. Humphrey & H. Humphrey, Trans.). New York: Appleton-Century-Crofts.

Jones, K. L. (1997). *Smith's recognizable patterns of human malformations* (5th ed.). Philadelphia: W.B. Saunders.

Kaiser, A. P., Yoder, P. J., & Keetz, A. (1992). Evaluation milieu training. In S. F. Warren & J. Reichle (Eds.), *Causes and effects in communication and language intervention* (pp. 9–47). Baltimore: Brookes.

Kanfer, F. H. (1980). Self-management methods. In F. H. Kanfer & A. P. Goldstein (Eds.), *Helping people change* (2nd ed., pp. 334–389). New York: Pergamon Press.

Kanner, L. (1943). Autistic disturbances of affective contact. *Nervous Child, 2,* 217–250.

Kanner, L. (1948). *Child psychiatry.* Springfield, IL: Charles C Thomas.

Kanner, L. (1964). *A history of the care and study of the mentally retarded.* Springfield, IL: Charles C Thomas.

Karoly, P., & Kanfer, F. H. (Eds.). (1982). *Self-management and behavior change: From theory to practice.* New York: Pergamon Press.

Kazdin, A. E. (1975). *Behavior modification in applied settings.* Homewood, IL: Dorsey.

Kazdin, A. E. (2001). *Behavior modification in applied settings* (6th ed.). New York: Wadsworth.

Keen, D., Sigafoos, J., & Woodyatt, G. (2001). Replacing prelinguistic behaviors with functional communication. *Journal of Autism and Developmental Disabilities, 22,* 407–423.

Koegel, R. L., & Frea, W. D. (1993). Treatment of social behavior in autism through the modification of pivotal skills. *Journal of Applied Behavior Analysis, 26,* 369–377.

Koegel, R. L., O'Dell, M. C., & Koegel, L. K. (1987). A natural language teaching package for nonverbal autistic children. *Journal of Autism and Developmental Disorders, 17,* 187–200.

Koegel, R. L., Schreibman, L., Good, A., Cerniglia, L., Murphy, C., & Koegel, L. K. (1989). *How to teach pivotal behavior to children with autism: A training manual.* Santa Barbara, CA: University of California.

Krantz, P. J., MacDuff, M. T., & Mc Clannahan, L. E. (1993). Teaching children with autism to initiate to peers: Effects of a script fading procedure. *Journal of Applied Behavior Analysis, 26,* 121–132.

LaBelle, C. A., & Charlop-Christy, M. H. (2003). Using analog functional analysis to assess changing functions in the problem behaviors of children with autism. *Journal of Positive Behaviors, 5,* 202–211.

Laushey, K. M., & Heflin, L. J. (2000). Enhancing the social skills of kindergarten children with autism through the training of multiple peers as tutors. *Journal of Autism and Developmental Disabilities, 30,* 183–193.

Lee, J. K., Larson, S. A., Lakin, K. C., Anderson, L., Lee, N. K., & Anderson, D. (2001). Prevalence of mental retardation and developmental disabilities: Estimates from the 1994/1995 national health interview survey disability supplements. *American Journal on Mental Retardation, 106,* 231–252.

Leland, H. (1991). Adaptive behavior scales. In J. L. Matson & J. A. Mulick (Eds.), *Handbook of mental retardation* (pp. 234–251). New York: Pergamon Press.

Lewis, F. M., Murdoch, B. E., & Woodyatt, G. C. (2007). Linguistic abilities in children with autism spectrum disorder. *Research in Autism Spectrum Disorders, 1,* 85–100.

Leyfer, O. T., Folstein, S. E., Bacalman, S., Davis, N. O., Dinh, E., Morgan, J., et al. (2006). Comorbid psychiatric disorders in children with autism: Interview development and rates of disorders. *Journal of Autism and Developmental Disorders, 36,* 849–861.

Liaupsin, C. J., & Scott, T. M. (2008). Disruptive behavior. In R. J. Morris & N. Mather (Eds.), *Evidence-based interventions for students with learning and behavioral challenges.* New York: Routledge.

Liu, X., Hubbard, J. A., Faber, R. A., & Adams, J. B. (2006) Sleep disturbances and correlates of children with autism spectrum disorder. *Child Psychiatry and Human Development, 27,* 179–191.

Lloyd, K. W., Hallahan, D. P., Kauffman, J. M., & Keller, C. E. (1998). Academic problems. In R. J. Morris & T. R. Kratochwill (Eds.), *The practice of child therapy* (3rd ed., pp. 167–198). Needham Heights, MA: Allyn & Bacon.

Losh, M., Adolphs, R., Poe, M. D., Couture, S., Penn, D., Baranek, G. T., et al. (2009). Neuropsychological profile in autism and the broad autism profile. *Archives of General Psychiatry, 66*, 518–526.

Lovaas, O. I. (1977). *The autistic child*. New York: Irvington.

Lovaas, O. I. (1987). Behavioral treatment and normal education and intellectual functioning in young autistic children. *Journal of Consulting and Clinical Psychology, 55*, 3–9.

Lovaas, O. I., & Buch, G. (1992). Editor's introduction. *Research in Developmental Disabilities, 13*, 1–8.

Lovaas, O. I., & Bucher, B. D. (Eds.). (1974). *Perspectives in behavior modification with deviant children*. Englewood Cliffs, NJ: Prentice-Hall.

Lovaas, O. I., Berberich, J. P., Perloff, B. F., & Schaeffer, B. (1966). Acquisition of imitative speech by schizophrenic children. *Science, 151*, 705–707.

Lovaas, O. I. (2003). *Teaching individuals with developmental delays*. Austin, TX: Pro-Ed.

Luce, S. C., Christian, W. P., Anderson, S. R., Troy, P. J., & Larsson, E. V. (1992). Development of a continuum of services for children and adults with autism and other severe behavior disorders. *Research in Developmental Disabilities, 13*, 9–25.

Luckasson, R., Borthwick-Duffy, S., Buntinx, W. H. E., Coulter, D. L., Craig, E. M., Reeve, A., et al. (2002). *Mental retardation: Definition, classification, and systems of supports* (10th ed.). Washington, DC: AAMR.

Luftig, R. L., & Muthert, D. (2005). Patterns of employment and independent living of adult graduates with learning disabilities and mental retardation of an inclusionary high school vocational program. *Research in Developmental Disabilities, 26*, 317–325.

MacDuff, G. S., Krantz, P. J., & McClannahan, L. E. (1993). Teaching children with autism to use photographic activity sheets: Maintenance and generalization of complex response chains. *Journal of Applied Behavior Analysis, 26*, 89–97.

MacMillan, D. L. (1982). *Mental retardation in school and society*. Boston: Little, Brown.

MacMillan, D. L., Gresham, F. M., & Siperstein, G. N. (1993). Conceptual and psychometric concerns about the 1992 AAMR definition of mental retardation. *American Journal on Mental Retardation, 98*, 325–335.

Madsen, K. M., Hviid, A., Vestergaard, M., Schendel, D., Wohlfahrt, J., Thorsen, P., et al. (2002). A population-based study of measles, mumps, and rubella vaccination in autism. *New England Journal of Medicine, 347*, 1477–1482.

Mahoney, W., Statmari, O., MacLean, J. E., Bryson, S. E., Bartolucci, G., Walter, S. D., et al. (2001). Reliability and accuracy of differentiating pervasive developmental disorder subtypes. *Journal of the American Academy of Child and Adolescent Psychiatry, 40*, 820–827.

Mash, E. J., & Wolfe, D. A. (1999). *Abnormal child psychology*. New York: Wiley.

Matson, J. L. (1995). Comments on Gresham, MacMillan, and Siperstein's paper "Critical Analysis of the 1992 AAMR Definition: Implications for School Psychology." *School Psychology Review, 10*, 20–23.

Matson, J. L., & Coe, D. A. (1992). Applied behavior analysis: Its impact on the treatment on mentally retarded emotionally disturbed people. *Research in Developmental Disabilities, 13*, 171–187.

Matson, J. L., & McCartney, J. R. (Eds.). (1981). *Handbook of behavior modification with the mental retarded*. New York: Plenum.

Matson, J. L., & Wilkins, J. (2008). Nosology and diagnosis of Asperger's syndrome. *Research in Autism Spectrum Disorders, 2*, 228–300.

Matson, J. L., Laud, R. B., & Matson, M. L. (Eds.). (2004). *Behavior modification for persons with developmental disabilities: Treatments and supports*. Kingston, NY: NADD Press.

Matson, J. L., Sevin, J. A., Box, M. L., Francis, K. L., & Sevin, B. M. (1993). An evaluation of two methods for increasing self-initiated verbalizations in autistic children. *Journal of Applied Behavior Analysis, 26*, 389–398.

Matson, J. L., Terlonge, C., & Minshawi, N. F. (2008). Children with intellectual disabilities. In R. J. Morris & T. R. Kratochwill (Eds.), *The practice of child therapy* (4th ed., pp. 337–361). New York: Lawrence Erlbaum & Associates.

McEachin, J. J., Smith, T., & Lovaas, I. O. (1993). Long term outcome for children with autism who received early intensive behavioral treatment. *American Journal of Mental Retardation, 97*, 359–372.

McGee, G. G., Krantz, P. J., & McClannahan, L. E. (1985). The facilitative effects of incidental teaching on preposition use by autistic children. *Journal of Applied Behavior Analysis, 18*, 17–31.

McLaren, J., & Bryson, S. E.(1987). Review of recent epidemiological studies of mental retardation: Prevalence, associated disorders and etiology. *American Journal of Mental Retardation, 92,* 243–254.

Meichenbaum, D., & Genest, M. (1980). Cognitive behavior modification: An integration of cognitive and behavioral methods. In F. H. Kanfer & A. P. Goldstein (Eds.), *Helping people change* (2nd ed., pp. 390–422). New York: Pergamon Press.

Migliore, A., & Butterworth, J. (2008). Trends in outcomes of the vocational rehabilitation program for adults with developmental disabilities. *Rehabilitation Counseling Bulletin, 52,* 35–44.

Miller, L. J. (2003). Empirical evidence related to therapies for sensory processing impairments. *National Association of School Psychologists Communique, 31*(5) 34–36.

Minderaa, R. B., Anderson, G. M., Volkmar, F. R., Harcherick, D., Akkerhuis, G. W., & Cohen, D. J. (1989). Whole blood serotonin and tryptophan in autism: Temporal stability and the effects of medication. *Journal of Autism and Developmental Disorders, 19,* 129–136.

Morris, R. J. (1976). *Behavior modification with children: A systematic guide.* Cambridge, MA: Winthrop.

Morris, R. J. (1985). *Behavior modification with exceptional children: Principles and practices.* Glenview, IL: Scott-Foresman.

Morris, R. J., & Kratochwill, T. R. (2008). Historical context of child therapy. In R. J. Morris & T. R. Kratochwill (Eds.), *The practice of child therapy* (4th ed., pp. 1–5). New York: Lawrence Erlbaum & Associates.

Morris, R. J., & McReynolds, R. A. (1986). Behavior modification with special needs children: A review. In R. J. Morris & B. Blatt (Eds.), *Special education: Research and trends* (pp. 66–130). New York: Pergamon Press.

Morrison, R. S., Sainato, D. M., Benchaaban, D., & Endo, S. (2002). Increasing play skills of children with autism using activity schedules and correspondence training. *Journal of Early Intervention, 25,* 58–72.

Mount, R. H., Hastings, R. P., Reilly, S., Cass, H., & Chjarman, T. (2003). Toward a behavioral phenotype for Rett syndrome. *American Journal on Mental Retardation, 108,* 1-12.

National Research Council. (2001). *Education children with autism.* Washington, DC: National Academy Press.

New York State Association for Retarded Children v. Rockefeller, 357 F. Supp. 752 (1973).

Newschaffer, C. J., Croen, L. A., Reaven, J., Reynolds, A. M., Rice, C. E., Schendel, D., et al. (2007). The epidemiology of autism spectrum disorders. *Annual Review of Public Health, 28,* 235–258.

Newschaffer, C. J., Falb, M. D., & Gurney, J. G. (2005). National autism prevalence trends from the United States special education data. *Pediatrics, 111,* 277–282.

Nirje, B. (1969). The normalization principle and its human management implications. In R. B. Kugel & W. Wolfensberaer (Eds.), *Changing patterns in residential services for the mentally retarded* (pp. 179–195). Washington, DC: President's Commission on Mental Retardation.

Odom, S. L., & Strain, P. S. (1984). Classroom based social skills instruction for severely handicapped preschool children. *Topics in Early Childhood Special Education, 4,* 97–116.

Odom, S. L., Brown, W. H., Frey, T., Karasu, N., Smith-Canter, L. L., & Strain, P. S. (2003). Evidence-based practices for young children with autism: Contributions for single-subject design research. *Focus on Autism and Other Developmental Disabilities, 18,* 166–175.

Odom, S. L., Hoyson, M., Jamieson, B., & Strain, P. S. (1985). Increasing handicapped preschoolers' peer social interactions: Cross-setting and component analysis. *Journal of Applied Behavior Analysis, 18,* 3–16.

Online Mendelian Inheritance in Man. (n.d.). Trademarked by Johns Hopkins University. Retrieved from http://www.ncbi.nlm.nih.gov/entrez/query.fcgi?db=OMIM.

Oswald, D. P., & Sonenklar, N. A. (2007). Medication use among children with autism spectrum disorders. *Journal of Child and Adolescent Psychopharmacology, 17,* 348-355.

Ozonoff, S., Goodlin-Jones, B. L., & Solomon, M. (2007). Autism spectrum disorders. In E. J. Mash & R. A. Barkley (Eds.) *Assessment of childhood disorders* (4th ed., pp. 487–525). New York: Guilford.

Pennington, B. F. (2009). *Diagnosing learning disorders* (2nd ed.). New York: Guilford.

Pennington, B. F., McGrath, L. M., & Peterson, R. L. (2009a). Intellectual disability. In B. F. Pennington (Ed.), *Diagnosing learning disorders* (2nd ed., pp. 181–226). New York: Guilford.

Pennington, B. F., McGrath, L. M., & Peterson, R. L. (2009b). Autism spectrum disorder. In B. F. Pennington (Ed.), *Diagnosing learning disorders* (2nd ed., pp. 108–151). New York: Guilford.

Pennsylvania Association for Retarded Children v. Commonwealth of Pennsylvania, 334 F. Supp. 1257 (1971).

Perel, I. (1992). Deinstitutionalization at a large facility: A focus on treatment. *Research in Developmental Disabilities, 13,* 81–86.

Perry, R., & Meiselas, K. (1988). Autism and schizophrenia: Pharmacotherapies. In J. L. Matson (Ed.), *Handbook of treatment approaches in childhood psychopathology* (pp. 301–325). New York: Plenum.

Peterson, F. M., & Martens, B. K. (1995). A comparison of behavioral interventions reported in treatment studies and programs for adults with developmental disabilities. *Research in Developmental Disabilities, 16,* 27–42.

Pierce, K. C., & Schreibman, L. (1994). Teaching daily living skills to children with autism in unsupervised settings through pictorial serf-management. *Journal of Applied Behavior Analysis, 27,* 471–481.

Rapin, I., & Katzman, R. (1998). Neurobiology of autism. *Annals of Neurology, 43,* 7–14.

Reilly, C., Nelson, D. L., & Bundy, A. C. (1983). Sensorimotor versus fine motor activities in eliciting vocalizations in autistic children. *The Occupational Therapy Journal of Research, 3,* 199–211.

Retrieved July 9, 2003, from http://search.epnet.com/direct.asp?an=3584132&db=aph.

Rimland, B. (1964). *Infantile autism.* New York: Appleton-Century-Crofts.

Rimm, D. C., & Masters, J. C. (1979). *Behavior therapy: Techniques and empirical findings.* New York: Academic Press.

Ritvo, E. R., Freeman, B. J., Mason-Brothers, A., Mo, A., & Ritvo, A. (1985). Concordance for one syndrome autism in 40 pairs of affected twins. *American Journal of Psychiatry, 142,* 64–77.

Ritvo, E. R., Spence, M. A., Freeman, B. J., Mason-Brothers, A., Mo, A., & Marzarita, M. L. (1985). Evidence of autosomal recessive inheritance in 46 families of multiple incidences of autism. *American Journal of Psychiatry, 142,* 187–192.

Ritvo, R. A., Ritvo, E. R., Guthrie, D., & Ritvo, M. J. (2008). Clinical evidence that Asperger's disorder is a mild form of autism. *Comprehensive Psychiatry, 49,* 1-5.

Rusch, F. R., McKee, M., Chadsey-Rausch, J., & Renzaglia, A. (1988). Teaching a student with severe handicaps to self-instruct: A brief report. *Education and Training of the Mentally Retarded, 23,* 51–58.

Safran, J. S. (2002). Supporting students with Asperger's syndrome in general education. *Teaching Exceptional Children, 34,* 60–66.

Safran, S. P. (2001). Asperger's syndrome: The emerging challenge to special education. *Exceptional Children, 67,* 151–160.

Salkever, D. S. (2000). Activity status, life satisfaction and perceived productivity for young adults with developmental disabilities. *Journal of Rehabilitation, 66,* 4–13.

Schaefer, H. H., & Martin, P. L. (1969). *Behavioral therapy.* NY: McGraw-Hill.

Scheerenberger, R. C. (1987). *A history of mental retardation.* Baltimore: Brookes.

Schopler, E. (1965). Early infantile autism and receptor processes. *Archives of General Psychiatry, 13,* 327–335.

Schopler, E. (1996). Are autism and Asperger's syndrome different labels or different disabilities? *Journal of Autism & Developmental Disabilities, 26,* 109–110.

Schopler, E., & Reichler, R. J. (1971). Psychobiological referents for the treatment of autism. In D. W. Churchill, G. P. Alpern, & M. K. DeMyer (Eds.), *Infantile autism* (pp. 327–335). Springfield, IL: Charles C. Thomas.

Schopler, E., Mesibov, G. B., & Hearsey, K. (1995). Structured teaching in the TEACCH system. In E. Schopler & G. B. Mesibov (Eds.), *Learning and cognition in autism* (pp. 243–268). New York: Plenum.

Shapiro, E. (1981). Self-control procedures with the mentally retarded. In M. Hersen, R. M. Eisler, & P. M. Miller (Eds.), *Progress in behavior modification* (Vol. 12, pp. 265–297). New York: Academic Press.

Shapiro, E. S. (1986). Behavior modification: Self-control and cognitive procedures. In R. P. Banett (Ed.), *Severe behavior disorders in the mentally retarded* (pp. 259–276). New York: Plenum.

Shaw, S. R. (2002, October). A school psychologist investigates sensory integration therapies: Promise, possibility, and the art of placebo. *Communique, 31,* 5–6.

Simonoff, E., Pickles, A., Charman, T., Loucas, T., Baird, G., & Chandler, S. (2008). Psychiatric disorders in children with autism spectrum disorders: Prevalence, comorbidity, and associated factors in a population-derived sample. *Journal of the American Academy of Child and Adolescent Psychiatry, 47,* 921–929.

Skinner, B. F. (1938). *The behavior of organisms.* New York: Appleton-Century-Crofts.

Skinner, B. F. (1953). *Science and human behavior.* New York: Macmillan.

Smith, T., Mruzek, K. W., & Mozingo, D. (2005). Sensory integrative therapy. In J. W. Jacobson, R. M. Foxx, & J. A. Mulick (Eds.), *Controversial therapies for developmental disabilities* (pp. 331–350). Mahwah, NJ: Erlbaum.

Smith, T., Parker, T., Taubman, M., & Lovaas, O. I. (1992). Transfer of staff retraining from workshops to group homes: A failure to generalize across settings. *Research in Developmental Disabilities, 13,* 57–71.

Sparrow, S. S., Cicchetti, D. V., & Balla, D.A. (2005). *Vineland-II: Vineland adaptive behavior scales* (2nd ed.). Circle Pines, MN: AGS.

Stacey, C. L., & DeMartino, M. F. (Eds.). (1957). *Counseling and psychotherapy with the mentally retarded.* Glencoe, IL: Free Press.

Stehli, A. (1992). *Sound of a miracle: A child's triumph over autism.* Roxbury, CT: Georgiana Organization.

Stevenson, R. E., Schwartz, C. E., & Schroer, R. J. (2000). *X-linked mental retardation.* Oxford, England: Oxford University Press.

Strain, P. S., Ken, M. M., & Ragland, E. U. (1979). Effects of peer-mediated social initiations and prompting/reinforcement procedures on the social behavior of autistic children. *Journal of Autism and Developmental Disorders, 9,* 41–54.

Szatmari, P. (2000). Children with autism spectrum disorder: Medicine today and in the new millennium. *Focus on Autism & Other Developmental Disabilities, 15,* 138–146.

Tanguay, P. M. (2000). Pervasive developmental disorders: A ten year review. *Journal of the American Academy of Child and Adolescent Psychiatry, 39,* 1079–1095.

Tharp, R. G., &Wetzel, R. J. (1969). *Behavior modification in the natural environment.* New York: Academic Press.

Thompson, T., & Grabowski, J. (Eds.). (1972). *Behavior modification of the mentally retarded.* New York: Oxford University Press.

Tsai, L. Y. (2000). Children with autism spectrum disorder: Medicine today and in the new millennium. *Focus on Autism & Other Developmental Disabilities, 15,* 138–147.

Tsai, L. Y. (2006). Autistic disorders. In M. Dulcaan & J. Weiner (Eds.) *Essentials of child and adolescent psychiatry.* Arlington, VA: American Psychiatric.

U.S. Department of Education. (2002). *Twenty-fourth annual report to congress on the implementation of the individuals with disabilities act.* Washington, DC: U.S. Government Printing Office.

Ullmann, L., & Krasner, L. (Eds.). (1965). *Case studies in behavior modification.* New York: Holt.

Ulrich, R., Stachnik, T., & Mabry, J. (1966). *Control of human behavior.* Glenview, IL: Scott Foresman and Company.

Volkmar, F. R., State, M., & Klin, A. (2009). Autism and autism spectrum disorders: Diagnostic issues for the coming decade. *Journal of Child Psychology and Psychiatry and Allied Disciplines, 50,* 108–115.

Wacker, D. P., & Berg, W. K. (1988). Behavioral habilitation of students with severe handicaps. In J. C. Witt, S. N. Elliott, & F. M, Gresham (Eds.), *Handbook of behavior therapy in education* (pp. 719–737). New York: Plenum.

Waterhouse, L. (2008). Autism overflows: Increasing prevalence and proliferating theories. *Neuropsychology Review, 18,* 273–286.

Watson, L. (1973). *Child behavior modification.* New York: Pergamon Press.

Wetzel, R. J. (1992). Behavior analysis of residential program development. *Research in Developmental Disabilities, 13,* 73–80.

White, S., O'Reilly, H., & Frith, U. (2009). Big heads, small details and autism. *Neuropsychologia, 47,* 1274–1281.

Williams, D. (1992). *Nobody, nowhere: The extraordinary life of an autistic.* New York: Times Books.

Williams, D. E., Kirkpatrick-Sanchez, S., & Crocker, W. T. (1994). A long-term follow-up of treatment for severe self-injury. *Research in Developmental Disabilities, 15,* 487–501.

Williams, J. G., Higgins, J. P. T., & Brayne, C. E. G. (2006). Systematic review of prevalence studies of autism spectrum disorders. *Archives of Disease in Childhood, 91,* 8–15.

Wing, L., & Potter, D. (2002). The epidemiology of autistic spectrum disorders: Is the prevalence rising? *Mental Retardation and Developmental Disabilities Research Review, 8,* 131–151.

Witwer, A. N., & Lecavalier, L. (2008). Examining the validity of autism spectrum disorder subtypes. *Journal of Autism and Developmental Disorders, 38,* 1611–1624.

Wolfensberger, W. (1969). The origin and nature of our institutional models. In R. B. Kugel & W. Wolfensberger (Eds.), *Changing patterns in residential services for the mentally retarded* (pp. 59–171). Washington, DC: President's Commission on Mental Retardation.

Wolfensberger, W. (1972). *The principle of normalization in human services.* Washington, DC: National Institute on Mental Retardation.

Wood, L., Lasker, J., Siegel-Causey, E., Beukelman, D., & Ball, L. (1998). An input framework for augmentative and alternative communication. *Augmentative and Alternative Communication, 14,* 261–267.

World Health Organization. (1992). *Manual of the international classification of diseases, injuries, and causes of death* (Vol. 1). Geneva: World Health Organization.

Wright, E. B. (1987). Developmental disabilities. In C. R. Reynolds & L. Mann (Eds.), *Encyclopedia of special education* (Vol. 1, pp. 486–488). New York: Wiley Interscience.

Wyatt v. Stickney, 325 F. Supp. 781 (1971).

Yeargin-Allsopp, M., Rice, C., Karapurkar, T., Doernberg, N., Boyle, C., & Murphy, C. (2003). Prevalence of autism in a US metropolitan area. *Journal of the American Medical Association, 289*, 49–55.

Zeev, B. B., Bebbington, A., Ho, G., de Klerk, N., Vecksler, M., Christodoulou, J., et al. (2009).The common BDNF polymorphism may be a modifier of disease severity in Rett syndrome. *Neurology, 72*, 1242–1247.

Zigler, E., & Hodapp, R. M. (1986). *Understanding mental retardation*. New York: Cambridge University Press.

14

Neuromuscular Disorders

Jeffrey M. Cohen, MD, Marissa Cohler, MD, and Ludmilla Bronfin, MD

This chapter will familiarize the reader with the most common disorders involving the neuromuscular system. Neuromuscular disorders are a group of disorders that can affect any part of the nerve or muscle. They include diseases of the motor neuron (anterior horn cell), the peripheral nerve, the neuromuscular junction, and the muscle itself (Figure 14.1). We will focus on representative disorders affecting the various components of the neuromuscular system. We first describe disorders of the anterior horn cell (amyotrophic lateral sclerosis, spinal muscular atrophy, and poliomyelitis). These diseases result in degeneration of motor neurons in the brain, spinal cord, and periphery, ultimately leading to muscle weakness and atrophy. Next, we discuss diseases of the peripheral nerve, both acquired (e.g., mononeuropathy multiplex) and hereditary (e.g., Charcot-Marie-Tooth disease [CMT]). Our next section will focus on neuromuscular junction disorders, of which myasthenia gravis (MG) is representative. Finally, we discuss myopathies, diseases that solely involve the muscle. Myopathies are divided into congenital myopathies, dystrophic myopathies, myotonic myopathies, inflammatory myopathies, and endocrine myopathies. We end this chapter with a discussion of the role of exercise in neuromuscular disorders.

Anatomically, the initial segment of the motor peripheral nerve is located in the spinal cord and is known as the motor neuron or anterior horn cell (Figure 14.2). The motor cell body occupies the ventral gray matter. The motor peripheral nerve supplies efferent motor impulses to muscles. For the sensory system, the sensory cell body is known as the dorsal root ganglion. Sensory nerves convey sensory stimuli from skin and deep structures back to the spinal cord.

MOTOR NEURON DISEASES/ ANTERIOR HORN CELL DISEASES

Amyotrophic Lateral Sclerosis

Amyotrophic lateral sclerosis (ALS), also known as Lou Gehrig's disease, is a progressive degenerative disorder of motor neurons (anterior horn cells) in the motor cortex, brainstem, and spinal cord. It involves both upper motor neurons (UMN) in the motor cortex (corticospinal and corticobulbar tracts) and brainstem (tectospinal, rubrospinal) as well as lower motor neurons (LMN) in the brainstem and spinal cord. The coexistence of both UMN and LMN findings is the distinctive feature of ALS.

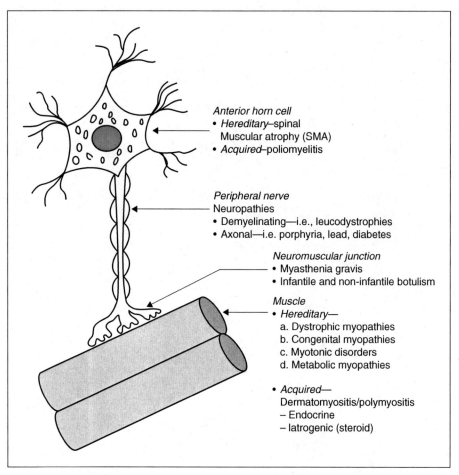

Anterior horn cell
- *Hereditary*–spinal
  Muscular atrophy (SMA)
- *Acquired*–poliomyelitis

Peripheral nerve
Neuropathies
- Demyelinating—i.e., leucodystrophies
- Axonal—i.e. porphyria, lead, diabetes

Neuromuscular junction
- Myasthenia gravis
- Infantile and non-infantile botulism

Muscle
- *Hereditary*—
  a. Dystrophic myopathies
  b. Congenital myopathies
  c. Myotonic disorders
  d. Metabolic myopathies

- *Acquired*—
  Dermatomyositis/polymyositis
  – Endocrine
  – Iatrogenic (steroid)

FIGURE 14.1 Anatomical breakdown of disorders of the lower motor neuron. *Source:* Sara J. Cuccurullo. Physical Medicine and Rehabilitation Board Review (New York: Demos, 2004). Copyright © 2004 by Demos Medical Publishing. Reprinted by permission of the publisher.

Epidemiology

ALS is the most common, disabling, and fatal motor neuron disease among adults (Bello-Haas, Florence, & Krivickas, 2008). The incidence of ALS peaks between the ages 55 and 75. ALS may present in sporadic or familial forms. Sporadic ALS has an annual incidence of about 1–2 per 100,000 and is more common in men (Brooks, 1998). Risk factors are thought to include excessive physical activity, smoking, electric shock, exposure to pesticides, and military service. However, many of these associations have been found to be weak and inconsistent (Armon, 2004; Haley, 2003; Horner et al., 2003; Weisskopf et al., 2005). Familial ALS represents 5–10% of all ALS cases. Familial ALS is usually autosomal dominant and has been found to be associated with a point mutation on the superoxide dismutase-1 (*SOD1*) gene in 25% of the cases. The mean age of onset of familial ALS is 47, 10 years younger than those who develop sporadic ALS. In familial ALS, the ratio of men to women is 1:1.

Clinical Features

Weakness has been found to be the presenting symptom in 60% of patients with ALS. Other clinical features include muscle cramps, fasciculations, and respiratory and swallowing difficulties. They may be the result of upper motor neuron involvement, lower motor neuron

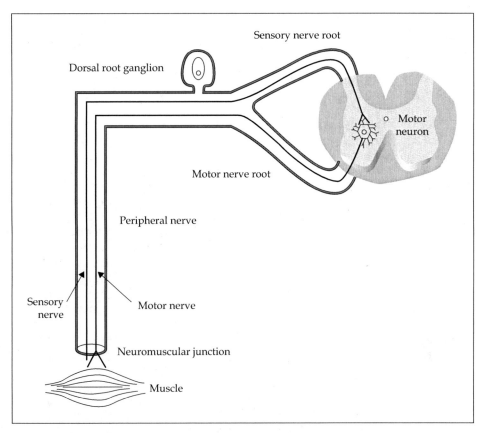

FIGURE 14.2 Peripheral nervous system pathway. Reprinted from *Easy EMG*, Julie Silver, "What is an EMG?", p. 2, Copyright 2004, with permission from Elsevier.

involvement, or a combination of the two. Upper motor neuron degeneration results in muscle weakness, spasticity, and pathological reflexes. Muscle weakness presents as difficulty with skillful movements and dexterity. This is usually described by a patient as "clumsiness" or "stiffness" of the extremities. As the UMN's degenerate, they no longer inhibit the LMN, resulting in increased LMN firing. This mechanism is responsible for the increased muscle stretch reflexes, spasticity, and clonus associated with UMN degeneration. The loss of brainstem UMN inhibition results in spasticity that is most prominent in upper extremity flexors and lower extremity extensors. Pathologic reflexes are present in normal infants and are lost as the central nervous system matures. However, in a degenerative process such as ALS, when UMN's are lost, these reflexes can reappear. The Babinski's sign (the big toe moves toward the top of the foot and the other toes fan out after the sole of the foot has been firmly stroked) and Hoffmann's sign (thumb flexion in response to a quick forceful flexion of the third finger) are examples of these pathological reflexes.

Pseudobulbar palsy is the result of an upper motor neuron lesion affecting the corticobulbar pathways. This leads to impairment of the function of the lower cranial nerves IX, X, XI, and XII that control the muscles of eating, swallowing, and talking. Pseudobulbar palsy is often associated with brisk jaw jerk and gag reflexes. Symptoms include difficulty with mastication, articulation, and deglutition. Aspiration of food and liquids into the lung may result leading to the development of pneumonia and laryngospasm. Another feature of pseudobulbar palsy in ALS is difficulty controlling emotions, which results in spontaneous laughter or crying that is out of proportion to the emotional stimuli.

Lower motor neuron degeneration results in muscle atrophy, flaccid weakness, hyporeflexia, and fasciculations. Weakness is more prominent in LMN degeneration than in UMN degeneration. As noted previously, whereas upper motor neuron degeneration produces stiffness and loss of dexterity, LMN degeneration leads primarily to weakness. The weakness is typically painless. The lower motor neuron degeneration often spreads to involve anterior horn cells bilaterally resulting in bilateral arm and leg weakness. Muscle atrophy is associated with LMN weakness and is a prominent feature of ALS.

Muscle cramps are another common feature of ALS. The mechanism for muscle cramps is not entirely clear but may relate to axonal hyperexcitability. Muscle cramps commonly occur in the calves, and, less commonly, in the thighs, abdomen, jaw, and neck. Fasciculations are one of the most well-known features of ALS. Fasciculations are caused by a spontaneous discharge of the entire motor unit (a motor neuron and the associated muscle fibers it innervates). The mechanism is felt to be similar to that of muscle cramps. Fasciculations are not painful and are often noticed by a clinician as a rapid and irregular twitching movement of the skin. Fasciculations may be enhanced by tapping lightly with a finger over the muscle. It is important to note that fasciculations are also common in people without neuromuscular disorders (benign fasciculations) and are rarely the initial presenting sign of ALS.

Lower motor neuron degeneration in the brainstem (medulla) results in bulbar palsy. Bulbar palsy is associated with atrophy and fasciculations of the tongue, absent jaw and gag reflexes, dysarthria, and dysphagia. Often patients have a mixture of pseudobulbar (UMN) palsy and bulbar (LMN) palsy. Patients with bulbar palsy have difficulty moving their tongues or opening or closing their mouths (due to weakness of the muscles of mastication innervated by cranial nerve V). The bulbar palsy may result in dysarthria or difficulty in articulating words, caused by impairment of the muscles used in speech. The dysarthric speech typically has a nasal quality and may progress to complete anarthria, where speech may be completely lost. Weakness of cranial nerves V, IX, X, and XII produces dysphagia. In ALS, difficulty with swallowing is usually more prominent with liquids than solids. In addition, ALS patients often report that increased time is necessary to eat a meal. As the disease progresses, the ability to cough diminishes, which may lead to aspiration. Drooling is a common sign of bulbar palsy.

Symptoms of respiratory insufficiency usually occur later in the disease. However, respiratory failure may be a presenting symptom of ALS and is associated with a poor prognosis. Early symptoms of respiratory insufficiency in ALS patients include difficulty lying flat in a bed, morning headaches, and exertional dyspnea. Following a patient's forced vital capacity (FVC) is important for monitoring the progression of respiratory failure.

Specific Treatment

In 1995, riluzole (Rilutek) became the first drug approved by the Food and Drug Administration for treating ALS. This drug is reported to prolong survival and may slow the disease progression in patients with ALS (American Academy of Neurology Quality Standards Subcommittee, 1997). It is estimated to provide a 9% increase in the probability of surviving 1 year and adds approximately 2 months to patient survival (Miller, Mitchell, Lyon, & Moore, 2002). It is the only approved drug for treatment of ALS.

Riluzole may be more beneficial when given in the early stages of the disease. Therefore, riluzole should be prescribed as soon as the diagnosis is established. The standard dosage is 50 mg twice a day. A transient elevation of serum transaminases (enzymes whose elevation may indicate liver damage) and rarely leukopenia (a condition in which the number of white blood cells circulating in the blood is abnormally low) have been reported in patients on riluzole. Thus, when administering the drug, complete blood counts and liver function tests must be performed every month for the first 3 months and every 3 months thereafter. Generally, riluzole is an easily tolerated medication in terms of side effects. Other drugs that have been investigated for possible usefulness in ALS include neurontin (Kalra, Cahman, Caramanos, Genge, & Arnold, 2003) and lithium (Fornai et al., 2008).

Symptomatic Treatment and Rehabilitation

Most of the clinical symptoms in patients with ALS are caused directly by the degenerating motor neurons and include muscle paralysis, atrophy, cramps, fasciculations, and loss of key motor functions. Other clinical stigmata include depression, anxiety, insomnia, and joint pains secondary to contracture. Symptomatic treatment is very important for patients with ALS because, as mentioned earlier, specific pharmacotherapy in ALS is limited. Quinine sulfate 325 mg twice a day is the most effective treatment option for muscle spasms and cramps (Borasio, Voltz, & Miller, 2001). Baclofen and tizanidine are used for excess muscle spasticity that causes incoordination and discomfort. Excess salivation (sialorrhea) may be treated with amitriptyline, atropine, botulinum toxin injection, glycopyrronium, or hyoscyamine (Phukan & Hardiman, 2009). A combination of dextromethorphan and quinidine (30 mg/30 mg) is effective in reducing uncontrollable pathologic laughter and crying secondary to pseudobulbar palsy and results in improved quality of life as well (Brooks et al., 2004).

Rehabilitation for patients with ALS requires a comprehensive approach. It is best achieved by an interdisciplinary team consisting of a physiatrist, neurologist, pulmonologist, nurse, physical therapist, occupational therapist, speech pathologist, psychologist, orthotist, dietician, and social worker (Sufit, 1997). The goals for patients with ALS are to improve function and quality of life, while maintaining independence for as long as possible. Psychological support throughout the disease process is crucial.

Physical therapy incorporates both active and passive exercises, the extent of which depends on the patient's muscle strength and tolerance. Exercises to maintain range of motion and improve strength and endurance are employed. It has been shown that moderate levels of exercise result in significantly better function and quality of life in patients with ALS, without adverse events, as compared to patients not engaged in an exercise program (Bello-Haas et al., 2007). The education of patients and caregivers is an important component of the rehabilitation process.

The ankle-foot orthosis (AFO) is the most frequently used brace in patients with ALS. In the early stages of ALS, ambulation with an AFO and a cane may be sufficient to maintain ambulation in patients with gait difficulties. However, as the disease progresses, a walker and ultimately a wheelchair are required. Whether to use a regular manual wheelchair or a motorized wheelchair depends on the individual needs of the patient.

Occupational therapy to improve upper extremity function for activities of daily living is a key component of the rehabilitation process. Patients are evaluated for assistive and adaptive equipment. Orthoses such as wrist extensor supports, mobile arm supports, and thumb splints as well as specialized eating utensils and holders are helpful for patients with arm and hand weakness. For head extension weakness, a soft cervical collar may provide effective support.

Instruction in energy conservation techniques and work simplification principles is an important component of occupational therapy. Successful rehabilitation also includes evaluating the patient's home. Home equipment can preserve patient independence and safety. Home adaptations include raised toilet seats and chair lifts for homes with stairs.

Dysarthria can make verbal communication difficult or impossible. Speech and language therapists provide strategies to enhance the intelligibility of speech such as reducing background noise, facing the listener, and slowing the rate of speech. A newer option for those with extremely limited communication skills is a gaze communication system (Daly & Wolpaw, 2008). It tracks the patient's eye movements and projects them onto a screen, allowing the user to spell a message for speech or text output.

A major principle in ALS care is that patients must be followed closely in order to detect impending problems with nutrition or respiration. Because of the development of dysphagia, patients are at high risk for aspiration. Altering food consistencies, high-calorie food supplements, and percutaneous endoscopic gastrotomy placement are essential steps in the prevention of aspiration while maintaining nutritional status.

Home care is necessary when the patient's condition severely deteriorates. Hospice provides comfort care to patients and their families (Borasio & Voltz, 1997).

Prognosis

Most patients die between 2 and 4 years after the onset of the symptoms. However, a significant proportion of ALS patients (20%) live beyond 5 years after onset. A better prognosis is associated with younger age of onset, spinal onset, UMN or LMN involvement, absent respiratory impairment, fewer fasciculations, a long interval from onset to the diagnosis, milder muscle involvement, normal amplitude motor action potentials on nerve conduction studies, and psychological well-being (Mitsumoto, 1997). Low serum chloride levels are associated with a poorer prognosis. Certain types of *SOD1* mutations are associated with short or long survival rates. Accurately predicting prognosis for any one individual patient is impossible. Patients and their families may have difficulty recognizing and accepting the poor prognosis of ALS. It is imperative to discuss advance directives early on in the disease course and to revisit the issue frequently. The timeliness of this conversation is paramount given that many patients eventually become incapable of communicating their wishes for end-of-life care. A health care proxy who will make decisions based on the patient's wishes should also be chosen. Palliative care is primarily directed toward improving the quality of life for dying patients. Treatment to relieve pain and use of opioids is recommended to relieve significant discomfort.

Poliomyelitis

This disease affects anterior horn cells and eventually destroys them. It is caused by a neurotropic enterovirus. The disease may result in severe disability due to LMN involvement.

Epidemics of poliomyelitis were commonplace worldwide until the introduction of the Salk vaccine between 1953 and 1956. Only a few cases of acute poliomyelitis have been seen in developed countries over the past 40 years. Because most of the patients in North America who had poliomyelitis acquired it before the mid-1950s, the youngest of these patients are now at least 50 years of age. Half the patients with spinal polio recover fully, one quarter recover with mild disability, and the remaining quarter are left with severe disability (Freeman, Johnson, Freeman, & Brown, 2004). Functional consequences in the older population include impaired mobility and difficulty performing skillful activity of daily living due to residual weakness, contractures, and skeletal deformities (such as scoliosis). Some of those affected are wheelchair-bound for life.

Between 25% and 50% of individuals who survive paralytic polio in childhood develop postpolio syndrome (PPS) later in life (National Institute of Neurological Disorders and Stroke, 2008). In this syndrome, patients develop symptoms such as muscle weakness and extreme fatigue, often decades after recovering from the acute infection. PPS is characterized by new weakening and fatigue in muscles that were previously affected by the polio infection and also in muscles that were seemingly unaffected (Trojan & Cashman, 2005). The main impact of PPS is on mobility-related activities affecting one's daily routine.

Spinal Muscular Atrophy

Spinal muscle atrophy (SMA) comprises a group of inherited disorders caused by degeneration of the motor neurons (anterior horn cells) in the brain stem and spinal cord. In contrast to ALS, there is no upper motor neuron involvement. There are three subtypes of SMA, each of which have an autosomal recessive inheritance and are linked to chromosome 5q13 (Freeman et al., 2004). SMA Type I (Werdnig-Hoffman Disease or Severe SMA) occurs due to the degeneration of the anterior horn cells of the spinal cord. It presents within the first 2 months of life with generalized hypotonia and symmetrical weakness. In addition to the hypotonia and weakness, infants present with a weak cry as well as sucking, swallowing, and respiratory difficulties.

Labored breathing during feeding, dysphagia, and frequent aspiration are common. On examination, there is symmetrical weakness, with the lower extremities more involved than the upper extremities and proximal muscles more involved than distal. Infants assume a "frog-leg" position when supine with the lower extremities abducted and externally rotated. Diaphragmatic breathing occurs due to intercostal and abdominal muscle weakness and relatively preserved diaphragmatic function. The prognosis is poor due to respiratory infections and the majority of patients die of pneumonia within the first year, with most of the remaining individuals dying within 3 years.

SMA Type II (Intermediate SMA) typically presents between the ages of 6 and 12 months and is also due to degeneration of anterior horn cells of the spinal cord. Symmetrical weakness of the legs (proximal greater than distal) is the cardinal clinical sign. Children are able to sit unsupported but have difficulty standing and walking. Associated features include a progressive kyphoscoliosis and a restrictive lung disease which are seen late in the first decade of life. The disease is slowly progressive and the long-term prognosis depends on respiratory function. Rehabilitation focuses on early achievement of standing posture in a standing frame, promotion of ambulation with appropriate orthoses, management of scoliosis through bracing and appropriate surgical referral, and maintenance of respiratory function.

SMA Type III (Kugelberg–Welander syndrome or mild SMA) is also due to degeneration of the anterior horn cells of the spinal cord. It has a variable age of onset: from the second year of life through adolescence and into adulthood. Presenting symptoms include difficulty with running, jumping, and climbing stairs. The cardinal clinical signs include proximal weakness, with the lower extremities more involved than the upper extremities, and difficulty arising from the floor (Gower's sign). A waddling gait with pelvic drop and lateral trunk lean over the stance phase side (compensated Trendelenberg gait) due to hip abductor weakness occurs. Fasciculations of the limb muscles and thoracic wall muscles are common, and scoliosis is frequent. Long-term prognosis depends on respiratory function but is generally good. Rehabilitation is aimed at the maintenance of ambulation through the use of appropriate orthotic devices, the management of scoliosis, and the maintenance of respiratory function.

PERIPHERAL NERVE DISEASES

Peripheral nerve diseases may involve one nerve (mononeuropathy) or multiple nerves (polyneuropathy). They may manifest as muscle atrophy, hyporeflexia, areflexia, and/or sensory impairment. Hyporeflexia or areflexia occur early in neuropathy and persist indefinitely, even after the return of motor power. This hyporeflexia must be differentiated from the markedly slowed reflexes of myxedema and the areflexia of muscles involved by a myopathy.

All modalities of sensation are typically impaired in peripheral neuropathies. Dissociation of sensory loss—where only one component is involved—is rare. Several patterns of dissociated sensory loss are worth highlighting.

In subacute combined degeneration (vitamin B12 deficiency related) and in spinocerebellar degeneration, such as Friedreich's ataxia, large-diameter primary sensory neurons degenerate early. Such patients lose touch-pressure, vibration, and joint-position sense but retain pain, light touch, and temperature sensation.

In contrast, in a variety of small-fiber neuropathies, the opposite is true. In amyloidosis, Fabry's disease, Tangier's disease, autonomic and diabetic neuropathy, and hereditary sensory neuropathy type I, pain sensation and thermal discrimination may be lost before touch-pressure, vibration, and joint-position sense.

Mononeuropathy

Mononeuropathies may present suddenly or have an insidious, slowly progressive onset. Mononeuropathies, which have a sudden onset, regardless of the nerve affected, location, etiology, or severity, are almost always manifested pathophysiologically as conduction failure secondary to a conduction block caused by demyelination. In contrast, chronic, slowly progressive mononeuropathies most often manifest as conduction failure due to axon loss. There are a few exceptions to this in which focal demyelination occurs. The most common exception is carpal tunnel syndrome, in which focal demyelination resulting in conduction slowing is the characteristic presentation.

Entrapment neuropathies occur when peripheral nerves are injured by mechanical pressure or ischemia at the points where they pass through rigid anatomical canals or beneath tight ligamentous or fascial bands, or where they enter, exit, or pass through muscle. Postoperative neuropathy may be the result of compression, traction, or ischemia (Dawson & Krarup, 1989). An example is entrapment neuropathy of the common peroneal nerve due to compression from positioning during surgery. Entrapment nerve trauma is more likely to occur when inflammation or degeneration is present in adjacent joints and tendons, as may happen in rheumatoid arthritis, myxedema, or acromegaly. It also occurs more commonly in nerves that lie in shallow grooves, allowing them to be easily compressed or traumatized repeatedly. The presence of an underlying peripheral neuropathy often renders nerves more susceptible to compressive injury (Atroshi, Gummesson, Johnsson, & Sprinchorn, 1999).

Mononeuropathy is commonly the result of injury. Because of the dramatic events associated with a fracture, nerve injuries are often overlooked. The nerve is usually injured by the sharp edge of a bone. However, the nerve may also be injured by soft tissue structures that crush or stretch the nerve. Hemorrhage or exudates into a restricted space, particularly near a joint, may compress the nerve. In fractures of the head of the humerus, the radial and ulnar nerves are most frequently involved. Intercostal neuropathy most commonly results from rib fractures. Fractures of the pelvis in the region of the sacroiliac joint may involve the sacral plexus. Hip fracture or dislocation may cause sciatic nerve injury. Fractures of the femur or pelvis may result in femoral nerve injury.

Trauma to nerves in athletes can be categorized by the types of sports involved (Sicuranza & McCue, 1992). Injuries to the brachial plexus commonly occur in motorcycle accidents, football, hockey, golf, acrobatics, and diving. The long thoracic nerve may be injured in wrestling, swimming, and tennis. The ulnar nerve is injured in bicycling, rowing, boxing, wrestling, football, and hockey. The radial nerve is injured in boxing, football, and hockey. The suprascapular nerve is injured in acrobatics, volleyball, baseball, and bowling. In the lower extremities, the lumbosacral plexus may be injured in diving, football, or acrobatics. The sciatic nerve is usually injured in golf or volleyball. Runners may experience peroneal nerve entrapment at the portion of the nerve that travels under the fibrous edge of the peroneus longus muscle. Male bicycle riders may experience numbness of the penis and scrotum because of the pressure of a hard saddle on the pudendal nerve.

A variety of occupations may be associated with peripheral nerve involvement. For example, craftsmen, such as jewelers, engravers, and machinists, who hold their tools tightly and exert hard pressure on the palm, suffer injury to the deep palmar branch of the ulnar nerve.

Nerve palsy may develop during sleep, especially after large doses of narcotics, sedatives, or alcohol. Developmental anomalies, an impaired nutritional state, and the surface on which the patient sleeps play a role in the development of the nerve palsy. The nerves affected most often are the radial and the peroneal. Radial paralysis may result from sleeping with an arm hanging over the back of a chair (Saturday night palsy), resting with the head of another lying on the arm (bridegroom's paralysis), or resting one's head on his/her own arm. If the patient is in the habit of sleeping with arms raised above the head, the median, axillary, musculocutaneous, and long thoracic nerves may become involved due to stretching or compression. In the lower extremity, the bones of the contralateral leg may compress the common peroneal nerve if the patient has slept while seated with the knees crossed.

Birth trauma can result in a brachial plexus injury. The upper arm is involved most frequently, and the lower arm less so. Erb's palsy results when injury occurs to the upper trunk of the brachial plexus and/or the C5–C6 cervical roots. It occurs in vertex presentations at birth when the head is pulled laterally to free the shoulders from the pelvis. The classic manifestation is the *Waiter's tip* position with the affected arm adducted, internally rotated, extended, pronated, and the wrist flexed. Paralysis of the lower arm (Klumpke's paralysis) results when an injury occurs to the C8–T1 nerve roots or lower trunk of the brachial plexus. It occurs from overextension of the arm in cases of face or breech presentation during birth or from traction on the axilla in vertex presentation (Dodds & Wolfe, 2000). Patients present with wasting of the small hand muscles and a claw hand deformity (Figure 14.3).

Awareness of the potential for the development of compression neuropathies can lead to a decrease in their incidence. Medical measures can prevent or reduce the severity of the deficit. Care in securing the arms and in providing protective pads has decreased the incidence of injury to the ulnar and radial nerves from hard surfaces during anesthesia. Fortunately, physical therapy and time usually suffice to bring about recovery in many patients.

Mononeuritis Multiplex

In mononeuritis multiplex, peripheral nerves become involved sequentially. Typically, the patient develops weakness, paresthesias, and dysesthetic pain in the distribution of a peripheral nerve. Later, symptoms occur in the distribution of an additional nerve. A key feature is that the neurologic deficits are asymmetric. Mononeuritis multiplex develops in diseases that produce a necrotizing angiitis (polyarteritis nodosa, rheumatoid arthritis, Wegener's granulomatosis, Churg–Strauss syndrome) but may also be seen in diabetes mellitus, inflammatory-demyelinating disorders, or a more benign vasculopathy.

When mononeuritis multiplex develops in a patient with rheumatoid arthritis or a systemic disease involving collagen vascular tissue, a necrotizing angiopathy should be suspected. The sedimentation rate is usually elevated, above 50 mm/hour, and there is a raised titer to nuclear antibodies.

Multiple cutaneous nerve involvement, as occurs in leprosy, is generally distinguishable from the causes of mononeuritis multiplex listed earlier. In lepromatous leprosy, the discrete loss of pain and sensitivity to temperature over a region of skin coincides with a depigmented area.

Brachial Plexus Neuropathy

The annual incidence of brachial plexus neuropathy is 1.64/100,000. The disorder is more common in men, and the incidence is highest between the third and seventh decades (Russell & Windebank, 1994).

Brachial plexopathy begins suddenly with pain. The pain is located in the region of the shoulder, but may radiate down the lateral arm. The pain is severe and constant and may be

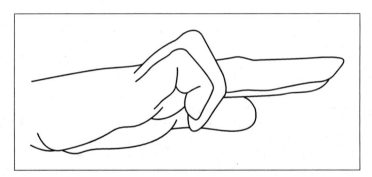

FIGURE 14.3 Ulnar claw hand. *Source:* Sara J. Cuccurullo. Physical Medicine and Rehabilitation Board Review (New York: Demos, 2004). Copyright © 2004 by Demos Medical Publishing. Reprinted by permission of the publisher.

described as sharp, stabbing, or aching. It is exacerbated by coughing, sneezing, and, in rare instances, by neck motion. It is accompanied by the rapid development of muscle weakness and wasting. Weakness primarily involves the deltoid, supraspinatus, infraspinatus, serratus anterior, biceps, and triceps. Complete unilateral limb paralysis has been reported. Plexus involvement in bilateral cases is usually not symmetric. Sensory loss is much less prominent than are pain and muscle weakness.

Magnetic resonance imaging scans of the brachial plexus are performed to exclude a mass lesion and are usually normal.

The etiology of this condition is unknown, though an allergic or autoimmune mechanism has been suspected. The prognosis is good. There is improvement in muscle strength within the first months after symptom onset with 90% recovery within 3 years. A few patients are left with minimal neurologic deficits. Recurrences are rare.

There is no evidence that steroids alter the course of this disease, although in some patients, steroids may result in relief of pain. Analgesics are needed for pain relief. Early rehabilitation is important in order to prevent the development of shoulder joint restrictions of range of motion and to improve muscle strength.

Polyneuropathy

A polyneuropathy is a disease affecting multiple peripheral nerves simultaneously. Polyneuropathies typically are characterized by symmetrical, bilateral distal motor, and sensory impairment with a graded increase in severity distally. The pathological processes affecting peripheral nerves include degeneration of the axon, myelin, or both. The various forms of polyneuropathy are categorized by the type of nerve affected (e.g., sensory, motor, or autonomic), by the distribution of nerve injury (e.g., distal vs. proximal), by the nerve component primarily affected (e.g., demyelinating vs. axonal), by etiology, and by the pattern of inheritance.

Acquired Polyneuropathies

DIAGNOSIS. In determining the type of polyneuropathy present, the patient's medical, social, and occupational history can provide clues. Information about infections to which the patient was exposed to, medications taken, drugs used, and exposure to industrial poisons should be ascertained.

The type of onset and clinical course of the disease helps to determine the type of neuropathic process. An acute or subacute onset is typical of the inflammatory immune-mediated neuropathies, various toxins, and poisons, as well as metabolic conditions such as acute intermittent porphyria. A recurrent course is seen in chronic inflammatory polyradiculoneuropathies, in intermittent poisoning, and in acute intermittent porphyria. A slowly progressive course is typical of many inherited motor and sensory neuropathies. It is necessary to know which population of neurons are affected in order to properly diagnose a peripheral polyneuropathy.

In inflammatory motor polyradiculoneuropathy, as is seen in Guillain–Barré syndrome, the muscle weakness that occurs tends to be symmetric. In this disease, spinal fluid examination revealing elevated protein levels is helpful in determining the diagnosis.

Symptoms of paresthesia, hyperalgesia, tightness, aching, and burning are indicative of sensory neuropathy. These symptoms represent excessive neural activity related to the damaged fibers or regenerated sprouts. Many mixed neuropathies also begin with these same sensory symptoms, even though motor and autonomic symptoms are also present. Diabetes mellitus, uremia, B_{12} deficiency, and hypothyroidism are common examples of mixed metabolic neuropathies.

Many toxic and medication-related neuropathies can begin with sensory symptomatology and then progress to include motor symptoms. In arsenic and thallium-related neuropathies, gastrointestinal upset is often followed by a painful, burning, distal neuropathy with weakness. In thallium neuropathy, these symptoms are also associated with hair loss. Amyloidosis often presents with sensory symptoms.

Carcinomatous sensory neuropathy may begin with symptoms from loss of both large- and small-fiber function. Patients become unsteady and, in addition, have hyperalgesia, tight band-like constrictions around toes and ankles, and hyperpathia.

Autonomic dysfunction in peripheral neuropathy can be varied and disabling. Acquired autonomic neuropathies are present in inflammatory immune-mediated neuropathy, α-lipoprotein deficiency (Tangier's disease), and in diabetes mellitus. Symptoms include dysfunction of tear production, temperature deregulation, dysphagia, and crampy abdominal pain. Impaired heart rate and blood pressure regulation are often found in patients with diabetes. The most troublesome symptom of dysautonomia is postural hypotension. The patient's blood pressure falls on standing. Impotence may develop in the male. This symptom is commonly reported in various types of amyloidosis and in diabetes mellitus (Bastron & Thomas, 1981). Dysautonomia is a major feature in the Riley–Day syndrome, a recessively inherited disorder in Jewish children.

METHODS OF INVESTIGATION. Nerve conduction and electromyography (EMG) should be done in all patients suspected of having a peripheral neuropathy (Dumitru, 1995). Spinal fluid is helpful in documenting protein elevation, malignant cells, or an elevation of gamma globulin. Biopsy of nerve tissue may help to determine an underlying process. Laboratory evaluation is helpful in the differential diagnosis of peripheral neuropathy and should include fasting and postprandial blood sugar, serum protein electrophoresis, 24-hour urine protein electrophoresis, serum lipids, and tissue estimation of specific heavy metals, medications, or toxins. DNA studies are necessary to diagnose inherited neuropathies (Dyck, Giannini, & Lais, 1993).

REHABILITATION. Common functional impairments include impaired gait and balance due to decreased strength and sensation in the lower extremities (especially the feet and ankles). In addition, decreased grip strength and sensation in the hands may result in difficulty performing activities of daily living. Peripheral neuropathies are rarely curable, but the symptoms are controllable through rehabilitation. The goals of rehabilitation are to maximize functional capacity, prolong or maintain independent function, inhibit or prevent physical deformity, and provide access to full integration into society with a good quality of life. The prescription of low impact aerobics such as swimming, walking, and stationary bicycling can help to reduce fatigue and improve physical functioning. Gentle stretching before and after workouts can maintain flexibility and reduce muscle cramps induced by exercise (Carter, 2005). At the same time, patients with peripheral neuropathy should generally avoid high-resistance exercise as they are more prone to overwork weak muscles (Kilmer, McCrory, Wright, Aitkens, & Bernauer, 1994). They should also be advised not to over-exercise as the risk of muscle damage and dysfunction may be significant (Carter et al., 1994).

Many patients will require some form of bracing or orthotics for their lower extremities (Paulson & Kilmer, 2001). A plastic polypropylene orthosis is often prescribed and preferred over the heavier, more cumbersome double-upright metal AFO. Metal bracing is, however, appropriate for patients with fluctuating edema, as they can accommodate changes in limb diameter as swelling waxes and wanes (Boninger & Leonard, 1996). Bracing can also be helpful when peripheral neuropathies involve the upper extremities. These braces may be static (rigid and supportive without allowing movement) or dynamic (supportive while allowing some movement). Custom-fitted orthotics and orthopedic shoes are imperative for preventing neuropathic arthropathy and foot ulceration.

Assistive and adaptive equipment can improve patient safety and quality of life. Canes or crutches benefit patients with an ataxic or antalgic gait. Wheeled walkers or quad (four-point) canes provide an increased area of support and facilitate mobility. Equipment for the bathroom, including handheld showers, bathtub benches, raised toilet seats, and grab bars, enhance safety.

PHARMACOLOGICAL MANAGEMENT. There are several drugs available to manage neuropathic pain. Gabapentin is the first-line agent and has a more favorable side effect profile than other older medications in the same class (e.g., carbamazepine, phenytoin, valproate). Pregabalin is also used to manage neuropathic pain. Tricyclic antidepressants, such as amitriptyline and nortriptyline, are also mainstays of treatment.

Inherited Polyneuropathies

CHARCOT-MARIE-TOOTH DISEASE. CMT is the most common human hereditary peripheral neuropathy, with a prevalence of 1 in 2,500 people (Skre, 1974). It comprises a large group of inherited neuropathies caused by genetic errors that result in the absence of proteins necessary for normal nerve function. This results in dysfunction in either the outer myelin sheath or the axon of the nerve cell (Shy, Dyck, Chance, Lupski, & Klein, 2005). CMT Type I (CMT1), which has an autosomal dominant inheritance, is the most common type of CMT, affecting 75% of CMT patients (Jani-Acsadi, Krajewski, & Shy, 2008). It is a demyelinating neuropathy characterized by a reduction in nerve conduction velocity (NCV) due to a partial or complete loss of the myelin sheath. CMTX, caused by a mutation carried on the X-chromosome, accounts for 10–20% of CMT patients (Ionasescu, Burns, Searby, & Ionasescu, 1988). It is also a demyelinating neuropathy with reduced NCV (Jani-Acsadi et al., 2008).

CMT Type II (CMT2) has an autosomal dominant inheritance (except CMT2B1) and affects approximately 22% of CMT patients (Ionasescu, Ionasescu, & Searby, 1993). It primarily affects the axon of the nerve cell and is characterized by reduced compound muscle action potential amplitudes on electrodiagnostic testing. In contrast to CMT1 and CMTX, the nerve conduction velocities are normal or only slightly reduced.

In most respects, the clinical phenotype of CMT2 patients is similar to patients with CMT1 and CMTX. Symptoms usually begin in late childhood or early adulthood. Patients present with distal weakness and atrophy that typically begins in the feet and calves and later affects the hands. The initial symptom is often a foot drop causing difficulty with ambulation. Atrophy of muscles below the knee can give rise to a "stork leg" or "inverted bottle" appearance of the legs. Patients also present with distal sensory loss and absent reflexes. Weakness in the hands and forearms tend to occur later as the disease progresses. Patients also suffer from skeletal deformities such as scoliosis or foot deformities such as pes cavus (high arch foot) and hammer toes (Shy et al., 2005).

Most patients with CMT will require physical or occupational therapy. The prescription of appropriate braces (orthotics) for the ankle can promote independent ambulation in patients with a foot drop. Occupational therapy to improve fine motor skills and to evaluate for adaptive equipment is essential for those with distal upper extremity involvement. Few high-quality studies exist regarding rehabilitation of patients with CMT. One study by Lindeman et al. (1995) demonstrated improved walking ability following 24 weeks of strength training. Genetic counseling is also essential in the management of patients with CMT.

There is currently no standard pharmacological treatment for CMT. However, a parallel group double-blind study of neurotrophin-3 has shown promising benefit with respect to the Neuropathy Impairment Score (Sahenk et al., 2005). Another promising therapy is vitamin C (Passage et al., 2004). It has been found that chronic treatment with vitamin C is a very effective treatment for mice overexpressing PMP22, the gene implicated in CMT. The treated mice not only had disease progression halted, but also had partial reversal of the CMT phenotype. Human trials with vitamin C are currently in progress (Pareyson et al., 2006). To date, small trials of exercise training, creatine monohydrate, orthoses, and purified bovine ganglioside injections have shown no significant benefit in people with CMT (Young, De Jonghe, Stogbauer, & Butterfass-Bahloul, 2008).

DISEASES OF THE NEUROMUSCULAR JUNCTION

Myasthenia Gravis

MG is the most common disorder of neuromuscular transmission. It is an acquired autoimmune disease characterized by the presence of antibodies directed against acetylcholine receptors (AChR). This results in impaired neuromuscular transmission. Clinically, it is manifested by fluctuating and fatiguable weakness. The weakness may be limited to a few muscles, such as the extraocular muscles (the muscles that control the movements of the eye), or it may be generalized. The weakness is often worse with activity and improved by rest.

Epidemiology

MG is a fairly common disorder with an incidence of 1–2 per 100,000 population and a prevalence of 20–50 per 100,000 population (Gold & Schneider-Gold, 2008). Although the incidence has not changed significantly, the prevalence has increased over the last 45 years, most likely due to longer life spans and improved therapies. There is no racial predominance.

Almost all cases occur sporadically, and familial clusters are rare. Patients are classified on the basis of age and the presence or absence of thymoma (Freeman et al., 2004). In patients without a thymoma, there is a female predominance under the age of 40 years (75%) and an increased association with human leukocyte antigen (HLA)-A1, B8, and DRw3 antigens. Men predominate over the age of 40 years (60%), and there is an increased association with HLA-A3, B7, and DRw2 antigens.

Pathogenesis

The reduction and blockade of AChR on the postsynaptic membrane of the neuromuscular junction by AChR antibodies play a major role in the pathogenesis of MG. The precipitating factors remain unknown. The implication of these antibodies in the neuromuscular abnormalities of MG is based on several lines of evidence. These include the presence of AChR modulating or blocking antibodies in 85–90% of patients (Meriggioli, 2009), and the beneficial effects of plasmapheresis in improving clinical symptoms (Gold & Schneider-Gold, 2008).

The thymus gland appears to play a central role in the evolution of the disease as well as in its treatment. Thymic hyperplasia has been reported to occur in 65% of myasthenic patients and thymoma in up to 15%. There is a beneficial effect of thymectomy, especially in younger patients (Gutmann, Crosby, Takamori, & Martin, 1972).

Clinical Presentation

Clinically, the initial presentation of MG may involve weakness of the extraocular muscles, facial muscles, bulbar muscles, neck musculature, and extremities. Patients may present with nasal or slurred speech (dysarthria), with upper eyelid weakness (ptosis), with double vision (diplopia), or with difficulty swallowing (dysphagia). When the extremities are affected, the proximal muscles are usually more severely involved than the distal ones. The disease does not involve cardiac or smooth muscle, nor is there an alteration of cognitive skills, coordination, sensation, or tendon reflexes.

Extraocular muscle weakness can result in any combination of gaze abnormality. Ptosis may involve one or both eyelids. The fluctuating eyelid ptosis and extraocular muscle weakness does not occur in other illnesses. Facial weakness causes the patient to have an expressionless look. In severe cases, the patient may have to support his or her jaw manually because of the weakness of the jaw muscles. Nasal or slurred speech results from the weakness of the tongue and soft palate. Weakness of the muscles responsible for coughing and swallowing leads to dysphagia with choking and aspiration of food and secretions. Keeping the airway patent sometimes proves difficult, and fatigue of respiratory muscles leads to dyspnea at rest or with exertion.

Weakness can be provoked by exertion, exposure to heat, infections, or emotional upset. Pregnancy causes a variable response, but the postpartum period is more likely to be associated with an exacerbation of the symptoms described earlier.

Myasthenic crisis is most commonly provoked by a respiratory infection or a major surgical procedure. Predictors of a crisis include a poor vital capacity due to respiratory muscle weakness and an inability to keep the airway patent.

Diagnosis

The distribution and fluctuating nature of the weakness, especially when it involves the extraocular and bulbar muscles, is characteristic of MG. The dramatic improvement following the intravenous injection of the rapidly acting acetylcholinesterase inhibitor edrophonium (Tensilon test) further helps to confirm the diagnosis. The presence of serum AChR antibodies is highly specific for MG. Electrodiagnostic testing is also helpful to confirm the diagnosis and rule out other neurological conditions. Repetitive nerve stimulation studies exhibiting more than 10% decline in amplitude are significant for pathology.

The use of radiographic studies (chest x-ray and chest computed tomography scans) is important in the evaluation and identification of those patients with thymoma. Assessment of antinuclear antibodies, rheumatoid factor, thyroid function studies, and vitamin B_{12} levels assist in the identification of associated autoimmune disorders.

Differential Diagnosis

The differential diagnosis includes the progressive external ophthalmoplegias, oculopharyngeal dystrophy, amyotrophic lateral sclerosis, progressive bulbar palsy, motor axonopathies, Lambert–Eaton syndrome (Castaigne et al., 1977), botulism, congenital myasthenic syndromes, intracranial mass lesions compressing cranial nerves, and the intranuclear ophthalmoplegia of multiple sclerosis. Clinical features and laboratory studies help a discerning clinician to differentiate among these disorders.

Treatment

The aim of treatment in MG is to improve the neurological symptoms, the patient's quality of life, and survival. Anticholinesterase medications are given as the initial therapy. Pyridostigmine (Mestinon) is the most commonly used. These medications inhibit the action of acetylcholinesterase, allowing acetylcholine to remain longer at the neuromuscular junction. This increases the ability to generate a muscle action potential. The usual starting dose of pyridostigmine is 30–60 mg every 4 hours. Side effects include abdominal cramps and diarrhea.

Thymectomy is now widely used early in the course of MG. Patients who undergo thymectomy have significantly greater rates of remission and improvement compared with those who do not undergo this procedure. Furthermore, they have a significantly greater survival (Bachmann et al., 2009). Currently, thymectomy is recommended for almost all patients under the age of 50–55 years, except for those with only ocular involvement.

Prednisone therapy is a mainstay in the treatment of MG in those patients over the age of 50, and may be useful in those younger patients in whom anticholinesterase medication and/ or thymectomy have not been sufficiently effective. It is being used more frequently in patients who have only ocular MG. Alternate-day therapy with 60–100 mg of prednisone is an effective and popular form of treatment with fewer potential side effects. Improvement usually occurs over several months and is followed by a gradual taper of the medicine. Long-term use is often modified with the addition of immunosuppressant agents such as azathioprine, cyclophosphamide, or cyclosporine (Gold et al., 2008). Azathioprine (2–3 mg/kg) may be initiated at the same time as prednisone, and has few side effects at this low dose. Cyclosporin A at 100–200 mg per day is another option for long-term immunosuppressive therapy. Other therapies used to treat MG patients, especially during exacerbations of the disease, include plasmapheresis and high-dose intravenous immune globulins. Plasmapheresis is a procedure in which abnormal antibodies are removed from the blood. It is a relatively safe, but expensive, treatment modality and is usually reserved for the treatment of a myasthenic crisis or for preparing a patient for a surgical procedure such as a thymectomy (Dau, 1982). The improvement produced by a course of plasmapheresis may range from mild, lasting for a few days, to marked, persisting for 3–6 weeks. Complications include hypotension, bleeding, sepsis, and embolism. It is not known whether there is a synergistic effect with plasmapheresis and immunosuppressive drugs. The use of high-dose intravenous immune globulin temporarily modifies the immune system and provides the body with normal antibodies from donated blood.

There are several off-label pharmacological options for those who do not respond to, or who suffer intolerable side effects from, the aforementioned treatments. They can also be used for those with very severe MG (Gold et al., 2008). Mycophenolate mofetil at 1,000–2,000 mg per day and methotrexate at 7.5–15 mg per week have been shown to be effective in several well-documented case studies. Cyclophosphamide is reserved for the most severely affected and treatment-refractory patients. Finally, tacrolimus and rituximab have shown some promise for the treatment of MG, but there is still very limited experience with them at this point.

Impending myasthenic crisis requires immediate treatment. In this setting, medications that adversely affect neuromuscular transmission should be used with caution. These include aminoglycoside antibiotics, procainamide, quinidine, β-adrenergic blocking agents, and lithium. Magnesium should be avoided. Respiratory failure requires endotracheal intubation, careful bronchopulmonary care, and mechanical ventilation in an intensive care unit. The FVC is the most commonly followed pulmonary function parameter. Myasthenic crises are usually self-limited, and spontaneous recovery is expected within a few days or weeks. Exercise therapies such as inspiratory muscle training, diaphragmatic breathing, and pursed lips breathing help improve pulmonary function and respiration (Fregonezi, Resqueti, Guell, Pradas, & Casan, 2005).

Prognosis

The prognosis for patients with MG has improved dramatically over the past 50 years with the mortality decreasing to 7%, and with 90% of patients either in remission, improved, or unchanged. The improvement in prognosis is a result of new treatment approaches including early thymectomy, immunosuppressive drug therapy, and short-term immunotherapies (plasmapheresis, intravenous immunoglobulins). It is also a result of advances in respiratory care including the availability of positive pressure ventilators, sophisticated intensive care equipment, and the evolution of new therapeutic modalities.

MUSCLE DISEASES

Muscle disease classification includes congenital myopathies, dystrophic myopathies, myotonic myopathies, inflammatory myopathies, and metabolic myopathies. Muscle weakness is the most common sign of muscle disease. However, patients with muscle disease often do not initially report muscle weakness. Clinicians should look for clues that suggest a reduction in physical activity. They should assess muscle function by observing the patient's ability to perform simple directed motor tasks such as having the patient transfer from sit to stand position to evaluate proximal lower extremity strength.

Congenital Myopathies

Congenital myopathies are disorders that are delineated on the basis of characteristic morphologic features. They include central core disease, multicore disease, nemaline myopathy, centronuclear myopathy, congenital fiber type disproportion, reducing body myopathy, fingerprint body myopathy, myopathies with tubular aggregates, and Type 1 myofiber.

The congenital myopathies often present in early infancy as the "floppy infant" syndrome. Fortunately, many of these infants have a relatively benign course with the weakness and hypotonia remaining static or even improving. However, some infants have a progressive course leading to early death from respiratory complications.

In those patients whose symptoms begin in early childhood, muscular weakness and hypotonia are often accompanied by skeletal anomalies such as a high-arched palate, pectus excavatum (caved-in or sunken appearance of the chest), kyphoscoliosis, and dislocated hips. Occasionally, this disorder begins in late childhood or adult life. When diagnosed in adults, the congenital myopathies are usually asymptomatic or only mildly progressive.

EMG generally shows nonspecific myopathic features, and the serum muscle enzymes are only mildly elevated or normal. Muscle biopsy reveals the characteristic morphological features.

Dystrophic Myopathies

The dystrophic myopathies are hereditary myopathies characterized by progressive muscle degeneration. These include dystrophin-deficient muscular dystrophies, congenital muscular dystrophies, limb girdle muscular dystrophies, fascioscapular muscular dystrophies, oculopharyngeal muscular dystrophies, distal muscular dystrophies, and Emery–Dreifuss muscular dystrophy (EDMD).

Duchenne Muscular Dystrophy

EPIDEMIOLOGY AND ETIOLOGY. Duchenne muscular dystrophy (DMD), or pseudo-hypertrophic muscular dystrophy, was first described in the mid-1800s. The incidence of DMD is about 30 per 100,000 live male births (Bonilla et al., 1988). DMD is transmitted by an X-linked recessive inheritance. It results from an abnormality at the *Xp21* gene loci, which codes for the plasma protein dystrophin, an important cytoskeletal protein localized to the inner surface of the sarcolemma membrane. The *Xp21* gene is an extremely large gene, which may account for its high rate of spontaneous mutations. The magnitude of dystrophin deficiency correlates with clinical severity. A quantity of dystrophin which is less than 3% of normal is diagnostic of DMD (Freeman et al., 2004).

CLINICAL FEATURES. DMD does not become clinically apparent until the age of 2–4 years. Initial manifestations include a delay in walking, frequent falls, and difficulty climbing stairs. The earliest weakness is seen in the neck flexors during the preschool years. Cardinal clinical signs include proximal muscle weakness with the lower extremities more involved than the upper ones, prominence of the calves (pseudohypertrophy of calf muscles), toe walking due to heel cord contractures, difficulty arising from the floor (Gower's sign), waddling type gait (due to hip abductor weakness), and an increasingly lordotic posture (due to hip extensor weakness).

Between the ages of 8 and 12 years, there is a steady and progressive decline in functional motor capability. The average age of wheelchair dependency is 10 years with a range of 7–13 years. Following wheelchair confinement, the development of contractures and kyphoscoliosis accelerates. Contractures typically affect the hip and knee flexors, iliotibial band, and ankle plantarflexors as well as the elbow and wrist flexors. Scoliosis in DMD typically occurs in the second decade and significant scoliosis (more than 20–30 degrees) is seen in 85–90% of patients. Significant scoliosis can result in difficulties with seating and positioning and can exacerbate underlying restrictive lung disease. Bracing is known to be ineffective to stop the progression of scoliosis in these children. Spinal stabilization is recommended to correct significant spinal deformity and pelvic obliquity as well as to prevent further progression (Hahn, Hauser, Espinosa, Blumenthal, & Min, 2008).

Increasing thoracic muscle weakness produces respiratory insufficiency. Patients develop a restrictive lung disease that initially is manifested by expiratory muscle weakness and difficulty coughing and clearing secretions. Ultimately, they can develop inspiratory muscle weakness, CO_2 retention, and respiratory failure (Freeman et al., 2004). Monitoring of the FVC is essential in assessing respiratory function. The use of noninvasive means of ventilatory support such as bidirectional positive airway pressure has been found to be helpful in improving respiratory function and quality of life.

Dystrophin also has been identified in cardiac Purkinje fibers, and nearly all patients older than 13 years demonstrate electrocardiography (EKG) abnormalities. Cardiomyopathy is usually first noted when the child is older than 10 years. Cardiomyopathy and systolic dysfunction are poor prognostic factors.

DIAGNOSIS. A presumptive clinical diagnosis of DMD can be made in boys between the ages of 3 and 5 years who present with the classic clinical findings described earlier. Confirmatory studies include a screening blood test for serum creatine kinase (CK). In children aged 3–5 with DMD, the CK can be elevated on the order of 10,000–30,000. By late adolescence, when skeletal muscle destruction is nearly complete, serum CK may decrease to near-normal levels. EMG demonstrates a myopathic pattern. Muscle biopsy reveals replacement of muscle fiber by fat and connective tissue and evidence of hypertrophied fibers, degenerating fibers, and atrophied fibers. Genetic studies (gene deletion studies using the polymerase chain reaction technique) can detect the presence of a dystrophin-deficient abnormality. However, gene studies cannot distinguish between the Duchenne and Becker clinical subtypes of muscular dystrophy. This requires a muscle biopsy with quantitative dystrophin analysis. As noted earlier, a quantity of dystrophin that is less than 3% of normal is diagnostic of DMD. In Becker's muscular dystrophy, dystrophin is present at 20–80% of normal levels (Freeman et al., 2004).

TREATMENT. At present, the management of DMD utilizes an interdisciplinary approach involving physical therapy, occupational therapy, bracing, and surgery. Prevention of fixed deformities by passive stretching is a mainstay of treatment. Attention should be given to the Achilles tendon to prevent an equinovarus deformity. Active exercise should be allowed as much as possible. However, children should not exercise to the point of exhaustion or the point where they develop muscle pains. The application of knee-ankle-foot orthoses allows the child to stand and walk when his own muscles are not strong enough to accomplish this. Referral to an orthopedic surgeon is advisable when tightness of the heel cords become severe enough to make walking difficult; a simple percutaneous release of the Achilles tendon may be all that is needed. Prompt surgical intervention for a progressing scoliotic curvature is essential. Respiratory function can be improved through chest physiotherapy to develop an effective abdominal assisted cough, through incentive spirometry to improve vital capacity, and through inspiratory resistive training.

The use of corticosteroids, prednisone, and deflazacort can be beneficial in the treatment of DMD. Multiple class I studies have demonstrated that prednisone can be beneficial for boys between 5 and 15 years of age with DMD (Manzur, Kuntzer, Pike, & Swan, 2008). Prednisone has been demonstrated to have a beneficial effect on arm and leg function, muscle strength, timed function tests, and FVC. It is typically prescribed at a dose of 0.75 mg/kg/day as treatment. The class I studies that evaluated daily prednisone treatment found that the most common side effects were weight gain and the development of a cushingoid facial appearance, beginning after 6–18 months of treatment. There was no significant increase in the number of patients developing hypertension, diabetes mellitus, gastrointestinal bleeding, psychosis, compression fractures, or cataracts.

Myoblast (muscle stem cell) transfer has been proposed as a technique to replace dystrophin, the skeletal-muscle protein that is deficient in DMD (Mouly et al., 2005). Donor myoblasts injected into muscles of affected patients can fuse with host muscle fibers, thus contributing their nuclei, which are potentially capable of replacing deficient gene products. However, to date, controlled trials involving the transfer of myoblasts into patients with DMD have been unsuccessful.

Becker Muscular Dystrophy

Becker muscular dystrophy (BMD) was recognized as a benign form of X-linked dystrophy in the 1950s. BMD occurs one tenth as often as DMD. Both BMD and DMD result from defects in the same dystrophin gene loci, *Xp21* (Freeman et al., 2004).

Patients present with weakness between the ages of 5 and 15, later than they do in DMD. The pattern of muscular involvement is similar to that of DMD, with proximal muscle weakness greater than distal muscle weakness. Presenting symptoms include difficulty with running or climbing steps. Cardinal clinical signs are proximal muscle weakness, pseudo-hypertrophy of the calves, increased lordosis, and a waddling gait. Approximately 75% have EKG abnormalities, and cardiac involvement may lead to cardiomyopathy.

Laboratory studies reveal serum CK levels that are markedly elevated (similar levels to those with DMD). EMG demonstrates myopathic features. Dystrophin is present at 20–80% of normal levels or is found at normal levels but with abnormal function.

BMD has a slowly progressive, variable course. Patients typically walk through the late teen years, and patients tend to live twice as long as those with the Duchenne subtype. Life expectancy is dependent upon the degree of progression and the extent of cardiopulmonary involvement.

Congenital Muscular Dystrophy

Congenital muscular dystrophy is a heterogeneous group of disorders that become manifest at birth. Affected infants present with flaccidity, weakness, and/or fixed joint deformities (in relation to intrauterine posture). Weakness is greater proximally than distally and often involves the facial muscles. Variable sucking, swallowing, and respiratory difficulties are noted. Associated features include the development of hip dislocations and scoliosis.

The course of the disease is variable. Many cases remain static or show functional improvement over time. In severe cases, death occurs due to respiratory failure. Treatment is symptomatic, including aggressive physical therapy to prevent contracture formation.

Limb Girdle Muscular Dystrophy

Limb girdle muscular dystrophy (LGMD) is a clinically and genetically diverse group of disorders manifested by proximal weakness (hip and shoulder girdle) and lacking the symptoms of the other dystrophies (Shields, 1994). An autosomal dominant variety of LGMD with later onset (second to fourth decade) has been mapped to chromosome 5. The serum creatine phosphokinase, EMG, and muscle biopsy findings vary from mild to severe. There is no disease-specific treatment.

Facioscapulohumeral Muscular Dystrophy

Facioscapulohumeral muscular dystrophy (FSHMD) is an autosomal dominant inherited dystrophy. The genetic defect has been mapped to chromosome 4. The age of onset is variable, from early childhood to adult life.

Clinically, weakness primarily involves the facial, shoulder girdle and humeral muscles. Weakness initially occurs in the face, and affected muscles include the orbicularis oculi, orbicularis oris, and zygomaticus. Patients have difficulty whistling. Shoulder girdle weakness typically develops next, primarily involving the periscapular and pectoralis muscles. Patients have difficulty bringing their arms to the level of their face and raising them above their head. Posterior and lateral scapular winging occurs due to weakness of the periscapular muscles. Humeral involvement, with wasting and weakness of the biceps and triceps, may produce a characteristic "Popeye" appearance due to the relative prominence of the forearm (Freeman et al., 2004).

Mild restrictive lung disease occurs in approximately 50% of patients. Cardiac complications are rare.

Laboratory studies reveal serum CK levels that are elevated in most patients, but may be within normal limits. The EMG typically demonstrates nonspecific myopathic features in the involved muscles.

Life expectancy, in general, is not adversely affected. There is no specific treatment for FSHMD. Physical therapy and bracing are employed symptomatically. Some patients benefit from surgical fixation of the scapula to facilitate arm abduction.

Oculopharyngeal Muscular Dystrophy

Oculopharyngeal muscular dystrophy (OPMD) is an autosomal dominant disorder. The genetic abnormality in OPMD has been located to chromosome 14. Originally associated with individuals of French-Canadian extraction, OPMD has now been found in a variety of nationalities. The disease manifests later in life, during the fourth to sixth decade.

Initial symptoms are upper eyelid weakness (ptosis) and difficulty swallowing (dysphagia). As the disease progresses, weakness involves other extraocular and proximal skeletal muscles. Dysphagia is the most serious manifestation. Double vision is uncommon. Cardiac muscle is not involved.

Serum CK is generally normal, but may be mildly increased. EMG studies may show mild myopathic features.

Patients are at risk for malnutrition and aspiration. Treatment of OPMD consists of symptomatic measures such as glasses with eyelid crutches, blepharoplasty, cricopharyngeal myotomy, and surgical placement of feeding tubes.

Distal Muscular Dystrophy

Distal myopathies are exceptions to the general rule that myopathies affect mainly proximal muscles. Serum CK is generally normal, or only mildly increased. EMG demonstrates myopathic features that are more prominent in distal muscles. While no specific treatment is available, patients may benefit from the use of AFOs.

Emery–Dreifuss Muscular Dystrophy

EDMD is an X-linked disorder that is clinically distinct from the Duchenne and Becker types of dystrophy. It affects only males, and onset is in adolescence or early adulthood (Freeman et al., 2004).

Clinically, affected men develop progressive muscle weakness and wasting in a humeroperoneal distribution (biceps, triceps, gastrocnemius, and peroneal muscles). This disease is associated with prominent early contractures of the spine, elbows, and ankles. Patients develop contractures of the cervical and lumbar extensor muscles resulting in limitations of neck and trunk flexion. Contractures of the elbow flexors results in limitations of elbow extension. Tightness of the Achilles tendons results in an equinus positioning of the feet and toe walking. EDMD also causes varying degrees of proximal girdle weakness. Patients present with difficulty walking or running or with complaints of spine rigidity.

Cardiac involvement can present with atrial rhythm disturbances, conduction defects, and occasionally complete heart block with sudden death.

No specific treatment is available. Management includes the promotion of ambulation and the prevention of joint contractures or their progression. Cardiac pacemaker placement may be required in patients with severe cardiac involvement. The course of the disease is very slowly progressive although cardiac involvement can be life-threatening.

Myotonic Dystrophies

Myotonic dystrophy is a slowly progressive, dominantly inherited myopathic disorder that usually manifests itself in the third or fourth decade but occasionally appears early in childhood. The genetic defect has been localized to the long arm of chromosome 19 in the type 1 disorder (Brook et al., 1992).

Myotonic dystrophy is characterized clinically by myotonia (a marked delay in muscle relaxation after a contraction). This can be demonstrated by delayed relaxation of the hand after a sustained grip. Patients also exhibit percussion myotonia: thumb adduction following percussing the thenar muscle with a reflex hammer. Patients have characteristic distal muscle weakness and atrophy. Atrophy of the masseter muscles causes what is known as a "hatchet face." Other clinical features include cataracts, frontal baldness, testicular atrophy, diabetes mellitus, cardiac abnormalities, and intellectual changes. Systemic involvement of the disorder is manifested by hypothyroidism, insulin resistance and diabetes, hypofunction of the adrenal glands, and hypogonadism (Kurihara, 2005).

Myotonic dystrophy is diagnosed by the characteristic clinical picture in combination with EMG findings, which reveal myotonic discharges in addition to findings suggestive of myopathy.

Treatment

For treatment of myotonia, sodium channel blockers such as phenytoin are used (Kurihara, 2005). Phenytoin is preferred over other drugs in this class, such as quinine sulfate or procainamide, which can have undesirable effects on cardiac conduction. Unfortunately, even if the myotonia is reduced, sodium channel blockers tend to reduce muscle power and contribute further to muscle weakness (Kurihara, 2005). Dehydroepiandrosterone sulfate, an intravenous steroid given daily, has shown promise in a pilot study to reduce myotonia while maintaining strength (Sugino et al., 1998). Modafinil may be used for excessive daytime sleepiness and has been shown to be effective without cardiovascular complications (MacDonald, Hill, & Tarnopolsky, 2002). In addition, treatment with gene therapy is on the horizon and therapeutic trials in vitro have been successful (Furling et al., 2003).

There is sparse literature on rehabilitation for patients with myotonic dystrophy. A Cochrane Review concluded that moderate-intensity strength training in this population is not harmful. However, there is insufficient evidence to establish that it offers benefit (van der Kooi, Lindeman, & Riphagen, 2005). Another meta-analysis failed to demonstrate that strength training has a significant effect on people with myotonic dystrophy (Sackley et al., 2009).

Inflammatory Myopathies

The inflammatory myopathies are a heterogeneous group of diseases (Dalakas, 1991). These include the idiopathic inflammatory myopathies and a smaller group caused by identifiable bacterial, mycotic, and viral pathogens. Polymyositis (PM) and dermatomyositis (DM) are generally considered to be multisystem autoimmune diseases. This interpretation is supported by the increased prevalence of certain HLA groups among patients with these inflammatory myopathies, the relatively frequent association with other immunologically mediated disorders, and the favorable response in many patients to immunosuppressive therapy. Microscopically, the association is supported by the results of immunohistochemical and immunocytochemical studies that have been performed on muscle biopsy specimens.

Polymyositis

PM can occur at any age, but it is most common in adults. Women are affected more often than men. The disease begins insidiously, and progresses gradually over a period of weeks to months. There may be spontaneous remissions and relapses.

Symmetrical proximal weakness involving the hip girdle musculature followed by the shoulder girdle is the major clinical manifestation. Neck flexor weakness is seen. Affected muscles are often tender, painful, and swollen. Dysphagia is common and results from involvement of pharyngeal and esophageal muscles. Cardiac involvement, such as cardiomyositis, may lead to congestive heart failure. Respiratory dysfunction caused by interstitial lung disease is found in about 10% of patients.

Serum CK is generally elevated when the disease is active but may decline during remission. Myoglobinuria (muscle breakdown products appearing in the urine) occurs. The erythrocyte sedimentation rate is often elevated, but does not correlate with disease activity. EMG demonstrates a mixture of fibrillations and brief, small amplitude, polyphasic potentials (myopathic pattern). Muscle biopsy shows a variable number of necrotic myofibers.

Dermatomyositis
The distribution of muscle weakness, laboratory findings, and electromyographic abnormalities in DM is similar to that encountered in patients with PM. Skin lesions are the main clinical features that distinguish DM from PM. Most common are a heliotrope discoloration of the eyelids and an erythematous rash over the face, neck, and chest.

DM is more common in children than adults. Malignant neoplasms, especially carcinomas of the lung, breast, and gastrointestinal tract, may occur with adult cases of DM. Muscle biopsy specimens show a distinctive pattern of myofiber atrophy described as perifascicular.

Treatment of Inflammatory Myopathies
The treatment of both PM and DM is similar. High-dose daily oral prednisone (1 mg/kg) is a common initial therapeutic strategy to reduce the burden of inflammation as quickly as possible. Once weakness has begun to resolve, the prednisone dosage is gradually tapered to limit toxicity. Steroids are begun in conjunction with a maintenance drug such as azathioprine or methotrexate for a "steroid-sparing" effect and to prevent relapses during prednisone tapering (Hengstman, van den Hoogen, & van Engelen, 2009). If the disease is not under control with azathioprine or methotrexate, high-dose intravenous immune globulin can be effective (Saito et al., 2008). If this fails to control the disease process, and the patient's condition is rapidly deteriorating, other therapies such as rituximab, tacrolimus, and mycophenolate mofetil have shown promise in small studies (Chung, Genovese, & Fiorentino, 2007; Hassan, Ven der Net, & Van Royan-Kerkhof, 2008; Pisoni, Cuadrado, Khamashta, Hughes, & D'Cruz, 2007). Patients with severe pulmonary involvement are treated acutely with high-dose intravenous methylprednisone. Results may be improved by administering pulsed intravenous cyclophosphamide and cyclosporin A (Kameda et al., 2005).

Beyond medications, exercise and nutritional supplements can reduce morbidity. Many patients and physicians are afraid to initiate an exercise program due to the fear that it might induce a relapse. However, studies have demonstrated the safety and efficacy of submaximal exercise programs to improve endurance in patients with chronic PM or DM (Alexanderson, 2009). Patients with chronic disease can tolerate intensive resistive training which results in improved muscle strength and endurance. Exercise training should begin at a low intensity and increase as muscle function improves. Isotonic muscle training at a submaximal level has been found to improve muscle strength and respiratory function. It has not been found to induce relapses of the disease (Varju, Petho, Kutas, & Czirjak, 2003). Strengthening exercises, in combination with aerobic exercises, have been shown to have a positive effect on body functions as well as on the level of activity participation in patients with inflammatory myopathies (Wiesinger et al., 1998). In addition, as treatment with high-dose corticosteroids predisposes these patients to a reduced bone density, loss of skeletal muscle mass, and type II diabetes, physical activity is especially important. The intensity of exercise can be adapted to the level of disease activity, the degree of muscle impairment, and the aerobic capacity.

In addition, combining physical exercise programs with oral creatine supplementation in the first 6 months following the acute phase of PM/DM can lead to superior outcomes (Chung et al., 2007).

Metabolic Myopathies
The metabolic myopathies are a heterogeneous group of disorders affecting all aspects of muscle metabolism. These include carbohydrate myopathies, lipid myopathies, mitochondrial myopathies, endocrine myopathies, and myalgic syndromes. The endocrine myopathies often have a treatable cause.

ENDOCRINE MYOPATHY. Muscle dysfunction is identified in a wide variety of endocrine disorders. Myopathy occurs frequently in hyperthyroidism. Muscle weakness, cramps, pain, and stiffness are common complaints, though objective muscle weakness is uncommon. The serum CK is generally not elevated. Nonspecific myopathic features are commonly found on EMG and in muscle biopsy specimens. Symptoms resolve with successful treatment of the underlying thyroid disorder.

Patients with hyperparathyroidism may have mild generalized muscle weakness. Clinically, hyperparathyroid myopathy presents with proximal weakness and wasting, occasional bulbar weakness, and preserved or even brisk reflexes. Serum CK is usually normal.

Muscle weakness, fatigue, and cramping are also frequent symptoms in patients with Addison's disease. Occasionally, the associated weakness is severe and it may be episodic. Treatment requires glucocorticoid and mineralocorticoid replacement and correction of the associated electrolyte abnormalities.

Patients with hyperaldosteronism may present with attacks of periodic paralysis and associated hypokalemia. Muscle weakness is a symptom in over 70% of these patients, but will cease if the underlying cause is corrected.

Muscle weakness occurs frequently in Cushing's syndrome and in patients exposed to glucocorticoids. The muscle weakness of steroid myopathy is typically insidious in onset and affects primarily proximal muscles. Serum CK is usually normal. EMG may show minor myopathic changes.

EXERCISE AND NEUROMUSCULAR DISEASE

With neuromuscular diseases, it is often beneficial to provide low levels of physical activity (not clearly defined as exercise) that can slowly improve endurance. Aerobic training can improve the cardiopulmonary status of patients with neuromuscular disease; however, the intensity and type of training prescribed depends on the type, stage, and severity of the disease. Research studies have shown that individuals who are mildly affected by their disease can significantly benefit from exercise. Exercise can help reverse the deconditioning caused by the neuromuscular disease and yield such positive health benefits as maintaining a healthy weight, improving energy, and boosting self-esteem. Unfortunately, persons with more severe forms of their disease may not respond as well to aerobic exercise (Abresch, Han, & Carter, 2009).

When prescribing strengthening programs to patient with neuromuscular diseases, one should begin before significant weakness has evolved and focus on muscles with greater than antigravity strength. It is important to periodically monitor muscle strength to assess for possible overwork weakness, especially in unsupervised programs. This can be accomplished using quantitative strength measures (e.g., a handheld dynamometer).

Most current knowledge about exercise training in neuromuscular disease is based on short-term, uncontrolled or nonrandomized studies with few subjects. There is a need for more high-quality, randomized controlled trials with large sample sizes analyzing the effects of exercise training on rehabilitation. Future research will enhance our understanding of and confidence in the role of exercise and physical activity as an integral part of the rehabilitation of people with neuromuscular disorders.

SUMMARY

Neuromuscular disorders are a complex group of disorders that afflict both the young and the old. Those affected are often in the prime of their life. These disorders are often progressive and sometimes fatal. They may result in weakness and impaired mobility as well as in difficulty performing basic self-care skills. The impact on one's quality of life can be devastating. As such, management of these disorders requires an interdisciplinary team of specialists encompassing physiatrists; nurses; physical, occupational, and speech therapists; psychologists; vocational counselors; and social workers. These diseases, although not curable, do respond to rehabilitation. An effective rehabilitation program is critical not only for maintaining a patient's quality of life but also for optimizing one's physical and psychosocial function.

REFERENCES

Abresch, R. T., Han, J. J., & Carter, G. T. (2009). Rehabilitation management of neuromuscular disease: The role of exercise training. *Neuromuscular Disease, 11*, 7–21.

Alexanderson, H. (2009). Exercise effects in patients with adult idiopathic inflammatory myopathies. *Current Opinions in Rheumatology, 21*, 158–163.

American Academy of Neurology Quality Standards Subcommittee. (1997). Practice advisory on the treatment of amyotrophic lateral sclerosis with riluzole: Report of the quality. *Neurology, 49*, 657–659.

Armon, C. (2004). Occurrence of amyotrophic lateral sclerosis among Gulf War veterans. *Neurology, 62*, 1027.

Atroshi, I., Gummesson, C., Johnsson, R., & Sprinchorn, A. (1999). Prevalence of carpal tunnel syndrome in a general population. *JAMA, 282*, 153.

Bachmann, K., Burkhardt, D., Schreiter, I., Kaifi, J., Schurr, P., Busch, C., et al. (2009). Thymectomy is more effective than conservative treatment for myasthenia gravis regarding outcome and clinical improvement. *Surgery, 145*, 392–398.

Bastron, J. A., & Thomas, J. E. (1981). Diabetic polyradiculopathy: Clinical and electromyographic findings in 105 patients. *Mayo Clinic Proceedings, 56*, 725.

Bello-Haas, V. D., Florence, J. M., Kloos, A. D., Scheirbecker, J., Lopate, G., Hayes, S. M., et al. (2007). A randomized controlled trial of resistance exercise in individuals with ALS. *Neurology, 68*, 2003–2007.

Bello-Haas, V. D., Florence, J. M., & Krivickas, L. S. (2008). Therapeutic exercise for people with amyotrophic lateral sclerosis or motor neuron disease. *Cochrane Database of Systematic Reviews*, CD005229.

Bonilla, E., Samitt, C. E., Miranda, A. F., Hays, A. P., Salviati, G., DiMauro, S., et al. (1988). Duchenne muscular dystrophy: Deficiency of dystrophin at the muscle cell surface. *Cell, 54*, 447–452.

Boninger, M. L., & Leonard, J. A., Jr. (1996). Use of bivalve ankle-foot orthosis in neuropathic foot and ankle lesions. *Journal of Rehabilitation Research and Development, 33*, 16–19.

Borasio, G. D., & Voltz, R. (1997). Palliative care in amyotrophic lateral sclerosis. *Journal of Neurology, 244*(Suppl. 4), S11–S17.

Borasio, G. D., Voltz, R., & Miller, R. G. (2001). Palliative care in amyotrophic lateral sclerosis. *Neurologic Clinics, 19*, 829.

Brook, J. D., McCurrach, M. E., Harley, H. G., Buckler, A. J., Church, D., Aburatani, H., et al. (1992). Molecular basis of myotonic dystrophy: Expansion of a trinucleotide (CTG) repeat at the 3′ end of a transcript encoding a protein kinase family member. *Cell, 68*, 799–808.

Brooks, B. R. (1998). Clinical epidemiology of ALS. In J. E. Riggs (Ed.), *Neurology clinics* (Vol. 14, pp. 399–420). Philadelphia: W. B. Saunders.

Brooks, B. R., Thisted, R. A., Appel, S. H., Bradley, W. G., Olney, R. K, Berg, J. E., et al. (2004). Treatment of pseudobulbar affect in ALS with dextromethorphan/quinidine: A randomized trial. *Neurology, 63*, 1364.

Carter, G. T. (2005). Rehabilitation management of peripheral neuropathy. *Seminars in Neurology, 25*, 229–237.

Carter, G. T., Kikuchi, N., Abresch, R. T., Walsh, S. A., Horasek, S. J., & Fowler, W. M., Jr. (1994). Effects of exhaustive concentric and eccentric exercise on murine skeletal muscle. *Archives of Physical Medicine and Rehabilitation, 75*, 555–559.

Castaigne, P., Rondot, M., Fardeau, M., Cathala, H. P., Ribadeau-Dumas, J. L., & Dudognon, P. (1977). Lambert-Eaton myasthenic syndrome: Clinical electrophysiological, histologic and ultrastructural studies. *Reviews in Neurology (Paris), 133*, 513.

Chung, Y. L., Alexanderson, H., Pipitone, N., Morrison, C., Dastmalchi, M., Ståhl Hallengren, C., et al. (2007). Creatine supplements in patients with idiopathic inflammatory myopathies who are clinically weak after conventional pharmacologic treatment: Six-month, double-blind, randomized, placebo-controlled trial. *Arthritis and Rheumatism, 57*, 694–702.

Chung, L., Genovese, M. C., & Fiorentino, D. F. (2007). A pilot trial of rituximab in the treatment of patients with dermatomyositis. *Archives of Dermatology, 143,* 763–767.

Dalakas, M. C. (1991). Polymyositis, dermatomyositis, and inclusion-body myositis. *New England Journal of Medicine, 325,* 1487–1498.

Daly, J. J., & Wolpaw, J. R. (2008). Brain–computer interfaces in neurological rehabilitation. *Lancet Neurology, 7,* 1032–1043.

Dau, P. C. (1982). Plasmapheresis in myasthenia gravis. *Progress in Clinical Biological Research, 8,* 265–285.

Dawson, D. M., & Krarup, C. (1989). Perioperative nerve lesions. *Archives of Neurology, 46,* 1355.

Dodds, S. D., & Wolfe, S. W. (2000). Perinatal brachial plexus palsy. *Current Opinions in Pediatrics, 12,* 40.

Dumitru, D. (1995). *Electrodiagnostic medicine.* Philadelphia: Hanley & Belfus.

Dyck, P. J., Giannini, C., & Lais, A. (1993). Pathologic alterations of nerves. In P. J. Dyck, P. K. Thomas, J. W. Griffin, P. A. Low, & J. Podusco (Eds.), *Peripheral neuropathy* (3rd ed., p. 514). Philadelphia: W. B. Saunders.

Fornai, F., Longone, P., Cafaro, L., Kastsiuchenka, O., Ferrucci, M., Manca, M. L., et al. (2008). Lithium delays progression of amyotrophic lateral sclerosis. *Proceedings of the National Academy of Sciences of the United States of America, 105,* 2052–2057.

Freeman T. L., Johnson, E., Freeman, E. D., & Brown, D. P. (2004). Electrodiagnostic medicine and clinical neuromuscular physiology. In S. J. Cuccurullo (Ed.), *Physical medicine and rehabilitation board review* (pp. 295–308). New York: Demos Medical.

Fregonezi, G. A., Resqueti, V. R., Guell, R., Pradas, J., & Casan, P. (2005). Effects of 8 week, interval-based inspiratory muscle training and breathing retraining in patients with generalized myasthenia gravis. *Chest, 128,* 1524–1530.

Furling, D., Doucet, G., Langlois, M. A., Timchenko, L., Belanger, E., Cossette, L., et al. (2003). Viral vector producing antisense RNA restores myotonic dystrophy myoblast functions. *Gene Therapy, 10,* 795–802.

Gold, R., & Schneider-Gold, C. (2008). Current and future standards in treatment of myasthenia gravis. *Neurotherapeutics, 5,* 535–541.

Gutmann, L., Crosby, T. W., Takamori, M., & Martin, J. D. (1972). The Eaton-Lambert syndrome and autoimmune disorders. *American Journal of Medicine, 53,* 354.

Hahn, F., Hauser, D. Espinosa, N., Blumenthal, S., & Min, K. (2008). Scoliosis correction with pedicle screws in Duchenne muscular dystrophy. *European Spine Journal, 17*(2), 255–261.

Haley, R. W. (2003). Excess incidence of ALS in young Gulf War veterans. *Neurology, 61,* 750.

Hassan, J., Ven der Net, J. J., & Van Royan-Kerkhof, A. (2008). Treatment of refractory juvenile dermatomyositis with tacrolimus. *Clinical Rheumatology, 27,* 1469–1471.

Hengstman, G. J. D., van den Hoogen, F. J. J, & van Engelen, B. G. M. (2009). Treatment of the inflammatory myopathies: Update and practical recommendations. *Expert Opinion on Pharmacotherapy, 10,* 1183–1190.

Horner, R. D., Kamins, K. G., Feussner, J. R., Grambow, S. C., Hoff-Lindquist, J., Harati, Y., et al. (2003). Occurrence of amyotrophic lateral sclerosis among Gulf War veterans. *Neurology, 61,* 742.

Ionasescu, V. V., Burns, T. L., Searby, C., & Ionasescu, R. (1988). X-linked dominant Charcot-Marie-Tooth neuropathy with 15 cases in a family genetic linkage study. *Muscle Nerve, 11,* 1154–1156.

Ionasescu, V. V., Ionasescu, R., & Searby, C. (1993). Screening of dominantly inherited Charcot-Marie-Tooth neuropathies. *Muscle Nerve, 16,* 1232–1238.

Jani-Acsadi, A., Krajewski, K., & Shy, M. E. (2008). Charcot-Marie-Tooth neuropathies: Diagnosis and management. *Seminars in Neurology, 28,* 185–194.

Kalra S., Cahman N. R., Caramanos Z., Genge, A., & Arnold, D. L. (2003). Gabapentin therapy for amyotrophic lateral sclerosis: Lack of improvement in neuronal integrity shown by MR spectroscopy. *American Journal of Neuroradiology, 24*(3), 476–480.

Kameda, H., Nagasawa, H., Ogawa, H., Sekiguchi, N., Takei, H., Tokuhira, M., et al. (2005). Combination therapy with corticosteroids, cyclosporin A, and intravenous pulse cyclophosphamide for acute/subacute interstitial pneumonia in patients with dermatomyositis. *The Journal of Rheumatology, 32,* 1719–1726.

Kilmer, D. D., McCrory, M. A., Wright, N. C., Aitkens, S. G., & Bernauer, E. M. (1994). The effect of a high resistance exercise program in slowly progressive neuromuscular disease. *Archives of Physical Medicine and Rehabilitation, 75,* 560–563.

Kurihara, T. (1995). New classification and treatment for myotonic disorders. *Internal Medicine, 44,* 1027–1032.

Lindeman, E., Leffers, P., Spaans, F., Drukker, J., Reulen, J., Kerckhoffs, M., et al. (1995). Strength training in patients with myotonic dystrophy & hereditary motor & sensory neuropathy: A randomized clinical trial. *Archives of Physical Medicine and Rehabilitation, 76,* 612–620.

MacDonald, J. R., Hill, J. D., & Tarnopolsky, M. A. (2002). Modafinil reduces excessive somnolence and enhances mood in patients with myotonic dystrophy. *Neurology, 59,* 1876–1880.

Manzur, A. Y., Kuntzer, T., Pike, M., & Swan, A. (2008). Glucocorticoid corticosteroids for Duchenne muscular dystrophy. *Cochrane Database of Systematic Reviews, 23*(1), CD003725.

Meriggioli, M. N. (2009). Myasthenia gravis with anti-acetylcholine receptor antibodies. *Frontiers of Neurology and Neuroscience, 26,* 94–108.

Miller, R. G., Mitchell, J. D., Lyon, M., & Moore, D. H. (2002). Riluzole for amyotrophic lateral sclerosis (ALS)/motor neuron disease (MND). *Cochrane Database of Systematic Reviews,* CD001447.

Mitsumoto, H. (1997). Diagnosis and progression of ALS. *Neurology, 48*(Suppl. 4), S2–S8.

Mouly, V., Aamiri, A., Perie, S., Mamchaoui, K., Barani, A., Bigot, A., et al. (2005). Myoblast transfer therapy: Is there any light at the end of the tunnel? *Acta Myologica, 24*(2), 128–133.

Pareyson, D., Schenone, A., Fabrizi, G. M., Santoro, L., Padua, L., Quattrone, A., et al. (2006). A multi-center, randomized, double-blind, placebo-controlled trial of long-term ascorbic acid treatment in Charcot-Marie-Tooth disease type 1A (CMT-TRIAAL): The study protocol. *Pharmacological Research, 54,* 436–441.

Passage, E., Norreel, J. C., Noack-Fraissignes, P., Sanguedolce, V., Pizant, J., Thirion, X., et al. (2004). Ascorbic acid treatment corrects the phenotype of a mouse model of Charcot-Marie-Tooth disease. *Nature Medicine, 10,* 396–401.

Paulson, L. E., & Kilmer, D. D. (2001). Orthotic management in peripheral neuropathy. *Physical Medicine and Rehabilitation Clinics of North America, 12,* 433–445.

Phukan, J., & Hardiman, O. (2009). The management of amyotrophic lateral sclerosis. *Journal of Neurology, 256,* 176–186.

Pisoni, C. N., Cuadrado, M. J., Khamashta, M. A., Hughes, G. R., & D'Cruz, D. P. (2007). Myocophenolate mofetil treatment in resistant myositis. *Rheumatology (Oxford), 46,* 516–518.

Post-Polio Syndrome Fact Sheet. (2008). In National Institute of Neurological Disorders and Stroke. Retrieved from http://www.ninds.nih.gov

Russell, J. W., & Windebank, A. J. (1994). Brachial and lumbar neuropathies. *Bailliere's Clinical Neurology, 3,* 173–191.

Sackley, C., Disler, P. B., Turner-Stokes, L., Wade, D. T., Brittle, N., & Hoppitt, T. (2009). Rehabilitation interventions for foot drop in neuromuscular disease. *Cochrane Database of Systematic Reviews,* CD003908.

Sahenk, Z., Nagaraja, H. N., McCracken, B. S., King, W. M., Freimer, M. L., Cedarbaum, J. M., et al. (2005). NT-3 promotes nerve regeneration and sensory improvement in CMT1A mouse models and in patients. *Neurology, 65,* 681–689.

Saito, E., Koike, T., Hashimoto, H., Miyasaka, N., Ikeda, Y., Hara, M., et al. (2008). Efficacy of high-dose intravenous immunoglobulin therapy in Japanese patients with steroid-resistant polymyositis and dermatomyositis. *Modern Rheumatology, 18,* 34–44.

Shields, R. W. (1994). Limb girdle syndromes. In A. G. Engel & C. Franzini-Armstrong (Eds.), *Myology, basic and clinical* (2nd ed., pp. 1258–1274). New York: McGraw-Hill.

Shy, M. E., Dyck, P. J., Chance, P. F., Lupski, J. R., & Klein, C. J. (2005). Hereditary motor and sensory neuropathies. In P. J. Dyck, & P. K. Thomas (Eds.). *Peripheral neuropathy* (pp. 1623–1658). Philadelphia: W. B. Saunders.

Sicuranza, M. J., & McCue, F. C., III. (1992). Compressive neuropathies in the upper extremity of athletes. *Hand Clinic, 8,* 263.

Skre, H. (1974). Genetic and clinical aspects of Charcot-Marie-Tooth disease. *Clinical Genetics, 6,* 98–118.

Sufit, R. (1997). Symptomatic treatment of ALS. *Neurology, 48*(Suppl. 4), S15–22.

Sugino, M., Ohsawa, N., Ito, T., Ishida, S., Yamasaki, H., Kimura, F., et al. (1998). A pilot study of dehydroepiandrosterone sulfate in myotonic dystrophy. *Neurology, 51,* 586–589.

Trojan, D., & Cashman, N. (2005). Post-poliomyelitis syndrome. *Muscle Nerve, 31*(1), 6–19.

van der Kooi, E. L., Lindeman, E., & Riphagen, I. (2005). Strength training and aerobic exercise training for muscle disease. *Cochrane Database of Systematic Reviews,* CD003907.

Varju, C., Petho, E., Kutas, R., & Czirjak, L. (2003). The effect of physical exercise following acute disease exacerbation in patients with dermato/polymyositis. *Clinical Rehabilitation, 17,* 83–87.

Weisskopf, M. G., O'Reilly, E. J., McCullough, M. L., Calle, E. E., Thun, M. J., Cudkowicz, M., et al. (2005). Prospective study of military service and mortality from ALS. *Neurology, 64,* 32.

Wiesinger, G. F., Quittan, M., Aringer, M., Seeber, A., Volc-Platzer, B., Smolen, J., et al. (1998). Improvement of physical fitness and muscle strength in polymyositis/dermatomyositis patients in a training programme. *British Journal of Rheumatology, 37,* 196–200.

Young, P., De Jonghe, P., Stogbauer, F., & Butterfass-Bahloul, T. (2008). Treatment for Charcot-Marie-Tooth disease. *Cochrane Database of Systematic Reviews, Issue 1,* Art no.: CD006052.

15

Musculoskeletal Disorders

Joseph E. Herrera, DO, FAAPMR, Jung Woo Ma, MD,
and Pete-Gaye Nation, MD

INTRODUCTION

Musculoskeletal disorders (MSDs) are ergonomic injuries affecting muscles, nerves, tendons, joints, cartilage, or spinal discs. Injuries caused by slips, trips, falls, motor vehicle accidents, or similar incidents are not considered MSDs (Bureau of Labor Statistics, 2008). Occupational overuse syndrome (OOS), cumulative trauma disorder (CTD), and repetitive strain injury (RSI) are other terms used to describe MSDs (Boocock et al., 2009). Although these terms offer a strictly physical cause for MSD, the World Health Organization (WHO) noted that MSDs occur due to multiple factors. These include physical, workplace organization, psychosocial, individual, and sociocultural. It is the factors other than the physical that make treating MSDs challenging.

MSDs are the leading sources of work-related injuries, days away from work, and workers compensation claims. It affects the overall workforce and has proven to be a major economic concern. In the United States, MSDs represent 40% of compensated cases and costs between $45 and $54 billion per year (Denis, St-Vincent, Imbeau, Jetté, & Nastasia, 2008). According to the Bureau of Labor Statistics (BLS), in 2007, the incidence rate of injuries due to MSD for all industries is 35 cases per 10,000 workers. Nursing aides, orderlies, and attendants had 44,930 days-away-from-work and a rate of 465 cases per 10,000 workers. Laborers and freight, stock, and material movers experienced the highest number of days-away-from-work, with 79,000 in 2007. The median number of days-away-from-work for all industries was 7 days in 2007. Mining had a median of 27 days-away-from-work, which is four times the median for all industries. The age of the worker also affects the number of days-away-from-work. Workers of age 65 and older experienced the longest absences from work with a median of 16 days. Workers of age 16–24 had a median of 4 days-away-from-work (Bureau of Labor Statistics, 2008).

The most common MSDs occur to the low back, shoulder, and wrist. Injuries to these areas result in 20 mean days away from work (Bureau of Labor Statistics, 2008). Repetitive injuries result in the following diagnosis: lumbago, lumbar strain sprain, lumbar radiculopathy, lumbar degenerative disc disease (DDD), shoulder tendinopathy, rotator cuff syndrome, shoulder joint disorder, carpal tunnel syndrome (CTS), and median nerve disorder. Although there are other conditions that result in work-related disability, this chapter will focus on the most common MSDs affecting the working population.

LOW BACK PAIN

Low back pain (LBP) remains the leading cause of work-related disability and loss of productivity (Ammendolia et al., 2009; Bureau of Labor Statistics, 2008; Stewart, Ricci, Chee, Morganstein, & Lipton, 2003; Waddell, 2004). The lifetime prevalence of LBP ranges from 54% to 80% (Hardt, Jacobsen, Goldberg, Nickel, & Buchwald, 2008; Manchikanti, Singh, Datta, Cohen, & Hirsch, 2009; Shelerud, 2006). Spinal pain remains the most common cause of disability for workers younger than 45 years. In the general population, prevalence of LBP is 12–30% and the incidence is 51–70%. In the occupational (working) population the type of work performed dictates the overall incidence. For example, 35% of sedentary workers injure their low back, whereas heavy laborers experience a rate of 47%. Interestingly, 10% of workers with LBP consume 75–80% of medical costs and compensation payments (Bureau of Labor Statistics, 2008; Shelerud, 2006). In the United States, 1% of adults are disabled temporarily, and 1% are disabled chronically as a result of LBP at any one time. Approximately 400,000 compensated back injuries occur each year (Andersson, 1998; Bureau of Labor Statistics, 2008; Deyo & Tsui-Wu, 1987; Frymoyer & Cats-Baril, 1991; Shelerud, 2006), accounting for a significant overall economic impact on disability.

According to recent data published by the BLS, the total number of MSDs reported was 1,158,870, in 2007. Back pain accounted for 471,920, or 41% of the total number of MSD-related injuries. The industries most affected are those involved in lifting and pushing. Health care workers were most affected, occurring primarily from lifting and transferring patients. Miners were the second most common group affected (Bureau of Labor Statistics, 2008).

Etiology and Role of the Workplace Physical Activities

LBP is a disorder with multiple etiologies. Although the physical component receives most of the attention, there are several factors that can make treating back pain confusing and ambiguous. Those factors include occupational, nonoccupational, emotional, and psychosocial issues (Cohen, Argoff, & Carragee, 2008; Feyer et al., 2000; Mannion, Dolan, & Adams, 1996; Truchon, Côté, Fillion, Arsenault, & Dionne, 2008). Specific job activities such as pulling, pushing, carrying, prolonged standing, and sitting are obvious risk factors for back pain. Somewhat less obvious activities, such as monotonous repetitive movement, job load, and stress, can also be associated with back pain (Hardt et al., 2008; Manchikanti et al., 2009). Seemingly simple activities, such as operating a motor vehicle, has been shown to increase the incidence of pain and spinal degeneration, which is believed to be due to the vibration that is transmitted to the spine (Kelsey & Hardy, 1975).

Nonoccupational risk factors for back pain include gender, age, obesity, and smoking. Women have been found to be more susceptible to back pain as compared with men (Bureau of Labor Statistics, 2008; Nagi, Burk, & Potter, 1965). Age has a role in return to work from an injury. On average, workers 65 years and older take three times longer to return to work as compared with workers aged 24–65 (Bureau of Labor Statistics, 2008). There are several studies that associate obesity with LBP. The combination of increase in weight and the shift of the center of gravity anteriorly places increased stress on the spine, predisposing a person to injury (Böstman, 1993; Deyo & Bass, 1989; Wai, Rodriguez, Dagenais, & Hall, 2008). Smoking has been found to increase the amount of neuropeptides that are responsible for pain. Neuropeptides are neuronal signaling molecules that influence the activity and function of the brain. Substance P and PGE2 are examples of inflammatory neuropeptides that increase the perception of pain. Substance P is increased in the cerebrospinal fluid of smokers, likely contributing to worker disability. Compounding the adverse impact of smoking is the fact that the amount of β-endorphins, also known as the "feel good" neuropeptides, are decreased in smokers (Böstman, 1993; del Arbol et al., 2000; Deyo & Bass, 1989; Vaerøy, Helle, Førre, Kåss, & Terenius, 1988; Wai et al., 2008).

Emotional and psychosocial factors play an important role in onset of back pain and return to work from such an injury. Psychological factors such as depression, anxiety, fear of movement, somatization are all risk factors for back pain. Somatization disorder is a condition in which a person has physical symptoms that are caused by psychological problems, and no physical cause can be found. Job satisfaction and happiness in the work place has also been found to be a key predictor for length of time out due to an injury. The number of days out of work increases if these psychological components are present and if job satisfaction is low (Cohen et al., 2008; Feyer et al., 2000).

Pathophysiology/Clinical Presentation

Diagnosing and finding a definitive pain generator in the lumbar spine is a challenging but important process. A thorough history and neuromusculoskeletal physical examination provide important clinical clues that will guide treatment and distinguish between emergent and nonemergent cases. In 85% of patients that present with LBP, the definitive pain generator is not identified (Deyo, Cherkin, Conrad, & Volinn, 1992). These challenges stem from the weak association of symptoms to physical examination findings, pathological changes, and imaging. Diagnosis depends on the history and physical examination findings and ranges from lumbar strain/sprain, myalgia, lumbar radiculopathy, lumbar DDD, sacroiliac (SI) joint dysfunction, and lumbar spondylosis. The multiple possible sources of pain make it challenging for the clinician to narrow it to one source, thus making a definitive diagnosis even more difficult.

There are multiple potential sources of pain in the lumbar spine. Acute pain that is localized to the low back region is most often caused by lumbar sprain/strain. The patient may present with pain localized to the lower back with or without muscle spasm (Mense & Simons, 2001). Lumbar sprain indicates an injury to the musculature, whereas lumbar strain points to ligamentous injury. Distinguishing between the two possible sources is difficult and ultimately with no clinical benefit as it will not impact treatment options (Anonymous, 1987; Meleger & Krivickas, 2007).

When pain localized to the lumbar region lasts for more than a few weeks, further investigation is needed to determine its cause, which may include facet-mediated pain, fracture, or discogenic pain. Facet joints, also known as the zygoapophaseal joints, are the small joints that connect one vertebral body to another vertebral body. There are two joints per spinal level that provide stability and allow limited movement of the spine. The joints can be a source of pain due to degenerative changes (also known as facet arthrosis and spondylosis), fracture, or dislocation. If the joints are compromised, spondylolisthesis, which is the slippage of one vertebral body on another, can occur leading to an unstable spine. Discogenic pain refers to spinal discs that are found to be painful. Discs are located between two vertebral bodies and consist of the outer layers of fibers known as the annulus fibrosis and an inner jelly-like substance known as the nucleus pulposis. Degenerative changes and/or tears to the layer of fibers can cause the disc to be a source of pain.

Pain that is localized to the spine is mediated through the sinuvertebral nerves and the posterior rami of the spinal nerves. The sinuvertebral nerves supply structures within the spinal canal. These nerves arise from the rami communicantes and enter the spinal canal by way of the intervertebral foramina. Branches ascend and descend one or more levels interconnecting with the sinuvertebral nerves from other levels and innervating the anterior and posterior longitudinal ligaments, the anterior and posterior portion of the dura mater, and blood vessels, among other structures. This system also may supply nociceptive branches to degenerated intervertebral disks. Branches of the posterior rami of the spinal nerves provide nociceptive fibers to the fascia, ligaments, periosteum, and facet joints (Groen, Baljet, & Drukker, 1990).

Pain that radiates into the lower extremity indicates nerve root impingement. Nerve root impingement commonly occurs from compromised discs but can also occur from ligament hypertrophy, facet arthrosis, and spondylolisthesis. When symptoms include neurological findings, such as weakness, paresthesias, numbness, tingling, and bowel and bladder compromise, immediate investigation is indicated. Radiating or radicular pain is mediated not by the sinuvertebral nerves or the posterior rami of the spinal nerves but rather by compression of nerves as they enter or leave the spine. Two major factors are involved in the generation of radicular-based radiating pain: compression and inflammation (Devereaux, 2009). Compressive forces result from displaced intervertebral disc, hypertrophied ligaments, and/ or facet spondylosis. Compressive forces also produce nerve injury and release of inflammatory factors that mediate pain. Other inflammatory factors, such as substance P are also released from the nucleus pulposis causing further neural injury.

Diagnostic Studies

Diagnostic tests are a compliment to a thorough history and physical examination, the latter two dictating which tests to order. Diagnostic tests range from plain X-rays, magnetic resonance imaging (MRI), electromyography nerve conduction studies (EMG/NCS), and interventional procedures such as discograms and medial branch blocks. X-rays and MRIs are the most common diagnostic imaging tools used to diagnose lumbar-related disorders. However, they often reveal abnormalities that have no bearing on patient symptoms, as several studies show that asymptomatic patients will have abnormal findings in both imaging modalities, making a carefully obtained history and physical examination extremely important (Jensen et al., 1994; van Tulder, Assendelft, Koes, & Bouter, 1997; Videman et al., 2003). MRIs are most useful when imaging correlates to the patient's symptoms and clinical findings. For example, a herniated disc found on an MRI that corresponds to neurological findings such as weakness and specific patterns of sensory deficits helps to confirm the diagnosis. EMG/NCS is a very sensitive test that detects abnormalities in the nerves and the muscles. It is useful in diagnosing peripheral nerve injuries, neuropathies, radiculopathies, and plexopathies. Injuries to nerves that result from pathology of the spine may be confirmed by EMG/NCS, particularly if patient symptoms and physical examination findings correspond to their results. If positive it further confirms diagnosis. EMG/NCS is most useful when trying to differentiate the cause of pain from multiple possibilities, such as peripheral neuropathy, brachial plexopathy, or myopathy.

Differentiating LBP from facet mediated and discogenic is difficult. The difficulty arises from the sensitivity of both X-rays and MRIs in detecting pathology not associated with patient symptoms. Both facet spondylosis and disc degeneration are often seen on MRIs and X-rays in asymptomatic patients. Interventional procedures such as discography and medial branch blocks are useful tools that will help to confirm the diagnosis. Lumbar discography is used to diagnose discogenic pain and was first described by Lindblom (1948). Using fluoroscopic guidance, a needle is introduced into the disc's nucleus pulposis and then injected with contrast dye. The dye increases the pressure in the disc. If the patient's familiar pain is reproduced, it is believed that the disc is the source of pain. Because of the various techniques with which this tool was used, it had fallen out of favor. More recent stringent criteria, such as the use of a pressure manometer and the absence of any sedation, increases the reliability of the test (Lee, Derby, Chen, Seo, & Kim, 2004; Seo et al., 2007). The pressure manometer measures the pressure within the disc as the dye is being injected. Discography is useful in guiding treatment, such as the need for surgical intervention

Comparative medial branch blocks are used to diagnose facet-mediated pain. The medial branches are the nerve fibers that innervate each individual facet joint. Each joint is innervated by two separate medial branches, for example, the L4–5 facet joint is innervated by the L3 and L4 medial branches. Performing a nerve block with the use of lidocaine or bupivicaine will anesthetize the nerve fibers. If the patient experiences pain relief after the block, the facet joint that was targeted is believed to be the source of pain. Pain relief is indicative of a positive test. This test will guide treatment (Leonardi, Pfirrmann, & Boos, 2006; Pevsner, Shabat, Catz, Folman, & Gepstein, 2003; Sehgal, Dunbar, Shah, & Colson, 2007).

Treatment, Return to Work, Prevention

Treatment options for back pain depend on clinical presentation and severity. For most acute back pain treatment with medications such nonsteriodal antiinflammatory drugs (NSAIDs), analgesics, muscle relaxants, opioids, and physical therapy are more than sufficient. Eighty percent of acute symptoms resolve within days to a week (Andersson, 1998; Deyo & Bass, 1989; Deyo & Tsui-Wu, 1987; Deyo et al., 1992). Most workers with back injuries usually return to work within 4–7 days (Bureau of Labor Statistics, 2008; Deyo & Tsui-Wu, 1987). When the pain lasts for a prolonged period of time and the patient fails conservative treatment, spinal interventions and surgery become the option.

Spinal intervention options for treatment of LBP include epidural steroid injections, facet joint injections, medial branch blocks, and SI joint injections. Surgical options include discectomy, fusion, and laminectomy. The use of these options to address spinal-mediated pain is useful, but caution should be taken when progressing to more aggressive treatment modalities as emotional and psychosocial issues may be adversely impacting outcomes in certain cases. A multidisciplinary approach that involves psychiatry, physical therapy, and traditional spinal care is ideal to address the multifaceted nature of pain in these cases. If the pain is refractory to the aforementioned treatment, options such as acupuncture, osteopathic manipulation, and massage therapy may provide some benefit.

Return to work after completion of treatment can be difficult. Developing a treatment plan with realistic expectations is usually the key. Educating the patient that return to work with residual symptoms is acceptable (Waddell & Burton, 2001). For example, it is not unusual for patients to return to work with restrictions and while continuing treatment. Restrictions may range from limited lifting, pushing, and pulling. However, return to work is impacted by job-specific activities. Therefore, a detailed history of job-specific responsibilities is important. A functional capacity evaluation (FCE) may be needed to evaluate other work options that patients may have if their current job responsibilities do not allow them to return. The FCE is performed by a licensed physical therapist and is a standardized way to collect information regarding the patient's physical abilities to determine whether or not they can return to their job.

Although an accurate diagnosis and thoughtful treatment plan is important, the best option is injury prevention. Prevention usually occurs with education of proper lifting and ergonometric evaluation. Ergonometric evaluations ensure the proper position of equipment to minimize any work-related injuries. Correct computer monitor height and appropriate seating are examples of changes that may result from an ergonometric evaluation. Worksite physical activity programs seem to be a feasible way of conducting primary prevention. Both strength training and all-round physical exercise have proven effective for relieve of musculoskeletal pain symptoms (Burton, Balagué, & Cardon, 2005; Nikander, 2006; Proper, 2003).

SHOULDER PAIN

Shoulder injuries account for the second most common cause of MSDs (Bureau of Labor Statistics, 2008). MSDs involving shoulder injuries encompass a wide array of disorders that are frequently encountered in the medical arena. Shoulder injuries include a variety of disorders including, but not limited to, shoulder impingement syndrome, labral tears, synovitis, rotator cuff tendonitis or tendinopathy, and rotator cuff tears. Shoulder impingement syndrome results from mechanical compression of the rotator cuff tendons under the acromion, particularly when the shoulder is internally rotated and forwardly flexed. Rotator cuff injuries comprise a continuum of disorders ranging from tendinitis to complete tears.

Epidemiology

Shoulder MSDs are multifactorial in origin. They may be associated with both occupational and nonoccupational factors. Occupational-related shoulder injuries are a rapidly emergent problem resulting in disability (Frost & Andersen, 1999). Currently, it is ranked the second most common work-related medical condition following low back disorders (Bureau of Labor Statistics, 2008; Frost & Andersen, 1999). In the United States, shoulder injuries account for approximately 56% to 65% of all occupational related injuries. It has a widely reported prevalence rate, ranging from 5% to 40%, with rapidly emerging incidence levels (Bureau of Labor Statistics, 2008; Frost & Andersen, 1999). The projected medical cost incurred secondary to shoulder disorder is exorbitant and estimated to be approximately 1–2 billion dollars annually. Appropriate preventative steps and interventions need to be instituted to properly manage these injuries. Ergonometric evaluation of the work place and patient education are a few ways to help patients prevent injury.

Pathophysiology of Rotator Cuff Injuries

Rotator cuff disorders can be divided into primary and secondary causes. Primary causes can be attributed to the patient's underlying anatomy, such as outlet impingement, compromised microvascular supply, and age-related degeneration. Outlet impingement refers to changes that have occurred to the acromioclavicular (AC) joint. The AC joint is the bony roof that sits above the rotator cuff muscles. Arthritic changes to the AC joint can cause injury to the muscle. Age-related degeneration is associated with intrinsic tendinopathy. As one ages there is an increased frequency of partial-thickness and full-thickness tears of the cuff muscles. These degenerative changes are commonly observed in workers who execute overhead activity, such as seen with painters and plumbers. The superficial side of the supraspinatus tendon, also known as the bursal side, maintains a higher blood supply compared with the side of the muscle that is above the glenohumeral articular surface. This difference in blood supply may be attributed to the increased incidence of articular surface tears compared with bursal tears (Frost & Andersen, 1999; Svendsen, 2004). Rotator cuff muscles may be susceptible to a decrease in intramuscular circulation due to increased intramuscular pressures along the articular surface (Yamaguchi et al., 2006). Secondary sources include glenohumeral instability.

Exposure to work-related activities and time to onset of new symptoms has been studied in an effort to identify the association between the cause of pain and the effect of specific activities related to pain. It is theorized that the initial onset of symptoms may be correlated with the daily and or extent of exposure to elevated shoulder postures, which may then lead to shoulder injury. In the Kilbom and Persson (1987) study, shoulder posture was identified as a work exposure factor that served as a significant predictor of severe shoulder injury at the 1- and/or 2-year follow-up evaluations. In addition, results of the study revealed that change in status included problems of the shoulder and also was associated with disorders of the neck and arm.

Risk Factors for Rotator Cuff Injuries

Risk factors associated with rotator cuff injuries are multifactorial and encompass numerous aspects, including patient-related facets (age, supraspinatus anatomy, and preexisting pathologies), and work-related features (repetitive stress, posture, arm positions, force/lifting requirements, and segmental vibration). Repetitive shoulder stressors relate to work activities characterized by a cycle, which is defined as one episode of flexion, extension, and abduction. Repetitive stresses can be described as frequency of shoulder flexion or abduction, the number of objects managed at any one time, the number of tasks repeated within distinct cycle, short cycle time/repeated tasks within cycle, or the characterization of repetitive work or repetitive arm movements. The study by English et al. (1995) demonstrated evidence of association between repetition, awkward posture, and shoulder tendonitis (Ohlsson et al., 1994, 1995). Furthermore, English's study confirmed a significant association between diagnosed shoulder disorders and repeated shoulder rotation with elevated arm postures. In addition, studies by Bjelle, Hagberg, and Michaelson (1981) and Ohlsson et al. (1995) demonstrated noteworthy and positive associations between the prevalence of shoulder disorders and the frequency of upper arm movements exceeding 60° of flexion or abduction.

As noted previously, there exist significant and positive relationships between repetitive movement and shoulder disorders. Another study by Herberts et al. theorized that rotator cuff muscles may develop increased intramuscular pressures at relatively low contraction levels. These high intramuscular pressures may possibly result in impaired intramuscular circulation. Increased pressure in rotator cuff muscles with resultant increased pressure on the supraspinatus tendon may activate distinct events related to impaired microcirculation. It is hypothesized that repeated or sustained episodes of muscle ischemia result in localized cell death and persistent inflammation, leading to small areas of cell death and shoulder tendonitis (English et al., 1995; Kilbom & Persson, 1987; Ohlsson et al., 1995).

Jobs associated with increased vibratory exposure, such as rock blasters, brick layers, foremen, and riveters are believed to be at risk for developing shoulder injuries. Comprehensive review of the literature reveals that there is inadequate evidence relating to the association between shoulder tendinitis and exposure to segmental vibration. Occupations associated with increased vibration exposure also place a large, static load on shoulder muscles so that the effects of forceful shoulder muscle exertions could not be separated from vibration. The difficulty in separating muscle contraction from vibration limits the studies ability to show a relationship with vibration and shoulder pathology (Burdorf & Monster, 1991).

Diagnosis

Obtaining a proper and detailed history is vital in diagnosing rotator cuff injuries. The practitioner has to rule out other pathologies including, but not limited to referred, cervical neck pain or cardiac sources of pain. One has to identify the patient's chief complaint and acquire more detailed information: handedness, onset, location, duration, exacerbating/alleviating symptoms, and radiation of pain. In addition, one should inquire about weakness, numbness, catching/popping of shoulder, instability, night pain, pain when lying on affected arm, and range of motion. It is imperative to gather some social history/occupational history information. Some patients may have tried alternative treatment options prior to seeking medical evaluation so it is beneficial to identify these sources of treatment modalities such as ice or heat; medications such as acetometaphin, NSAIDs, aspirin; physical therapies; injections; or surgical interventions. One should follow a systematic approach when performing the physical examination: inspection, palpation, range of motion, manual muscle strength testing, sensation, reflexes and special testing.

Diagnosis Studies

Radiologic studies can be invaluable in diagnosing rotator cuff disorders. The initial workup should entail X-rays of the shoulder. MRI is highly sensitive and specific in identifying rotator cuff (RTC) injuries. Disadvantages of MRI include cost and the necessity of the patient to remain absolutely still during the study. Ultrasound (US) is an alternate study that may be considered. It is of low cost and extremely precise in identifying RTC (Middleton, 2004; Teefey, Middleton, Bauer, Hildebolt, & Yamaguchi, 2000; Teefey et al., 2004).

Treatment

Treatment of rotator cuff injuries involves a multimodal approach ranging from conservative measures such as medications and physical therapy to invasive procedures including surgery. Medications utilized in the treatment of RTC include acetometaphin and NSAIDS. If the patient is refractory to oral medications, one may consider providing a subacromial corticosteroid injection, while cautiously avoiding direct injection into the RTC tendons. The ultimate goal of physical therapy is to strengthen both the RTC and the muscles that stabilize the scapula (rhomboids, levator scapulae, trapezius, and serratus anterior). Surgery is indicated in individuals with RTC tears who fail to demonstrate decreased pain and or improved function over a 6 month period while participating in a rehabilitation program.

Return to work following treatment depends on the severity of the injury, handedness of the individual, and job requirements. If the dominant hand is affected, this will increase days away from work. Also important to note that return to work will be postponed for months if surgery is performed. On average, when surgery is not required, the return to work following a shoulder injury ranges from 5 to 9 days (Bureau of Labor Statistics, 2008; Bjelle et al., 1981; Svendsen et al., 2004; Yamaguchi et al., 2006).

CARPAL TUNNEL SYNDROME

CTS is the most common entrapment neuropathy, accounting for approximately 90% of cases (Aroori & Spence, 2008). It results from an entrapment of the median nerve at the wrist as it passes through the carpal tunnel, the region where the hand joins the wrist. CTS causes burning pain associated with tingling and numbness in the distribution of median nerve distal to the wrist and may produce functional impairment of the hand. In the United States, approximately 1 million adults are estimated to have CTS annually requiring medical attention (Aroori & Spence, 2008). Palmer and Hanrahan (1995) estimated that between 400,000 and 500,000 cases of CTS require operative treatment annually, and its economic cost exceeds $2 billion per year (Aroori & Spence, 2008).

The prevalence of CTS is estimated between 1% and 5% in the general population (Atroshi et al., 1999; De Krom et al., 1992). However, the incidence and prevalence rates are reported higher among workers in certain occupations that involve high force/pressure and the repetitive use of vibrating tools. The BLS identifies CTS as the leader in the amount of lost work time among major disabling injuries (Bureau of Labor Statistics, 2002b). Their 1995 report stated that approximately five individuals out of 10,000 workers missed work due to job-related CTS (Bureau of Labor Statistics, 1995). In 1999, the median number of days absent from work due to CTS was reported to be 27 days (Bureau of Labor Statistics, 2001). In addition, the number was highest for CTS when compared with any other major disabling illnesses and injuries (Bureau of Labor Statistics, 2001). Tanaka, Wild, Cameron, and Freund reported in 1997 that an estimated population prevalence of CTS was 53 cases per 10,000 workers, and 20% of these individuals were absent from work because of the disease.

Etiology and Role of the Workplace Physical Activities

CTS is generally believed to be caused by increased pressure in the carpal tunnel that compresses the median nerve and is associated with a variety of underlying medical conditions. These include, but are not limited to, pregnancy, renal dysfunction, gout, pseudogout infection, collagen disorders, rheumatoid arthritis, diabetes, hypothyroidism, obesity, trauma, and hemodialysis. According to the review by Tanaka et al. (1995), approximately half of the cases of CTS are associated with physical workplace factors, such as repetitive motions of the hand. Brian and Wright (1947) first implied that CTS may be associated with certain occupations, such as grinders, cashiers, meat packers, workers sewing car seats, aircraft engineers, and small part assembly liners. Einhorn and Leddy (1996) reported a higher incidence of CTS in workers in certain industries that require repetitive use of the hands and wrist, in comparison with the general population (5% vs. 1%). Forst, Andersen, and Nielsen (1998) and Rosecrance, Cook, Anton, & Merlino (2002) reported a prevalence of CTS up to 10% among workers in slaughterhouse and apprentice construction, respectively. Despite these findings, the contributions of occupational physical activities in its etiology are not fully understood.

In recent years, numerous epidemiological studies have examined the relationship of occupational factors with the development of CTS. Most of these reviews concluded that physical workplace factors are one of the important causes of CTS (National Institute for Occupational Safety and Health, 1997). The National Institute for Occupational Safety and Health (NIOSH) reviewed more than 30 epidemiological studies that addressed the association of physical workplace factors with CTS in 1997. NIOSH found a positive association between highly repetitive, forceful, and vibratory work and CTS (National Institute for Occupational Safety and Health, 1997).

Rempel (1995) hypothesized that repetitive hand activities may cause a substantial increase in the pressure in the carpal tunnel, resulting in damage to the median nerve through edema and fibrosis. Substantial load on the fingertip with the wrist in a neutral position can also increase the pressure in the tunnel by 10 fold. In addition, Chiang et al. (1994) reported a statistically significant dose-response relationship CTS with increasing levels of force and repetition. With many supporting data, NIOSH concluded that there was evidence of a positive association between highly repetitive work alone or forceful work alone and CTS and strong evidence between a combination of forceful hand/wrist exertion and repetitiveness and CTS (National Institute for Occupational Safety and Health, 1997).

Wrist posture has been also studied for a possible cause of CTS. This hypothesis was based upon an observation that typing with the wrist in 45° of extension can result in an acute pressure in the carpal tunnel that is 15 times greater than the normal resting pressure with the wrist in a neutral position (National Institute for Occupational Safety and Health, 1997). One of the possible mechanisms suggested by Skie, Zeiss, Ebraheim, and Jackson (1990) stated that flexed wrist postures may reduce the area of the carpal tunnel, thus potentially increasing pressure in the tunnel resulting in increasing the risk of development of CTS. There are limited studies that address wrist posture as the sole cause of CTS (National Institute for Occupational Safety and Health, 1997). Most studies did not separate the posture variables from other work factors such as forceful exertion (Rempel, 1995). Therefore, NIOSH concluded that there was insufficient evidence in the current epidemiological literature to demonstrate that awkward postures alone are associated with CTS (National Institute for Occupational Safety and Health, 1997).

Vibration is another factor that has been suspected to be associated with development of CTS. Chatterjee, Barwick, and Petrie (1982) studied rock drillers and found a significant difference in signs and symptoms of CTS and nerve conduction study measurements between study subjects and controls. Cannon, Bernacki, and Walter (1981) found that use of vibrating tools in combination with forceful and repetitive hand motions was associated with a greater incidence of CTS than was repetitive motion alone. Although the mechanism by which vibration causes CTS is not clear, it may be that vibration exposure is usually accompanied by exposure to forceful and repetitive motions (National Institute for Occupational Safety and Health, 1997). Vibration may cause impaired sensation in the hands leading to an increase in the amount of force exerted during manipulative tasks. It may also directly injure the peripheral nerves or digital arteries, producing symptoms of paresthesia (National Institute for Occupational Safety and Health, 1997). Lundborg et al. (1987) demonstrated that vibration caused epineural edema in the sciatic nerve in rats. After reviewing nine studies, NIOSH concluded that there was evidence supporting an association between exposure to vibration and CTS (National Institute for Occupational Safety and Health, 1997).

Pathophysiology

The exact pathogenesis of CTS is uncertain. Aroori and Spence (2008) mentioned in their review some of the popular theories in the literature. They include mechanical compression, microvascular insufficiency, and vibration theories. First, the mechanical compression theory attributes the symptoms of CTS to compression of the median nerve in the carpal tunnel mediated by several factors such as overuse, repeated or prolonged wrist extension, and prolonged grasping of tools. Second, the microvascular insufficiency theory suggests that the lack of blood supply to the median nerve causes scar and fibrous tissue and eventually causing ischemia of the median nerve. Third, the vibration theory proposes that long-term use of vibrating tools causes the symptoms of CTS via median nerve injury due to edema in the outer coating of the nerve fibers known as the epineurium or direct injury of the nerve's axons.

Clinical Features

Patients typically complain of an intermittent numbness and tingling also known as paresthesias in the distribution of median nerve distal to wrist. They may awaken with pain or tingling that may be relieved with hanging their hand out of bed or shaking it vigorously. Symptoms of nocturnal paresthesia in the distribution of the median nerve are reported to be 51–96% sensitive and 27–68% specific which makes it a great screening question while taking the patients history (Aroori & Spence, 2008). Patients may also present with weakness in the hand and pain radiating to the forearm. Physical examination may reveal atrophy of the muscles in the palm closest to the thumb and weakness of thumb abduction.

Diagnosis

The diagnosis of CTS is mainly based on clinical signs and symptoms and NCS. Physical examination maneuvers specific to CTS include Phalen's and Tinel's test. Phalen's test is performed with the position of both hands in the "reversed prayer position." Both hands are flexed and the dorsum of each hand are touching. The position is held for 90 seconds to see if the symptoms are reproduced. Tinel's test is performed by tapping over the carpal tunnel. The test is positive if the symptoms are reproduced. The sensitivity and specificity of the Phalen's sign are reported to be 68% and 73% respectively, and those of the Tinel's sign to be 50% and 77%, respectively (MacDermid & Wessel, 2004). Alternative useful diagnostic tests are electrodiagnostic studies, US, and MRI. High-resolution US has been used widely in the evaluation of CTS. El Miedany et al. concluded that US is comparable to electrodiagnostic studies in the diagnosis of CTS (Aroori & Spence, 2008). Although MRI is an accurate diagnostic tool, it is only recommended when NCS are equivocal.

Treatment

Treatment options for CTS can be divided into surgical and nonsurgical. Most patients (82%) respond to conservative therapy. However, the recurrence rate after 1 year is reported up to 80%, in which case surgical intervention may be necessary (Stahl, Yarnitsky, Volpin, & Fried, 1996). Nonsurgical options include wrist splinting, NSAIDs, oral steroids, local injection of corticosteroids, ergonomic modifications, yoga and so on. O'Connor, Marshall, and Massy-Westropp (2003) in the recent Cochrane review concluded that a significant short-term benefit could be obtained with oral steroids, wrist splinting, local US therapy and yoga. However, the authors found no evidence of benefit with hand brace, exercises, usage of ergonomic keyboards, oral diuretics, and oral NSAIDs (O'Connor et al., 2003). A corticosteroid injection has been shown to have a statistically significant benefit in CTS (Girlanda et al., 1993; Sevim et al., 2004). Definitive treatment consists of surgical division of transverse carpal ligament that releases pressure on the median nerve. Surgery is indicated in patients with symptoms that do not respond to conservative measures and in those with severe nerve entrapment. A long-term success rate from surgery is reported of cases in more than 75% of cases (Girlanda et al., 1993).

Disability and Worker's Compensation

CTS, depending on its symptoms, can result in severe disability. The annual number of CTS claims increased steadily until 1993 and then declined to relatively stable values through year 2000. Daniell, Fulton-Kehoe, Chiou, and Franklin (2005) reported that compensation for lost work was provided in 65% of claims and for permanent partial disability in 29% of claims. They also found that compensation tended to be more frequent in claims where a diagnosis of CTS was made late in the claim. The median cost of a CTS claim was $5,605 ($9,738 with surgery and $1,197 without surgery). Again, claim costs increased as the CTS diagnosis occurred later in the course of the claim (Daniell et al., 2005).

Return to Work Following CTS

De Kesel, Donceel, and De Smet (2008) reported that work-related features such as repetitive movements and heavy manual handling activity influenced more on return to work than personal, pathological, or surgical features. Katz et al. (1997) showed that economic and psychosocial variables have a strong influence upon return to work. They also suggested in their 1995 article that efforts to enhance return to work following carpal tunnel release should be multidimensional (clinical, demographic, economic, and workplace factors) to reduce work absence (Katz et al., 2005). Work hardening and multidisciplinary occupational rehabilitation also seem to play roles in enhancing return to work. The work hardening program is a highly structured, goal oriented program designed to return patients back to work. Work hardening is associated with 83% of patients returning to work following treatment (Flinn-Wagner, Mladonicky, & Goodman, 1990). Evidence has shown that workers who receive multidisciplinary occupational rehabilitation are significantly more likely to return to work compared with those who receive "usual treatment" (74% vs. 40%) and are also more likely to return to full-time work (91% vs. 50%) (Feuerstein & Zastowny, 1996). Bonzani, Millender, Keelan, and Mangieri (1997) found that the psychosocial classification and current employment status are the most important factors in prolonging disability among workers.

Primary Prevention of Work-Related CTS

Lincoln et al. (2000) in their meta-analysis of 24 studies concluded that although several reports suggested beneficial effects of preventive interventions such as ergonomic programs, alternative keyboard supports, and mouse and tool redesign, their roles as the primary prevention of CTS remains inconclusive. CTS is one of the most common occupational MSDs and considered the leader in the amount of lost work time among major disabling injuries. In order to reduce disability and economic burden associated with this condition, it is important to make an accurate diagnosis and to initiate appropriate treatment promptly. Furthermore, more research will be necessary to identify personal and workplace factors that can be incorporated into the primary prevention of CTS.

CONCLUSION

MSDs are a major problem which affects the employee, employer, and the economy. The difficulty of treating MSDs, whether it is back pain, shoulder pain, or CTS, is the multifactorial issues that surround each condition. Although effective treatment options may be in place for the physical disorder, the overall treatment of each condition is complicated by nonoccupational, emotional, and psychsocial factors. The ideal treatment includes a multidisciplinary approach coupled with effective communication regarding treatment goals and outcomes. Prevention through education and ergonometric evaluation of workstations is ideal. Unfortunately, the ideal is rarely achieved. Overall, the incidence and prevalence of MSDs in the United States continues and deserves continued diligent medical attention.

REFERENCES

Ammendolia, C., Cassidy, D., Steensta, I., Soklaridis, S., Boyle, E., Eng, S., et al. (2009). Designing a workplace return-to-work program for occupational low back pain: An intervention mapping approach. *BMC Musculoskeletal Disorders, 9, 10*, 65.

Andersson, G. B. (1998). Epidemiology of low back pain. *Acta Orthopaedica Scandinavica, 281 (Suppl),* 28–31.

Anonymous. (1987). Scientific approach to the assessment and management of activity-related spinal disorders: A monograph for clinicians. Report of the Quebec Task Force on Spinal Disorders. *Spine, 12*, S1–S59.

Aroori, S., & Spence, R. A. (2008). Carpal tunnel syndrome. *Ulster Medical Journal, 77*, 6–17.

Atroshi, I., Gummesson, C., Johnsson, R., Ornstein, E., Ranstam, J., & Rosen, I. (1999). Prevalence of carpal tunnel syndrome in a general population. *Journal of the American Medical Association, 282*, 153–158.

Bjelle, A., Hagberg, M., & Michaelson, G. (1981). Occupational and individual factors in acute shoulder-neck disorders among industrial workers. *British Journal of Industrial Medicine, 38*, 356–363.

Bonzani, P. J., Millender, L., Keelan, B., & Mangieri, M. G. (1997). Factors prolonging disability in work-related cumulative trauma disorders. *Journal of Hand Surgery. American Volume, 22*, 30–34.

Boocock, M. G., Collier, J. M., McNair, P. J., Simmonds, M., Larmer, P. J., & Armstrong, B. (2009). A framework for the classification and diagnosis of work-related upper extremity conditions: Systematic review. *Seminars in Arthritis and Rheumatism, 38*, 296–311.

Böstman, O. M. (1993). Body mass index and height in patients requiring surgery for lumbar intervertebral disc herniation. *Spine (Phila Pa 1976), 18*, 851–854.

Brian, W. R., & Wright, A. D. (1947). Spontaneous compression of both median nerves in the carpal tunnel. *Lancet, 1*, 277–282.

Burdorf, A., & Monster, A. (1991). Exposure to vibration and self-reported health complaints of riveters in the aircraft industry. *Annals of Occupational Hygiene, 35*, 287–298.

Bureau of Labor Statistics. (1995). Washington, DC: BLS.

Bureau of Labor Statistics. (2001). *News: Lost-work time injuries and illnesses: Characteristics and resulting time away from work.* United States: BLS.

Bureau of Labor Statistics. (2002b). *Nonfatal cases involving days away from work: Selected characteristics.* Washington, DC: BLS.

Bureau of Labor Statistics. (2008). *"News U.S. Department of Labor" survey of occupational injuries and illnesses in cooperation with participating state agencies.* USDL 08–1716. Washington, DC: BLS.

Burton, A. K., Balagué, F., & Cardon, G.; COST B13 Working Group on European Guidelines for Prevention in Low Back Pain, et al. (2005). How to prevent low back pain. *Best Practice and Research. Clinical Rheumatology, 19*, 541–555.

Cannon, L. J., Bernacki, E. J., & Walter, S. D. (1981). Personal and occupational factors associated with carpal tunnel syndrome. *Journal of Occupational Medicine, 23*, 255–258.

Chatterjee, D. S., Barwick, D. D., & Petrie, A. (1982). Exploratory electromyography in the study of vibration-induced white finger in rock drillers. *British Journal of Industrial Medicine, 39*, 89–97.

Chiang, H., Ko, Y., Chen, S., Yu, H., Wu, T., & Chang, P. (1994). Prevalence of shoulder and upper-limb disorders among workers in the fish-processing industry. *Scandinavian Journal of Work, Environment and Health, 19*, 126–131.

Cohen, S. P., Argoff, C. E., & Carragee, E. J. (2008). Management of low back pain. *BMJ, 337*, 2718.

Daniell, W. E., Fulton-Kehoe, D., Chiou, L. A., & Franklin, G. M. (2005). Work-related carpal tunnel syndrome in Washington state workers' compensation: Temporal trends, clinical practices, and disability. *American Journal of Industrial Medicine, 48,* 259–269.

De Kesel, R., Donceel, P., & De Smet, L. (2008). Factors influencing return to work after surgical treatment for carpal tunnel syndrome. *Occupational Medicine (London), 58,* 187–190.

De Krom, M. C., Knipschild, P. G., Kester, A. D., Thijs, C. T., Boekkooi, P. F., & Spaans, F. (1992). Carpal tunnel syndrome: Prevalence in the general population. *Journal of Clinical Epidemiology, 45,* 373–376.

del Arbol, J. L., Muñoz, J. R., Ojeda, L., Cascales, A. L., Irles, J. R., Miranda, M. T., et al. (2000). Plasma concentrations of beta-endorphin in smokers who consume different numbers of cigarettes per day. *Pharmacology, Biochemistry and Behavior, 67,* 25–28.

Denis, D., St-Vincent, M., Imbeau, D., Jetté, C., & Nastasia, I. (2008). Intervention practices in musculoskeletal disorder prevention: A critical literature review. *Applied Ergonomics, 39,* 1–14.

Devereaux, M. (2009). Low back pain. *Medical Clinics of North America, 93,* 477–501.

Deyo, R. A., & Tsui-Wu, Y.-J. (1987). Descriptive epidemiology of low back pain and its related medical care in the United States. *Spine, 12,* 264–268.

Deyo, R. A., & Bass, J. E. (1989). Lifestyle and low-back pain. The influence of smoking and obesity. *Spine (Phila Pa 1976), 14,* 501–506.

Deyo, R. A., Cherkin, D., Conrad, D., & Volinn, E. (1992). Cost, controversy, crisis: Low back pain and the health of the public. *Annual Review of Public Health, 12,* 141–155.

Einhorn, N., & Leddy, J. P. (1996). Pitfall of endoscopic carpal tunnel release. *Orthopedic Clinics of North America, 27,* 373–380.

English, C. J., Maclaren, W. M., Court-Brown, C., Hughes, S. P., Porter, R. W., Wallace, W. A., et al. (1995). Relations between upper limb soft tissue disorders and repetitive movements at work. *American Journal of Industrial Medicine, 27,* 75–90.

Feuerstein, M., & Zastowny, T. (1996). Occupational musculoskeletal disorders: A multidisciplinary approach. In: R. J. Gatchel, D. Turk (Eds.), *Psychological approaches to pain management: A practitioner's handbook* (pp. 458–485). New York: Guilford Press.

Feyer, A. M., Herbison, P., Williamson, A. M., de Silva, I., Mandryk, J., Hendrie, L., et al. (2000). The role of physical and psychological factors in occupational low back pain: A prospective cohort study. *Journal of Occupational and Environmental Medicine, 57,* 116–120.

Flinn-Wagner, S., Mladonicky, A., & Goodman, G. (1990). Characteristics of workers with upper extremity injuries who make a successful transition to work. *Journal of Hand Therapy, 3,* 51–55.

Frost, P., & Andersen, J. H. (1999). Shoulder impingement syndrome in relation to shoulder intensive work. *Journal of Occupational and Environmental Medicine, 56,* 494–498.

Frost, P., Andersen, J. H., & Nielsen, V. K. (1998). Occurrence of carpal tunnel syndrome among slaughterhouse workers. *Scandinavian Journal of Work, Environment and Health, 24,* 285–292.

Frymoyer, J., & Cats-Baril, W. (1991). An overview of the incidence and costs of low back pain. *Orthopedic Clinics of North America, 22,* 263–271.

Girlanda, P., Dattola, R., Venuto, C., Mangiapane, R., Nicolosi, C., & Messina, C., et al. (1993). Local steroid treatment in idiopathic carpal tunnel syndrome: Short- and long-term efficacy. *Journal of Neurology, 240,* 187–190.

Groen, G., Baljet, B., & Drukker, J. (1990). Nerves and nerve plexuses of the human vertebral column. *American Journal of Anatomy, 188,* 282–296.

Hardt, J., Jacobsen, C., Goldberg, J., Nickel, R., & Buchwald, D. (2008). Prevalence of chronic pain in a representative sample in the United States. *Pain Medicine, 9,* 803–812.

Jensen, M. C., Brant-Zawadzki, M. N., Obuchowski, N., Modic, M. T., Malkasian, D., Ross, J. S., et al. (1994). Magnetic resonance imaging of the lumbar spine in people without back pain. *New England Journal of Medicine, 331,* 69–73.

Katz, J. N., Amick, B. C., Keller, R., Fossel, A. H., Ossman, J., Soucie, V., et al. (2005). Determinant of work absence following surgery for carpal tunnel syndrome. *American Journal of Industrial Medicine, 47,* 120–130.

Katz, J. N., Keller, R. B., Fossel, A. H., Punnett, L., Bessette, L., Simmons, B. P., et al. (1997). Predictors of return to work following carpal tunnel release. *American Journal of Industrial Medicine, 31,* 85–91.

Kelsey, J. L. & Hardy, R. J. (1975). Driving of motor vehicles as a risk factor for acute herniated lumbar intervertebral disc. *American Journal of Epidemiology, 102,* 63–73.

Kilbom, A., & Persson, J. (1987). Work technique and its consequences for musculoskeletal disorders. *Ergonomics, 30,* 273–279.

Lee, S. H., Derby, R., Chen, Y., Seo, K. S., & Kim, M. J. (2004). In vitro measurement of pressure in inter-vertebral discs and annulus fibrosus with and without annular tears during discography. *The Spine Journal, 4,* 614–618.

Leonardi, M., Pfirrmann, C. W., & Boos, N. (2006). Injection studies in spinal disorders. *Clinical Orthopaedics and Related Research, 443,* 168–182.

Lincoln, A. E., Vernick, J. S., Ogaitis, S., Smith, G. S., Mitchell, C. S., & Agnew, J. (2000). Interventions for the primary prevention of work-related CTS. *American Journal of Preventive Medicine, 18(Suppl.),* 37–50.

Lindblom, K. (1948). Diagnostic puncture of the intervertebral disc in sciatica. *Acta Orthopaedica Scandinavica, 17,* 213–239.

Lundborg, G., Dahlin, L. B., Danielsen, N., Hansson, H. A., Necking, L. E., & Pyykko, I. (1987). Intraneural edema following exposure to vibration. *Scandinavian Journal of Work, Environment and Health, 13,* 326–329.

MacDermid, J. C., & Wessel, J. (2004). Clinical diagnosis of carpal tunnel syndrome: A systematic review. *Journal of Hand Therapy, 17,* 309.

Manchikanti L, Singh, V., Datta, S., Cohen, S. P., & Hirsch, J. A. (2009). Comprehensive review of epidemiology, scope, and impact of spinal pain. *Pain Physician, 12,* E35–E70.

Mannion, A. F., Dolan, P., & Adams, M. A. (1996). Psychological questionnaires: Do "abnormal" scores precede or follow first-time low back pain? *Spine, 21,* 2603–2611

Meleger, A. L., & Krivickas, L. S. (2007). Neck and back pain: Musculoskeletal disorders. *Neurologic Clinics, 25,* 419–438.

Mense, S., & Simons, D. (2001). *Muscle pain: Understanding its nature, diagnoses and treatment.* Baltimore, MD: Lippincott Williams & Wilkins. pp. 117–118.

Middleton, W. D., Payne, W. T., Teefey, S. A., Hildebolt, C. F., Rubin, D. A., & Yamaguchi, K. (2004). Sonography and MRI of the shoulder: Comparison of patient satisfaction. *AJR. American Journal of Roentgenology, 183,* 1449–1452.

Nagi, S. Z., Burk, R. D., & Potter, H. R. (1965). Back disorders and rehabilitation achievement. *Journal of Chronic Diseases, 18,* 181–197.

National Institute for Occupational Safety and Health. (1997). *Musculoskeletal disorders and workplace factors. A critical review of epidemiologic evidence for work-related musculoskeletal disorders of the neck, upper extremity, and low back. Chapter 5-Hand/wrist musculoskeletal disorders (Carpal tunnel syndrome): Evidence for work-relatedness.* Atlanta, GA: National Institute for Occupational Safety and Health, CDC.

Nikander, R., Mälkiä, E., Parkkari, J., Heinonen, A., Starck, H., & Ylinen, J. (2006). Dose-response relationship of specific training to reduce chronic neck pain and disability. *Medicine and Science in Sports and Exercise, 38,* 2068–2074.

O'Connor, D., Marshall, S., & Massy-Westropp, N. (2003). Non-surgical treatment (other than steroid injection) for carpal tunnel syndrome. *Cochrane Database of Systemic Reviews, 1,* CD003219.

Ohlsson, K., Attewell, R. G., Pålsson, B., Karlsson, B., Balogh, I., Johnsson, B., et al. (1995). Repetitive industrial work and neck and upper limb disorders in females. *American Journal of Industrial Medicine, 27,* 731–747.

Ohlsson, K., Hansson, G. A., Balogh, I., Strömberg, U., Pålsson, B., Nordander, C., et al. (1994). Disorders of the neck and upper limbs in women in the fish processing industry. *Journal of Occupational and Environmental Medicine, 51,* 826–832.

Palmer, D. H., & Hanrahan, L. P. (1995). Social and economic costs of carpal tunnel surgery. *Instructional Course Lectures, 44,* 167–172.

Pevsner, Y., Shabat, S., Catz, A., Folman, Y., & Gepstein, R. (2003). The role of radiofrequency in the treatment of mechanical pain of spinal origin. *European Spine Journal, 12,* 602–605.

Proper, K. I., Koning, M., van der Beek, A. J., Hildebrandt, V. H., Bosscher, R. J., & van Mechelen, W. (2003). The effectiveness of worksite physical activity programs on physical activity, physical fitness, and health. *Clinical Journal of Sport Medicine, 13,* 106–117.

Rempel, D. (1995). Musculoskeletal loading and carpal tunnel pressure. In S. L. Gordon, S. J. Blair, L. J. Fine (Eds.), *Repetitive motions disorders of the upper extremity* (pp. 123–133). Rosemont, IL: American Academy of Orthopaedic Surgeons.

Rosecrance, J. C., Cook, T. M., Anton, D. C., & Merlino, L. A. (2002). Carpal tunnel syndrome among apprentice construction workers. *American Journal of Industrial Medicine, 42,* 107–116.

Sehgal, N., Dunbar, E. E., Shah, R. V., & Colson, J. (2007). Systematic review of diagnostic utility of facet (zygapophysial) joint injections in chronic spinal pain: An update. *Pain Physician, 10,* 213–228.

Seo, K. S., Derby, R., Date, E. S., Lee, S. H., Kim, B. J., & Lee, C. H., et al. (2007). In vitro measurement of pressure differences using manometry at various injection speeds during discography. *The Spine Journal, 7,* 68–73.

Sevim, S., Dogu, O., Camdeviren, H., Kaleagasi, H., Aral, M., Arslan, E., et al. (2004). Long-term effectiveness of steroid injections and splinting in mild and moderate carpal tunnel syndrome. *Neurological Sciences, 25,* 48.

Shelerud, R. A. (2006). Epidemiology of occupational low back pain. *Clinics in Occupational and Environmental Medicine, 5,* 501–528.

Skie, M., Zeiss, J., Ebraheim, N. A., & Jackson, W. T. (1990). Carpal tunnel changes and median nerve compression during wrist flexion and extension seen by magnetic resonance imaging. *Journal of Hand Surgery, 15A,* 939.

Stahl, S., Yarnitsky, D., Volpin, G., & Fried, A. (1996). Conservative therapy in carpal tunnel syndrome. *Harefuah, 130,* 241–243.

Stewart, W. F., Ricci, J. A., Chee, E., Morganstein, D., & Lipton, R. (2003). Lost productive time and cost due to common pain conditions in the US workforce. *Journal of the American Medical Association, 290,* 2443–2454.

Svendsen, S. W., Bonde, J. P., Mathiassen, S. E., Stengaard-Pedersen, K., & Frich, L. H. (2004). Work related shoulder disorders: Quantitative exposure-response relations with reference to arm posture. *Journal of Occupational and Environmental Medicine, 61,* 844–853.

Tanaka, S., Wild, D. K., Cameron, L., & Freund, E. (1997). Association of occupational and nonoccupational risk factors with the prevalence of self-reported carpal tunnel syndrome in a national survey of the working population. *American Journal of Industrial Medicine, 32,* 550–556.

Tanaka, S., Wild, D. K., Seligman, P. J., Halperin, W. E., Behrens, V. J., & Putz-Anderson, V. (1995). Prevalence of work-related carpal tunnel syndrome among U.S. workers: Analysis of the occupational health supplement data of 1988. National Health Interview Survey. *American Journal of Industrial Medicine, 27,* 451–470.

Teefey, S. A., Middleton, W. D., Bauer, G. S., Hildebolt, C. F., & Yamaguchi, K. (2000). Sonographic differences in the appearance of acute and chronic full-thickness rotator cuff tears. *Journal of Ultrasound in Medicine, 19,* 377–378.

Teefey, S. A., Rubin, D. A., Middleton, W. D., Hildebolt, C. F., Leibold, R. A., & Yamaguchi, K. (2004). Detection and quantification of rotator cuff tears: Comparison of ultrasonographic, magnetic resonance imaging and arthroscopic findings in seventy-one consecutive cases. *Journal of Bone and Joint Surgery. American Volume, 86,* 708–716.

Truchon, M., Côté, D., Fillion, L., Arsenault, B., & Dionne, C. (2008). Low-back-pain related disability: An integration of psychological risk factors into the stress process model. *Pain, 137,* 564–573.

Vaerøy, H., Helle, R., Førre, O., Kåss, E., & Terenius, L. (1988). Elevated CSF levels of substance P and high incidence of Raynaud phenomenon in patients with fibromyalgia: New features for diagnosis. *Pain, 32,* 21–26.

van Tulder, M. W., Assendelft, W. J., Koes, B. W., & Bouter, L. M. (1997). Spinal radiographic findings and nonspecific low back pain. A systematic review of observational studies. *Spine, 22,* 427–434.

Videman, T., Battie, M. C., Gibbons, L. E., Maravilla, K., Manninen, H., & Kaprio, J., et al. (2003). Associations between back pain history and lumbar MRI findings. *Spine, 28,* 582–588.

Waddell, G., & Burton, A. K. (2001). Occupational health guidelines for the management of low back pain at work: Evidence review. *Occupational Medicine (London), 51,* 124–135.

Waddell, G. (2004). *The back pain revolution.* 2nd ed. Edinburgh, United Kingdom: Churchill Livingstone.

Wai, E. K., Rodriguez, S., Dagenais, S., & Hall, H. (2008). Evidence-informed management of chronic low back pain with physical activity, smoking cessation, and weight loss. *The Spine Journal, 8,* 195–202. Review.

Yamaguchi, K., Ditsios, K., Middleton, W. D., Hildebolt, C. F., Galatz, L. M., & Teefey, S. A. (2006). The demographic and morphological features of rotator cuff disease. A comparison of asymptomatic and symptomatic shoulders. *Journal of Bone and Joint Surgery. American Volume, 88,* 1699–1704.

16

Pediatric Disorders: Cerebral Palsy and Spina Bifida

Joan T. Gold, MD, and David Salsberg, PsyD, DABPS

INTRODUCTION

Physically challenged children present with a variety of developmental and neuromuscular disabilities that are often difficult to diagnose, hard to remediate, and impossible to cure. These are accompanied by psychological and neuropsychological issues that also require major on-going interventions to maximize functional potentials. The restrictions imposed by such a disability may not permit the patient the motoric control or the experiences to acquire skills at the same rate as the typically developing child. Accordingly, secondary developmental delays may occur (Missuna & Pollack, 1991). Medical complications unique to the underlying diagnosis, with frequent hospitalizations and surgeries, social isolation, parental dependency, and financial burdens are stressors for patients, parents, and siblings (Worley, Rosenfeld, & Liscomb, 1991a, 1991b).

It is the purpose of this chapter to discuss cerebral palsy and spina bifida, two of the more common handicapping conditions of childhood, and the strategies that allow for appropriate medical treatment and rehabilitation. This information permits the health professional to serve as an advocate for optimization of care, prevention of complications, referral to early intervention programs, and placement of the child in the least restrictive school setting. Additionally, potentially abusive and neglectful behaviors of parents and caretakers may be circumvented (Benedict, White, Wulff, & Hall, 1990).

This chapter will address the wide range of emotional challenges that face children diagnosed with chronic medical disorders and disabilities. Children with spina bifida and cerebral palsy require attention to their psychological issues and neuropsychological challenges to facilitate both rehabilitation courses and general functioning within a community setting (Gerring et al., 2008; Pellock, 2004; Max et al., 2002). Significant family stressors and multicultural factors have an impact upon the child's developmental growth (Morison, Bromfield, & Cameron, 2003). The holistic care of children with disabilities requires a multidisciplinary approach that fully integrates the child's developmental, cognitive, and psychological issues, as well as family and cultural dynamics, in addition to the medical presentation (Spates, Samaraweera, Plaiser, Souza, & Otsui, 2007).

CEREBRAL PALSY

Cerebral palsy is a descriptive clinical term that denotes a group of static encephalopathies of diverse etiologies resulting from nonprogressive lesions of the brain sustained in the pre-, peri-, or postnatal periods. The disorder is characterized by abnormalities in muscle tone, muscle control and movement, and postures, of which spasticity is the most common type of presentation, occurring in 65–80% of cases. Secondary dysfunction and deformities occur, but there is not the frank regression in function seen with neurodegenerative disorders, such as the leukodystrophies. Other symptoms of cerebral dysfunction, such as learning disabilities, mental retardation, and seizures, may be seen, but it is the motoric dysfunction that is essential to the diagnosis of the condition (Ingram, 1955).

Incidence

The incidence of cerebral palsy in the past 20 years has remained at 2 cases per 1000 births in the United States (Nelson & Ellenberg, 1986), with approximately 400,000 patients currently being affected. There was a concern that with survival of more medically fragile, lower birth weight infants, the incidence may have increased, despite advances in intrapartum monitoring that can herald fetal distress (albeit with a false-positive rate approaching 99.8%) (Grant, O'Brien, Joy, Henessy, & MacDonald, 1989; Stanley & Blair, 1991; Vohr & Msall, 1997). However, more recent studies do not support this and greater proportion of lower birth weight infants are surviving unscathed, with better management of their brain injury, chronic lung disease, and sepsis (Hack & Costello, 2008). The cases that do occur may also be less severe with a reduction in the number of cases of quadriplegia, a relative increase in the numbers of spastic diplegia, and an overall reduction in the incidence of later seizure disorders (Sigurdardottir, Halldorsdottir, Thorkelsson, Thorarensen, & Vik, 2009). A further reduction in incidence may not be easily forthcoming as prenatal etiologies in a majority of cases (Ford, Kitchen, Doyle, Richards, & Kelly, 1990) cannot be clinically identified. Intervention may be required in a greater percentage of the population as more than 40% of the group may require special education services, although they are not specifically diagnosed with cerebral palsy.

Etiology and Risk Factors

Cerebral palsy was first described by Little in 1843 in infants born prematurely; they developed increased tone and incoordination primarily affecting the lower extremities, or what is now termed as spastic diplegia. With changes in medical treatment, a reduced association with dystocia (difficult labor), erythroblastosis (Rh-negative blood incompatibility), and encephalitis, and an increased association with multiple births, prematurity, acquired hydrocephalus (following intracranial hemorrhage and antenatal infection), and trauma have been noted (Capute, Shapiro, & Palmer, 1981). Accordingly, fewer patients are affected with the writhing movement disorder of athetosis, seen with erythroblastosis and subsequent deposition of abnormal hemoglobin pigments into the basal ganglia, and a greater number of patients have diffuse cerebral dysfunction, with spasticity and cognitive dysfunction.

Etiology can be identified in up to 71% of quadriplegics (those patients with equal involvement of all four extremities) and 40% of nonquadriplegics (Naeye & Peters, 1989). A gestational age of less than 32 of 40 weeks is the greatest predictor for the development of cerebral palsy, although children born at 34–36 weeks gestation still have a threefold risk of incurring cerebral palsy (Petrini et al., 2009). Other risk factors, such as maternal mental retardation, birth weight of less than 2001 g, presence of congenital malformations, and symptomatic intoxications such as fetal alcohol syndrome, support a largely prenatal etiology (Coorsen, Msall, &

Duffy, 1991; Ellenberg & Nelson, 1981). Factors that result in chronic antenatal hypoxia with brain injury include maternal anemia, preeclampsia/gestational hypertension, a drop in third-trimester blood pressure, postterm delivery, and multiple births (Nelson, 1989). These events have a high association with the presence of congenital malformations.

A prenatal etiology for cerebral palsy has been identified in up to 50–60% of patients (Hom, 1982; Naeye & Peters, 1989), most presenting with hypotonia, ataxia, or hemiplegia (unilateral limb involvement). In utero infections, in association with maternal fever during labor (Nelson, 1998), have been demonstrated as one of the predisposing factors in the etiology of cerebral palsy. Inflammatory markers such as cytokines and interferon levels of cord blood are frequently elevated in the population of patients who progress to have spastic diplegia (Nelson, 1998; Rousset et al., 2008).

Thrombotic events in utero, which are really early onset ischemic strokes, may also explain many cases of cerebral palsy. Analysis of cord blood levels for Protein S and Protein C deficiencies, conditions that predispose to hypercoagulability, and in utero stroke may be of value in patients who are subsequently diagnosed as having the hemiplegic variety of cerebral palsy (Gibson, Mac Lennan, Goldwater, & Dekker, 2003). Identification of a parental coagulopathy or other serological markers could potentially provide for early designation of a population at risk, with more prompt and effective initiation of early intervention therapeutic services and for the development of a preventative protocol (Kraus, 1997).

A perinatal etiology has been identified in only about 10–15% of cases although placental abruption, cord prolapse, and uterine rupture when they do occur can be significant (Nelson, 2008). Factors thought to be characteristic of birth asphyxia, such as meconium staining and fetal distress, are more often the result of nonasphyxial disorders that have been present as chronic stressors in the pregnancy and clinically may not have a way of being identified, tracked, or ameliorated (Nelson, 1989). True perinatal asphyxia may be related to obstetrical complications such as placental abruption, nuchal cord, or meconium aspiration. Such an etiology is often accompanied by seizures in the newborn period and evidence of other organ system dysfunction due to anoxia such as cardiac, renal, and/or hepatic dysfunction. Other perinatal etiologies include central nervous system bleeding (Williams, Lewandowski, Coplan, & D'Eugenio, 1987) and meningeal infections. Patients in this group are most likely to be spastic.

A postnatal etiology occurs in about 10% of patients (Holm, 1982). Factors include head trauma, of an accidental or inflicted (abusive) nature, central nervous system infections, and cerebrovascular accidents. Such patients are likely to be hemiparetic. A mixed etiology occurs in about 7% of cases (Hom, 1982). In some cases, there may be multifactorial factors that result in cumulative risk.

Neonatal indicators for the development of static encephalopathy include intracranial hemorrhage, seizures, microcephaly (small head size), hyper- or hypotonia, abnormal suck/cry/grasp reflexes, jitteriness, temperature instability, and feeding difficulties (Nelson & Ellenberg, 1979). Apgar scores that reflect immediate neonatal status are not as predictive as once thought (Nelson & Ellenberg, 1981). Periventricular hemorrhage in association with attenuation of the white matter about the ventricles (periventricular leukomalacia or PVL) with formation of cysts, which can be demonstrated on head ultrasound or other neuroimaging studies, correlates with the development of cerebral palsy (Graham, Levene, & Trounce, 1987). PVL is associated with birth trauma, asphyxia and respiratory failure, cardiopulmonary defects, premature birth/low birth weight with associated immature cerebrovascular development, and lack of appropriate autoregulation of cerebral blood flow in response to hypoxic–ischemia insult. Other pertinent findings on neuroimaging may include lesions of the basal ganglia, cortical and subcortical lesions, malformations, and focal infarcts (Bax, Tydeman, & Flodmark, 2006).

Brain cells known as oliogodendrocytes are vulnerable to the exposure of free-radical chemicals that are liberated during these events. They are further compromised by poor circulation and the presence of cytokines that are seen with inflammation and infection. If this process is identified earlier and better delineated by newer imaging studies, such as diffusion imaging and other studies, which are not yet routinely available or demonstrated as the standard of care, it is possible to develop treatment that would have more direct efficacy on treating the brain injury. Such options could potentially include use of drugs that reverse the effects of free-radicals and other inflammatory chemicals such as the use of interleukin-10 (Bell & Hallenback, 2002; Mesples, Plaisant, & Gressens, 2003; Rezaie & Dean, 2002).

Delineation of an etiology may imply a specific clinical presentation and prognosis that permits parents to be supplied with an overview of the child's potential outcome. Counseling of parents that actions during the time of conception and pregnancy are most likely unrelated to the development of the cerebral palsy permits feelings of guilt to be assuaged and promotes better acceptance of the child.

Functional Presentation

Cerebral palsy is classified on the basis of etiology, muscle tone, and the anatomical distribution of neurological abnormalities (Perlstein, 1952). Pyramidal or spastic (clasp-knife) cerebral palsy is the most common. Resistance is noted when muscles are stretched rapidly beyond a critical point. Associated hyperreflexia, up-going plantar responses (toes move upward in response to stimulation of the plantar surface of the foot), prolonged contraction of muscles, inability to isolate fine motor movements, co-contractions of agonist and antagonist muscles, and misfiring of muscles during ambulation resulting in gait abnormalities are found. Quadriplegia occurs in about 20% of these cases, with diffuse cortical involvement, and, in the most disabled, widespread atrophy occurs with cavity formation and decreased white matter density. Hemiplegia occurs in about 30% and is associated with atrophy/gliosis of the cerebral hemisphere opposite the side of muscle weakness, likely caused by a vascular disturbance. Liquifaction necrosis may occur, resulting in a porencephalic cyst (Mannino & Traunor, 1983).

Diplegics, who comprise more than 50–65% of this population, are generally, but not exclusively, premature infants who have undergone significant intraventricular hemorrhages (Blair & Stanley, 1990; Hagberg & Hagberg, 1989). The periventricular areas have cortical radiations to the lower extremities, which are more involved with spasticity than the upper extremities; this differentiates these patients from quadriplegics, in whom all extremities are involved to the same degree. Diplegia, and cerebral palsy, in general, in premature infants is most correlated with periventricular leukomalacia as discussed above, and is demonstrable on head ultrasound, computed tomography (CT) scan, and MRI studies. The severity of these findings seems to correlate with the degree of the child's sensorimotor involvement. Infants in this group, who also demonstrate thalamic lesions, are more likely to have severe motor and cognitive dysfunction (Yokochi, 1997). Monoplegia and triplegia (affecting one and three limbs, respectively) are rare. Bilateral involvement is the most common presentation, occurring in 75% of preterm and 45% of term patients (Hagberg & Hagberg, 1996).

Extrapyramidal or nonspastic types of cerebral palsy are responsible for about 20% of cases. Patients who have athetosis or rigidity have basal ganglia dysfunction that account for their movement disorders. Ataxic patients have difficulties with balance and position sense, resulting from cerebellar pathology. Diagnostic work-up is most important with ataxias, as posterior fossa brain tumors and degenerative inherited diseases, such as ataxia telangiectasia and Friedrich's ataxia, may have similar presentations.

Hypotonic patients have widespread damage to cortical and subcortical areas, so spasticity cannot be mounted as a response, and they have the poorest prognosis for cognitive and motor function. Some hypotonic patients may become athetoid with time. The remaining cases have mixed features (i.e., diffuse cerebral involvement and impaired motor function).

Differential Diagnosis

Up to 40% of patients with an initial diagnosis of cerebral palsy have been incorrectly diagnosed. Other disorders that present with gross motor delays, aberrant tone, and abnormal movement patterns include mental retardation, neurodegenerative disorders, hydrocephalus, subdural effusions, slowly growing brain tumors, spinal cord lesions, muscular dystrophy, spinal muscular atrophy, and congenital cerebellar ataxias. Obviously, prognosis, inheritance patterns, and treatment vary widely in these disorders.

Investigations that may be helpful in substantiating or excluding the diagnosis of cerebral palsy include the following: CT or MRI scans to assess structural lesions, ultrasound of the head to exclude the possibility of intraventricular hemorrhage, lumbar puncture to exclude elevated protein in the cerebral spinal fluid that is seen in association with neurodegenerative disorders, serum uric acid and blood and urine assays for amino and organic acids to exclude congenital metabolic disorders, viral and parasitic titers (TORCH) to exclude the possibility of an intrauterine-acquired infection, and chromosomal studies to exclude such abnormalities, especially in dysmorphic children. Recent studies have begun to investigate the usefulness of diffusion tensor imaging (DTI) and fiber tracking in delineating the primary and secondary degenerative changes in cerebral white matter and deep grey matter in patients with cerebral palsy and to explore any possible reorganization of the axonal architecture

Associated Medical Problems

Mental retardation co-exists in 50–60% of patients with cerebral palsy, communication and learning disorders in 40–50%, visual problems, including strabismus and myopia, in 50%, deafness in 6–16%, seizure disorders in 33–38%, and orthopedic deformities in 50% (Robinson, 1973). Visual problems are not only important in terms of learning and school-related tasks, but also affect head and hand movements that influence gross motor coordination including ambulation and self-care skills.

Generalized seizures are most common in patients with quadriplegia, and partial seizures are most common in those patients with hemiplegia (Carlson, Hagberg, & Olssom, 2003). Electroencephalograms and visual- and auditory-evoked potentials are helpful in delineation of such problems. The superimposed seizures and medication effects also increase the risk of behavioral problems and need for counseling in this population (Carlsson, Olsson, Hagberg, & Beckung, 2008).

The parietal lobe syndrome is characterized by hemiplegia, limb length discrepancies (the upper extremity being more affected), and sensory deficits as manifested by reduced two-point discrimination, stereognosis, and graphesthesia (Staheli, Duncan, & Schafer, 1960). A less common triad, seen with erythroblastosis-related disease, includes kernicterus (bilirubin deposition from red blood cell breakdown in the basal ganglia) with resultant athetosis, hearing loss, and paralysis of upward gaze. This is less commonly seen due to a reduction in the incidence of athetoid cerebral palsy but can still be demonstrated in the older cerebral palsied population.

Oropharyngeal incoordination may result in poor oral intake, with failure to thrive, occasionally necessitating placement of a gastrostomy tube for caloric supplementation (Vaughn, Neilson, & O'Dwyer, 1988). Misdirected swallowing and gastroesophageal reflux may result in aspiration pneumonias (Drvaric, Roberts, Burke, King, & Falterman, 1987; Gisel & Patrik, 1988). Poor hand function, pooling of saliva, and abnormal muscle tone can result in poor dental hygiene and malocclusion (Rosenstein, 1982). Restrictive pulmonary disease may result from hypertonicity, and scoliosis may further limit endurance (Rothman, 1978). Bladder spasticity and sphincteric incoordination, rather than cognitive limitations, may result in urinary incontinence and may be responsive to uropharmacological and behavioral management

(Keating, McCarron, James, Gruenberg, & Lonczak, 1985; McNeal, Hawtrey, Wolraich, & Mapel, 1983).

Orthopedic complications include the development of limb contractures and deformities, dislocations, especially at the hips, and scoliosis due to prolonged muscle imbalance. All of these conditions may require medical and therapeutic attempts at normalization of tone and/or surgical interventions as described below. Fractures may occur in these patients as a result of osteopenia concomitant with spasm and secondary effects of anticonvulsant administration (Lingam & Joester, 1994). In nonambulatory, quadriplegic children, lumbar spine bone mineral density may be decreased by as much as 58%, and up to 39% of the patients may suffer nontraumatic hip fractures (King, Levin, Schmidt, Oestreich, & Heubi, 2003). Prolonged periods of immobilization following orthopedic procedures may exacerbate this tendency with up to a 34% loss in bone mineral density occurring over a 4–6-week period (Szalay, Harriman, Eastlund, & Mercer, 2008). Initial studies suggest that the use of bisphosphonate infusions (Pamidronate) may be helpful in treatment of this complication (Henderson, Lark, & Kecskemethy, 2002). Oral agents need to be considered carefully, as they usually require the patient to sit upright for at least 1 hour, which is potentially difficult in this population. Dietary deficiencies may also require supplementation with calcium and vitamin D.

The long-term effects of sedentary lifestyle not of their choosing may have an effect not only on bony fragility of patients with cerebral palsy, but on overall health, sense of well-being, and cardiovascular fitness as well (Morris, 2008), although specific studies in this area are lacking.

Clinical Findings and Prognostic Indicators

Cerebral palsy may be difficult to identify in a patient who is younger than 1 year. Although gross motor milestones may be delayed, hypertonicity, movement disorders, and early hand dominance may have not yet occurred (Levine, 1980). Although the brain lesion that results in the encephalopathy is static, the child's neurological appearance may vary with growth and mediation of the brain. The infant with spastic quadriparesis is generally identified by 5 months of age; diplegics are not identified until 12 months of age, on average, and hemiplegics at 21 months (Harris, 1989). Difficulty in diagnosis is compounded by the plasticity of the immature nervous system, with compensatory branching of the corticospinal tract fibers (Farmer, Harrison, Ingram, & Stephens, 1991), allowing cerebral palsy to "disappear" in up to 55% of cases (Tardorff, 1986). Labeling an infant as "high-risk" may result in overinterpretation of normal physical findings (Ashton, Piper, Warren, Stewin, & Byrne, 1991).

Motor development in the subtypes of cerebral palsy varies, but common denominators exist (Bobath & Bobath, 1975). Abnormal positioning of the hands, hypertonicity of the neck extensors, inability to isolate lower extremity movements (i.e., an all-flexor or all-extensor pattern), difficulty in bringing the elbows across midline suggestive of increased tone, poor head control, microcephaly, abnormal deep tendon reflexes, persistence of grasp reflexes, and up-going plantar responses beyond 12 months of age are all suspect findings. Lack of symmetrical movement and early onset of hand dominance are suggestive of a hemiparesis. Not only may gross motor activities be delayed, but when performed, they may be carried out in an abnormal way, often with utilization of abnormal, stereotypical primitive reflexes to initiate the movement (see below). The use of head arching to initiate rolling and crawling on the abdomen with both legs being flexed simultaneously rather than on all fours in a reciprocal manner are two examples of these behaviors. In the absence of frankly abnormal gross motor movements or reflex abnormalities, the lack of variation of limb movements may also be a finding indicative of a static encephalopathy (Bruggink et al., 2008).

Major support for the diagnosis of cerebral palsy is given by the persistence of primitive reflexes. These subcortical reflexes are normally suppressed by 6 months of age. They can always be summoned but are modulated by more advanced learned motor activities. When these reflexes occur each time a child is placed in a position, they interfere with that child's ability to change position, and to assume and maintain an antigravity position. These reflexes include the symmetric and asymmetric (fencer) tonic neck reflexes, the tonic labyrinthine response, positive support reaction, and the Moro (startle) response. Postural reactions such as head and neck righting responses may be delayed or absent. The persistence of more than one reflex beyond 2 years of age, in association with the child's inability to sit, is negatively associated with future ambulation (Capute, 1978; Sala & Grant, 1995). Conversely, the ability of the child to sit by 2 years correlates with a good prognosis for ambulation. More recently, identification of certain patterns of antigravity movements, such as head lifting, sitting with upper extremity support, and ambulating 10 steps, may stratify the cerebral palsied population into five different types of patients where motor development can be more definitely assessed (Palisano, Rosenbaum, Walter, & Hanna, 1997). However, these studies are preliminary and should not be utilized as a way of limiting therapeutic services or other medical interventions at this time.

Children who do not ambulate by 7–8 years are usually unable to do so, unless limited therapeutic services have not been provided prior to this time. Ninety-eight percent of hemiplegics, 75% of diplegics, and 50% of quadriplegics will ambulate according to studies performed in the past (Molnar & Gordon, 1976). Of those patients with quadriplegia, 25% will be independent, 50% will require assistance, and 25% will utilize wheelchairs as their means of community ambulation. Most patients with the ataxia variant of cerebral palsy will ambulate. Hypotonic and rigid patients have the poorest prognosis for ambulation (Molnar, 1979). These studies were performed prior to newer interventions such as selective dorsal rhizotomy and placement of intrathecal Baclofen pumps; it is yet to be determined if such interventions will result in significant alterations of these prognostic parameters. Children ambulate abnormally because of static and dynamic muscle dysfunction (Sutherland, 1984). Gaits are energy-inefficient, resulting in fatigability and limited endurance (Mossberg, Linton, & Friske, 1990).

Fine motor, personal-social, and language skills may also be impaired to a variable degree. The Amiel-Tison scale, Milani-Comparetti scale, Denver Developmental Screening Test, and the Bayley Scale of Infant Development III are some of the tools that have been developed for documentation and tracking of these dysfunctions. Periodic neuropsychological evaluations to include nonverbal measures as appropriate and the assessment of social, personality, and educational functioning are recommended.

Therapeutic Interventions

Direct treatment for cerebral palsy is for the most part unavailable. However, use of certain physical supports and medications has recently indicated that potential for change and effective treatment is possible. Treatment trials of total body and head cooling for the reduction of effects of hypoxic ischemic encephalopathy have suggested potential reduction in both death and disability (Eicher, Wagner, & Katikaneni, 2004; Shah, Ohlsson, & Perlman, 2007). The use of extracorporeal membrane oxygenation in patients with severe respiratory distress syndrome has been demonstrated as having additional efficacy over traditional ventilatory support, and although these infants are at risk, they have improved survival and need further assessments as to later neuropsychological outcomes (Wagner et al., 2007).

Certain pharmacological agents have been demonstrated to modulate the stressors that may result in a static encephalopathy and appear to be of statistical benefit. The use of prenatal glucocorticoids (dexathamethasone) treatment administered to mothers of preterm infants may reduce the risk of intraventricular hemorrhage and periventricular leukomalacia. The protective effect may occur due to direct stabilization of the vasculature of the fetal brain and a reduction of the acid–base fluctuations that ensue with reduced/aborted respiratory distress syndrome for which these steroids are administered. The risk of the development of cerebral palsy in such a group may be reduced from 22% to 10% (Salakor et al., 1997). Research has also suggested that the use of free-radical scavengers and blockers of receptors of excitatory amino acids could limit the tissue damage that is sustained by neonates with perinatal asphyxia (Vannucci, 1990). Magnesium sulfate, which is used to protect mothers from the hypertension associated with preeclampsia, may also offer a protective effect by acting as a vasodilator to the fetal brain (Hirtz & Nelson, 1998; Rouse et al., 2008) although results of some of these studies are somewhat equivocal (Galvin, 1998). Indomethacin, a nonsteroidal antiinflammatory agent used in the treatment of infants to close a patent ductus arteriosus, has also been recently utilized as a neuroprotective agent to decrease the risk of intraventricular hemorrhage in premature neonates. Other trials are in progress but are not yet in widespread use (Degos, Loron, Mantz, & Gressens, 2008).

Other secondary treatments include therapy, tone-altering medications, provision of adaptive equipment to enhance patients' level of function, and orthopedic and neurosurgical procedures that correct deformities and normalize tone, as discussed below (Diamond, 1986; Lord, 1984; Ronan & Gold, 2007).

Therapeutic systems share the goals of maintenance of joint range, prevention of contractures, normalization of tone, improvement in interaction with the environment, postural control, assumption of antigravity postures, development of muscular control and coordination, and education of the family (Deaver, 1956; Kottke, Halpern, Easton, Ozel, & Burrill, 1978). Many systems are axiomatic, being based on the concept of neuroplasticity in the child, avoidance of abnormal movement patterns, and the importance of sensorimotor learning in cognitive development (Matthews, 1988). Controlled studies are difficult to design, as parents are unwilling to assign their child to a nontreatment group (Guyatt et al., 1986; Martin & Epstein, 1976; Tirosh & Rabino, 1989). It has also been problematic to document the clinical effectiveness of early intervention programs, but there is a strong sense of the clinical validity of such treatment (Palmer et al., 1990; Resnick, Eyler, Nelson, Eitman, & Bucciarelli, 1987). Meta-analyses of such interventions have revealed that when services were initiated in at-risk infants prior to 6 months of age, an improvement of 9–13 points in IQ testing results. The developmental stimulation, rather than physical therapy alone, may be responsible for enhancement of gross motor and cognitive skills (Palmer, Shapiro, & Wachtel, 1988). This is a rationale offered by proponents of the system of conductive education (Hill, 1990). Systems have been proposed by Rood, Knott and Voss, Brunstrom, Temple Fay, and Dolman-Delacato (patterning) (Halpern, 1984), but the Bobath type of treatment generally prevailed in this setting, although motor learning theory may recently be preempting this type of intervention. According to Bobath principles, by placing the affected child in a position in which the effects of abnormal tone and postures are deemphasized, voluntary muscular control may develop, in a proximal-to-distal fashion, paving the way for more functional activities, and the use of the upper extremities for something other than support (Finnie, 1974). Secondary reductions in tone may result in improvement in oromotor control, feeding, speech, and respiration (Nwaobi & Smith, 1986). Motor learning treatment is a more task-directed application where the child learns by limb placement and repetition of the motor tasks required (Tscharnuter, 2002; Valvano, 2004).

Other systems have been developed to deal with the visual-manual and spatial learning difficulties that may co-exist (Bachrach & Greenspun, 1990). Additional options include training the patient in age-appropriate self-care skills and behavior modification. Traditionally, strengthening programs were felt to be contraindicated in spastic conditions such as cerebral palsy, as such efforts were thought to re-enforce the patterns of spasticity that already existed. However, newer studies do not support this notion. Strengthening has been documented as resulting in improvement of hip and knee strength, gait pattern marked by a reduction in crouching and better control of walking speed, and in Gross Motor Functional Measurement ratings (Andersson, Grooten, Hellsten, Kaping, & Mattson, 2003). Similar efficacy has also been recently demonstrated for upper extremity function with use of an arm cranking device (Unnithan et al., 2007).

Efficacy not only exists for younger patients, but teenagers and even patients in the fifth decade have shown demonstrable improvements without negative effects or increases in Ashworth scores (a spasticity measurement scale) (Damiano, Kelly, & Vaughn, 1995; Damiano, Vaughn, & Abel, 1995). Therefore, neurological maturation or cessation of growth is not a contraindication to efficacy of services. However, most adults with cerebral palsy need to be educated as to maintaining their own physical regimen to maintain both endurance and range of motion while preventing pain (Gorter et al., 2009), with more formal therapeutic interventions indicated in response to a more generalized change in their physical status, injury, or surgical intervention.

Abstracted from the experience with adult hemiplegic patients who have had strokes, constraint-induced movement therapy has been used in a small group of hemiplegic children, but current experience is still anecdotal (Pierce, Daly, Gallaghger, Gershkoff, & Schaumburg, 2002). However, it is advisable that children selected for such treatment be chronologically/ cognitively at least at the 6–7-year level so that these efforts are not perceived as being punative. Although there are clinical proponents, the efficacy of other treatments, such as hyperbaric oxygenation, use of the Adeli suit for proximal stabilization (Bar-Haim et al., 2006), craniosacral therapy, massage, acupuncture and acupressure, hippotherapy, and aquatherapy, has not been scientifically substantiated (Hurvitz, Leonard, Ayyangar, & Nelson, 2003; Fragala-Pinkham, Dumas, Barlow, & Pasternak, 2009). Parental perceptions of improvement may not be in accordance with more objectifying measures (Duncan, Barton, Edmonds, & Blashill, 2004).

A variety of modalities, including shaking and cold, are believed to exert effects at the level of the vestibular receptors, muscle spindles, and the Golgi tendon apparatus. Nerve and motor point blocks and biofeedback have also been used (Halpern, 1982; Kassover, Tauber, Au, & Pugh, 1986). Nerve blocks in contrast to motor point blocks not only resulted in weakness, but concurrent, and undesirable sensory deficits/dysesthesias and are therefore used less frequently.

Botulinum A toxin, derived from denatured Clostridium, injected into the muscles of cerebral palsied patients has been shown to transiently reduce spasticity for a period of about 4 months by decreasing acetylcholine release at motor nerve endings thereby blocking neuromuscular transmission in a controlled fashion. This temporary reduction in tone may permit reduction of dynamic deformities such as talipes equinus by reducing tone in spastic gastrocnemius muscles, knee flexion contractures by injection into the hamstrings, and reduction in scissoring following injection into hip adductors. Strengthening of agonist muscle groups also assists in improvement of gait and function. Both upper and lower extremity muscles may be treated. Total dosage for injections at multiple sites should not exceed 6–10 units/kg. The treatment has the advantage of specifically targeting certain areas, rather than globally reducing tone so that loss of trunk and proximal control are much less of a concern. Tendon-lengthening procedures may be deferred on this basis until the patient is older, but it is uncertain if such interventions will reduce the total number of surgical interventions that the patient will eventually require (Korman, Mooney, Smith, Goodman, & Mulvaney, 1993). However, studies in animal models suggest that when given early in development, it may promote growth of muscles, altering the development of contractures (Cosgrove & Graham, 1994). Other studies suggest that injection of Botox in conjunction with serial casting of lower extremity deformities may approach the results obtained from percutaneous tendon lengthenings (Glantzman, Kim, Swaminathan, & Beck, 2004) or selective dorsal rhizotomy (see below), although the number of injection sites (Satila et al., 2008) and protocols vary widely, making analysis of results difficult (Molenaers, Desloovere, & DeCat, 2001; Kelly, MacKay-Lyons, Berryman, Hyndman, & Wood, 2008). The advantages of this treatment are the relative ease of administration, although younger children may require sedation when deeper muscles are injected, and development of usually only mild side effects, which include local soreness to muscles and generalized transient myalgias. More serious, but infrequent, side effects include an association with aspiration pneumonia in patients with pseudobulbar palsy and spastic quadriparesis, global muscle weakness and atrophy (Ansved, Odergren, & Borg, 1997), urinary and fecal incontinence, development of antibodies not associated with clinical disease (Goschel, Wohlfarth, Frevert, Dengler, & Bigalke, 1997), possible potentiation of weakness seen with aminoglycoside antibiotics and depolarizing agents, and acute allergic reactions (Preiss, Condie, Rowley, & Graham, 2003).

The use of oral medications, including diazepam, dantrolene sodium, baclofen, and tizandine, can be tried to reduce tone. Although these may be effective, diazepam has central, sedative effects, is habit forming, and is relatively undesirable in patients who may already have cognitive limitations. It has, however, been reported to decrease tone and improve lower extremity range and spontaneous movements without daytime drowsiness in cerebral palsied children (Mathew, Mathew, Thomas, & Antonisamy, 2005). Dantrolene, which reduces tone by modulating calcium regulation into muscles, is metabolized by the liver, and thus is not a good option for children who may be concurrently prescribed anticonvulsant medications, which are also metabolized by the same route, potentially placing a child at risk for hepatic dysfunction (Zarfonte, Lornard, & Elovic, 2004). Baclofen may also have a sedative effect when used orally. Tizanidine is a newer drug that works on α-adrenergic nerve endings; it is similar to an antihypertensive medication from which it is derived, and therefore, blood pressure needs to be monitored carefully with its introduction. Reduction of nocturnal spasms in children with spastic quadriparesis has been reported with its use (Tanaka et al., 2004).

Appropriate prescription of seating devices for nonambulatory patients permits positioning in an upright manner, improved eye contact, enhanced interaction with the environment, decreased effect of hypertonicity (which pushes the patient out of the chair and adducts the hips), and enhanced feeding, respiration, and ability to use communication devices (Bergen & Colangelo, 1982). Helmets, bed rails, and cushions are used to prevent injury.

Orthotics are prescribed to prevent progression of deformities, provide stability, and enhance function (Gold, 1991). Traditional leather and metal braces have given way to custom-molded plastic orthoses that are lighter and more easily control angular (varus/valgus) deformities. Full control, hip-knee-ankle-foot orthoses are generally used for positioning, but are too heavy for functional ambulation. Variations of these devices exclude the medial metal uprights and thigh cuffs and may be helpful for children with toe walking and dynamic internal rotation at the hips. Ankle-foot orthoses are indicated to improve ankle dorsiflexion and control equinus deformities. Spring-assisted devices are generally contraindicated as rapid stretch may exacerbate spasticity. Orthoses used to maintain muscle length must be worn for at least 6 hours per day to achieve a physiological effect (Tardieu & Lespargot, 1988). The use of tone-reducing orthoses with full footplates and the toes maintained in extension (Bronkhorst & Lamb, 1987; Hinderer & Harris, 1988) may have a direct effect on muscle ultrastructure with resultant increase in sarcomere (muscle unit) length (Tardieu, de la Tour, Bret, & Tardieu, 1982). It is important to discuss these findings with parents/guardians, so that compliance with the recommended wearing schedule is achieved. Ankle-foot orthoses may have hinges incorporated at the ankles to allow for active ankle dorsiflexion and to facilitate movements from sitting to standing (Wilson, Haideri, Song, & Telford, 1997). Orthoses that extend to just above the ankles (supramalleolar orthoses) can control foot alignment, but do not control the ankle joints (Carlson, Vaughan, Damiano, & Abel, 1997). The long-term effect of orthoses in reducing deformity and need for subsequent surgical intervention is controversial (Crenshaw et al., 2000; Sankey, Anderson, & Young, 1989) .

Total contact splinting and use of serial casting are other orthotic options that can be considered for tone reduction and improvement in range. Neoprene garments to improve sensory feedback and proximal stability have also recently been used. There have been some preliminary reports of reduction of peripheral tone and improved quality of gait pattern with their use (Siracusa, Taylor, Geletka, & Overby, 2005).

For maximally involved children, the use of a walking frame with casters provides trunk alignment and support, in conjunction with hip-knee-ankle orthoses. Although functional ambulation is not possible with such devices, their utilization permits tolerance of the upright posture, increased weight bearing, and a sense of movement for the child, which may be psychologically rewarding (Stallard, Major, & Farmer, 1996). Similarly, body-weight supported treadmill training has been explored as a means of enhancing reciprocal stepping patterns as a preliminary activity to prepare for ambulation (Dieruf et al., 2009; Eisenberg, Zuk, Carmeli, & Katz-Leuer, 2009).

Threshold electrical stimulation can be utilized as an adjunct to traditional therapeutic interventions. Low-intensity transcutaneous stimulation can be applied to a variety of weak, superficial muscles, nocturnally. Theoretically, the resultant increase in blood flow to these muscles at a time when growth hormone levels are highest encourages their growth. This permits the traditional strengthening efforts applied during the day to be more effective. Improvement in gait (enhanced tibialis anterior function, better balance, and improved gait pattern) has been demonstrated in a few studies (Hazelwood, Brown, Rowe, & Salter, 1994; Pape et al., 1993; Seifart, Unger, & Burger, 2009). However, the long-term effect of this treatment and any possible associated reduction in the subsequent need for surgical intervention have not yet been demonstrated.

Given the multiple potential interventions and confounding clinical variables that exist, truly objective research design is extremely difficult. The use of standardized testing and functional scales may serve as an adjunct in such studies, permitting the patient to be compared to his/her own pretreatment performance. Such measurement tools include measurement of torque/resistance to passive stretch as an indicator of spasticity, the Gross Motor Function Measure (Wei et al., 2006), the Wee-F.I.M. or functional independence measure for patients younger than 7 years (Sanders et al., 2006), the Pediatric Evaluation of Disability Inventory (PEDI) (Hayley, Ludlow, & Coster, 1993), and the Ashworth scale for clinically reproducible measurement of spasticity (Clopton et al., 2005).

Surgical Options

Prevention of deformities resulting from inequalities in muscle tone and strength in association with fixed posturing due to the influence of retained positive primitive reflexes is the best treatment option; however, orthopedic surgery should not be perceived as a failure of previous treatment, but rather as an adjunct to achievement of therapeutic goals. The muscles of spastic patients with cerebral palsy are too short, with chronic increases in tone possibly resulting in reduced sarcomere length and abnormal connectin protein (Graham & Selber, 2003). With inability of the muscles to relax, imbalances occur between the growth of the long bones and the muscle tendons resulting in secondary structural deformities (Ziv, Blackborn, Rang, & Koresk, 1984). Subluxation and early-onset osteoarthritis with regression in function, not associated with an actual decline in neurological status may occur. Hence, early and efficient surgical interventions are warranted (Frieden & Lieber, 2003) and may permit less invasive soft tissue rather than bony surgery (osteotomies) to be performed. Conversely, early tendon releases may initially interfere with acquisition of motor milestones and mobility, and may increase the need for repeat surgery as the child grows. Psychological support services to both parents and child, to cope with fears and expectations, are most important. At least 6 months of extensive postoperative physical rehabilitation may be required to see signs of functional improvement because of transient deconditioning (Reimers, 1990), with reduction of muscle strength and readjustment of the body to a new muscle length–tension ratio. The separation of the parent from the child and the financial burdens encountered are other factors to be considered.

A full discussion of the orthopedic deformities and their surgical treatment may be found in several excellent texts (Bleck, 1987; Samilson, 1981). Common lower extremity deformities include hip flexion contractures, femoral anteversion with medial rotation of the legs, hip adduction with subluxation, pelvic asymmetry with secondary scoliosis, hamstring spasticity with hyphosis and knee flexion contractures, and equinovarus or equinvalgus deformities, with hemiplegia and diplegia, respectively. Typical upper extremity deformities include internal rotation contractures of the shoulders, flexion contractures at the elbows, wrist flexion contractures, ulnar deviation, finger flexion contractures, and thumb-in-palm deformities. For dependent patients, surgery may be performed to facilitate perineal care, reduce pain association with dislocation, and correct pelvic asymmetry that may exacerbate scoliosis and reduce supported sitting tolerance (Carr & Gage, 1987; Cooperman, Bartucci, Dietrick, & Miller, 1987). For children with better gross motor function, surgery is indicated to improve lower extremity alignment and correct a progressively crouched gait, scissoring, and other gait abnormalities that result in poor balance and easy fatigability due to excessive energy expenditure.

Procedures include adductor tenotomies and varus derotation osteotomies of the femurs. Previously, these patients were confined in extensive plaster casts postoperatively, but this is now less commonly used resulting in fewer cases of secondary skin breakdown, and earlier mobilization, weight bearing, and rehabilitation without an increased rate of complication (Schafer, McCarthy, & Josephic, 2007). Hamstring lengthenings are performed to correct knee flexion contractures, avoiding overlengthening, which could result in hyperextension at the knees (Gage, 1990) that would require another procedure (rectus femoris transfer) to be performed. Achilles tendon lengthenings are the most commonly performed procedure; with correction of the equinus deformity, toe walking is corrected, a stable base of support on a flat foot is established, and walking speed and stride length are increased (Shapiro & Susa, 1990). A posterior tibialis tendon transfer may be indicated to correct equinovarus and to elevate the foot when walking. For more resistant deformities at the foot, an extraarticular (Grice) procedure or other arthrodesis may be required (Fulford, 1990). Computerized gait analysis may be utilized to assess surgical indications and outcomes (Narayanan, 2007). The techniques of the lower extremity surgical procedures have not changed considerably in the recent past, but surgeries are more frequently performed at multiple levels at the same time to reduce both anesthetic exposures and rehabilitation admissions, while maximizing functional correction (Graham & Harvey, 2007). With growth, there may be a recurrence of deformities necessitating reoperation with an overall recurrence rate of about 10–15% per level.

Bony procedures about the hips are associated with the development of heterotopic ossification (bone growth outside of skeletal tissue) in about 25% of cases, and the hardware usually needs to be removed after 1 year to prevent stress fractures and pain.

Surgery for the upper extremities is performed less frequently, as improved outcomes may be limited by cognitive and sensory impairments. Procedures include release of the internal rotators of the shoulder, release of the biceps tendon and anterior capsulotomy to correct elbow flexion contractures, transfer of wrist flexors to function as wrist extensors, and release of the thumb-in-palm deformity (Mital & Sakellarides, 1981). Spinal fusion may be required to control scoliosis. Luque and other newer spinal instrumentations permit some patients to forgo prolonged immobilization in a body jacket (Lonstein & Akbamia, 1983).

Neurosurgical procedures to restore function and to control associated intractable seizures by resection of localized focus of electrical abnormalities are newer adjuncts in the care of the cerebral palsied patient. Implantation of a cerebellar pacemaker had been utilized in the past for tone modulation, but is not currently used in any large numbers (Penn, Mykleburst, Gottlieb, Agarwal, & Etzel, 1980).

The selective dorsal rhizotomy procedure to decrease lower extremity tone and to secondarily permit for development of isolated lower extremity tone and improvement in gait has been utilized for more than 20 years. Spinal nerve rootlets that have been determined as being electrically abnormal (Cahan & Kundi, 1987) are surgically lesioned in purely spastic children without clinical evidence of a progressive neurological disorder. With modulation of abnormal sensory input, there is a resetting of muscle spindle sensitivity with a reduction in tone. Electromyographic monitoring is used intraoperatively to assess which of the spastic rootlets should be lesioned, although responses may be less consistent than previously thought. In conjunction with a well-delineated postoperative program, improvements in tone, range, posture, sitting balance, and gait occurs in 85–90% of appropriately selected candidates (Abbott, Johann-Murphy, & Gold, 1991; Peacock & Staudt, 1991) to a greater extent than would be anticipated on the basis of physical therapy intervention alone (Steinbok, Reiner, Beauchamp, Armstrong, & Cochrane, 1997). Improvement in gait is characterized by increased dynamic range-of-motion at the hips, improved velocity of ambulation, and improved stride length (Thomas, Aiona, Pierce, & Piatt, 1996). Over time, this may result in a decreased need for Achilles tendon lengthenings, adductor releases, and hamstring releases, and may not affect the subsequent rates of ankle-foot operations, femoral osteotomies, and ilipsoas releases in these patients (Chicoine, Park, & Kaufman, 1997). An improvement of 12.1 versus 4.4 points in children treated with physical therapy alone has been documented on the gross motor function measure at 6–12 months postoperatively. Although not a specific indication for performance of the procedure, secondary improvements in upper extremity function and reduction in bladder spasticity may also result (Sweetser, Badell, Schneider, & Badlin, 1995). Energy efficiency is improved in over half of the patients. Recurrence of spasticity and deterioration of gait with adolescence is prevented in a majority of cases (Nordmark et al., 2008). Complications may include dysesthesias, sensory deficits, and, on long-term follow-up, spinal stenosis (Gooch & Walker, 1996). Despite the documented improvements, 66–75% of patients undergoing rhizotomy will still require additional orthopedic surgery.

The effect of anoxia on the spinal cord has been described (Clancy, Sladsky, & Rorke, 1989; Harrison, 1988), thus lending credence to the use of baclofen (Young & Delwaide, 1981). Baclofen is a derivative of the inhibitory neurotransmitter γ-aminobutyric acid, which inhibits excitatory neurotransmission in the brain and spinal cord. This results in secondary inhibition of excitatory neurotransmitters and reduces muscle tone. This medication may also be administered intrathecally (Albright, Cervi, & Singletary, 1991), via a surgically implantable and programmable pump, allowing for titration and reversal of dosage with reduced risk of medication-induced side effects (Albright, 1996). The implementation of this treatment is more suitable in patients with less satisfactory underlying strength, which may require some spasticity for antigravity/ambulatory activities, and in older patients. Documented benefits in hamstring motion, upper extremity function, ambulation (Gerszten, 1997), and activities of daily living (ADL) have been associated with this treatment (Albright, Barron, Fasisck, Polinko, & Janosky, 1993), and possibly a reduction in the need for subsequent orthopedic surgical interventions from 58% to 21% in one population studied (Armstrong, Steinbok, & Cochrane, 1997). It may be implanted even when there is anticipated need for subsequent posterior spinal fusion for scoliosis treatment (Borowski, Shah, Littleton, Dabney, & Miller, 2008). Complications of this device include long-term reliance upon the device with need for approximately monthly refills of the reservoir in which the medication is housed, risk of catheter breakage and infection, risk of acute baclofen withdrawal if the pump is not refilled on a timely and regular basis or because of pump failure, risk of exacerbation of seizure disorders, loss of ability to assume and maintain antigravity positions, and possibly an increased risk of aspiration pneumonia when utilized in the most physically involved patients (Sgoros & Seri, 2002). Selective dorsal rhizotomy, which reduces tone by surgical lesioning of sensory input at the spinal cord level (Fasano, Barolat-Romana, Zeme, & Squazzi, 1979), may also be utilized to this goal, as detailed above.

Psychological, Vocational, and Medical Problems of Adults

Therapeutic services may enhance acquisition of gross motor skills, but cognitive improvement and emotional maturity are more elusive to treat. The severity of the physical disability does not correlate with the physical or psychological health of the parents (Wallender,

Babani, Varni, Banis, & Wilcox, 1989). Sibling and spousal support are pertinent predictors of achieving mental health and improvement in physical performance (Craft, Lakin, Oppliger, Clancy, & Vanderlinder, 1990). Despite similar interest and enjoyment in extracurricular activities as their typically developing peers, activities are significantly limited in children with cerebral palsy (Engel-Yeter, Jarus, Anaby, & Law, 2009). Lives of 50–90% of adolescents with cerebral palsy (and spina bifida) may be characterized by dependence on parents for personal care, lack of responsibility for home chores, lack of information about sexuality, and limited participation in social activities and sexual relationships (Blum, Resnick, Nelson, & St. Germaine, 1991; Hirtz, 1989; Murphy, Molnar, & Lankasky, 2000). This does not encourage independent living, marriage, or employment. In one optimistic study, up to 68% of adults with cerebral palsy were able to live independently (Michelsen, Uldall, Hansen, & Madsen, 2006). Only 30–50% of cerebral palsy patients are employed full-time at maturity; diplegics and hemiplegic patients are more successful (Bleck, 1987; Michelsen, Uldall, Mette, & Madsen, 2005). Other positive factors relating to employability include independence in ADL, ability to ambulate, being female, and enrollment in a nonrestrictive high school setting (Magill-Evans, & Restall, 1991; Sillanpaa, Piekkala, & Pisira, 1982; Tobimatsu & Nakamura, 2000). Therefore, it is important to assess the ability of adult patients to perform instrumental ADL, which include money management, travel training, and meal planning (van der Dussen, Nieuwstraten, Roebroeck, & Stam, 2001).

Transition to adulthood for cerebral palsy patients and those with other chronic diseases of childhood is extremely difficult as services are lacking and physicians treating adult patients may be unfamiliar with their disorders. This is a happy situation for which planning had not occurred, as 90% of patients with cerebral palsy will now live into adulthood. Education of both patients to familiarize themselves with the details of their history and to learn advocacy skills when parents are no longer able to provide these services may take years to learn (Donkervoort, Wiegerink, van Meeteren, Stam, & Roebroeck, 2009; Young, 2007).

It has not been established what therapeutic services are necessary for adult cerebral palsy patients to maintain their function. It is sobering to acknowledge that deterioration in gait in the presence of a static encephalopathy may begin prior to 14 years of age, and is manifested by an increase in double-support time and a decrease in knee, ankle, and pelvic motion (Johnson, Damiano, & Abel, 1997). Because of this deterioration, only 20% of adult patients with cerebral palsy will be independent ambulators, 40% will ambulate with assistance, and 40% will be nonambulatory, although 75% of these patients will retain their independence in ADL (Anderson & Mattson, 2001; Brown, Bontempo, & Turk, 1992). Medical complications in an aging population (Bachrach & Greenspun, 1990) include cervical and lumbar radiculopathies (Ebura et al., 1990; Reese, Msall, & Owens, 1991), carpal tunnel syndrome (Alvarez, Larkin, & Roxborough, 1981), and arthritis at major joints, each of which may require surgical intervention for restoration of function. Specifically, cervical disc disease is eight times more frequent in the adult athetoid patient than in the general patient (Harade et al., 1996). There is an overall 63% incidence of degenerative arthritis, especially at the hips, in cerebral palsy patients younger than 50 years (Bajelidze, Beithur, Littlerton, Dabney, & Miller, 2008). Chronic pain may occur in up to 84% of the adult population, which may require direct and indirect management, including treatment of increased spasticity (Engel, Kartin, & Jensen, 2002; Turk, Scandale, Rosenbaum, & Weber, 2001). Seizure disorders persist into adulthood. Neurogenic bladder and unrecognized problems with toileting accessibility may also be problematical. Referral sources for provision of gynecological care, especially in provision of mammograms to nonambulatory patients may be sorely lacking. Little in the way of organized and proactive treatment is available for this population (Murphy, Molnar, & Lankasky, 1995). As activity decreases, there may be a greater mortality in this population due to ischemic heart disease, compounded by difficulty with communication and lack of family supervision once placement options have been sought (Strauss, Cable, & Shavelte, 1999), and an increased incidence of deep vein thromboses also related to inactivity (Rapp & Torres, 2000).

Despite potential complications, 90% survival into adulthood is seen with cerebral palsy (Evans, Evans, & Alberman, 1990). Earlier demise occurs in patients who have severe mental deficiency, are totally dependent, have poorly controlled seizures, require gastrostomy feeding, have no means of communication, and whose secondary illnesses are primarily respiratory in nature (Evans & Alberman, 1990; Maudsley, Hultor, & Pharoah, 1999). Recently, the poor prognostic implication of gastrostomy tube placement has come under review, and does not appear to auger quite the dire prognosis as when placed in the elderly. One study indicated that 83% of the pediatric population in whom gastrostomy placement occurs survive 2 years, 75% survive 7 years, and there is family satisfaction with quality of life in 90% (Smith, Camfield, & Camfield, 1999). There have been some studies to suggest that an increased susceptibility to infection exists not only on a neuromuscular basis, but on a biological basis as well. Some patients have been noted to have fewer soluble interleukin-2 receptors and lymphocyte proliferative and lytic responses, resulting in reduced resistance to an infectious agent. Demise is often coincident with the "aging-out" of parents and relocation from the home to an institutional facility (Eyman & Grossman, 1990). These findings should prompt the reexamination of public policies for provision of medical benefits to handicapped adults whose parents wish them to retain the family domicile and other financial assets that would permit home-based care.

SPINA BIFIDA

Spina bifida, or myelomeningocele, denotes a condition in which there are congenital abnormalities of the vertebral elements in association with extrusion of abnormally formed neural elements. Patients present with various degrees of lower-extremity motor and sensory deficits concomitant with variable bowel and bladder control, hydrocephalus, and other medical problems. The resultant condition impinges on normal motor development and may alter fine motor, perceptual, linguistic, and cognitive function. A discussion of treatment strategies reflects not only technical advancements but also the changes in the advocacy for the treatment of the physically challenged child. This is a congenital but not a static disorder, in which progressive neurological dysfunctions may occur over time in up to 40% of patients (Spindel, Bauer, & Dryon, 1987).

Anatomical Abnormalities

Failure of fusion of the posterior elements of the lumbosacral spine without associated neurological abnormalities is known as spina bifida occulta and occurs in 20–25% of the general population (without overt or open spina bifida). Should such findings be noted in a patient with incontinence, cavus (high-arched) feet, and/or hairy tuft or hemangioma over the lower spine, an associated malformation of the spinal cord may be present, which can readily be documented on a magnetic resonance imaging (MRI) study. A terminal myelocystocele is a closed defect that presents with a lumbosacral fat-containing mass comprised of cerebrospinal fluid and neural tissue, which will require surgical intervention. It may be associated with abnormal development of the lower spine, genitalia, bowel, bladder, kidneys, and opening of the abdominal wall, such as an omphalocele. It is not generally associated with hydrocephalus. Ambulatory compromise may require interventions similar to those in the more typical form of spinal dysraphism (Choi & Mc Comb, 2000).

In the most severe of open spina bifida, there are abnormally formed neural elements with cystic structures within the spinal cord. Patients present with findings of both upper and lower motor neuron dysfunction, such as weakness, spasticity, and low tone (Stark & Baker, 1967). Defects at the lumbosacral level are the most common; thoracic and cervical lesions occur less frequently. Because of the resultant lack of normal innervation, varying degrees of paralysis of the lower extremities occurs, and there are secondary and often severe orthopedic deformities that occur due to the imbalance of muscular forces.

The Lorber Criteria and Their Abandonment

In the past, severely deformed infants with myelomeningocele died, without treatment, from meningitis, hydrocephalus, and/or renal failure because of the desire not to prolong the lives of children who were cognitively subnormal, nonambulatory, and chronically ill. The mortality rate within the first month of life was 63% and 89% by the sixth month. Lorber (1971) advised no treatment for those infants who would be totally plegic in the lower extremities, had severe hydrocephalus, had severe kyphoscoliosis that would not permit an erect posture, and/or had severe congenital malformations such as exstrophy of the bladder or congenital heart disease. He felt that only 18% of the population would be ambulatory, cognitively normal, and able to earn an income. The initial study did not recognize that the survivors would be more compromised than necessary (McLaughlin & Shurtleff, 1979), or that there was an inability to predict which of the cognitively normal patients would be sacrificed by the lack of treatment. Adoption of these criteria implied that a life in a wheelchair was one without quality. These and other assumptions have recently proved invalid with more advanced treatments, as noted below (Khoury, Erickson, & James, 1982; Mc Clone, Dias, Kaplan, & Sommers, 1985).

Neurosurgery in the neonate to drain the collection of excessive cerebrospinal fluid associated with hydrocephalus can result in restoration of a relatively normal head circumference and reexpansion of the cerebral mantle. With appropriate treatment, a 5-year survival rate of 86% has been reported, however, patients with brain stem dysfunction had a greater mortality (Worley, Schuster, & Oakes, 1996). The severe gibbus deformity (sharply angulated toward flexion of the spine) associated with kyphoscoliosis may be surgically corrected (Linter & Lindseth, 1994), as may other congenital anomalies. Mental retardation is not intrinsic to spina bifida or to the Arnold-Chiari malformation, which results in hydrocephalus. Up to 75% of patients with spina bifida manifesta have normal intelligence (McClone, Czyzewski, Raimondi, & Somers, 1985), but the incidence of learning disabilities will be high, with arithmetic and design copying skills frequently being compromised (Wills, Holmbeck, Dillon, & McClone, 1990). Functional bowel and bladder continence may ideally be achieved in 80% of school-aged children. Eighty percent of school-aged children will be community ambulators. Only 10–15% of patients will require supportive care as adults. The emotional and psychological costs for delaying treatment are high. Hence, early and aggressive treatment of these infants is now the rule.

Incidence, Embryology, and Etiology

The incidence of spina bifida manifesta in the United States is approximately 2 cases per 10,000 births, which represents a decline of more than 27–50% over the past decades (Lary & Edmonds, 1996; Meyer & Siega-Riz, 2002). This is largely attributable to the supplementation of grain products, such as cereal with folic acid, for women of child-bearing age. The decline has been greatest in mothers older than 30 years, those who have had a high-school education, whose medical care was not Medicaid funded, and who were non-Hispanic Caucasians.

Although folic acid supplementation and possibly vitamin B_{12} plays a role in prevention, the etiology for neural tube defects is likely multifactorial, including a genetic basis. The undefined insult to the embryo occurs at 21–26 days of gestation, when the neural tube that will become the central nervous system is invaginating. Early theories suggested that there was a failure of fusion or disruption of the tissue columns caused by abnormalities in the cerebral spinal fluid pressure (Streeter, 1942). More recently, studies from animal models have revealed a group of developmental genes, termed homeobox genes, which direct the segmental development of the nervous system. In mammals, the Hox genes have been demonstrated to encode positions from the top of the brain to the lower spinal cord. Another similar group of genes has been described as assisting in differentiation of the ventral from the dorsal spinal cord. Mechanisms that damage gene function may affect the process of nervous system development, resulting in myelomeningocele and the related Chiari II malformation responsible for hydrocephalus; clinically, this may explain the mechanism in at least 15% of patients with spina bifida (Mc Clone, 1998).

The incidence of neural tube defects can be reduced by up to 86% by the intake of 0.4 mg/day folic acid in the periconceptual period. Decreased folate and increased total homocystiene levels have been documented in the mothers of such patients. This metabolically may result in a decrease in methionine formation, which results in abnormal gene transcription and impairment of neural tube differential and closure (Botto & Yang, 2000; Veland, Hosted, Schneede, Refsum, & Vollset, 2001).

Control of obesity (maternal weight less than 31 kg/m^2) prior to conception may play a role in this and other congenital anomalies, which does not appear to be directly related to dietary deficiencies (Stothard, Tennant, Bell, & Rankin, 2009). Other factors that have been implicated include maternal hyperthermia, other dietary deficiencies, use of valproate by epileptic women during pregnancy, and presence of certain chronic maternal diseases such as diabetes (Khoury et al., 1982; Leck, 1974; Padmanabhan, 2006). There is a 5% risk of recurrence of another infant with spina bifida with subsequent pregnancies, and in all spina bifida patients who produce offsprings.

Prenatal diagnosis can be made by ultrasound (Robinson, Hood, Adam Gibson, & Ferguson-Smith, 1980). Prenatal anatomical levels as determined on high-resolution ultrasound can be reliably utilized to discuss functional motor outcome with the parents (Coniglio, Anderson, & Ferguson, 1996). Analysis of amniotic fluid and/or maternal serum for elevated α-fetoprotein, a substance that is liberated by fetal blood vessels of the uncovered neural elements, is also indicative of the disorder. Analyses are performed in the second trimester so that termination of pregnancy, if desired, is possible. False-positive results may occur in association with gastrointestinal malformations (Milunsky & Alpert, 1976a, 1976b). Anencephaly and skin-covered lesions cannot be identified by chemical analysis, so ultrasound is very important. These tests were not consistently performed in pregnancy so that in previous decades, the majority of cases were not diagnosed in utero. Of all neural tube defects so identified, 39.9% result in termination of pregnancy. For those pregnancies that go to completion, a caesarian section is indicated in fetuses with functional lower-extremity movements to lessen the risk of trauma to the exposed neural elements and hydrocephalus head.

Antenatal and Neonatal Treatment

In utero repair of myelomeningocele is still a new option for attempting to reduce subsequent neurological dysfunction, being available in only three centers in the United States at present. Interposition of latissimus dorsi flaps over the neurological lesion or other techniques may prevent further in utero damage to the spinal cord and nerve roots or damage that occurs at the time of delivery (Meuli et al., 1997; Meuli-Simmen, Meuli, Adzick, & Harrison, 1997). Interventions have been attempted both laparoscopically and by robotic intervention (Bruner & Tulipan, 2005). The procedure may also lessen the risk for subsequent ventriculoperitoneal placement. Infusion of neural stem cells at the site of the open neural placode has been utilized in animal models (Fauza, Jennings, Teng, & Synder, 2008). In utero treatment of hydrocephalus has also been attempted. Both these treatment options may result in premature delivery, so there is a risk of trading one developmental disability for another given the current state of the art (Chervenak & McCullough, 2002).

The deformities of spina bifida manifesta are obvious at birth. The spinal defect is generally closed at 24–48 hours, and a ventriculoperitoneal shunt is required in a total of 80% of patients at a variable time thereafter. In the period proceeding surgical intervention, the infant should be transferred to a tertiary care facility where a multidisciplinary team is available, kept abdomen-down in a warmer, and placed on prophylactic intravenous antibiotics to prevent central nervous system infection. The patient should be assessed for other congenital abnormalities and urological and orthopedic assessments should also be performed (Alexander & Steig, 1989). The hiatus from birth to surgical treatment permits parents to be supplied with information about their child's condition, which will facilitate their ability to select suitable treatment options (Charney, 1990). Pediatricians who are unfamiliar with the diagnosis may offer an unnecessarily dire prognosis (Siperstein, Wolraich, Reed, & O'Keefe, 1988). Parents should handle the infant as soon as possible and be familiarized with range-of-motion techniques, learn how to deal with the infant's insensate skin, and be instructed in intermittent urinary catheterization if this is indicated (Boytim, Davidson, Charney, & Melchionne, 1991).

The Arnold-Chiari Malformation and Hydrocephalus

The Arnold-Chiari II malformation, seen in up to 90% of patients with spina bifida (Badell-Ribera, Swinyeard, Greenspan, & Deaver, 1964) is characterized by a downward displacement of a portion of the cerebellum through the foramen magnum into the spina canal, with secondary compression of the fourth ventricle and development of hydrocephalus (Lemire, 1988). Untreated, this condition results in progressive expansion of the ventricles, with compression of cerebral tissue, spasticity, retardation, blindness, dysphagia, apnea, and death (Charney, Rorke, Sutton, & Schut, 1991). A shunt is placed from the ventricles into the peritoneal space to decompress the hydrocephalus. Shunted patients and those in whom shunting is not required have normal intelligence quotients (IQ of 95 and 102, respectively). However, for each episode of bacterial ventriculitis, there is a 10–15 point decrement in the IQ, with an average score of 72 (Hunt & Holmes, 1976). Shunt surgery may also be complicated by breakage, distal blockage, nephritis, and hydrocele. Patients requiring shunt revision after the age of 2 years may have a poorer prognosis for overall cognitive function (Hunt, Oakeshold, & Kerry, 1999) and for memory skills that correlate with subsequent functional independence and quality of life.

New imaging studies of the brain, such as DTI, may be of value in providing noninvasive estimation of potential intellectual involvement (Hasan, Sankar et al., 2008) and have demonstrated abnormalities of the association pathways needed for sustained concentration to task and higher intellectual function in some patients (Hasan, Eluvathingal et al., 2008). This is important information to derive and needs to be correlated with psychometric testing, given the risk for learning disabilities and modifications of therapeutic and school program, which may subsequently be indicated for these patients (Burmeister et al., 2005; Vinck, Maassen, Mullaart, & Rotteveel, 2006).

A newly developed alternative for the management of hydrocephalus is endoscopic third ventriculostomy. At present, its application may be best suited for patients older than 6 months. Long-term shunt dependence with later complications may thereby be avoided (Teo & Jones, 1996).

Seizures may occur in up to 21% of patients with spina bifida. Underlying additional structural anomalies of the brain such as encephalomalacia, agenesis of the corpus callosum, and/ or calcifications predispose to this complication (Talwar, Baldwin, & Hornblatt, 1995; Yoshida et al., 2005).

Neurological Level: Functional Implications

The performance of a neurological examination in the neonate is challenging because of lack of cooperation and existence of spinal shock (Chiaramonte, Horowitz, Kaplan, & Brock, 1986). Stimulation of the arms and the upper trunk rather than of the lower extremities may more reliably evoke volitional rather than reflexogenic movements (Stark & Baker, 1967).

Somatosensory-evoked potentials may also be used to document the level of innervation. This determination is crucial, as it will indicate, with good reliability, ambulatory status and risk for the development of orthopedic deformities, those patients with the lowest sacral levels of spinal involvement having the best prognosis (DeSouza & Carroll, 1976). Further delineation of prognosis involves the determination of strength of the musculature at a given level (McDonald, Jaffe, Mosca, Shurtleff, & Menalaus, 1991a, 1991b), especially the strength of the hip flexors and knee extensors and the presence of scoliosis, which may occur in up to 50% of this population (Drennan, 1976). Factors of lesser importance include age, sitting balance, height, sex, motivation, presence of spasticity, adequacy of bracing, appropriateness of orthopedic surgery, and motor planning abilities (Asher & Olsen, 1983). Infants with a thoracic level lesion will have no voluntary movements in their lower extremities. With training and correction of lower extremity contractures, 50% of this group become therapeutic or community ambulators in childhood, with extensive bracing (Charney, Melchionni, & Smith, 1991; Shafer & Dias, 1983). As the child matures, increasing weight, upward displacement of the center of gravity, and underlying trunk and respiratory muscle dysfunction cause increasing energy expenditure (Findley & Agre, 1988). By adulthood, this group is usually reliant on wheelchairs for mobility but is capable of independent transfers, dressing, bowel and bladder management, and being employed (Carroll, 1977). Despite the transient nature of their ambulation, walking should be attempted to provide patients with vertical orientation, permit performance of tabletop activities in standing, improve respiratory excursion and urinary drainage, and lessen the possibilities of skin breakdown, contractures, and osteoporosis-related fractures (Dosa et al., 2007).

Patients with innervation at the first three lumbar levels have motor power in hip flexors and adductors (which bring the legs to midline), and to a variable degree in the knee extensors. There is no ability to extend or abduct the hips or to move the feet. At this level, there is the highest risk of hip dislocation, given the imbalance of muscle pull. Hip dislocation may be an impediment to continued ambulation, especially if the hips are stiff or if the dislocation is unilateral resulting in leg length discrepancy, pelvic obliquity, and progressive scoliosis (Crandall, Birkeback, & Wintor, 1989; Curtis, 1973). Iliopsoas transfers (Sharrard, 1964) were routinely performed in the past to prevent hip flexion contractures, but this limited patients' abilities to flex at hips and ascend stairs, and therefore it is currently rarely performed. Osteotomies of the femoral heads for treatment of subluxation are performed to restore symmetry about the hips, but are not obligatory for ambulation to be achieved (Sherk, Uppal, Lane, & Melchionni, 1991). Release of hip flexion contractures of greater than 30° can also be considered in this group (Frawley, Broughton, & Menalaus, 1996). Infants may be provided with foot drop splints to prevent progressive equinus deformities and may require hip abduction devices to maintain stability at those joints.

In nonambulatory children with high-level lesions, unilateral hip dislocations may cause little functional disability, and surgical intervention is less frequently indicated than in the years past. In ambulatory patients with lower-level lesions, leg-length discrepancy and its effect on functional problems mandate surgical correction (Fraser, Bourke, Broughton, & Menalaus, 1995). Patients with higher-level lesions are generally braced with full-control devices necessitated not only by their lower extremity weakness, but also by their hydrocephalus-related hypotonia. They can be supplied with a standing device known as a parapodium at about 18 months (Letts, Fulford, Eng, & Robinson, 1976). A spina bifida car can also be provided for independent mobility (Charney, Rorke, et al., 1991). By 2–3 years, hip-knee-ankle-foot orthoses can be provided and gait training with a rollator commenced (Lough & Nielsen, 1986). Alternatively, an Orlau parawalker (a type of standing frame with a swivel base) can be considered (Major, Stollard, & Farmer, 1997). Depending on praxis and eye-hand coordination, crutches may be supplied at 4–5 years, with household and some community ambulation anticipated. Reciprocating gait orthosis (with cables) may help to facilitate ambulation and reduce energy consumption by up to 50% in this group when compared with the use of traditional knee-ankle-foot orthoses used with a four-point gait (Cuddeford et al., 1997).

With full innervation at the fourth lumbar level, knee extensors are stronger, and patients may be advanced to knee-ankle-foot orthoses. Some patients may have imbalance between knee flexors and extensors, requiring surgical release of the hamstrings to improve gait (Marshall, Broughton, Menelaus, & Graham, 1996). With innervation at the fifth lumbar level, muscle power about the hips is more balanced. The ankle dorsiflexors, but not the plantar flexors, are functioning, usually resulting in calcaneal deformities with ambulation occurring on insensate feet that increases the risk of skin breakdown at these sites. Thus, an indication arises for transfer of the tibialis anterior muscles, which normally dorsiflex the foot, to a more posterior location, so that weight bearing can be achieved in a plantargrade manner. Foot deformities such as planovalgus may occur at this and other levels. Triple arthrodesis (subtalar fusion to stabilize inversion/eversion) may be performed at about 12 years of age, when the feet are relatively grown. Other surgical procedures considered for correction of valgus deformities provide correction with less rigidity (Abraham, Lubicky, Sanger, & Millar, 1996).

Patients with such lower-lumbar lesions can be anticipated to pull to standing by 1 year and ambulate in the community with or without orthoses despite gait deviations. For patients with sacral level lesions, only minor foot deformities are anticipated. These patients may require shoe modifications or ankle-foot orthoses, but would be able to ambulate without them. They are, however, expected to have bowel and bladder incontinence because of involvement of nerves that normally regulate these functions. It is very important to follow up patients with such low lesions as almost one third may show a decline in ambulatory abilities over time, occurring because of skin breakdown, osteomyelitis, and the need for amputation in association with underrecognized tethering of the spinal cord and syringomyelia, as discussed below (Brinker et al., 1994).

Scoliosis and Tethering of the Spinal Cord

Management of a paralytic spinal curvature is difficult. As posterior vertebral elements are lacking, surgical fixation with metal rods usually has to be performed both anteriorly and posteriorly (Banta & Park, 1983). Surgical procedures require a period of immobilization, but less so with the development of newer hardware systems. Patients need to be observed post-operatively for further neurological compromise and the development of pseudoarthroses (movement in areas where bones should be solid). Unchecked, scoliosis causes restrictive pulmonary disease with decreased endurance. The uneven posture that results causes a disturbance in the sitting balance, necessitating the use of the upper extremities as tripods. The listing to one side, especially in tandem with hip dislocation, may result in formation of intractable skin breakdown due to asymmetries of pressure distribution.

Scoliosis may occur in response to unequal innervation of the paraspinal muscles and may be compounded by vertebral abnormalities, but rapid progression may herald the development of neurological complications. Prior to the development of MRI, many of these conditions went undetected, and many childhood ambulators were using wheelchairs by adolescence. Other factors that may negatively affect ambulatory performance include obesity, joint stiffness with arthritic changes, and lack of motivation.

The two primary conditions responsible for the deterioration in function and often seen with progression of scoliosis are tethering of the spinal cord and syringomyelia. Tethering is caused by scar tissue that holds the spinal cord firmly in place, placing it at risk for repeated microtrauma brought on by spinal flexion and extension (Yamada, Zinke, & Saunders, 1981). Patients exhibit decreased lower extremity strength, spasticity frequently associated with a crouched gait, dysesthesias or progressive sensory deficit, pain over the neural placode (site of the residual spinal deformity), and/or decompensation of a previously well-managed neurogenic bowel and bladder (Peacock, Arens, & Berman, 1987). MRI studies and somatosensory-evoked potentials may be helpful in providing objective evidence of the changes noted on physical examination (Li, Albright, Sclabassi, & Pang, 1996). Urodynamics and perineal-evoked potentials are also useful diagnostic tools in demonstrating change in neurological function (Torre et al., 2002). Surgical release of the tether can result in restoration of function or can stop further neurological progression in most cases (Clancy, et al., 1989; Reigel, 1983). Surgical techniques should permit the neural elements to remain free in the cerebrospinal fluids, preventing the risk of retethering (Zide, Constantini, & Epstein, 1995). An expanding fluid-filled cyst may distend the cord at any level, and may be associated with increasing weakness and sensory deficits, frequently involving the upper extremities. This is known as syringomyelia; it can be treated by surgical drainage of the cyst and placement of a shunt at that level into the peritoneum.

Therapeutic Assessment and Intervention

Assessment should include evaluation and description of joint contractures and deformities, neurological level and muscle power, presence, location, and extent of pressure sores, and mobility and ability of patients to perform self-care skills. Treatment includes gentle, active-assistive range-of-motion exercises for the lower extremities, strengthening of innervated musculature, transfer training, gait training, and instruction in self-care skills. Physical activity programs aimed at improving cardiovascular fitness and strength may improve the self-image of the physically challenged child or adolescent (Andrade, Kramer, Garber, & Longmuir, 1991).

In general, infants with myelomeningocele are less active (Morrow, 1995). This coupled with low tone, weakness, and upper extremity dysfunction provides compelling reasons for referral to an early intervention program. Initial studies of patients so referred suggest subsequent enhancement of functional ambulatory and cognitive abilities so that educational mainstreaming is more likely to occur.

Hypo- or hypertonia may exist in the trunk and upper extremities in association with hydrocephalus. Even children with sacral lesions may present in this manner and require early institution of therapeutic services. The infant should be encouraged to assume antigravity positions, such as quadruped with weight bearing on extended forearms. These attempts may have to be augmented by placing the child over a bolster in prone position and/or by provision of a scooter board. Care must be taken that devices are padded so that secondary skin irritation does not occur. As the child progresses, a bolster can be utilized to work on trunk and abdominal strengthening and sitting balance. Later, a standing table can be used. Depending on the neurological level, the child can then progress to rising from sitting to half-kneeling, and from half-kneeling to standing, utilizing adaptive equipment, as needed.

Appropriate orthoses are either of metal and leather or newer custom-molded plastic variety (Krebs, Edelstein, & Fishman, 1988). Whereas the former devices permits accommodation for dependent edema if problematic, the latter are lighter and often considered more cosmetic. Ambulation, especially with hip-knee-ankle-foot orthoses, is energy-inefficient, with caloric expenditures about six times greater than normal. The use of reciprocating gait orthoses should therefore be considered to reduce energy consumptions and improve endurance (McCall & Schmidt, 1986). More recently, it has been felt that use of such devices is a trade-off, and more conventional bracing might permit for rapid increases in speed required for activities such as crossing the street.

Upper extremity dysfunction and perceptual-motor problems correlate with both the severity of hydrocephalus and the level of the lesion. With the development of increased intracranial pressure, there is stretching of the motor and sensory fibers that surround the enlarged ventricles seen with the Arnold-Chiari malformation, and this may be compounded by abnormalities of the cervical nerve roots (Hwang, Kentish, & Burns, 2002). Hand function should be assessed in terms of preference, tactile discrimination, kinesthetic awareness, ability to conform to certain positions and to perform activities including page turning, stacking of blocks and checkers and the speed with which these activities are carried out, grasp, manipulation of small objects, handling of feeding utensils, graphesthesia, and two-point discrimination (Brunt, 1980; Grimm, 1976; Wallace, 1973). Older children must be assessed in terms of figure copying, graphomotor skills, and academic difficulties. Letter reversals and difficulty in sequencing of tasks are not uncommon. Visual problems of astigmatism, nystagmus, and hyperopia seen in association with hydrocephalus may be contributory factors (Mankinen-Heikkinen & Mustonene, 1987). Remediation of perceptual-motor difficulties may require use of occupational therapy and special education services (Gluckman & Barling, 1980). Upper extremity dysfunction may adversely affect the ability to use crutches (Radke & Gosky, 1981; Wallace, 1973), accounting for discrepancies in ambulation, which occur among patient of the same neurological level.

ADL skills in spina bifida patients are likely to be below age-level norms (Sousa, Gordon, & Shurtleff, 1976). This may be related to dysfunction of praxis, motor planning, parental overprotection, and time constraints. Preparation for adulthood and independent living may be restricted by these factors rather than by lack of intelligence. The development of standardized assessments of self-care, such as the Functional Independence Measure for Children (Wee-FIM) (Granger, Hamilton, & Kayton, 1987) and the PEDI (Feldman, Haley, & Coryell, 1990), help to pinpoint deficiencies that require remediation.

Up to 61% of spina bifida patients may have strabismus. There is a high incidence of amblyopia as well, likely related to the presence of hydrocephalus. Such deficits require treatment, and their amelioration may permit better upper extremity and perceptual motor function (Bigan, 1995). Exacerbation of such findings may indicate need for reassessment of ventriculoperitoneal shunt malfunction.

Respiratory problems may occur as a result of brain stem dysfunction, either on the basis of a congenital malformation or as a result of repeated traction on that area. Loss of central ventilatory function may present with stridor, intermittent loss of consciousness, and apnea. Initially, stridor may be misinterpreted as a manifestation of reactive airway disease. Sleep studies with an analysis of respiratory gases document the lack of chemoregulatory ability, which can result in hypercarbia and anoxia (Swaminathan et al., 1989). Positive pressure or frank respiratory support may be required, in association with a tracheotomy necessitated by vocal cord paralysis, noting that some children gradually improve over time. Some centers advocate a posterior decompression of the cervical spine, although ultimate survival may not be improved with this intervention (Worley et al., 1996). Similarly, brain stem dysfunction may lead to oromotor incoordination, feeding difficulties, and aspiration.

Speech and language dysfunction arise from the various central structural abnormalities associated with spina bifida. Developmental as well as acquired lesions of the cerebellum result in a disruption of motor speech skills. There is resultant dysfluency, ataxia, dysarthria, and abnormality in the rate of speech or prosody, and alteration of intelligibility and vocal intensity. Abnormalities of the corpus callosum may result in difficulty in comprehension and in pragmatic speech, language skills, and use of idioms (Huber-Okrainec, Blaser, & Dennis, 2004) with relative preservation of grammar and lexicon (Fletcher, Barnes, & Dennis, 2002). More specifically, these deficits are characterized by echolalia/repetition, excessive use of social phrases in conversation, and overfamiliarity, in what has been termed the "cocktail party syndrome" (Tew, 1979). These patients may appear to function on a superficial basis better than they actually perform. Therapeutic efforts are indicated in these children to develop pragmatic, step-by-step verbal skills. These skills are prerequisites for instruction in dressing, learning the sequencing required to master self-catheterization, and other ADL tasks.

Bowel and bladder incontinence results from lack of innervation at the sacral levels, with paralysis and incoordination of the bladder and urinary sphincter on the basis of upper and lower motor neuron involvement (Verhoef, Lurvink, et al., 2005). Urinary incontinence, stasis, and reflux of urine back into the kidneys may result in chronic infections with a potential for urosepsis, chronic renal acidosis, hypertension, renal failure, and death (Mundy, Shah, Borzyskowski, & Saxton, 1985). Until about 30 years ago, upper urinary tract deterioration as characterized by hydronephrosis, hypertension, and decreased renal function was felt to be inevitable, resulting in surgical correction with an ileal conduit (an interposed loop of bowel to serve as a biological reservoir in which to contain urine). Currently, intermittent catheterization is the mainstay of treatment, decreasing the risk of infection and stasis, and permitting functional urinary continence (Petersen, 1987) and maintenance of good renal function (Pecker, Damber, Hjalman, Sjodin, & Von Zeigbergk, 1997). Catheterization may be required in infancy to prevent hydronephrosis, which can be present in up to 81% of patients by 5 years of age (Charney, Synder, & Melchionni, 1991; Kari, Safdar, Jamjoon, & Anshasi, 2009). Earlier initiation of catheterization may also prevent irreversible bladder dysfunction and reduce the number of children requiring bladder augmentation from 27% to 11% (Iwu, Baskin, & Kogan, 1997). Dependent upon sitting balance, hand function, and cognitive skills, self-catheterization can begin as early as 5 years (Smith, 1991). Perceptual problems may make the technique difficult to learn; anatomically correct dolls, coloring books, and other simple visual aides can facilitate training.

Continence can be further enhanced by use of uropharmacological agents. Drugs can be used that relax bladder tone to prevent uncontrolled and untimely voiding whereas other medications improve contraction of the urinary sphincter that prevents leakage. Low-dose oral antibiotic therapy may be clinically indicated to prevent recurrent infections, although research support of this recommendation is lacking. In males, external collecting devices can be used as a back-up measure, but females must rely upon diapers or pads. Attention should be paid to the development of latex allergies that may occur in up to 35% of spina bifida patients, possibly related to prolonged and repeated exposures to the material from multiple surgeries and intermittent catheterizations (Slater, 1989), as well as a disease-associated propensity for latex sensitization (Eiwgger et al., 2006). Allergic manifestations are not only those of reactive airway disease, but include urticaria and anaphylaxis. The average time from exposure to development of symptoms is from 1.5 to 9 years, with an average of 5.6 years, with the incidence being proportionate to the number of prior surgical procedures (Obojski et al., 2002). Avoidance of latex-containing items in this population and the maintenance of a latex-free operating room in major medical centers are advised. Patients should be provided with emergency identification bracelets that denote their allergies and other relevant medical problems. When emergent procedures need to be performed under less than optimal circumstances, premedication with steroids and gastrointestinal prophylaxis should occur.

Yearly renal ultrasound studies and blood tests to monitor renal function are mandatory. Surgical techniques include bladder augmentation to increase bladder capacity between catheterizations and the placement of an artificial urinary sphincter (Kaplan, 1985). In patients with some residual sensation, biofeedback techniques may also be successful (Kaplan & Richard, 1988). Low-intensity transcutaneous therapeutic electrical stimulation may be a method for achieving urinary and fecal incontinence (Balcom, Wintrak, Blifield, Rauen, & Langenstroer, 1997). Bowel continence is generally managed by the use of stool softeners, diet, and suppositories or enemas given at a consistent time. The olfactory stigma of an incontinent child may result in ostracism and is a compelling reason for the early implementation of an effective bowel and bladder program. If the regimen is not successful, surgical interventions such as performance of a modified antegrade continence enema procedure utilizing the appendix for the stoma in a majority of cases is also a possibility (Sinha, Grewal, & Ward, 2008).

Until recently, endocrinological dysfunction has been overlooked in this population. Up to 15% of patients may have reduction in grown hormone levels as manifested by a decrease in longitudinal height and arm span. This is likely hydrocephalus-related, with secondary pressure effects being exerted on the hypothalamus, and/or pituitary gland (Hochhaus, Butenandl, Schwarz, & Ring-Mrozik, 1997). Higher-level spina bifida lesions may result in a greater degree of growth impairment (Rotenstein & Riegel, 1996). Not only are such reductions in height stigmatizing, but the associated changes in bony maturation may alter the standard surgical timetable. Supplementation of growth hormone is a treatment option, although its long-term effect in terms of accentuating linear growth, elevating the center of gravity, and increasing the incidence of symptomatic tethering of the spinal cord has not yet been determined (Gold, 1996).

General pediatric care may be compromised in this group given the 20-fold increase in frequency of hospitalizations for surgery, acute intercurrent infections, and other medical problems. Up to 25% of pediatric patients may be deficient in routine immunizations despite provision of multiple subspecialty medical services, augmented by parental concern with regard to pertussis vaccine administration due to coexistent neurological dysfunction. Accordingly, an immunization history is an important part of each clinic visit (Raddish, Goldman, Kaplan, & Perrin, 1998).

Given the increased longevity of the spina bifida patient and the possibility of late complications, it is essential that team management is continued throughout the adult years. Without such transdisciplinary services, well over half of the patients might not receive any specialized services, and some patients might receive no medical care at all (Kaufman et al., 1994). With consistent, on-going care, potentially preventable complications including pyelonephritis, sepsis, progressive paralysis due to cord-tethering, and osteomyelitis and amputation may be prevented (Calado, & Loff, 2002; Rowe & Jadhav, 2008). With comprehensive care for adult patients that includes monitoring for these and other problems, such as cardiovascular diseases, upper extremity dysfunction due to prolonged wheelchair use-induced rotator cuff injuries, and possible increased risk of colorectal cancer (Tomlinson, & Sugarman, 1995), specific interventions can be performed that decrease their impact on overall health and function. However, provision of care is not idealized, and transition issues that include instruction in medical conditions and self-advocacy skills are difficult to access and require preparation over many years (Greenly, Coakley, Holmbeck, Jandasek, & Wills, 2006). Parents should be proactive and develop a system of home-based medical records and treatment timelines that can be transferred to their teen or adult children when appropriate (Osterland, Dosa, & Smith, 2005).

Considerations for Adults

In the setting of multiple physical and medical problems, it is admirable that patients with spina bifida can function as well as has been described. Acknowledgement of psychological differences in myelomeningocele patients may be seen as early as in the preschool period. Figure drawings by such children reveal fewer portrayals of lower extremities than in the general population. Children tend to rate themselves as significantly different in terms of physical and cognitive competence, but not on maternal or peer acceptance (Mobley, Harless, & Miller, 1996). Most patients without hydrocephalus are independent in ADL skills except for bladder control regardless of their neurological level, as are patients with neurological levels at L2 or below, despite the presence of hydrocephalus (Verhoeft et al., 2006).

The secondary disability of social isolation results from the time allocated to medical care and hospitalizations, augmented by parental overprotectiveness, with mothers exhibiting this tendency to a greater extent than the fathers (Hombeck et al., 2002). Thus, by mid-childhood, children so afflicted have up to a fourfold risk of developing a psychiatric disorder, primarily neurotic in nature. Hence, early intervention, socialization, and family counseling are warranted (Connell & McConnel, 1981). Dorner (1976, 1977) detailed the social dysfunction of the group. Teenagers were found to be lonely and unhappy, and have limited exposure to the typically developing population, sexual experiences, and community resources. Despite attempts at comprehensive interventions and care, newer studies reflect similar findings (Buran, Mc Daniel, & Bree, 2002; Cate, Kennedy, & Stevenson, 2002), although some life satisfaction studies are more promising (Barf et al., 2007). Academic achievement may be somewhat improved on the basis of mainstreaming (Borjeson & Logergren, 1990; Lord, Varzis Behrman, Wicks, & Wicks, 1990). Participation in sporting activity is also limited (Buffart et al., 2008).

Instruction in sexual and reproductive function by physicians is reported to occur in only 25% of male and 68% of female patients (Cardenas, Topolski, White, McLaughlin, & Walker,

2008). Adult males with spina bifida have decreased understanding of sexual function, decreased fertility, and difficulty in maintaining erections, with only 52% of such patients reporting sexual satisfaction (Verheof et al., 2005). Conversely, females often achieve fertility early because of their hydrocephalus. Pregnant females may be predisposed to premature labor due to a contracted pelvis and urinary tract abnormalities. Ventriculoperitoneal shunts may have an increased incidence of dysfunction during this period. If a C-section is indicated for delivery, then prophylactic antibiotics should be given and peritoneal irrigation should be performed (Rietber & Lindhout, 1993). Sexual education in either circumstance is exceedingly important.

Despite good cognitive skills and educational opportunities, it is not uncommon for more than 60% of patients to remain in the homes of their parents past maturity (Young et al., 2006). This may not only be a sign of prolonged emotional dependence, but may be an economic necessity as well, for less than 50% of adults are likely to be employed (Castree, & Walker, 1981; Magill-Evans, Galambos, Darrah, & Nickerson, 2008), with about 20% being placed in a sheltered workshop environment (van Mechelen, Verheof, van Asbeck, & Post, 2008). Functional numeracy but not functional literacy skills appear to be correlated with a better chance for employment (Dennis & Barnes, 2002) and for quality of life, in general (Hetherington, Dennis, Barnes, Drake, & Gentili, 2006). The survival rate for the majority of patients with spina bifida now exceeds 90% of the total population. This provided the medical community with a mandate to expand the range of services available to such adults.

General Psychological and Neuropsychological Considerations

Although there are certainly psychological and neuropsychological issues that are unique to the individual diagnoses of cerebral palsy and spina bifida (as enumerated above), there are also some general considerations that apply to both diagnoses.

As with all aspects of children's care, discussion of medical interventions must also address relevant psychological issues. Family expectations, relationships, and reactions clearly play a significant role in the trajectory of the child's development of sense of self, resilience, and adjustment to disability and medical interventions (Aran, Shalev, Biran, & Gross-Tsur, 2007). Family dynamics, support networks, coping resources, and adaptations to disability must be carefully assessed and addressed on an individualized basis as families react and respond to illness and disability in a myriad of ways (Greening & Stoppelbein, 2007).

With children who have congenital and/or developmental disabilities, families may need guidance regarding when they should realistically expect more from their child in terms of autonomy and resilience. This is especially difficult with children and adolescents who are actually dependent on their caregivers for so many basic ADL. Medical and therapeutic staff need to understand the familial perspective by including them as members of the team, by modifying their preconceived notions of absolute "right and wrong," and by avoiding the use of such judgmental labels as "enmeshed" and "infantilizing" (Zaccario, Salsberg, et al., in press). Connecting with parents and patients psychologically and emotionally and helping them move forward appropriately will ultimately culminate in better treatment outcome for the child (Spates et al., 2007). It is not uncommon for parents to be reluctant to push their children toward independence as a mixed result of fear, protection, and doubt. An adolescent developmental level is especially challenging as separation and individuation issues become particularly salient during that time for even typically developing children. For example, adolescents with a developmental disability may no longer be comfortable with their parents assisting them with toileting and bathing skills, despite years of compliance and continued necessity (Zaccario, Salsberg, Gordon, & Bilginer, in press). Although children and adolescents can be remarkably resilient and deficits in self-concept cannot be assumed just by the presence of a disability (Shields, Murdoch, Loy, Dodd, & Taylor, 2006), careful consideration does need to be given to their emotional functioning.

The medical and therapeutic staff must be attuned to the goals and expectations of a child with a disability, as well as those of their parents, even when these goals may not coincide with what seems medically or therapeutically important. For example, a teenager with spina bifida who is integrated into the community and quite functional with the motorized wheelchair, may not share the therapeutic goal of working on upright ambulation, partly because his awkward gait and slower speed could actually make him feel more disabled (Zaccario, Salsberg, et al., in press).

Given the unique stressors associated with pediatric illness and disability, it is not unusual for young patients and their parents to require repeated instructions and an integrated effort among treatment team members to appropriately and clearly understand disseminated information. Single meetings may not give families enough time to process information and to ask appropriate follow-up questions. Emotionally, they may be too angry, sad, stressed, and/ or overwhelmed to properly understand information stated by a clinician on a single occasion. Consistent repetition of diagnostic, prognostic, and treatment information by multiple members of a treatment team can be an effective means of communicating information more thoroughly and respectfully to a family in crisis (Zaccario, Salsberg, et al., in press).

Commensurate with the rehabilitation model approach to treatment, it is also essential to consider cultural factors and multicultural perspectives when working with pediatric populations and their families (Hanson & Kerkhoff, 2007) as these perspectives can also affect how families deal with such issues as regarding authority, assertiveness, emotional expressiveness, and reactions to pain. Overall, understanding and appreciating the emotional and psychological issues of the individual child and family in the context of cultural background is critical for the delivery of optimal patient care and treatment outcome. Patient care also needs to be appropriately formulated based upon the individual child's developmental level and needs. Referrals to mental health professionals (depending on the medical setting, this could include the departments of child-life, psychology, psychiatry, and/or social work) should be made as appropriate to assist a family and the medical team; but these referrals also need to be made in a supportive, well-timed, and culturally sensitive manner. The therapeutic value of these referrals should be explained thoroughly to the family and framed not in the context of psychopathology, but rather as additional tools to promote optimal care of the affected child (Zaccario, Salsberg, et al., in press).

A neuropsychological consultation and evaluation should be considered for children diagnosed with spina bifida or cerebral palsy at various intervals throughout their childhood and adolescence (Gordon, Salsberg, & McCaul, 2001). Specifically, academic transitions, school-mandated triennial evaluations, postsurgical follow-ups, and reintegration of hospitalized patients into the community setting are examples of appropriate occasions for neuropsychological assessments. A properly trained psychologist (Warschausky, Kaufman, & Steirs, 2008) should be able to choose and adapt testing batteries to best serve these medically complex patients; to consider medical, neuropsychological, and psychiatric diagnoses when formulating cases and making recommendations; and to write reports that will be informative to referring physicians, treating therapists, patient families, and school personnel. When a full neuropsychological assessment is indicated for either pediatric inpatients or outpatients the following neurocognitive domains are surveyed: intellectual abilities; verbal and language skills; visual-spatial, sensorimotor, and visuomotor skills; attention, memory, and learning; executive functioning; adaptive skills; and preacademic and/or academic abilities (Baron, 2000). In addition, but just as essential, an analysis of social-emotional functioning for the comprehensive assessment of medically fragile, neurologically impaired, and/or developmentally challenged patients is required. Specifically, an evaluator needs to consider the following domains: mood and affect; clarity of thinking and reality testing; self-perception and self-esteem; interpersonal relatedness and perception of others; and coping resources and stress tolerance (Zaccario, Salsberg, et al., in press).

A crucial aspect of testing, with regard to this population, for an evaluating psychologist is the creation of appropriate and salient recommendations to parents, physicians, treating therapists, and school personnel in feedback sessions and in comprehensive neuropsychological reports. The neuropsychological report is often the primary tool utilized in aftercare programs and schools to reintegrate the recovering child or adolescent in the home and school environment. Therefore, recommendations need to be relevant, clearly written, and feasible for implementation (Maedgen & Semrud-Clikeman, 2007). They typically include educational placement suggestions; academic and classroom modifications; assistive technology; aftercare rehabilitative treatment (occupational, physical, and speech and language therapy); psychotherapy; counseling and group therapy; behavior modification plans; cognitive remediation; medical or professional follow-up; and suggestions for future assessments and reevaluations. It is crucial that the evaluating psychologist be not only well versed with the child's myriad of needs but also prepared to practically advise the family and the school system on implementation of recommendations (Zaccario and Salsberg, et al, in press). As such, a psychologist should understand the rights afforded to children by federal law governing special education, namely The Individuals with Disabilities Education Act (IDEA, 1990, 1997, 2004).

REFERENCES

Abbott, R., Johann-Murphy, M., & Gold, J. T. (1991). Selective functional rhizotomy for the treatment of spasticity in children. In M. Sindou (Ed.), *Neurosurgery for spasticity* (pp. 149–157). New York: Springer-Verlag.

Abraham, E., Lubicky, J. P., Sanger, M. N., & Millar, E. A. (1996). Supramalleolar osteotomy for angle valgus in myelomeningocele. *Journal of Pediatric Orthopaedics, 16*, 774–781.

Albright, A. L. (1996). Baclofen in the treatment of cerebral palsy. *Journal of Child Neurology, 11*, 77–83.

Albright, A. L., Barron, W. B., Fascik, D., Polinko, P., & Janosky, J. (1993). Continuous intrathecal baclofen infusion for spasticity of cerebral origin. *Journal of the American Medical Association, 270*, 2475–2477.

Albright, A. L., Cervi, A., & Singletary, J. (1991). Intrathecal baclofen for spasticity in cerebral palsy. *Journal of the American Medical Association, 265*, 1418–1422.

Alexander, M. A., & Steig, N. L. (1989). Myelomeningocele: Comprehensive treatment. *Archives of Physical Medicine and Rehabilitation, 70*, 637–641.

Alvarez, N., Larkin, C., & Roxbrough, J. (1981). Carpal-tunnel syndrome in athetoid-dystonic cerebral palsy. *Archives of Neurology, 39*, 311–326.

Andersson, C., Grooten, W., Hellsten, M., Kaping, K., & Mattson, E. (2003). Adults with cerebral palsy: Walking ability after progressive strength training. *Developmental Medicine and Child Neurology, 45*, 220–228.

Andersson, C., & Mattson, E. (2001). Adults with cerebral palsy: Survey describing problems, needs, and resources with special emphasis on locomotion. *Developmental Medicine and Child Neurology, 43*, 76–82.

Andrade, C. K., Kramer, J., Garber, M., & Longmuir, P. (1991). Changes in self-concept, cardiovascular endurance, and muscle strength of children with spina bifida aged 8 to 13 years in response to a 10-week physical activity program: A pilot study. *Child Care Health Development, 17*, 183–196.

Ansved, T., Odergren, T., & Borg, K. (1997). Muscle fiber atrophy in leg muscles after botulinum type A treatment of cervical dystonia. *Neurology, 48*, 1440–1442.

Aran, R., Shalev, S., Biran, G., & Gross-Tsur, V. (2007). Parenting style impacts on quality of life in children with cerebral palsy. *Journal of Pediatrics, 151*, 56–60.

Armstrong, R. W., Steinbok, P., & Cochrane, D. D. (1997). Intrathecally administered baclofen for the treatment of children with spasticity of cerebral origin. *Journal of Neurosurgery, 87*, 409–414.

Asher, M., & Olsen, J. (1983). Factors affecting the ambulatory status of patients with spina bifida cystica. *Journal of Bone and Joint Surgery, 65-A*, 350–356.

Ashton, B., Piper, M. C., Warren, S., Stewin, L., & Byrne, P. (1991). Influence of medical history of assessment of at-risk infants. *Developmental Medicine and Child Neurology, 33*, 412–418.

Bachrach, S., & Greenspun, B. (1990). Care of the adult with myelomeningocele. *Delaware Medical Journal, 62*, 1287–1295.

Badell-Ribera, A., Swinyeard, C., Greenspan, L., & Deaver, G. (1964). Spina bifida with myelomeningocele: Evaluation of rehabilitation potential. *Archives of Physical Medicine and Rehabilitation, 45*, 443–453.

Bajelidze, G., Beithur, M., Littlerton, A. G., Dabney, K., & Miller, F. (2008). Diagnostic evaluation using whole-body technetium bone scan in children with cerebral palsy and pain. *Journal of Pediatric Orthopaedics, 28,* 112–117.

Balcom, A. H., Wintrak, M., Blifeld, T., Rauen, K., & Langenstroer, P. (1997). Initial experience with home therapeutic electrical-stimulation for continence in the myelomeningocele population. *Journal of Urology, 158,* 1272–1276.

Banta, J. V., & Park, S. M. (1983). Improvement in pulmonary function in patients having combined anterior and posterior spine fusion for myelomeningocele scoliosis. *Spine, 8,* 765–770.

Barf, H. A., Post, M. W. M., Verhoef, M., Jennekens-Schickel, A., Gooskens, R., & Prevo, A. (2007). Life satisfaction of young adults with spina bifida. *Developmental Medicine and Child Neurology, 49,* 458–463.

Baron, I. S. (2000). Clinical implications and practical applications of child neuropsychological evaluations. In K. O. Yeates, M. D. Ris, & H. G. Taylor (Eds.), *Pediatric neuropsychology: Research, theory, and practice.* New York: Guilford.

Bar-Haim, S., Harries, N., Belokopytov, M., Frank, A., Copeliovitch, L., Kaplanski, J., et al. (2006). Comparison of efficacy of Adeli suit and neurodevelopmental treatment of children with cerebral palsy. *Developmental Medicine and Child Neurology, 48,* 325–330.

Bax, M., Tydeman, C., & Flodmark, O. (2006). Clinical and MRI correlates of cerebral palsy: The European cerebral palsy study. *Journal of the American Medical Association, 296,* 1602–1608.

Bell, M. J., & Hallenbeck, E. (2002). Effects of intrauterine inflammation on developing rat brain. *Journal of Neuroscience Research, 70,* 570–579.

Benedict, M. I., White, R. B., Wulff, L. M., & Hall, B. J. (1990). Reported maltreatment in children with multiple disabilities. *Child Abuse Neglect, 14,* 207–217.

Bergen, A. F., & Colangelo, C. (1982). *Positioning of the client with central nervous system deficits: The wheelchair and other adaptive equipment.* Valhalla, NY: Valhalla Rehabilitation.

Bigan, A. W. (1995). Strabismus associated with meningomyelocele. *Journal of Pediatric Ophthalmology Strabismus, 32,* 309–314.

Blair, E., & Stanley, F. (1990). Intrauterine growth retardation and spastic cerebral palsy: 1. Association with birth weight for gestational age. *American Journal of Obstetrics and Gynecology, 162,* 229–237.

Bleck, E. E. (1987). Orthopedic management of cerebral palsy. In *Clinical developmental medicine* (Vol. 99/100). Oxford, England: MacKeith.

Blum, R. W., Resnick, M. D., Nelson, R., & St. Germaine, A. (1991). Familiar and peer issues among adolescents with spina bifida and cerebral palsy. *Pediatrics, 88,* 280–285.

Bobath, B., & Bobath, K. (1975). *Motor development in the different types of cerebral palsy.* London: Heineman.

Borjeson, M. C., & Logergren, J. (1990). Life conditions of adolescents with myelomeningocele. *Developmental Medicine and Child Neurology, 32,* 698–706.

Borowski, A. E., Shah, S., Littleton, A., Dabney, K., & Miller, F. (2008). Baclofen pump implantation and spinal fusion in children: Techniques and complications. *Spine, 33,* 1995–2000.

Botto, L. D., & Yang, Q. (2000). Ethylene tetrahydrofolate reductase gene variants and congenital anomalies. A HuGE review. *American Journal of Epidemiology, 151,* 862–877.

Boytim, M. J., Davidson, R. S., Charney, E., & Melchionne, J. B. (1991). Neonatal fractures in myelomeningocele patients. *Journal of Pediatric Orthopaedics, 11,* 28–30.

Brinker, M. R., Rosenfeld, S. R., Feiwell, R., Granger, S. P., Mitchell, D. C., & Rice, J. C. (1994). Myelomeningocele at the sacral level. *Journal of Bone and Joint Surgery, 76-A,* 1293–1300.

Bronkhorst, A. J., & Lamb, G. A. (1987). Orthosis to aid in the reduction of lower extremity spasticity. *Orthotics and Prosthetics, 41,* 23–28.

Brown, M. C., Bontempo, A., & Turk, M. A. (1992). *Secondary consequences of cerebral palsy: Adults with cerebral palsy in New York state.* Albany, NY: Developmental Disabilities Planning Council.

Bruggink, L. M., Einspieler, C., Butcher, P. R., Stremmelaar, E. F., Prechtl, H., & Bos, A. F. (2008). Quantitative aspects of the early motor repertoire in preterm infants: Do they predict minor neurological dysfunction at school age? *Early Human Development, 85,* 25–36.

Bruner, J. P., & Tulipan, N. (2005). Intrauterine repair of spina bifida. *Clinical Obstetrics and Gynecology, 48,* 942–955.

Brunt, A. (1980). Characteristics of upper limb movements in a sample of myelomeningocele children. *Perceptual Motor Skills, 51,* 431–437.

Buffart, L. M., van der Ploeg, H., Bauman, A. E., Van Asbeck, F. W., Stam, H. J., Roebroeck, M. E., et al. (2008). Sports participation in adolescents and young adults with myelomeningocele and its role in total physical activity behaviour and fitness. *Journal of Rehabilitation Medicine, 40,* 702–708.

Buran, C. F., Mc Daniel, A., & Bree, T. J. (2002). Needs assessment in a spina bifida program: A comparison of the perceptions by adolescents with spina bifida and their parents. *Clinical Nurse Specialist, 16,* 256–262.

Burmeister, R., Hannay, H. J., Copeland, K., Fletcher, J. M., Boudousquale, A., & Dennis, M. (2005). Attention problems and executive functions in children with spina bifida and hydrocephalus. *Child Neuropsychology, 11,* 265–283.

Cahan, L. D., & Kundi, M. S. (1987). Electrophysiological studies in selective dorsal rhizotomy for spasticity in children with cerebral palsy. *Applied Neurophysiology, 50,* 459–460.

Calado, E., & Loff, C. (2002). The "failures" of spina bifida transdisciplinary care. *European Journal of Pediatric Surgery, 12,* 525–526.

Capute, A. J. (1978). *Primitive reflex profile.* Baltimore: University Park Press.

Capute, A. J., Shapiro, B. K., & Palmer, F. B. (1981). Spectrum of developmental disabilities. *Orthopedic Clinics of North America, 12,* 3–22.

Cardenas, D. D., Topolski, T. D., White, C. J., McLaughlin, J. F., & Walker, W. O. (2008). Sexual functioning in adolescents and young adults with spina bifida. *Archives of Physical Medicine and Rehabilitation, 89,* 31–35.

Carlson, W. E., Vaughn, C. L., Damiano, D. L., & Abel, M. F. (1997). Orthotic management of gait in spastic diplegia. *American Journal of Physical Medicine and Rehabilitation, 76,* 216–225.

Carlsson, M., Hagberg, G., & Olssom, I. (2003). Clinical and etiological aspects of epilepsy in children with cerebral palsy. *Developmental Medicine and Child Neurology, 45,* 371–376.

Carlsson, M., Olsson, I., Hagberg, G., & Beckung, E. (2008). Behavior in children with cerebral palsy with and without epilepsy. *Developmental Medicine and Child Neurology, 50,* 784–789.

Carr, C., & Gage, J. R. (1987). The fate of the non-operated hip in cerebral palsy. *Journal of Pediatric Orthopaedics, 7,* 262–267.

Carroll, N. C. (1977). The orthotic management of spina bifida children: Present status, future goals. *Prosthetics and Orthotics International, 1*(1) 39–42.

Castree, J., & Walker, J. H. (1981). The young adult with spina bifida. *British Medical Journal, 283,* 1040–1042.

Cate, I. M. P., Kennedy, C., & Stevenson, J. (2002). Disability and quality of life in spina bifida and hydrocephalus. *Developmental Medicine and Child Neurology, 44,* 317–322.

Charney, E. B. (1990). Parental attitudes toward management of newborns with myelomeningocele. *Developmental Medicine and Child Neurology, 32,* 14–19.

Charney, E. B., Melchionni, J. B., & Smith, D. R. (1991). Community ambulation by children with myelomeningocele and high-level paralysis. *Journal of Pediatric Orthopaedics, 11,* 579–582.

Charney, E. B., Rorke, L. B., Sutton, L. N., & Schut, L. (1991). Management of Chiari II complications in infants with myelomeningocele. *Journal of Pediatrics, 111,* 371–374.

Charney, E. B., Synder, H. M., & Melchionni, J. B. (1991). Upper urinary tract deterioration with myelomeningocele. *Developmental Medicine and Child Neurology, 33*(Suppl. 64), 18–37.

Chervenak, R. A., & McCullough, L. B. (2002). A comprehensive ethical framework for fetal research and its application to fetal surgery for spina bifida. *American Journal of Obstetrics and Gynecology, 187,* 10–14.

Chiaramonte, R. M., Horowitz, R. M., Kaplan, G. M., & Brook, W. A. (1986). Implications of hydronephrosis in newborns with myelodysplasia. *Journal of Urology, 136,* 427–429.

Chicoine, M. R., Park, T. S., & Kaufman, B. A. (1997). Selective dorsal rhizotomy and rates of orthopaedic surgery in children with spastic cerebral palsy. *Journal of Neurosurgery, 86,* 34–39.

Choi, S. H., & McComb, J. G. (2000). Long-term outcome of terminal myelocystocele patients. *Pediatric Neurosurgery, 32,* 86–91.

Clancy, R. R., Sladsky, J. T., & Rorke, L. B. (1989). Hypoxic-ischemia spinal cord injury following perinatal asphyxia. *Annals of Neurology, 25,* 185–189.

Clopton, N., Dutton, J., Featherston, T., Grigsby, A., Mobley, J., Melvin, J. (2005). Interrater and intrarater reliability of the Modified Ashworth Scale in children with hypertonia. *Pediatric Physical Therapy, 17,* 268–274.

Coniglio, S. J., Anderson, S. M., & Ferguson, J. E. (1996). Functional motor outcome in children with myelomeningocele. Correlation with anatomic prenatal ultrasound. *Developmental Medicine and Child Neurology, 38,* 675–680.

Connell, H. M., & McConnel, T. S. (1981). Psychiatric sequelae in children treated operatively for hydrocephalus in infancy. *Developmental Medicine and Child Neurology, 23,* 505–517.

Cooperman, D. R., Bartucci, E., Dietrick, E., & Millar, E. A. (1987). Hip dislocation in spastic cerebral palsy: Long-term consequences. *Journal of Pediatric Orthopaedics, 7,* 268–276.

Coorsen, E. A., Msall, M. E., & Duffy, L. C. (1991). Multiple minor manifestations as a marker for prenatal etiology of cerebral palsy. *Developmental Medicine and Child Neurology, 33,* 730–736.

Cosgrove, A. P., & Graham, H. K. (1994). Botulinum toxin A prevents the development of contractures in the hereditary spastic mouse. *Developmental Medicine and Child Neurology, 36,* 379–385.

Craft, M. J., Lakin, J. A., Oppliger, R. A., Clancy, G. M., & Vander Linden, D. W. (1990). Siblings as change agents for promoting the functional status of children with cerebral palsy. *Developmental Medicine and Child Neurology, 32,* 1049–1057.

Crandall, R. C., Birkeback, C. R., & Wintor, B. R. (1989). The role of hip location and dislocation in the functional status of the myelodysplastic patient. *Orthopedics, 12,* 675–683.

Crenshaw, S., Herzog, R., Castagno, P., Richards, J., Miller, F., Michaloski, G., et al. (2000). The efficacy of tone-reducing splints in children with spastic diplegic cerebral palsy. *Journal of Pediatric Orthopaedics, 20,* 210–216.

Cuddeford, T. J., Freeling, R. P., Thomas, S. S., Aniona, M. D., Rex, D., Sirolli, H., et al. (1997). Energy consumption in children with myelomeningocele: A comparison between reciprocating gait orthosis and hip-knee-ankle-foot orthosis ambulators. *Developmental Medicine and Child Neurology, 39,* 239–242.

Curtis, B. H. (1973). The hip in the myelomeningocele child. *Clinical Orthopaedics and Related Research, 90,* 11–21.

Damiano, D. L., Kelly, L. E., & Vaughn, C. L. (1995). Effects of quadriceps femoris muscle strengthening on crouch gait in children with spastic diplegia. *Physical Therapy, 75,* 658–667.

Damiano, D. L., Vaughn, C. L., & Abel, M. F. (1995). Muscle response to heavy resistance exercise in children with spastic cerebral palsy. *Developmental Medicine and Child Neurology, 37,* 731–739.

Deaver, G. (1956). Cerebral palsy: Methods of beating the neuromuscular disability. *Archives of Physical Medicine and Rehabilitation, 37,* 363–378.

Degos, V., Loron, G., Mantz, J., & Gressens, P. (2008). Neuroprotective strategies for the neonatal brain. *Anesthesia and Analgesia, 106,* 1670–1680.

Dennis, N., & Barnes, M. (2002). Math and numeracy in young adults with spina bifida and hydrocephalus. *Developmental Medicine and Child Neurology, 41,* 141–155.

De Souza, L. L., & Carroll, N. (1976). Ambulation of the braced myelomeningocele patient. *Journal of Bone and Joint Surgery, 58-A,* 1112–1118.

Diamond, N. (1986). Rehabilitation strategies for the child with cerebral palsy. *Pediatric Annals, 15,* 230–236.

Dieruf, K., Burtner, P., Provost, B., Phillips, J., Bernitsky-Beddingfield, A., Sullivan, K. J. (2009). A pilot study of quality of life in children with cerebral palsy after intensive body weight-supported treadmill training. *Pediatric Physical Therapy, 21,* 45–52.

Donkervoort, M., Wiegerink, D., van Meeteren, J., Stam, H., & Roebroeck, M. (2009). Transition to adulthood: Validation of the Rotterdam Transition Profile for young adults with cerebral palsy and normal intelligence. *Developmental Medicine and Child Neurology, 51,* 53–62.

Dorner, S. (1976). Adolescents with spina bifida: How they view their situation. *Archives of Disease in Childhood, 51,* 439–444.

Dorner, S. (1977). Sexual interest and activity in adolescents with spina bifida. *Journal of Child Psychology, 18,* 220–237.

Dosa, N. P., Eckrich, M., Katz, D. A., Turk, M., & Liptak, G. S. (2007). Incidence, prevalence, and characteristic of fractures in children, adolescents, and adults with spina bifida. *Journal of Spinal Cord Medicine, 30,* S5–S9.

Drennan, J. C. (1976). Orthotic management of the myelomeningocele spine. *Developmental Medicine and Child Neurology, 18,* 97–103.

Drvaric, D. M., Roberts, J. M., Burke, S. W., King, A. G., & Falterman, K. (1987). Gastroesophageal evaluation in totally involved cerebral palsy patients. *Journal of Pediatric Orthopaedics, 7,* 187–190.

Duncan, R., Barton, I., Edmonds, E., & Blashill, B. M. (2004). Parental perceptions of the therapeutic efficacy of osteopathic manipulation or acupuncture in children with spastic cerebral palsy. *Clinical Pediatrics, 43,* 349–353.

Ebara, S., Yamazaki, Y., Harada, T., Hosono, N., Morimoto, Y., Tang, L., et al. (1990). Motion analysis of the cervical spine in athetoid cerebral palsy. *Spine, 15,* 1097–1103.

Eicher, D. J., Wagner, C. L., & Katikaneni, L. P. (2004). Moderate hypothermia in neonatal encephalopathy: Efficacy outcomes. *Journal of Pediatric Neurology, 32,* 11–17.

Eisenberg, S., Zuk, L., Carmeli, E., & Katz-Leuer, M. (2009). Contribution of stepping while standing to function and secondary conditions among children with cerebral palsy. *Pediatric Physical Therapy, 21,* 79–85.

Eiwegger, T., Dehlink, E., Schwindt, J., Popmberger, G., Reider, N., Frigo, E., et al. (2006). Early exposure to latex products mediates latex sensitization in spina bifida but not in other diseases with comparable latex exposure rates. *Clinical and Experimental Allergy, 36,* 1242–1246.

Ellenberg, J. H., & Nelson, K. B. (1981). Early recognition of infants at risk for cerebral palsy. Examination at age 4 months. *Developmental Medicine and Child Neurology, 23,* 705–714.

Engel, J. M., Kartin, D., & Jensen, M. D. (2002). Pain treatment in persons with cerebral palsy. Frequency and helpfulness. *Journal of Physical Medicine and Rehabilitation, 81,* 291–296.

Engel-Yeger, B., Jarus, T., Anaby, D., & Law, M. (2009). Differences in patterns of participation between youth with cerebral palsy and typically developing peers. *American Journal of Occupational Therapy, 63,* 96–104.

Evans, D. M., & Alberman, E. (1990). Certified cause of death in children and young adults with cerebral palsy. *Archives of Disease in Childhood, 66,* 325–329.

Evans, D. M., Evans, J. W., & Alberman, E. (1990). Cerebral palsy: Why we must plan for survival. *Archives of Disease in Childhood, 65,* 1329–1333.

Eyman, R. K., & Grossman, H. J. (1990). The life expectancy of profoundly handicapped people with mental retardation. *New England Journal of Medicine, 323,* 584–589.

Farmer, S. F., Harrison, L. M., Ingram, D. A., & Stephens, J. A. (1991). Plasticity of central motor pathways in children with hemiplegic cerebral palsy. *Neurology, 41,* 1505–1510.

Fasano, V. A., Barolat-Romana, G., Zeme, S., & Suazzi, A. (1970). Electrophysiological assessment of spinal circuits in spasticity by direct dorsal root stimulation. *Neurosurgery, 4,* 146–151.

Fauza, D. O., Jennings, R. W., Teng, Y. D., & Synder, E. Y. (2008). Neural stem cell delivery to the spinal cord in an ovine model of fetal surgery for spina bifida. *Surgery, 144,* 367–373.

Feldman, A. B., Haley, S. M., & Coryell, J. (1990). Concurrent and construct validity of the Pediatric Evaluation of Disability Inventory. *Physical Therapy, 70,* 602–610.

Ficter, M. A., Dornseifer, U., Henke, J., Schenider, K., Kovacs, L., Biemer, E., et al. (2005). Fetal spina bifida repair—Current trends and prospects of intrauterine neurosurgery. *Fetal Diagnostic Therapy, 23,* 271–286.

Findley, T. W., & Agre, J. C. (1988). Ambulation of the adolescent with spina bifida: Oxygen costs of mobility. *Archives of Physical Medicine and Rehabilitation, 69,* 855–861.

Finnie, N. R. (1974). *Handling the young cerebral palsied child at home.* New York: E.P. Dutton.

Fletcher, J. M., Barnes, M., & Dennis, M., (2002). Language development in children with spina bifida. *Seminars in Pediatric Neurology, 9,* 201–208.

Ford, G. W., Kitchen, W. H., Doyle, L. W., Richards, A. L., & Kelly, E. (1990). Changing diagnosis of cerebral palsy in very low birth weight children. *American Journal of Perinatology, 7,* 178–181.

Fragala-Pinkham, M., Dumas, H., Barlow, C., & Pasternak, A. (2009). An aquatic physical therapy program at a pediatric rehabilitation hospital: A case series. *Pediatric Physical Therapy, 21,* 68–78.

Fraser, R. K., Bourke, H. M., Broughton, N. S., & Menalaus, M. B. (1995). Unilateral dislocation of the hip in spina bifida: A long-term follow-up. *Journal of Bone and Joint Surgery, 77-B,* 299–302.

Frawley, P. A., Broughton, N. S., & Menalaus, M. B. (1996). Anterior release for fixed flexion deformity of the hip in spina bifida. *Journal of Bone and Joint Surgery, 78-B,* 299–302.

Frieden, J., & Lieber, R. (2003). Spastic muscle cells are shorter and stiffer than normal cells. *Muscle and Nerve, 26,* 157–164.

Fulford, G. E. (1990). Surgical management of ankle and foot deformities in cerebral palsy. *Clinical Orthopaedics and Related Research, 253,* 55–61.

Gage, J. R. (1990). Surgical treatment of knee dysfunction in cerebral palsy. *Clinical Orthopaedics and Related Research, 253,* 45–54.

Galvin, K. A. (1998). Postinjury magnesium sulfate treatment is not markedly neuroprotective for striatal medium spiny neurons after perinatal hypoxic/ischemia in the rat. *Pediatrics Research, 44,* 740–745.

Gerring, J. P., Brady, K. D., Chen, A., Vasa, R., Grados, M., Bandeen-Roche, K. J., et al. (1998). Premorbid prevalence of ADHD and development of secondary ADHD after closed head injury. *Journal of the American Academy of Child and Adolescent Psychiatry, 37,* 647–654.

Gertszten, P. C. (1997). Effect on ambulation of continuous intrathecal baclofen infusion. *Pediatric Neurosurgery, 27,* 40–44.

Gibson, C. S., Mac Lennan, A. H., Goldwater, P. N., & Dekker, G. A. (2003). Antenatal causes of cerebral palsy: Association between inherited thrombophilias, viral, and bacterial infections, and inherited susceptibilities to infection. *Obstetric and Gynecological Surgery, 58,* 209–220.

Gisel, E. G., & Patrick, J. (1988). Identification of children with cerebral palsy unable to maintain a normal nutritional state. *Lancet, 1,* 283–286.

Glantzman, A. M., Kim, H., Swaminathan, K., & Beck, T. (2004). Efficacy of botulinum toxin A, serial casting, and combined treatment for spastic equinus: A retrospective analysis. *Developmental Medicine and Child Neurology, 46,* 807–811.

Gluckman, S., & Barling, J. (1980). Effect of remedial program on visual-motor perception in spina bifida children. *Journal of General Psychology, 136,* 195–200.

Gold, J. T. (1991). Orthotic management and rehabilitation of the foot and ankle in the neurologically impaired child. In M. H. Jahss (Ed.), *Disorders of the foot and ankle.* Philadelphia: W.B. Saunders.

Gold, J. T. (1996). Growth hormone treatment of children with neural tube defects (Letter; comment). *Journal of Pediatrics, 129,* 177.

Gooch, J. L., & Walker, M. L. (1996). Spinal stenosis after total lumbar laminectomy for selective dorsal rhizotomy. *Pediatric Neurosurgery, 25,* 28–30.

Gordon, R., Salsberg, D., & McCaul, P. (2001). Neuropsychological assessment of childhood stroke. *Loss, Grief & Care, 9,* 61–82.

Gorter, H., Holty, L., Rameckers, E., Hans, J., & Rob, O. (2009). Changes in endurance and walking ability through functional physical therapy training in children with cerebral palsy. *Pediatric Physical Therapy, 21,* 31–37.

Gosechel, J., Wohlfarth, K., Frevert, J., Dengler, R., & Bilgalke, T. T. (1997). Botulinum A toxin therapy: Neutralizing and non-neutralizing antibodies—Therapeutic consequences. *Experimental Neurology, 147,* 96–102.

Graham, H. K., & Harvey, A. (2007). Assessment of mobility after multi-level surgery for cerebral palsy. *Journal of Bone and Joint Surgery, 89,* 993–994.

Graham, H. K., & Selber, P. (2003). Musculoskeletal aspects of cerebral palsy. *Journal of Bone and Joint Surgery, 85-B,* 157–166.

Graham, L., Levene, M. I., & Trounce, J. Q. (1987). Prediction of cerebral palsy in very low birth weight infants: Prospective ultrasound study. *Lancet, 2,* 593–596.

Granger, C. V., Hamilton, B. B., & Kayton, R. (1987). *Guide to the use of the Functional Independence Measure for Children (WeeFIM) of the Uniform Data Set for Medical Rehabilitation.* Buffalo, NY: Research Foundation, State University of New York.

Grant, A., O'Brien, N., Joy, M. T., Hennessy, E., & Mac Donald, D. (1989). Cerebral palsy among children born during the Dublin randomized trial of intrapartum monitoring. *Lancet, 2,* 1233–1236.

Greening, L., & Stoppelbein, L. (2007). Brief report: Pediatric cancer, parental coping style, and risk for depressive, posttraumatic stress and anxiety symptoms. *Journal of Pediatric Psychology, 32,* 1272–1277.

Greenley, R. N., Coakley, R. M., Holmbeck, G. N., Jandasek, B., & Wills, K. (2006). Condition-related knowledge among children with spina bifida: Longitudinal changes and predictors. *Journal of Pediatric Psychology, 31,* 828–839.

Grimm, R. A. (1976). Hand preference and tactile perception in a group of children with myelomeningocele. *American Journal of Occupational Therapy, 30,* 234–250.

Guyatt, G., Sackett, D., Taylor, D. W., Chong, J., Roberts, R., & Dugsley, S. (1986). Determining optimal therapy: Randomized trials in individual patients. *New England Journal of Medicine, 314,* 889–892.

Hack, M., & Costello, D. W. (2008). Trends in the rates of cerebral palsy associated with neonatal intensive care of preterm children. *Clinical Obstetrics and Gynecology, 51,* 763–774.

Hagberg, B., & Hagberg, G. (1989). The changing panorama of cerebral palsy in Sweden: 5 The birth year period 1979–82. *Acta Paediatrica Scandinavica, 78,* 283–290.

Hagberg, B., & Hagberg, G. (1996). The changing panorama of cerebral palsy: Bilateral spastic forms in particular. *Acta Paediatrica Scandinavica, 415,* 48–52.

Halpern, D. (1982). Duration of relaxation after intramuscular neurolysis with phenol. *Journal of the American Medical Association, 247,* 1473–1476.

Halpern, D. (1984). Therapeutic exercises for cerebral palsy. In J. V. Basmajiani (Ed.), *Therapeutic exercises* (pp. 118–143). Baltimore, MD: Williams & Wilkins.

Hanson, S. L., & Kerkhoff, T. R. (2007). Ethical decision making in rehabilitation: Consideration of Latino cultural factors. *Rehabilitation Psychology, 52,* 409–420.

Harade, T., Ebara, S., Anwar, M. M., Okawa, A., Kajiura, I., Kiroshima, K., et al. (1996). The cervical spine in athetoid cerebral palsy: A radiological study of 180 patients. *Journal of Bone and Joint Surgery, 78-B,* 613–619.

Harris, S. R. (1989). Early diagnosis of spastic diplegia, spastic hemiplegia, and quadriplegia. *American Journal of Disease in Childhood, 143,* 1356–1360.

Harrison, A. (1988). Spastic cerebral palsy: Possible interneuronal contributions. *Developmental Medicine and Child Neurology, 30,* 760–780.

Hasan, K. M., Eluvathingal, T. J., Kramer, L. A., Ewing-Cobbs, L., Dennis, M., Fletcher, J. M. (2008). White matter microstructural abnormalities in children with spina bifida myelomeningocele and hydrocephalus: A diffusions tensor tractography study of the association pathways. *Journal of Magnetic Resonance Imaging, 27,* 700–709.

Hasan, K. M., Sankar, A., Halphen, C., Kramer, L. A., Ewing-Cobbs, L., Dennis, M., et al. (2008). Quantitative diffusion tensor imaging and intellectual outcomes in spina bifida. *Journal of Neurosurgery and Pediatrics, 2,* 75–82.

Hayley, S. M., Ludlow, L. H., & Coster, W. J. (1993). Pediatric evaluation of disability inventory. *Physical Medicine and Rehabilitation of North America, 4,* 529–540.

Hazlewood, M. I., Brown, J. K., Rowe, P. J., & Salter, P. M. (1994). The use of therapeutic electrical stimulation in the treatment of hemiplegic cerebral palsy. *Developmental Medicine and Child Neurology, 36,* 661–673.

Henderson, R. C., Lark, R. K., & Kecskemethy, H. (2002). Bisphosphonates to treat osteopenia in children with quadriplegic cerebral palsy: A randomized clinical trial. *Journal of Pediatrics, 141,* 644–651.

Hetherington, R., Dennis, M., Barnes, M., Drake, J., & Gentili, F. (2006). Functional outcome in young adults with spina bifida and hydrocephalus. *Child's Nervous System, 22,* 117–124.

Hill, A. E. (1990). Conductive education for physically handicapped children. *Ulster Medical Journal, 59,* 41–45.

Hinderer, K. A., & Harris, S. R. (1988). Effects of tone reducing versus standard plaster casts on gait improvement in children with cerebral palsy. *Developmental Medicine and Child Neurology, 30,* 370–377.

Hirtz, D. G., & Nelson, K. (1998). Magnesium sulfate and cerebral palsy in premature infants. *Current Opinion in Pediatrics, 10,* 131–137.

Hirtz, M. (1989). Patterns of impairment and disability related to social handicap in young people with cerebral palsy and spina bifida. *Journal of Biosocial Science, 21,* 1–12.

Hochhaus, R., Butenandl, O., Schwarz, H. P., & Ring-Mrozik, E. (1997). *European Journal of Pediatrics, 156,* 597–601.

Holm, V. A. (1982). The causes of cerebral palsy. *Journal of the American Medical Association, 247,* 1473–1475.

Hombeck, G. N., Johnson, S. Z., Wills, K. E., McKernon, W., Rose, B., Erklin, S., et al. (2002). Observed and perceived parental overprotection in relation to psychosocial adjustment in preadolescents with a physical disability: The mediation role of behavioral autonomy. *Journal of Consulting and Clinical Psychology, 70,* 96–110.

Huber-Okrainec, J., Blaser, S. E., & Dennis, M. (2004). Idiom comprehension deficits in relation to corpus callosum agenesis and hypoplasia in children with spina bifida meningomyelocele. *Brain Language, 93,* 349–368.

Hunt, G. M., & Holmes, A. E. (1976). Factors relating intelligence in treated cases of spina bifida cystica. *American Journal of Disease in Children, 130,* 823–827.

Hunt, G. M., Oakesholt, P., & Kerry, S. (1999). Link between the CSF shunt and achievement in adults with spina bifida. *Journal of Neurology, Neurosurgery, and Psychiatry, 67,* 591–595.

Hurvitz, E. A., Leonard, C., Ayyangar, R., & Nelson, V. S. (2003). Complementary and alternative medicine use in families of children with cerebral palsy. *Developmental Medicine and Child Neurology, 45,* 364–370.

Hwang, R., Kentish, M., & Burns, Y. (2002). Hand positioning in children with spina bifida myelomeningocele. *Australian Journal of Physiotherapy, 48,* 17–22.

Individuals with Disabilities Education Act of 1990, Public Law 101–476. U.S. Statutes at Large (1990).

Individuals with Disabilities Education Act of 1997, Public Law 105–17. (IDEA Reauthorized), U.S. Statutes at Large (1997).

Individuals with Disabilities Education Improvement Act of 2004, Public Law 108–446. (IDEA Reauthorized), U.S. Statutes at Large 118 (2004):2647.

Ingram, T. S. S. (1955). Early manifestations and course of diplegia in childhood. *Archives of Disease in Childhood, 30,* 244–250.

Iwu, H. Y., Baskin, L. S., & Kogan, B. A. (1997). Neurogenic bladder dysfunction due to myelomeningocele: Neonatal versus childhood treatment. *Journal of Urology, 157,* 2295–2297.

Johnson, D. C., Damiano, D. L., & Abel, M. F. (1997). The evolution of gait in childhood and adolescent cerebral palsy. *Journal of Pediatric Orthopaedics, 17,* 392–396.

Kaplan, W. E. (1985). Management of myelomeningocele. *Urologic Clinics of North America, 12,* 930191.

Kaplan, W. E., & Richard, I. (1988). Intravesicle bladder stimulation in myelodysplasia. *Journal of Urology, 140,* 1282–1284.

Kari, J. A., Safdar, O., Jamjoon, R., & Anshasi, W. (2009). Renal involvement in children with spina bifida. *Saudi Journal of Kidney Disease Transplant, 20,* 102–105.

Kassover, M., Tauber, C., Au, J., & Pugh, J. (1986). Auditory biofeedback in spastic diplegia. *Journal of Orthopedics Research, 4,* 246–249.

Kaufman, B. A., Terbrock, A., Winters, N., Ito, J., Klosterman, A., & Park, T. S. (1994). Disbanding a multidisciplinary clinic: Effects on health care of myelomeningocele patients. *Pediatric Neurology, 21,* 36–44.

Keating, J. C., McCarron, K., James, J., Gruenberg, J., & Lonczak, R. S. (1985). Urobehavioral intervention in the rehabilitation of lower urinary tract dysfunction: A case report. *Journal of Manipulative and Physiological Therapeutics, 8,* 185–189.

Kelly, B., MacKay-Lyons, M. J., Berryman, S., Hyndman, J., & Wood, E. (2008). Assessment protocol for serial casting after botulinum toxin A injections to treat equinus gait. *Pediatric Physical Therapy, 20,* 233–241.

Khoury, M. J., Erickson, J. D., & James, L. M. (1982). Etiologic heterogenicity of neural tube defects: Clues from epidemiology. *American Journal of Epidemiology, 115,* 538–548.

King, W., Levin, R., Schmidt, R., Oestreich, A., & Heubi, J. E. (2003). Prevalence of reduced bone mass in children and adults with spastic quadriplegia. *Developmental Medicine and Child Neurology, 45,* 12–16.

Korman, L. A., Mooney, J. F., Smith, B., Goodman, A., & Mulvaney, T. (1993). Management of cerebral palsy with botulinum-A toxin: Preliminary investigations. *Journal of Pediatric Orthopaedics, 13,* 489–495.

Kottke, F. J., Halpern, D., Easton, J. K. M., Ozel, A. T., & Burrill, C. A. (1978). The training of coordination. *Archives of Physical Medicine and Rehabilitation, 59,* 567–578.

Kraus, F. T. (1997). Cerebral palsy and thrombi in placental vessels of the fetus: Insights from litigation. *Human Pathology, 28,* 246–248.

Krebs, D. E., Edelstein, J. E., & Fishman, S. (1988). Comparison of plastic/metal and leather/metal knee-ankle-foot orthoses. *American Journal of Physical Medicine, 67,* 175–185.

Lary, J. M., & Edmonds, L. D. (1996). Prevalence of spina bifida at birth—United States 1983–1990: A comparison of two surveillance systems. *Morbidity Mortality Weekly Reports CDC Surveillance Summaries, 45,* 15–26.

Leck, I. (1974). Causation of neutral tube defects; Clues from epidemiology. *British Medical Bulletin, 30,* 158–163.

Lemire, R. J. (1988). Neural tube defects. *Journal of the American Medical Association, 259,* 558–562.

Letts, R. M., Fulford, D., Eng, B., & Robinson, D. A. (1976). Mobility aids for the paraplegic child. *Journal of Bone and Joint Surgery, 58-A,* 38–41.

Levine, M. S. (1980). Cerebral palsy diagnosis in children over 1 year of age: Standard criteria. *Archives of Physical Medicine and Rehabilitation, 61,* 385–392.

Li, V., Albright, A. L., Sclabassi, R., & Pang, D. (1996). The role of somatosensory evoked potentials in the evaluation of spinal cord retethering. *Pediatric Neurosurgery, 24,* 126–133.

Lintner, S. A., & Lindseth, R. E. Kyphotic deformity in patients—Who have myeloemingocele: Operative treatment and long-term follow up. *Journal of Bone and Joint Surgery, 76-A,* 1301–1307.

Lonstein, J. E., & Akbamia, B. (1983). Operative treatment of spinal deformities in patients with cerebral palsy or mental retardation. *Journal of Bone and Joint Surgery, 63-A,* 43–57.

Lorber, J. (1971). Results of treatment of myelomeningocele: An analysis of 524 selected cases with special reference to possible selection for treatment. *Developmental Medicine and Child Neurology, 13,* 279–303.

Lord, J. P. (1984). Cerebral palsy: A clinical approach. *Archives of Physical Medicine and Rehabilitation, 65,* 542–556.

Lord, J. P., Varzos, N., Behrman, B., Wicks, J. G., & Wicks, D. (1990). Implications of mainstream classrooms for adolescents with spina bifida. *Developmental Medicine and Child Neurology, 32,* 20–29.

Lough, L. K., & Nielsen, D. J. (1986). Ambulation of children with myelomeningocele: Parapodium versus parapodium with Orlau swivel modification. *Developmental Medicine and Child Neurology, 28,* 489–497.

Maedgen, J. W., & Semrud-Clikeman, M. (2007). Bridging neuropsychological practice with education. In S. J. Hunter & J. Donders (Eds.), *Pediatric neuropsychological intervention: A critical review of science and practice.* Cambridge: Cambridge University Press.

Magill-Evans, J., Galambos, N., Darrah, J., & Nickerson, C. (2008). Predictors of employment for young adults with developmental motor disabilities. *Work, 31,* 433–442.

Magill-Evans, J. E., & Restall, G. (1991). Self-esteem of persons with cerebral palsy: From adolescence to adulthood. *American Journal of Occupational Therapy, 45,* 819–825.

Major, R. E., Stollard, J., & Farmer, S. E. (1997). A review of 42 patients of 16 years and over using the Orlau Parawalker. *Prosthetics and Orthotics International, 21,* 147–152.

Mankinen-Heikkinen, A., & Mustonene, E. (1987). Ophthalmologic changes in hydrocephalus. *Acta Ophthalmologica, 65,* 81–86.

Mannino, F. L., & Traunor, D. (1983). Stroke in neonates. *Journal of Pediatrics, 102,* 605–609.

Marshall, P. D., Broughton, N. S., Menelaus, M. B., & Graham, H. K. (1996). Surgical release of knee flexion contractures in myelomeningocele. *Journal of Bone and Joint Surgery, 78-B,* 912–916.

Martin, J. E., & Epstein, L. H. (1976). Evaluating treatment effectiveness in cerebral palsy. *Physical Therapy, 56,* 285–293.

Mathew, A., Mathew, C., Thomas, M., & Antonisamy, B. (2005). The efficacy of diazepam in enhancing motor function in children with spastic cerebral palsy. *Journal of Tropical Medicine and Hygiene, 51,* 109–113.

Matthews, D. (1988). Controversial therapies in the management of cerebral palsy. *Pediatric Annals, 17,* 762–765.

Maudsley, G., Hultor, J. L., & Pharoah, P. (1999). Cause of death in cerebral palsy: A descriptive study. *Archives of Disease in Childhood, 81,* 390–394.

Max, J. E., Mathews, K., Lansing, A. E., Robertson, B. A. M., Fox, P. T., Lancaster, J. L., et al. (2002). Psychiatric disorders after childhood stroke. *Journal of the American Academy of Child and Adolescent Psychiatry, 41,* 555–562.

McCall, R. E., & Schmidt, W. T. (1986). Clinical experiences with the reciprocating gait orthosis in myelodysplasia. *Journal of Pediatric Orthopaedics, 16,* 157–161.

McClone, D. G. (1998). The biological resolution of malformations of the central nervous system. *Neurosurgery, 43,* 1375–1380.

McClone, D. G., Cyzewski, D., Raimondi, A., & Sommers, M. (1985). Central nervous system infections as a limiting factor in the intelligence of children with myelodysplasia. *Pediatrics, 70,* 338–342.

McClone, D. G., Diaz, L., Kaplan, W., & Sommers, R. (1985). Concepts in the management of spina bifida. *Concepts in Pediatrics and Neurosurgery, 5,* 97–106.

McDonald, C. M., Jaffe, K. M., Mosca, V. S., Shurtleff, D. B., & Menalaus, M. B. (1991a). Ambulatory outcome of children with myelomeningocele: Effect of lower extremity strength. *Developmental Medicine and Child Neurology, 33,* 482–490.

McDonald, C. M., Jaffe, K. M., Mosca, V. S., Shurtleff, D. B., & Menalaus, M. B. (1991b). Modifications to the traditional description of neurosegmental innervation in myelomeningocele. *Developmental Medicine and Child Neurology, 33,* 473–481.

McLaughlin, J. F., & Shurtleff, D. B. (1979). Management of the newborn with myelodysplasia. *Clinical Pediatrics, 18,* 463–476.

McNeal, D., Hawtry, C. E, Wolraich, M. L., & Mapel, J. R. (1983). Symptomatic neurogenic bladder in a cerebral palsy population. *Developmental Medicine and Child Neurology, 25,* 612–621.

Mesples, B., Plaisant, F., & Gressens, P. (2003). Effects of interleukin-10 on neonatal excitotoxic brain lesions in mice. *Brain Research, 141,* 25–32.

Meuli, M., Meuli-Simmens, C., Hutchins, G. M., Seiler, M. J., Marrison, M. R., & Adzick, N. S. (1997). The spinal cord lesion in human fetuses with myelomeningocele. Implications for fetal surgery. *Journal of Pediatric Surgery, 32,* 448–452.

Meuli-Simmens, C., Meuli, M., Adzick, N. S., & Harrison, M. R. (1997). Latissimus dorsi flap procedures to cover myelomeningocele in utero: A feasibility study in human fetuses. *Journal of Pediatric Surgery, 32,* 1154–1156.

Meyer, R. E., & Siega-Riz, A. M. (2002). Sociodemographic patterns in spina bifida with prevalence trends—North Carolina, 1995–1999. *Morbidity Mortality Weekly Report, 51,* 12–15.

Michelsen, S. I., Uldall, P., Hansen, T., & Madsen, M. (2006). Social integration of adults with cerebral palsy. *Developmental Medicine and Child Neurology, 48,* 643–649.

Michelsen, S. I., Uldall, P., Mette, A., & Madsen, M. (2005). Education and employment prospects in cerebral palsy. *Developmental Medicine and Child Neurology, 47,* 511–517.

Milunsky, A., & Alpert, E. (1976a). Prenatal diagnosis of neural tube deficits: l. Problems and pitfalls: Analysis of 2495 cases using the alpha-fetoprotein assay. *Journal of Obstetrics and Gynecology, 48,* 1–5.

Milunsky, A., & Alpert, E. (1976b). Prenatal diagnosis of neural tube deficits: 2. Analysis of false positive and false negative alpha-fetoprotein results. *Journal of Obstetrics and Gynecology, 48,* 6–12.

Missuna, C., & Pollack, N. (1991). Play deprivation in children with physical disabilities: The role of the occupational therapist in preventing secondary disability. *American Journal of Occupational Therapy, 45,* 882–888.

Mital, M. A., & Sakellardies, H. (1981). Surgery of the upper extremity in the retarded individual with spastic cerebral palsy. *Orthopedic Clinics of North America, 12,* 127–136.

Mobley, C. E., Harless, L. S., & Miller, K. L. (1996). Self-perception of preschool children with spina bifida. *Journal of Pediatric Neurosurgery, 11,* 217–224.

Molenaers, G., Desloovere, K., & DeCat, J. (2001). Single event multi-level botulinum toxin type A treatment and surgery: Similarities and differences. *European Journal of Neurology, 8,* 88–97.

Molnar, G. E. (1979). Cerebral palsy prognosis and who to judge it. *Pediatric Annals, 8,* 10–24.

Molnar, G. E., & Taft, L. T. (1977). Pediatric rehabilitation: Part I. Cerebral palsy and spinal cord injuries. *Current Problems in Pediatrics, 7,* 6–11.

Morison, J. E., Bromfield, L. M., & Cameron, H. J. (2003). A therapeutic model for supporting families of children with a chronic illness or disability. *Child and Adolescent Mental Health, 8,* 125–130.

Morris, P. J. (2008). Physical activity recommendations for children and adolescents with chronic disease. *Current Sports Medicine Reports, 7,* 353–358.

Morrow, J. D. (1995). Temperament in the infant with myelomeningocele. *Journal of Pediatric Nursing, 10,* 99–104.

Mossberg, K. A., Linton, K. A., & Friske, K. (1990). Ankle-foot orthoses: Effect on energy expenditure of gait in spastic diplegic children. *Archives of Physical Medicine and Rehabilitation, 71,* 490–494.

Mundy, A. R., Shah, P. J. R., Borzyskowski, M., & Saxton, H. M. (1985). Sphincter behavior in myelomeningocele. *British Journal of Urology, 57,* 647–651.

Murphy, K. P., Molnar, G. E., & Lankasky, K. (1995). Medical and functional status of adults with cerebral palsy. *Developmental Medicine and Child Neurology, 37,* 1075–1084.

Murphy, K. P., Molnar, G. E., & Lankasky, K. (2000). Employment and social issues in adults with cerebral palsy. *Archives of Physical Medicine and Rehabilitation, 81,* 807–811.

Naeye, R. L., & Peter, E. C. (1989). Origins of cerebral palsy. *American Journal of Disease in Childhood, 143,* 1154–1160.

Narayanan, U. G. (2007). The role of gait analysis in the orthopaedic management of ambulatory cerebral palsy. *Current Opinion in Pediatrics, 19,* 38–43.

Nelson, K. B. (1989). Relationship of intrapartum and delivery events to long-term neurologic outcome. *Clinical Perinatology, 16,* 995–1007.

Nelson, K. B. (1998). Neonatal cytokines and coagulation factors in children with cerebral palsy. *Annals of Neurology, 44,* 665–675.

Nelson, K. B. (2008). Causative factors in cerebral palsy. *Clinical Obstetrics and Gynecology, 51,* 749–762.

Nelson, K. B., & Ellenberg, J. H. (1979). Neonatal signs as a predictor of cerebral palsy. *Pediatrics, 64,* 2–14.

Nelson, K. B., & Ellenberg, J. H. (1981). Apgar scores as predictors of cerebral palsy. *Pediatrics, 68,* 36–46.

Nelson, K. B., & Ellenberg, J. H. (1986). Antecedents of cerebral palsy. *New England Journal of Medicine, 315,* 81–86.

Nordmark, E., Josenby, A. L., Lagergren, J., Anderson, G., Stromblad, L. G., Westbom, L. (2008). Long-term outcomes five years after selective dorsal rhizotomy. *BMC Pediatrics, 8,* 54–69.

Nwaobi, O. M., & Smith, P. D. (1986). Effects of adaptive seating on pulmonary function in children with cerebral palsy. *Developmental Medicine and Child Neurology, 28,* 351–354.

Obojoski, A., Chodorski, J., Borg, W., Medal, W., Fal, A. M., & Malolepsz, Y. (2002). Latex allergy and sensitization in children with spina bifida. *Pediatrics Neurosurgery, 37,* 262–266.

Osterlund, C. S., Dosa, N. P., & Smith, C. A. (2005). Mother knows best: Medical record management for patients with spina bifida during the transition from pediatric to adult care. *AMIA Proceedings,* 580–584.

Padmanabhan, R. (2006). Etiology, pathogenesis, and prevention of neural tube defects. *Congenital Anomalies, 46,* 55–67.

Palisano, R. J., Rosenbaum, P. L., Walter, S. D., & Hanna, S. (1997). Development and reliability of a system to classify gross motor function in children with cerebral palsy. *Developmental Medicine and Child Neurology, 39,* 214–223.

Palmer, F. B., Shapiro, B. K., Allen, M. C., Mosher, B. S., Bilker, S. A., Harryman, S. E., et al. (1990). Infant stimulation curriculum for infants with cerebral palsy: Effects on infant temperament, parent infant interaction and home environment. *Pediatrics, 85,* 411–415.

Palmer, F. B., Shapiro, B. K., & Wachtel, R. C. (1988). Effects of physical therapy on cerebral palsy. *New England Journal of Medicine, 318,* 803–808.

Pape, K. E., Kirsch, S. E., Galil, A., Boultron, J. E., White, M. A., & Chipman, M. (1993). Neuromuscular approach to the motor deficits of cerebral palsy: A pilot study. *Journal of Pediatric Orthopaedics, 13,* 628–633.

Peacock, W. J., Arens, L. J., & Berman, B. (1987). Cerebral palsy spasticity: Selective posterior rhizotomy. *Pediatric Neuroscience, 13,* 61–66.

Peacock, W. J., & Staudt, L. A. (1991). Functional outcomes following selective posterior rhizotomy for children with cerebral palsy. *Journal of Neurosurgery, 74,* 380–385.

Pecker, R., Danver, J. E., Hjalmas, K., Sjodin, J. G., & Von Zweibergk, M. (1997). The urological fate of young adults with myelomeningocele: A three decade follow-up study. *European Urology, 32,* 213–217.

Pellock, J. M. (2004). Defining the problem: Psychiatric and behavioral comorbidity in children and adolescents with epilepsy. *Epilepsy & Behavior, 5*(Suppl. 3), 3–9.

Penn, R. D., Mykleburst, B. M., Gottlieb, G. L., Agarwal, G. C., & Etzel, M. E. (1980). Chronic cerebellar stimulation for cerebral palsy. *Journal of Neurosurgery, 53,* 160–169.

Perlstein, M. A. (1952). Infantile cerebral palsy: Classification and clinical correlations. *Journal of the American Medical Association, 149,* 30–37.

Petersen, T. (1987). Management of urinary incontinence in children with myelomeningocele. *Acta Neurologica Scandinavica, 75,* 52–55.

Petrini, J., Dias, T., McCormick, M., Massolo, M., Green, N., & Escobar, G. (2009). Increased risk of adverse neurological development of later preterm infants. *Journal of Pediatrics, 154,* 169–176.

Pierce, S. R., Daly, K., Gallagher, K. G., Gershkoff, A. M., & Schaumburg, S. W. (2002). Constraint-induced therapy for a child with hemiplegic cerebral palsy: A case report. *Archives of Physical Medicine and Rehabilitation, 83,* 1462–1463.

Preiss, R. A., Condie, D. N., Rowley, D. I., & Graham, H. K. (2003). The effects of botulinum toxin (BTX-A) on spasticity of the lower limb and gait in cerebral palsy. *Journal of Bone and Joint Surgery, 85-B,* 943–948.

Raddish, M., Goldman, D. A., Kaplan, D. C., & Perin, J. M. (1998). The immunization status of children with spina bifida. *American Journal of Diseases of Children, 147,* 849–853.

Radke, J., & Gosky, G. A. (1981). Hearing and speech screening in a hydrocephalus myelodysplasia population. *Spina Bifida Therapy, 3,* 25–26.

Rapp, C. E., & Torres, M. M. (2000). The adult with cerebral palsy. *Archives of Family Medicine, 9,* 466–472.

Reese, M. E., Msall, M. E., & Owens, S. (1991). Acquired cervical spine impairment in young adults with cerebral palsy. *Developmental Medicine and Child Neurology, 33,* 153–156.

Reigel, D. H. (1983). Tethered spinal cord. *Concepts Pediatric Neurosurgery, 4,* 142–164.

Reimers, J. (1990). Functional changes in the antagonists after lengthening of the agonists in cerebral palsy. *Clinical Orthopaedics and Related Research, 253,* 3037.

Resnick, M. B., Eyler, F. D., Nelson, R. M., Eitman, D. V., & Bucciarelli, R. L. (1987). Developmental intervention for low birth weight infants: Improved early developmental outcome. *Pediatrics, 80,* 68–74.

Rezaie, P., & Dean, A. (2002). Periventricular leukomalacia, inflammation and white matter lesions within the developing nervous system. *Neuropathology, 22,* 106–132.

Rietberg, C. C., & Lindhout, D. (1993). Adult patients with spina bifida cystica. *European Journal of Obstetrics, Gynecological Reproductive Biology, 52,* 63–70.

Robinson, H. P., Hood, V. D., Adam, H. D., Gibson, A. A. M., & Ferguson-Smith, M. A. (1980). Diagnostic ultrasound: Early detection of fetal neural tube defects. *Obstetrics and Gynecology, 56,* 705–710.

Robinson, R. O. (1973). The frequency of other handicaps in children with cerebral palsy. *Developmental Medicine and Child Neurology, 15,* 305–316.

Ronan, S., & Gold, J. T. (2007). Nonoperative management of spasticity in children. Child's Nervous System. *Children's Nervous System, 23,* 943–956.

Rosenstein, S. N. (1982). *Dentistry in cerebral palsy and related handicapping conditions.* Springfield, IL: Charles. C. Thomas.

Rotenstein, D., & Riegel, D. H. (1996). Growth hormone treatment of children with neural tube defects; Results from 6 months to 6 years. *Journal of Pediatrics, 128,* 184–189.

Rothman, J. G. (1978). Effects of respiratory exercise on the vital capacity and forced volume in children with cerebral palsy. *Physical Therapy, 58,* 421–425.

Rouse, D., Hirtz, D., Thom, E., Varner, M., Spong, C. Y., Mercer, B. M., et al. (2008). A randomized controlled trial of magnesium sulfate for the prevention of cerebral palsy. *New England Journal of Medicine, 359,* 895–905.

Rousset, C. I., Kassem, J., Olivier, P., Chalon, S., Gressens, P., & Saliba, E. (2008). Antenatal bacterial endotoxin sensitizes the immature rat brain to postnatal excitotoxic injury. *Journal of Neuropathology and Experimental Neurology, 67,* 994–1000.

Rowe, D. E., & Jadhav, A. L. (2008). Care of the adolescent with spina bifida. *Pediatric Clinics of North America, 55,* 1359–1374.

Sala, D. A., & Grant, A. D. (1995). Prognosis for ambulation in cerebral palsy. *Developmental Medicine and Child Neurology, 37,* 1020–1026.

Salakor, P. T., Sajaniemi, N., Hallvack, H., Kari, A., Rila, H., & von Wednt, L. (1997). Randomization study of the effects of antenatal dexamethasone on growth and development of premature children at the corrected age of two years. *Acta Paediatrica, 86,* 294–298.

Samilson, R. L. (1981). Current concepts of surgical management in the lower extremities in cerebral palsy. *Clinical Orthopaedics and Related Research, 158,* 99–113.

Sanders, J. O., McConnell, S. L., King, R., Landford, A., Montpetit, K., Gates, P., et al. (2006). A prospective evaluation of the Wee FIM in patients with cerebral palsy undergoing orthopaedic surgery. *Journal of Pediatric Orthopaedics, 26,* 542–546.

Sankey, R. J., Anderson, D. M., & Young, J. A. (1989). Characteristics of ankle-foot orthoses for management of the spastic lower limb. *Developmental Medicine and Child Neurology, 31,* 466–471.

Satila, H., Pietkainen, T., Hsalo, T., Lehtonen-Katy, P., Salu, M., Haataja, R., et al. (2008). Botulinum toxin type A injections into the calf muscles for treatment of spastic equinus in cerebral palsy: A randomized trial comparing single and multiple injection sites. *American Journal of Physical Medicine and Rehabilitation, 87,* 386–394.

Schaefer, M. K., McCarthy, J. J., & Josephic, K. (2007). Effects of early weight bearing on the functional recovery of ambulatory children with cerebral palsy after bilateral proximal femoral osteotomy. *Journal of Pediatric Orthopaedics, 27,* 668–670.

Seifart, A., Unger, M., & Burger, M. (2009). The effect of lower limb functional electrical stimulation on gait of children with cerebral palsy. *Pediatric Physical Therapy, 21,* 23–30.

Sgoros, S., & Seri, S. (2002). The effect of intrathecal baclofen on muscle co-contraction in children with spasticity of cerebral origin. *Pediatric Neurosurgery, 37,* 225–230.

Shafer, M. F., & Dias, L. S. (1983). *Myelomeningocele: Orthopaedic treatment.* Baltimore, MD: Williams & Wilkins.

Shah, P. S., Ohlsson, A., & Perlman, A. (2007). Hypothermia to treat neonatal hypoxic ischemic encephalopathy. *Archives of Pediatrics and Adolescent Medicine, 161,* 951–958.

Shapiro, A., & Susa, K. Z. (1990). Pre-operative and post-operative gait evaluation in cerebral palsy. *Archives of Physical Medicine and Rehabilitation, 71,* 236–240.

Sharrard, W. J. W. (1964). Posterior iliopsoas transplantation in the treatment of paralytic dislocation of the hip. *Journal of Bone and Joint Surgery, 46-B,* 426–444.

Sherk, H. H., Uppal, G. S., Lane, G., & Melchionni, J. (1991). Treatment versus non-treatment of hip dislocations in ambulatory patients with myelomeningocele. *Developmental Medicine and Child Neurology, 33,* 491–494.

Shields, N., Murdoch, A., Loy, Y., Dodd, K. J., & Taylor, N. F. (2006). A systematic review of the self-concept of children with cerebral palsy compared with children without disability. *Developmental Medicine & Child Neurology, 48,* 151–157.

Sigurdardottir, S., Halldorsdottir, M., Thorkelsson, T., Thorarensen, O., & Vik, T. (2009). Trends in prevalence and characteristics of cerebral palsy among Icelandic children born 1990 to 2003. *Developmental Medicine and Child Neurology, 51,* 356–363.

Sillanpaa, M., Piekkala, P., & Pisira, H. (1982). The young adult with cerebral palsy and his chances of employment. *International Journal of Rehabilitation Research, 5,* 467–476.

Sinha, C. K., Grewal, A., & Ward, H. C. (2008). Antegrade continence enema (ACE); Current practice. *Pediatric Surgery International, 24,* 685–688.

Siperstein, G. N., Wolraich, M. L., Reed, D., & O'Keefe, P. (1988). Medical decisions and prognostications of pediatricians for infants with myelomeningocele. *Journal of Pediatrics, 113,* 835–840.

Siracusa, C., Taylor, M., Geletka, B., & Overby, A. (2005). Effectiveness of biomechanical intervention in children with cerebral palsy. *Pediatric Physical Therapy, 17,* 83–84.

Slater, J. E. (1989). Rubber anaphylaxis. *New England Journal of Medicine, 320,* 1126–1129.

Smith, K. A. (1991). Bowel and bladder management of the child with myelomeningocele in the school setting. *Journal of Pediatric Health Care, 4,* 175–180.

Smith, S., Camfield, C., & Camfield, D. (1999). Living with cerebral palsy and tube feeding: A population-based follow-up study. *Journal of Pediatrics, 135,* 307–310.

Sousa, J. C., Gordon, L. H., & Shurtleff, D. B. (1976). Assessing the development of daily living skills in patients with spina bifida. *Developmental Medicine and Child Neurology, 37*(Suppl. 18), 134–143.

Spates, C. R., Samaraweera, N., Plaiser, B., Souza, T., Otsui, K. (2007). Psychological impact of trauma on developing children and youth. *Primary Care: Clinics in Office Practice, 34,* 387–405.

Spindel, M. R., Bauer, S. B., & Dyron, I. M. (1987). The changing lesion in myelodysplasia. *Journal of the American Medical Association, 258,* 1630–1633.

Staheli, L. T. L., Duncan, W. R., & Schaefer, E. (1960). Growth alterations in the hemiplegic child. *Clinical Orthopaedics and Related Research, 60,* 205–212.

Stallard, J., Major, R. E., & Farmer, S. E. (1996). The potential for ambulation by severely handicapped cerebral palsy patients. *Prosthetics and Orthototics International, 20,* 122–128.

Stanley, F., & Blair, E. (1991). Why we have failed to reduce the frequency of cerebral palsy? *Medical Journal of Australia, 154,* 623–626.

Stark, G. D., & Baker, G. C. W. (1967). The neurological involvement of the lower limb in myelomeningocele. *Developmental Medicine and Child Neurology, 9,* 178–184.

Steinbok, P., Reiner, A. M., Beauchamp, R., Armstrong, R. W., & Cochrane, D. D. (1997). A randomized clinical trial to compare selective posterior rhizotomy plus physiotherapy with physiotherapy alone in children with spastic diplegic cerebral palsy. *Developmental Medicine and Child Neurology, 39,* 178–184.

Stothard, K. J., Tennant, P., Bell, R., & Rankin, J. (2009). Maternal overweight and obesity and the risk of congenital anomalies. A systemic review and meta-analysis. *Journal of the American Medical Association, 301,* 636–650.

Strauss, D., Cable, W., & Shavelte, R. (1999). Causes of excess mortality in cerebral palsy. *Developmental Medicine and Child Neurology, 41,* 580–585.

Streeter, G. L. (1942). Developmental horizons in human embryos: Description of age group XI: 13 to 20 somites, and age group XII, 21–29 somites. *Contributions in Embryology, 30,* 211–245.

Sutherland, D. H. (1984). *Gait disorders of childhood and adolescence.* Baltimore, MD: Williams & Wilkins.

Swaminathan, S., Patton, J. Y., Ward, S. D. L., Jacobs, R. A., Sargent, C. W., & Keens, T. G. (1989). Abnormal control of ventilation in adolescents with myelodysplasia. *Journal of Pediatrics, 115,* 898–903.

Sweetser, P. M., Badell, A., Schneider, S., & Badlin, G. H. (1995). Effects of sacral dorsal rhizotomy on bladder function in patients with spastic cerebral palsy. *Neuroradiology and Urodyanamics, 14,* 57–64.

Szalay, E. A., Harriman, D., Eastlund, B., & Mercer, D. (2008). Quantifying postoperative bone loss in children. *Journal of Pediatric Orthopaedics, 28,* 320–323.

Talwar, D. D., Baldwin, N. A., & Hornblatt, C. (1995). Epilepsy in children with myelomeningocele. *Pediatric Neurology, 13,* 29–32.

Tanaka, H. M., Fukada, I., Miyamoto, A., Oka, R., Cho, K., Fujieda, K. (2004). Effects of tizanidine for refractory sleep disturbance in disabled children with spastic quadriparesis. *No to Hattatsu, 36,* 455–460.

Tardieu, C., de la Tour, H., Bret, N. D., & Tardieu, G. (1982). Muscle hypoextensibility in children with cerebral palsy. *Archives of Physical Medicine and Rehabilitation, 63,* 97–110.

Tardieu, C., & Lespargot, A. (1988). For how long must the soleus muscle be stretched each day to prevent contracture? *Developmental Medicine and Child Neurology, 30,* 3019.

Tardoff, K. (1986). Spontaneous remission in cerebral palsy. *Neuropediatrics, 17,* 19–22.

Teo, C., & Jones, R. (1996). Management of hydrocephalus by endoscopic third ventriculostomy in patients with myelomeningocele. *Pediatric Neurosurgery, 25,* 57–63.

Tew, B. (1979). The "cocktail party syndrome" in children with hydrocephalus and spina bifida. *British Journal of Disorders of Communication, 14,* 89–101.

Thomas, S. S., Aiona, M. D., Pierce, R., & Piatt, J. H. (1996). Gait changes in children with spastic diplegia after selective dorsal rhizotomy. *Journal of Pediatric Orthopaedics, 16,* 474–452.

Tirosh, E., & Rabino, S. (1989). Physiotherapy for children with cerebral palsy. *American Journal of Diseases in Childhood, 143,* 551–553.

Tobimatsu, Y., & Nakamura, R. (2000). Retrospective study of factors affecting employability of individuals with cerebral palsy in Japan. *Tohoku Journal of Experimental Medicine, 192,* 291–299.

Tomlinson, P., & Sugarman, I. D. (1995). Complications in shunts in adults with spina bifida. *American Journal of Diseases in Childhood, 143,* 551–553.

Torre, M., Planche, D., Louis-Borrione, C., Sabiani, F., Lena, G., & Guys, J. M. (2002). Value of electrophysiological assessment after surgical treatment of spinal dysraphism. *Journal of Urology, 168,* 1759–1763.

Tscharnuter, I. (2002). Clinical application of dynamic theory concepts according to Tscharnuter Akademie for Movement Organizations (TAMO) therapy. *Pediatric Physical Therapy, 14,* 29–37.

Turk, M., Scandale, J., Rosenbaum, P. F., & Weber, R. J. (2001). The health of women with cerebral palsy. *Physical Medicine and Rehabilitation Clinics of North America, 12,* 153–166.

Unnithan, V., Katsmanis, G., Evangelinou, C., Kosmas, C., Kandrali, I., & Kellis, E. (2007). Effect of strength and aerobic training in children with cerebral palsy. *Medicine and Science in Sports and Exercise, 39,* 1902–1909.

Valvano, J. (2004). Activity-focused motor interventions for children with neurological conditions. *Physical and Occupational Therapy in Pediatrics, 24,* 79–107.

Van der Dussen, L., Nieustraten, W., Roebroeck, M., & Stam, H. J. (2001). Functional level of young adults with cerebral palsy. *Clinical Rehabilitation, 15,* 84–91.

Van Mechelen, M. C., Verheof, M., van Asbeck, F., & Post, M. W. M. (2008). Work participation among young adults with spina bifida in the Netherlands. *Developmental Medicine & Child Neurology, 50,* 772–777.

Vannucci, R. C. (1990). Experimental biology of cerebral hypoxic ischemia: Relationship of perinatal brain damage. *Pediatric Research, 27,* 317–326.

Vaughn, C. W., Neilson, P. D., & O'Dwyer, N. J. (1988). Motor control deficits in oro-facial muscles in cerebral palsy. *Journal of Neurology and Neurosurgical Psychiatry, 51,* 534–539.

Veland, P. M., Hosted, S., Schneede, J., Refsum, H., & Vollset, S. (2001). Biological and clinical implications of MTHFR C677T polymorphism. *Trends in Pharmacological Science, 22,* 195–201.

Verhoef, M., Barf, H. A., Post, M. W. M., van Asbeck, F., Rob, H., & Arie, J. H. (2006). Functional independence among young adults with spina bifida, in relation to hydrocephalus and level of lesion. *Developmental Medicine and Child Neurology, 48,* 114–119.

Verhoef, M., Barf, H. A., Vroege, J. A., van Asbeck, F. W., Gooskens, R. H., Prevo, A. J. (2005). Sex education, relationships, and sexuality in young adults with spina bifida. *Archives of Physical Medicine and Rehabilitation, 86,* 979–987.

Verhoef, M., Lurvink, M., Barf, H. A., Post, M. W. M., van Asbeck, F. W. A., Gooskens, R. H. J. M., et al. (2005). High prevalence of incontinence among young adults with spina bifida: Description, prediction and problem perception. *Spinal Cord, 43,* 331–340.

Vinck, A., Maassen, B., Mullaart, R., & Rotteveel, J. (2006). Arnold-Chiari II malformation and cognitive functioning in spina bifida. *Journal of Neurology, Neurosurgery, and Psychiatry, 77,* 1083–1086.

Vohr, B. R., & Msall, M. E. (1997). Neuropsycholgical and functional outcomes of very low birth weight infants. *Seminars in Perinatology, 21,* 202–220.

Wagner, K., Risnes, I., Berntsen, T., Skaro, A., Ramberg, B., Vandvik, I. H., et al. (2007). Clinical and psychosocial follow-up of children treated with extracorporeal membrane oxygenation. *Annals of Thoracic Surgery, 84,* 1349–1355.

Wallace, S. J. (1973). The effect of upper-limb function on mobility of children with myelomeningocele. *Developmental Medicine and Child Neurology, 15,* 84–91.

Wallender, J. K., Babani, L., Varni, J. W., Banis, H. T., & Wilcox, K. T. (1989). Family resources as resistance factors for psychological maladjustment in chronically ill and handicapped children. *Journal of Pediatric Psychology, 14,* 157–173.

Wallender, J. L., Varni, J. W., Babani, L., Deltaan, C. V., Wilcox, K. T., & Banis, J. T. (1989). The social environment and the adaptation of mothers of physically handicapped children. *Journal of Pediatric Psychology, 14,* 371–387.

Warschausky, S., Kaufman, J. P., & Stiers, W. (2008). Training requirements and scope of practice in rehabilitation psychology and neuropsychology. *Journal of Pediatric Rehabilitation Medicine: An Interdisciplinary Approach, 1,* 61–65.

Wei, S., Su-juan, W., Yuan-Gui, L., Hong, Y., Xiu-Juan, X. U., & Xiao-Mei, S. (2006). Reliability and validity of the GMFM-66 in 0–3-year old children with cerebral palsy. *American Journal of Physical Medicine and Rehabilitation, 85,* 141–147.

Williams, M. D., Lewandowski, L. J., Coplan, J., & D'Eugenio, D. B. (1987). Neurodevelopmental outcome of preschool children born preterm with and without intracranial hemorrhage. *Developmental Medicine and Child Neurology, 29,* 243–249.

Wills, K. E., Holmbeck, G. N., Dillon, K., & McClone, D. G. (1990). Intelligence and achievement in children with myelomeningocele. *Journal of Pediatrics Psychology, 15,* 161–176.

Wilson, H., Haideri, M. E., Song, K., & Telford, D. (1997). Ankle foot orthosis for preambulatory children with spastic diplegia. *Journal of Pediatric Orthopaedics, 17,* 370–376.

Worley, G., Rosenfeld, L. R., & Lipscomb, J. (1991a). Financial counseling for families of children with chronic disabilities. *Developmental Medicine and Child Neurology,* 679–689.

Worley, G., Rosenfeld, L. R., & Lipscomb, J. (1991b). Influence on survival of cervical laminectomy for children with meningomyelocele who have potentially lethal brainstem dysfunction due to the Chiari II malformation. *Developmental Medicine and Child Neurology, 33*(Suppl. 64), 19–26.

Worley, G., Schuster, J. M., & Oakes, W. J. (1996). Survival at 5 years of a cohort of newborn infants with myelomeningocele. *Developmental Medicine and Child Neurology, 38,* 816–822.

Yamada, S., Zinke, D. E., & Saunders, D. (1981). Pathophysiology of tethered cord syndrome. *Journal of Neurosurgery, 54,* 494–503.

Yokochi, K. (1997). Thalamic lesions revealed by M.R.I. associated with periventricular leukomalacia and clinical profiles of suspect. *Acta Paediatrica Scandinavica, 86,* 493–496.

Yoshida, F., Morioka, T., Hashiguchi, K., Kawamura, T., Miyagi, Y., Nagata, S., et al. (2006). Epilepsy in patients with spina bifida in the lumbosacral region. *Neurosurgical Review, 29,* 327–332.

Young, N. L. (2007). The transition to adulthood for children with cerebral palsy: What do we know about their health care needs? *Journal of Pediatric Orthopaedics, 27,* 476–479.

Young, R. R., & Delwaide, P. J. (1981). Drug therapy: Spasticity. *New England Journal of Medicine, 304,* 28–43.

Young, N. L., Mc Cormick, A., Mills, W., Barden, W., Law, M., Wedge, J., et al. (2006). The transitions study: A look at youth and adults with cerebral palsy, spina bifida, and acquired brain injury. *Physical and Occupational Therapy in Pediatrics, 26,* 25–45.

Zaccario, M., Salsberg, D., Gordon, R., & Bilginer, L. (in press). Psychological and neuropsychological issues in the care of children with disabilities. *Journal of Pediatric Rehabilitation Medicine.*

Zarfonte, R., Lornard, L., & Elovic, E. (2004). Antispasticity medications: Uses and limitations of enteral therapy. *American Journal of Physical Medicine and Rehabilitation, 83,* s50–s66.

Zide, B., Constantini, S., & Epstein, F. J. (1995). Prevention of recurrent tethered spinal cord. *Pediatric Neurosurgery, 22,* 111–1143.

Ziv, I., Blackborn, N., Rang, M., & Koresk, J. (1984). Muscle growth in normal and spastic mice. *Developmental Medicine and Child Neurology, 26,* 94–99.

17

Geriatric Rehabilitation

Monwara Hassan, MD, Adrian Cristian, MD,
and Teina Daley, OTR/L, CHT

INTRODUCTION

The increasing growth of the age 65 and older population affects many aspects of our society, challenging policymakers, families, businesses, and health care providers to meet the needs of aging individuals. The U.S. population aged 65 and older are the largest consumers of medical care. Their health care needs will be even greater as we move through the 21st century.

DEMOGRAPHICS

Improvements in health care have resulted in an increased life expectancy for the U.S. population. The average life expectancy today is more than 78 years compared with 72 and 49 years in 1985 and 1900, respectively.

In 2007, 37.9 million Americans, aged 65 and older, lived in the United States, accounting for nearly 13% of the total population; 1.5 million lived in nursing facilities, comprising 4% of all people in this age group. The population of adults aged 85 years or older has grown from just over 100,000 in 1900 to 5.3 million in 2006 (U.S. Census Bureau, 2006). The U.S. Census Bureau has projected that this population could grow to nearly 21 million by 2050. The "baby boomers" (those born between 1946 and 1964) will start turning 65 in 2011, and the number of older people will increase dramatically during the 2010–2030 period. The older population in 2030 is projected to be twice as large as in 2000, growing from 35 million to 71.5 million and representing nearly 20% of the total U.S. population (Figure 17.1). Gender disparities are also present as evidenced by the fact that 75% of older nursing home residents are women.

These demographic changes pose unique challenges to the U.S. health care system, the expenses of which reached $2.4 trillion in 2008 or 17% of gross domestic product (GDP) (Conwell & Cohen, 2002; Keehan, Lazenby, Zezza, & Catlin, 2004; Stanton, 2005). These expenses are projected to grow to $4.3 trillion by 2017, eventually reaching 20% of the GDP.

In 2002, the population aged 65 or older consumed 37% of the health care expenses. Elderly people suffer from various chronic debilitating conditions, which contribute to this significant consumption of health care. Chronic diseases such as heart disease, stroke, cancer, and diabetes are among the most common and costly diseases in this age group.

A National Long-Term Care Survey in 1999 showed the overall prevalence of age-related chronic disability in the U.S. population aged 65 and older was 19.7% (Manton & Gu, 2001). In

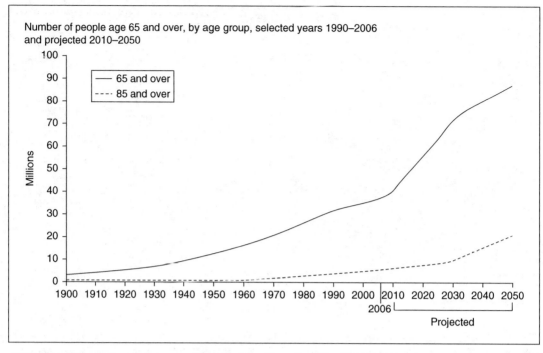

FIGURE 17.1   U.S. population age 65 and older. *Note:* Data for 2010–2050 are projections of the population. (*Reference population:* These data refer to the resident population.) *Source:* U.S. Census Bureau, Decennial Census, Population Estimates and Projections.

discussing the impact of aging and chronic diseases, it is important to understand the definitions of impairment, activity limitation, and participation restriction. According to the World Health Organization (WHO), "an *impairment* is a problem in body function or structure; an *activity limitation* is a difficulty encountered by an individual in executing a task or action; while a *participation restriction* is a problem experienced by an individual in involvement in life situations" (WHO, 2010).

Living with a chronic illness can have a negative impact on the quality of life of the affected individual, contributing to a decline in function and challenges to remaining an active member in the community. Forty-two percent of people age 65 and older living in a community settings reported a functional limitation in performing activities of daily living (ADLs) and instrumental activities of daily living (IADLs).

In a recent survey, 12% of the population age 65 and older living at home had difficulty performing one or more IADLs (but no ADL limitation). Eighteen percent had difficulty with 1–2 ADLs, 5% had difficulty with 3–4 ADLs, and 3% had difficulty with 5–6 ADLs (Figure 17.2).

Incidences of functional limitations are similar in those living in the nursing homes (Hing, Sekscenski, & Strahan, 1989). Women living in nursing homes require more assistance with daily activities than men. Incidence of these limitations is 2.6 times more in people aged 85 and older.

AGING-RELATED CHANGES

Normal changes in the human body associated with aging are briefly discussed in the following sections. Although physiological, these age-related changes predispose to various disease conditions, functional limitation, falls, and quality of life.

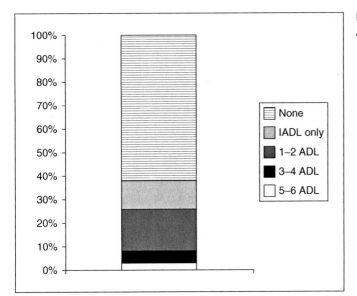

FIGURE 17.2 Incidence of IADL/ADL limitation at age 65 or older.

Cardiovascular System

A number of anatomical and physiological changes occur with aging, particularly left ventricular hypertrophy, decrease in the size of the sinoatrial and atrioventricular nodes due to a loss of cells, calcification, irregularity of endothelial cells, increased amount of connective tissue, and lipid deposits in the blood vessels contributing to atherosclerosis. These changes can lead to hypertension, cardiac arrhythmia, and increased susceptibility to myocardial infarction and stroke. However, the cardiac output of the aging heart remains normal at rest.

Pulmonary System

With aging, the compliance of the chest wall decreases due to several factors such as stiffening and calcification of costal cartilage, decreased elasticity of the thoracic cage, decreased disc height of thoracic vertebrae, and increased thoracic kyphosis. There is also a decrease in elastic recoil of the lung. All of these changes are thought to be responsible for a decrease in vital capacity and an increase in functional residual capacity and residual volume. Decrease in pulmonary function results in poor performance and endurance.

Skin

The moisture content of the skin, rate of epidermal renewal, elasticity, sebum secretion, vascular supply, hair and nail growth, sensitivity to touch, pain, and temperature all decrease, making the skin more vulnerable to damage and disease. Decreased subcutaneous fat and poor capillary function, increase the risk of developing pressure ulcers. Age-related changes in thermoregulation along with drugs and disease condition predisposes to both hypothermia and hyperthermia.

Gastrointestinal System

Aging-related changes in the gastrointestinal system include pharyngeal muscle weakness, reduction in stomach acid production, delay in emptying time, and reduction in the absorption of calcium, vitamin D, and iron. Constipation is common and diverticulosis can be seen in about one-third of healthy adults older than 65 years and two-thirds of adults older than 80 years. GI system changes may result in malabsorption and malnutrition with subsequent anemia, osteoporosis, and so on.

Genitourinary System

Renal mass (i.e., glomerular tubules) and blood flow decreases by 6–10% every 10 years beginning in the fourth decade of life. As a result there is a 40% reduction in kidney function by age 70 even in the absence of kidney disease. This can have significant implications when prescribing medications that are cleared by the kidneys; therefore, appropriate renal dosing is important. Prostate enlargement is also common in older men.

Endocrine System

The function of hypothalamus, pituitary gland, and end organs like the thyroid, parathyroid, adrenal, and gonads as well as the pancreas change with age. Decreased feedback inhibition of the hypothalamic–pituitary–adrenal axis can result in imbalance of growth hormone, thyroid production, and decreases in estrogen and testosterone production. Age-related endocrine dysfunctions put elderly people at risk of osteoporosis, osteoarthritis (OA), and diabetes.

Neurological System

Aging-related changes involve both central and peripheral nervous system. Visual, auditory, motor, and sensory system changes are important as they cause changes in quality of life and limitation of function. However, changes in cognitive function with normal aging are minimal (Shock et al., 1984). Changes in the eyes include small irregular pupils with a diminished reaction to light and near reflexes, and reduced ocular range of motion on convergence and upward gaze. Motor changes include the presence of tremors, short-stepped and/ or broad-based gait with diminished associated movement, dysmetria, dysdiadochokinesia, and prolonged reaction time. Sensory changes are manifested by diminished vibratory sense in the feet and hands in addition to reduced proprioception and increased threshold for light touch, pain, and temperature. Muscle stretch reflexes are often either reduced or absent with impaired righting reflexes.

Musculoskeletal Changes

As people age, there is a 40% decline in lean muscle mass from age 30 to 80. Testosterone and growth hormone decline result in a shift of balance between muscle protein synthesis and breakdown. As a result, muscle strength and bone density decrease. OA develops as a result of disordered equilibrium between breakdown and repair of joint tissues.

PATIENT ASSESSMENT

A comprehensive assessment consists of the chief complaint, history of present illness, medical history, and review of systems, allergies, psychosocial assessment (including an evaluation for substance abuse), disability history, and physical examination. History taking is a critical component of patient assessment. A careful and comprehensive evaluation of the older adults is imperative to both identifying the clinical problems and subsequently determining the appropriate rehabilitation plan. Because of various age-related sensory limitations (such as vision, hearing), obtaining a history can be challenging in the older population. Interview sessions should be individualized based on patient's ability; however, information from other sources (physician, family members, or home aide) may be needed. It is important to include an evaluation for the presence of depression since the incidence of depression is 10–15% in community-dwelling elderly and even higher in institutionalized population. The geriatric depression screen is helpful in identifying underlying depression (Brink et al., 1982). Medications should be routinely reviewed since "polypharmacy" in the elderly can be associated with adverse side effects and drug–drug interactions.

There are older adults living with various disabilities acquired throughout their lives such as amputation of a lower extremity, stroke, brain injury, and multiple sclerosis. In assessing them, clinicians should also perform a disability history with emphasis on the following elements: (a) disability-related symptoms such as impaired communication and swallowing, insomnia, pain, falls and near falls, bowel/bladder dysfunction, and spasticity; (b) disability-associated psychosocial issues such as anxiety, depression, aging caregivers, financial difficulties, and gaps in home health care and ability to manage their finances; (c) assessment of mobility aids such as prostheses, orthotics, and wheelchairs and presence of adaptive equipment in the home such as grab bars, raised toilet seat, and tub bench (Cristian, 2006).

Physical Examination

A thorough physical examination should include patient's vital signs, and assessment of essentially all systems previously mentioned in age-related changes section.

Neurological evaluation should include examination of cognition, cranial nerves, sensation, proprioception, motor strength, reflexes, tone, balance, and gait. The mini-mental status examination is useful and an easily administered screening tool at the bedside (Folstein, Folstein, & McHugh, 1975). A score of ≥24 out of 30 is considered normal in population aged >65 years. Score <24 is associated with delirium, dementia, or severe depression.

Musculoskeletal examination should focus on presence of deformities, range of motion limitations, muscle strength, contractures, and tender areas in the spine and extremities.

Functional Assessment

As part of a comprehensive assessment, it is important for clinicians to evaluate and treat the older adult's ability to participate in daily functional activities, such as self-care, mobility, and community activities. Deficit areas are identified and appropriate treatment goals and plans are made to improve the functional level of independence.

Examples of functional activities that should be evaluated in older adults are as follows: (1) mobility; (2) ADL; and (3) IADL, such as the ability to use the telephone, manage money, take medications, shop, and prepare meals and leisure activities. The level of dependence or independence can be quantified using a validated instrument such as the Functional Independence Measure (FIM) scale (Table 17.1) (Center for Functional Assessment Research, 1993). The FIM instrument assesses the following areas: (1) self-care (grooming, bathing, dressing, feeding, and toileting); (2) sphincter control (bowel and bladder management); (3) mobility and transfer (bed–chair–wheelchair–toilet–tub–shower); (4) locomotion (walk/wheelchair, stairs); (5) communication (comprehension, expression); and (6) social cognition (social integration, memory, and problem solving).

Basic ADLs can also be assessed by the Katz Index and IADLs by the Lawton Scale (Katz, Downs, Cash, & Grotz, 1970; Lawton & Brody, 1969).

TABLE 17.1   FIM Instrument Scoring

Level of Function	Score	Definition
Independence	7	Complete independence (timely, safely)
	6	Modified independence (device used)
Modified independence	5	Supervision
	4	Minimal assistance (subject performs >75% of tasks)
	3	Moderate assistance (subject performs 50–74% of tasks)
	2	Maximal assistance (subject performs 25–49% of tasks)
Complete dependence	1	Total assistance (subject performs <25% of tasks)

Source: Copyright © 1993 Uniform Data System for Medical Rehabilitation, a division of UB Foundation Activities, Inc. Reprinted with permission.

GENERAL PRINCIPLES OF GERIATRIC REHABILITATION

Rehabilitation professionals are commonly asked to evaluate and participate in the treatment of older adults with a variety of diagnoses as outlined in Table 17.2.

The main goals of geriatric rehabilitation are to maximize function and to minimize disability thereby returning the individual to the highest level of independence that is attainable. This is often accomplished via a multidisciplinary team of rehabilitation professionals that typically includes a physiatrist, psychologist, physical therapist, occupational therapist, speech pathologist, rehabilitation nurse, social worker, and recreational therapist.

Once impairments and limitations are identified, goals are set by the team members and a treatment plan is initiated and reviewed at appropriate time intervals. The rehabilitation of the older adult can occur in a variety of settings such as acute inpatient rehabilitation units, subacute facilities, outpatient, and home-based rehabilitation programs.

Evidence to support the role of rehabilitation medicine in the care of older adults has been reviewed by Cruise, Sasson, and Lee (2006). Higher therapy intensity was associated with better outcomes as they relate to length of stay and functional improvement for patients who have stroke, orthopedic conditions, and cardiovascular and pulmonary conditions and are receiving rehabilitation in a skilled nursing facility setting (Jette, Warren, & Wirtalla, 2005). Older adults with hip fractures receiving rehabilitation in inpatient rehabilitation facilities do better functionally compared with skilled nursing facilities (Munin, Seligman, & Dew, 2005). Subacute rehabilitation facilities are better at returning stroke patients to the community as

TABLE 17.2   Diagnoses Commonly Encountered in the Rehabilitation of Older Adults

1	Osteoarthritis
2	Coronary artery disease
3	Congestive heart failure
4	Chronic obstructive pulmonary disease
5	Diabetes mellitus
6	Osteoporosis
7	Fractures
8	Joint replacement
9	Stroke

compared with nonrehabilitation nursing homes (Kramer, 1997). Whereas acute rehabilitation is more expensive than subacute rehabilitation, it has shown greater functional gains with the same discharge disposition (Keith, Wilson, & Gutierrez, 1995). Even home-based programs have been shown to improve functionality among physically frail older adults living at home (Gill et al., 2002). Therefore, a fiscally responsible individualized rehabilitation program tailored to the need of the patient is pertinent to recovery.

Underlying diseases such as hypertension, diabetes, coronary artery diseases (CADs), osteoporosis, congestive heart failure, chronic renal failure, chronic obstructive pulmonary disease, depression, and cancer are common in older adults and need to be adequately treated so that the geriatric patient can safely undergo a rehabilitation program.

Exercise in the Elderly

The benefits of exercise in preventing illness and injury, and limiting functional loss and disability in elderly were reviewed by Frankel, Bean, and Frontera (2006). There are four basic components to the exercise prescription: (1) progressive resistance training (PRT); (2) endurance training; (3) balance training; and (4) flexibility training. An exercise program has been shown to improve daily function, reduce disability, reduce blood pressure, improve lipid profiles, lower cardiac mortality, reduce stroke-associated weakness, reduce pain and improve function in OA and rheumatoid arthritis, and reduce risk of fall (Frankel et al., 2006).

Whereas there are many benefits to exercise in the elderly, clinicians should be aware that exercise can pose dangers as well. Contraindications to exercise in the older adult include (a) acute medical illness, (b) unstable angina (a condition in which the heart does not get enough blood flow and oxygen, a prelude to a heart attack), (c) end-stage congestive heart failure, (d) severe cardiac valve disease, (e) unstable arrhythmia, (f) systolic blood pressure at baseline of 200 mmHg or greater and/or diastolic blood pressure of 110 mmHg or greater, (g) large or expanding aneurysm, (h) cerebral aneurysm, (i) acute retinal hemorrhage or recent eye surgery, (j) severe behavioral disturbance, or (k) severe dementia. It is prudent to obtain appropriate medical clearance for these conditions prior to the start of a rehabilitation program.

Once an older patient has been medically cleared to participate in exercise, appropriate precautions in high-risk patients are recommended. Examples include the following: (a) monitoring vital signs (pulse, heart rate, and oxygen saturation) before, during, and immediately after exercise; (b) heart rate at 60–70% of maximal heart rate (ideally determined via cardiac stress test); (c) moderate level of intensity on Borg scale of the rate of perceived exertion (RPE). RPE ranges from 6 to 20, where 6 means "no exertion at all" and 20 means "maximal exertion." A rating of 11–13 on the Borg scale suggests that physical activity is being performed at a moderate level of intensity. The rating is a subjective measure based on the physical sensations a person experiences during physical activity, including increased heart rate, increased respiration or breathing rate, increased sweating, and muscle fatigue; (d) use of supplemental oxygen in patients that require it; (e) monitoring for fatigue and providing judicious rest periods; and (f) control pain prior to exercise. Treating therapists should also be made aware if a patient is at risk for fracture, falls, seizure, or hypoglycemia. They should also be informed of any weight-bearing precautions or restrictions to range of motion.

Progressive Resistance Training

PRT consists of moving the major joints repeatedly through the full range of motion several times weekly, with or without some form of resistance. A typical program is performed two to three times per week and ranges in intensity from low in deconditioned patients to moderately high intensity in more active older adults. Key muscle groups in the lower extremities such as the hip flexors, hip extensors, knee extensors, ankle dorsiflexors, ankle plantar flexors, and the triceps in the upper extremities should be emphasized. It is also important to add task-specific exercises that mimic real-life scenarios and improve functionality. Liu and Latham (2009) reviewed 121 trials with 6,700 participants to evaluate progressive resistance strength training for improving physical function in older adults. Overall, this review suggests that PRT has a small but significant effect on improving physical function (complex activities), a small to moderate effect on decreasing some impairments and functional limitations, and a large effect on increasing strength. In addition, there is some preliminary evidence, which suggests that PRT might reduce pain in older people with OA.

Endurance Training

Endurance is the ability to maintain a given level of exercise over time or to perform a given task repeatedly without fatigue that prevents further such activity. Endurance training program is usually performed for 30 minutes five times per week at 60–70% of maximal age-predicted heart rate (calculated from the formula: $208 - 0.7 \times age$) (Tanaka, Monahan, & Seals, 2001) or based on cardiac stress test results in high-risk patients. Examples of endurance training include treadmill and stationary cycling; however, it is important to take into account patient's preferences as well (i.e., square dancing) to encourage continued participation. The benefits of an endurance training program include (1) reduced resting blood pressure, (2) improved lipid profiles, (3) improved insulin sensitivity, and (4) improved functionality. It is recommended that patients with underlying cardiac problems be medically cleared to participate in an exercise program.

Balance Training

A balance training program can be beneficial as part of a fall prevention program and some examples include tai chi, high-velocity ankle exercises, and weighted vest exercises (Li, Harmer, Fisher, & McAuley, 2004; Richardson, Sandman, & Vela, 2001; Shaw & Snow, 1998; Tsang & Hui-Chan, 2005; Wolf, Coogler, & Xu, 1997). The goals are to progressively challenge the base of support as tolerated. Ideally, exercises should be performed on most days of the week.

Flexibility Program

Decreased flexibility is common in the elderly and can lead to contractures around joints. It is important to stretch the major joints of the upper and lower extremities daily. Typical program consists of four to five repetitions each held for 30 seconds apiece.

Exercise in Older Adults With Disabilities

Older adults aging with physical disabilities such as spinal cord injury, brain injury, multiple sclerosis and lower limb amputations face significant challenges (Li et al., 2004; Rimmer, 2005). This is due to a combination of several factors: (a) the impairments caused by their underlying disability; (b) normal aging-related changes; and (c) existing comorbidities such as CAD, obesity, OA, and diabetes. As a result, activities that were easier to accomplish at a younger age (i.e., transfers, wheelchair propulsion, and ambulation with a prosthesis) are now more difficult. There appears to be a vicious cycle of disability, physical inactivity, development of secondary conditions, and functional loss leading to further disability.

Exercise can help reverse some of these conditions and also help with the performance of ADLs with less effort. However, there are certain key principles that should be considered when prescribing exercise in this population: (1) clinicians should use precautions to ensure that the exercises do not increase the risk of injury (i.e., osteoporotic fractures in osteopenic bones, pressure ulcers over bony prominences, and skin breakdown in residual limb); (2) caution should be used when prescribing exercise in people with progressive diseases such as amyotrophic lateral sclerosis and progressive multiple sclerosis, because they may not tolerate exercise as well; (3) patience and consistency should be used in adults with cognitive impairments; (4) adults with neurogenic bowel and bladder should void prior to the exercise session; and (5) wheelchair users should use gloves, padded push rims, and leg-securing devices to avoid repetitive stress injuries.

ASSISTIVE AND ORTHOTIC DEVICES

The aging process can often make performing ADLs difficult for older adults. It may become difficult for the patient to reach items from the floor due to decreased range of motion of the upper extremities or impaired balance. Extending the reach with lengthened devices can increase the level of independence for ADLs. Weakness of the lower extremities or impaired standing balance may also impact the patient's ability to safely transfer on or off surfaces of low to average height from the floor. Showering and bathing are tasks that require considerable energy, and provision of shower chairs and other bathtub devices can make this task less taxing for the patient. Table 17.3 lists commonly used adaptive and assistive devices, which may be beneficial to the geriatric population.

Commonly used orthotics such as neck collars, elbow splints, wrist splints, lumbosacral corsets, knee braces, and ankle foot orthoses can be of help in supporting, protecting, and assisting weakened limbs and painful joints.

Wheelchairs

Accessibility within the home and the outside environment is a major concern for the elderly who can often become homebound or even bed bound. Provision of an appropriate mobility device can ensure that the geriatric population has access to medical services and is able to maintain health and quality of life.

There are many different types of wheelchairs prescribed for older adults with physical disabilities. It is important for clinicians to perform a thorough evaluation of the patient's

TABLE 17.3 *Assistive Devices*

Adaptive/Assistive Device	Use/Purpose Device
Long reacher	Extend reach to self-care items, reduce bending
Long shoe horn	Extend reach to remove shoes
Long dressing stick	Extend reach to don/doff garments
Long handled sponge/brush	Extend reach to wash body
Sock aide	Extend reach to don socks
Button hook and zipper pull	Hook to assist with buttoning and zipping
Elastic shoe laces	Eliminate the need for lace tying
Raised toilet seat with armrests	Reduce effort required for transfer on/off seat
Shower chair	Reduce effort required by sitting for showers
Tub transfer bench	Eliminate need for stepping over tub for transfers
Hand-held shower	Allows easy showering while sitting
Wall grab bars	Sturdy support structure to hold when transferring
Built-up handles on grooming and feeding tools	Improve grip when grasp is limited and weak

underlying medical condition, physical condition, mobility needs, and lifestyle in order to identify the appropriate seating and mobility devices that will meet the older person's needs.

In review of the medical history, clinicians should check for the presence of cardiopulmonary disease, neurological disorders such as multiple sclerosis, stroke, progressive neuromuscular disease, and history of lower extremity amputation. This will alert the team of special seating and mobility needs that are usually required for that population, such as amputee supports and axles, hemi-height wheelchairs, and advanced electronics for progressive disorders.

The physical condition of the elderly is also assessed to help in the determination of the most appropriate device. The elderly patient needs to have intact cognition to learn the functionality of the device, as well as good vision and hearing so that the mobility device will be operated with good safety judgment to protect self and others within the environment. Upper and lower extremity strength and range of motion is important to determine whether the elderly person will be able to reach and operate the switches and controls of the device, as well as tolerate sitting in the chair for prolonged periods. Features of the device may need to be adjusted to accommodate for the presence of deformities and contractures of the hips, knees, and ankles, such as the seat back angle, position of the front rigging and foot plate, and type of cushion. This will help to prevent further development of contractures and deformities, pain in the back and extremities, prevention of pressure ulcers, and maintenance of skin integrity. Assessing trunk control and level of transfers help to determine which device would be suitable for the elderly to reduce the risk of falls. Special switches and controls or seating accessories may be required to address increased tone/spasticity in the upper and lower extremities and impaired hand dexterity. Knowledge of the older person's lifestyle will help the clinician provide a device that will allow the older person to function within his or her environment. Social history will be obtained from the elderly patient and/or caregiver about the social support systems (lives alone or with family/friend, home health aide); current living accommodations (private home with stairs, wheelchair-accessible building); method of transportation (car, taxi, bus/train, and ambulette) and which device will be used; ability to perform self-care tasks and IADLs. A home evaluation is often helpful to assess for wheelchair-accessibility barriers for entering and moving about the home, the presence of clutter, bulky furniture, narrow doorways and hallways, poor lighting, and safe and sheltered location to store, and charge the device if needed.

Once a decision has been made that a wheelchair is indicated, it is helpful to refer the patient to a wheelchair clinic, which is staffed by therapists and physiatrists with experience in prescribing wheelchairs. During the assessment, a recommendation is made by the team and discussed with the elderly patient based on the aforementioned evaluation. Upon agreement, the patient is fitted for the recommended device, which may be a manual or motorized wheelchair, powered scooter, specialized cushion, and/or wheelchair accessories.

There are three basic types of mobility devices commonly used in older adults: (a) manual wheelchairs; (b) motorized scooters; and (c) motorized wheelchairs.

Manual Wheelchairs
Primarily issued for patients whose ambulation is compromised by limb or joint issues of the upper and lower extremities and/or poor trunk control and other postural issues. Manual wheelchairs additionally can be equipped with a tilt-in-space option to allow adjustment of the seat position while maintaining a fixed seat angle. This could be beneficial in patients at high risk for pressure ulcers and difficulty in performing pressure relief techniques as it changes pressure over specific areas while reducing shear forces as the chair is tilted.

Motorized Scooter
Recommended for patients with compromised endurance secondary to cardiopulmonary conditions or significant OA in the lower extremities that limits their ability to ambulate for long distances. Patients need to have intact cognition to operate the scooter safely and have good trunk control since they need to be able to transfer on/off the scooter independently.

Motorized Wheelchair

Recommended for patients who have either lost a limb or have significant spasticity or poor trunk control that requires significant support from the wheelchair.

SELECTED TOPICS

Falls and Fractures

Among adults older than 65 years, falls are the leading cause of accidental death (National Center for Injury Prevention and Control, 2003) and the seventh leading cause of death from complications of fractures, such as deep venous thrombosis, pulmonary embolism, fat embolism, disseminated intravascular coagulation, and pressure sores, which may be complicated by septicemia. In a recent report from Centers for Disease Control and Prevention, 1.6 million seniors were treated in emergency departments for fall-related injuries and 353,000 were hospitalized. Death rates from falls rise exponentially with increasing age for both sexes and in all racial groups. Incidence of falls is greater in nursing home residents (67%) than healthy community-dwelling elders (33%) aged >65 years. Seventy percent of emergency department visits in elderly population are due to falls. Until age 75, falls occur more frequently in women; however, the frequency is the same for both genders thereafter (Beers et al., 2000).

Falls threaten the independence of elderly people and produce a cascade of individual and socioeconomic consequences. It is essential to assess and identify risk factors during either routine physical examination or after acute injury in addition to initiating appropriate interventions to decrease the risk of future falls and fall-related injuries.

In elderly people, most falls occur indoors and during usual activities such as walking. Indoor falls are common in the bathroom, bedroom, stairs, and kitchen. Ten percent of falls occur on stairs, with the first and last steps being the most dangerous (Morley & Colberg, 2007). Descending down stairs is more perilous than ascending up stairs. Curbs and steps are common sites of falls outdoors. In institutional settings, the most common sites of falls are the bedside (during transfers into or out of bed) and the bathroom. Falls can cause fractures, soft-tissue injury, and can be associated with secondary complications such as dehydration, pressure ulcers, deep vein thrombosis, pneumonia, and rhabdomyolysis. In elderly population, 10–20% of falls result in soft-tissue injuries and 3–5% result in a fracture.

Presence of osteoporosis makes elderly people more vulnerable to fracture with the most common sites of fractures being the humerus, wrist, pelvis, and hip. The quality of life and individual's functionality can deteriorate after a fall. Fallophobia, also commonly known as the fear of falling, can lead to an avoidance of ambulation and performance of key ADLs, which can lead to social isolation. Hip fracture is the most serious injury resulting from falls in the elderly with greatest likelihood of morbidity and mortality. More than 250,000 hip fractures occur each year in the United States in people older than 65 with 5% of hip fractures resulting in death during hospitalization. Fifty percent of the elderly who were able to walk before a hip fracture cannot do so after the fracture, and 50% are unable to live independently after the hip fracture. Mortality consequent to hip fractures ranges from 12% to 67% year after the injury. The risk of hip fractures due to falls doubles with use of certain antipsychotic and long-acting benzodiazepine drugs, which are listed in Table 17.4.

The cause of falls in the elderly is usually due to a combination of factors, which can be either intrinsic or extrinsic (Steinweg, 1997). These factors are outlined in Table 17.5. It is prudent to consider these factors when evaluating a patient with a history of falls or near falls.

Elderly people often do not report falls and should therefore be asked open-ended questions about the most recent falls or near falls. As part of their physical examination, the "get-up-and-go" and the "timed up and go (TUG)" tests can be very useful (Mathias, Nayak, & Isaacs, 1986; Podsiadlo & Richardson, 1991). The TUG test provides a measure of motor skills essential for independent living. The test consists of measuring the time it takes a person to stand from a standard armchair, walk 3 meters, turn 180°, walk back to the chair, and sit

TABLE 17.4 *Drugs Contributing to Risk of Fall*

Mechanism	Drugs
Reduce alertness or retard central processing	Opioids Psychoactive drugs (antidepressants, long-acting benzodiazepines and phenothiazines)
Impair cerebral perfusion	Vasodilator (antihypertensive) Antiarrhythmics Diuretics
Contribute to direct vestibular toxicity	Aminoglycosides High-dose loop diuretics
Induce extrapyramidal syndromes	Phenothiazines

down. More than 16 seconds performing this task predicts an increased risk of falling in community-dwelling older adults.

A recent review found the following interventions likely to be beneficial in preventing falls in elderly people: (a) muscle strengthening; (b) balance training; (c) home hazard modification (Table 17.6) (Lin & Lane, 2005; Tideiksaar, 1989, 1996); (d) withdrawal of psychotropic medications; and (e) 15-week tai chi program (Gillespie et al., 2003). Vitamin D supplementation has been shown to reduce osteoporosis and improve neuromuscular function leading to a decrease in the number of falls, and therefore, a decline in the number of fractures (Chapuy

TABLE 17.5 *Etiological Factors Contributing to Falls in Elderly Population*

Intrinsic factors	Changes in postural control
	  Decreased proprioception
	  Slower righting reflexes
	  Decreased muscle tone and strength
	  Increased postural sway

	Changes in gait
	  Lower foot swing height
	  Slower gait

	Declining visual abilities
	  Depth perception
	  Clarity
	  Dark adaptation
	  Color sensitivity
	  Declining visual fields
	  Visuospatial function
	  Increased sensitivity to glare

Extrinsic factors	Poor lighting in commonly traveled areas of home Slick or irregular floor surfaces Furnishings that are too low or too high Unsafe stairways Bathroom fixtures that are too low or too high or that do not have arm support Loose rugs
Situational factors	Walking in stocking feet or in footwear with high heels Rushing to the bathroom (especially at night when not fully awake or when lighting may be inadequate) Rushing to answer the telephone

TABLE 17.6 *Home Assessment*

Kitchen safety: Gas stove should be checked for leaks. Floor area by sink should be kept dry. Use nonskid floor mat. Commonly used dishes and utensils should be kept at arm's length so that the older adult does not have to climb on step stools. Use hand-held reacher.

Bathroom safety: Grab bars in appropriate places, raised toilet seat, nonslip surfaces for shower or bath tub; hand-held shower hose and head.

Stairs: Should be well lit; if there is carpeting on stairs it should be securely fastened; dark, patterned carpeting should be removed. Consider reflective tape on noncarpeted steps.

Heating and air conditioning: Systems should be checked regularly and properly maintained.

Hot water heater: The controls should be accessible and easy to read.

Emergency actions and evacuation route: Emergency numbers should be on or near the telephone. There should be a means of exit in case of emergency.

Electrical cords: Frayed cords or cords lying across hallways or walking paths should be replaced.

Lighting and night lights: Commonly traveled areas should be well lit (i.e., route from the bedroom to the bathroom).

Fire and smoke detectors and fire extinguishers: Fire extinguishers should be present and accessible. Fire and smoke detectors should be present. Batteries for fire alarms should be changed regularly.

Loose carpets and throw rugs: Loose carpets and throw rugs should be secured or removed.

Tables, chairs, and other furniture: Furniture should be sturdy and well balanced. Tables and chairs with legs sticking out or wobbly legs should be removed.

et al., 1992; Staud, 2005). Other interventions that can be useful include gait training with an appropriate assistive device, pain management, and corrective glasses for patients with visual impairments, evaluation of wheelchairs, prostheses and orthotics for proper fit and function, and consideration for the use of hip protectors.

Educating a patient about what to do after a fall is equally important to prevent subsequent injury. Some recommended techniques include (a) turning from the supine to prone position, (b) crawling to a strong support surface, (c) use of an emergency response system, and (d) consider having a telephone on the floor (American Geriatrics Society, 2010; Eillespie et al., 2003).

Pain Assessment and Management in Older Adults

Pain is very common in older adults and is often multifactorial. The most common origins of pain in the elderly are from degenerative conditions of the musculoskeletal system and neuropathic pain, although other sources include fractures, ischemia, and cancer. Pain is common in both the community and nursing home settings. It can affect quality of life, performance of ADL, and be associated with depression and anxiety (Cristian, Thomas, Nisenbaum, & Jeu L, 2005).

Assessment of pain in the elderly can be challenging for a variety of reasons such as difficulties arising from communication disorders and cognitive impairment. In addition, there may be fears about need for invasive tests to diagnose the sources of the pain as well as the treatments themselves. As a result, older adults may not report pain. Nevertheless, it is important for clinicians to enquire about the characteristics of pain (i.e., location, quality, intensity, radiation, frequency, duration, pattern, alleviating, and aggravating factors), impact of pain on functionality, previous diagnostic tests, as well as treatments and their outcomes. The assessment of pain should include a thorough neuromusculoskeletal examination, as well as a focused cognitive evaluation. It is important also to evaluate wheelchairs, orthotics, and prosthesis whenever indicated for proper fit and use.

Pain management can be very challenging in the older adult due to factors such as reduced kidney and liver function and reduced GI peristalsis that alter drug metabolism and absorption. Adverse effects from polypharmacy are a real concern, and therefore, a careful review of current medications and possible drug–drug interactions with analgesics is advised. Clinicians can consider other methods to reduce pain such as topical agents, modalities such as heat, ice, exercise for weakness, bracing of painful body parts, and injections whenever indicated, thus decreasing the chances of undesired drug effects.

In prescribing medications for pain, it is advised to choose drugs with the fewest side effects, abide by the adage "start low and go slow," treat as many symptoms with same agent, anticipate side effects (i.e., opioid-induced constipation), and use renal and liver dosing whenever indicated.

Aging With a Disability

Adults with physical disabilities sustained earlier in life such as spinal cord injuries, multiple sclerosis, and polio are living longer lives due to advances in medical, nursing, and rehabilitative care. However, because they are living longer, they face new challenges in aging with their disabilities that can impact on their well-being and independence.

Some of these challenges include (a) accelerated aging of key organs and systems due to the cumulative stresses placed on them from years of daily activities such as wheelchair propulsion (e.g., shoulder elbow and wrist injuries) and living with neurogenic bowel and bladder, (b) narrower margin of good health due to decreased functional organ reserve and chronic infections such as urinary tract infections and pneumonia, (c) increased risk of comorbidities such as obesity, CAD, and diabetes associated with a sedentary lifestyle, (d) fatigue, (e) depression, (f) substance abuse, (g) osteoporosis and related fractures, and (h) pain from degenerative conditions of the musculoskeletal system and neuropathies.

These changes can lead to a functional decline so that activities that were easier to perform at an earlier age are now more difficult to perform (e.g., transfers, wheelchair propulsion, pressure relief techniques, and bladder catheterizations). Functional decline can lead to an increased need for assistance from home health aides at a time when finances and resources for transportation may be diminishing. The increased needs can also take a toll on aging caregivers who may find it difficult to provide the additional care required.

The challenges to health care providers is in maintaining an optimal level of good health and the maximal level of independence achievable to adults aging with disabilities. This is best accomplished by proactively anticipating problems associated with aging in this population and using a combination of medical, nursing, and rehabilitative interventions to address them (Bartels & Omura, 2005; Capoor & Stein, 2005; Stern, 2005).

Traumatic Brain Injury in the Elderly

Although traumatic brain injury (TBI) is very common in young adults, there is a second peak in incidence that occurs in adults older than 65 years (Flanagan, Hibbard, Riordan, & Gordon, 2006). Falls are a major cause of TBI in the elderly and subdural hematomas (SDH) are common in this population. An SDH can occur from even seemingly trivial injuries because of shearing of bridging veins in the atrophied brain. It has been reported that it can be difficult for clinicians to differentiate between cognitive impairment due to brain injury or dementia. One distinction has been that older adults with TBI can learn and retain, whereas those with dementia do not. TBI may occur from occupational injury, motor vehicle accident, sports injury, gunshot wound, or other act of violence, including military combat. In a recent review of the literature, the Institute of Medicine concluded that there was sufficient evidence of a causal relationship between TBI and neurological (seizures and dementia) and psychiatric disorders (depression and PTSD) in addition to psychosocial problems (aggressive behaviors and unemployment) (Institute of Medicine, 2008).

Older adults with TBI can make gains in their rehabilitation, but it often requires a longer period of time. They may also be less able to take care of themselves than their younger counterparts. They are also at increased risk of depression and suicidal ideation, which clinicians should be aware of and intervene as needed.

Pharmacological interventions in the elderly with TBI require careful consideration regarding compliance, polypharmacy, and undesired effects. Many medications are centrally acting and may result in worsening of preexisting TBI-related problems such as impairments in balance and cognition. It has also been suggested that some individuals with TBI are more sensitive to medications, indicating again that clinicians should "start low and go slow."

The Older Amputee

The age-related incidence of lower limb amputation in persons older than 80 years has increased, although most patients who experience a lower limb amputation are between 51 and 69 years old. More than 1.5 million people in the United States live with some form of major limb amputation and there are approximately 50,000 new cases annually.

Lower limb amputation is eight times more common than upper limb amputation. Peripheral vascular disease (PVD) and diabetes are common causes of lower limb amputations in older adults. Additional comorbidities such as CAD, end-stage renal disease (ESRD), and multiple revascularization attempts prior to the lower limb amputation can make the older amputee frailer and deconditioned, even before he or she learns to use a prosthesis. Older amputees are also at risk for contralateral limb amputation and their 5-year survival rate has been estimated to be between 35% and 40% (Frieden, 2005).

There are three common types of lower limb amputations: (a) partial foot, (b) transtibial (also commonly referred to as below knee amputation), and (c) transfemoral (above knee amputation).

The assessment of the older amputee should focus on the individual's previous level of function and level of independence and management of existing comorbidities such as CAD, PVD, and ESRD. It is also important to ask about recent weight gain or weight loss since these can have an impact on prosthetic fit. Pain is also a common complaint in older amputees. Some common examples include residual limb pain from poor prosthetic fit, phantom pain, ischemia, and musculoskeletal sources arising in the spine and lower extremity joints. Clinicians should also enquire about the presence of depression.

The physical examination should assess cognition, vision, upper and lower limb range of motion of major joints, muscle strength, and an evaluation of the cardiopulmonary system. The examination of the residual limb should include inspection for evidence of skin breakdown, palpation of tender areas, measurement of range of motion, and testing of muscle strength. The contralateral limb should also be assessed for evidence of skin breakdown. Functional evaluation should include transfers and hopping with an appropriate assistive device with and without prosthesis. The prosthesis should also be evaluated for evidence of wear and tear and poor alignment.

Treatment

The treatment of the amputee should ideally begin before the amputation surgery itself. An amputee care team consisting of a physiatrist, physical therapist, occupational therapist, psychologist, and prosthetist should prepare the patient preoperatively through psychological counseling, upper and lower body strengthening, mobility training, and treatment of underlying pain. Treatment begins with appropriate goal setting keeping in mind that older amputees have different expectations and deconditioned older amputees may need a slower and less intense program emphasizing reconditioning and functional restoration. It is interesting to note that older amputees exhibit less depression and fewer psychological symptoms when compared with younger amputees (Frank, 1984). Cardiopulmonary precautions should be adhered to whenever indicated and cardiac clearance is advised in cardiac patients. A typical rehabilitation program consists of: (1) upper and lower body strengthening (targeting key muscle groups such as the triceps, hip flexors and extensors, and knee extensors); (2) gait, balance, and endurance training; (3) ADL training with appropriate adaptive devices; (4) fall prevention; and (5) pain management. Residual limb care and appropriate techniques to minimize risk of further limb loss should also be a part of the treatment plan. Choice of prosthetic components should be a balance between patient's preference for his/her lifestyle, level of function, and safety.

The Older Adult With Parkinson's Disease

Parkinson's disease (PD) is a chronic degenerative movement disorder characterized by abnormal involuntary movements (dyskinesia), alteration in muscle tone, and disturbances in body posture. It is a frequent cause of motor disability in people older than 60 years. Common clinical presentations of this syndrome include tremor, muscle rigidity, akinesia, gait disturbance, and loss of postural reflexes. Elderly patients with PD commonly present with gait dysfunction and akinesia, whereas young patients often present with tremor-predominant disease.

Clinical manifestations of PD are believed to be caused by the loss of dopaminergic cells in the pars compacta of the substantia nigra and the subsequent loss of nigrostriatal dopaminergic modulation of the neural mechanism for movement control (Obeso, Rodriguez, & DeLong, 1997). Although the exact cause of PD is unknown, many researchers believe that a combination of several factors such as free radicals, accelerated aging, environmental toxins, and genetic predisposition are involved in the development of PD.

The rehabilitation program of an older adult with PD typically consists of the following: (1) flexibility and strength training of the lower and upper extremities; (2) gait training with an appropriate assistive device; (3) posture training; (4) balance training; (5) evaluation and training in the use of adaptive devices for ADL; (6) home hazard evaluation to minimize the risk of falling; (7) swallowing and communication evaluation and treatment; and (8) evaluation and treatment of neurogenic bowel and bladder.

Patient Safety in Geriatric Rehabilitation

Older adults undergoing rehabilitation are often at high risk for medical errors due to the following reasons: (1) reduced kidney and liver function increases their risk for medication-related side effects and drug interactions; (2) multiple comorbidities; and (3) impaired cognition and communication (Cristian, 2009).

There are four basic types of medical errors: (1) failure to diagnose; (2) failure to provide adequate treatment; (3) failure to prevent a problem before it starts; and (4) poor communication between providers—especially at points of transition in medical care such as transfers from an acute medical service to a rehab unit.

To minimize the risk of medical errors and maximize patient safety, some general recommendations include:

I. *MEDICATIONS:* The right medication should be ordered at the right time, using the right dose with the right unit of measurement. Medication orders should be checked for legibility, accuracy, appropriate abbreviations, and appropriate placement of decimal points. Appropriate dosing should also take into account kidney and liver impairment. Clinicians should also be wary of "sound-alike" and "look-alike" medications.

2. *COMMUNICATION:* Communication between providers is especially important at transition points in care, and all efforts should be made to minimize distractions during this critical period. Providers should ensure that complete medical records are available and that there is appropriate communication between providers about the patient's care

3. *HAND WASHING:* Older adults are susceptible to infections, and a simple and very effective method of reducing this risk by health care providers is to wash their hands. Hands should be washed for a period of 15 seconds with antibacterial soap between patients and before and after gloves are applied.

CONCLUSION

As the number of older adults continues to increase, rehabilitation will continue to have a significant role in their overall health and improvement of the quality of their lives. The goals of geriatric rehabilitation are to maximize function and minimize disability in an often frailer population with multiple comorbidities. An interdisciplinary team approach that uses the principles described in this chapter provides an important cornerstone of a geriatric rehabilitation program.

REFERENCES

American Geriatrics Society. (2010). *Guideline for the prevention of falls.* Retrieved from www.american geriatrics.org

Bartels, M. N., & Omura, A. (2005). Aging in polio. *Physical Medicine and Rehabilitation Clinics of North America, 16,* 197–218.

Beers, M. H, Jones, T. V., Berkwits, M., Kaplan, J. L., Porter, R., et al. (Eds.). (2000). Falls. In *Merck Manual of Geriatrics* (3rd ed.). Whitehouse Station, NJ: Merck Research Laboratories. http://www.merck.com/pubs/mm_geriatrics/sec2/ch20.htm.

Brink, T. L., Yesavage, J. A., Lum, O., Heersema, P., Adey, M. B., & Rose, T. L. (1982). Screening tests for geriatric depression. *Clinical Gerontologist, 1,* 37–44.

Capoor, J., & Stein, A. B. (2005). Aging with spinal cord injury. *Physical Medicine and Rehabilitation Clinics of North America, 16,* 129–161.

Center for Functional Assessment Research. (1993). *Guide for the Uniform Data Set for Medical Rehabilitation (Adult FIM). Version 4.0.* Buffalo, NY: State University of New York at Buffalo.

Chapuy, M. C., Arlot, M. E., Duboeuf, F., Brun, J., Crouzet, B., Arnaud, S., et al. (1992). Vitamin D and calcium to prevent hip fractures in elderly women. *New England Journal of Medicine, 327,* 1637–1642.

Conwell, L. J., & Cohen, J. W. *Characteristics of people with high medical expenses in the U.S. civilian non-institutionalized population, 2002. Statistical Brief #73. March 2005.* Agency for Healthcare Research and Quality, Rockville, MD. Retrieved April 7, 2006 from http://www.meps.ahrq.gov/mepsweb/data_files/publications/st73/stat73.pdf

Cristian, A. (2006). The Assessment of the older adult with a physical disability: A guide for clinicians. *Clinics in Geriatric Medicine, 22,* 221–238.

Cristian, A. (2009). Patient safety in medical management of adults with neurologic disabilities. New York: Demos.

Cristian, A., Thomas, J., Nisenbaum, M., & Jeu, L. (2005). Practical considerations in the assessment and treatment of pain in adults with physical disabilities. *Physical Medicine and Rehabilitation Clinics of North America, 16,* 57–90.

Cruise, C. M., Sasson, N., & Lee, M. H. M. (2006). Rehabilitation Outcomes in the Older Adults. *Clinics in Geriatric Medicine, 22,* 257–267.

Flanagan, S. R., Hibbard, M. R., Riordan, B., & Gordon, W. A. (2006). Traumatic brain injury in the elderly: Diagnostic and treatment challenges. *Clinics in Geriatric Medicine, 22,* 449–468.

Folstein, M. F., Folstein, S. E., & McHugh, P. R. (1975). Mini-mental state. A practical method for grading the cognitive state of patients for the clinician. *Journal of psychiatric research, 12,* 189–198.

Frank, R. G., Kashani, J. H., Kashani, S. R., Wonderlich, S. A., Umlauf, R. L., & Ashkanazi, G. S. (1984). Psychological response to amputation as a function of age and time since amputation. *British Journal of Psychiatry, 144,* 493–497.

Frankel, J. E., Bean, J. F., & Frontera, W. R. (2006). Exercise in the Elderly: Research and Clinical Practice. *Clinics in Geriatric Medicine, 22,* 239–256.

Frieden, R. (2005). The geriatric amputee. *Physical Medicine and Rehabilitation Clinics of North America, 16,* 179–196.

Gill, T. M., Baker, D. I., Gottschalk, M., Peduzzi, P. N., Allore, H., & Byers, A. (2002). A program to prevent functional decline in physically frail elderly persons living at home. *New England Journal of Medicine, 347,* 1068–1074.

Gillespie, L. D., Gillespie, W. J., Robertson, M. C., Lamb, S. E., Cumming, R. J., & Rowe, B. H. (2003). Interventions for preventing falls in elderly people. *Cochrane Database Systematic Review* (4):CDOOO340.

Hing, E., Sekscenski, E., & Strahan, G. (1989). The national nursing home survey: 1985 summary for the United States. *Vital and Health Statistics series 13, 97,* 1–249.

Institute of Medicine. (2008, December). *Gulf War and Health,* Vol. 7: Long-term consequences of traumatic brain injury. Washington, DC: Author.

Jette, D. U., Warren, R. L., & Wirtalla, C. (2005). The relation between therapy intensity and outcomes of rehabilitation in skilled nursing facilities. *Archives of Physical Medicine and Rehabilitation, 86,* 373–379.

Katz, S., Downs, T. D., Cash, H. R., & Grotz, R. C. (1970). Progress in the development of the index of ADL. *Gerontologist, 1,* 20–30.

Keehan, S. P., Lazenby, H. C., Zezza, M. A., & Catlin, A. C. (2004). Age Estimates in the National Health Accounts. *Health Care Financing Review, 1.*

Keith, R. A., Wilson, D. B., & Gutierrez, P. (1995). Acute and subacute rehabilitation for stroke: A comparison. *Archives of Physical Medicine and Rehabilitation, 76,* 495–500.

Kramer, A. M., Steiner, J. F., Schlenker, R. E., Eilertsen, T. B., Hrincevich, C. A., Tropea, D. A., et al. (1997). Outcomes and costs after hip fracture and stroke: A comparison of rehabilitation settings. *Journal of the American Medical Association, 227,* 396–404.

Lawton, M. P., & Brody, E. M. (1969). Assessment of older people: Self-monitoring and instrumental activities of daily living. *Gerontologist, 9,* 179–186.

Li, F., Harmer, P., Fisher, K. J., & McAuley, E. (2004). Tai Chi: Improving functional balance and predicting subsequent falls in older persons. *Medicine and Science in Sports and Exercise, 36,* 2046–2052.

Lin, J., & Lane, J. M. (2005). Falls in the elderly population. *Physical Medicine and Rehabilitation Clinics of North America, 16,* 109–128.

Liu, C. J., & Latham, N. K. (2009). Progressive resistance strength training for improving physical function in older adults. *Cochrane Database of Systematic Reviews,* Issue 3. Art. No.: CD002759.

Manton, K. G., & Gu, X. (2001). Changes in the prevalence of chronic disability in the United States black and nonblack population above age 65 from 1982 to 1999. *Proceedings of National Academy of Sciences, 98,* 6354–6359.

Mathias, S., Nayak, U. S., & Isaacs, B. (1986). Balance in elderly patients: The "get up and go test." *Archives of Physical Medicine and Rehabilitation, 67,* 387–389.

Morley, J. E., & Colberg, S. R. (Eds.). (2007). *The science of staying young: 10 simple steps to slow the aging process.* Dubuque, IA: McGraw-Hill.

Munin, M.C., Seligman, K., & Dew, M. A. (2005). Effect of rehabilitation site on functional recovery after hip fracture. *Archives of Physical Medicine and Rehabilitation, 86,* 367–372.

National Center for Injury Prevention and Control, 2003, http://www.cdc.gov/ncipc/factsheets/falls.htm

Obeso, J. A., Rodriguez, M. C., & DeLong, M. R. (1997). Basal ganglia pathophysiology. A critical review. *Advances in Neurology, 74,* 3–18.

Podsiadlo, D., & Richardson, S. (1991). The timed "up and go": A test of basic functional mobility for frail elderly persons. *Journal of the American Geriatrics Society, 39,* 142–148.

Richardson, J. K., Sandman, D., & Vela, S. (2001). A focused exercise regimen improves clinical measures of balance in patients with peripheral neuropathy. *Archives of Physical Medicine and Rehabilitation, 82,* 205–209.

Rimmer, J. H. (2005). Exercise and physical activity in persons aging with a physical disability. *Physical Medicine and Rehabilitation Clinics of North America, 16,* 41–55.

Shaw, J. M., & Snow, C. M. (1998). Weighted vest exercise improves indices of fall risk in older women. *The Journals of Gerontology. Series A, Biological Sciences and Medical Sciences, 53,* M53–M58.

Shock, N. W., Greulich, R. C., Costa, P. T., Andres, R., Lakatta, E. G., Arenberg, D., et al. (1984). *Normal Human Aging: The Baltimore Longitudinal Study of Aging.* U.S. Department of Health and Human Services., Bethesda, MD: NIH.

Stanton, M. W. The high concentration of U.S. health care expenditures. (2005). *Research in Action, Issue 19.*

Staud, R. (2005). Vitamin D: More than just affecting calcium and bone. *Current Rheumatology Reports, 7,* 356–364.

Steinweg, K. (1997). The changing approach to falls in the elderly. *American Family Physician, 56,* 1815–1822.

Stern, M. (2005). Aging with multiple sclerosis. *Physical Medicine and Rehabilitation Clinics of North America, 16,* 219–234.

Tanaka, H., Monahan, K. D., & Seals, D. R. (2001). Age-predicted maximal heart rate revisited. *Journal of the American College of Cardiology, 37,* 153–156.

Tideiksaar, R. (1989). Home safe home: Practical tips for fall-proofing. *Geriatric Nursing, 10,* 280–284.

Tideiksaar, R. (1996). Preventing falls: How to identify risk factors, reduce complications. *Geriatrics, 51,* 43–50,53.

Tsang, W. W. N., & Hui-Chan, C. W. Y. (2005). Comparison of muscle torque, balance, and confidence in older Tai Chi and healthy adults. *Medicine and Science in Sports and Exercise, 37,* 280–289.

U.S. Census Bureau, 2006.

Wolf, S. L., Coogler, C., & Xu, T. (1997). Exploring the basis for Tai Chi Chuan as a therapeutic exercise approach. *Archives of Physical Medicine and Rehabilitation, 78,* 886–892.

World Health Organization. (2010). Retrieved from www.who.int/topics/disabilities/en/

18

Introduction to Peripheral Vascular Disorders

Glenn R. Jacobowitz, MD

Peripheral vascular disease (PVD) encompasses not only diseases of arteries and veins but also multiple underlying medical conditions such as coronary artery disease, diabetes, and renal insufficiency that are associated with, and are often the cause of, the vascular pathology. Such a broad range of diseases involves the entire body, literally from the head to toe. The brain, abdominal viscera, lungs, and upper and lower extremities are all end organs affected by vascular disease. It is not uncommon for one patient to manifest different aspects of vascular disease. There are various functional presentations that must be recognized. After treatment of PVD, patients are often left with disabilities that require extensive rehabilitation, both physical and psychological. Ambulation and activities of daily living must often be relearned after either revascularization or amputation of an extremity. Cerebrovascular disease may lead to central cognitive and/or motor deficits. A wide range of services may be required for these patients, including physical therapy, occupational therapy, and psychosocial support. In addition, rehabilitation physicians and staff must be aware of the chronic nature of PVD. In the rehabilitation phase of recovery, these patients may have recurrence of their disease (e.g., leg ischemia and transient ischemic attack), which must be recognized and expeditiously treated. Therefore, it is critical for the rehabilitation physician and other rehabilitation providers to have an understanding of the functional presentation and treatment of PVD.

The broad scope of PVD may be separated into several areas. A practical organization should include (1) lower extremity peripheral arterial occlusive disease, (2) cerebrovascular disease, (3) venous disease, and (4) peripheral and abdominal arterial aneurysmal disease. All these entities are associated with specific medical presentations, indications for operation, treatment modalities, recovery regimens, and disabilities that warrant separate attention and will therefore be reviewed individually.

FUNCTIONAL PRESENTATION

Lower Extremity Peripheral Arterial Occlusive Disease

There are several disease processes, associated disorders, and degrees of disability related to lower extremity PVD. The most common is atherosclerotic occlusive disease. Patients with chronic lower extremity ischemia have been divided into two groups. The first group includes patients with intermittent claudication who are considered to have a good prognosis, benign course, and low rate of amputation or need for surgical intervention. In contrast, the second group includes patients with limb-threatening ischemia. These patients have been believed to have a poor prognosis with almost certain amputation if no intervention is performed. The definition of limb-threatening ischemia is rest pain or the presence of gangrene in the extremity.

In the past, the presence of limb-threatening ischemia was the primary indication for surgical intervention and appropriate angiographic studies. However, because the diagnostic and interventional armamentarium has expanded in recent years, previous indications for intervention and imaging have been re-evaluated. The advent of balloon angioplasty, intra-arterial stenting, thrombolytic agents, and endovascular prostheses has revolutionized the treatment of PVD. Imaging techniques, including both conventional angiography and magnetic resonance angiography (MRA), have significantly improved. Now, there are many treatment options for vascular disease, including noninvasive modalities that may carry less risk for the debilitated patient. Physicians caring for patients with vascular disease should be aware of these options and the indications for their use.

The term claudication is derived from the Latin verb "to limp" or "to be lame." Claudication occurs when there is inability to mount an appropriate augmentation of blood supply in response to exercise. It consists of three essential features: the pain is in a functional muscle unit; it is reproducibly precipitated by a consistent amount of exercise; and it is promptly relieved by cessation of exercise. At least 10% of the population above the age of 70 and 1–2% of younger patients have intermittent claudication (Peabody, Kannel, & McNamara, 1974). However, the majority of these patients can be treated nonoperatively. A thorough understanding of the natural history of lower extremity ischemia and the available treatment options form the basis of sound clinical decision making.

The most important studies on the natural history of intermittent claudication have focused not only on patient history but also on objective evidence of arterial obstruction by arteriography or noninvasive means such as ankle-brachial blood pressure indices. Some of these studies document up to 80% of such patients remaining stable or improving over 2.5–6 years (Imparato, Kim, Davidson, & Crowley, 1975; Jonason & Ringquiest, 1985). Other studies have shown only 40–60% of claudication improvement over time (Cronenwett et al., 1984; Rosenbloom et al., 1988). Risk factors for worsening ischemia include cigarette smoking and diabetes. The single worst prognostic factor is the severity of arterial occlusive disease at the time of initial presentation (Cronenwett et al., 1984; Imparato et al., 1975; Jonason & Ringquiest, 1985; Rosenbloom et al., 1988).

Limb-threatening ischemia occurs when resting blood flow is unable to meet baseline metabolic demands because of arterial occlusion. Clinically, this presents as rest pain (typically in the most distal portion of the extremity such as the forefoot or toes), ulceration, or gangrene. The pain is typically exacerbated by elevation of the extremity and alleviated by placing the leg in a dependent position from which arterial pressure is increased by gravity. Ischemic ulceration may occur when minor traumatic lesions fail to heal because of inadequate blood flow. Gangrene occurs when arterial blood flow is so poor that areas with the least perfusion undergo spontaneous necrosis (Figure 18.1).

The assumption that rest pain or tissue loss results in uniform limb loss is not entirely valid, as shown by several studies using nonoperative therapy (Rivers, Veith, Ascer, & Gupta, 1986; Schuler et al., 1984). Chronic ischemia represents a spectrum of levels of disease from fairly benign, mild intermittent claudication to the gangrenous extremity. The likelihood of limb loss remains related to the severity of ischemia at initial presentation, as measured both angiographically (injecting contrast dye into the artery and visualizing the areas of blockage) and through arterial Doppler signals (noninvasive measurements of blood pressure at the ankle). Absent Doppler signals carry a poor prognosis for the limb in question if no intervention is performed (Felix, Siegel, & Gunther, 1987).

The success of exercise and cessation of smoking make this nonoperative therapy the first treatment option in patients with intermittent claudication. An additional reason is the

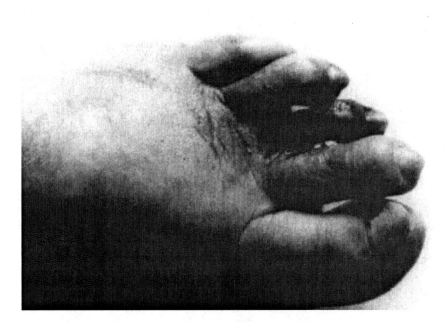

FIGURE 18.1
Gangrene of the left third toe resulting from ischemia.

observation (although controversial) that a failed bypass graft may acutely induce limb-threatening ischemia or ultimately obligate a higher level of amputation than a nonoperated limb (Dardik, Kahn, Dardik, Sussman, & Ibrahim, 1982; Schlenker & Wolkoff, 1975). Operative management is thus reserved for threatened limb loss as determined by clinical and angiographic parameters.

The less invasive modalities of percutaneous angioplasty and stent placement have significantly broadened the scope of treatable conditions, particularly for debilitated patients. Limb-threatening ischemia can often be treated with these measures, frequently with the patient under local anesthesia, which minimizes risk. Advancements in catheter and stent technology have allowed vascular specialists to treat lesions in the popliteal and tibial arteries, as well as more proximal lesions in the iliac and femoral vessels. These included smaller-diameter balloons and stents as well as wires and devices that can effectively cross long areas of chronic occlusion in vessels. Several studies have shown that amputation-free survival in patients with critical limb ischemia is similar in patients treated with balloon angioplasty compared with those treated with open bypass (Adam et al., 2005; Romiti, et al., 2008).

Extracranial Cerebrovascular Disease

Cerebrovascular disease may include disease of the aortic arch, carotid arteries, or the vertebrobasilar system. Although individuals with cerebrovascular disease may be asymptomatic, functional presentations may include a transient ischemic attack (e.g., amaurosis fugax or other neurological deficit resolving within 24 hours) or a completed stroke. Depending on the degree of disability, patients may require varying degrees of rehabilitation and support services. It is extremely important to evaluate the extracranial circulation in patients presenting for rehabilitation after strokes so that further strokes may be prevented, when possible, by surgical or medical intervention.

The diagnosis and treatment of extracranial cerebrovascular disease begin at the aortic valve. The decrease in annual stroke rate in the United States has paralleled the increase in the frequency of carotid endarterectomy (Lamparello & Riles, 1975). Currently, more than 100,000 carotid endarterectomies are performed annually in this country. During the past 40 years, the safety of carotid surgery has improved, with most large centers reporting perioperative morbidity and mortality rates of less than 2%. Indications for extracranial cerebral revascularization have been well defined for both symptomatic and asymptomatic patients in large prospective, randomized trials. The North American Symptomatic Carotid Endarterectomy Trial established that symptomatic patients with more than 70% diameter reduction of the internal carotid artery have a significant reduction in the incidence of stroke with surgery when compared with medical management alone (North American Symptomatic Carotid Endarterectomy Trial Collaborators, 1991). Similarly, the Asymptomatic Carotid Atherosclerosis Study demonstrated better stroke prevention in patients with more than 60% stenosis treated with endarterectomy versus those treated medically (The Executive Committee for the Asymptomatic Carotid Atherosclerosis Study, 1995). As noted above, these patients may present after completed strokes, with a history of a transient ischemic attack, or they may be asymptomatic, with carotid stenoses detected on duplex examinations performed as part of a workup for a bruit heard on physical examination or for nonspecific neurological symptoms.

Upper extremity ischemia is also often related to aortic arch disease. Emboli (blood clots that travel from one part of the body to another) to the hands or fingers may originate in the chambers of the heart, aortic arch, or axillary and subclavian arteries. Transesophageal echocardiography and aortic arch and upper extremity angiography are the tests of choice for identifying a potential source of emboli. MRA may also be useful. Functional presentation is similar to that in the lower extremity with sudden onset of pain and cyanosis of the distal hand or fingers. Pulses may be absent. Collateral circulation of the upper extremity is usually excellent, often allowing the hand to remain viable during workup.

In the last decade, significant advancements have been made in the technology and efficacy of carotid artery stenting. This is a less invasive procedure that can be performed under local anesthesia by means of a femoral arterial puncture. Long-term results are still not available, but there seems to be a benefit from carotid stenting, particularly for high-risk surgical patients (Yadav, 2002). This includes patients with significant medical comorbidities, anatomically inaccessible lesions, and radiation-induced carotid stenosis (Veith et al., 2001). It is not uncommon for patients undergoing rehabilitation to have significant medical comorbidities, and the risks and benefits of carotid stenting versus carotid endarterectomy should be considered. Early results of carotid stenting had higher rates of periprocedural strokes, but this complication has been significantly reduced with the advent of balloon- and umbrella-type cerebral protection devices that are temporarily deployed during the procedure to prevent distal embolization of plaque material. More recent trials have shown results that are more disparate, with some showing that carotid artery stenting is not superior or even equivalent to carotid endarterectomy (Mas et al., 2006; SPACE Collaborative Group, 2006).

Venous Disease

Patients with venous disorders frequently exhibit a chronic course and are not often markedly improved by surgical procedures. Chronic venous insufficiency (CVI) is the most common form of venous disease, and nonoperative therapy remains the mainstay of treatment. The other form of venous disease seen commonly, especially in the nonambulatory patient, is acute deep venous thrombosis. This is more sudden in onset and requires systemic anticoagulation or, occasionally, placement of a vena-caval filter, and more rarely, mechanical or pharmacological thrombolysis with catheter-directed therapy. These two forms of venous disease will be discussed separately.

CVI: Anatomy, Etiology, Function, and Treatments

The venous anatomy consists of a superficial and a deep system. In the lower extremity, the longest superficial vein, the great saphenous vein, is located anterior to the medial malleolus and courses along the medial aspect of the leg until it reaches the saphenofemoral junction in the medial aspect of the proximal thigh. The short saphenous vein is located in the posterior calf and most commonly drains into the popliteal vein. Connecting the superficial system to the deep system are the perforating veins. The functional presentation of CVI includes swelling, pain, and ulceration of the lower extremity. This is due to valvular incompetence of the venous system, resulting in increased hydrostatic pressure. Typically, CVI presents as swelling of the distal lower extremity with thickening of the subcutaneous tissue in the perimalleolar "gaiter" distribution. Mild CVI is associated with mild-to-moderate ankle edema. Often, the patients complain of a feeling of heaviness or pain in the legs. This mild form of insufficiency is usually limited to the superficial veins. Moderate CVI has hyperpigmentation of the skin caused by hemosiderin deposition in the subcutaneous tissue, moderate nonpitting edema, and subcutaneous fibrosis without ulceration. Severe CVI is associated with ulceration, eczematoid skin changes (stasis dermatitis), and severe edema. Extensive involvement of the deep venous system and diffuse loss of valvular function are present. These different stages of venous disease are now well described in a uniform classification system called the CEAP classifications, which includes clinical, etiological, anatomical, and pathophysiological descriptions (Eklof et al., 2004). The clinical classifications are listed in Table 18.1, and examples are shown in Figures 18.2a and 18.2b.

Bed rest and limb elevation have universally been accepted as effective therapy for CVI. However, they are impractical for most patients, particularly those in a rehabilitation program promoting ambulation. Effective therapy must control the symptoms of CVI, promote healing, and prevent recurrence of venous stasis ulcers while allowing for normal ambulation.

Several studies have shown the benefits of compression stockings in the treatment of CVI and venous ulceration (Dinn & Henry, 1992; Mayberry, Moneta, & Taylor, 1991). Cellulitis may be associated with CVI and often requires oral or intravenous antibiotic therapy. Hydrocortisone cream may help surround stasis dermatitis. Typical compression stockings have 30–40 Torr of elastic compression at the level of the ankle, which gradually decreases more proximally. This type of stocking may be used with normal arterial circulation. If arterial circulation is compromised, a stocking with less compression must be used to permit adequate circulation. In addition, ACE bandages may be used. There are multiple brands of compression stockings in the market, with different designs to make application possible for the patient with disability.

Acute Deep Venous Thrombosis

Acute deep venous thrombosis may occur in the upper or, more commonly, the lower extremity. In the upper extremity, thrombus may occur in the axillosubclavian vein, and the most common causes are thoracic outlet syndrome and catheter-related thrombosis. Under most circumstances, one or more of the features of Virchow's triad for venous thrombosis is present. The triad includes endothelial injury (as by a catheter), stasis (as by thoracic outlet obstruction), or a hypercoagulable state (as with some malignancies).

Functional presentation of upper extremity deep venous thrombosis includes swelling of the extremity, usually to the level of the axilla, and prominence of the subcutaneous veins

TABLE 18.1   *CEAP Clinical Classification*

Class 0	No venous disease
Class 1	Telangiectasias of reticular veins
Class 2	Varicose veins
Class 3	Edema
Class 4	Skin changes
Class 5	Healed ulcer
Class 6	Open ulcer

a
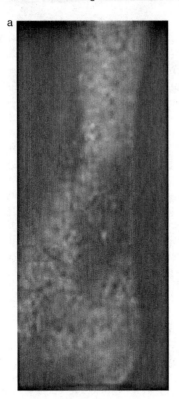

b
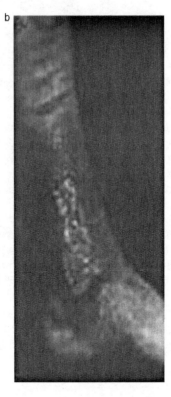

FIGURE 18.2   (a) CEAP Class 5 (healed ulcer) and (b) CEAP Class 6 (open ulcer).

over the shoulder girdle and the anterior chest wall, which become engorged with collateral venous flow due to obstruction of the deep vein (Figure 18.3). Pain of an aching or stabbing type may include the shoulder and axilla but can also be felt in the arm. These classic symptoms are particularly common in patients who thrombose acutely because of thoracic

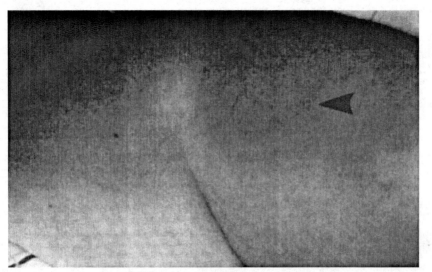

FIGURE 18.3 Swollen proximal left upper arm in patient with axillosubclavian thrombosis. Arrow shows engorged subcutaneous veins over anterior shoulder.

outlet compression. This can occur after weightlifting or similar exertional activity with the upper extremity. Axillosubclavian vein thrombosis may also present after sleeping, probably because of sleeping with the arm overhead (with the thoracic outlet partially obstructed).

Initial diagnosis of axillosubclavian vein thrombosis is by venous duplex examination. If this is negative and there is a high clinical index of suspicion, then a venogram should be performed. Similarly, if the duplex is positive and thrombolytic therapy is being considered, venography is indicated. The reported incidence of pulmonary embolism with untreated upper extremity deep venous thrombosis is about 9–12% (Becker, Philbrick, & Walker, 1991). Patients should be treated with heparin anticoagulation followed by a 3–6-month course of warfarin. Persistent symptoms are least likely in patients with catheter-related thrombosis. Chronic symptoms (arm swelling with exercise) occur in about 38% of patients treated with anticoagulation and 15% receiving thrombolytic therapy (intra-arterial urokinase infusion) compared with 64% receiving no therapy (Becker et al., 1991). When axillosubclavian vein thrombosis is recognized, a vascular surgeon should be consulted to further direct therapy. Unless contraindicated, anticoagulation should be started promptly to prevent further propagation of thrombus. If thrombolysis is performed, currently available techniques include mechanical thrombectomy catheters and tissue plasminogen activator infusion.

The signs and symptoms of lower extremity deep venous thrombosis are similar to those of upper extremity deep venous thrombosis. They include swelling of the limb, prominence of superficial veins, and pain that is usually dull in character. Unfortunately, physical examination is often falsely negative in patients with acute deep venous thrombosis and falsely positive in patients with symptoms related to conditions other than deep venous thrombosis (Goodacre, Sutton, & Sampson, 2005).

The acute complication of deep venous thrombosis is pulmonary embolism, and the late complication is the post-thrombotic syndrome. This syndrome is that of chronic swelling and venous insufficiency due to valvular damage that occurs from the thrombus. Anticoagulation will reduce the risk for pulmonary embolus from approximately 25%, if left untreated, to less than 5% (Hyers, Hull, & Weg, 1992). In patients with a contraindication to anticoagulation, a vena-caval filter may be placed (usually percutaneously) that prevents the embolus from reaching the pulmonary vessels. These devices will lower the incidence of pulmonary embolus to 2–4%.

Abdominal Aortic and Peripheral Arterial Aneurysmal Disease

Abdominal aortic aneurysm (AAA) is defined as a focal dilation of the aorta of at least 50% greater than the expected normal diameter (Johnston et al., 1991) (Figure 18.4). The main complication of AAA is rupture, for which the mortality may exceed 90%. The 5-year risk of rupture for AAA 5 cm or greater in diameter ranges from 25% to 40%. This may be as high as 20% per year for aneurysms more than 7 cm in diameter. Aneurysms measuring between 4 and 5 cm in diameter have lower 5-year rupture rates of about 3–12% (Brown, Pattenden, & Gutelius, 1992). Aneurysms less than 4 cm in diameter have a rupture rate of about 2%. Overall elective surgical mortality is about 2–4% (Ernst, 1993). Therefore, repair of AAA is reserved for asymptomatic aneurysms more than 5 cm in diameter, symptomatic aneurysms (abdominal or back pain), or a ruptured AAA. Rarely, laminated thrombus from the inner lining of an aneurysm sac may embolize to the lower extremities. This is also an indication for repair regardless of aneurysm diameter. Standard surgical repair is by replacement of the aneurysmal segment with a synthetic graft, usually Dacron. Recent technological advances have included the successful use of transfemorally placed vascular endografts that exclude the aneurysmal segment from arterial pressure. This method of endovascular repair has been shown to be effective in preventing AAA rupture with reduced patient morbidity and mortality (Arko et al., 2002; Zarins et al., 1999). Debilitated patients who were at prohibitive risk for standard surgical repair are now often considered for the less invasive endovascular repair. Hospital stay is often as short

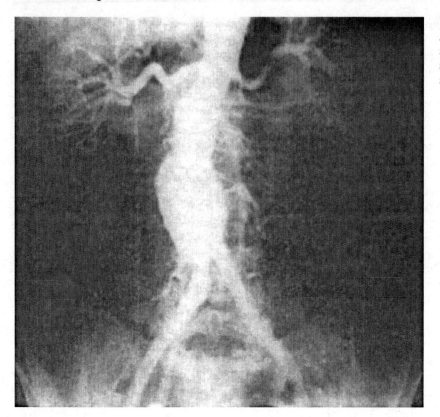

FIGURE 18.4
Angiogram of an infrarenal abdominal aortic aneurysm.

as 2 days, and patients can resume oral intake within 1 day. Long-term complications include endoleaks that occur when the endovascular graft does not completely seal off the aneurysm sac. These endoleaks can often be treated with additional endovascular maneuvers, but they require continued follow-up imaging with computed tomography (CT) or duplex scanning.

AAA usually presents as a finding on routine physical examination (pulsatile abdominal mass) or as an incidental finding on a radiological study (abdominal ultrasound, CT scan, or magnetic resonance image) obtained for other reasons. Any aneurysm more than 3 cm in diameter should be brought to the attention of an internist or vascular surgeon who can follow-up the patient with yearly ultrasound examination to monitor the aneurysm size. Average annual growth of AAA is about 0.4 cm in diameter per year.

Popliteal artery aneurysms (PAA) are the most common peripheral artery aneurysm. There is a strong association of PAA with AAA. A patient with a unilateral PAA has a 50% chance of having a contralateral PAA and a 30% chance of having an AAA. More than 90% of PAAs occur in men (Szilagyi, Schwartz, & Reddy, 1981).

A popliteal artery is considered aneurysmal if its diameter exceeds 2 cm or 1.5 times the diameter of the proximal, nonaneurysmal segment. The clinical presentation is variable. Almost 30% of PAAs are symptomatic. They are usually found on physical examination (pulsatile mass or wide pulse at the popliteal fossa) or incidentally on ultrasound, CT scan, or magnetic resonance imaging of the popliteal fossa. Results of surgical management in this group of patients are excellent. Although ruptures are rare, symptomatic PAAs usually present with distal embolization to the tibial arteries. This embolization is often severe, with lower-limb ischemia occurring in up to 70% of patients and amputation rates as high as 20% (Reilly, Abbott, & Darling, 1983). Elective repair of all PAAs is recommended because of the high rate of limb loss once these aneurysms become symptomatic. Recent advances in available devices and techniques have also made endovascular repair of PAAs possible with good short-term results (Tielliu et al., 2005).

PSYCHOLOGICAL AND VOCATIONAL IMPLICATIONS

PVD can leave patients with severe vocational impairment and psychological stress. Partial or complete amputation of a limb, and the ramifications of strokes, can be tremendously disabling, both physically and psychologically.

Two thirds of all lower extremity amputations are currently performed as a result of complications of PVD or diabetes. As a result, a majority of lower extremity amputations are performed by vascular surgeons. The purpose of amputation is to remove gangrenous tissue, relieve pain, obtain primary healing of the most distal amputation possible, and obtain maximum rehabilitation after amputation.

It has been shown that the greatest chance of successful ambulation is with expeditious rehabilitation, either by immediate postoperative prosthesis or by accelerated conventional programs using temporary prosthesis until a permanent prosthesis can be made (Folsum, King, & Rubin, 1992). Advantages of early ambulation include decreased hospital time, increased rates of rehabilitation, a reduction in the complications of amputation, and an improvement in the psychological outcome of the patient after amputation (Bradway, Racy, & Malone, 1984). Early ambulation alleviates a sense of loss and inadequacy experienced by many amputees.

It is clear that a full rehabilitation team provides the best outcome. This should include the rehabilitation physician, prosthetist, patient's family, physical and occupational therapists, social services, and community services.

PVD is present in many patients who have had strokes, and it is the common underlying cause of those strokes. Fortunately, the perioperative stroke rate for carotid endarterectomy in most major centers is less than 3%. However, many patients present with a completed stroke before carotid endarterectomy, and the operation serves only to prevent further infarction. As a result, many patients with PVD, and in particular those with extracranial cerebrovascular disease, may require rehabilitation for stroke.

Major factors affecting rehabilitation of stroke victims include motivation and family support (Evans & Northwood, 1983). In addition, depression may be a significant complication of stroke that can inhibit patient motivation (Parikh, Lipsey, & Robinson, 1987). Anxiety and fear are also common among stroke victims, which can be eased by an empathetic rehabilitation team. The recovery of physical function and motor skills is often enhanced by emotional stability of the patient. In turn, the return of function enhances psychosocial functioning. Thus, psychosocial, recreational, and vocational interventions must all be provided. Peer support may also be extremely helpful. All of these services should be provided in the setting of a directed stroke rehabilitation program, which has been shown to enhance functional ability beyond that of natural recovery (Kalra, 1994).

Age alone probably does not play a major role in determining the recovery of a patient with stroke. However, it may be associated with significant medical comorbidities (such as PVD), which may make recovery more difficult. Consequently, older patients may have longer recovery times and require increased psychosocial support.

CONCLUSION

Patients with PVD usually have multiple medical problems, and the nature of their disease may be chronic and involve multiple organ systems. The high incidence of limb surgery, limb loss, and stroke make patients with PVD in particular need of rehabilitation medicine and services. The chronic nature of PVD requires the rehabilitation team to be keenly aware of its functional presentation because recurrences or progression of disease are not uncommon. In addition, advances in minimally invasive endovascular techniques have increased treatment options for debilitated patients who are not candidates for conventional open surgical interventions. It is only with a full range of physical and psychological rehabilitation services are that patients with PVD may be completely treated.

REFERENCES

Adam, D. J., Beard, J, D., & Cleveland, T., Bell, J., Bradbury, A. W., Forbes, J. F., et al. BASIL trial participants. (2005). Bypass versus angioplasty in severe ischemia of the leg (BASIL): Multicentre, randomized controlled trial. *Lancet, 366,* 1925–1934.

Arko, F. W., Lee, W. A., Hil, B. B., Olcott, C., Dalman, D. L., Harris, E. J., et al. (2002). Aneurysm-related death: Endpoint analysis for comparison of open and endovascular repairs. *Journal of Vascular Surgery, 36,* 297–304.

Becker, D. M., Philbrick, J. T., & Walker, F. B. (1991). Axillary and subclavian venous thrombosis: Prognosis and treatment. *Archives of Internal Medicine, 151,* 1934–1943.

Bradway, J. P., Racy, J., & Malone, J. M. (1984). Psychological adaptation to amputation. *Orthotics and Prosthetics, 38,* 46–50.

Brown, P. M., Pattenden, R., & Gutelius, J. R. (1992). The selective management of small abdominal aortic aneurysms: The Kingston study. *Journal of Vascular Surgery, 15,* 21–27.

Cronenwett, J. L., Warner, K. G., Zelenock, G. B., Whitehouse, W. M., Graham, L. M., Lindenhauser, S. M., et al. (1984). Intermittent claudication: Current results of non-operative management. *Archives of Surgery, 119,* 430–436.

Dardik, H., Kahn, M., Dardik, I., Sussman, B., & Ibrahim, I. (1982). Influence of failed bypass procedures on conversion of below-knee to above-knee amputation levels. *Surgery, 91,* 64–69.

Dinn, E., & Henry, M. (1992). Treatment of venous ulceration by injection sclerotherapy and compression hosiery. *Phlebology, 7,* 23–26.

Eklof, B., Rutherford, R. B., Bergan, J. J., Carpentier, P. H., Gloviczki, P., Kistner, R. L., et al. (2004). American Venous Forum International Ad Hoc Committee for Revision of the CEAP Classification. Revision of the CEAP classification for chronic venous disorders: Consensus statement. *Journal of Vascular Surgery, 40,* 1248–1252.

Ernst, C. B. (1993). Abdominal aortic aneurysm. *New England Journal of Medicine, 328,* 1167–1173.

Evans, R. L., & Northwood, L. (1983). Social support needs in adjustment to stroke. *Archives of Physical Medicine and Rehabilitation, 64,* 61–64.

Felix, W. R. Jr., Siegel, B., & Gunther, N. L. (1987). The significance for morbidity and mortality of Doppler absent pedal pulses. *Journal of Vascular Surgery, 5,* 849–855.

Folsum, D., King, T., & Rubin, J. (1992). Lower extremity amputation with immediate postoperative prosthetic placement. *American Journal of Surgery, 164,* 320–323.

Goodacre, S., Sutton, A. J., & Sampson, F. C. (2005). Meta-analysis: The value of clinical assessment in the diagnosis of deep venous thrombosis. *Annals of Internal Medicine, 143,* 129–139.

Hyers, T. M., Hull, R. D., & Weg, J. G. (1992). Antithrombotic therapy for venous thromboembolic disease. *Chest, 102*(suppl.), 408–425.

Imparato, A. M., Kim, G. E., Davidson, T., & Crowley, J. G. (1975). Intermittent claudication: Its natural course. *Surgery, 78,* 795–799.

Johnston, K. W., Rutherford, R. B., & Tilson, M. D. (1991). Suggested standards for reporting on arterial aneurysms. *Journal of Vascular Surgery, 13,* 452–458.

Jonason, T., & Ringquiest, I. (1985). Factors of prognostic importance for subsequent rest pain in patients with intermittent claudication. *Acta Medica Scandinavica, 218,* 27–33.

Kalra, L. (1994). The influence of stroke unit rehabilitation on functional recovery from stroke. *Stroke, 25,* 821–825.

Lamparello, P. J., & Riles, T. S. (1975). MR angiography in carotid stenosis: A clinical perspective. *MRI Clinics of North America, 3,* 455–465.

Mas, J. L., Chatellier, G., Beyssen, B., Branchereau, A., Moulin, T., Becquemin, J-P., et al. (2006). Endarterectomy versus stenting in patients with symptomatic severe carotid stenosis. *New England Journal of Medicine, 355,* 1660–1671.

Mayberry, J. C., Moneta, G. L., & Taylor, L. M. (1991). Fifteen-year results of ambulation compression therapy for chronic venous ulcers. *Surgery, 109,* 573–581.

North American Symptomatic Carotid Endarterectomy Trial Collaborators. (1991). Beneficial effect of carotid endarterectomy in symptomatic patients with high-grade stenosis. *New England Journal of Medicine, 325,* 445–453.

Parikh, R. M., Lipsey, J. R., & Robinson, R. G. (1987) Two-year longitudinal study of post-stroke mood disorders: Dynamic changes in correlates of depression at one and two years. *Stroke, 18,* 579–584.

Peabody, C. N., Kannel, W. B., & McNamara, P. M. (1974). Intermittent claudication—Surgical experience. *Archives of Surgery, 109,* 693–697.

Reilly, M. K., Abbott, W. M., & Darling, R. C. (1983). Aggressive surgical management of popliteal artery aneurysms. *American Journal of Surgery, 145,* 498–502.

Rivers, S. P., Veith, F. J., Ascer, E., & Gupta, S. K. (1986). Successful conservative therapy of severe limb threatening ischemia: The value of nonsympathectomy. *Surgery, 99,* 759–762.

Romiti, M., Albers, M., Brochado-Neto, F. C., Durazzo, A. E., Pereira, C. A., De Luccia, N. (2008). Meta-analysis of infrapopliteal angioplasty for chronic critical limb ischemia. *Journal of Vascular Surgery, 47,* 975–981.

Rosenbloom, M. S., Flanigan, D. P., Schuler, J. J., Meyer, J. P., Durham, J. P., Edrup-Jorgensen, J., et al. (1988). Risk factors affecting the natural history of claudication. *Archives of Surgery, 123,* 867–870.

Schlenker, J. D., & Wolkoff, J. S. (1975). Major amputation after femoropopliteal bypass procedures. *American Journal of Surgery, 129,* 495–499.

Schuler, J. J., Flanigan, D. P., Holcroft, J. W., Ursprung, J. J., Mohrland, J. S. A., & Pyke, J. (1984). Efficacy of prostaglandin E1 in the treatment of lower extremity ischemic ulcers secondary to peripheral vascular occlusive disease: Results of a prospective randomized double-blind multicenter clinical trial. *Journal of Vascular Surgery, 1,* 160–170.

SPACE Collaborative Group, Ringleb, P. A., Allenberg, J., Bruckmann, H., et al. (2006). 30-day results from the SPACE trial of stent-protected angioplasty versus carotid endarterectomy in symptomatic patients: A randomised non-inferiority trial. *Lancet, 368,* 1239–1247.

Szilagyi, D. E., Schwartz, R. I., & Reddy, D. L. (1981). Popliteal arterial aneurysms. *Archives of Surgery, 116,* 724–728.

The Executive Committee for the Asymptomatic Carotid Atherosclerosis Study. (1995). Endarterectomy for asymptomatic carotid artery stenosis. *Journal of the American Medical Association, 273,* 1421–1428.

Tielliu, I. F., Verhoeven, E. L., Zeebregts, C. J., Prins, T. R., Span, M. M., & van den Dungen, J. J. (2005). Endovascular treatment of popliteal artery aneurysms: Results of a prospective cohort study. *Journal of Vascular Surgery, 41,* 561–567.

Veith, F. J., Amor, M., Ohki, T., Beebe, H. G., Bell, P. R., Bolia, A., et al. (2001). Current status of carotid bifurcation angioplasty and stenting based on a consensus of opinion leaders. *Journal of Vascular Surgery, 33*(Suppl. 2), S111–S116.

Yadav, J., for the SAPPHIRE Investigators. (2002). Stenting and angioplasty with protection in patients at high risk for endarterectomy: The SAPPHIRE study. *Circulation, 106,* 2986–2989.

Zarins, C. K., White, R. A., Schwarten, D., Kinney, K., Dietrich, E. B., Hodgson, K. J., et al., for the Investigators of the Medtronic AneuRx Multicenter Clinical Trial. (1999). AneuRx stent graft vs. open surgical repair of abdominal aneurysm: Multicenter prospective clinical trial. *Journal of Vascular Surgery, 29,* 292–308.

19

Limb Deficiency

Jeffrey M. Cohen, MD, and Joan E. Edelstein, PT, MA, FISPO

INTRODUCTION

This chapter will familiarize the reader with limb deficiencies affecting both the upper and lower extremity. A limb deficiency is defined simply as a complete or partial loss of a limb. It can be congenital (present at birth) or acquired. In the first section of the chapter, we will focus on limb deficiency affecting the lower extremity. This section will be further subdivided into sections on etiology, levels of amputation, and pre- and postoperative management of the lower-limb amputee. We will end this section with a discussion of lower-limb prosthetics and prosthetic training. The second portion of the chapter will focus on the individual with an upper extremity limb deficiency. It too will be subdivided into sections on etiology, amputation levels, pre- and postoperative management, and prostheses and prosthetic training.

Amputation surgery is a procedure that dates to prehistoric times (Murdoch & Wilson, 1996). The earliest literature discussing amputation is contained within the Babylonian code of Hammurabi 1700 B.C.E. In 385 B.C.E, Plato's *Symposium* mentions therapeutic amputation of the hand and foot. Hippocrates in *De Articularis* provides the earliest description of amputation for vascular gangrene, cautioning that amputation should be at the edge of the ischemic tissue, with the wound left open to allow healing by secondary intent. The ensuing centuries have led to refinements in surgery technique, hemostasis (control of bleed), perioperative conditions, and anesthesia. Today, approximately 140,000 new amputations are performed annually in the United States. The number of persons estimated by be living with limb loss in this country is 1.7 million (Ziegler, MacKenzie, Ephraim, Travison, & Brookmeyer, 2008).

LOWER LIMB DEFICIENCY

Etiology

There are multiple etiologies for lower-limb deficiency. The major categories are vascular disease (pertaining to the blood vessels), trauma, malignancy, and congenital absence (Dillingham, Pezzin, & MacKenzie, 2002). Each year, the majority of new amputations occur due to complications of the vascular system. Over the past 30 years, dysvascular amputations have increased by 27%. In contrast, amputations secondary to trauma and cancer have decreased by 50%. The incidence of congenital (present at birth) limb *deficiency has remained stable.*

Dysvascular

Lower-limb deficiency is most commonly due to vascular disease (82%; Dillingham et al., 2002). Vascular disease can manifest as an episode of acute arterial insufficiency leading to gangrene. It can also present as progressive small-vessel occlusion leading to ulcers over pressure points, infection of the skin (cellulitis) and bone (osteomyelitis), as well as gangrenous changes in the distal lower extremities. Individuals with vascular disease may undergo a series of procedures in an attempt to salvage the involved limb (e.g., attempts at revascularization, multiple debridements, toe and foot amputations). Ultimately, limb removal may be required for uncontrollable soft tissue or bone infection, nonreconstructable disease with persistent tissue loss, or unrelenting rest pain due to muscle ischemia.

An estimated 65,000 lower-limb amputations are performed each year in the United States for adults with vascular disease. The majority are due to complications from diabetes mellitus (Boulton, Kirsner, & Vileikyte, 2004). Diabetes mellitus has a prevalence of 7% in the general population and the prevalence increases to 18.3% in those older than age 60. A twofold increased risk for leg lesions, including gangrene, exists among persons with diabetes (Diabetes Control and Complications Research Group, 1993). About 85% of all lower limb amputations in diabetics are preceded by a foot ulcer. The more proximal the amputation is, the higher the mortality. In 1965, the ratio of above-knee to below-knee amputations was 70:30. By 1990, the ratio had become 30:70, as better diagnostic and surgical procedures increased the probability of retaining the knee joint. Of those with a dysvascular amputation, 15–28% undergo a contralateral limb amputation within 3 years.

Trauma

Trauma is the primary etiology in 18% of cases of lower-limb deficiency (Dillingham et al., 2002). Traumatic limb loss is most often secondary to motor vehicle or industrial accidents. It usually occurs among young men. Such accidents can result in a direct limb transsection or an open fracture with associated nerve injury, soft tissue loss, and ischemia. Limb-salvage techniques, if feasible, are attempted initially in patients who eventually have traumatic limb loss. However, salvage may require multiple surgical procedures at a very high cost in time and money. Often, despite these attempts, the individual is left with a painful, nonfunctional limb that ultimately will require amputation surgery.

Malignancy

In 0.9% of persons with lower-limb deficiency, malignancy is the primary etiological factor (Dillingham et al., 2002). For persons with malignant bone tumors, advanced limb-salvage surgery has replaced amputation as the initial treatment. The patient is referred for amputation only if limb salvage has been excluded as an option.

Congenital

Congenital limb deficiencies comprise 0.8% of cases of lower-limb deficiency. In children, congenital limb deficiencies are more common than acquired deficiencies. They occur as a result of the failure of the formation of part or all of a limb bud. The first trimester is the critical time for limb formation with the bud occurring at 26 days and differentiation through the 8th week of gestation (Rossi, Alexander, & Cuccurullo, 2004). The etiology is often unclear, but teratogenic agents, for example, thalidomide and radiation exposure, and maternal diabetes are risk factors.

Levels of Amputation

In 1989, the International Standards Organization (ISO) adopted a series of standards for terminology intended for descriptive use in prosthetics and orthotics (Schuch & Pritham, 1994). This standard applies to acquired amputation levels. It consists of terms relating to external limb prostheses and wearers of these prostheses. The standards replaced the previous

American practice of using the terms above, below, or through the involved joint, for example, above knee and below knee. The current terminology uses the adjectives *trans, disarticulation,* and *partial* to describe amputation levels. The adjective *trans* is used when the amputation is across the axis of a long bone, for example, transfemoral/transhumeral. In cases, where the amputation is through two contiguous bones, for example, tibia and fibula, only the larger bone is identified, for example, transtibial. When the amputation is through the center of a joint (between long bones), the descriptor is *disarticulation,* for example, knee disarticulation, ankle disarticulation, and so on. The term *partial* describes amputations of the foot distal to the ankle joint and amputations of the hand distal to the wrist. Thus, in the current terminology, any amputation distal to the ankle level is referred to as a partial foot amputation. The single exception is the use of the term *forequarter amputation* for amputations of the upper limb at the scapulothoracic and the sternoclavicular joints. Figure 19.1 (Schuch & Pritham, 1994) depicts acquired amputation levels, the ISO terms, and, where applicable, the previous terms. Table 19.1 (Uustal & Baerga, 2004) provides a detailed description of levels of amputation.

Management of Lower Limb Deficiency

Management of a person undergoing lower-limb amputation surgery can be divided into pre- and postoperative phases. The preoperative phase helps to prepare the patient both physically and psychologically for the upcoming surgery. The postoperative phase focuses on wound healing, edema control, contracture prevention, and pain management. This is the time to prepare the residual limb for prosthetic fitting.

Preoperative Management

The time to start thinking about rehabilitation is the day that amputation is considered. When an amputation is anticipated, rehabilitation clinicians have an opportunity to help prepare the patient physically and psychologically. Ideally, discussions should involve the surgeon,

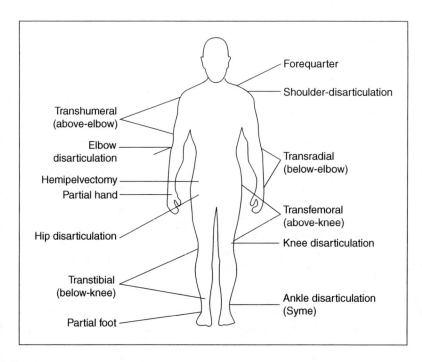

FIGURE 19.1 A depiction of acquired amputation levels, the new ISO terms, and where applicable, the previously accepted standards. *Source:* Schuch, C. M., & Pritham, C. H. (1994). International Forum—International Standards Organization Terminology: Application to Prosthetics and Orthotics. *Journal of Prosthetics and Orthotics, 6,* 29. Reprinted by permission of the publisher.

TABLE 19.1   *Levels of Amputation-Lower Limb*

Level	Anatomical Description	Details
Partial foot	Amputation distal to the ankle level	■ Preserves the ankle dorsiflexors and plantarflexors allowing for a functional weight-bearing foot.
Ankle disarticulation	Amputation through the ankle joint	■ Maintains nearly all limb length and preserves the heel pad, providing an excellent weight bearing limb. ■ Bulbous residual limb. ■ May not be appropriate for dysvascular patients as requires healthy plantar heel skin.
Transtibial	Amputation through the tibia and fibula	■ Lower mortalities and higher healing rate (80–90%) compared with the transfemoral level.
Knee disarticulation	Amputation through the knee joint	■ Patient supports weight through the end of the amputation limb. ■ Slight difference in thigh lengths when the patient sits.
Transfemoral	Amputation through the femur	■ Higher mortality rates and lower healing rate compared with the transtibial level.
Hip disarticulation	Amputation through the hip joint	■ Most patients are adolescents or young adults with bone tumors.
Transpelvic	Amputation through any portion of the pelvis	■ Most patients are adolescents or young adults with bone tumors.

Source: Adapted from Cuccurullo, S. J. (2004). *Physical medicine and rehabilitation board review.* New York: Demos Medical Publishing. Copyright © 2004 by Demos Medical Publishing. By permission of the publisher.

physiatrist, physical therapist, occupational therapist, prosthetist, psychologist, and social worker. If possible, a visit by a rehabilitated person with a similar level of amputation can be of tremendous benefit, reducing anxiety and fear for the patient and family (Marzen-Groller & Bartman, 2005).

Preoperative assessment of the patient includes an evaluation of the individual's strength, endurance, range of motion, and ambulatory status. The presence of any joint contracture (shortening of a muscle or tendon making passive stretching difficult) should be noted. A major component of the preoperative management is patient education. The likely exercise program is reviewed and a series of range of motion and strengthening exercises is initiated. Training in ambulation with crutches or a walker on level surfaces and stairs is also begun if the patient is medically stable. In addition, education about prostheses is helpful. Early involvement of a psychologist is critical. New amputees' feelings run the gamut of apprehension, depression, and anger, with adjustment and grief reactions common. Stages of survival, recovery, and reintegration have been described (Van Dorsten, 2004).

Many amputees report that the preoperative meeting with the rehabilitation team was critical to their making informed decisions and adjusting to life postoperatively. Patient education with exposure to actual prostheses and amputee peers reduces fear, shortens recovery time, and maximizes the rehabilitation effort (Hakimi, Eftekhari, & Czerniecki, 2008).

Postoperative Medical Management
The postoperative medical management of persons undergoing lower-limb amputation surgery focuses on promoting wound healing, controlling edema, and managing pain.

WOUND HEALING. Wound healing requires scrupulous attention to wound cleanliness and optimal nutrition. Well-nourished patients have an 86% success rate for wound healing after amputation, while malnourished individuals have an 85% failure rate (Dickhaut, DeLee, & Page, 1984). In addition, anemia should be corrected, along with optimizing glycemic control in diabetic patients.

EDEMA CONTROL. Controlling limb edema (swelling due to excessive accumulation of fluid in body tissues) is necessary to facilitate wound healing, reduce pain, and prepare the limb for prosthetic fitting. The ideal shape for a transtibial residual limb is cylindrical, whereas the ideal shape for a transfemoral residual limb is somewhat conical. To control edema and promote limb shaping, rigid, semirigid, and soft dressings are used.

Rigid Dressing. A rigid dressing is a cast made of plaster or fiberglass that is suspended by a waist belt or shoulder harness. A removable rigid dressing is made in two pieces so it can be removed easily to allow for wound inspection. If removed, however, the dressing must be replaced within minutes to prevent edema reaccumulation. Removable rigid dressings help control edema, leading to rapid residual limb shrinkage and a reduction in postoperative pain (Hakimi et al., 2008). The rigid dressing promotes healing by protecting the residual limb from trauma and helps to desensitize the limb. In the case of transtibial amputations, the dressing also prevents knee flexion contractures.

Semirigid Dressing. Several types of semirigid postoperative dressings are available to control edema and facilitate healing. The Unna paste dressing uses a bandage permeated with zinc oxide, gelatin, glycerin, and calamine oxide. It is generally applied directly on the skin, although it may be wrapped over a soft elastic dressing (Hakimi et al., 2008). Unna semirigid dressings are more effective than elastic dressings in facilitating healing and preparing the limb for prosthetic fitting (Wong & Edelstein, 2000). In addition, amputees treated with an Unna dressing are more likely to ambulate with a prosthesis upon discharge from a rehabilitation facility (Wong & Edelstein, 2000).

Soft Dressing. Soft dressings are of two forms: elastic bandages and elastic shrinker socks. Elastic bandages are inexpensive and lightweight, but must be reapplied multiple times daily because the bandage loosens as the patient moves about. Bandages are ineffective if patients fail to master the proper wrapping technique. The preferred technique is a figure-of-eight method, which uses diagonal turns. If poorly applied, elastic bandages can cause circumferential constriction with distal edema. Elastic shrinkers are easier to apply and provide uniform compression. However, if not adequately suspended by a waist belt, they too can lead to skin damage and limb constriction.

PAIN MANAGEMENT. Pain can lead to significant disability, difficulty performing daily living skills, and a diminished ability to tolerate one's prosthesis. A careful evaluation to determine the exact source of pain is necessary as it may originate from bone, muscle, nerve, or skin. Pain can be categorized as residual limb pain or phantom-limb pain.

Residual Limb Pain. Residual limb pain is a local pain that originates from the residual limb. It may be due to pressure on adherent scars or a neuroma (nerve ending left exposed during surgery). It may also originate from bone spurs or from a poorly fitting prosthesis. In addition, it may represent intermittent claudication (pain that is caused by inadequate blood flow to the leg muscles). Residual limb pain may also be an indication of a local tumor recurrence in patients who had undergone an amputation for tumor removal. Incisional pain tends to resolve as the wound heals.

Phantom Sensation and Phantom Pain. In addition to postoperative pain, most patients experience phantom sensations, the feeling that the amputated limb is still present. These sensations are produced by brain networks that are normally triggered by continuous input from the extremity prior to its amputation. Once the limb is removed, this input is replaced by phantom sensations. These sensations manifest as nonpainful mild tingling. They are common, with an incidence of 80–100% in amputees immediately postoperatively. Only 10% of patients develop it after 1 month (Hakimi et al., 2008). The phenomenon of "telescoping," the sensation that the phantom limb has shrunk (i.e., the toes are at the ankle and the foot is at the knee), often accompanies phantom sensations. The intensity of phantom sensation typically diminishes over time, but some awareness can persist throughout the patient's lifetime.

Phantom pain is the sensation of pain originating from the amputated portion of the extremity. It may be related to neuronal deafferentiation hyperexcitability. Deafferentation is a loss of sensory input from a portion of the body due to the elimination or interruption of sensory-nerve fibers. After deafferentation, alterations in the functional properties of the dorsal horn of the spinal cord occur, and may underlie the occurrence of abnormal sensations referred to the denervated body part (Ovelmen-Levitt, 1988). Phantom pain is most often characterized as a cramping, squeezing, burning, or a sharp, shooting pain (Flor, 2002). It may accompany phantom sensation. Phantom pain usually develops within the first postoperative month, and it is most intense immediately after the amputation. It may be diffuse, through the phantom limb, or localized to a single nerve distribution. It is usually worse at night or after the limb has been in a dependent position and can be exacerbated by anxiety and stress. Phantom pain tends to diminish over time, and chronic phantom pain is rare, reported by less than 5% of the total amputee population. Of those complaining about phantom limb pain, only 14% report it is severely limiting (Ehde et al., 2000).

There are many treatments for phantom pain that have varying levels of success. Overall, therapeutic regimens have less than a 30% long-term efficacy (Czerniecki & Ehde, 2003). In light of this, an interdisciplinary approach to the treatment of phantom pain encompassing physical, pharmacological, and psychological means is often most effective. Treatment measures that create increased peripheral input can provide at least temporary relief. Such measures include desensitization techniques (massaging or gently tapping the residual limb), consistent wearing of a prosthesis as well as the use of transcutaneous electrical nerve stimulation (TENS). TENS is the application of electrical current through the skin for pain control. In addition, treatment aimed at reducing neuromas and infections also diminishes phantom pain. Psychological interventions such as hypnosis, biofeedback, behavioral therapy, relaxation therapy, and voluntary control of the phantom limb (mental imaging) have also met with varying levels of success.

Unlike postsurgical pain, phantom pain does not respond well to opioid medications. Phantom pain is best treated with low doses of anticonvulsants (pregabalin, gabapentin, carbamazepine) that stabilize the nerve's ability to depolarize. Antidepressants (duloxetine, nortriptyline, amitryptyline) can be effective and also improve sleep. Interventional treatments such as nerve blocks, epidural blocks, chemical sympathectomy, or other neurosurgical procedures are reserved for refractory cases. They have poor long-term success.

Postoperative Rehabilitation Management
Early aggressive and comprehensive rehabilitation after limb amputation is necessary for a good functional and psychological outcome. Rehabilitation that begins soon after surgery has many advantages, including minimizing residual and phantom-limb pain and improving prosthetic ambulation (Friedmann, 1990).

PHYSICAL THERAPY. Contractures affect prosthetic fitting and patient function. Maintaining range of motion, especially in the proximal joints of the affected limb, is critical to a successful, functional outcome. Absence of a residual limb contracture correlates with successful prosthetic ambulation (Munin et al., 2001). For the transtibial amputee, the focus is on preventing a knee-flexion contracture. To accomplish this, strategies include avoiding placing a pillow under the knee, limiting sitting for prolonged periods, and maintaining aggressive pain control. Patients benefit from wearing a soft- or rigid-knee splint when sitting. They should keep the knee extended on a board placed under the wheelchair cushion; the board extends to the distal end of the amputation limb. The transfemoral amputee is prone to the development of hip flexion and abduction contractures. A transfemoral amputation results in the unopposed pull of the iliopsoas, gluteus medius/minimus, and deep external rotator muscles; pulling the hip into a position of flexion; abduction; and external rotation. The transfemoral amputee should avoid placing a pillow under the thigh or standing with the residual limb resting on a crutch handle, to prevent hip flexion contractures. In addition, the transfemoral amputee should avoid placing a pillow between the legs when in bed or in a wheelchair, to prevent hip abduction contractures. Other preventive strategies include placing the patient in a prone or side-lying position on a firm mattress, three times daily for 15 minutes each, if clinically feasible. The lower-limb amputee should be encouraged to actively extend the hip on the amputated side while flexing the contralateral limb.

Physical conditioning is essential for the lower-limb amputee, especially for those with cardiovascular or vascular compromise. Improving aerobic capacity has a direct impact on the potential for functional ambulation, even for the frailest patients. Endurance activities such as wheelchair propulsion, single-limb ambulation with an appropriate assistive device and upper-limb ergometry improve the patient's cardiovascular status in preparation for prosthetic training.

To function successfully with one's prosthesis requires good upper-body strength, adequate hip and knee stability, as well as good trunk control, posture, and balance. Strengthening programs for the upper body focus on the biceps, triceps, and latissimus dorsi. A lower-limb strengthening program for the transfemoral amputee emphasizes the gluteal muscles on both the intact and amputated sides. In transtibial amputees, the focus is on strengthening the gluteal muscles, the hamstrings, and quadriceps muscles. These strengthening exercises help facilitate transfers from the sitting to standing position and ambulation (Rheinstein, Wong, & Edelstein, 2006).

OCCUPATIONAL THERAPY. Occupational therapy helps the patient achieve functional independence in activities of daily living. Occupational therapists also evaluate the patient for appropriate assistive and adaptive equipment. They assess the patient's home environment to maximize patient independence and safety. Wheelchair prescription emphasizes the importance of ordering a chair with a posteriorly placed axle to prevent rearward tipping and swing-out leg rests to facilitate transferring in and out of the wheelchair.

PSYCHOLOGICAL THERAPY. Continued involvement of a psychologist is necessary throughout the postoperative period. The psychologist should follow the patient through the immediate postamputation period, through the prosthetic training period and as the patient attempts to reintegrate into society. New amputees have to deal not only with the physical ordeal of the amputation but also with its impact on interpersonal relationships, careers, and the stresses of daily living. The patient must learn to come to terms with an altered self-image. The psychologist helps the new amputee live with these realities and recognize that he or she is still basically the same person as prior to the surgery.

VOCATIONAL REHABILITATION. Not only is training for physical mobility and independence in activities of daily living necessary post amputation, but return to school or work, especially in the younger population, is important too. Employment is central to well-being, as it enlarges one's social environment and can provide a stable income. Aims of vocational rehabilitation should be to shorten the time between the amputation and the return to work and to adapt the workplace to any limitations imposed by the amputation.

Success in job reintegration is associated with a younger age, a higher educational level, and wearing a more comfortable prosthesis (Schoppen et al., 2001). Amputees who changed to a physically less-demanding type of work following their amputation have a greater success rate in returning to work. In addition, amputees who have returned to work have been noted to experience greater job satisfaction than their able-bodied peers (Schoppen et al., 2002). Job satisfaction among unilateral lower-limb amputees could be improved by workplace modifications, depending on the functional capabilities of the person and the functional demands of the job. Vocational satisfaction can also be improved by utilizing vocational rehabilitation programs, especially for those people with additional medical problems.

Prosthetics

Candidacy

When evaluating a patient as a potential prosthetic candidate, multiple factors must be considered. This is especially true in the elderly dysvascular patient who may have such comorbidities as diabetes mellitus, kidney disease, cardiovascular disorder, respiratory disease, arthritis, neuropathy, and impaired vision. Each patient should undergo a thorough musculoskeletal and functional evaluation to assess the person's suitability for prosthetic ambulation. Factors such as amputation level, cardiovascular status, cognitive ability, as well as the person's mobility goals, are considered in determining whether a patient is a candidate for prosthetic rehabilitation.

Energy Requirements/Functional Outcome

In assessing a lower-limb amputee's potential for prosthetic ambulation, one must be aware of the energy requirements involved. As the level of amputation proceeds from distal (e.g., transtibial) to more proximal, (e.g., transfemoral), the energy required to ambulate a fixed distance increases. In addition, the walking speed decreases. Table 19.2 (Uustal & Baerga, 2004) depicts the increased energy requirements above normal required for traumatic amputees of different amputation levels to ambulate over a fixed distance. Of note, traumatic bilateral transtibial amputees actual exert less extra effort to ambulate than do unilateral transfemoral amputees. This finding emphasizes the importance of retaining the anatomical knee whenever possible.

The etiology of the amputation also influences energy cost (Table 19.3; Uustal & Baerga, 2004). Individuals whose amputations are due to trauma walk faster and use less energy than dysvascular amputees (Su, Gard, Lipschultz, & Kuiken, 2008). This difference in performance may result partly from age-related changes and partly from concurrent cardiovascular disease. Dysvascular amputees tend to be older and have lower energy reserves (MacNeill, Devlin, Pauley, & Yudin, 2008). In the dysvascular amputee, the energy source for walking may be anaerobic rather than the more efficient aerobic metabolic pathways. Due

TABLE 19.2 *Energy Expenditure of Traumatic Amputees—Level of Amputation*

Level of Amputation	Increased Energy Expenditure Above Normal (%)
Transtibial	20–25
Bilateral transtibial	41
Transfemoral	60–70
Transtibial/transfemoral	118
Bilateral transfemoral	>200

Source: Adapted from Cuccurullo, S. J. (2004). *Physical medicine and rehabilitation board review.* New York: Demos Medical Publishing. Copyright © 2004 by Demos Medical Publishing. By permission of the publisher.

TABLE 19.3   *Energy Expenditure—Traumatic vs. Vascular Amputations*

Level of Amputation	Increased Energy Expenditure Above Normal (%)
Transtibial	
Traumatic	25
Vascular	40
Transfemoral	
Traumatic	68
Vascular	100

Source: Adapted from Cuccurullo, S. J. (2004). *Physical medicine and rehabilitation board review.* New York: Demos Medical Publishing. Copyright © 2004 by Demos Medical Publishing. By permission of the publisher.

to the increased energy demands, long-term use of bilateral transfemoral prostheses in the dysvascular population is rare. In contrast, the typically younger traumatic amputee has a larger cardiac and respiratory functional reserve capacity. A significant number of traumatic bilateral transtibial amputees are successful prosthetic users.

A well-fitting prosthesis that results in a satisfactory gait, not requiring crutches or a walker, significantly decreases physiological energy demands. For individuals with unilateral transtibial or transfemoral amputations, regardless of their age or etiology of amputation, the energy cost of walking with a prosthesis is less than that expended when walking without a prosthesis using crutches or a walker (Waters & Mulroy, 1999; Wu, Chen, & Lin, 2001). This difference, however, is not significant in dysvascular amputees, as the great majority require an assistive device (cane, walker, or crutches) to ambulate, which in turn increase energy requirements. Bilateral amputees fitted with a pair of prostheses incorporating multiaxial ankles (McNealy & Gard, 2008) or microprocessor C-leg-knee units (Perry, Burnfield, Newsam, & Conley, 2004) have demonstrated greater gait efficiency.

The findings regarding energy consumption are confirmed by many other studies that demonstrate a more active functional outcome among those with more distal amputations and those with a traumatic, rather than dysvascular, etiology (Asano, Rushton, Miller, & Deathe, 2008; Aulivola et al., 2004; Bilodeau, Hebert, & Destrosiers, 2000; Brunelli et al., 2006; Bussmann, Schrauwen, & Stam, 2008; Chen et al., 2008; Davies & Datta, 2003; Deans, McFadyen, & Rose, 2008; Dillingham & Pezzin, 2008; Dillingham, Pezzin, MacKenzie, & Burgess, 2001; Dougherty, 2001, 2003; Fletcher et al., 2001; Gailey, Allen, Castles, Kucharik, & Roeder, 2008; Gauthier-Gagnon, Grise, & Potvin, 1999; MacKenzie et al., 2004; Nehler et al., 2003; Pezzin, Dillingham, & MacKenzie, 2000; Pezzin, Dillingham, MacKenzie, Ephraim, & Rossbach, 2004; Schoppen et al., 2002, 2003). The functional outcome of patients who sustained tumor-related amputations has been found to be very positive. Most were independent ambulators (Kauzlaric, Kauzlaric, & Kolundzic, 2007) with employment, income, marital status, and health comparable to the general nondisabled population (Hoffman, Saltzman, & Buckwalter, 2002).

Terminology

A *prosthesis* is a replacement for a body part, including false teeth, heart valves, hip replacements, and artificial limbs. Limb prostheses are made by *prosthetists* who are skilled in prosthetic design, materials, and methods of fitting so that patients are comfortable and obtain the maximum function from their prostheses. The prosthetist works closely with the physician and physical therapist.

The major purpose of a limb prosthesis is to restore the appearance and function of the missing limb. Because no prosthesis fulfills these goals completely, the patient and the rehabilitation team must determine which compromises are most acceptable. Nevertheless, Medicare regulations (HCFA Common Procedure Coding System, 2001), which are not limited to the elderly, specify which components will be reimbursed, depending on the physician's assessment of the patient's current or anticipated level of function. Medicare requires the physician to categorize the amputee's potential by designating a *K level*. The K level will limit the amputee to certain prosthetic components, depending on their potential activity level. The following K levels apply to persons with unilateral transtibial and transfemoral amputations.

- **Level 0**: The amputee does not have the ability or potential to ambulate or transfer safely. Prosthesis is not appropriate, usually because of dementia or very poor cardiopulmonary function.
- **Level 1**: Household ambulator. Ability or potential to use a prosthesis for transfers or ambulation on level surfaces at a fixed speed. SACH (solid ankle, cushion heel) or single-axis foot for transtibial and transfemoral prostheses and knee units, excluding fluid-controlled ones, are covered.
- **Level 2**: Limited community ambulator. Ability or potential for traversing low environmental barriers, such as curbs, stairs, and uneven surfaces. Flexible keel or a multiaxial foot, as well as an axial rotation unit, are covered for transtibial and transfemoral prostheses. Knee units excluding fluid-controlled units are covered.
- **Level 3**: Community ambulator. Ability or potential for ambulation with various speeds; ability to traverse most environmental barriers involves vocational, therapeutic, or exercise activity beyond simple walking. Energy storing feet, including Flex-Foot, and a rotation unit are permitted. Pneumatic and hydraulic knee units, with or without electronic control, are covered.
- **Level 4**: Child, active adult, or athlete. Ability or potential to exceed basic ambulation skills, and participate in activities of high impact, stress, or energy levels. Any of the feet, rotators, and knee units are covered.

Transtibial Prostheses

The transtibial prosthesis (Figure 19.2) consists of four parts, namely, a prosthetic foot, shank, socket, and suspension. Many options are available for each of these parts. The unique combination for each patient should enable the individual to stand and walk with reasonable comfort, appearance, and efficiency. Walking involves supporting weight on the prosthesis during *stance phase* when all or a part of the foot contacts the floor, as well as clearing the floor during *swing phase*.

All *prosthetic feet* share several characteristics. They resemble the size and general shape of the human foot, in sizes suitable for young children to large adults. They enable the wearer to stand. Feet enable stance phase, providing a slight amount of plantar flexion when the wearer first contacts the floor; this motion contributes to stability when balancing over the prosthesis. Later in stance phase, feet simulate dorsiflexion, which normally

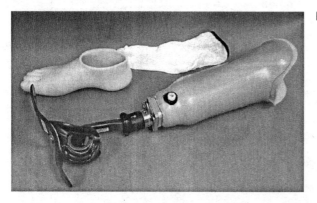

FIGURE 19.2   Transtibial prosthesis.

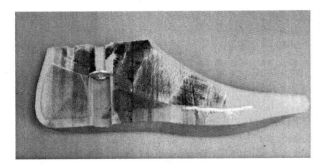

FIGURE 19.3 SACH (solid ankle, cushion heel) foot.

occurs at the metatarsophalangeal joints. In swing phase, feet remain in neutral position, allowing the wearer to clear the floor without dragging the prosthetic forefoot. No prosthetic feet permit tip toeing, nor do they provide sensory feedback.

The most frequently used foot is the SACH (solid ankle, cushion heel) foot (Figure 19.3). The solid ankle, known as the keel, is usually wooden; it extends from the top of the foot to a point corresponding to the base of the toes. This basic foot suits people who limit their walking to moving about the home. Other feet substitute flexible material for the keel; such feet adapt more readily to irregular terrain. The single-axis foot has a transverse axle that enables slight plantar flexion and dorsiflexion during stance phase; the ease of motion is influenced by rubber bumpers in front and in back of the axle (Figure 19.4).

Some prosthetic feet store energy in early- and mid-stance and return the stored energy to the patient in late stance. These dynamic, energy-responsive feet, such as the Flex-Foot, contribute to a springy, lively walking pattern appropriate for people who walk vigorously indoors and outdoors (Hafner, 2005; Hsu, Nielsen, Lin-Chan, & Shurr, 2006; Marinakis, 2004; Underwood, Tokuno, & Eng, 2004; Zmitrewicz, Neptune, Walden, Rogers, & Bosker, 2006). A few feet are multiaxial, providing mediolateral and transverse plane motion, in addition to limited plantar and dorsiflexion; they adapt well to cobblestones and similar surfaces (Marinakis, 2004). Some feet permit adjustments to accommodate shoes having various heel heights.

The section of the prosthesis located immediately above the foot is the shank (shin) that supports the wearer's weight. An exoskeletal shank is hard-shell shaped and is colored to resemble the intact leg. An endoskeletal shank is a central pylon covered with foam material carved to duplicate the contours of the opposite leg; it is covered with hosiery that matches the patient's skin color. The endoskeletal shank permits minor adjustments after the prosthesis is

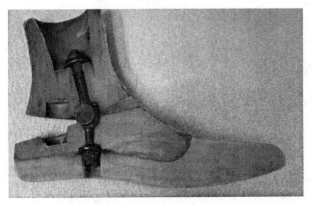

FIGURE 19.4 Single-axis foot. Posterior bumper removed.

fabricated and is somewhat lighter in weight as compared with the exoskeletal version. The foam cover, however, is not as durable as the hard shell. Either type of shank may include an axial rotation unit which absorbs shock in the transverse plane. A vertical shock absorber may also be included in an endoskeletal shank. Shock absorbers shield the skin and anatomic joints on the amputated side from impact and are thus indicated for active wearers (Berge, Czerniecki, & Klute, 2005; Gard & Konz, 2003).

The most important part of any prosthesis is the *socket* that surrounds the amputation limb. The upper part of an exoskeletal shank encases the socket. If the prosthesis has an endoskeletal shank, the socket will be placed above the pylon. Sockets are custom made of plastic, either a combination of flexible thermoplastic and rigid plastic, or entirely rigid. A popular design is the patellar tendon bearing design that features a marked indentation in the upper part of the front of the socket intended to support a fair amount of load on the patellar tendon (ligament). Another option is the total surface bearing design, which has slightly smoother contours (Selles, Janssens, Jongenengel, & Bussmann, 2005). Both types contact all portions of the amputated limb to maximize the contact area, thus minimizing unit pressure. Sockets are frequently equipped with a resilient liner to cushion the body part. Patients often wear cotton or wool socks inside the socket. Alternatively, vigorous walkers may prefer a silicone or urethane liner, which reduces friction that occurs as the amputation limb moves slightly within the socket during walking (Baars & Geertzen, 2005).

In order that the prosthesis may stay securely on the patient's limb during the swing phase of walking and when the wearer is climbing stairs, some form of *suspension* is required. Options include a leather or fabric cuff attached to the socket; the cuff wraps around the lower portion of the thigh. Athletic individuals generally prefer pin suspension; they wear a silicone liner that has a metal pin at the lower end. The pin locks into a receptacle at the bottom of the socket. A few use vacuum suspension. Some people augment suspension with an elastic sleeve that extends from the lower thigh to the upper part of the socket. Others attach a forked strap to the socket; the upper part of the strap has elastic webbing that attaches to a waist belt. Two other modes of suspension are extensions of the socket, namely, supracondylar and supracondylar/suprapatellar, both of which cover more of the upper part of the amputation limb. A few patients require a thigh corset that is attached to the socket by a pair of metal side bars.

Once the components of the prosthesis are selected, the prosthetist measures the patient's limb in order to construct the socket. The limb may be wrapped in plaster of Paris to form a cast that the prosthetist will use to create a model of the limb as the basis of the socket. Alternatively, the prosthetist may take electronic measurements to enable computer-aided design and computer-aided manufacture of the socket. In either case, the resulting socket should fit comfortably, protecting sensitive areas from excessive loading. The prosthetic foot is then fitted to a temporary shank, and the socket is attached to the shank. The temporary shank enables the prosthetist to align the prosthesis, namely, altering the relation of the parts of the prosthesis. Alignment contributes to the comfort and stability that the patient will achieve with the prosthesis. The alignment is then transferred to the permanent shank. Finally, the suspension is attached, unless it is part of the upper contour of the socket.

Transfemoral Prostheses

The transfemoral prosthesis consists of five parts: a prosthetic foot, shank, knee unit, socket, and suspension (Figure 19.5). As with the transtibial prosthesis, many options are available for each of these parts.

The same choices of *prosthetic foot* and *shank* as previously described are available for the transfemoral prosthesis. Athletically inclined patients walk more efficiently with energy-storing feet (Graham, Datta, Heller, & Howitt, 2007).

The *knee unit* transmits body weight from the upper parts of the prosthesis to the shank and foot. All knee units bend to permit patients to sit comfortably. Most units also allow the shank to oscillate during the swing phase of walking. The most critical parts of knee units relate

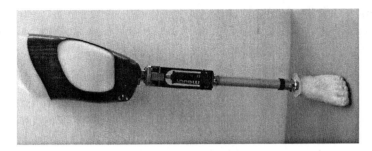

FIGURE 19.5 Transfemoral prosthesis.

to the wearer's stability when standing and during stance phase, and the individual's ease of progressing through swing phase. Stance-phase stability is influenced by the alignment of the prosthesis. A patient who is very unsteady may require a manually locked knee unit (Devlin et al., 2002). The prosthesis will be rigid during stance phase, maximizing stability. Unfortunately, the rigid prosthesis presents an unnatural appearance during swing phase. The wearer can unlock the knee when sitting. Alternative means of providing stance stability include various braking mechanisms. These resist knee-flexion during early stance, but permit knee motion during late stance and swing phase.

During swing phase, most knee units (with the exception of manually locked units) contain a friction mechanism to resist extreme knee flexion during early swing and abrupt knee extension at late swing. The individual who is expected to walk on a limited basis, primarily at home, will be well served by a friction mechanism consisting of a pair of clamps that can be tightened or loosened according to the patient's walking style. The clamps affect the ease with which the shank swings. More active people benefit from the more expensive pneumatic (air) and hydraulic (oil) units. Because air and oil are fluids, the units adjust automatically when the patient walks slowly or rapidly. Some hydraulic units incorporate stance control, providing very high resistance when the patient first strikes the floor with the prosthetic heel. The most sophisticated hydraulic units, such as the C-Leg, have electronic sensors which detect the wearer's walking speed, shank position, and the contour and texture of the walking surface. Wearers of microprocessor units exhibit smoother, more efficient gait, and report greater activity (Hafner, Willingham, Buell, Allyn, & Smith, 2007; Kahle, Highsmith, & Hubbard, 2008; Kaufman et al., 2008; Orendurff et al., 2006; Sapin, Goujon, de Almeida, Fode, & Lavaste, 2008; Segal et al., 2006; Seymour et al., 2007). The newest microprocessor units incorporate magnetized fluid rather than oil, with good clinical results (Johansson, Sherrill, Riley, Bonato, & Herr, 2005).

Sockets, as always, are custom made to fit the individual patient and are generally made of thermoplastic in a rigid plastic frame. The traditional design is quadrilateral, named for its four-sided contour; the patient supports a fair amount of weight on the posterior brim of the socket. An alternative is the ischial containment socket that covers the ischial tuberosity. Both types provide total contact of the amputation limb.

Most transfemoral sockets are *suspended* with suction. Pressure within the socket is lower than atmospheric pressure. Suction sockets have a one-way air expulsion valve to maintain the pressure difference. Full suction suspension is lightweight and does not require any straps or other attachments and thus permits the freest hip motion. The patient must have an amputation limb that does not fluctuate in volume in order to obtain good suspension with suction. Some people wear an elastic belt over the top of the prosthesis for extra support. Those who do have varying amounts of edema require additional suspension devices such as a Silesian webbing belt attached to the socket and surrounding the lower torso. The most rigid suspension is provided by a pelvic band, generally used with a more loosely fitting socket. The pelvic band is a belt with a rigid portion to which is attached a hinged metal or plastic upright joining the belt to the socket. The pelvic band limits mediolateral and rotational hip motions and is the heaviest suspension option.

Other Prostheses

Prostheses for people with *hip disarticulation* or *transpelvic amputation* (formerly known as hemipelvectomy) consist of a socket, hip unit, thigh section, knee unit, shank, and foot. The socket encases the lower torso and, depending on the extent of loss, may encroach on the lower ribs. The hip unit permits sufficient hip flexion so the individual can sit, as well as slight hip extension. Most units do not allow other hip motions. The thigh section is a foam-covered endoskeletal connection between the hip unit and the knee unit. Knee units, shanks, and feet are the same as used in transtibial and transfemoral prostheses.

The *knee disarticulation* prosthesis has a socket that may have an opening in the front, a knee unit similar to that used for transfemoral prostheses, and a shank and a foot that resemble those used for transfemoral prostheses.

Partial foot prostheses range from a *toe filler* in the shoe of the person who is missing one or more toes, to a full socket for those who have more extensive amputation. The ideal *transmetatarsal* prosthesis consists of a socket fitted to a modified prosthetic foot. A similar approach is used for individuals whose foot has been severed in the intertarsal region, such as Lisfranc (disarticulation between the metatarsals and the tarsals) and Chopart (disarticulation through the midtarsal joints). The *Syme's* prosthesis consists of a socket covering most of the leg and a specially designed prosthetic foot.

Bilateral prostheses resemble those for single amputations, except for foot size and leg length (Uellendahl, 2004). The patient will achieve greater stability by wearing a pair of prosthetic feet that are wider than the preamputation shoe size. Shorter prosthetic feet facilitate transferring weight forward during the stance phase of walking. Patients wearing bilateral prostheses consume more energy than do those wearing a unilateral prosthesis (Wright, Marks, & Payne, 2008). Individuals whose amputations were caused by trauma walked somewhat faster than those with vascular disease (Su et al., 2008). Reducing the height of the shanks also contributes to stability, placing the individual's center of gravity closer to the floor; this advantage, however, must be balanced against the cosmetic implications of reducing the wearer's height (MacNeill et al., 2008; McNealy & Gard, 2008; Perry et al., 2004; Wu et al., 2001).

Prosthetic Training

The basic elements of training are donning and doffing the prosthesis, standing and sitting in various chairs, and walking on a level surface, as well as caring for the amputation limb and the prosthesis. The patient can sit while donning the transtibial prosthesis, first applying a sock, then the socket liner, if present, and then placing the residual limb in the socket and fastening the cuff or corset. Pin suspension requires that the individual apply a silicone liner, which has a distal pin, onto the residual limb and then add socks as needed for a snug socket fit. The individual then pushes the residual limb into the socket so that the pin engages the locking mechanism. Donning the transfemoral socket is easiest if the patient removes the suction valve, lubricates the thigh with lotion, pushes the amputation limb into the socket, and installs the valve. Alternatively, the patient may apply tubular stockinet onto the thigh, then draw the end of the stockinet through the valve hole, and pull on the fabric while flexing and extending the contralateral hip and knee. After the stockinet has been pulled from the limb, the patient installs the valve and fastens any additional suspension, such as a Silesian belt or pelvic band.

To rise from a chair, the patient should place the sound (or stronger) leg closer to the chair, regardless of level of amputation. By extending both hips and knees, the individual comes to the standing position. Sitting also is easiest with the sound leg closer to the chair, so that the individual can feel the chair with the intact leg and can maneuver the center of gravity most easily.

Walking requires the ability to shift weight to the prosthesis in order to control the prosthetic foot. The transfemoral amputee learns to flex the prosthetic knee by flexing the hip and to extend the knee unit by hip extension (Bussmann et al., 2008; Isakov, Keren, & Benjuya, 2000; Jones, Bashford, & Mann, 1997; Miller, Speechley, & Deathe, 2001; Miller & Deathe, 2004; Nadollek, Brauer, & Isles, 2002; Nolan & Lees, 2000; Nolan et al., 2003; Rau, Bonvin, & de Bie, 2007; Vrieling et al., 2008a, 2008b). Beyond these rudimentary activities, more agile patients learn to climb stairs and ramps (Nair, Hanspal, Zahedi, & Saif, 2008; Paysant, Beyaert, Datie, Martinet, & Andre, 2006; Schmalz, Blumentritt, & Marx, 2007; Vickers, Palk, McIntosh, & Beatty, 2008), step over obstacles (Vrieling et al., 2007), drive a car (Boulias, Meikle, Pauley, & Devlin, 2006), and engage in a wide range of sports (Nolan & Lees, 2007; Nolan & Patritti, 2008; Nolan, Patritti, & Simpson, 2006; Rogers, Strike, & Wallace, 2004; Yazicioglu, Taskaynatan, Guzelkucuk, & Tugcu, 2007).

Special Considerations for Children

Congenital limb deficiencies are classified as transverse, similar in appearance to acquired amputation, and longitudinal, with both proximal absence and distal presence of portions of the limb (Fisk & Smith, 2004; Gaebler-Spira & Uellendahl, 1999; International Standards Organization, 1989; Stanger, 2000). Prenatal vascular disruption may be a significant causative factor (Boonstra, Rijnders, Groothoff, & Eisma, 2000).

Children's prostheses are simplified versions of adult limbs, with a more limited selection of components. Choice of components is governed by the developmental level of the child as well as the need to accommodate growth. Very young children begin walking by striking the ground with the entire sole, unlike the mature pattern of making initial contact with the heel, then transferring weight over the rest of the foot. Consequently, the first foot is likely to be the SACH foot, fitted to infants as early as 6 months. The first transtibial prosthesis will also have an exoskeletal shank, custom-made socket, and cuff suspension. Typically, the first transfemoral prosthesis does not have a knee unit and is usually suspended with a harness. Toddlers have a wider choice of feet. The smallest of more sophisticated foot and knee unit designs suit 10- to 12-year-olds. Electronic knee units suit older adolescents.

Increase in height can be accommodated with an endoskeletal shank and, for transfemoral prostheses, the shank and thigh sections. The outgrown pylon can be exchanged for a longer unit. Planning for the increasing girth and length of the amputation limb often includes initially fitting the child with one or two concentric sockets. When the innermost socket becomes tight, it can be discarded extending the duration of use of the prosthesis. An alternative approach involves fitting the child with a thermoplastic socket in an extra thick frame. Thermoplastic can be remolded by heating it and the thick walls of the frame ground slightly to accommodate the larger socket. Growth also requires periodically exchanging the prosthetic foot for one that matches the sound foot size. Functional outcome is excellent, with most children wearing their prostheses full time and engaging in age-appropriate activities (Nagarajan et al., 2003).

UPPER-LIMB DEFICIENCY

Etiology

In the United States, only 10% of all amputations involve the upper limb, most frequently below the elbow (Hakimi et al., 2008). The most frequent cause of upper-limb deficiency is trauma. Accidents involving machinery account for 40% of traumatic upper- and lower-limb amputations; these include 28% from power tools, 8.5% from firearms, and 8% from motor vehicle accidents. The second most common etiology for upper-limb deficiency is congenital absence. Among children, however, this is the most common cause of upper-limb deficiency.

The third most common etiology is oncological, particularly osseous tumors at the distal end of the humerus.

Levels of Amputation

Consistent with lower-limb amputation terminology, terms adopted by the International Standards Organization in 1989 apply to the upper extremity (Schuch & Pritham, 1994). Table 19.4 describes the levels of upper limb amputation (Uustal & Baerga, 2004).

Management of Upper-Limb Deficiency

Care of the patient with an upper-limb amputation is similar to that described for the lower limb. The major distinctions relate to the different functions performed by the arms and legs.

TABLE 19.4 *Levels of Amputation—Upper Limb*

Level	Anatomical Description	Details
Partial hand	Amputation distal to wrist level	■ Rarely fitted with a prosthesis. ■ Surgical reconstruction may be a more appropriate choice to preserve or enhance function, while maintaining sensation in the residual partial hand.
Wrist disarticulation	Amputation through the wrist joint, preserving the distal radius-ulnar articulation	■ Preserves full forearm supination and pronation. ■ Long bony leverage for lifting. ■ Poor cosmesis due to a bulbous residual limb.
Transradial	Amputation through the forearm: 1. Very short-residual limb length (<35%) 2. Short-residual limb length (35–55%) 3. Long-residual limb length (55–90%)	■ Allows a high level of functional recovery in the majority of cases. ■ Suitable for body-powered prostheses. ■ Suitable for physically demanding work. ■ Residual limb length of 60–70% is preferred for using an externally powered prosthesis.
Elbow disarticulation	Amputation through the elbow joint	■ Rapid surgery with decreased blood loss. ■ Improved prosthetic self suspension. ■ Good control of socket rotation on residual limb. ■ Poor cosmesis as needs external elbow mechanism
Transhumeral	Amputation through the humerus: 1. Humeral neck-residual limb length (<30%) 2. Short-residual limb length (30–50%) 3. Standard-residual limb length (50–90%)	■ Longer residual length associated with better prosthetic function.
Shoulder disarticulation	Amputation through the shoulder joint	■ Difficult to fit with a functional prosthesis.
Forequarter	Amputation of the entire arm and a portion of the shoulder girdle, thorax, or both	■ Difficult to fit with a functional prosthesis.

Source: Adapted from Cuccurullo, S. J. (2004). *Physical medicine and rehabilitation board review.* New York: Demos Medical Publishing. Copyright © 2004 by Demos Medical Publishing. By permission of the publisher.

The upper-limb amputation wound is generally smaller and thus faster to heal than a wound through the thigh or lower leg. Arms are rarely used to support weight, unlike standing on the legs. Most functional activities can be performed with one hand.

Preoperative Management
Most upper-limb amputations occur suddenly, without an extended preoperative period. Nevertheless, if at all possible, the rehabilitation team should meet with the patient and family to discuss the likely course of rehabilitation and the prosthetic possibilities. Peer support is especially valuable to enable the patient to accept the amputation and realize some of its functional implications.

To the extent feasible, the range of motion and strength of both arms and the trunk should be assessed. If the decision to amputate is made after attempts to salvage the limb, the amount of residual neurovascular damage should be determined.

Postoperative Medical Management
As with lower-limb amputations, postoperative medical management emphasizes wound healing, edema control, and pain management. The techniques are basically the same as already described. Although edema is much less a problem with the smaller body part and the generally younger age of the patient, some form of limb dressing is required. Rigid and semirigid dressings are effective in controlling edema, thereby accelerating healing and reducing pain. Some patients have the alternative soft elastic bandage or shrinker dressing. Pain is likely to be a greater issue with loss of any portion of the upper limb. In addition to residual limb pain, the patient is likely to complain about phantom pain and sensation. The hand is much more emotionally significant than the foot and the brain has a larger cortical representation for the hand. The same treatments to control pain, as described for the lower limb, are used.

Postoperative Rehabilitation Management
Early, aggressive, and comprehensive rehabilitation after upper limb amputation is necessary to achieve a good functional and psychological outcome. Ideally, the patient should be treated in a rehabilitation facility that specializes in the care of persons with upper-limb deficiency (Gajewski & Granville, 2006; Smurr, Gulick, Yancosek, & Ganz, 2008). Most clinicians see many fewer such patients; thus, it is difficult to acquire substantial experience. The psychologist and social worker play a major role in rehabilitating children born with limb loss and the adults who acquire an upper limb amputation.

Maintaining range of motion is key to achieving a successful, functional outcome. The patient with a transradial (below-elbow) amputation should work actively to preserve forearm pronation and supination. Otherwise, the individual will have to rely extensively on a mechanism to alter the position of the prosthetic replacement of the hand. The transradial amputee is also vulnerable to elbow flexion contractures. With transhumeral (above-elbow) amputations, the concern focuses on maintaining maximum shoulder range of motion and strength. High-level amputations also alter posture, compromising appearance and respiration (Meier & Atkins, 2004).

Prosthetics

Transradial Prostheses
Although no prosthesis can replace the dexterity and sensitivity of the human hand, many options are available to provide the patient with a useful assistive device. Prostheses for the forearm (below-elbow, transradial) amputations include a terminal device, wrist unit, socket, suspension, and control system (Figure 19.6). These prostheses are suitable for people with wrist disarticulations as well as forearm absence to a point just below the anatomic elbow.

Replacement for the missing hand is known as a *terminal device (TD)*. The most common TDs are a prosthetic hand and a hook. Neither provides tactile feedback nor the infinite range of normal hand postures. The *hand* TD resembles the shape, size, and color of the human hand, generally restoring the appearance of the wearer. The two basic types of prosthetic hands are *passive* and *active*. Both are usually covered by a silicone glove that matches the patient's skin color. Some people wear rings and a watch to enhance the life-like appearance. Passive hands, although they lack interior mechanism, are useful, aiding the wearer to stabilize objects, such as a parcel, or a bank check while the user signs it. Inasmuch as most daily activities can be performed with one hand, the person who wears a passive hand can present a convincing appearance. Active hands have a mechanism that allows the wearer to open and close three or more fingers. In most models, the thumb, index, and middle finger move at the base of the finger; the ring and little fingers are passive. The joints within the fingers usually do not move.

Hook TDs have two fingers, one or both of which can move. Hook fingers are more slender than prosthetic hand fingers, thus making it easier for the wearer to see the object being handled. Hooks are usually made of aluminum or steel, with several shape options. They are less expensive than hands, more durable, and lighter in weight. Grasping small objects is less difficult with a hook, while larger items are easier to manage with the larger surface area of the hand. In daily use, most people learn to function with either type of TD.

Movement may be *voluntary opening* (VO) requiring the wearer to open the device voluntarily by action of an attached cable. Relaxing the tension on the cable causes the VO TD to close fully. Grasp force is determined by the mechanism. Alternatively, the TD may be *voluntary closing* (VC). The wearer exerts tension on the cable to close the fingers the desired distance with the intended force, within the limits of the mechanism. Relaxing cable tension causes the TD to open fully. The wearer determines the grasp force, within a much broader range than with a VO TD. Most daily activities can be accomplished with either a VO or a VC TD (Fraser, 1999).

Electric TDs have both VO and VC capabilities. The TD or other components are activated by a battery-powered motor. Electric hands and hooks give most wearers the versatility of directly controlling both the opening and closing of the TD. The motor is controlled either with a *switch* usually placed in the harness that suspends the prosthesis or by means of muscle contraction in the amputation limb. The latter design describes *myoelectric* TDs. The patient wears a socket fitted with one or two sets of electrodes. The electrodes detect the

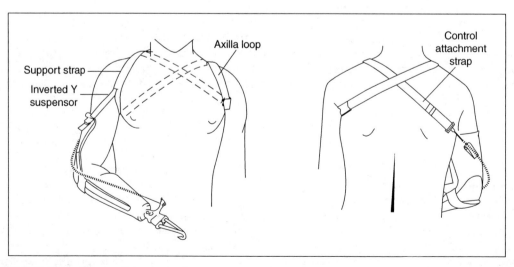

FIGURE 19.6 Transradial prosthesis.

wearer's contraction of the appropriate muscle and transmit the minute electrical signal to a miniature processor which transforms the signal to a form which can activate a motor. The socket is worn without a sock and thus must fit snugly so that each electrode has adequate skin contact. The transradial prosthesis that has a myoelectric TD often does not need a harness (Uellendahl & Riggo-Heelan, 2000; Williams, 2004).

As compared with cable-operated TDs, electric ones are considerably heavier, more expensive, more fragile, and require periodic battery recharging (Edelstein & Berger, 1993; Pylatiuk, Schulz, & Doderline, 2007). Nevertheless, children and adults fitted with myoelectric prostheses wore them for most of the day and preferred them to cable-operated ones.

A *wrist unit* is the receptacle for the TD, permitting interchanging TDs if the wearer has several of them. Wrist units enable the wearer to rotate the TD to place it in any angle of pronation, midposition, and supination. Some patients require a *wrist flexion unit*, in addition to the basic wrist unit. The flexion unit offers several positions of palmar flexion, facilitating placing the TD at the midline of the body. Patients who can abduct and rotate the shoulder can position the TD at the head and torso and thus generally do not need a flexion unit. Most wrist units and flexion units are passive, without cable or electrode control. The wearer uses the opposite hand or leans against a rigid surface to nudge the unit into the desired position.

The transradial *socket* encases the amputation limb. If the limb is relatively long, the upper margin of the socket lies below the elbow. A shorter limb requires a *supracondylar* socket that covers the lower part of the arm. People who wear myoelectric TDs may also be fitted with a supracondylar socket that eliminates the need for a harness to suspend the prosthesis.

Provision for *suspension* is essential. Either the patient will have a supracondylar socket or a Dacron webbing harness to resist the weight of the prosthesis. The most common harness is called *figure of eight* because it resembles the numeral. The harness provides an attachment for the TDs cable, if present. Because a myoelectric TD incorporates electrodes rather than a cable, there is no need for a cable attachment to a harness.

The transradial *control system* enables the wearer to operate the TD. Cable control is achieved when the wearer puts tension on the cable connecting the TD to the harness. Flexing the shoulder on the amputated side causes the TD to move, whether VO or VC. Relaxing the shoulder muscles produces the opposite action. When buttoning a shirt or performing other activities close to the body, the patient will abduct the scapula on the amputated side to tense the cable. Electric switch control is similar, because the switch is usually located in the harness. Myoelectric control involves contracting the appropriate muscle, usually the forearm extensor muscles to open the TD and the forearm flexor muscles to close the TD.

Transhumeral Prostheses

Prostheses for the arm (above-elbow, transhumeral) amputations include a terminal device, wrist unit, forearm section, elbow unit, socket, suspension, and control system.

TD and wrist unit options are identical with those for transradial prostheses. Component weight, however, becomes more important because the patient has a rather poor ability to lift heavy units. The *forearm section* is a plastic shell that replaces the length of the missing forearm. Its lower end is attached to the wrist unit and the upper end joins the elbow unit.

The *elbow unit* is a hinge that permits the patient to place the TD in place. Most elbow units have a cable-controlled locking mechanism. The mechanism alternates locking and unlocking in the same manner that a light switch alternates lighting and darkening a lamp. The transhumeral prosthesis also has a passive turntable with which the wearer can rotate the forearm to the desired position.

As with all sockets, the transhumeral *socket* is plastic, custom made, contacting all portions of the amputation limb. For those with a relatively long amputation limb, the upper margin of the socket lies near the shoulder. Short limbs need a socket that covers part of the chest.

Transhumeral prostheses are *suspended* with a harness, usually a figure-of-eight harness similar to that used on transradial prostheses. The transhumeral harness has additional straps to aid suspension and to enable controlling more components.

Control of the transhumeral prosthesis is usually *dual control*, with two cables attached to the harness. The longer cable extends from the back of the harness, past the elbow, to the TD. When the elbow unit is unlocked, tension on this cable causes the elbow hinge to flex. When the elbow unit is locked, the same cable operates the TD, whether VO or VC. The shorter cable runs from the front of the harness to the elbow lock cable. Most patients exert tension on this cable by lowering the shoulder and simultaneously extending the shoulder in order to lock the elbow. The first motion locks the elbow; the second motion in the same direction unlocks the elbow, in an alternating manner. When the patient wishes to move an object from the table to a shelf, the first step is to flex the elbow with the long cable, angling the prosthesis so the TD reaches the shelf. The next step is to lock the elbow with the short cable. The final step is to lean over the table, grasp the object with the long cable, stand upright, and release the object on the shelf. Fortunately, most practical activities do not require elbow motion. The patient flexes and locks the elbow unit and then can perform many TD maneuvers in the same way as someone wearing a transradial prosthesis.

Some patients are fitted with a *hybrid prosthesis*, which includes a myoelectric TD and a cable-controlled elbow unit. The electrodes are fitted into the socket.

A recent development is targeted muscle reinnervation involving the surgical transfer of nerves from the amputation limb to alternative muscle sites that can be used to control a transhumeral prosthesis (Kuiken et al., 2009). The technology is still experimental; components are not yet available commercially.

Other Prostheses

Partial hand prostheses are available; however, most people who are missing one or more fingers opt not to wear prostheses because the prosthesis covers sensate skin. Some people want cosmetic fingers to restore a more attractive appearance.

Elbow disarticulation prostheses are similar to transhumeral ones, except that the elbow unit is simpler. The patient has the full length of the upper arm and thus can transmit shoulder rotation to the rest of the prosthesis, eliminating the need for a turntable. The prosthesis still requires dual control to operate the elbow hinge, elbow lock, and TD.

Very high levels include *humeral neck amputation* (a very small portion of the upper arm remains), *shoulder disarticulation*, and *forequarter amputation* (absence of the entire arm and some portion of the shoulder girdle and rib cage). Prostheses are cumbersome because they must cover part of the chest. Except for humeral neck amputations, the prostheses also include a passive shoulder joint. Other components and control systems are similar to those for the transhumeral prosthesis. Those with unilateral amputations have a very high rejection rate for these prostheses.

The principal difference between *unilateral* and *bilateral prostheses* is the harness. The unilateral figure-of-eight harness is modified so that the cables from both prostheses can be attached to the harness, thereby enabling the wearer to control both prostheses. Some people prefer to wear matching TDs, while others trade the functional versatility of having two different TD designs for the abnormal appearance. The only contraindicated fitting is a pair of passive hands. People have been successfully fitted with one or both active hands, whether controlled via cable or myoelectrically, as well as various pairs of hooks or hook–hand combinations. The remainder of each prosthesis, including the control system, is the same as for unilateral fitting. Individuals who have a very high amputation may prefer to wear only a prosthesis on the longer amputation limb.

Prosthetic Training

A temporary prosthesis restores some bimanual function and helps the patient to adjust to his or her new reality. If the dominant hand has been amputated, then efforts to change dominance should begin as early as possible. Although some people choose to write with the prosthesis, other tasks involving fine manipulation, such as buttoning, are easier to accomplish with the remaining hand. If both hands are amputated, then early restoration of independent function with or without temporary prostheses is imperative for the patient's emotional health and self-care. The patient learns to depend on visual cues rather than the tactile and proprioceptive feedback that prostheses lack.

Physically, most people with well-healed upper-limb amputations are candidates for a prosthesis. Nevertheless, the individual's emotional status must be considered, as well as available funding, particularly if an electric or myoelectric prosthesis is sought.

CONTROLS TRAINING. The transradial prosthesis has two mechanisms that the patient must control, namely, the terminal device and the wrist unit. If the terminal device is cable operated, the patient should flex the shoulder on the amputated side to apply tensile stress to the cable that, in turn, transmits the stress to the terminal device, whether voluntary opening or voluntary closing (Atkins, 2004). After this skill is well established, the patient learns to operate the terminal device by scapular abduction; this motion is essential for using the terminal device close to the body. If the prosthesis has a myoelectric terminal device, the patient is taught to contract the appropriate muscle to open the terminal device, typically the flexors; extensor contraction usually closes the terminal device.

Most wrist units are passively operated. The patient learns to turn the unit to position the terminal device in the desired position, whether pronation, midposition, or supination. If the unit has a locking mechanism, the wearer is taught how to unlock it, turn the unit, then lock it. Wrist flexion units are generally passive, requiring the patient to nudge its control lever to position the terminal device in the appropriate degree of palmar flexion.

USE TRAINING. Use training refers to instructing the patient in the most basic skills required to function with an upper-limb prosthesis. The purpose of a unilateral prosthesis is to assist the sound hand. Consequently, use training involves presenting the patient with activities that ordinarily are performed bimanually. Most dressing, grooming, eating, and writing activities are accomplished with one hand. The prosthesis is helpful in managing zippers, donning socks and shoes, squeezing toothpaste onto the toothbrush, cutting meat with a knife and fork, cutting paper with scissors, and similar activities.

Vocational and Avocational Activities

Young adults who sustain an upper-limb amputation should be directed to specialized vocational training. This enables the individual either to return to his or her original job or be trained for a new occupation with minimal dependence on adaptive equipment. Amputation is not a deterrent to driving an automobile (Fernandez, Lopez, & Navarro, 2000). Simple adaptations in technique or equipment enable many people to engage in a wide range of sports, from archery to windsurfing (Radocy & Furlong, 2004).

Functional Outcome

Upper-limb prostheses are much more likely to be rejected, as compared with lower-limb prostheses (Raichle et al., 2008). Prosthetic restoration of the appearance and function of the hand is much less successful than that of the leg and foot. With usual clothing, the hand is more visible than the leg. Individuals with bilateral amputations or unilateral transradial amputation are more likely to wear prostheses than those with unilateral transhumeral or higher amputations (Wright, Hagen, & Wood, 1995). Those with a congenital limb deficiency are more likely to wear a prosthesis than those with an acquired amputation (Gaine, Smart, & Bransby-Zachary, 1997). One investigator noted that fewer than half of patients wore their prostheses (Davidson, 2002), while others report higher utilization (Biddiss & Chau, 2007; Dudkiewicz, Gabrielov, Seiv-Ner, Zelig, & Heim, 2004). Greater acceptability of transradial and wrist disarticulation prostheses suggests that patients derive sufficient function from them, while those with higher amputations dislike the weight of the prosthesis and the relative complexity of operating the elbow unit.

Special Considerations for Children

Infants are likely to be fitted with an infant passive hand or a plastic-coated hook at approximately 6 months of age. The first transradial prosthesis will lack a wrist unit, while the initial transhumeral prosthesis will have a passive elbow unit. Both will be suspended with a harness designed to prevent the youngster from removing the prosthesis. Early fitting accustoms the child to bimanual function, such as holding a large stuffed toy or ball. The prosthesis also prevents the infant from relying on the tactile sensation of the anatomic limb. Passive hands with flexed fingers are manufactured to facilitate crawling. At about 12 months of age, most children can learn to operate TD cable control. Those as young as 18 months old can control a myoelectric TD. The delicate mechanism needs to be shielded from such hazardous environments as water, sand, and high-impact play. Most 3-year-olds can use a cable-controlled elbow unit (Shaperman, Landsberger, & Setoguchi, 2003).

Provision for enlarging the socket is important for children's prostheses. As with the lower-limb counterpart, the socket may be either several concentric encasements or a thermoplastic socket in a thick frame. Socket fit is particularly important for those fitted with myoelectric control. Maintaining length symmetry is not as critical for upper-limb prostheses as compared with lower-limb devices. Nevertheless, for aesthetic reasons, the prosthesis should approximate the length of the sound arm. A forearm section resembling an endoskeletal shank facilitates lengthening.

Training the infant involves establishing a consistent wearing schedule, providing opportunities for bimanual usage, and recognizing when prosthetic adjustments are needed (Patton, 2004). Older children engage in a wide range of sports, sometimes utilizing specialized terminal devices (Walker, Coburn, Cottle, Burke, & Talwalkar, 2008; Webster, Levy, Bryant, & Prusakowski, 2001).

Outcome studies suggest that children are likely to wear multiple prostheses to perform specific activities and may prefer simpler prostheses to myoelectric ones (Crandall & Tomhave, 2002).

SUMMARY

Loss of a limb produces a permanent disability that can have a devastating effect on a person's self-image, self-care, and mobility. New amputees have to deal not only with the physical ordeal of the amputation but also its impact on interpersonal relationships, careers, and the stresses of daily living. To handle these challenges, the amputee requires a devoted interdisciplinary team of experts, with each member playing a vital role in the amputee's recovery. This team of physicians, nurses, physical and occupational therapists, psychologists, recreational therapists, vocational counselors, social workers, and certified prosthetists helps the amputee overcome the many physical and emotional barriers he or she faces. Rehabilitation following an amputation helps the amputee come to terms with an altered self-image, live with the new realities, and return to the highest level of function and independence possible.

REFERENCES

Asano, M., Rushton, P., Miller, W. C., & Deathe, B. A. (2008). Predictors of quality of life among individuals who have a lower limb amputation. *Prosthetics and Orthotics International, 32,* 231–243.

Atkins, D. (2004). Functional skills training with body-powered and externally powered prostheses. In R. H. Meier & D. J. Atkins (Eds.), *Functional restoration of adults and children with upper extremity amputation* (pp. 139–158). New York: Demos Medical Publishing.

Aulivola, B., Hile, C. N., Hamdan, A. D., Sheahan, M. G., Veraldi, J. R., Skillmanm, J. J., et al. (2004). Major lower extremity amputation: Outcome of a modern series. *Archives of Surgery, 139,* 393–399.

Baars, E. C. T., & Geertzen, J. H. B. (2005). Literature review of the possible advantages of silicon liner socket use in trans-tibial prostheses. *Prosthetics and Orthotics International, 29,* 27–37.

Berge, J. S., Czerniecki, J. M., & Klute, G. K. (2005). Efficacy of shock-absorbing versus rigid pylons for impact reduction in transtibial amputees based on laboratory, field, and outcome metrics. *Journal of Rehabilitation Research and Development, 42*, 795–808.

Biddiss, E., & Chau, T. (2007). Upper-limb prosthetics: Critical factors in device abandonment. *American Journal of Physical Medicine and Rehabilitation, 86*, 977–987.

Bilodeau, S., Hebert, R., & Destrosiers, J. (2000). Lower limb prosthesis utilization by elderly amputees. *Prosthetics and Orthotics International, 24*, 126–132.

Boonstra, A. M., Rijnders, L. J., Groothoff, J. W., & Eisma, W. H. (2000). Children with congenital deficiencies or acquired amputations of the lower limbs: Functional aspects. *Prosthetics and Orthotics International, 24*, 19–27.

Boulias, C., Meikle, B., Pauley, T., & Devlin, M. (2006). Return to driving after lower-extremity amputation. *Archives of Physical Medicine and Rehabilitation, 87*, 1183–1188.

Boulton, A. J., Kirsner, R. S., & Vileikyte, L. (2004). Clinical practice. Neuropathic diabetic foot ulcers. *New England Journal of Medicine, 351*, 48–55.

Brunelli, S., Averna, T., Porcacchia. P., Paolucci, S., DiMeo, F. B., & Traballesi, M. (2006). Functional status and factors influencing the rehabilitation outcomes of people affected by above-knee amputation and hemiparesis. *Archives of Physical Medicine Rehabilitation, 87*, 995–1000.

Bussmann, J. B., Schrauwen, H. J., & Stam, H. J. (2008). Daily physical activity and heart rate response in people with a unilateral traumatic transtibial amputation. *Archives of Physical Medicine and Rehabilitation, 89*, 430–434.

Chen, M. C., Lee, S. S., Hsieh, Y. L., Wu, S. J., Lai, C. S., & Lin, S. D. (2008). Influencing factors of outcomes after lower-limb amputation: A five-year review in a plastic surgical department. *Annals of Plastic Surgery, 61*, 314–318.

Crandall, R. C., & Tomhave, W. (2002). Pediatric unilateral below-elbow amputees: Retrospective analysis of 34 patients given multiple prosthetic options. *Journal of Pediatric Orthopedics, 22*, 380–383.

Czerniecki, J. M., & Ehde, D. M. (2003). Chronic pain after lower extremity amputation. *Critical Reviews in Physical and Rehabilitation Medicine, 15*, 3–4.

Davidson, J. (2002). A survey of the satisfaction of upper limb amputees with their prostheses, their lifestyles, and their abilities. *Journal of Hand Therapy, 15*, 62–70.

Davies, D., & Datta, D. (2003). Mobility outcome following unilateral lower limb amputation. *Prosthetics and Orthotics International, 27*, 186–190.

Deans, S. A., McFadyen, A. K., & Rose, P. J. (2008). Physical activity and quality of life: A study of a lower-limb amputee population. *Prosthetics and Orthotics International, 32*, 186–200.

Devlin, M., Sinclair, L. B., Colman, D., Parsons, J., Nizio, H., & Campbell, J. E. (2002). Patient preference and gait efficiency in a geriatric population with transfemoral amputation using a free-swinging versus a locked prosthetic knee joint. *Archives of Physical Medicine and Rehabilitation, 83*, 246–249.

Diabetes Control and Complications Research Group. (1993). The effect of intensive treatment of diabetes on the development and progression of long-term complications in insulin-dependent diabetes mellitus. *New England Journal of Medicine, 329*, 977–986.

Dickhaut, S. C., DeLee, J. C., & Page, C. P. (1984). Nutritional status: Importance in predicting wound healing after amputation. *Journal of Bone and Joint Surgery, 66A*, 71–75.

Dillingham, T. R., & Pezzin, L. E. (2008). Rehabilitation setting and associated mortality and medical stability among persons with amputations. *Archives of Physical Medicine and Rehabilitation, 89*, 1038–1045.

Dillingham, T. R., Pezzin, L. E., & MacKenzie, E. J. (2002). Limb amputation and limb deficiency: Epidemiology and recent trends in the United States. *Southern Medical Journal, 95*, 875–883.

Dillingham, T. R., Pezzin, L. E., MacKenzie, E. J., & Burgess, A. R. (2001). Use and satisfaction with prosthetic devices among persons with trauma-related amputations: A long-term outcome study. *American Journal of Physical Medicine and Rehabilitation, 80*, 563–571.

Dougherty, P. J. (2001).Transtibial amputees from the Vietnam War: Twenty-eight-year follow-up. *Journal of Bone and Joint Surgery, 83A*, 383–390.

Dougherty, P. J. (2003). Long-term follow-up of unilateral transfemoral amputees from the Vietnam war. *Journal of Trauma, 54*, 718–723.

Dudkiewicz, I., Gabrielov, R., Seiv-Ner, I., Zelig, G., & Heim, M. (2004). Evaluation of prosthetic usage in upper limb amputees. *Disability & Rehabilitation, 26*, 60–63.

Edelstein, J. E., & Berger, N. (1993). Performance comparison among children fitted with myoelectric and body-powered hands. *Archives of Physical Medicine and Rehabilitation, 74*, 376–380.

Ehde, D. M., Czerniecki, J. M., Smith, D. G., Campbell, K. M., Edwards, W. T., Jensen, M. P., et al. (2000). Chronic phantom sensations, phantom pain, residual limb pain and other regional pain after lower limb amputation. *Archives of Physical Medicine and Rehabilitation, 81*, 1039–1044.

Fernandez, A., Lopez, M. J., & Navarro, R. (2000). Performance of persons with juvenile-onset amputation in driving motor vehicles. *Archives of Physical Medicine and Rehabilitation, 81*, 288–291.

Fisk, J. R., & Smith, D. G. (2004). The limb-deficient child. In D. G. Smith, J. W. Michaels, & J. H. Bowker (Eds.), *Atlas of amputations and limb deficiencies* (3rd ed., pp. 773–777). Rosemont, IL: American Academy of Orthopaedic Surgeons.

Fletcher, D. D., Andrews, K. L., Butters, M. A., Jacobsen, S. J., Rowland, C. M., & Hallett, J. W. (2001). Rehabilitation of the geriatric vascular amputee patient: A population-based study. *Archives of Physical Medicine and Rehabilitation, 82*, 776–779.

Flor, H. (2002). Phantom–limb pain: Characteristics, causes and treatment. *Lancet Neurology, 1*, 182–189.

Fraser, C. M. (1999). An evaluation of the use made of cosmetic and functional prostheses by unilateral upper limb amputees. *Prosthetics and Orthotics International, 22*, 216–223.

Friedmann, L. (1990). Rehabilitation of the lower extremity amputee. In F. J. Kottke & J. F. Lehmann (Eds.), *Krusen's handbook of physical medicine and rehabilitation* (4th ed., pp. 1024–1969). Philadelphia, PA: W. B. Saunders Company.

Gaebler-Spira, D., & Uellendahl, J. (1999). Pediatric limb deficiencies. In G. Molnar (Ed.), *Pediatric rehabilitation* (3rd ed., pp.331–350). Philadelphia, PA: Hanley & Belfus.

Gailey, R., Allen, K., Castles, J., Kucharik, J., & Roeder, M. (2008). Review of secondary physical conditions associated with lower-limb amputation and long-term prosthetic use. *Journal of Rehabilitation Research and Development, 45*, 15–30.

Gaine, W. J., Smart, C., & Bransby-Zachary, M. (1997). Upper limb traumatic amputees: Review of prosthetic use. *Journal of Hand Surgery, 22*, 73–76.

Gajewski, D., & Granville, R. (2006). The United State Armed Forces Amputee Care Program. *Journal of American Academy of Orthopedic Surgeons, 14*, S183–S187.

Gard, S. A., & Konz, R. J. (2003). The effect of a shock-absorbing pylon on the gait of persons with unilateral transtibial amputation. *Journal of Rehabilitation Research and Development, 40*, 109–124.

Gauthier-Gagnon, C., Grise, M. C., & Potvin, D. (1999). Enabling factors related to prosthetic use by people with transtibial and transfemoral amputation. *Archives of Physical Medicine and Rehabilitation, 80*, 706–713.

Graham, L. E., Datta, D., Heller, B., & Howitt, J. (2007). A comparative study of conventional and energy-storing prosthetic feet in high-functioning transfemoral amputees. *Archives of Physical Medicine and Rehabilitation, 88*, 801–806.

Hafner, B. J. (2005). Perceptive evaluation of prosthetic foot and ankle systems. *Journal of Prosthetics and Orthotics, 17*, 842–846.

Hafner, B. J., Willingham, L. L., Buell, N. C., Allyn, K. J., & Smith, D. G. (2007). Evaluation of function, performance, and preference as transfemoral amputees transition from mechanical to microprocessor control of the prosthetic knee. *Archives of Physical Medicine and Rehabilitation, 88*, 207–217.

Hakimi, K., Eftekhari, N., & Czerniecki, J. (2008). Amputation rehabilitation: Epidemiology, preprosthetic management and complications. In B. J. O'Young, M. A. Young, & S. A. Stiens (Eds.), *Physical medicine and rehabilitation secrets* (3rd ed., pp. 267–276). Philadelphia, PA: Mosby Elsevier.

HCFA Common Procedure Coding System. (2001). Washington: US Government Printing Office [Chapter 5.3.].

Hoffman, R. D., Saltzman, C. L., & Buckwalter, J. A. (2002). Outcome of lower extremity malignancy survivors treated with transfemoral amputation. *Archives of Physical Medicine and Rehabilitation, 83*, 177–182.

Hsu, M. J., Nielsen, D. H., Lin-Chan, S. J., & Shurr, D. (2006). The effects of prosthetic foot design on physiologic measurements, self-selected walking velocity, and physical activity in people with transtibial amputation. *Archives of Physical Medicine and Rehabilitation, 87*, 123–129.

International Standards Organization. (1989). *ISO 8548–1; Prosthetics and orthotics-Limb deficiencies. Part 1: Method of describing limb deficiencies present at birth*. Geneva, Switzerland: Author.

Isakov, E., Keren, O., & Benjuya, N. (2000). Trans-tibial amputee gait: Time-distance parameters and EMG activity. *Prosthetics and Orthotics International, 24*, 216–220.

Johansson, J. L., Sherrill, D. M., Riley, P. O., Bonato, P., & Herr, H. (2005). A clinical comparison of variable-damping and mechanically passive prosthetic knee devices. *American Journal of Physical Medicine and Rehabilitation, 84*, 563–575.

Jones, M. E., Bashford, G. M., & Mann, J. M. (1997). Weight bearing and velocity in trans-tibial and trans-femoral amputees. *Prosthetics and Orthotics International, 21*, 183–186.

Kahle, J. T., Highsmith, M. J., & Hubbard, S. L. (2008). Comparison of nonmicroprocessor knee mechanism versus C-Leg on Prosthesis Evaluation questionnaire, stumbles, falls, walking tests, stair descent, and knee preference. *Journal of Rehabilitation Research and Development, 45*, 1–14.

Kaufman, K. R., Levine, J. A., Brey, R. H., McCrady, S. K., Padgett, D. J., & Joyner, M. J. (2008). Energy expenditure and activity of transfemoral amputees using mechanical and microprocessor-controlled prosthetic knees. *Archives of Physical Medicine and Rehabilitation, 89*, 1380–1385.

Kauzlaric, N., Kauzlaric, K. S., & Kolundzic, R. (2007). Prosthetic rehabilitation of persons with lower limb amputation due to tumour. *European Journal of Cancer Care, 16*, 238–243.

Kuiken, T. A., Li, G., Lock, B. A., Lipschultz, R. D, Miller, L. A. Stubblefield, K. A., et al. (2009). Targeted muscle reinnervation for real-time myoelectric control of multifunction artificial arms. *Journal of American Medical Association, 301*, 619–628.

MacKenzie, E. J., Bosse, M. J., Castillo, R. C., Smith, D. G., Webb, L. X., Kellam, J. F., et al. (2004). Functional outcomes following trauma-related lower-extremity amputation. *Journal of Bone and Joint Surgery: American Volume, 86A*, 1636–1645.

MacNeill, H. L., Devlin, M., Pauley, T., & Yudin, A. (2008). Long-term outcomes and survival of patients with bilateral transtibial amputations after rehabilitation. *American Journal of Physical Medicine and Rehabilitation, 87*, 189–196.

Marinakis, G. N. (2004). Interlimb symmetry of traumatic unilateral transtibial amputees wearing two different prosthetic feet in the early rehabilitation stage. *Journal of Rehabilitation Research and Development, 41*, 581–590.

Marzen-Groller, K., & Bartman, K. (2005). Building a successful support group for post-amputation patients. *Journal of Vascular Nursing, 23*, 42–45.

McNealy, L. L., & Gard, S. A. (2008). Effect of prosthetic ankle units on the gait of persons with bilateral trans-femoral amputations. *Prosthetics and Orthotics International, 32*, 111–126.

Meier, R. H., & Atkins, D. J. (Eds.) (2004). *Functional restoration of adults and children with upper extremity amputation.* New York: Demos Medical Publishing.

Miller, W. C., & Deathe, A. B. (2004). A prospective study examining balance confidence among individuals with lower limb amputation. *Disability and Rehabilitation, 26*, 875–881.

Miller, W. C., Speechley, M., & Deathe, B. (2001). The prevalence and risk factors of falling and fear of falling among lower extremity amputees. *Archives of Physical Medicine and Rehabilitation, 82*, 1031–1037.

Munin, M. C., Guzman, M. C. E., Boninger, M. L., Fitzgerald, S. G., Penrod, L. E., & Singh, J. (2001). Predictive factors for successful early prosthetic ambulation among lower-limb amputees. *Journal of Rehabilitation, Research and Development, 38*, 379–384.

Murdoch, G., & Wilson, A. B. (Eds.). (1996). *Amputation: Surgical practice and patient management.* St. Louis, MO: Butterworth-Heinemann Medical.

Nadollek, H., Brauer, S., & Isles, R. (2002). Outcomes after trans-tibial amputation: The relationship between quiet stance ability, strength of hip abductor muscles and gait. *Physiotherapy Research International, 7*, 203–214.

Nagarajan, R., Neglia, J. P., Clohisy, D. R., Yasui, Y., Greenberg, M., Hudson, M., et al. (2003). Education, employment, insurance, and marital status among 694 survivors of pediatric lower extremity bone tumors: A report from the Childhood Cancer Survivor Study. *Cancer, 97*, 2554–2564.

Nair, A., Hanspal, R. S., Zahedi, M. S., Saif, M., & Fisher, K. (2008). Analyses of prosthetic episodes in lower limb amputees. *Prosthetics and Orthotics International, 32*, 42–49.

Nehler, M. R., Coll, J. R., Hiatt, W. R., Regensteiner, J. G., Schnickel, G. T., Klenke, W. A., et al. (2003). Functional outcome in a contemporary series of major lower extremity amputations. *Journal of Vascular Surgery, 38*, 7–14.

Nolan, L., & Lees, A. (2000). The functional demands on the intact limb during walking for active trans-femoral and trans-tibial amputees. *Prosthetics and Orthotics International, 24*, 117–125.

Nolan, L., & Lees, A. (2007). The influence of lower limb amputation level on the approach in the amputee long jump. *Journal of Sports Sciences, 25*, 393–401.

Nolan, L., & Patritti, B. L. (2008). The take-off phase in transtibial amputee high jump. *Prosthetics and Orthotics International, 32*, 160–171.

Nolan, L., Patritti, B. L., & Simpson, K. J. (2006). A biomechanical analysis of the long-jump technique of elite female amputee athletes. *Medicine and Science in Sports and Exercise, A38*, 1829–1835.

Nolan, L., Wit, A., Dudzinski, K., Lees, A., Lake, M., & Wychowanski, M. (2003). Adjustments in gait symmetry with walking speed in trans-femoral and trans-tibial amputees. *Gait & Posture, 17,* 142–151.

Orendurff, M., Segal, A. D., Klute, G. K., McDowell, M. L. Pecoraro, J. A., & Czerniecki, J. M. (2006). Gait efficiency using the C-leg. *Journal of Rehabilitation Research and Development, 43,* 239–246.

Ovelmen-Levitt, J. (1988). Abnormal physiology of the dorsal horn as related to the deafferentation syndrome. *Applied Neurophysiology, 51,* 104–116.

Patton, J. G. (2004). Training the child with a unilateral upper-extremity prosthesis. In R. H. Meier & D. G. Atkins (Eds.), *Functional restoration of adults and children with upper extremity amputation* (pp. 297–316). New York: Demos Medical Publishing.

Paysant, J., Beyaert, C., Datie, A. M., Martinet, N., & Andre, J. J. (2006). Influence of terrain on metabolic and temporal gait characteristics of unilateral transtibial amputees. *Journal of Rehabilitation Research and Development, 43,* 153–160.

Perry, J., Burnfield, J. M., Newsam, C. J., & Conley, P. (2004). Energy expenditure and gait characteristics of a bilateral amputee walking with C-leg prostheses compared with stubby and conventional articulating prostheses. *Archives of Physical Medicine and Rehabilitation, 85,* 1711–1717.

Pezzin, L. E., Dillingham, T. R., & MacKenzie, E. J. (2000). Rehabilitation and the long-term outcomes of persons with trauma-related amputations. *Archives of Physical Medicine and Rehabilitation, 81,* 292–300.

Pezzin, L. E., Dillingham, T. R., MacKenzie, E. J., Ephraim, P., & Rossbach, P. (2004). Use and satisfaction with prosthetic limb devices and related services. *Archives of Physical Medicine and Rehabilitation, 85,* 723–729.

Pylatiuk, C., Schulz, S., & Doderline, L. (2007). Results of an Internet survey of myoelectric prosthetic hand users. *Prosthetics and Orthotics International, 31,* 362–370.

Radocy, R., & Furlong, A. (2004). Recreation and sports adaptations. In R. H. Meier & D. J. Atkins (Eds.), *Functional restoration of adults and children with upper extremity amputation* (pp. 251–274). New York: Demos Medical Publishing.

Raichle, K. A., Hanley, M. A., Molton, I., Kadel, N. J., Campbell, K., Phelps, E., et al. (2008). Prosthesis use in persons with lower- and upper-limb amputation. *Journal of Rehabilitation Research and Development, 45,* 961–972.

Rau, B., Bonvin, F., & de Bie, R. (2007). Short-term effect of physiotherapy rehabilitation on functional performance of lower limb amputees. *Prosthetics and Orthotics International, 31,* 258–270.

Rheinstein, J., Wong, C. K., & Edelstein, J. E. (2006). Post-operative management. In K. Carroll & J. E. Edelstein (Eds.), *Prosthetics and patient management: A comprehensive clinical approach* (pp. 15–31). Thorofare, NJ: Slack.

Rogers, J. P., Strike, S. C., & Wallace, E. S. (2004). The effect of prosthetic torsional stiffness on the golf swing kinematics of a left and a right-sided trans-tibial amputee. *Prosthetics and Orthotics International, 28,* 121–131.

Rossi, R., Alexander, M., & Cuccurullo, S. (2004). Pediatric rehabilitation. In S. J. Cuccurullo (Ed.), *Physical medicine and rehabilitation boardreview* (pp. 645–741). New York: Demos Medical Publishing.

Sapin, E., Goujon, H., de Almeida, F., Fode, P., & Lavaste, F. (2008). Functional gait analysis of trans-femoral amputees using two different single-axis prosthetic knees with hydraulic swing-phase control: Kinematic and kinetic comparison of two prosthetic knees. *Prosthetics and Orthotics International, 32,* 201–218.

Schmalz, T., Blumentritt, S., & Marx, B. (2007). Biomechanical analysis of stair ambulation in lower limb amputees. *Gait & Posture, 25,* 267–278.

Schoppen, T., Boonstra, A., Groothoff, J. W., deVries, J., Goeken, L. N., & Eisma, W. H. (2001). Factors related to successful job reintegration of people with a lower limb amputation. *Archives of Physical Medicine and Rehabilitation, 82,* 1425–1431.

Schoppen, T., Boonstra, A., Groothoff, J. W., deVries, J., Goeken, L. N., & Eisma, W. H. (2002). Job satisfaction and health experience of people with a lower-limb amputation in comparison with healthy colleagues. *Archives of Physical Medicine and Rehabilitation, 83,* 628–634.

Schoppen, T., Boonstra, A., Groothoff, J. W., deVries, J., Goeken, L. N., & Eisma, W. H. (2003). Physical, mental, and social predictors of functional outcome in unilateral lower-limb amputees. *Archives of Physical Medicine and Rehabilitation, 84,* 803–811.

Schuch, C. M., & Pritham, C. H. (1994). International Forum—International Standards Organization Terminology: Application to Prosthetics and Orthotics. *Journal of Prosthetics and Orthotics, 6,* 29–33.

Segal, A. D., Orendurff, M. S., Klute, G. K., MacDowell, M. L., Pecoraro, J. A., & Shofer, J. (2006). Kinematic and kinetic comparisons of transfemoral amputee gait using C-Leg and Mauch SNS prosthetic knees. *Journal of Rehabilitation Research and Development, 43*, 857–870.

Selles, R. W., Janssens, P. J., Jongenengel, C. D., & Bussmann, J. B. (2005). A randomized controlled trial comparing functional outcome and cost efficiency of a total surface-bearing socket versus a conventional patellar tendon-bearing socket in transtibial amputees. *Archives of Physical Medicine and Rehabilitation, 86*, 154–161.

Seymour, R., Engbretson, B., Kott, K., Ordway, N., Brooks, G., Crannell, J. et al. (2007). Comparison between the C-Leg microprocessor-controlled prosthetic knee and nonmicroprocessor-controlled prosthetic knees: A preliminary study of energy expenditure, obstacle course performance and quality of life survey. *Prosthetics and Orthotics International, 31*, 51–61.

Shaperman, J., Landsberger, S., & Setoguchi, Y. (2003). Early upper limb prosthetic fitting: When and what do we fit? *Journal of Prosthetics and Orthotics, 15*, 11–19.

Smurr, L. M., Gulick, K., Yancosek, K., & Ganz, O. (2008). Managing the upper extremity amputee: A protocol for success. *Journal of Hand Therapy, 21*, 160–175.

Stanger, M. (2000). Limb deficiencies and amputations. In S. K. Campbell, D. W. Vander Linden, & R. J. Palisano (Eds.), *Physical therapy for children* (2nd ed., pp. 370–397). Philadelphia, PA: W. B. Saunders Company.

Su, P. F., Gard, S. A., Lipschultz, R. D., & Kuiken, T. A. (2008). Differences in gait characteristics between persons with bilateral transtibial amputations, due to peripheral vascular disease and trauma, and able-bodied ambulators. *Archives of Physical Medicine and Rehabilitation, 89*, 1386–1394.

Uellendahl, J. E., & Riggo-Heelan, J. (2000). Prosthetic management of the upper limb deficient child. *Physical Medicine and Rehabilitation: State of the Art Reviews, 11*, 221–235.

Uellendahl, J. E. (2004). Bilateral upper limb prostheses. In D. G. Smith, J. W. Michael, & J. H. Bowker (Eds.), *Atlas of amputations and limb deficiencies* (3rd ed., pp. 311–326). Rosemont, IL: American Academy of Orthopedic Surgeons.

Underwood, H. A., Tokuno, C. D., & Eng, J. J. (2004). A comparison of two prosthetic feet on the multi-joint and multi-plane kinetic gait compensations in individuals with unilateral trans-tibial amputation. *Clinical Biomechanics (Bristol, Avon), 19*, 609–616.

Uustal, H., & Baerga, E. (2004). Prosthetics and orthotics. In S. J. Cuccurullo (Ed.), *Physical medicine and rehabilitation board review* (pp. 409–487). New York: Demos Medical Publishing.

Van Dorsten, B. (2004). Integrating psychological and medical care: Practice recommendations for amputation. In R. H. Meier & D. J. Atkins (Eds.), *Functional restoration of adults and children with upper extremity amputation* (pp. 73–88). New York: Demos Medical Publishing.

Vickers, D. R., Palk, C., McIntosh, A. S., & Beatty, K. T. (2008). Elderly unilateral transtibial amputee gait on an inclined walkway: A biomechanical analysis. *Gait & Posture, 27*, 518–529.

Vrieling, A. H., van Keeken, H. G., Schoppen, T., Otten, E., Halbertsma, J. P., Hof, A. L., et al. (2007). Obstacle crossing in lower limb amputees. *Gait & Posture, 26*, 587–594.

Vrieling, A. H., van Keeken, H. G., Schoppen, T., Otten, E., Halbertsma, J. P., Hof, A. L., et al. (2008a). Gait initiation in lower limb amputees. *Gait & Posture, 27*, 423–430.

Vrieling, A. H., van Keeken, H. G., Schoppen, T., Otten, E., Halbertsma, J. P., Hof, A. L., et al. (2008b). Uphill and downhill walking in unilateral lower limb amputees. *Gait & Posture, 28*, 235–242.

Walker, J. L., Coburn, T. R., Cottle, W., Burke, C., & Talwalkar, V. R. (2008). Recreational terminal devices for children with upper extremity amputations. *Journal of Pediatric Orthopedics, 28*, 271–273.

Waters, R. L., & Mulroy, S. (1999). The energy expenditure of normal and pathological gait. *Gait & Posture, 9*, 207–231.

Webster, J. B., Levy, C. E., Bryant, P. R., & Prusakowski, P. E. (2001). Sports and recreation for persons with limb deficiency. *Archives of Physical Medicine and Rehabilitation, 82*, S38–S44.

Williams, T. W. (2004). Control of powered upper extremity prostheses. In R. H. Meier & D. J. Atkins (Eds.), *Functional restoration of adults and children with upper extremity amputation* (pp. 207–224). New York: Demos Medical Publishing.

Wong, C. K., & Edelstein, J. E. (2000). Unna and elastic postoperative dressings: Comparison of their effects on function of adults with amputation and vascular disease. *Archives of Physical Medicine and Rehabilitation, 81*, 191–198.

Wright, D. A., Marks, L., & Payne, R. C. (2008). A comparative study of the physiological costs of walking in ten bilateral amputees. *Prosthetics and Orthotics International, 32*, 57–67.

Wright, T. W., Hagen, A. D., & Wood, M. B. (1995). Prosthetic usage in major upper extremity amputations. *Journal of Hand Surgery, 20*, 619–622.

Wu, Y. J., Chen, S. Y., & Lin, M. C. (2001). Energy expenditure of wheeling and walking during prosthetic rehabilitation in a woman with bilateral transfemoral amputations. *Archives of Physical Medicine and Rehabilitation, 82,* 265–269.

Yazicioglu, K., Taskaynatan, M. A., Guzelkucuk, U., & Tugcu, I. (2007). Effect of playing football (soccer) on balance, strength, and quality of life in unilateral below-knee amputees. *American Journal of Physical Medicine and Rehabilitation, 86,* 800–805.

Ziegler, G. K., MacKenzie, E. J., Ephraim, P. L., Travison, T. G., & Brookmeyer, R. (2008). Estimating the prevalence of limb loss in the United States: 2005 to 2050. *Archives of Physical Medicine and Rehabilitation, 89,* 422–429.

Zmitrewicz, R. J., Neptune, R., Walden, J. G., Rogers, W. E., & Bosker, G. W. (2006). The effect of foot and ankle prosthetic components on braking and propulsive impulses during transtibial amputee gait. *Archives of Physical Medicine and Rehabilitation, 87,* 1334–1339.

20

Organ Transplantation and Rehabilitation

Jeffrey M. Cohen, MD, Mark Young, MD, and Bryan O'Young, MD

INTRODUCTION

Life-saving treatment of disease by organ transplantation has become a standard part of medical practice. The past 25 years have seen considerable advances in the field of organ transplantation. This has been the result of advances in surgical techniques, technological improvements, and the discovery of potent immunosuppressive drugs that reduced rejection of the grafted organ. Today, there are more than 19 transplantable organ systems. The focus of this chapter will be on the four most common solid organ transplants seen in rehabilitation medicine: liver, renal, cardiac, and pulmonary.

LIVER TRANSPLANTATION

Liver transplantation is the therapeutic option of choice for patients with acute and chronic end-stage liver disease. Liver disease can be either acute (fulminant or subfulminant failure) or chronic (decompensated cirrhosis). In the pretransplantation era, liver failure was nearly universally fatal, with mortalities from fulminant hepatic failure of 80–90% and 1-year mortality in decompensated cirrhosis of more than 50%. The first attempts at human liver transplantation were made in 1963 by Starzl and colleagues (Starzl, Klintmalm, Porter, Iwatsuki, & Schroter, 1981; see also Keeffe, 2001). However, the first successful liver transplantation was not achieved until 1967 (Keeffe, 2001). Over the past several decades, liver transplantation has evolved from being primarily an experimental procedure with limited success, to a routine operation that provides excellent survival rates for patients with irreversible acute or chronic end-stage liver disease. Presently, survival rate of patients who had liver transplantation is more than 85% at 1 year and more than 70% at 5 years (Koffron & Stein, 2008).

The development of immunosuppressive agents was a critically important step in the growth of solid organ transplantation. The early 1980s witnessed the discovery of cyclosporine, which led to an increased survival rate after liver transplantation, from 30% to more than 70% (Starzl et al., 1981). The development of newer immunosuppressive agents such as tacrolimus was associated with further improvements in 1-year graft and patient survival rates. Its use was associated with fewer episodes of acute cellular and steroid-resistant rejection (The U.S. Multicenter FK 506 Liver Study Group, 1994).

Indications

Patients with liver failure who undergo liver transplantation fall into two major categories: acute fulminant hepatic failure and chronic liver failure (Table 20.1; Rudow and Goldstein, 2008). This population varies greatly in terms of the extent of their debility. Acute fulminant hepatic failure may be the result of a toxic ingestion (e.g., acetaminophen overdose) or secondary to viral hepatitis. As the liver failure occurs suddenly, in otherwise healthy patients, these patients often present with limited functional deficits. In contrast, patients experiencing chronic liver failure have usually lived with their disease for a number of years. They have experienced a generalized decline in their functional abilities resulting in a state of severe deconditioning and fatigue. Chronic liver failure is most commonly secondary to chronic hepatitis C and alcoholic liver disease (Keeffe, 2001). Other etiologies of chronic liver

TABLE 20.1 *Indications for Liver Transplant*

1. Acute liver failure
Drug induced
Toxins
Hypersensitivity
Fulminant hepatitis/necrosis

2. Chronic liver failure

Cholestatic disorders
Primary biliary cirrhosis
Biliary atresia
Alagille syndrome
Familial cholestasis
Secondary biliary cirrhosis
Primary sclerosing cholangitis

Parenchymal cirrhosis
Cryptogenic cirrhosis
Chronic hepatitis B and C
Alcoholic cirrhosis
Congenital hepatic fibrosis
Autoimmune hepatitis

Metabolic liver disease
Metabolic defect in the liver resulting in end-stage liver disease:
Alpha1 antitrypsin deficiency
Wilson's disease
Tyrosinemia
Cystic fibrosis
Familial amyloidosis

Malignancies
Hepatocellular carcinoma
Hepatoblastoma
Hemangioendothelioma (confined to the liver)
Cholangiocarcinoma (new research protocols)

Vascular disease
Budd-Chiari syndrome
Portal vein thrombosis
Giant hepatic hemangioma

Source: Rudow, D. L., & Goldstein, M. J. (2008). Critical care management of the liver transplant recipient. *Critical Care Nursing Quarterly*, 31, 233. Reprinted by permission of the publisher.

failure include hepatitis B, primary biliary cirrhosis, primary sclerosing cholangitis, autoimmune hepatitis, cholestatic disorders (disorders in which the excretory function of the liver is compromised), metabolic diseases such as hemochromatosis and Wilson's disease, and hepatocellular carcinoma. In the pediatric population, the most common indications for liver transplantation are biliary atresia and alpha 1-antitrypsin deficiency.

Types of Liver Transplantation

Liver transplantation involves the replacement of a diseased or injured liver with a new organ (allograft). The allograft mostly involves any one of the following: taking a whole organ from a deceased donor, a split liver graft from a deceased donor, or a partial graft from a live donor. Living donor-liver transplantation is a planned surgical procedure in which a healthy donor donates part of his or her liver.

Selection for Liver Transplantation

The following factors are assessed in order to determine whether a patient is suitable for liver transplantation: etiology and stage of the liver disease, patient's psychosocial status, and potential contraindications to surgery. Clinically, the following conditions warrant consideration for liver transplantation (Lopez & Martin, 2006):

1. Fulminant hepatic failure (severe impairment of liver function in the absence of preexisting liver disease)
2. Intractable ascites (an abnormal accumulation of fluid in the abdomen)
3. Refractory encephalopathy (changes in consciousness, mentation, and behavior seen in patients with advanced liver disease due to the accumulation of wastes from protein breakdown)
4. Recurrent variceal bleeding (bleeding from dilated or variceal veins, usually esophageal varices, due to end-stage liver failure)
5. Severe deficits in the ability of the liver to perform its synthetic functions (production of the protein albumin and clotting factors). This leads to severe malnutrition and defects in the ability of the blood to clot in the usual time period.

Contraindications to liver transplantation include uncontrolled infection, metastatic hepatobiliary or extrahepatic cancers, the presence of AIDS (as posttransplant immunosuppression accelerates the course of AIDS), multiorgan failure, and irreversible brain damage (Koffron & Stein, 2008).

Pre-Liver Transplantation Medical Issues

Laboratory abnormalities commonly associated with hepatocellular dysfunction include anemia and leukopenia (a lower-than-normal amount of white blood cells, also known as leukocytes, in the blood), which places an individual at an increased risk of infection. Other laboratory abnormalities include thrombocytopenia (abnormally low number of platelets in the bloodstream) and an increased prothrombin time—a measure of the amount of time it takes for the liquid portion of one's blood (plasma) to clot.

Whereas a minority of patients (e.g., those with acute fulminant liver failure) will have only a few days of physical inactivity prior to transplantation, the majority live with their diseased liver for a prolonged period of time before transplantation occurs. They present as severely malnourished and deconditioned. The following are some of the salient features to watch out for, when working with chronically debilitated liver-failure patients prior to transplantation.

Cachexia

The etiology of cachexia (severe muscle wasting) in liver disease is multifactorial. Cirrhosis of the liver is considered a catabolic disease and can lead to profound loss of muscle mass. The prevalence of cachexia has been found to be as high as 80% in patients with cirrhosis (Harrison, McKiernan, & Neuberger, 1997). Because of the dysfunction of the diseased liver in glycogen storage and gluconeogenesis, muscle protein and fat are broken down for energy use. These result in weakness and weight loss because the need to use protein and fat for energy further decreases protein's availability for muscle maintenance. Other contributing factors to cachexia and protein-energy malnutrition are anorexia (decreased dietary intake) and malabsorption (steatorrhea). Diseased bile ducts results in reduced synthesis and secretion of bile salts into the intestines, making fat and fat-soluble vitamin absorption difficult. Fat malabsorption, or steatorrhea, occurs and is prevalent in 40–50% of cirrhotic patients (Munoz, 1991). Cachexia has been found to be predictive of poor outcomes after liver transplantation (Vintro, Krasnoff, & Painter, 2002).

Osteoporosis

Osteoporosis is a disease characterized by a decrease in bone mass and density. It is the most common bone disorder in persons with chronic liver disease, with a prevalence documented as 15–40% (Crosbie, Freaney, McKenna, & Hegarty, 1999). Ingestion of alcohol can directly and indirectly promote bone loss. In addition, poor diet and physical inactivity contribute further to the deterioration of bone. Absorption of vitamin D and calcium may be reduced in liver disease (Li et al., 2000). The incidence of fractures has been reported to be as high as 30% in persons awaiting liver transplantation (Diamond, Stiel, Wilkinson, & Posen, 1990). Persons who have a low bone-mineral density (BMD) prior to liver transplantation are at an even greater risk of fracture after transplantation, which results in significantly increased morbidity and mortality (Keogh et al., 1999).

Exercise Limitations

Patients with chronic liver disease experience a prolonged period of weakness and fatigue resulting in deconditioning. This is expressed as decreased oxygen uptake, decreased muscle strength, and poor endurance. These patients have been found to have a reduced VO_2 max (the maximal volume of oxygen that can be utilized in 1 minute during maximal exercise). Patients with chronic liver disease have been found to have a VO_2 max that is 40% less than predicted for sedentary healthy individuals of the same age and sex (Beyer et al., 1999). In addition, muscle strength in these patients has been found to be 30% of age-predicted levels (Beyer, Aadahl, Strange, Mohr, & Kjaer, 1995). Inactivity and bed rest results in the disuse of muscles (primarily postural and weight-bearing muscles) that leads to a deterioration of muscle structure and function (Saltin et al., 1968). In addition, patients with cirrhosis often have severe edema (swelling of soft tissues as a result of excess water accumulation) and ascites that negatively affects their ability to move in bed, to transfer, and to ambulate. The adverse effects of physical inactivity and bed rest not only exacerbate the complications of cachexia/muscle wasting and bone loss but also have been correlated with posttransplant success (Carithers, 2000).

Pre-Liver Transplantation—Rehabilitation Program

Goals of Therapy

Rehabilitation therapy in patients with end-stage liver disease is directed at improving a patient's physical functioning and quality of life (QOL). This must be supplemented by appropriate nutritional care. It is critical to institute rehabilitation therapy as soon as possible to maintain relatively healthy levels of physical functioning and to improve survival before and after transplantation. Patients who have been wasting muscle at a higher rate have a poorer prognosis after transplantation (Selberg et al., 1997).

Physical Activity

To prevent the significant physical deconditioning associated with reduced physical activity while waiting for a transplant, a pretransplantation rehabilitation program is instituted. Disuse weakness and atrophy are most effectively treated by prevention. Therefore, a program of graded isometric exercises aimed at restoring muscle mass and strength is employed. Contraction of a muscle at 20–30% of maximal strength for a few seconds daily will maintain its strength (Kohzuki et al., 2000). Contractures of joints are best prevented by the institution of an exercise program that involves a range of motions and gentle stretching exercises. Exercise programs instituted in the preoperative period can reduce the cardiovascular risk and the extent of osteoporosis and muscle wasting after liver transplantation (Vintro et al., 2002).

Nutrition

Careful nutritional monitoring, frequent nutritional reassessment, and provision of adequate calories are essential in the pre-liver transplantation patient. Individualized dietary counseling should be offered to all patients. Nutrient-dense foods, nutritional supplements, and smaller, more frequent meals during the day are recommended. Megestrol acetate has been used successfully in patients with end-stage liver disease for appetite stimulation (Gurk-Turner, 1997). Parenteral nutrition may be indicated in some cases. Liver-transplant candidates should be encouraged to consume foods high in calcium and vitamin D, and if consumption is low, supplementation is recommended.

Psychological Issues

Psychological and social work support services play an important role in the pretransplantation assessment. Assessment of the patient's lifestyle, psychological stability, and family support are key factors that can help predict a patient's ability to function following liver transplantation. This is particularly true in patients with a history of drug and alcohol abuse. Relapse into alcohol abuse has been found to occur in up to 30% of liver transplantation patients (Dew et al., 2008). The ability of a patient to abstain from alcohol posttransplantation is predicted by an ability to abstain from alcohol for at least 6 months before transplantation, a stable employment history, and a strong family/friend support structure (Koffron & Stein, 2008). In light of the high relapse rate, the need for continued psychological support posttransplant is essential.

Post-Liver Transplantation Medical Issues

Complications of Liver Transplantation

Most life-threatening complications associated with liver transplantation occur within the perioperative period and include primary graft malfunction (graft failure in the immediate postoperative period with no obvious cause), acute rejection episodes, severe infections, and technical complications such as hepatic artery thrombosis and biliary leaks (Table 20.2). Long-term morbidity and mortality after liver transplantation, in contrast, are mainly the result of the adverse effects of the immunosuppressive medications prescribed to prevent rejection (Benten, Staufer, & Sterneck, 2009).

REJECTION. The risk of liver rejection is highest (40%) during the first 3–6 months after transplantation and decreases significantly afterwards (Lopez & Martin, 2006). Acute (cellular) hepatic allograft rejection is an attempt by the immune system to attack and destroy the transplanted liver; it typically occurs 7–14 days posttransplantation but can also occur earlier or later. Rejection is most commonly manifested by fever, malaise, right upper-quadrant pain or tenderness, graft enlargement, and diminished graft function. A rise in bilirubin and transaminase levels is observed. With early detection, most acute rejection episodes can be

TABLE 20.2 *Complications of Liver Transplant*

Graft dysfunction	Neurologic complication
Primary nonfunction	Neuropathy
Preservation injury	Seizure
Small for size	Coma
Syndrome	Encephalopathy
Rejection	Aphasia
Vascular thrombosis	Tremors
Hepatic artery thrombosis	Central pontine
Portal vein thrombosis	Myelinolysis
Biliary complications	Electrolyte imbalance
Stricture	Hyponatremia
Leaks	Hypokalemia
Infection	Hyperkalemia
Bacterial	Hypocalcemia
Viral	Hypophosphoremia
Fungal	Hypoglycemia
Opportunistic	Hyperglycemia
Nosocomial	Hypomagnesium
Latent	Pulmonary
Recurrent	Mechanical ventilation
Gastrointestinal	Pneumonia
Ileus	Pleural effusion
Ulcer	Pneumothorax
Gastrointestinal bleeding	Pulmonary
Diarrhea	Hypertension
Drug interactions	Hypoxia
Interference with cytochrome P 3A4	

Source: Rudow, D. L., & Goldstein, M. J. (2008). Critical care management of the liver transplant recipient. *Critical Care Nursing Quarterly, 31*, 238. Reprinted by permission of the publisher.

treated successfully by augmentation of existing immunosuppressive medications or high doses of steroids. Chronic rejection that occurs months to years posttransplantation results in progressive jaundice and graft dysfunction and may require retransplantation.

ELECTROLYTE IMBALANCES. Electrolyte imbalances are a very common metabolic problem after liver transplantation. These include abnormally low concentrations of sodium, potassium, calcium, phosphorous, and magnesium in the blood. They can also manifest as abnormally high concentrations of potassium and glucose in the blood (Rudow & Goldstein, 2008). A low serum magnesium level potentiates cyclosporine (an immunosuppressive drug) neurotoxicity and may result in seizures. As a result, efforts are made to keep the magnesium level high enough to prevent this complication. Careful laboratory monitoring of electrolytes is necessary.

MUSCULOSKELETAL COMPLICATIONS. Post-liver transplantation, issues of continued muscle loss, osteoporosis, and fatigue continue. The most common posttransplantation complaints by patients include the following: muscle weakness, fatigue, and bone/joint discomfort (Beyer et al., 1995). A study by van Ginneken and colleagues (2007) found that of 96 liver-transplant patients, 66% were fatigued and 44% were severely fatigued during the posttransplantation phase. They noted that the patients experienced physical fatigue and reduced activity levels rather than mental fatigue and reduced motivation. They reasoned that fatigue after liver transplantation might be reduced by rehabilitation programs focusing on improving activity patterns and physical fitness.

NEUROLOGICAL COMPLICATIONS. Neurological complications are a common effect posttransplantation (Rudow & Goldstein, 2008). Pretransplant encephalopathy can manifest postoperatively as disorientation and somnolence. This condition typically resolves as liver function returns to normal. Additional neurological manifestations include headaches, seizures, delirium, coma, and stroke. In addition, patients who have undergone liver transplantation are prone to developing neuropathies. The frequency and causes of generalized neuromuscular weakness after liver transplantation has been studied (Campellone, Lacomis, Giuliani, & Kramer, 1998). Researchers prospectively performed detailed neurological examinations on 100 liver-transplant recipients and found that 10% of these individuals had developed focal peripheral nerve lesions during the postoperative period. Ulnar neuropathy was the most common mononeuropathy and was felt to result from intraoperative compression or postoperative trauma in the region of the elbow. The authors felt that this finding warranted the use of empiric elbow padding intraoperatively. Of note, they reported no incidences of brachial plexopathy in their patient population. Brachial plexopathy, which is the most common neurological complication in surgical patients, is felt to be due to excessive traction on the brachial plexus from hyperabduction of the arm during surgery. The authors felt that the absence of this complication in their series was due to the strict adherence to maintaining the patient's arms at less than 90° abduction during surgery.

Complications Secondary to Immunosuppressive Use

Maintenance immunosuppression is usually achieved by using the calcineuron inhibitors (cyclosporine A or tacrolimus) and corticosteroids. These may be combined with newer anti-metabolite compounds (e.g., mycophenolate-cellcept) with the goal of decreasing steroid and/or calcineurin inhibitor use (Koffron & Stein, 2008).

Cyclosporine toxicity is manifested by tremulousness, hypertension, hyperkalemia, and nephrotoxicity. The most common cause of a rise in blood urea nitrogen (BUN) and creatinine levels after transplantation is cyclosporine toxicity. This improves with a reduction in its dosage. Cyclosporine also has neurotoxic effects, including seizures, paranoid delusions, and hallucinations. As noted previously, a low serum magnesium level potentiates cyclosporine neurotoxicity and may result in seizures.

Tacrolimus is a macrolide antibiotic that shares many characteristics with cyclosporine. Like cyclosporine, tacrolimus toxicity is manifested by nephrotoxicity and neurotoxicity. Nephrotoxicity is related to high levels of the drug and improves with dosage reduction. Manifestations of neurotoxicity may range from mild symptoms (tremors, insomnia, somnolence, headaches) to severe complications (seizures, obtundation, coma). These symptoms are related to high doses of the drug and improve with dosage reduction. Tacrolimus levels are monitored daily by obtaining trough levels.

Corticosteroids are routinely used, following solid organ transplantation to prevent rejection. Long-term steroid use is associated with complications such as refractory hypertension, diabetes, osteoporosis, fractures, hip necrosis, cataracts, and obesity. The introduction of tacrolimus has enabled maintaining patients on lower doses of prednisone.

Antiproliferative drugs include azathioprine, mycophenolate mofetil, and sirolimus and work by inhibiting mitosis, and hence, proliferation of lymphocytes.

As immunosuppressive agents have significant toxicities, other medications are often added to prevent infections. Maintenance prophylaxis for infections is instituted for 3–12 months posttransplantation. These medications include trimethoprim-sulfamethoxazole and dapsone (prophylactic antibiotics to prevent *Pneumocystis carinii* pneumonia), acyclovir (to inhibit herpes viruses), ganciclovir (to inhibit cytomegalovirus), and clotrimazole and/or nystatin (to control fungal infections such as *Candida*).

Post-Liver Transplantation—Rehabilitation Program

Physical Rehabilitation

The goal of physical activity after liver transplantation is to reverse the musculoskeletal changes resulting from inactivity and bed rest. Physical therapy should be instituted immediately after the transplant recipient has been surgically stabilized. Restoration of muscle mass and strength, beginning with graded isometric exercises, as well as aerobic conditioning exercises are implemented.

Beyer and colleagues (1999) evaluated the effects of a fitness program on 23 men and 15 women before and at 6 months posttransplantation. Posttransplantation patients participated in a supervised exercise program that consists of aerobic and muscle-strengthening exercises for 1 hour twice a week over 8–24 weeks. Exercise capacity increased 43% and knee extensor/flexor strength increased 60–100% by 6 months after transplantation. However, these patients still remained 10–20% below age-matched controls, an indication of how deconditioned they were pretransplantation. All patients were independent in functional activity of daily living skills at 6 months posttransplantation. The authors concluded that a supervised post-liver transplant exercise program improves physical fitness, muscle strength, and functional performance in persons with chronic liver disease.

Studies have also shown that highly trained liver-transplant recipients are capable of achieving high levels of physical functioning. Sixteen liver-transplant recipients tested at the 1996 U.S. Transplant Games were found to achieve exercise capacities that were 101% of age-predicted normal levels (Painter et al., 1997). In addition, long-term liver-transplant recipients who reported participation in regular physical activity had higher scores on health-related QOL scales than those who were inactive. Also, physically active patients had less hypertension and fewer orthopedic complaints (Painter, Krasnoff, Paul, & Ascher, 2001).

Psychological Issues

As noted earlier, due to the high relapse rate in patients with a history of drug and alcohol abuse posttransplantation, the need for close, continued psychological support is essential.

Nutrition

Following successful liver transplantation, the albumin level slowly rises to normal levels. As it normalizes, the generalized edema that patients experience posttransplantation begins to disappear. Posttransplantation nutritional therapy should include a diet that is moderate in protein intake. Nutritional recommendations should also include a diet that reduces the risk of osteoporosis and promotes bone synthesis. Osteoporosis is common after transplantation with the greatest amount of bone loss occurring between 3 and 12 months posttransplantation (McCaughan & Feller, 1994). Dietary calcium and vitamin D intakes should reach 1.0–1.5 g and 400–800 units/daily, respectively. In addition, diets should be low in fat, low in sodium, and high in vegetables and fruits (Weseman & McCashland, 1998).

Post-Liver Transplantation—Outcomes

As patient survival rates after liver transplantation continue to rise, there has been an increased emphasis on measuring successful outcomes by improvements in patient functional status and QOL. A retrospective study on 55 liver transplantation patients found that significant functional gains as measured by the Functional Independence Measure (FIM) instrument could be achieved in an acute inpatient rehabilitation program (Cortazzo, Helkowski, Pippin, Boninger, & Zafonte, 2005). All patients had improvements in their FIM scores with an average gain of 26 points. In addition, the majority of patients were discharged home after acute rehabilitation. The authors also found that patients admitted to the rehabilitation unit with lower albumin levels remained in rehabilitation longer and made less significant gains in therapy based on FIM efficiency (the amount of FIM gained per day in rehabilitation). They felt that this finding reinforces the need to emphasize good nutrition both before and after liver transplantation to potentially improve functional gains. In addition, the authors noted several comorbidities in their patient population that had rehabilitation implications. They found that 12 patients (22%) developed neuropathies with 5 requiring bracing (4 ankle-foot orthoses and 1 volar wrist-extension splint). They also found that 4 patients (7%) had symptomatic osteoporotic spine compression fractures, with 3 of them requiring spinal bracing. The authors recommended weight-bearing exercises to help maintain/increase bone mass in this population.

A survey to determine the functional and vocational outcomes of patients 3 years post-liver transplantation at the University of Pittsburgh Medical Center found that 61% of patients reported severe impairments in endurance prior to transplantation (Robinson, Switala, Tarter, & Nicholas, 1990). However, only 6% reported endurance impairments after transplantation. Three years after transplantation, 39% were working full time and 26% were homemakers. Overall, the patients were largely independent in activities of daily living (ADL) skills and mobility, had improved endurance, and returned to work despite physical limitations. Another survey of 166 patients who underwent liver transplantation at Rush-Presbyterian-St. Lukes Medical Center in Chicago found that at 1 year posttransplantation, nearly all patients were able to perform basic ADL (Nicholas, Oleske, Robinson, Switala, & Tarter, 1994). In addition, the percentage of patients with severely impaired endurance had decreased from 43.9% pretransplantation to 8.0% following the transplant. A retrospective study of 203 adult liver-transplant patients found that 57% of those surveyed were employed and 43% were unemployed at least 9 months posttransplantation (Adams, Ghent, Grant, & Wall, 1995). Older recipients and those who were continuously out of the workplace for several years pretransplantation were the least likely to return to gainful employment.

Summary

Liver transplantation is the only definitive treatment modality for end-stage liver disease (Abbasoglu, 2008). With the advances in technical skills, improvements in immunosuppressive drugs, and the management of postoperative complications, liver transplantation has become the standard treatment for many patients with acute fulminant liver failure and chronic liver disease. Today, the major constraint to meeting the demand for liver transplants is the availability of donated (cadaver) organs. Raising public awareness of the shortage of organs for donation and the use of living-donor liver transplants are the two major efforts currently underway to alleviate the organ shortage.

RENAL TRANSPLANTATION

Renal transplantation is the treatment of choice for patients with end-stage renal disease (ESRD). Renal or kidney transplantation is a surgical procedure during which a diseased kidney is replaced by a healthy kidney from another person. It is classified as deceased-donor (formerly cadaveric) or living-donor transplantation, depending on the source of the recipient organ. Living-donor transplantations are further classified as living related (if a biological relationship exists between the donor and recipient) or living unrelated. Since the first transplantation of a kidney from one human to another in 1954, renal transplantation has evolved from essentially an experimental procedure to one which is now commonplace and has excellent survival rates. In the United States, in 2004, first-time recipients of a deceased-donor renal transplant had 1-year patient and graft survival rates of 95% and 88%, respectively (Colm & Pascual, 2004). First-time recipients of a living-donor transplant had 1-year patient- and graft-survival rates of 98% and 94%, respectively.

Improvements in the success rate of renal transplantation reflect improvements in immunosuppressive regimens, antimicrobial prophylaxis, surgical and medical care, as well as improvements in cross-matching tests (pretransplantation in-vitro assays to detect donor antibodies to recipient human leukocyte antigens). Long-term graft survival (beyond the first year) has not improved to the same extent as early survival. The principal causes of renal allograft loss beyond the first transplantation year are cardiovascular disease, infection, and malignancy. As such, one primary area of research interest is on renal transplantation strategies that aim to improve long-term outcomes by preventing and treating cardiovascular disease, infection, bone disease, and neoplasia.

Indications

The indication for kidney transplantation is ESRD, regardless of the primary cause. This is defined as a decrease in the glomerular filtration rate from 20% to 25% of normal state. Diabetes remains the leading cause of ESRD in the United States and worldwide (Colm & Pascual, 2004). Other diseases leading to serious kidney dysfunction and for which renal transplants may be required include congenital renal obstructive disorders leading to hydronephrosis, congenital nephrotic syndrome, Alport syndrome, polycystic kidney disease, glomerulonephritis, as well as autoimmune conditions such as systemic lupus erythematosus and Goodpasture's syndrome.

Pre-Renal Transplantation Rehabilitation Issues

Diminished Exercise Tolerance

Patients with compromised renal function have a markedly impaired exercise tolerance. This impaired physical performance not only interferes with their ability to perform physical tasks such as climbing stairs but also interferes with their ability to perform leisure-time exercise. A majority of patients with impaired renal function are unable to work due to their impaired energy status. Their reduced physical fitness is characterized by reduced flexibility, coordination disturbances, as well as decreased muscular strength and endurance (Fuhrmann & Krause, 2004). The mechanisms behind this reduced work capacity are not fully known, but are felt, in part, to be due to years of reduced activity level prior to transplantation. The decline in physical fitness parallels the progression of the renal disease. Patients with renal disease awaiting transplantation have been found to have a decreased maximal oxygen uptake (VO_2 max; Robertson et al., 1990). Oxidative metabolism is impaired in their skeletal muscles, which is most likely caused by impaired exchange of oxygen between muscle and blood (Young & Stiens, 2006). Erythropoetin treatment has been found to increase the VO_2 max by 20–30%. However, despite treatment with erythropoietin and a restoration of a normal hemoglobin concentration, the VO_2 max remained lower than normal (Kjaer et al., 1996).

Muscle Weakness and Atrophy

Patients with ESRD exhibit weakness in both their proximal and distal musculature. The cause of this weakness is felt to be a combination of muscle atrophy, a decreased ability of the muscle to generate strength, and a reduced capacity of the nervous system to activate motor units (Juskowa et al., 2006). These patients have been found to have a reduced muscle strength in their legs, which contributes to a reduced physical performance (Bohannon, Smith, Hull, Palmeri, & Barnhard, 1995). In addition, deficiencies of vitamin D and parathyroid hormone contribute to stiffening of periarticular soft tissue that additionally limits the motor capacity of these patients.

Pre-Renal Transplantation Rehabilitation Program

Studies of hemodialysis patients engaged in an exercise program have shown that training has multiple beneficial effects. Training has been shown to result in an increase in physical work capacity (VO$_2$ max) and muscle strength (Painter et al., 1986). The Borg Rating of Perceived Exertion (RPE) scale is a simple method of rating perceived exertion. The scale ranges from 6 to 20 (6 = no exertion at all to 20 = maximal exertion; Borg, 1982). The Borg RPE scale is recommended for monitoring the training of patients with ESRD (Fuhrmann & Krause, 2004). Physical exercise has also been shown to increase the hematocrit level, improve the lipid profile, lower the requirement for antihypertensive medications, and normalize insulin sensitivity (Goldberg et al., 1986). It essentially modifies factors known to be associated with atherogenesis and cardiovascular disease in hemodialysis patients. In addition to its physiological benefits, exercise has been found to improve depressed mood in hemodialysis patients (Carney et al., 1987).

Post-Renal Transplantation Medical Issues

When working with the patient following renal transplantation, the rehabilitation team must be aware of the most common complications that occur during the postoperative period. These include the following.

Transplant Rejection
As discussed earlier in this chapter, rejection is the normal reaction of the body to a foreign object. When a new kidney is placed in the body, the body sees the kidney as a threat and the host immune system produces antibodies to reject the new organ. Kidney rejection is often preceded by symptoms of malaise and anorexia. Clinical signs of kidney-transplant rejection that arise in the postoperative period include elevated temperature, decreased urine output, edema (usually beginning in the hands or feet), a sudden increase in weight (3–5 pounds in a 24-hour period) as well as tenderness at the graft site. Laboratory findings include a leukocytosis (elevation in the white blood cell count) as well as elevated blood urea nitrogen (BUN) and creatinine levels (Young & Stiens, 2006).

To prevent rejection, immunosuppressants are used to suppress the immune system from rejecting the donor kidney. The most commonly used antirejection medications following renal transplantation are cyclosporine and tacrolimus. A combination of agents is often utilized to achieve adequate immunosuppression, without the need for toxic doses of any one agent (Colm & Pascual, 2004). As the risk of acute rejection is greatest in the early posttransplantation period, more intensive immunosuppression is given early and is progressively lowered in the following weeks and months. Immunosupressant medications must be taken for the rest of a patient's life.

Infections
The transplantation procedure and subsequent immunosuppression increase the risk of serious infections. In the first month after transplantation, infections of the surgical wound, lungs, urinary tract and those involving vascular catheters are most common. Between 1 and 6 months posttransplantation, however, weeks of intense immunosuppresion increase the risk of opportunistic infections from microorganisms such as cytomegalovirus, Epstein–Barr virus, and *P. carinii*. Prophylactic measures for infections posttransplantation include antiviral prophylaxis (for 1–3 months) and prophylaxis against *P. carinii* (trimethoprim-sulfamethoxazole, for 6–12 months), similar to those with liver transplantation.

Bleeding
Bleeding is uncommon post-renal transplantation (Humar, Denny, Matas, & Najarian, 2003). When it occurs, it is usually due to small blood vessels in the renal hilum that had not been ligated during surgery. Meticulous hemostasis during the operation can help to prevent this complication. Close observation of a patient's vital signs and hematocrit is necessary in the early postoperative period to detect bleeding. A falling hematocrit, hypotension, or tachycardia can alert the clinician to the possibility of bleeding. Most small perirenal

hematomas are asymptomatic. However, large hematomas can produce significant flank pain and lower-extremity swelling due to venous or ureteral obstruction and may require surgical exploration.

Post-Renal Transplantation Rehabilitation Issues

When prescribing a rehabilitation program for a patient following a renal transplant, one must be cognizant of several important physiological factors in this patient population. The renal transplant recipient's capacity for exercise remains quite limited. This is due to the presence of anemia as well as increased stresses on the cardiovascular system. The presence of anemia results in a reduction in the patient's blood oxygen-carrying capacity. In addition, the sodium and water retention that accompanies renal failure results in an increase in circulatory volume. As this volume increases, it places greater stresses on the cardiovascular system (Young & Stiens, 2006). This leads to a worsening of hypertension and hypertrophy of the cardiac muscle, which in turn lead to a decrease in compliance and stiff ventricles. The VO_2 max decreases and is found to be in the range of only 75–80% of that observed healthy control-group subjects (Krull, Schulze-Neick, Hatopp, Offner, & Brodehl, 1994).

In addition, the patient's reduced BMD continues to be a major problem after transplantation. This is a result of suboptimal kidney function and the superimposed effects of steroids on bone. A reduction in BMD has been found in 60% of patients in the first 18 months after renal transplantation (Colm & Pascual, 2004), with pathological fractures commonly occurring post-renal transplantation. The estimated fracture rate after transplantation is 2% per year in nondiabetic patients, 5% per year in diabetic patients, and 12% per year in pancreas–kidney recipients. It is also important to note that there is a high incidence of muscle/tendon injuries in the posttransplant population (Agarwal & Owen, 1990) that is felt to be due to a combination of metabolic and immunological factors, as well as the administration of corticosteroids. Together, these factors impair the mechanical properties of connective tissue, placing patients at a higher risk for overuse injuries.

Post-Renal Transplantation Rehabilitation Program

Rehabilitation after renal transplantation seeks to improve the patient's physical and psychological fitness. The goal is to achieve a level of activity that permits maintenance of an active lifestyle. The rehabilitation program focuses on stretching exercises, repetitive low-level resistance exercises, and aerobic exercises. The initiation of an exercise program post-transplantation can result in an improvement in an individual's exercise capacity and cardiac function (Kempeneers et al., 1988). Exercise training, in addition to improving exercise capacity, is also felt to improve insulin resistance in these patients (Christiansen et al., 1996). When prescribing a rehabilitation program for post-renal transplantation patients, care should be given to close monitoring of blood pressure. Although patients may be normotensive at rest, they respond to exercise with a higher-than-normal blood pressure that indicates an inappropriately high systemic vascular resistance (Scott, Hay, Higenbuttam, Evans, & Calne, 1990). In addition, care should be taken during exercise training to not overload tendons in order to prevent tendon rupture (Agarwal & Owen, 1990). Renal-transplant patients who engaged in a structured rehabilitation program showed significant improvements in respiratory function (peak expiratory flow) as well as range of motion in the radiocarpal joint when compared with post-renal transplant controls (Korbiewska, Lewandowska, Juskowa, & Bialoszewski, 2007). The rehabilitation program focused on strengthening exercises for the abdominal muscles, upper and lower extremities, breathing exercises, coordination, and relaxation exercises. The authors concluded that there is a need to establish rehabilitation programs for patients who have undergone successful renal transplantation. Juskowa and colleagues

(2006) in a randomized-controlled clinical trial of exercise training after renal transplantation found a positive correlation between muscle strength and improved graft function in the group receiving rehabilitation compared with the control group. A prospective, randomized-controlled study by Painter and coworkers (2002b) examined the effects of exercise intervention on health-related fitness (exercise capacity, muscle strength, body composition) and QOL in patients following renal transplantation. Their data showed that the group undergoing an exercise training program exhibited improved cardiopulmonary fitness, increased muscle strength, and less limitations in physical functioning compared with the control group that persisted for at least 12 months posttransplantation. The authors felt that exercise recommendations should be part of the routine medical treatment of patients during the posttransplantation phase, in order to optimize overall health and achieve the best-possible outcomes.

Post-Renal Transplantation Outcomes

As the survival rate following renal transplantation continues to improve, there has been an increased focus on health-related quality of life (HRQL). It has been shown that patients following successful transplantation exhibit a significantly higher HRQL compared to patients on dialysis (Fujisawa et al., 2000). Overbeck and colleagues (2005) evaluated QOL in 76 transplant patients compared with 65 patients with ESRD and awaiting transplantation. Their data demonstrated a considerable improvement in the QOL in the transplant patients. However, despite the improved QOL, levels of unemployment remained high, emphasizing the need for vocational rehabilitation in this patient population. Neipp and coworkers (2006) in a retrospective study found that 15 years posttransplantation, patients continued to exhibit a satisfactory HRQL. Renal-transplant patients who were employed reported a significantly improved HRQL in areas such as physical functioning, physical pain, vitality, social functioning, and mental health. The authors stress that vocational rehabilitation following transplantation is of utmost importance among long-term survivors and is associated with improved HRQL.

Summary

Renal transplantation is a life-extending procedure. The typical patient with renal failure will live 10–15 years longer with a kidney transplant than one maintained on dialysis (Wolfe et al., 1999). This gain in years of life has been found to be even greater for younger patients. However, even 75-year-old recipients gain an average 4 more years of life. Patients who have undergone a kidney transplant have been found to have more energy, a less restricted diet, and fewer complications compared with those who stay on conventional dialysis. Studies have also shown that the longer a patient is on dialysis prior to transplantation, the less time the kidney transplant will survive. Thus, there is a need for the rapid referral to a transplant program for the population of patients with ESRD.

CARDIAC TRANSPLANTATION

The role of rehabilitation medicine in both the preoperative preparation and postoperative functional aftercare of persons who have undergone cardiac transplantation continues to grow in significance (Young & Stiens, 2002). Physical restoration of persons who have undergone complex cardiac-transplant procedures is an important priority of the rehabilitation team and has emerged as a global rehabilitation priority (Ring, 2004).

Cardiac transplantation is a surgical procedure utilized for persons with end-stage heart failure, severe heart-muscle disease, and irreversible coronary-artery disease associated with multiple myocardial infarctions that have proven unresponsive to medical or surgical management. According to the United Network for Organ Sharing and the American Heart

Association (AHA) statistics, a total of 2,210 heart transplantations were performed through-out the United States in 2007 (American Heart Association, 2009). Demographically, 73.7% of cardiac transplants were performed on men and 26.3% on women; 19.9% were performed on persons aged 35–49 and 54% on people aged 50 years or older (AHA, 2009). According to sta-tistics updated on May 30, 2008, 1-year survival rate was 85.5% for women and 87.5% for men, whereas the 5-year survival rate was 67.4% for women and 72.3% for men.

Following the initial cardiac transplant procedure performed in 1967, the 90-day survival rate of patients has improved dramatically (Solomon et al., 2004). Because of improvements in organ availability and surgical capacity in the United States, the waiting list of candidates declined by 45% (i.e., from 2,414 in 1997 to 1,327 in 2006). This trend continues. Documented outcomes are improving with transplant-recipient survival exceeding 92% at 3 months 88% at 1 year (Mulligan et al., 2008), and 85% at 5 years (Deuse et al., 2008). Recently, reports of "20-year survivors" indicate that this group requires ongoing treatment for a variety of comorbid medical conditions, including hypertension (87%), allograft vasculopathy (43%), diabetes (14%), and malignancy (44%; Deuse et al., 2008).

Several important trends have contributed to the growing success of cardiac transplanta-tion. The development of technologically improved and inventive methods of "buying time" for preoperative heart-transplant candidates who remain on the waiting list has facilitated survivorship. Novel approaches, once thought inconceivable such as the left ventricular assist devices (LVAD) and the temporary artificial heart (TAH) have significantly contributed to decreased morbidity and mortality (Copeland et al., 2004; Lahpor, 2009). The recent introduc-tion of a "wearable" pneumatic driver technology for powering the artificial heart outside the hospital has improved outcomes and is thought to represent a "bridge to life" (International Society for Heart and Lung Transplantation, 2009). It is predicted that post-cardiac-transplant survival rates will continue to improve with judicious patient selection, improvements in surgical techniques, reduced rejection rates, and ongoing rehabilitation efforts.

Indications

End-stage congestive heart failure (CHF) that has proven refractory to traditional medical therapy is a major indication for heart transplantation. Often end-stage CHF necessitating transplant is preceded by a history of idiopathic cardiomyopathy, viral myocarditis, ischemic heart disease, or valve dysfunction (Joshi & Kevorkian, 1997; Latlief & Young, 1994).

Selection

Comprehensive evaluation of the patient prior to cardiac transplantation encompasses assess-ments of circulatory impairments, exercise tolerance, and performance, as well as a determi-nation of comorbid conditions that affects heart function and physical functionality (D'Amico, 2005). Improvement in the functional ability and QOL of this patient population is predicated on a comprehensive team approach, by using a dedicated cardiac-transplant team of medi-cal professionals—cardiologist, transplant surgeon, physiatrist, nurse, physical therapists, occupational therapists, psychologists, and social worker—who play an active, integrated, and meaningful role. This comprehensive assessment also necessitates direct patient input regarding expectations so that the rehabilitation program can be individualized to maxi-mize the patient's potential. Successful cardiac transplant outcomes are often dependent on identifying candidates who demonstrate sufficient physical capacity and endurance reserves. Careful selection of patients with achievable goals will improve the odds of maximally ben-efiting cardiac-transplant candidates who receive a transplanted heart and who later receive rehabilitation (Solomon et al., 2004). During the period of heart procurement, implantation of LVAD and other "bridge-to-transplant" devices such as the TAH can improve tolerance for activity and allow preliminary rehabilitation. (Gammie, Edwards, Griffith, Pierson, & Tsao,

2004; Rao et al., 2003). Multiple criteria are generally utilized for cardiac transplant candidate selection (Tayler & Bergin, 1995).

Post-Cardiac Transplantation Medical Issues/Complications

The cardiac rehabilitation team must be intimately familiar with the complications associated with cardiac transplantation surgery. This will enable safe and timely recognition and treatment of complications that arise that can ultimately adversely affect patients' functional outcomes. Comprehensive and longitudinal coordination of care and dialogue between the team members, including the cardiac surgeon, the cardiologist, and the physiatrist, is essential for ensuring an appropriate rehabilitation outcome.

One of the major posttransplant complications is allograft failure that occurs due to organ rejection. Other complications include pulmonary hypertension, neurological sequelae such as metabolic encephalopathy and stroke, and infections and side effects caused by immuno-suppressive agents. In a study of cardiac-transplant recipients on an inpatient rehabilitation unit, several salient secondary complications were identified, including hypertension, nutritional limitations, neuromuscular deficits, and compression fractures (Joshi & Kevorkian, 1997). Stress fractures of the weight-bearing extremities have also been observed (Lucas & Einhorn, 1993), which, in most cases, are attributable to steroid-induced osteoporosis. The likelihood of this complication can be reduced through monitoring vitamin D levels and preventive supplementation of vitamin D (1,000–2,000 units/daily).

Rejection

After the posttransplant patient has achieved circulatory and vascular stability, a continued goal is prevention of rejection. It is important to remember that the cardiac-transplant recipient is less immunologically depressed than the kidney-transplant patient. Prolonged uremia associated with renal failure accounts for this difference. Acute rejection in heart transplantation is a major complication that may be predicted by onset of a constellation of symptoms, including fulminant exacerbation of CHF, increased peripheral edema, premature atrial contractions, a diastolic gallop, and a sudden, marked reduction in exercise capacity.

Chronic rejection can also progress with accelerated graft atherosclerosis (Dandel et al., 2003; Von Scheidt, Kembes, Reichart, & Erdmann, 1993). At 1-year posttransplantation, 10–15% of patients have developed accelerated graft atherosclerosis, which increases by 35–50% by the fifth postoperative year (Drexler & Schroeder, 1994; Shiba et al., 1994). After heart transplantation, the heart is no longer innervated by the autonomic nervous system, leading to a process called denervation. Denervation produces an upregulation of muscarinic receptors, which facilitates increased calcium influx in the coronary arteries of the transplanted heart. This causes diffuse, circumferential narrowing of the arterial luminal diameters. This type of coronary artery disease has a major negative effect on the long-term survival of cardiac-transplant patients. To reduce/prevent the complication of graft atherosclerosis, the treatment plan should include educating the patients about the complication, regular arterial monitoring of atheroscerois, and proper use of medication. Recent scientific investigations suggest that this condition can be prevented and improved with calcium-channel blockers (Shiba et al., 2004; Schroeder et al., 1993).

Pulmonary Hypertension

During the early postoperative phase, a frequently encountered complication is the inability of the transplanted right ventricle to cope with preexisting pulmonary hypertension. Pulmonary hypertension can be due to chronic right-sided heart failure. It may also be due to cyclosporine-induced renal vasoconstriction (Greenberg et al., 1987; McGiffin, Kirklin, & Nafiel, 1985; O'Connell et al., 1992). Medical management of pulmonary hypertension includes using alternative cyclosporine dosing regimens, as well as the use of calcium-channel antagonists and angiotensin-converting enzyme inhibitors to promote arteriolar dilation (Bunke & Ganzel, 1992; Legault, Olgilvie, Cardella, & Leenen, 1993; Valentine et al., 1992). It is important that the rehabilitation professional be aware that, throughout the physical restoration process, blood pressures should be closely monitored and used as a guide for antihypertensive therapy (Painter et al., 2002a). This is achievable most of the time without interrupting the exercise-therapy regimen. Timely and appropriate medical management of the hypertensive state encourages full participation in the rehabilitative process to achieve functional improvements in patients.

Neurological Complications
Neurological complications following cardiac transplantation include metabolic encephalopathy, stroke, central nervous system infection, seizures, and psychosis. Most commonly, these complications present during the acute posttransplant period, though they can also occur during the rehabilitative/restorative phase, long after the original transplant surgery (Sliwa & Blendonohy, 1988). Common etiologies for stroke posttransplantation include particulate embolism, air embolism, or inadequacy of perfusion arising from the transplantation procedure. During the postoperative phase, the rehabilitation team led by the physiatrist should conduct a careful review of mental status, perceptual sensations, and motor function of the patients, to ensure neurological integrity.

Infection
The leading cause of death in post-cardiac transplant patients is infection (Miller et al., 1994; Vaska, 1993). Common types of infections include mediastinitis, pneumonia, urinary tract infections, and intravenous catheter-induced sepsis (Hosenpud, Novick, Breen, & Daily, 1994; Miller et al., 1994; Vaska, 1993). When such problems arise, they tend to develop during the first 2 years following the cardiac transplant (Braith et al., 2000; Mills, 1994). Bacterial and viral infections account for 47% and 41% of infections, respectively. Infections caused by fungus and protozoa comprise 12% of posttransplant morbidity.

Post-Cardiac Transplantation Rehabilitation Factors

Physiology and Function of a Transplanted Heart
Developing a rehabilitation program for a transplant patient requires a thorough understanding of the physiology of the transplanted heart and the impact of exercise on cardiac dynamics. The normal heart is innervated and strongly influenced by the autonomic nervous system that exerts both chronotropic (affecting the heart rate) and inotropic effects (affecting the force of muscular contractions; Auerbach et al., 1999; Beck, Barnard, & Schrire, 1969). The sympathetic nervous system serves to enhance venous return, stroke volume, and cardiac output. With orthotropic heart transplantation, there is complete denervation of the heart, which leads to a loss of the autonomic nervous system control mechanism. Since the transplanted heart is denervated, it consequently achieves a maximal heart rate more slowly than a normal heart. The transplanted heart modulates its heart rate primarily through a response to circulating catecholamines and to a limited extent via partial and inconsistent, gradual, sympathetic reinnervation (Bernardi et al., 2007; Wenting et al., 1987). The denervated heart has a higher than normal resting heart rate, which can be controlled by carotid massage, the Valsalva maneuver, and body inclination (Leenen, Davies, & Fourney, 1995; Wechsler, Giardina, Sciacca, Rose, & Barr, 1995). The physiological explanation for the higher-than-normal heart rate is the loss of vagal tone associated with denervation (Savin, Haskell, Schroeder, & Stinson, 1980). Following an exercise session or mobility activity, the heart-transplant patient experiences a more gradual return to baseline. Notwithstanding the denervated status of the transplanted heart, cardiac output will typically increase in response to dynamic total body activity, promoting venous return and increasing stroke volume through increased preload volume of blood filling the left ventricle (Bernardi et al., 2007).

For the cardiac-transplant patient participating in rehabilitation, there are a host of physiological adaptations that take place. As the patient gradually begins exercise, a slight increase in heart rate is immediately observable and can be attributed to the Bainbridge reflex (Shaver, Leon, Gray, Leonard, & Bahnson, 1969), which is an increase in heart rate in response to increased pressure in the veins entering the right heart or the increased rate of ventricular work. This acceleration will continue for 3–5 minutes. This gradual, ongoing increase in heart rate continues into the recovery period and may contribute to a slower-than-normal return to preexercise heart rate (Martin, Gaucher, Pupa, & Seaworth, 1994). It is essential to advise the patient that he or she should first warm-up and then gradually increase the intensity of activities. It is generally recognized that the peak heart rate achieved during maximal exercise is significantly lower in cardiac-transplant recipients than in age-matched control participants (Leenen et al., 1995; Martin et al., 1994). The transplanted heart compensates for output demand primarily by increasing stroke volume. The resting stroke volume of patients with transplanted hearts is less than that of individuals without transplantation (Kavanagh et al., 1988). Despite this, cardiac output is virtually normal (Kavanagh et al., 1988; Kavanagh & Yacoub, 1992; Meyer et al., 1994). Most heart recipients experience a rapid increase in stroke volume of about 20% when they begin their exercise regimen (Leenen et al., 1995; Meyer et al., 1994). Subsequent increases in stroke volume or cardiac output during prolonged submaximal exercise are mediated by inotropic responses to circulating catecholamines (Kao et al., 1995; Kavanagh & Yacoub, 1992; Keteyian et al., 1994; Leenen et al., 1995). Following gradual conditioning, higher-intensity training can be achieved in a period of over 15 months to achieve athletic capabilities in some younger transplant recipients (Rajendran, Pandurangi, Mullasari, Gomathy, & Rao, 2006).

Since heart-transplant patients display an unusual catecholamine-driven cardioacceleratory response to exercise, empiric exercise prescriptions based on target heart rates have limited utility and are not recommended (Borg, 1982; Greenberg et al., 1987; Kavanagh & Yacoub, 1992). The effect of transplantation on blood pressure is that both systolic and diastolic blood pressures are higher than expected, but pulse pressure, that is, the difference between the maximum systolic blood pressure and the minimum diastolic blood pressure in one heart beat, is essentially normal at rest (Greenberg et al., 1985). Diastolic blood pressure may decline early in submaximal exercise because of reduced peripheral resistance (Greenberg et al., 1985; Griepp, Stinson, Dong, Clark, & Shumway, 1971; Joshi & Kevorkian, 1997; Kao et al., 1995). The peak systolic blood pressure is less than that of individuals without cardiac transplants, but diastolic blood pressure is not significantly different.

Following heart transplantation, patients consume less oxygen during submaximal exercise than do normal controls (Kavanagh & Yacoub, 1992; Keteyian et al., 1994; Paterson, Cunningham, Pickering, Babcock, & Boughner, 1994; Squires, 1991). Oxygen consumption at the anaerobic threshold is also considerably lower than that of age-matched normal individuals (Kavanagh & Yacoub, 1992; Paterson et al., 1994; Squires, 1991). According to Braith and Edwards (2000), the decrement in peak oxygen consumption seen in transplant recipients is due in part to architectural alterations in skeletal muscle. Skeletal-muscle myopathy associated with the heart-failure syndrome produces atrophy, decreased mitochondrial counts, and decreased oxidative enzymes. Corticosteriods also promote muscle atrophy and thinning that affect primarily Type II fibers; cyclosporine further decreases oxidative enzymes (Braith & Edwards, 2000).

Post-Cardiac Transplantation Rehabilitation Outcomes

Early in the history of cardiac transplantation, it was considered inadvisable to start an exercise protocol immediately following the surgery. However, new research suggests a vitally important role for the initiation of exercise therapy beginning at least as soon as a month after transplant surgery (Braith & Edwards, 2000; Valentine et al., 1992). Benefits that accrue from this include improved strength, enhancement of aerobic capacity (Lampert, Mettauer,

Hoppeler, Charloux, & Charpentier, 1998; Ville et al., 2002), and improved physical work capability.

Increasing evidence suggests that supervised exercise programs (Stewart, Badenhop, Brubaker, Keteyian, & King, 2003) should be a standard of care for heart-transplant patients (Kobashigawa et al., 1999; Le Jemtel, 2003). Studies in the rehabilitation literature have focused on the hemodynamic responses to upright exercise after cardiac transplantation, as well as the cardiovascular response to gait training and ambulation in hemiparetic heart recipients (Sliwa, Andersen, & Griffin, 1990; Sliwa & Blendonohy, 1988). Kobashigawa and colleagues (1999) evaluated 27 cardiac-transplant patients who were randomly divided into two groups (structured exercise and nonstructured exercise). The structured exercise group of 14 patients were assigned to participate in a 6-month aerobics exercise program involving sitting-to-standing exercises. Each patient in the structured exercise group worked with a physical therapist and had a customized program of muscular strength and aerobics training. The second group of 13 patients (nonstructured exercise group) received only written instructions about exercises to do at home, with no supervised sessions. All 27 patients were tested for muscle strength, aerobic capacity, and flexibility within 1 month of receiving a heart transplant and tested again 6 months later. Although all patients showed an improvement in all areas, those in the structured-exercise group showed significantly better results. Muscle strength, measured by the number of times a patient could stand from a sitting position repetitively for 1 minute, improved 125% for the structured-exercise group (from a mean of 10.6 times per minute to a mean of 23.9 times). The nonstructured exercise group of patients who had received only written instructions showed an 18% gain, increasing from 10.4 times per minute to 12.3. Aerobic capacity, tested by peak oxygen consumption, increased 49% in the group receiving formal exercise training, compared to just 18% in the nonstructured-exercise group.

Aerobic capabilities as measured by VO_2 max have been shown to increase from 12% to 49%, with cardiovascular exercises done 3 times per week over 7–11 months (Braith et al., 2000). Training with a cycle ergometer and limiting intensity to 15 on the Borg scale prevents excessive exertion. In the alternative, exercise can be dosed in time and rate on the cycle (Shephard, Kavanagh, Mertens, & Yacoub, 1996). It is generally held that cardiac-transplant survivors can perform exercise and physical training routines and achieve improvements comparable to those achieved by normal individuals of similar age (Kjaer, Beyer, & Secher, 1999). Aerobic cardiovascular-conditioning programs and exercise regimens emphasizing endurance tasks have also been shown to improve the ability of heart-transplant patients to achieve higher levels of participation in ADL (Mettauer et al., 2005).

A regularly scheduled practical exercise regimen that can be carried out in a group setting is generally suggested for heart-transplant recipients. The fellowship and support that occurs with group exercise is valuable for transplant patients. In general, patients tolerate exercise well after cardiac transplantation (Kobashigawa et al., 1998), and progressive resistance training is also a beneficial aspect of treatment (Oliver et al., 2001; Quittan et al., 2001; Shephard et al., 1996; Tegtbur, Pethig, Machold, Haverich, & Busse, 2003; Wiesinger et al., 2001). Resistance training should not begin until 6–8 weeks after transplantation, permitting time for sternum healing and corticosteroid tapering (Tegtbur, Busse, Jung, Pethig, & Haverich, 2005). A controlled study designed to determine the effect of resistance exercise training on bone metabolism in heart-transplant recipients revealed that as soon as 2 months after heart transplantation, about 3% of whole-body BMD has been lost, due to decreases in trabecular bone (Streiff et al., 2001). Six months of resistance exercise, consisting of low back exercises that isolate the lumbar spine and a regimen of variable resistance exercises, restored BMD toward pretransplantation levels. Research has suggested that resistance exercise is osteogenic and should be incorporated into the rehabilitation program after heart transplantation (Braith & Edwards, 2000). Progressive resistance exercise with lumbar extension and upper- and lower-limb resistance machines has been demonstrated to limit muscle mass loss (Braith, Welsch, Mills, Keller, & Pollock, 1998). The initial training resistance is set at 50% of the one repetition maximum, and repetitions are limited to 15 per session.

Although almost every cardiac-transplant patient faces the specter of graft rejection, it is rarely necessary to curtail the patient's exercise workout during episodes of moderate rejection. However, when the patient shows signs of new arrhythmias, hypotension, or fever, the physiatrist can abruptly adjust the exercise regimen to balance medical management with restorative rehabilitative services (Braith et al., 2000; Kevorkian, 1999). The patient's long-term prognosis generally becomes worse as rejection episodes increase in frequency and severity. Clinical and physiological monitoring of the patient and regular review of personal life and family goals is essential in maximizing the patient's prognosis, life plans, and family function (Moro et al., 2008). Patient and family education play a critical role in transplantation rehabilitation and should be considered a mainstay of medical management (Hummel, Michauk, Hetzer, & Fuhrmann, 2001).

Summary

Cardiac transplantation is an important and life-saving surgical intervention used for persons with severe heart muscle disease, end-stage heart failure, and irreversible coronary artery disease associated with multiple myocardial infarctions that have proven unresponsive to medical, surgical, or conservative management. Recent research has demonstrated the critical importance of the application of early exercise initiation following heart transplantation. As outlined in this chapter, a variety of important benefits result from cardiac rehabilitation transplant programs. These include optimization of aerobic capacity, enhanced physical endurance, and vocational capability, as well as improved psychosocial outlook. Rehabilitation team professionals have come to play an important role in this life-extending activity.

LUNG TRANSPLANTATION

The lung functionally serves as a physiological bellow that promotes oxygen acquisition from the atmosphere and carbon dioxide (CO_2) escape into the atmosphere. In respiratory failure, the level of oxygen in the blood becomes dangerously low and/or the level of CO_2 becomes dangerously high. There are two ways this can occur. Either the process by which oxygen and CO_2 are exchanged between blood and the alveoli is compromised, or the movement of air into and out of the lungs becomes dysfunctional. Through either process, chronic respiratory failure can lead to multiple impairments, including severe dyspnea and fatigue that can interfere with the person's ability to participate in ADL. In cases of progressive end-stage lung disease refractory to medical and rehabilitation management, lung transplantation becomes an essential and viable option in not only prolonging life but also improving one's ability to live meaningfully.

In 1963, Dr. James Hardy performed the first single-lung transplant at the University of Mississippi (Hardy, Webb, Dalton, & Walker, 1963). Although the patient died in 18 days, the transplant was considered a tremendous success after several decades of animal studies promising the feasibility of human-lung transplants. Since then, perfection of surgical technique and transplant technology has led to an increase in the number of lung-transplant surgeries conducted each year. The number of bilateral lung transplants has more than doubled over the last decade to 887 and represented 64% of the lung transplants done in 2008 (Mulligan et al., 2008). The International Society for Heart and Lung Transplantation and the St. Louis International Lung Transplantation Registry report 1-year survival rates of 71% and 5-year survival rates of 45% following lung transplantation. The median wait list time has dropped by 87% over the last decade (to 132 days, in 2006; Mulligan et al., 2008). To prevent or minimize transplant-related infection and organ rejection, improved screening methods for infection and tissue-matching techniques for tissue compatibility in organ donors have been developed. This has resulted in marked improvements in the survival rate of organ recipients

(American Transplant Congress, 2003). In addition, state-of-the-art developments in pharmacotherapy, including novel solutions for achieving immunosuppression by employing drugs with greater potency and diminished side effects, have notably improved patient outcomes. Within many medical centers, overall improvement in postsurgical transplantation care and antirejection and antiinfection treatment modes has allowed earlier transfer to the acute rehabilitation venue.

Indications

The most common indications for single-lung transplants are chronic obstructive pulmonary disease and idiopathic pulmonary fibrosis. Bilateral lung transplants are often performed for cystic fibrosis and pulmonary hypertension. Lung transplantation referrals are generally considered for patients with 1-second forced-expiratory ventilation (FEV_1) values of less than 30% of predicted, hypoxia manifested by $PO_2 < 60$ mmHg, or hypercarbia marked by $PCO_2 > 50$ mmHg (Palmer & Tapson, 1998). Workup for lung-transplant candidacy includes chest X-rays, computed tomography scans, and ventilation–perfusion scans. To assess for ischemia, cardiac assessment with catheterization or a chemical-stress test (persantine thalium) is used.

Pre-Lung Transplantation Rehabilitation Factors

A pulmonary rehabilitation program is established to document baseline functions and maximize performance prior to surgery. Oxygen saturations at rest and with exercise are determined with variable flow tanks and ambulatory oxygen saturation meters. Manual muscle testing identifies problem areas and guides a program of resistance exercise. Maximizing nutritional intake in these patients helps to improve postoperative outcomes (Hasse, 1997). Careful review of patient BMI, diet, and prealbumin and albumin levels is essential.

To assess pulmonary functional capacity, the rehabilitation team should quantify ventilatory effort, vital capacity, and FEV_1. Auscultation of the chest for wheezing and bronchial breath sounds is essential for assessment of the effectiveness of bronchodilators, mucociliary clearance, and expectoration efficiency (Downs, 1996). The 6-minute walk test (6MW) is a standard assessment tool used to measure exercise tolerance in patients with various pulmonary diseases. The patient is instructed to ambulate as fast as possible over a flat measured course for 6 minutes. Performance is maximized by adjusting oxygen saturations to stay above 90% and utilization of the most efficient ambulation pattern. Higher-level testing can utilize a cycle ergometer or treadmill. After an individualized plan is designed, patients are initially encouraged to exercise repeatedly for short periods to avoid prolonged breathlessness. Lung-transplant candidates with end-stage pulmonary disease frequently perform better with interval exercise training rather than continuous training, since less ventilatory demand is required. The goal of therapy is to gradually and incrementally decrease the number of required rest periods to enable the patient to achieve longer exercise durations and to reduce the amount of exercise-limiting symptoms. In general, each program should include instructions on efficient ventilation, expectoration, stretching, strengthening, and low-level aerobic endurance. An exercise program that gradually approaches and maintains 60% of peak heart rate can very effectively condition patients (Downs, 1996). Upper-limb exercise has been safely and effectively utilized in pulmonary rehabilitation programs, although it can contribute to dyspnea. In patients with severe pulmonary disease, upper-limb exercise can result in decreased exercise duration and dyssynchronous thoracoabdominal breathing, and hence should be prescribed cautiously.

Inspiratory muscle exercise training can also help to optimize function (Reid & Dechman, 1995). Energy conservation exercises can help the patient adjust to the low functional capacity caused by advanced pulmonary disease. Occupational therapy instruction can aid in the formulation of appropriate work-simplification strategies and energy-conservation measures. The identification of the optimal level of exercise intensity suitable for each patient is an important goal of the rehabilitation team. Target heart rates can be applied to patients with lung disease, a procedure similar to that followed in the case of patients with cardiac disease. However, the high resting-heart rates of this population must be taken into account. Exercise regimens using 60% of peak heart rate as a target, as determined by an exercise test, have been demonstrated to increase exercise tolerance (Biggar, Malen, Trulock, & Cooper, 1993; Bunzel & Laederach-Hofmann, 1999). Patients with severe lung disease typically do not attain predicted maximal heart rates, as exercise is limited by pulmonary rather than cardiac function. Traditional cardiac rehabilitation target exercise formulas, therefore, do not universally apply to the pulmonary rehabilitation patient (Butler, 1995).

The "dyspnea index" is a helpful and simple clinical tool for monitoring and prescribing exercise intensity in patients with dyspnea (Karam et al., 2003). Dyspnea can be assessed using this 5-level index that is based on the number of breaths the patient must take to count to 15. The index runs from Level 0, in which the patient can count to 15 in one breath, to Level 4, in which the patient is too short of breath to count. An alternative measure is the "dyspnea scale" in which the patient rates the degree of dyspnea during exercise (Biggar et al., 1993). A third alternative is the Borg RPE scale (Borg, 1982), which requires the patient to evaluate self-perceived effort during exercise.

Alterations in the patient's health status during the acute pretransplant period often occur due to deteriorating disease. As pulmonary reserves worsen, the pre-lung transplant patient might require abrupt cessation of exercise until he or she is deemed clinically stable to take up exercises (Biggar et al., 1993). Hospitalization might be required if the patient's lung function continues to decline. This deterioration should move the patient's name closer to the top of the transplant waiting list. Some lung-transplant programs require the patient to move closer to the operating center so that they can be more closely monitored (Egan, Kaiser, & Cooper, 1989; Egan et al., 1992).

Post-Lung Transplantation Medical Issues/Complications

Infection
Infection is the most common complication post-lung transplantation and can lead to premature death if not properly recognized and treated (Yun & Mason, 2009). Clinicians should be aware of common pathogens associated with infection. Cytomegalovirus is a common viral pathogen and generally appears 14–100 days postoperatively. The diagnosis of its infection can be made with bronchoscopic lavage and biopsy. Typical fungal pathogens include *Candida, Aspergillus,* and *Pneumocystis* (Arthurs et al., 2009).

Rejection
A majority of acute rejection episodes occur during the initial 3 months following transplantation. Chronic rejection can also occur and can manifest as a sudden decrease in FEV_1 (De Vito et al., 2004). This is known histologically as bronchiolitis obliterans, which may be exacerbated by gastroesophageal reflux (Corris & Christie, 2008). To prevent acute and chronic rejection, patients are commonly placed on triple drug immunosuppressant induction regimens, for example, basiliximab, daclizumab, and antithymocyte globulin. Patients are later discharged on baseline therapy that typically includes corticosteroids, tacrolimus, and an antimetabolite, such as azathioprine. The newer generation of immunosuppressant medications, tacrolimus, rapamycin, and leflunomide are very helpful in averting acute and/ or chronic rejection, although they have significant side effects (McShane & Garrity, 2009; Ng, Madsen, Rosengard, & Allan, 2009).

Post-Lung Transplantation Rehabilitation Program

The Transplanted Lung—Physiology and Function

The transplanted lung is denervated, which leads to impairments of the cough reflex, gas exchange, circulatory autoregulation, mucociliary clearance, and fluid balance. This can result in ineffective clearance of airway secretions, necessitating chest physical therapy. Lymphatic disruption contributes to fluid retention and congestion that hinders gas exchange and reduces lung compliance. Diaphragmatic dysfunction can also be present in lung-transplant recipients, which can be evaluated with electrodiagnostic studies (Biggar et al., 1993; Bunzel & Laederach-Hofmann, 1999; Chlan et al., 1998). Bed rest in these patients can cause orthostatic intolerance, reduced ventilation, increased resting heart rate, and decreased oxygen uptake (Saltin et al., 1968).

Rehabilitation Program

The goals of immediate postoperative rehabilitation are to minimize atelectasis, clear airway secretions, and normalize gas exchange. Altering the patient's position from supine position to a side-lying or upright position can increase drainage from chest tubes, as well as promote drainage of pulmonary secretions. The decreased mucociliary clearance associated with denervated lungs (Dolovich et al., 1987) can contribute to increased susceptibility to infection in the early postoperative period. Therefore, the patient should be assisted with airway clearance, beginning on the first postoperative day if the patient is stable. Patients who are mechanically ventilated can benefit from a combination of shaking (Pneumovest) and hyperinflation with a manual ventilation bag (Webber & Pryor, 1993).

Following extubation, the patient can use the active-cycle-of-breathing technique or use a flutter-valve device. Active-cycle-of-breathing technique uses alternate periods of breathing control, thoracic expansion exercises, and huffing with an open glottis in place of coughing to mobilize secretions. The flutter valve is a pipe-like device used to interrupt expiratory airflow and promote secretion mobilization with a combination of positive expiratory pressure and airway oscillation.

Secretion expectoration requires an effective cough, but such efforts are often hampered by incisional pain and bronchial sensory defects from denervation (Egan et al, 1989; Richard et al., 1955). Coughing technique can be improved using adequate pain-control measures and optimal positioning (Lannefors & Wollmer, 1992). The patient should be encouraged to sit upright during coughing, as this produces the greatest expiratory flow rates (Lannefors & Wollmer, 1992; Webber & Pryor, 1993). Huff coughing is performed without closing the glottis and has been shown to produce a larger volume of expired air at a higher flow rate of secretions than conventional coughing (Hietpas, Roth, & Jensen, 1979). Huffing produces a lower sound, vibrates the pharynx less, and patients may find this activity more comfortable after surgery. For patients unable to generate substantial airflow, the techniques of stacking breaths or positive pressure breathing, before the expulsion phase, can increase the effectiveness of a cough. Incisional pain can interfere with activity progression, deep-breathing exercises, and coughing (Webber & Pryor, 1993). Splinted coughing, with a pillow against the incision, can help reduce incisional pain. Patients may also complain of pain originating from the chest tube sites. Epidural analgesia can help in pain management and allow the patient to participate more enthusiastically in rehabilitation.

Progressive activity should be initiated on the first postoperative day, beginning with range of motion exercises (Palmer & Tapson, 1998). These can be advanced to transfers out of bed to a chair and then to ambulation. After the patient leaves the intensive care unit, rehabilitation should continue to focus on lung ventilation, mobilizing pulmonary secretions, and ventilation–perfusion matching to optimize the concentration of oxygen in the blood. Thoracic mobility can be improved by instructing the patient in chest and upper-extremity mobilization exercises (Butler, 1995; Downs, 1996). Breathing exercises should be incorporated into thoracic mobility and cardiovascular exercise programs, coughing and airway clearance techniques, and general activities.

As the patient progresses, a treadmill and cycle ergometer can be introduced into the exercise program, allowing the patient to improve cardiovascular endurance and strength and reduce the infection risk. Pulmonary transplant recipients can often reach exercise intensities comparable to fully able-bodied patients of similar ages (Palmer & Tapson, 1998). Denervation of the lungs does not impair the ability to increase ventilation during physical exertion, and most studies show that physical training results in improved endurance and strength (Kjaer et al., 1999). Before discharge from the hospital, the patient should progress to stair climbing, which is the hallmark of recovery, as advanced pulmonary disease typically has made it impossible for most patients to do this for a period of weeks to years.

Cardiopulmonary exercise testing has demonstrated areas of limitation in assessing exercise capacity after lung transplantation. Aerobic capacity, judged by maximal oxygen uptake, typically remains reduced by 32–60% of the predicted value in this patient population (Williams, Grossman, & Maurer, 1990). This reduction in aerobic capacity is thought to underlie the exercise limitations in lung-transplant patients. Abnormalities of gas exchange and ventilation perfusion are not thought to play a major role in the reduced exercise capacity of single-lung-transplant patients. Many other factors can contribute to reduced exercise reserve, including chronic deconditioning and muscle atrophy. Peripheral muscle work capacity is reduced following lung transplantation and is predominantly responsible for performance limitations of patients while exercising.

Post-Lung Transplantation Outcomes

Following lung transplantation, patients usually achieve considerable restoration of functional ability (Duarte et al., 2008). Compared to education alone, pulmonary rehabilitation has been shown to increase exercise performance and to decrease muscle fatigue and shortness of breath (Ries, Kaplan, Limberg, & Prewitt, 1995). Improvement in exercise tolerance has been demonstrated by an increase in 6-minute walk distances after transplantation (Biggar et al., 1993; Egan et al., 1992; Mal et al., 1994; Williams et al., 1990). One center reported that none of their lung transplant recipients had to terminate a maximal symptom-limited exercise test because of dyspnea, as the main complaint was lower-limb discomfort or pain (Howard, Iademarco, & Trulock, 1994).

After surgery has been performed and the recuperative process has been successful, the lung-transplant survivor faces the challenge of returning to work. Quite often, returning to work or homemaking duties helps to restore a critical sense of normalcy to the daily routine and helps to significantly bolster self-esteem and wellness (Petrucci et al., 2007). Fortunately, more than 90% of lung transplantation patients report satisfaction with their health while performing these tasks (Craven, Bright, & Dear, 1990). One leading study revealed a 37% employment rate among lung-transplant survivors (Paris et al., 1998). Employment status has not been shown to be correlated with the type of lung transplantation procedure performed (single or bilateral; Huddleston et al., 2002).

Summary

The process of rehabilitation following lung transplant is an essential component of restorative aftercare that can facilitate marked improvements in ADL and functional independence. Though the early goals of posttransplant rehabilitation are largely physiological, that is, promotion of normalized gas exchange, clearing of airway secretions and minimization of atelectasis, during the more advanced phase of pulmonary rehabilitation, patients are remobilized and encouraged to regain proficiency in ADL skills and functional self-sufficiency.

Ultimately, the lung-transplant patient is provided with opportunities for vocational reentry and employment as part of the rehabilitation cycle.

CONCLUSION

Advances in medical care and surgical techniques and technology within the past 25 years have significantly reduced morbidity and mortality in posttransplantation patients. Success can no longer be measured by the number of years after transplantation but by the quality of those years. Rehabilitation has never played a more important role in maximizing the potential of these patients. Transplant rehabilitation can add "life to years," serving as a vital complement to transplant surgery that adds "years to life."

REFERENCES

Abbasoglu, O. (2008). Liver transplantation: Yesterday, today and tomorrow. *World Journal of Gastroenterology, 14*, 3117–3122.

Adams, P. C., Ghent, C. N., Grant, D. R., & Wall, W. J. (1995). Employment after liver transplantation. *Hepatology, 21*, 140–144.

Agarwal, S., & Owen, R. (1990). Tendinitis and tendon rupture in successful renal transplant recipients. *Clinical Orthopaedics and Related Research*, (252), 270–275.

American Heart Association. (2009). *Heart transplants: Statistics.* Retrieved from http://www.american-heart.org/presenter.jhtml?identifier=4588

American Transplant Congress. (2003). The Fourth Joint American Transplant Meeting. May 30–June 04, 2003. Washington, DC.

Arthurs, S. K., Eid, A. J., Deziel, P. J., Marshall, W. F., Cassivi, S. D., Walker, R. C., et al. (2009, August 27). The impact of invasive fungal diseases on survival after lung transplantation. *Clinical Transplantation,* [Epub ahead of print].

Auerbach, I., Tenenbaum, A., Motro, M., Stroh, C. I., Har-Zahav, Y., & Fisman, E. Z. (1999). Attenuated responses of Doppler-derived hemodynamic parameters during supine bicycle exercise in heart transplant recipients. *Cardiology, 92*, 204–209.

Beck, W., Barnard, C. N., & Schrire, V. (1969). Heart rate after cardiac transplantation. *Circulation, 40*, 437–445.

Benten, D., Staufer, K., & Sterneck, M. (2009). Orthotopic liver transplantation and what to do during follow-up: Recommendations for the practitioner. *Gastroenterology and Hepatology, 6*, 23–36.

Bernardi, L., Radaelli, A., Passino, C., Falcone, C., Auguadro, C., Martinelli, L., et al. (2007). Effects of physical training on cardiovascular control after heart transplantation. *International Journal of Cardiology, 118*, 356–362.

Beyer, N., Aadahl, M., Strange, B., Kirkegaard, P., Hansen, B. A., Mohr, T., et al. (1999). Improved physical performance after orthotopic liver transplantation. *Liver Transplant Surgery, 5*, 301–309.

Beyer, N., Aadahl, M., Strange, B., Mohr, T., & Kjaer, M. (1995). Exercise capacity of patients after liver transplantation. *Medicine & Science in Sports & Exercise, 6*, S84.

Biggar, D. G., Malen, J. F., Trulock, E. P., & Cooper, J. D. (1993). Pulmonary rehabilitation before and after lung transplantation. In R. Kasaburi & T. L. Petty (Eds.), *Principles and practice of pulmonary rehabilitation* (pp. 459–467). Philadelphia: W. B. Saunders.

Bohannon, R. W., Smith, J., Hull, D., Palmeri, D., & Barnhard, R. (1995). Deficits in lower extremity muscle and gait performance among renal transplant candidates. *Archives of Physical Medicine and Rehabilitation, 76*, 547–551.

Borg, G. (1982). Psychophysical basis of perceived exertion. *Medicine & Science in Sports & Exercise, 14*, 377–381.

Braith, R. W., & Edwards, D. G. (2000). Exercise following heart transplantation. *Sports Medicine, 30*, 171–192.

Braith, R. W., Clapp, L., Brown, T., Brown, C., Schofield, R., Mills, R. M., et al. (2000). Rate-responsive pacing improves exercise tolerance in heart transplant recipients: A pilot study. *Journal of Cardiopulmonary Rehabilitation, 20*, 377–382.

Braith, R. W., Welsch, M. A., Mills, R. M. Jr., Keller, J. W., & Pollock, M. L. (1998). Resistance exercise prevents glucocorticoid-induced myopathy in heart transplant recipients. *Medicine & Science in Sports & Exercise, 30*, 483–489.

Bunke, M., & Ganzel, B. (1992). Effects of calcium antagonists on renal function in hypertensive heart transplant recipients. *Journal of Heart and Lung Transplantation, 2*, 1194–1199.

Bunzel, B., & Laederach-Hofmann, K. (1999). Long-term effects of heart transplantation: The gap between physical performance and emotional well-being. *Scandinavian Journal of Rehabilitation Medicine, 31*, 214–222.

Butler, B. B. (1995). Physical therapy in heart and lung transplantation. In E. Hillegas, & S. Sadowski, (Eds.), *Cardiopulmonary physical therapy* (3rd ed.) (pp. 404–422). St Louis, MO: Mosby–Year Book.

Campellone, J. V., Lacomis, D., Giuliani, M. J., & Kramer, D. J. (1998). Mononeuropathies associated with liver transplantation. *Muscle and Nerve, 21*, 896–901.

Carithers, R. L. Jr. (2000). Liver transplantation: American Association for the Study of Liver Diseases. *Liver Transplantation, 6*, 122–135.

Carney, R. M., Templeton, B., Hong, B. A., Harter, H. R., Hagberg, J. M., Schechtman, K. B., et al. (1987). Exercise training reduces depression and increases the performance of pleasant activities in hemodialysis patients. *Nephron, 47*, 194–198.

Chlan, L., Snyder, M., Finkelstein, S., Hertz, M., Edin, C., Wielinski, C., et al. (1998). Promoting adherence to an electronic home spirometry research program after lung transplantation. *Applied Nursing Research, 11*, 36–40.

Christiansen, E., Vestergaard, H., Tibell, A., Hother-Nielsen, O., Holst, J. J., Pedersen, O., et al. (1996). Impaired insulin-stimulated non-oxidative glucose metabolism in pancreas-kidney transplant recipients. Dose- response characteristics of insulin on glucose turnover. *Diabetes, 45*, 1267–1275.

Colm, C. M., & Pascual, M. (2004). Update in renal transplantation. *Archives of Internal Medicine, 164*, 1373–1388.

Copeland, J. G., Smith, R. G., Arabia, F. A., Nolan, P., Sethi, G. K., Tsau, P. H., et al. (2004). CardioWest Total Artificial Heart Investigators. Bridge to transplantation. *New England Journal of Medicine, 351*, 859–867.

Corris, P. A., & Christie, J. D. (2008). Update in transplantation 2007. *American Journal of Respiratory and Critical Care Medicine, 177*, 1062–1067.

Cortazzo, M. H., Helkowski, W., Pippin, B., Boninger, M. L., & Zafonte, R. (2005). Acute inpatient rehabilitation of 55 patients after liver transplantation. American *Journal of Physical Medicine & Rehabilitation, 84*, 880–884.

Craven, J. L., Bright, J., & Dear, C. L. (1990). Psychiatric, psychosocial and rehabilitative aspects of lung transplantation. *Clinics in Chest Medicine, 11*, 247–257.

Crosbie, O., Freaney, R., McKenna, M., & Hegarty, J. (1999). Bone density, vitamin D status and disordered bone remodeling in end-stage chronic liver disease. *Calcified Tissue International, 64*, 295–300.

D'Amico, C. L. (2005). Cardiac transplantation: Patient selection in the current era. *Journal of Cardiovascular Nursing, 20*(Suppl. 5), S4–S13.

Dandel, M., Wellnhofer, E., Hummel, M., Meyer, R., Lehmkuhl, H., & Hetzer, R. (2003). Early detection of left ventricular dysfunction related to transplant coronary artery disease. *Journal of Heart and Lung Transplantation, 22*, 1353–1364.

De Vito Dabbs, A., Hoffman, L. A., Swigart, V., Happ, M. B., Iacono, A. T., & Dauber, J. H. (2004). Using conceptual triangulation to develop an integrated model of the symptom experience of acute rejection after lung transplantation. *Advances in Nursing Science, 27*, 138–149.

Dew, M. A., DiMartini, A. F., Steel, J., De Vito Dabbs, A., Myaskovsky, L., Unruh, M., et al. (2008). Metaanalysis of risk for relapse to substance use after transplantation of the liver or other solid organs. *Liver Transplantation, 14*, 159–172.

Deuse, T., Haddad, F., Pham, M., Hunt, S., Valantine, H., Bates, M. J., et al. (2008). Twenty-year survivors of heart transplantation at Stanford University. *American Journal of Transplantation, 8*, 1769–1774.

Diamond, T., Stiel, D., Wilkinson, M., & Posen, J. R. (1990). Osteoporosis and skeletal fractures in chronic liver disease. *Gut, 31*, 82–87.

Dolovich, M., Rossman, C., Chambers, C., Grossman, R. F., Newhouse, M., The Toronto Lung Transplant Group, et al. (1987). Mucociliary function in patients following single lung or lung/heart transplantation. *American Review of Respiratory Disease, 135*, 363 [Abstract].

Downs, A. M. (1996). Physical therapy in lung transplantation. *Physical Therapy, 76*, 626–642.

Drexler, H., & Schroeder, J. S. (1994). Unusual forms of ischemic heart disease. *Current Opinion in Cardiology, 9,* 457–464.

Duarte, A. G., Terminella, L., Smith, J. T., Myers, A. C., Campbell, G., & Lick, S. (2008). Restoration of cough reflex in lung transplant recipients. *Chest, 134,* 310–316.

Egan, T. M., Kaiser, L. R., & Cooper, J. D. (1989). Lung transplantation. *Current Problems in Surgery, 26,* 673–752.

Egan, T. M., Westerman, J. H., Lambert, C. J. Jr., Detterbeck, F. C., Thompson, J. T., Mill, M. R., et al. (1992). Isolated lung transplantation for end-stage lung disease: A viable therapy. *Annals of Thoracic Surgery, 53,* 590–596.

Fujisawa, M., Ichikawa, Y., Yoshiya, K., Isotani, S., Higuchi, A., Nagano, S., et al. (2000). Assessment of health-related quality of life in renal transplant and hemodialysis patients using the SF-36 health survey. *Urology, 56,* 201.

Fuhrmann, I., & Krause, R. (2004). Principles of exercising in patients with chronic kidney disease, on dialysis and for kidney transplant recipients. *Clinical Nephrology, 61,* S14–S25.

Gammie, J. S., Edwards, L. B., Griffith, B. P., Pierson, R. N. 3rd, & Tsao, L. (2004). Optimal timing of cardiac transplantation after ventricular assist device implantation. *Journal of Thoracic and Cardiovascular Surgery, 127,* 1789–1799.

Goldberg, A. P., Geltman, E. M., Gavin, J. R. 3rd, Carney, R. M., Hagberg, J. M., Delmez, J. A., et al. (1986). Exercise training reduces coronary risk and effectively rehabilitates hemodialysis patients. *Nephron, 42,* 311–316.

Greenberg, A., Egel, J. W., Thompson, M. E., Hardesty, R. L., Griffith, B. P., Bahnson, H. T., et al. (1987). Early and late forms of cyclosporine nephrotoxicity: Studies in cardiac transplant recipients. *American Journal of Kidney Diseases, 9,* 12–22.

Greenberg, M. L., Uretsky, B. F., Reddy, P. S., Bernstein, R. L., Griffith, B. P., Hardesty, R. L., et al. (1985). Long-term hemodynamic follow-up of cardiac transplant patients treated with cyclosporine and prednisone. *Circulation, 71,* 487–494.

Griepp, R. B., Stinson, E. D., Dong, E. Jr., Clark, D. A., & Shumway, N. E. (1971). Hemodynamic performance of the transplanted human heart. *Surgery, 70,* 88–96.

Gurk-Turner C. (1997). Management of the metabolic complications of liver disease: An overview of commonly used pharmacological agents. *Support Line, 19,* 17–19.

Hardy, J. D., Webb, W. R., Dalton, M. L., & Walker, G. R., Jr. (1963). Lung homotransplantation in man. *Journal of the American Medical Association, 186,* 1065–1074.

Harrison, J., McKiernan, J., & Neuberger, J. M. (1997). A prospective study on the effect of recipient nutritional status on outcome in liver transplantation. *Transplant International, 10,* 360–374.

Hasse, J. M. (1997). Diet therapy for organ transplantation. A problem-based approach. *Nursing Clinics of North America, 32,* 863–880.

Hietpas, B., Roth, R., & Jensen, W. (1979). Huff coughing and airway patency. *Respiratory Care, 24,* 710–714.

Hosenpud, J. D., Novick, R. J., Breen, T. J., & Daily, O. P. (1994). Registry of the International Society for Heart and Lung Transplantation: Eleventh official report—1994. *Journal of Heart and Lung Transplantation, 13,* 561–570.

Howard, D. K., Iademarco, E. J., & Trulock, E. P. (1994). The role of cardiopulmonary exercise testing in lung and heart-lung transplantation. *Clinics in Chest Medicine, 15,* 405–420.

Huddleston, C. B., Bloch, J. B., Sweet, S. C., de la Morena, M., Patterson, G. A., & Mendeloff, E. N. (2002). Lung transplant in children. *Annals of Surgery, 236,* 270–276.

Humar, A., Denny, R., Matas, A. J., & Najarian, J. S. (2003). Great and quality of life outcomes in older recipients of a kidney transplant. *Experimental and Clinical Transplantation, 1,* 69–72.

Hummel, M., Michauk, I., Hetzer, R., & Fuhrmann, B. (2001). Quality of life after heart and heart-lung transplantation. *Transplantation Proceedings, 33,* 3546–3548.

International Society for Heart & Lung Transplantation. (2009). International Society for Heart and Lung Transplant ISHLT- 29th Annual Meeting and Scientific Sessions. Paris, France.

Joshi, A., & Kevorkian, C. G. (1997). Rehabilitation after cardiac transplantation. Case series and literature review. *American Journal of Physical Medicine & Rehabilitation, 76,* 249–254.

Juskowa, J., Lewandowska, M., Bartłomiejczyk, I., Foroncewicz, B., Korabiewska, I., Niewczas, M., et al. (2006). Physical rehabilitation and risk of atherosclerosis after successful kidney transplantation. *Transplantation Proceedings, 38,* 157–160.

Harrison, J., McKiernan, J., & Neuberger, J. M. (1997). A prospective study on the effect of recipient nutritional status on outcome in liver transplantation. *Transplant International, 10,* 360–374.

Kao, A. C., Van Trigt, P. R., Shaeffer-McCall, G. S., Shaw, J. P., Kuzil, B. B., Page, R. D., et al. (1995). Allograft diastolic dysfunction and chronotropic incompetence limit cardiac output response to exercise two to six years after heart transplantation. *Journal of Heart and Lung Transplantation, 14,* 11–22.

Karam, V., Castaing, D., Danet, C., Delvart, V., Gasquet, I., Adam, R., et al. (2003). Longitudinal prospective evaluation of quality of life in adult patients before and one year after liver transplantation. *Liver Transplantation, 9,* 703–711.

Kavanagh, T., & Yacoub, M. H. (1992). Exercise training in patients after heart transplantation. *Annals Academy of Medicine Singapore, 21,* 372–378.

Kavanagh, T., Yacoub, M. H., Mertens, D. J., Kennedy, J., Campbell, R. B., & Sawyer, P. (1988). Cardiorespiratory responses to exercise training after orthotopic cardiac transplantation. *Circulation, 77,* 162–171.

Keeffe, E. B. (2001). Liver Transplantation: Current status and novel approaches to liver replacement. *Gastroenterology, 120,* 749–762.

Kempeneers, G. L. G., Myburgh, K. H., Wiggins, T., Adams, B., van Zyl-Smit, R., & Noakes, T. D. (1988). The effect of an exercise training program on renal transplant recipients. *Transplantation Proceedings* 20(Suppl. 1), 381–386.

Keogh, J. B., Tsalamandris, C., Sewell, R. B., Jones, R. M., Angus, P. W., Nyulasi, I. B., et al. (1999). Bone loss at the proximal femur and reduced lean mass following liver transplantation: A longitudinal study. *Nutrition, 15,* 661–664.

Keteyian, S., Marks, C. R., Levine, A. B., Fedel, F., Ehrman, J., Kataoka, T., et al. (1994). Cardiovascular responses of cardiac transplant patients to arm and leg exercise. *European Journal of Applied Physiology, 68,* 441–444.

Kevorkian, C. G. (1999). Stroke rehabilitation and the cardiac transplantation patient. *New England Journal of Medicine, 340,* 976.

Kjaer, M., Beyer, N., & Secher, N. H. (1999). Exercise and organ transplantation. *Scandinavian Journal of Medicine & Science in Sports, 9,* 1–14.

Kjaer, M., Kelding, S., Engfred, K., Rasmussen, K., Sonne, B., Kirkegård, P., et al. (1996). Glucose homeostasis during exercise in humans with a liver or kidney transplant. *American Journal of Physiology, 268,* E636–E644.

Kobashigawa, J. A., Laks, H., Marelli, D., Moriguchi, J. D., Hamilton, M. A., Fonarow, G., et al. (1998). The University of California at Los Angeles experience in heart transplantation. *Clinical Transplantation,* 303–310.

Kobashigawa, J. A., Leaf, D. A., Lee, N., Gleeson, M. P., Liu, H., Hamilton, M. A., et al. (1999). A controlled trial of exercise rehabilitation after heart transplantation. *New England Journal of Medicine, 340*(12), 976.

Koffron, A., & Stein, J. A. (2008). Liver transplantation: Indications, pre-transplant evaluation, surgery, and post-transplant complications. *Medical Clinics of North America, 92,* 861–888.

Kohzuki, M., Abo, T., Watanabe, M., Goto, Y., Ohkohchi, N., Satomi, S., et al. (2000). Rehabilitating patients with hepatopulmonary syndrome using living-related orthotopic liver transplant: A case report. *Archives of Physical Medicine and Rehabilitation, 81,* 1527–1530.

Korbiewska, L., Lewandowska, M., Juskowa, J., & Bialoszewski, D. (2007). Need for rehabilitation in renal replacement therapy involving allogeneic kidney transplantation. *Transplantation Proceedings, 39,* 2776–2777.

Krull, F., Schulze-Neick, I., Hatopp, A., Offner, G., & Brodehl, J. (1994). Exercise capacity and blood pressure response in children and adolescents after renal transplantation. *Acta Paediatrica, 83,* 1296–1302.

Lampert, E., Mettauer, B., Hoppeler, H., Charloux, A., & Charpentier, A. (1998). Skeletal muscle response to short endurance training in heart transplant recipients. *Journal of the American College of Cardiology, 32,* 420–426.

Lannefors, L., & Wollmer, P. (1992). Mucus clearance with three chest physiotherapy regimens in cystic fibrosis: A comparison between postural drainage, PEP, and physical exercise. *European Respiratory Journal, 5,* 748–753.

Lahpor, J. R. (2009). State of the art: Implantable ventricular assist devices. *Current Opinion in Organ Transplantation, 14,* 554–559.

Latlief, G. A., & Young, M. A. (1994). Cardiac transplant rehabilitation in a post-partum woman. *Archives of Physical Medicine and Rehabilitation, 75,* 1040.

Le Jemtel, T. H. (2003). Review of a controlled trial of exercise rehabilitation after heart transplantation. *Transplantation Proceedings, 35,* 1513–1515.

Leenen, F. H., Davies, R. A., & Fourney, A. (1995). Role of cardiac beta 2- receptors in cardiac responses to exercise in cardiac transplant patients. *Circulation, 91,* 685–690.

Legault, L., Olgilvie, R. I., Cardella, C. J., & Leenen, P. H. (1993). Calcium antagonists in heart transplant recipients: Effects on cardiac and renal function and cyclosporine pharmacokinetics. *Canadian Journal of Cardiology, 9,* 398–404.

Li, S., Lue, W., Mobarhan, S., Nadir, A., Van Thiel, D., & Hagety, A. (2000). Nutrition support for individuals with liver failure. *Nutrition Reviews, 58,* 242–247.

Lopez, P. M., & Martin, P. (2006). Update on liver transplantation: Indications, organ allocation and long-term care. *Mount Sinai Journal of Medicine, 73,* 1056–1066.

Lucas, T. S., & Einhorn, T. A. (1993). Stress fracture of the femoral neck during rehabilitation after heart transplantation. *Archives of Physical Medicine and Rehabilitation, 74,* 1004–1006.

Mal, H., Sleiman, C., Jebrak, G., Messian, O., Dubois, F., Darne, C., et al. (1994). Functional results of single-lung transplantation for chronic obstructive lung disease. *American Journal of Respiratory and Critical Care Medicine, 149,* 1476–1481.

Martin, T. W., Gaucher, J., Pupa, L. E., & Seaworth, J. F. (1994). Response to upright exercise after cardiac transplantation. *Clinical Cardiology, 17,* 292–300.

McCaughan, G. W., & Feller, R. B. (1994). Osteoporosis in chronic liver disease: Pathogenesis, risk factors and management. *Digestive Diseases of Sciences, 12,* 223–231.

McGiffin, D., Kirklin, J. K., & Nafiel, D. C. (1985). Acute renal failure after heart transplantation and cyclosporine therapy. *Journal of Heart and Lung Transplantation, 4,* 396–399.

McShane, P. J., & Garrity, E. R. Jr. (2009). Minimization of immunosuppression after lung transplantation: Current trends. *Transplant International, 22,* 90–95.

Mettauer, B., Levy, F., Richard, R., Roth, O., Zoll, J., Lampert, E., et al. (2005). Exercising with a denervated heart after cardiac transplantation. *Annals of Transplantation, 10,* 35–42.

Meyer, M., Rahmel, A., Marconi, C., Grassi, B., Cerretelli, P., & Cabrol, C. (1994). Adjustment of cardiac output to step exercise in heart transplant recipients. *Zeitschrift für Kardiologie, 83*(Suppl. 3), 103–109.

Miller, L. W., Naftel, D. C., Bourge, R. C., Costanzo, M. R., Pitts, D., Rayburn, B., et al. (1994). Infection after heart transplantation: A multi-institutional study—Cardiac Transplant Research Database Group. *Journal of Heart and Lung Transplantation, 13,* 381–393.

Mills, R. M. Jr. (1994). Transplantation and the problems afterward including coronary vasculopathy. *Clinical Cardiology, 17,* 287–290.

Moro, J. A., Almenar, L., Martñez-Dolz, L., Agüero, J., Sánchez-Lázaro, I., Iglesias, P., et al. (2008). Support program for heart transplant patients: Initial experience. *Transplantation Proceedings, 40,* 3039–3040.

Mulligan, M. S., Shearon, T. H., Weill, D., Pagani, F. D., Moore, J., & Murray, S. (2008). Heart and lung transplantation in the United States 1997–2006. *American Journal of Transplantation, 8*(Part 2), 977–987.

Munoz, S. (1991). Nutritional therapies in liver disease. *Seminars in Liver Disease, 11,* 278–289.

Neipp, M., Karavul, B., Jackobs, S., Meyer zu Vilsendorf, A., Richter, N., Becker, T., et al. (2006). Quality of life in adult transplant recipients more than 15 years after kidney transplantation. *Transplantation, 81,* 1640–1644.

Ng, C.Y., Madsen, J. C., Rosengard, B. R., & Allan, J. S. (2009). Immunosuppression for lung transplantation. *Frontiers in Bioscience, 1,* 1627–1641.

Nicholas, J. J., Oleske, D., Robinson, L. R., Switala, J. A., & Tarter, R. (1994). The quality of life after orthotopic liver transplantation: An analysis of 166 cases. *Archives of Physical Medicine and Rehabilitation, 75,* 431–435.

O'Connell, J. B., Bourge, R. C., Costanzo-Nordin, M. R., Driscoll, D. J., Morgan, J. P., Rose, E. A., et al. (1992). Cardiac transplantation: Recipient selection, donor procurement, and medical follow-up—A statement for health professionals from the Committee on Cardiac Transplantation of the Council on Clinical Cardiology, American Heart Association. *Circulation, 86,* 1061–1079.

Oliver, D., Pflugfelder, P. W., McCartney, N., McKelvie, R. S., Suskin, N., & Kostuk, W. J. (2001). Acute cardiovascular responses to leg-press resistance exercise in heart transplant recipients. *International Journal of Cardiology, 81,* 61–74.

Overbeck, I., Bartels, M., Decker, O., Harms, J., Hauss, J., & Fangmann, J. (2005). Changes in quality of life after renal transplantation. *Transplantation Proceedings, 37,* 1618–1621.

Painter, P. L., Nelson-Worel, J. N., Hill, M. M., Thornbery, D. R., Shelp, W. R., Harrington, A. R., et al. (1986). Effects of exercise training during hemodialysis. *Nephron, 43,* 87–92.

Painter, P., Krasnoff, J., Paul, S., & Ascher, N. (2001). Physical activity and quality of life in long-term liver transplant recipients. *Liver Transplantation, 7,* 213–219.

Painter, P., Moore, G., Carlson, L., Paul, S., Myll, J., Phillips, W., et al. (2002a). Effects of exercise training plus normalization of hematocrit on exercise capacity and health-related quality of life. *American Journal of Kidney Diseases, 39,* 257–265.

Painter, P. L., Hector, L., Ray, K., Lynes, L., Dibble, S., Paul, S. M., et al. (2002b). A randomized trial of exercise training after renal transplantation. *Transplantation, 74,* 42–48.

Painter, P. L., Luetkemeier, M. J., Moore, G. E., Dibble, S. L., Green, G. A., Myll, J. O., et al. (1997). Health-related fitness and quality of life in organ transplant recipients. *Transplantation, 64,* 1795–1800.

Palmer, S. M., & Tapson, V. F. (1998). Pulmonary rehabilitation in the surgical patient. Lung transplantation and lung volume reduction surgery. *Respiratory Care Clinics of North America, 4,* 71–83.

Paris, W., Diercks, M., Bright, J., Zamora, M., Kesten, S., Scavuzzo, M., et al. (1998). Return to work after lung transplantation. *Journal of Heart and Lung Transplantation, 17,* 430–436.

Paterson, D. H., Cunningham, D. A., Pickering, J. G., Babcock, M. A., & Boughner, D. R. (1994). Oxygen uptake kinetics in cardiac transplant recipients. *Journal of Applied Physiology, 77,* 1935–1940.

Petrucci, L., Ricotti, S., Michelini, I., Vitulo, P., Oggionni, T., Cascina, A., et al. (2007). Return to work after thoracic organ transplantation in a clinically-stable population. *European Journal of Heart Failure, 9,* 1112–1119.

Quittan, M., Wiesinger, G. F., Sturm, B., Puig, S., Mayr, W., Sochor, A., et al. (2001). Improvement of thigh muscles by neuromuscular electrical stimulation in patients with refractory heart failure: A single-blind, randomized, controlled trial. *American Journal of Physical Medicine & Rehabilitation, 80,* 206–214, 215–216, 224.

Rajendran, A. J., Pandurangi, U. M., Mullasari, A. S., Gomathy, S., Rao, K. V. (2006). High intensity exercise training programme following cardiac transplant. *Indian Journal of Chest Diseases & Allied Sciences, 48,* 271–273.

Rao, V., Oz, M. C., Flannery, M. A., Catanese, K. A., Argenziano, M., & Naka, Y. (2003). Revised screening scale to predict survival after insertion of a left ventricular assist device. *Journal of Thoracic & Cardiovascular Surgery, 125,* 855–862.

Reid, W. D., & Dechman, G. (1995). Considerations when testing and training the respiratory muscles. *Physical Therapy, 75,* 971–982.

Richard, C., Girard, F., Ferraro, P., Chouinard, P., Boudreault, D., Ruel, M., et al. (1955). Acute postoperative pain in lung transplant recipients. *Annals of Thoracic Surgery, 77,* 1951–1955.

Ries, A. L., Kaplan, R. M., Limberg, T. M., & Prewitt, L. M. (1995). Effects of pulmonary rehabilitation on physiologic and psychosocial outcomes in patients with chronic obstructive pulmonary disease. *Annals of Internal Medicine, 122,* 823–832.

Ring, H. (2004). International Rehabilitation Medicine: Closing the Gaps and Globalization of the Profession. *American Journal of Physical Medicine & Rehabilitation, 83,* 667–669.

Robertson, H. T., Haley, N. R., Guthrie, M., Cardenas, D., Eschbach, J. W., & Adamson, J. W. (1990). Recombinant erythropoietin improves exercise capacity in anemic hemodialysis patients. American Journal of Kidney Diseases. *American Journal of Physical Medicine & Rehabilitation, 15,* 325–332.

Robinson, L. R., Switala, J., Tarter, R. E., & Nicholas, J. J. (1990). Functional outcome after liver transplantation: A preliminary report. *Archives of Physical Medicine and Rehabilitation, 71,* 426–427.

Rudow, D. L., & Goldstein, M. J. (2008). Critical care management of the liver transplant recipient. *Critical Care Nursing Quarterly, 31,* 232–243.

Saltin, B., Blomqvist, G., Mitchell, J., Johnson, R. J., Wildenthal, K., & Chapman, C. (1968). Response to exercise after bed rest and after training. *Circulation, 38*(Suppl. 5), 1–80.

Savin, W. M., Haskell, W. L., Schroeder, J. S., & Stinson, E. B. (1980). Cardiorespiratory responses of cardiac transplant patients to graded symptom limited exercise. *Circulation, 62,* 55–60.

Schroeder, J. S., Gao, S. Z., Alderman, E. L., Hunt, S. A., Johnstone, I., Boothroyd, D. B., et al. (1993). A preliminary study of diltiazem in the prevention of coronary artery disease in heart transplant recipients. *New England Journal of Medicine, 328,* 164–170.

Scott, J. P., Hay, I. F., Higenbuttam, C., Evans, D., & Calne, R.Y. (1990). Hypertensive exercise responses in cyclosporine treated normotensive renal transplant recipients. *Nephron, 56,* 143–147.

Selberg, O., Bottcher, J., Tusch, G., Pichlmayr, R., Henkel, E., & Muller, M. (1997). Identification of high and low-risk patients before liver transplantation: A prospective cohort study of nutritional and metabolic parameters in 150 patients. *Hepatology, 25,* 652–657.

Shaver, J. A., Leon, D. F., Gray, S. D., Leonard, J. J., & Bahnson, H. T. (1969). Hemodynamic observations after cardiac transplantation. *New England Journal of Medicine, 281,* 822–827.

Shephard, R. J., Kavanagh, T., Mertens, D. J., & Yacoub, M. (1996). The place of perceived exertion ratings in exercise prescription for cardiac transplant patients before and after training. *British Journal of Sports Medicine, 30,* 116–121.

Sliwa, J. A., Andersen, S., & Griffin, J. (1990). Cardiovascular responses to gait training and ambulation in a hemiparetic heart recipient. *Archives of Physical Medicine and Rehabilitation, 71,* 424–425.

Sliwa, J. A., & Blendonohy, P. M. (1988). Stroke rehabilitation in a patient with a history of heart transplantation. *Archives of Physical Medicine and Rehabilitation, 69,* 973–975.

Solomon, N. A., McGiven, J. R., Alison, P. M., Ruygrok, P. N., Haydock, D. A., Coverdale, H. A., et al. (2004). Changing donor and recipient demographics in a heart transplantation program: Influence on early outcome. *Annals of Thoracic Surgery, 77,* 2096–2102.

Squires, R. W. (1991). Exercise training after cardiac transplantation. *Medicine & Science in Sports & Exercise, 23,* 686–694.

Starzl, T. E., Klintmalm, G. B., Porter, K. A., Iwatsuki, S., & Schroter, G. P. (1981). Liver transplantation with use of cyclosporin A and prednisone. *New England Journal of Medicine, 305,* 266–269.

Stewart, K. J., Badenhop, D., Brubaker, P. H., Keteyian, S. J., & King, M. (2003). Cardiac rehabilitation following percutaneous revascularization, heart transplant, heart valve surgery, and for chronic heart failure. *Chest, 123,* 2104–2111.

Streiff, N., Feurer, I., Speroff, T., Davis, S. F., Butler, J., Chomsky, D., et al. (2001). The effects of rejection episodes, obesity, and osteopenia on functional performance and health-related quality of life after heart transplantation. *Transplantation Proceedings, 33,* 3533–3535.

Tayler, A., & Bergin, J. (1995). Cardiac transplantation for the cardiologist not trained in transplantation. *Annals of Thoracic Surgery, 129,* 578–592.

Tegtbur, U., Pethig, K., Machold, H., Haverich, A., & Busse, M. (2003). Functional endurance capacity and exercise training in long-term treatment after heart transplantation. *Cardiology, 99,* 171–176.

Tegtbur, U., Busse, M. W., Jung, K., Pethig, K., & Haverich, A. (2005). Time course of physical reconditioning during exercise rehabilitation late after heart transplantation. *Journal of Heart & Lung Transplantation, 24,* 270–274.

The U.S. Multicenter FK 506 Liver Study Group. (1994). A comparison of tacrolimus (FK 506) and cyclosporine for immunosuppression in liver transplantation. *New England Journal of Medicine, 331,* 1110–1115.

Valentine, H., Keogh, A., McIntosh, N., Hunt, S., Oyer, P., & Schroeder, J. (1992). Cost containment: Co-administration of diltiazem with cyclosporine, after heart transplantation. *Journal of Heart & Lung Transplantation, 2*(part 1), 1–7.

van Ginneken, B. T., van den Berg-Emons, R. J., Kazemier, G., Metselaar, H. J., Tilanus, H. W., & Stam, H. J. (2007). Physical fitness, fatigue and quality of life after liver transplantation. *European Journal of Applied Physiology, 100,* 345–353.

Vaska, P. L. (1993). Common infections in heart transplant patients. *American Journal of Critical Care, 2,* 145–156.

Ville, N. S., Varray, A., Mercier, B., Hayot, M., Albat, B., Chamari, K., et al. (2002). Effects of an enhanced heart rate reserve on aerobic performance in patients with a heart transplant. *American Journal of Physical Medicine & Rehabilitation, 81,* 584–589.

Vintro, A. Q., Krasnoff, J. B., & Painter, P. (2002). Roles of nutrition and physical activity in musculoskeletal complications before and after liver transplantation. *AACN Clinical Issues, 13,* 333–347.

Von Scheidt, W., Kembes, B. M., Reichart, B., & Erdmann, E. (1993). Percutaneous transluminal coronary angioplasty of focal coronary lesions after cardiac transplantation. *Journal of Clinical Investigation, 71,* 524–530.

Webber, B. A., & Pryor, J. A. (1993). Physiotherapy skills: Techniques and adjuncts. In B. A. Webber & J. A. Pryor (Eds.), *Physiotherapy for respiratory and cardiac problems* (pp. 116–127). Edinburgh: Churchill Livingstone.

Wechsler, M. E., Giardina, E. G., Sciacca, R. R., Rose, E. A., & Barr, M. L. (1995). Increased early mortality in women undergoing cardiac transplantation. *Circulation, 91,* 1029–1035.

Wenting, G. J., vd Meiracker, A. H., Simoons, M. I., Stroh, C. I., Har-Zahav, Y., & Fisman, E. Z. (1987). Circadian variation of heart rate but not of blood pressure after heart transplantation. *Transplantation Proceedings, 19,* 2554–2555.

Weseman, R. A., & McCashland, T. M. (1998). Nutritional care of the chronic post-transplant patient. *Topics in Clinical Nutrition, 13,* 27–34.

Wiesinger, G. F., Crevenna, R., Nuhr, M. J., Huelsmann, M., Fialka-Moser, V., & Quittan, M. (2001). Neuromuscular electric stimulation in heart transplantation candidates with cardiac pacemakers. *Archives of Physical Medicine and Rehabilitation, 82,* 1476–1477.

Williams, T. J., Grossman, R. F., & Maurer, J. R. (1990). Long-term functional follow-up of lung transplant recipients. *Clinics in Chest Medicine, 11,* 347–358.

Wolfe, R. A., Ashby, V. B., Milford, E. L., Ojo, A. O., Ettenger, R. E., Agodoa, L. Y., et al. (1999). Comparison of mortality in all patients on dialysis, patients on dialysis awaiting transplantation and recipients of a first cadaveric transplant. *New England Journal of Medicine, 341,* 1725–1730.

Young, M. A., & Stiens, S. A. (2006). Transplant Rehabilitation. In Braddom R. H. (Ed.), *Physical medicine and rehabilitation* (3rd ed.). Elsevier Health Sciences, (pp. 1443–1453). Philadelphia, PA: W. B. Saunders Co.

Young, M. A., & Stiens, S. A. (2002). Rehabilitation of the transplant patient. In B. J. O'Young, M. A. Young, & S. A. Stiens (Eds.), *PM&R secrets* (2nd ed.) (pp. 317–320). Philadelphia, PA: Hanley Belfus Inc.

Yun, J. J., & Mason, D. P. (2009). Lung transplantation: Past, present, and future. *Minerva Chirurgica, 64,* 37–44.

21

Psychiatric Disabilities

Marina Kukla, MS, and Gary R. Bond, PhD

The term *psychiatric disability* refers to a diagnosis of mental illness that prevents an individual from achieving age-specific goals. In the psychiatric literature, the term "severe mental illness" refers to a person with a diagnosable mental illness, who experiences difficulty in role functioning (e.g., those relating to employment, self-care, self-direction, interpersonal relationships, learning and recreation, independent living, and economic self-sufficiency), with these conditions persisting for a significant period of time (Goldman, 1984). The criterion for sufficient duration is usually met by at least one admission to a psychiatric hospital or other restrictive setting (e.g., group home) within a 5-year period. In this chapter, we use the term "severe psychiatric disability" to refer to what is also commonly referred to as severe mental illness (Schinnar, Rothbard, Kanter, & Jung, 1990).

Currently, the diagnostic standards in the field of mental health are codified in the *International Classification of Diseases and Related Health Problems* (ICD-10th revision; World Health Organization, 1992), which is used worldwide, and the *Diagnostic and Statistical Manual Version IV Text Revision* (*DSM-IV-TR*), which is used in the United States (American Psychiatric Association, 2000a). Both these diagnostic systems are critical sources of mental health and diagnostic information and they correspond closely in content. Because the *DSM-IV-TR* is used in the United States, we will refer to it in this chapter.

The *DSM-IV-TR* utilizes a descriptive, atheoretical stance toward classifying disorders. It attempts to define symptoms of psychiatric disorders based on observable criteria. To increase specificity, *DSM-IV-TR* uses a *multiaxial system* of diagnosis, by assessing five distinct dimensions: clinical syndromes (Axis I), personality disorders and mental retardation (Axis II), general medical conditions (Axis III), psychosocial stressors (Axis IV), and current level of functioning (Axis V). Psychiatric disabilities include Axis I (excluding substance use disorders) and personality disorders, although individuals with psychiatric disorders often have co-occurring disorders, such as substance use disorders. For funding and treatment purposes, substance use disorders and mental retardation are grouped separately by state and federal agencies.

Proper assessment of psychiatric disorders requires a trained diagnostician who administers a structured interview and has access to records of the patient's psychiatric history (First, Spitzer, Gibbon, & Williams, 1994). In practice, however, diagnoses are often made based on far less rigorous assessment procedures. Although important for treatment planning, particularly medication decisions, diagnosis is less relevant to rehabilitation planning than a functional assessment of the individual's strengths and weaknesses in specific environments (Anthony, Cohen, Farkas, & Gagne, 2002). This chapter first briefly describes the major psychiatric syndromes and then addresses the associated functional impairments that define the degree to which a psychiatric disorder can be disabling.

KEY PSYCHIATRIC DIAGNOSES

Information on psychiatric diagnosis is widely available in many sources, ranging from technical manuals (American Psychiatric Association, 2000a) to less technical but detailed sources such as abnormal psychology textbooks (Kring, Davidson, Neale, & Johnson, 2007), guides for the general public (Neugeboren, 2001; Torrey, 2001), personal accounts from those with a psychiatric illness, and journal accounts (Nasar, 1998; Sheehan, 1982). In the following sections, we provide a brief overview of several common major psychiatric illnesses.

Schizophrenia and Related Disorders

Given its debilitating symptoms and profound effect on the person, the family, and society, schizophrenia is considered the most severe of all mental illnesses. It is a complex disorder that affects individuals in diverse ways, including the ability to think clearly, to sort out and interpret incoming sensations, and to act decisively. Difficulties in social functioning (Mueser & Tarrier, 1998) and deficits in social skills are also common features of the disorder (Bellack, Mueser, Gingerich, & Agresta, 2004). Schizophrenia is a *psychotic* disorder that typically includes episodes of impaired reality, as indicated by disorientation and confusion, odd sensory experiences (e.g., hallucinations), false beliefs (e.g., delusions), and/or impairments in the emotional domain (e.g., affect flattening and depression). Schizophrenia is also considered a thought disorder, as individuals often display distortions in thought content (e.g., delusions) and language and thought processes (e.g., disorganized speech). The course of the illness is highly individualized. For some, there are acute episodes interspersed with normal or near-normal adjustment. In still other instances, the disturbance is relatively continuous, punctuated by periods of temporary improvement and deterioration.

Positive symptoms of schizophrenia include hallucinations (sensory experiences in the absence of any environmental stimuli), delusions (false and often bizarre beliefs, usually held firmly even in the face of disconfirming evidence), and disorganized speech. Hallucinations in schizophrenia may take several forms, including auditory, visual, tactile, and olfactory, although auditory, in the form of hearing voices, are by far the most common (Mueser, Bellack, & Brady, 1990). For instance, in an international study of schizophrenia, 74% of the sample reported auditory hallucinations (Sartorius, Shapiro, & Jablonsky, 1974). A more recent study corroborated this notion, with the finding that 65% of their sample of persons with schizophrenia experienced auditory hallucinations (Sharma, Dowd, & Janicak, 1999). Delusions range from innocuous confusions to extensive paranoid delusions involving perceived threats from conspiracies of seemingly unrelated people and events. Delusions often involve *ideas of reference*, where one attaches personal significance to unrelated activities of others (e.g., concluding that an overheard conversation between strangers refers to oneself). *Paranoid delusions* may be combined with *delusions of grandeur*, an exaggerated belief in one's own powers and sometimes the assumption of the identity of a famous person. *Thought broadcasting* (belief in the ability to transmit thoughts directly from one's mind to another person) and *thought insertion* (belief in the reception of thoughts in this fashion) are also positive symptoms of schizophrenia.

Negative symptoms of schizophrenia consist of patterns of nonresponsivity: passivity, a lack of spontaneity, *flat affect* (a lack of emotional expression), social withdrawal, a lack of motivation, and *anhedonia* (an inability to experience pleasure) (American Psychiatric Association, 2000b). The negative symptom of *ambivalence* (difficulty making decisions) may perpetuate a pattern of inaction. Flat affect is particularly common, present in about two-thirds of individuals with schizophrenia (Sartorius et al., 1974). Furthermore, negative symptoms are particularly distressing and are frequently present in early and more chronic phases of the disorder (Stahl & Buckley, 2007). In addition, these symptoms often interfere with psychosocial functioning, more so than other factors. For instance, the presence of negative affect and anhedonia are associated with poor social functioning in people with schizophrenia (Blanchard, Mueser, & Bellack, 1998).

Disorganized symptoms of schizophrenia manifest in different ways in both behavioral and language domains. Individuals with schizophrenia commonly experience disorganized behavior that may include childlike silliness and/or unpredictable agitation, difficulties performing activities of daily living (e.g., difficulties dressing oneself appropriately leading to a disheveled appearance and deficits in personal hygiene) and impairments in goal-directed behavior. Symptoms relating to disorganized speech include peculiar patterns of speech, such as *loose associations* (odd juxtaposition of topics and ideas), *neologisms* (invented words with private meanings), and *poverty of speech* (conversation conveying little information) (American Psychiatric Association, 2000). Persons with schizophrenia have difficulty with words that have more than one meaning; a word they interpret with the wrong meaning may lead them off on a tangent. They are also often baffled by simple analogies, as suggested by their poor performance in diagnostic tests, which require them to interpret common proverbs. Transfer of training from one context to another (e.g., applying skills learned in a hospital setting to a community setting) is often poor (Stein & Test, 1980).

Cognitive deficits associated with schizophrenia span a wide array of neurocognitive domains. Notable impairments are in the areas of verbal and nonverbal memory, working memory, attention, executive functions, and processing speed. A review of empirical studies including those that utilized both performance-based measures and neuroimaging indicates that persons with schizophrenia display deficits in all of these areas as compared with healthy control participants, with the largest deficits found in episodic memory and executive functioning (Reichenberg & Harvey, 2007). Furthermore, persons with schizophrenia range widely in their capacity to apply their intellectual abilities. After the onset of schizophrenia, they often do not attain or regain the level of accomplishment expected by their premorbid educational achievement. When the onset occurs in adolescence, not only is the individual's peer group affiliation often disrupted but also the educational process. Significant evidence suggests that cognitive functioning in schizophrenia is a predictor of functioning in important areas of life, such as the ability to work competitively in the community (Christensen, 2007; McGurk & Mueser, 2004) and the ability to function in a wide variety of social domains (Corrigan, Mueser, Bond, Drake, & Solomon, 2008).

A commonly accepted prevalence rate for schizophrenia is approximately 1% of the population at any time, but rates from epidemiological studies differ (Andreasen, 1984; Torrey, 2001). A review of major epidemiological studies concluded that schizophrenia occurs in all populations with a prevalence rate in the range of 1.4–4.6 per 1,000 (Jablensky, 2000). Recent evidence suggests that these prior estimates may be somewhat inflated, with current estimates found to be around a 0.7% prevalence rate (Beck, Rector, Stolar, & Grant, 2009). Incidence rates of schizophrenia are estimated to be between 7.7 and 43.0 per 100,000 (median value of 15.2 per 100,000) across geographical regions (McGrath et al., 2004). Other important factors that likely play a role in schizophrenia include ethnicity and urbanicity. Specifically, important differences are found across cultures; African Americans are significantly more likely to be diagnosed with schizophrenia as compared with other ethnic groups (Blow et al., 2004; Bresnahan et al., 2007). Cultural bias may influence the diagnosis of schizophrenia in African Americans (Whaley, 2004). Residing in an urban area and migrating from a rural area to an urban area are other significant risk factors leading to the development of the disorder (McGrath et al., 2004). The peak age of onset of schizophrenia is 15–30 years; however, approximately 15% of persons with the disorder may experience initial symptoms after age 45 (Harris & Jeste, 1988). Some studies have found that men are as likely as women to develop schizophrenia; however, more recent research suggests that rates of schizophrenia are higher in men than in women (McGrath et al., 2004). In addition, men are more likely to have their first psychiatric hospitalization before the age of 25, whereas the opposite is true after the age of 25.

Related diagnoses in the *DSM-IV-TR* include *schizophreniform disorder*, which applies when all the symptoms of schizophrenia are present, but the duration of the disorder is less than 6 months, and *schizoaffective disorder*, in which symptoms of schizophrenia are accompanied by prominent affective symptoms (depression and/or mania).

Mood Disorders

The two major types of mood disorders (also known as "affective disorders") are depressive disorders and bipolar disorders. Mood disorders are very common. The 1-year prevalence rates of mood disorders are 10.3% for *major depression*, 2.5% for *dysthymic disorder* (a chronic dysphoria or anhedonia not severe enough to meet the full criteria for major depression), and 1.3% for *bipolar disorder* (Kessler et al., 1994). During a lifetime, approximately 10–25% of women and 5–12% of men will suffer a *major depressive episode*. Bipolar disorders have a lifetime prevalence of 0.4–1.6% and affect men and women equally. The age of onset for depression is highly variable, whereas the age of onset for bipolar disorder is about 20 years (American Psychiatric Association, 2000). Furthermore, not all people with a mood disorder suffer long-term disability. As compared with other mood disorders, those with bipolar disorder tend to most likely experience significant impairments in functioning, which may include the periodic need for hospitalization (Corrigan et al., 2008).

The cognitive symptoms of depression include negative, pessimistic beliefs, distorted, negative self-image (including feelings of guilt and worthlessness), suicidal thoughts, and trouble concentrating (American Psychiatric Association, 2000). Whereas disordered thought in schizophrenia is often bizarre and puzzling, the distortions accompanying major depression are usually coherent, albeit often magnifying difficulties and jumping to distorted conclusions from incomplete information or selective attention to details. Beck (1967) has termed these distortions as *faulty logic*. Depression also includes physical symptoms such as lethargy, insomnia or hypersomnia, loss of appetite or overeating, and lack of sexual interest (American Psychiatric Association, 2000). Severe depression can be termed psychotic when it includes hallucinations or delusions (e.g., "I am dead"). Depression is probably the widest-ranging psychiatric disorder in terms of severity and duration. There are vexing diagnostic problems, for example, in deciding whether depressed feelings accompanying a difficult situation, such as physical disability or recent bereavement, qualify as a separate psychiatric diagnosis.

Bipolar disorder (previously known as "manic depression") differs symptomatically from major depression primarily by the presence of *mania*, an episode of elevated or irritable mood. Manic episodes last from several days to several months. In its most severe form, bipolar disorder involves frequent alternation between manic and depressive episodes (*rapid cycling*), but there are many different patterns including those in which either mania or depression rarely occurs. Persons experiencing a manic episode are expansive, unrealistically happy (although they can also be irritable when thwarted), impulsive, and easily distracted. They often have an exaggerated belief in their own abilities and make reckless decisions (e.g., extravagant purchases). Another common symptom is nonstop talking (*pressured speech*), even when others try to break in, or when no one is listening. Their conversation may show *flight of ideas* in which they quickly shift from one unfinished topic to another. Bipolar disorder is classified into two primary types: Bipolar I disorder and bipolar II disorder. Bipolar I disorder is the more severe form in which an individual experiences phases of depression and periods of severe, full-blown mania, which may include psychosis. Bipolar II disorder is hallmarked by periods of depression and periods of *hypomania*, which is a less severe form of the mania (American Psychiatric Association, 2000).

Anxiety Disorders

Affecting approximately 18% of the population in any given 12-month period (Kessler et al., 2005b) and 29% of people across a lifetime (Kessler et al., 2005a), anxiety disorders are the most prevalent of all psychiatric diagnoses. In contrast to psychotic disorders, persons with anxiety disorders usually recognize their symptoms and are not out of touch with reality. Hence, these disorders tend to be less severe as compared to the clinical syndromes just discussed (Kessler, Dupont, Berglund, & Wittchen, 1999). Anxiety disorders, however, frequently co-occur with other psychiatric disorders (Regier, Rae, Narrow, Kaelber, & Schatzberg, 1998).

One of the most debilitating anxiety disorders is *panic disorder*, which is characterized by sudden and unanticipated attacks of an imminent sense of doom, accompanied by symptoms such as increased heart rate, difficulty breathing, dizziness, and terror. In *DSM-IV-TR*, panic disorders are diagnosed as with or without *agoraphobia*, which may take the form of a fear of leaving home, even to do simple errands or to be employed outside the home. *Generalized anxiety disorder* (GAD) is a condition of constant worry and fretting across many situations. *Phobic disorders* are characterized by an intense fear of an object or situation representing no real danger. Phobic disorders run the gamut from childhood fears (e.g., of the dark), which often disappear spontaneously, to more pervasive and enduring conditions such as a social phobia, involving exaggerated shyness. *Obsessive–compulsive disorder* involves intrusive and recurring thoughts and impulses, known as *obsessions*, and ritualistic repetitions of illogical behaviors in response to these obsessions, known as *compulsions*. Finally, *posttraumatic stress disorder* (PTSD) is an extreme emotional reaction to a life trauma, such as combat, rape, or an accident, in which the individual reexperiences the feared event in nightmares and flashbacks. Symptoms include a reduced interest in previous activities, estrangement from others, poor concentration, and an inability to recall aspects of the trauma (American Psychiatric Association, 2000).

Personality Disorders

Personality disorders are defined by the presence of inflexible and maladaptive personality traits that cause significant functional impairment or subjective distress. Severe cases of personality disorders may be accompanied by brief psychotic symptoms.

Personality disorders are grouped into three clusters in *DSM-IV-TR*. The Odd/Eccentric Cluster consists of *paranoid personality disorder* (marked by pervasive and unwarranted suspiciousness and mistrust of others), *schizoid personality disorder* (marked by detachment from social relationships and a restricted range of expression of emotions), and *schizotypal personality disorder* (marked by social/interpersonal deficits due to eccentricities of cognition and/or behavior). The Dramatic/Emotional/Erratic Cluster consists of *antisocial personality disorder* (marked by violation of the rights of others without remorse), *borderline personality disorder* (marked by impulsivity and a pervasive pattern of instability of interpersonal relationships, self-image, and affects), *narcissistic personality disorder* (marked by exaggerated sense of self-importance and need for admiration), and *histrionic personality disorder* (marked by excessive emotionality and attention seeking). The Anxious/Fearful Cluster consists of *avoidant personality disorder* (marked by extreme social discomfort because of a pervasive fear of negative evaluation), *dependent personality disorder* (marked by submissive behavior due to an excessive need to be taken care of), and *obsessive–compulsive personality disorder* (marked by pervasive orderliness, perfectionism, and mental and interpersonal control).

FUNCTIONAL PRESENTATION OF PSYCHIATRIC DISABILITY

Psychiatric disabilities include a heterogeneous group of disorders. Even within a single diagnosis, wide variations in the severity of the illness and the success in coping with the symptoms exist; however, the pattern of symptoms within any one individual tends to be quite consistent. It is also important to note the distinction between the severity of psychiatric disabilities and those mental disorders that are less serious and do not cause disability. Specifically, most people who fit the criteria for a severe psychiatric disability have a diagnosis of schizophrenia, whereas a sizable minority have mood disorders, such as bipolar disorder. Severe cases of personality disorder or anxiety disorder also may fulfill these criteria. Some of the major functional impairments associated with severe psychiatric disabilities are described in the following text.

Difficulties Relating to Others

Many persons with psychiatric disabilities are withdrawn and avoid contact with others; one study reported that 75% were moderately to very isolated (Minkoff, 1978). They may lack assertiveness in even routine social transactions (e.g., receiving correct change at a store). Often, they are not inclined to initiate or continue conversations. Lack of spontaneity and other negative symptoms interfere with the formation and maintenance of intimate relationships. In most studies involving persons with severe psychiatric disabilities, the rate of those currently married is 20% or less (Rogers, Anthony, & Jansen, 1988), with particularly low rates reported for men with schizophrenia.

Not surprisingly, persons with psychiatric disabilities tend to have impoverished social networks, even early on in their disorder. For instance, a recent study found that newly diagnosed individuals with schizophrenia tend to have small social networks, and social network size was significantly correlated with current and premorbid social functioning (Horan, Subotnik, Snyder, & Nuechterlein, 2006). Often an immediate family member or mental health professional provides the only continuous social contact (Pescosolido, Wright, & Lutfey, 1999). Such relationships tend to be nonreciprocal. A person with a psychiatric disability may show little gratitude or awareness of the effort put forth by the caregiver even under conditions of extreme dependency (Torrey, Erdman, Wolfe, & Flynn, 1990).

Vulnerability to Stress

Persons with psychiatric disabilities often have limited tolerance to stress of any kind, for example, noise, inclement weather, and everyday hassles. They tend to function poorly in emotionally charged, critical social situations. In particular, persons with schizophrenia are much more likely to have an exacerbation of psychotic symptoms if they live in families with high expressed emotion, that is, families that are hostile and critical (Brown, Birley, & Wing, 1972). Similar findings have been reported for major depression and bipolar disorder (Mueser & Glynn, 1995). Stress is also believed to be an important mechanism in the underlying pathophysiology influencing the development of depression (Yulug, Ozan, Gönül, & Kilic, 2009).

Substance Abuse

Substance use disorder is the most common and clinically significant co-occurring disorder in psychiatric disabilities, affecting 50% of people with psychiatric disabilities at some time during their lifetime (Regier et al., 1990; Volkow, 2009). Substance use is a complicating factor in psychiatric disability because of its interaction with the mental illness and with psychotropic medications. Presence of a dual disorder of substance use with psychiatric disabilities has consistently been associated with negative outcomes including increased relapses and hospitalizations, housing instability and homelessness, violence, economic burden on the family, serious infections such as human immunodeficiency virus and hepatitis, treatment nonadherence (Drake & Brunette, 1998), as well as problems with the legal system, occupational dysfunction, and reduced access to health care (Compton, Weiss, West, & Kaslow, 2005).

Unemployment

Although most adults with psychiatric disabilities desire to work and feel that work is an important goal in their recovery (McQuilken et al., 2003), less than 15% of clients with psychiatric disabilities who are enrolled in community mental health programs are competitively

employed at any time (Rosenheck et al., 2006). Those who work often do so at t
the entitlements.

Poverty

Poverty is another common consequence of psychiatric disability (Draine, Salzer, Culhane, &
Hadley, 2002). Many persons with psychiatric disabilities are unable to meet basic needs, such
as those relating to housing, mental health care, transportation, and personal safety (Perese,
2007). Among people with severe psychiatric disabilities attending mental health programs,
80% or more typically have government entitlements as their main source of support (Rogers
et al., 1988).

Living Situation

Many people with psychiatric disabilities are not well integrated into community life and
most individuals are unsatisfied with their current living situation (Perese, 2007). Fortunately,
relatively few spend years in psychiatric hospitals, as was the case half a century ago. On the
other hand, only a minority are living independently. For example, among individuals with
schizophrenia, about 31% are living independently, 28% are living with a family member, 17%
are in supervised living (e.g., halfway houses), and 24% are in hospitals, nursing homes, jails/
prisons, shelters, or on the streets (Torrey, 2001). Among those counted as "living in the community" are many who are leading isolated, barren lives often without social or recreational
outlets (Segal & Aviram, 1978). Unfortunately, "successful discharges" from psychiatric hospitals often include individuals transferred to nursing homes (Grabowski, Aschbrenner,
Feng, & Mor, 2009) and supervised group home settings. Some observers have suggested that
in this process, many patients have not been deinstitutionalized but are *transinstitutionalized*.
Studies of homelessness further document the grim realities of psychiatric disabilities, as
research has shown that homeless individuals with psychiatric disabilities are more likely to
utilize inpatient and emergency services than outpatient services (Folsom, et al., 2005).

Criminal Justice Involvement

Incarcerated persons worldwide are significantly more likely to have a psychiatric diagnosis,
and are 10 times more likely to have antisocial personality disorder as compared with the
general population (Fazel & Danesh, 2002). Between one-quarter and one-half of all people
with psychiatric disabilities have contact with the criminal justice system at some point during the course of their disorder (Solomon, 2003). Of the 1.1 million individuals held in state
and federal prisons in 1995, the 1-year prevalence rates were 5% for schizophrenia, 6% for
bipolar disorder, and 9% for major depression (SAMHSA, 1997). In 1998, of those incarcerated
in American prisons and jails on any given day, approximately 284,000 (16%) were individuals
with psychiatric disabilities (Ditton, 1999). This was four times the number of people in state
mental hospitals throughout the country. Glied and Frank (2009) estimated that in 2006, 7%
of individuals with psychiatric disability in the United States had been incarcerated. Studies
have also found that incarcerated persons with psychiatric disabilities are more likely to be
homeless and have co-occurring substance abuse disorders (McNeil, Binder, & Robinson,
2005).

The widely held belief that mental illness leads to increased risk of violent behavior is a
damaging stereotype, reinforced by dramatic examples (e.g., the assassination attempt on
President Reagan by John Hinkley, who has a diagnosis of schizophrenia). Although rates
of violent behaviors in adults with psychiatric disabilities are higher than those with no
psychiatric diagnosis (Arseneault, Moffitt, Caspi, Taylor, & Silva, 2000; Swanson, Holzer,

t majority of individuals with psychiatric disabilities do not com-
violence does occur, it is often associated with substance abuse,
past violent victimization, and violence in the surrounding envi-
98; Swanson et al., 1990; Swartz et al., 1998). Therefore, usually it is
es *per se* that lead to assaultiveness, but its convergence with other
gnificantly increase the likelihood of violent behavior.

na

victimization of persons with psychiatric disabilities is a serious public health problem, as
they are 11 times more likely to be victimized by violence and crime than the general population (Teplin, McClelland, Abram, & Weiner, 2005). Between 43% and 81% of those with psychiatric disabilities report some type of victimization over their lifetime (Rosenberg et al.,
2001). Victimization of this group occurs in many forms, such as physical and sexual assaults,
verbal abuse, exploitation, bullying, threats, and theft, often at the hands of others in the community, caregivers, and even family members (Perese, 2007). In a large-scale survey, one-third
of men and women with schizophrenia reported severe physical or sexual assault in the past
year (Goodman et al., 2001). In addition, up to 53% of persons with psychiatric disabilities
report childhood sexual or physical abuse (Rosenberg et al., 2001). Given the high prevalence,
particularly among homeless women, interpersonal violence can be considered a normative
experience for people with psychiatric disabilities (Goodman, Dutton, & Harris, 1997).

Although often overlooked, PTSD is a common comorbid diagnosis in people with psychiatric disabilities, with prevalence rates for current PTSD diagnosis ranging between 29%
and 43% in some studies (Mueser et al., 1998; Rosenberg et al., 2001). Exposure to trauma and
the presence of PTSD are associated with poorer functioning in people with psychiatric disabilities, including more severe symptoms, poorer health, and higher rates of psychiatric and
medical hospitalization (Switzer et al., 1999).

Increased Risk for Suicide

Feelings of worthlessness and self-hatred are very common in persons with psychiatric disabilities and are associated with suicidal ideation and attempts (Harris & Barraclough, 1997).
The yearly suicide prevalence rate for major depression is approximately 0.29%, with similar
rates for bipolar disorder. Overall, the risk for suicide in mood disorders is 20–30 times that
of the general population (Tondo, Isacsson, & Baldessarini, 2003). Individuals who are hospitalized with mood disorders also show elevated mortalities from suicide, a finding that is
particularly strong for those with major depression rather than bipolar I or bipolar II disorder
(Angst, Stassen, Clayton, & Angst, 2002). The lifetime suicide rate for persons with schizophrenia has been estimated to be between 1.8% and 5.6% (Palmer, Pankratz, & Bostwick,
2005). Another review found suicide rates ranging from 8% to 10% in longitudinal studies of
patients with schizophrenia (Jobe & Harrow, 2005). The risk for suicide is particularly great
for those who are younger and newly diagnosed with the disorder (Palmer et al., 2005).

Environmental Influences

Although many of the characteristics described earlier are directly related to psychiatric
symptoms, they are also influenced by external factors (e.g., institutionalization and societal
attitudes). For example, the stultifying effects of hospital and nursing homes undoubtedly
reinforce the passivity and withdrawal so prominent in psychiatric disabilities (Goffman,
1961). At the societal level, the labeling process in mental illness is demoralizing and discriminatory (Estroff, 1989). Sometimes individuals with psychiatric disabilities internalize social

stigma, creating feelings of demoralization, reduced self-esteem, and barriers to self-empowerment and the attainment of important life goals (Corrigan et al., 2008). Moreover, employers attach more stigmas to psychiatric disabilities than to physical disabilities (Berven & Driscoll, 1981; Hazer & Bedell, 2000). In the housing domain, the NIMBY (not in my back yard) prejudice against persons with psychiatric disabilities is intense; group homes are particularly likely to meet with community resistance if located in conservative, middle-class neighborhoods (Segal & Aviram, 1978). Stigma and discrimination continue to be significant barriers to community integration (Corrigan et al., 2008; Hall, Graf, Fitzpatrick, Lane, & Birkel, 2003). Some have expressed hope that prominent individuals with mental illness can help combat stigma by public disclosure (Corrigan, 2003). Educational programs also may be used to reduce the stigma associated with psychiatric disabilities successfully (Corrigan et al., 2008).

PROGNOSIS

Schizophrenia—Long Term

The prognosis for schizophrenia is generally worse than for most other major psychiatric disorders. For many, it is a lifelong, disabling condition. However, contrary to an early misconception promulgated by Emil Kraepelin, the German psychiatrist who first identified a set of syndromes that served as a framework for the diagnosis, schizophrenia does not follow a relentlessly downward course; rather, it is quite heterogeneous in course and outcome based upon patient-related factors (e.g., age of onset, type of symptoms, and acuteness at onset) and other prognostic factors (Jobe & Harrow, 2005). Decline in psychosocial functioning typically plateaus approximately 5–10 years after onset of the disorder (McGlashan, 1988). Traditionally, the prognostic rule of thumb for schizophrenia has been that one-third are expected to show a sharp decline in functioning, one-third to achieve a marginal adjustment, and one-third to recover to essentially former levels of functioning (Jobe & Harrow, 2005). With appropriate community support and rehabilitation, a substantially larger percentage may approach former levels of functioning (Harding, Brooks, Ashikaga, Strauss, & Breier, 1987). In addition, the introduction and widespread use of antipsychotic drugs have helped to reduce relapse rates and decrease the severity of florid psychotic symptoms (Jobe & Harrow, 2005). Furthermore, among persons with schizophrenia, approximately one-half (and two-thirds of their families) recognize the prodromal symptoms (i.e., the warning signs of an impending psychotic episode specific to each individual) before their decompensation (Herz, 1984). Psychoeducational groups are designed to assist clients to recognize these symptoms and to employ coping strategies (e.g., reducing stress, seeking additional support).

Schizophrenia—Early Psychosis

Swift intervention and treatment early in the course of psychosis is important for recovery. Reviews of empirical studies have found that a longer duration of untreated first episode psychosis is associated with a poorer response to antipsychotic medications and a lower likelihood of functional and symptomatic recovery (Perkins, Gu, Boteva, & Lieberman, 2005). Duration of untreated psychosis is also positively correlated with the severity of negative symptoms (Perkins et al., 2005). Consistent with these results, another study found that a shorter duration of the first psychotic episode in schizophrenia was associated with full recovery and less symptomatology during the 5-year follow-up period (Robinson, Woerner, McMeniman, Mendelowitz, & Bilder, 2004). Several factors predict the likelihood of recovery and psychotic episode recurrence early on in the course of schizophrenia, including demographic variables, socioeconomic factors, family history, stress, and drug use (Corrigan et al., 2008). For instance, studies have found that drug use has a deleterious effect on functional outcomes and schizophrenia symptoms. Persons with schizophrenia who abuse illegal drugs and alcohol after their first psychotic episode are more likely to have future psychiatric hospitalizations and more psychotic symptoms compared with those who do not (Sorbara, Liraud, Assens, Abalan, & Verdoux, 2003). Studies have also found that 22–64% of individuals presenting with their first psychotic episode have a history of cannabis abuse and these individuals are at significantly increased risk for relapse, worse symptomatology, and suicidal behavior (Verdoux, Tournier, & Cougnard, 2005). While drug use is one factor that influences the course and outcome, problems related to early psychosis are complex, and researchers are only beginning to study and understand them.

Prognosis of Mood Disorders

Most people with major depression recover, with or without treatment. In a longitudinal study by Coryell and colleagues (1994), about 60% and 80% of both clinical and nonclinical populations who developed a major depressive episode recovered by 6 months and 1 year, respectively. A recent longitudinal study found that approximately half of participants with a depressive mood disorder (i.e., major depressive episode, dysthymic disorder) no longer reported symptoms that met the criteria for the diagnosis at the 3-year follow-up (Forsell, 2007). However, a substantial minority experience recurrent and chronic depression: The 2- and 6-month relapse rates are 20% and 30%, respectively (Belsher & Costello, 1988), and 22% of patients experience an episode persisting more than 1 year (Thornicroft & Sartorius, 1993). Another study found that between 42% (primary care patients) and 61% (psychiatric care patients) of participants with major depression reported experiencing at least one relapse across the 7-year follow-up period; 21–26%, respectively, of the two patient groups still met the criteria for major depressive disorder after 7 years (Poutanen et al., 2007). Between depressive episodes, persons with major depression may be highly functional and productive (e.g., as illustrated by the historical examples of Winston Churchill and Abraham Lincoln). With proper treatment, the prognosis is good for the majority of those who suffer from this mood disorder. Important age differences also exist with regard to the prognosis of major depression; older patients with depression are more likely to relapse and tend to have poorer response to antidepressant medications and more medical comorbidities as compared to middle-aged depressed persons (Mitchell & Subramaniam, 2005). Furthermore, bipolar disorders are generally far more debilitating and have greater relapse rates as compared to major depression (Angst, Gamma, Sellaro, Lavori, & Zhang, 2003); untreated, patients with bipolar disorders have a poor prognosis.

Prognosis of Anxiety Disorders

The long-term prognosis for anxiety disorders is generally favorable. Most people with GAD will achieve full recovery (i.e., free of symptoms) with proper treatment (Angst, Gamma, Baldwin, Ajdacic-Gross, & Rossler, 2009), although a few may have residual symptoms, such as somatic complaints (Rubio & Lopez-Ibor, 2007a). Persons with panic disorder also experience recovery across time (i.e., fewer panic attacks), although the course tends to be more chronic than that of GAD, as residual symptoms and somatizations are fairly common (Rubio & Lopez-Ibor, 2007b).

Prognosis of Personality Disorders

Personality disorders are, by definition, pervasive and enduring patterns of thinking, feeling, and behaving that typically remain quite stable over time. As such, we do not yet have many effective treatment strategies to help such individuals "recover" from a personality disorder, although with targeted interventions, promising functional improvements have been shown for some diagnoses such as borderline personality disorder (Linehan & Armstrong, 1991).

Specifically, in recent years, dialectical behavior therapy has been shown to be an effective treatment for borderline personality disorder, particularly regarding a reduction in suicide attempts (Linehan et al., 2006).

TREATMENT AND REHABILITATION

History of Treatment Approaches

Before the 1950s, numerous somatic treatments were used for psychiatric disabilities (Isaac & Armat, 1990). With the exception of electroconvulsive therapy, none of these proved to be effective and many were harmful. Psychiatric hospitalization in large state-run facilities providing little more than custodial care (and often neglect) was standard practice. Beginning in the 1950s, a combination of economic, legal, and humanitarian factors in addition to the widespread use of antipsychotic medications led to *deinstitutionalization,* the process of releasing patients from state hospitals (Talbott, 1978). The resident population of state and county mental hospitals, which peaked at 558,922 in 1955, declined to fewer than 60,000 by 1998 (Lamb & Bachrach, 2001). In 1963, the Community Mental Health Centers Act authorized the creation of a network of community mental health centers (CMHCs) with a broad mission to address the mental health needs of the nation, including the care and treatment of discharged patients with mental disorders (U.S. Congress, 1963). Altogether, 789 CMHCs were eventually funded, which provided the bulk of public mental health services for people with psychiatric disabilities (Torrey, 2001).

Initially, most CMHCs were unprepared to serve people with psychiatric disabilities for several reasons, including unrealistic expectations about the efficacy of medications (i.e., the assumption that medications alone would allow individuals to function in the community), poor planning (e.g., too few CMHCs to serve the large numbers of patients being released from hospitals), poor coordination and execution of services (e.g., lack of communication between hospitals and CMHCs; CMHCs were not taking responsibility for patients upon discharge from hospitals), and funding irregularities (Torrey, 2001). Finally, CMHCs failed to address a wide range of needs relating to housing, employment, socialization, and other areas of functioning discussed above. The phenomenon of *revolving-door* clients—those who return frequently to psychiatric hospitals—was one of the consequences of this limited treatment focus. More than half of all psychiatric patients released from state hospitals returned within 2 years (Anthony, Cohen, & Vitalo, 1978). Decades later, the problem of revolving-door clients still had not been fully solved with 250,000 short-term psychiatric hospitalizations in the United States annually (Weiden & Olfson, 1993). These trends suggested the need for new, comprehensive psychosocial approaches to augment traditional CMHC services (Talbott, 1978) and to complement pharmacological treatments.

Pharmacological Treatments

Medications for Schizophrenia
About two-thirds of people with schizophrenia benefit from antipsychotic medications, which include chlorpromazine (Thorazine), thioridazine (Mellaril), and haloperidol (Haldol). The efficacy of antipsychotic medications in reducing the relapse rate and the positive symptoms of schizophrenia is well established (Davis, 1980). Unfortunately, antipsychotics have troubling side effects, summarized by the mnemonic, THE SEA: tardive dyskinesia, hypotension, extrapyramidal symptoms, sedation, endocrine disturbances, and anticholinergic symptoms (Wittlin, 1988). *Tardive dyskinesia,* the most serious of the side effects, involves stereotyped, involuntary movements of the mouth and face. Occurring more commonly after long use of traditional antipsychotic drugs, it is usually irreversible. *Hypotension* refers to abnormally low

blood pressure, which may be experienced as dizziness. *Extrapyramidal* symptoms, prominent during the first week of drug treatment, include tremors of the arms, rigidity of extremities, *akinesia* (listlessness), and *akathisia* (internal restlessness). *Sedation* is experienced as drowsiness. *Endocrine disturbances* include sexual dysfunction and weight gain. *Anticholinergic* symptoms include dry mouth and blurred vision. These traditional antipsychotic medications may also cause increases in prolactin levels that may result in breast enlargement, which is particularly troubling in men. Treatment of side effects includes reducing dosage levels, changing medications, and, in the case of extrapyramidal symptoms, the use of antiparkinsonian drugs such as benztropine (Cogentin). Another limitation to traditional antipsychotics is their lack of effect on negative symptoms.

Beginning in 1990, several *atypical* antipsychotic drugs were developed and approved for use in the United States by the Food and Drug Administration (FDA). The year of FDA approval for six of these were as follows: clozapine (Clozaril), 1990; risperidone (Risperdal), 1994; olanzapine (Zyprexa), 1996; quetiapine (Seroquel), 1997; ziprasidone (Geodon), 2001; and aripiprazole (Abilify), 2002. Atypicals have been heavily marketed with great success by pharmaceutical companies (Wang, West, Tanielian, & Pincus, 2000). Early optimistic reports of significantly greater effectiveness with fewer side effects for atypical antipsychotics as compared to the traditional drugs generally have not been borne out (Lieberman et al., 2005). One important exception is clozapine, which is regarded as the most effective of the atypicals, as it is useful in patients who do not respond to other antipsychotic medications (McEvoy et al., 2006). However, clozapine is not the initial antipsychotic prescribed for schizophrenia because of its side effects. Clozapine requires frequent blood tests because of the risk of life-threatening *agranulocytosis* (a significant decrease in white blood cell counts). One major drawback of atypicals is that they are priced many times higher than traditional antipsychotics. Some atypical antipsychotics (particularly clozapine and olanzapine) have also been associated with clinically significant bodyweight gain (Allison et al., 1999), increasing the risk of medical comorbidity including diabetes, hypertension, cardiovascular disease, and high cholesterol (Henderson, 2002; Nasrallah, 2002).

Medications for Mood Disorders

A range of drugs have been used for treating mood disorders. Lithium is used to treat bipolar disorder particularly during the manic phases although it is also used by patients who have never had manic episodes. It is effective in 63–90% of all cases of mania (Noll, Davis, & DeLeon-Jones, 1985). Lithium is lethal in high doses; thus, patients require careful monitoring of their blood. More recently, anticonvulsant medications (e.g., carbamazepine) and atypical antipsychotic medications (e.g., risperidone, olanzapine, and aripiprazole) have been prescribed as treatments for acute and mixed phases in bipolar disorders, particularly for those patients who do not respond to or cannot tolerate lithium. Lamotrigine is often used as a maintenance therapy for bipolar disorder (Thase, 2008). Various antidepressant drugs have been used for major depression. Before the 1990s, the most common ones were the tricyclics including amitriptyline (Elavil) and imipramine (Tofranil) and monamine oxidase inhibitors (MAOIs), such as tranylcypormine (Parnate), isocarboxazid (Marplan), and phenelzine (Nardil). The side effects of the tricyclics include anticholinergic effects, sedation, and irregularities in the cardiovascular system, whereas the side effects of irreversible MAOIs include life-threatening hypertensive crisis facilitated by interactions between the drug and certain foods. Given their serious side effects, MAOIs are seldom prescribed today, in favor of other drug classes that have similar clinical effectiveness. A group of antidepressants known as *selective serotonin reuptake inhibitors* (SSRIs) including fluoxetine (Prozac), paroxetine (Paxil), sertraline (Zoloft), and escitalopram (Lexapro) have favorable side-effect profiles (Glod, 1996; Möller & Volz, 1996) and are currently widely prescribed for major depression and a wide array of other psychiatric disorders. A recent meta-analysis comparing the efficacy of various SSRIs found that sertraline and escitalopram had a favorable profile with regard to efficacy (i.e., treatment response) and acceptability (fewer patients stopped taking the medications) compared to other medications; the authors conclude that these drugs could be the best start-up treatments for moderate to severe major depression (Cipriani et al., 2009). Recently, mixed reuptake inhibitors that block the reuptake of seretonin and norepinephrine in the brain (e.g., venlafaxine [Effexor] and duloxetine [Cymbalta]) and drugs that inhibit dopamine and norepinephrine uptake (e.g., bupropion [Wellbutrin]) have been developed. These drugs have similar efficacy in treating depression as compared with the SSRIs; they may be useful in ameliorating chronic pain associated with depression, and some drugs (i.e., bupropion) may be more effective in treating refractory depression that cannot be helped by SSRIs (Mann, 2005).

Medications for Anxiety Disorders

Persons with anxiety disorders are often prescribed antianxiety drugs (also called *anxiolytics*) including diazepam (Valium), which falls in the class of drugs known as benzodiazepines and which at one time was the most frequently prescribed medication in the United States (Lickey & Gordon, 1991). Research on the psychopharmacology of anxiolytics has been rapidly expanding in recent years with the attempt to find specific agents to reduce the symptoms of specific disorders. For example, another benzodiazepine, alprazolam (Xanax), has been used for treating GAD, panic, and phobic disorders. Major drawbacks of the benzodiazepines are that they may lead to physical and psychological dependence and are dangerous if taken in combination with alcohol (Brunette, Noordsy, Xie, & Drake, 2003). Buspirone (BuSpar), which is often used to treat GAD, appears to avoid both of these problems. SSRIs are also commonly prescribed to treat anxiety disorders; they are particularly effective in treating panic disorder and social phobia, and are considered a first-line treatment for obsessive–compulsive disorder and PTSD (Bandelow et al., 2008).

Medication Nonadherence

Medication nonadherence is a major barrier to effective treatment of psychotic disorders with nearly half of the patients not taking drugs as prescribed (Lacro, Dunn, Dolder, Leckband, & Jeste, 2002). One review concluded that patients on antipsychotics took an average of 58% of the recommended amount, with higher adherence rates for patients on antidepressants (Cramer & Rosenheck, 1998). In addition, secretive or suspicious attitudes are characteristic of approximately two-thirds of all persons with schizophrenia (Sartorius et al., 1974). This same survey found that 97% of the sample population lacked insight about their illness. Indeed, people with schizophrenia often have little or no awareness that they have a mental illness or even that they have any problems at all. This lack of awareness often leads to nonadherence to the recommended treatment. Medication nonadherence is also a problem in patients with mood disorders. One review of empirical studies found that median prevalence rates for medication nonadherence in major depression and bipolar disorders ranges from 41% to 53%. The authors also identified risk factors for nonadherence, including attitudes (e.g., stigma) health beliefs, the degree of "choice" in treatment options, the quality of the doctor–patient relationship, and comorbid drug and alcohol use (Lingam & Scott, 2002).

Nonadherence to treatment regimens in psychiatric disabilities has serious consequences, often resulting in higher rates of relapse and rehospitalization and poorer community adjustment. Fundamental to any medication treatment is the identification of the optimal dosage level. Some research has suggested that with careful monitoring, the use of much lower dosage levels than usually prescribed can reduce side effects while retaining the positive effects of antipsychotics (Hogarty et al., 1988). Medication education (Corrigan et al., 2008; Wallace, Liberman, MacKain, Blackwell, & Eckman, 1992; Zygmunt, Olfson, Boyer, & Mechanic, 2002) and *behavioral tailoring* (i.e., fitting medication-taking into daily routines; Mueser et al., 2002) are strategies used to increase adherence. Another strategy to ensure adherence to antipsychotic medication is to substitute long-acting injectable forms of medications such as fluphenazine decanoate (Prolixin) for the usual oral administration (Kane, Woerner, & Sarantakos, 1986).

Medication Guidelines

In recent years, *practice guidelines* and *algorithms* have been developed to systematize knowledge about "best practices" in the pharmacological treatment of psychiatric disorders (Drake, Essock, & Bond, 2009). The best known of these approaches is the Texas Medication Algorithm Project (Miller et al., 1999). These guidelines incorporate evidence from clinical trials and expert consensus. Principles of evidence-based medication management include respecting and incorporating client preferences, accurate diagnosis and specification of target symptoms; choosing medication and dosage range supported by the research evidence; ongoing evaluation of changes in symptoms and side effects and modification recommended by the illness-specific guidelines (e.g., raising dosage, changing to another efficacious medication, and using an augmentation strategy); treatment of co-occurring syndromes; and the involvement of patient and family in treatment planning (Mellman et al., 2001). Medication practice guidelines for psychiatric disorders are evolving.

Psychotherapy

There is no single "best" therapeutic approach for persons with psychiatric disabilities, given the heterogeneity of the population. The literature demonstrating the efficacy of psychotherapy for relieving distress in persons with mild anxiety and depression is substantial (Lipsey & Wilson, 1993). The beneficial effect of cognitive behavioral therapy (CBT) in various conditions has been extensively documented. Specifically, CBT leads to symptom reduction in adult and childhood depression, GAD, panic disorder, social phobia, and PTSD, as hallmarked by large effects (Butler, Chapman, Forman, & Beck, 2006). Other effective treatments for mood disorders include mindfulness-based therapies (Kuyken et al., 2008), interpersonal therapy (Weissman, 2006), and behavioral activation techniques (Cuijpers, van Straten, & Warmerdam, 2007). Other evidence-based therapeutic interventions for anxiety disorders include behavioral techniques, such as exposure-based therapies (i.e., for treating PTSD; Bisson & Andrew, 2007) and systematic desensitization (i.e., for treating specific phobias; Choy, Fyer, & Lipsitz, 2007). CBT is also an effective adjunct to pharmacological treatment in schizophrenia. Empirical reviews have found that CBT is related to decreases in positive symptoms and fewer psychotic relapses (Turkington, Kingdom, & Weiden, 2006), as well as to a reduction in negative symptoms that may persist across time (Beck et al., 2009). Although the strongest evidence exists for the use of CBT in schizophrenia, other therapeutic techniques are also used, including supportive psychotherapy, biomedical model psychoeducation, personal therapy, and psychoanalytically oriented psychotherapy (Turkington et al., 2006). In addition, *motivational interviewing,* a set of techniques that tailors interventions to the client's readiness to change, has received increasing recognition as an important therapeutic tool (Miller & Rollnick, 2002) in schizophrenia and other psychiatric disorders. Intensive psychotherapeutic approaches emphasizing insight and exploration of childhood experiences are not helpful and are sometimes harmful for individuals with schizophrenia (Drake & Sederer, 1986).

Furthermore, all successful interventions encompass several "common factors." Effective interventions for people with psychiatric disabilities entail direct, unambiguous communication, supportive, noncritical attitudes, and a focus on problem-solving skills training (Mueser & Gingerich, 1994). The foundation for all successful interventions is a therapeutic relationship, or the relationship between the patient and the therapist. This relationship is ideally characterized by mutual respect, empathy, honesty, and unconditional positive regard (Turkington et al., 2006). This principle applies to people with psychiatric disabilities (McGrew, Wilson, & Bond, 1996), as well as to individuals with less severe psychiatric disorders.

Psychiatric Rehabilitation

Psychiatric rehabilitation addresses the many psychosocial challenges associated with psychiatric disabilities that are not adequately addressed by medication or psychotherapy alone, such as unemployment, isolation, vulnerability to stress, substandard living conditions, homelessness, and the heavy burden of caregiving on relatives. Psychiatric rehabilitation encompasses an array of practical psychosocial interventions that, in concert with pharmacological treatment, effectively promote recovery among people with severe psychiatric disabilities (to be referred as *consumers* for the rest of the chapter) (Corrigan et al., 2008).

Although psychiatric rehabilitation approaches vary, they embrace a common set of guiding principles (Bond & Resnick, 2000; Dincin, 1975; Pratt, Gill, Barrett, & Roberts, 1999). These principles include but are not limited to *individualized and comprehensive assessment, planning, and intervention; community integration* (helping consumers exit patient roles, treatment centers, segregated housing arrangements, and/or sheltered work); *pragmatism* (helping consumers with the practical problems in everyday life, with services organized around specific, tangible goals); *consumer choice* (as experts of their own illness, consumers are empowered to set their own goals and make informed decisions in their treatment and rehabilitation, and services are shaped to their preferences); *promoting hope* (focusing on consumer strengths, building their self-confidence, and instilling hope for recovery through a rehabilitation relationship); and *integration of treatment and rehabilitation*. These principles mirror the guiding principles for the field of rehabilitation in general.

In the 1970s, a national conference of mental health experts culminated in the conceptualization of a *community support program* (CSP) (Turner & TenHoor, 1978). The concept assumes that nontraditional roles for mental health providers are necessary for successful interventions for consumers with SMI including outreach to those not receiving services, assistance in housing and other basic needs, development of permanent support networks, vocational rehabilitation, and advocacy. The CSP model has had a dramatic effect on the way system planners conceptualize organizing services, supports, and opportunities to help consumers with SMI reach their full potential in the society. A number of approaches compatible with CSP principles have been developed, including the *clubhouse model, skills training*, and *self-help activities* associated with the consumer movement. Many of these approaches have achieved wide popularity but have lacked strong empirical support, although more recently, a number of practices have been systematically evaluated in randomized-controlled trials and consequently been designated as *evidence-based practices* (Drake, Merrens, & Lynde, 2005).

Clubhouse Model

The psychosocial approach known as the clubhouse originated with the Fountain House program in New York City (Beard, Propst, & Malamud, 1982). In the 1940s, the precursor to Fountain House was a self-help group for patients discharged from the state psychiatric hospital. Subsequently, the group sought a professional to serve as director of their center. Under his direction, the group evolved into an innovative program for helping consumers with psychiatric disabilities adjust to community living. Operating outside of the mental health system, the program became known as a *clubhouse* because its identity revolved around a central meeting place for "members" to socialize. Fountain House pioneered many innovations including two key vocational concepts: the *work-ordered day* and *transitional employment*. As part of the work-ordered day, members participate in prevocational work crews doing chores around the clubhouse. Transitional employment consists of temporary, part-time community jobs secured by the clubhouse staff. The clubhouse model emphasizes informal and experiential learning as opposed to more structured approaches found in skills training. Clubhouse programs are found throughout the United States and internationally (Macias, Jackson, Schroeder, & Wang, 1999), although the empirical literature supporting the effectiveness of this model is mostly observational.

Skills Training

The rationale for skills training is based on the findings that consumers with SMI often experience difficulties in interpersonal situations ranging from intimate relationships to everyday contacts in public settings. The goal of social skills training is to teach the component skills necessary for effective social interactions in a systematic manner. Typically, the steps in skills training are as follows: (1) give a rationale for learning the skill; (2) role-play the skill; (3) provide an exercise for the client to role-play the skill; (4) give specific positive and corrective feedback on the client's role-play; (5) practice the skill; and (6) give a homework assignment in a real-life situation (Mueser, Drake, & Bond, 1997). Although skills training typically focuses on social skills, it also has been used for a range of other skills needed for independent living. There is little doubt that well-defined skills including social skills can be taught to consumers with psychiatric disabilities (Kopelowicz, Liberman & Zarate, 2006). Some evidence suggests that skills training generalizes across real-world settings when skills are practiced and when individuals are encouraged and reinforced for using skills (Kopelowicz et al., 2006).

Consumer Movement

In the past two decades, the consumer movement has prompted major changes in the conception of mental health services. Advocates have insisted that individuals with mental illness should have equal access to societal and environmental resources, equal access to options and opportunities, and equal "location of life," that is, places where people live, work, play, and pray are the same regardless of the presence of mental illness (Ralph, 2000). An influential federal report echoes these themes (New Freedom Commission on Mental Health, 2003). Nationally, there is widespread interest in receiving training in the Wellness Action Recovery Plan (Copeland, 1997), a manual providing systematic tools for coping with symptoms and developing relapse prevention plans.

More than 500 mental health self-help groups have formed nationwide (Chamberlin, Rogers, & Sneed, 1989). These groups have been active in developing drop-in centers, which provide friendship, social and recreational activities, and concrete assistance (Mowbray, Chamberlain, Jennings, & Reed, 1988). Since its inception in 1979, the National Alliance on Mental Illness (NAMI), an organization for families, has grown to 1,200 state and local affiliates in the United States and a membership of 210,000 (NAMI, 2003).

Evidence-Based Practices

One of the most significant advances in the psychiatric rehabilitation field in recent years is the movement toward *evidence-based practices*, defined as a set of well-delineated interventions that have demonstrated effectiveness in rigorous empirical research (Drake, Goldman, et al., 2001). Six evidence-based practices have been endorsed by a national consensus panel of leading mental health researchers, advocates, and program directors for widespread adoption for the treatment and rehabilitation of psychiatric disabilities: *assertive community treatment* (ACT), *family psychoeducation, illness management and recovery* (IMR), *integrated dual disorders treatment* (IDDT), *medication management,* and *supported employment* (Mueser, Torrey, Lynde, Singer, & Drake, 2003). Controlled trials on these practices suggest specific benefits in the areas of reductions in rates of relapse, hospitalization, and substance use, better control of symptoms, and improvements in housing stability, employment, and overall quality of life. Medication management was discussed previously in the section "Pharmacological Treatments"; each of the remaining five evidence-based practices is briefly described in the following text.

Assertive Community Treatment

Developed in the 1970s by Stein and Test (1980), ACT is an intensive approach most appropriate for consumers with psychiatric disabilities whose needs have not been adequately met by more traditional, less intensive programs of treatment. Typical ACT clients have a chronic psychotic disorder (i.e., schizophrenia), experiencing numerous inpatient psychiatric hospitalizations in the past. ACT services are provided by a group of professionals representing various disciplines (e.g., psychiatry, nursing, case management, vocational and substance abuse specialists) who work as a team. They serve clients on an individual basis, with most contact occurring in consumers' homes and neighborhoods, rather than in agency offices. The ACT team maintains frequent contact with clients, typically averaging two visits per week. The nature of the contacts depends on the needs of a client on a given day. ACT teams help in such things as budgeting money, shopping, finding housing, and taking medications. ACT teams attempt to anticipate crises, for example, by paying attention to the warning signs of a relapse. It is common for ACT staff to provide service outside the traditional workday, often with 24-hour crisis coverage and weekend staffing. ACT programs exemplify assertive outreach in that staff members actively initiate contact with clients, rather than depending on clients to keep appointments. Another feature of ACT is its emphasis on continuity and consistency. Clients are not discharged from ACT teams, but continue to receive services on a time-unlimited basis (Test, 1992). The effectiveness of the ACT model has been well established; a review of 25 randomized controlled studies concluded that ACT clients experienced reduced psychiatric hospitalization, increased housing stability, and improved symptoms and subjective quality of life (Bond, Drake, Mueser, & Latimer, 2001). In addition, recent reviews have found strong evidence that homeless consumers of ACT services experience a reduction in homelessness and an improvement in psychiatric symptoms as compared with those receiving traditional case management services (Coldwell & Bender, 2007).

Family Psychoeducation

Family psychoeducation aims to achieve the best possible outcome for consumers with psychiatric disabilities, alleviate the stress in the family, and improve functioning of all family members through collaborative treatment. Controlled studies have shown a 25–75% reduction in relapse and rehospitalization rates among consumers with psychiatric disabilities whose families received psychoeducation. Although the existing models of family interventions vary, effective family psychoeducation programs share the following elements: basic psychoeducation about psychiatric disability and its management; training in communication and problem-solving skills; provision of emotional support, empathy, and hope; development of a social support network; and long-term, flexible interventions tailored to the needs of individual families (Dixon et al., 2001). In family psychoeducation, the term "family" is interpreted broadly to including anyone in the consumer's natural support system who is functioning as family. A recent review indicates that family psychoeducation not only reduces relapse rates and the number of psychiatric hospitalization, but also decreases expressed emotion in families and leads to better treatment compliance of consumers (Pfammatter, Junghan, & Brenner, 2006).

Illness Management and Recovery

The primary aim of IMR is to empower consumers with psychiatric disabilities to manage their illness, find their own goals for recovery, and make informed decisions about their treatment by teaching them the necessary knowledge and skills. IMR involves various interventions designed to help consumers improve their ability to overcome the debilitating effects of their illness on social and role functioning. The evidence-based components of IMR are psychoeducation, behavioral tailoring for medication, relapse prevention training, and coping skills training (Mueser et al., 2002). To teach these components effectively and to ensure that knowledge is put into practice, practitioners use various techniques including motivational, educational, and cognitive-behavioral strategies. Little research has yet to investigate IMR systematically; however, one randomized controlled trial found that consumers had better outcomes, were more informed about their illness, and had achieved greater progress toward their personal goals after participating in an IMR program (Hasson-Ohayon, Roe, & Kravertz, 2007).

Integrated Dual Disorders Treatment

As noted previously, about 50% of individuals with SMI have a comorbid substance use disorder; these consumers are said to have dual disorders, which are associated with various negative outcomes. In IDDT, the same clinicians or teams of clinicians working in one setting provide psychiatric and substance abuse interventions in a coordinated fashion. IDDT aims to help consumers learn to manage both illnesses so that they can pursue meaningful life goals. The critical ingredients of IDDT include assertive outreach, motivational interventions, and a comprehensive, long-term, staged, and individualized approach to recovery (Drake, Essock, et al., 2001). Contrary to traditional treatments for people with dual disorders, abstinence is not a prerequisite to assisting with consumer goals for stable housing or meaningful activity such as employment. Controlled studies have shown IDDT's effectiveness in reducing substance abuse, which in turn leads to improvement in other outcomes including symptoms, general functioning, housing stability, and treatment retention (Corrigan et al., 2008).

Supported Employment

Defined as paid work that takes place in normal work settings with ongoing support services, supported employment was developed originally for people with developmental disabilities as a more effective, humane, and cost-effective alternative to sheltered workshops (Wehman & Moon, 1988). The evidence-based principles of supported employment for individuals with psychiatric disabilities include the following principles: eligibility based on consumer choice, integration with mental health treatment, competitive employment as the goal, attention to consumer preferences, rapid job search (i.e., no requirements for completing extensive pre-employment assessment and training), and continuous follow-along support (Becker & Drake, 2003). Fifteen experimental studies and several quasi-experimental studies comparing supported employment to traditional vocational approaches (e.g., skills training preparation, sheltered workshops, transitional employment, and day treatment) suggest that more than 60% of clients with psychiatric disabilities enrolled in supported employment programs obtain jobs in the competitive employment market, compared to less than 20% of clients not receiving supported employment (Bond et al., 2007; Bond, Drake, & Becker, 2008; Twamley, Jeste, & Lehman, 2003).

Supported education refers to helping consumers with psychiatric disabilities obtain education and training to have the skills and credentials necessary for obtaining jobs with career potential (Moxley, Mowbray, & Brown, 1993). Although few studies have been conducted that have rigorously assessed supported education, there is emerging evidence that supported education combined with supported employment is effective in enhancing both educational and employment outcomes. This is particularly critical in young adults, as supported education and supported employment may be used to combat jointly the effects of early psychosis and preserve functioning as well as the attainment of life goals for this group (Corrigan et al., 2008).

Access

Consumers with psychiatric disabilities continue to have problems accessing effective services (Wang, Lane, Olfson, Pincus, Wells, & Kessler, 2005). Despite extensive evidence and expert agreement on effective practices, most mental health centers do not provide them (Lehman & Steinwachs, 1998). The number of exemplary programs in the United States is dwarfed by the size of the population in need. Underfunding of mental health services is one of the major factors in this disparity between need and program capacity. In an effort to disseminate the best practices of psychiatric rehabilitation, a national project developed standardized guidelines and training materials, and demonstrated that the toolkits in conjunction with systematic training and consultation can facilitate faithfully implementing each of evidence-based practices in routine mental health service settings (McHugo et al., 2007).

CONCLUSION

Psychiatric disorders can look very different from one another in terms of symptom presentation, course, and treatment. An encouraging shift in the collective mindset regarding the treatment of psychiatric disabilities has occurred, with an emphasis on the right and ability of individuals to pursue meaningful goals comparable to nondisabled persons.

Like individuals with other types of long-term illnesses, people with psychiatric disabilities want to manage their own illnesses, form and maintain meaningful social relationships, work in the community, and live in normal housing situations. With the help of pharmacological treatments, psychotherapy, and psychosocial rehabilitation services, consumers can feel better and attain these goals. Hence, the focus of psychiatric rehabilitation is not just to keep consumers stable and out of the hospital but also to assist and empower them in pursuing their personal aspirations, manage their illnesses, and develop independence and self-fulfillment. Progress has been made toward realizing these objectives, although many changes are needed in the mental health system before exemplary services are available to everyone who could benefit from them.

REFERENCES

Allison, D. B., Mentore, J. L., Heo, M., Chandler, L. P., Cappelleri, J. C., Infante, M. C., et al. (1999). Antipsychotic-induced weight gain: A comprehensive research synthesis. *American Journal of Psychiatry, 156*, 1686–1696.

American Psychiatric Association. (2000a). *Diagnostic and statistical manual of mental disorders: Fourth edition, Text Revision* (4th ed.). Washington, DC: Author.

American Psychiatric Association. (2000b).: Practice guideline for the treatment of patients with major depressive disorder (revision). *American Journal of Psychiatry, 157*(Suppl. 4), 1–45.

Andreasen, N. C. (1984). *The broken brain.* New York: Harper & Row.

Angst, J., Gamma, A., Baldwin, D. S., Ajdacic-Gross, V., & Rossler, W. (2009). The generalized anxiety spectrum: Prevalence, onset, course, and outcome. *European Archives of Psychiatry and Clinical Neuroscience, 259*, 37–45.

Angst, J., Gamma, A., Sellaro, R., Lavori, P. W., & Zhang, H. (2003). Recurrence of bipolar disorders and major depression. A life-long perspective. *European Archives of Psychiatry and Clinical Neuroscience, 253*, 236–240.

Angst, F., Stassen, H. H., Clayton, P. J., & Angst, J. (2002). Mortality of patients with mood disorders: Follow-up over 34–38 years. *Journal of Affective Disorders, 68*, 167–181.

Anthony, W. A., Cohen, M., Farkas, M. D., & Gagne, C. (2002). *Psychiatric rehabilitation* (2nd ed.). Boston: Center for Psychiatric Rehabilitation.

Anthony, W. A., Cohen, M. R., & Vitalo, R. (1978). The measurement of rehabilitation outcome. *Schizophrenia Bulletin, 4*, 365–383.

Arseneault, L., Moffitt, T. E., Caspi, A., Taylor, P. J., & Silva, P. A. (2000). Mental disorders and violence in a total birth cohort: Results from the Dunedin Study. *Archives of General Psychiatry, 57*(10), 979–986.

Bandelow, B., Zohar, J., Hollander, E., Kasper, S., Moller, H.-J., & WFSBP Task Force on Treatment Guidelines for Anxiety Obsessive–Compulsive and Post-Traumatic Stress Disorders-First Revision. (2008). World federation of societies of biological psychiatry (WFSBP) guidelines for the pharmacological treatment of anxiety, obsessive-compulsive and post-traumatic stress disorders—First Revision. *World Journal of Biological Psychiatry, 9*, 248–312.

Beard, J. H., Propst, R. N., & Malamud, T. J. (1982). The Fountain House model of rehabilitation. *Psychosocial Rehabilitation Journal, 5*(1), 47–53.

Beck, A. T. (1967). *Depression: Clinical, experimental, and theoretical aspects.* New York: Harper & Row.

Beck, A. T., Rector, N. R., Stolar, A., & Grant, P. (2009). *Schizophrenia: Cognitive theory, research and therapy.* New York: Guilford.

Becker, D. R., & Drake, R. E. (2003). *A working life for people with severe mental illness.* New York: Oxford Press.

Bellack, A. S., Mueser, K. T., Gingerich, S., & Agresta, J. (2004). *Social skills training for schizophrenia: A step-by-step guide* (2nd ed.). New York: Guilford.

Belsher, G., & Costello, C. G. (1988). Relapse after recovery from unipolar depression: A critical review. *Psychological Bulletin, 104,* 84–96.

Berven, N. L., & Driscoll, J. H. (1981). The effects of past psychiatric disability on employer evaluation of a job applicant. *Journal of Applied Rehabilitation Counseling, 12,* 50–55.

Bisson, J., & Andrew, M. (2007). Psychological treatment of post-traumatic stress disorder (PTSD). *Cochrane Database of Systematic Reviews, 18*(3).

Blanchard, J. J., Mueser, K. T., & Bellack, A. S. (1998). Anhedonia, positive and negative affect, and social functioning in schizophrenia. *Schizophrenia Bulletin, 24,* 413–424.

Blow, F. C., Zeber, J. E., McCarthy, J. F., Valenstein, M., Gillon, L., & Bingham, C. R. (2004). Ethnicity and diagnostic patterns in veterans with psychosis. *Social Psychiatry and Psychiatric Epidemiology, 39,* 841–851.

Bond, G. R., Drake, R. E., & Becker, D. R. (2008). An update on randomized controlled trials of evidence-based supported employment. *Psychiatric Rehabilitation Journal, 31,* 280–290.

Bond, G. R., Drake, R. E., Mueser, K. T., & Latimer, E. (2001). Assertive community treatment for people with severe mental illness: Critical ingredients and impact on patients. *Disease Management & Health Outcomes, 9,* 141–159.

Bond, G. R., & Resnick, S. G. (2000). Psychiatric rehabilitation. In R. G. Frank & T. Elliott (Eds.), *Handbook of rehabilitation psychology* (pp. 235–258). Washington, DC: American Psychological Association.

Bond, G. R., Salyers, M. P., Dincin, J., Drake, R. E., Becker, D. R., Fraser, V. V., et al. (2007). A randomized controlled trial comparing two vocational models for persons with severe mental illness. *Journal of Consulting and Clinical Psychology, 75*(6), 968–982.

Bresnahan, M., Begg, M. D., Brown, A., Schaefer, C., Sohler, N., Insel, B., et al. (2007). Race and risk of schizophrenia in a U.S. birth cohort: Another example of health disparity? *International Journal of Epidemiology, 36,* 751–758.

Brown, G. W., Birley, J. L., & Wing, J. K. (1972). Influence of family life on the course of schizophrenic disorders: A replication. *British Journal of Psychiatry, 121,* 241–258.

Brunette, M. F., Noordsy, D. I., Xie, H., & Drake, R. E. (2003). Benzodiazepine use and abuse among patients with severe mental illness and co-occurring substance use disorders. *Psychiatric Services, 54,* 1395–1401.

Butler, A. C., Chapman, J. E., Forman, E. M., & Beck, A. T. (2006). The empirical status of cognitive-behavioral therapy: A review of meta-analyses. *Clinical Psychology Review, 26,* 17–31.

Chamberlin, J., Rogers, J. A., & Sneed, C. S. (1989). Consumers, families, and community support systems. *Psychosocial Rehabilitation Journal, 12*(3), 93–106.

Choy, Y., Fyer, A. J., & Lipsitz, J. D. (2007). Treatment of specific phobia in adults. *Clinical Psychology Review, 27,* 266–286.

Christensen, T. O. (2007). The influence of neurocognitive dysfunctions on work capacity in schizophrenia patients: A systematic review of the literature. *International Journal of Psychiatry in Clinical Practice, 11,* 89–101.

Cipriani, A., Furukawa, T. A., Salanti, G., Geddes, J. R., Higgins, J. T. P., Churchill, R., et al. (2009). Comparative efficacy and acceptability of 12 new-generation antidepressants: A multiple-treatments meta-analysis. *Lancet, 373,* 746–758.

Coldwell, C. M., & Bender, W. S. (2007). The effectiveness of assertive community treatment for homeless populations with severe mental illness. *American Journal of Psychiatry, 164,* 393–399.

Compton, M. T., Weiss, P. S., West, J. C., & Kaslow, N. J. (2005). The associations between substance use disorders, schizophrenia-spectrum disorders, and Axis IV psychosocial problems. *Social Psychiatry and Psychiatric Epidemiology, 40,* 939–946.

Copeland, M. E. (1997). *Wellness recovery action plan.* Brattleboro, VT: Peach.

Corrigan, P. W. (2003). Beat the stigma: Come out of the closet. *Psychiatric Services, 54,* 1313.

Corrigan, P. W., Mueser, K. T., Bond, G. R., Drake, R. E., & Solomon, P. (2008). *Principles and practice of psychiatric rehabilitation. An empirical approach.* New York: Guilford.

Coryell, W., Akiskal, H. S., Leon, A. C., Winokur, G., Maser, J. D., Mueller, T. I., et al. (1994). The time course of nonchronic major depressive disorder. Uniformity across episodes and samples. National Institute of Mental Health Collaborative Program on the Psychobiology of Depression—Clinical studies. *Archives of General Psychiatry, 51,* 405–410.

Cramer, J. A., & Rosenheck, R. (1998). Compliance with medication regimens for mental and physical disorders. *Psychiatric Services, 49,* 196–201.

Cuijpers, J., van Straten, A., & Warmerdam, L. (2007). Behavioral activation treatments of depression: A meta-analysis. *Clinical Psychology Review, 27,* 318–326.

Davis, J. M. (1980). Antipsychotic drugs. In H. I. Kaplan, A. M. Freedman, & B. J. Sadock (Eds.), *Comprehensive textbook of psychiatry* (Vol. 3, pp. 2257–2289). Baltimore: Williams & Wilkins.

Dincin, J. (1975). Psychiatric rehabilitation. *Schizophrenia Bulletin, 1*, 131–147.

Ditton, P. J. (1999). *Bureau of Justice statistics special report: Mental health treatment of inmates and probationers.* Washington, DC: U.S. Department of Justice.

Dixon, L., McFarlane, W. R., Lefley, H., Lucksted, A., Cohen, M., Falloon, I., et al. (2001). Evidence-based practices for services to families of people with psychiatric disabilities. *Psychiatric Services, 52*, 903–910.

Draine, J., Salzer, M. S., Culhane, D. P., & Hadley, T. R. (2002). Role of social disadvantage in crime, joblessness, and homelessness among persons with serious mental illness. *Psychiatric Services, 53*, 565–573.

Drake, R. E., & Brunette, M. F. (1998). Complications of severe mental illness related to alcohol and drug use disorders. In M. Galanter (Ed.), *Recent developments in alcoholism, Vol. 14: The consequences of alcoholism* (pp. 285–299). New York: Plenum.

Drake, R. E., Essock, S. M., & Bond, G. R. (2009). Implementing evidence-based practices for people with schizophrenia. *Schizophrenia Bulletin, 35*, 704–713.

Drake, R. E., Essock, S. M., Shaner, A., Carey, K. B., Minkoff, K., Kola, L., et al. (2001). Implementing dual diagnosis services for clients with severe mental illness. *Psychiatric Services, 52*, 469–476.

Drake, R. E., Goldman, H. H., Leff, H. S., Lehman, A. F., Dixon, L., Mueser, K. T., et al. (2001). Implementing evidence-based practices in routine mental health service settings. *Psychiatric Services, 52*(2), 179–182.

Drake, R. E., Merrens, M. R., & Lynde, D. W. (Eds.). (2005). *Evidence-based mental health practice: A textbook.* New York: WW Norton.

Drake, R. E., & Sederer, L. I. (1986). The adverse effects of intensive treatment of chronic schizophrenia. *Comprehensive Psychiatry, 27*, 313–326.

Estroff, S. E. (1989). Self, identity, and subjective experiences: In search of the subject. *Schizophrenia Bulletin, 15*, 189–196.

Fazel, S., & Danesh, J. (2002). Serious mental disorder in 23000 prisoners: A systematic review of 62 surveys. *Lancet, 359*, 545–550.

First, M. B., Spitzer, R. L., Gibbon, M., & Williams, J. B. (1994). *Structured clinical interview for axis I DSM-IV disorders—Patient edition (SCID-I/P, Version 2.0).* New York: Biometric Research Department, New York State Psychiatric Institute.

Folsom, D. P., Hawthorne, W., Lindamer, L., Gilmer, T., Bailey, A., Golshan, S., et al. (2005). Prevalence and risk factors for homelessness and utilization of mental health services among 10,340 patients with serious mental illness in a large public mental health system. *American Journal of Psychiatry, 162*, 370–376.

Forsell, Y. (2007). A three-year follow-up of major depression, dysthymia, minor depression, and subsyndromal depression: Results from a population-based study. *Depression and Anxiety, 24*, 62–65.

Glied, S. A., & Frank, R. G. (2009). Better but not best: Recent trends in the well-being of the mentally ill. *Health Affairs, 28*, 637–648.

Glod, C. A. (1996). Recent advances in the pharmacotherapy of major depression. *Archives of Psychiatric Nursing, 10*, 355–364.

Goffman, E. (1961). *Asylums: Essays on the social situation of mental patients and other inmates.* Chicago: Aldine.

Goldman, H. H. (1984). Epidemiology. In J. A. Talbott (Ed.), *The chronic mental patient: Five years later* (pp. 15–31). Orlando, FL: Grune & Stratton.

Goodman, L. A., Dutton, M. A., & Harris, M. (1997). The relationship between violence dimensions and symptom severity among homeless, mentally ill women. *Journal of Traumatic Stress, 10*, 51–70.

Goodman, L. A., Salyers, M. P., Mueser, K. T., Rosenberg, S. D., Swartz, M., Essock, S. M., et al. (2001). Recent victimization in women and men with severe mental illness: Prevalence and correlates. *Journal of Traumatic Stress, 14*, 615–632.

Grabowski, D. C., Aschbrenner, K. A., Feng, Z., & Mor, V. (2009). Mental illness in nursing homes: Variations across states. *Health Affairs, 28*, 689–700.

Hall, L. L., Graf, A. C., Fitzpatrick, M. J., Lane, T., & Birkel, R. C. (2003). *Shattered lives: Results of a national survey of NAMI members living with mental illness and their families.* Arlington, VA: NAMI/TRIAD (Treatment/Recovery Information and Advocacy Data Base).

Harding, C. M., Brooks, G. W., Ashikaga, T., Strauss, J. S., & Breier, A. (1987). The Vermont longitudinal study of persons with severe mental illness: II. Long-term outcome of subjects who retrospectively met DSM-III criteria for schizophrenia. *American Journal of Psychiatry, 144*, 727–735.

Harris, E. C., & Barraclough, B. (1997). Suicide as an outcome for mental disorders: A meta-analysis. *British Journal of Psychiatry, 170*, 205–228.

Harris, M. J., & Jeste, D. V. (1988). Late-onset schizophrenia: An overview [comment]. *Schizophrenia Bulletin, 14*, 39–55.

Hasson-Ohayon, I., Roe, D., & Kravertz, S. (2007). A randomized controlled trial of the effectiveness of the illness management and recovery program. *Psychiatric Services, 58*, 1461–1466.

Hazer, J. T., & Bedell, K. V. (2000). Effects of seeking accommodation and disability on preemployment evaluations. *Journal of Applied Social Psychology, 30*, 1201–1223.

Henderson, D. C. (2002). Diabetes mellitus and other metabolic disturbances induced by atypical antipsychotic agents. *Current Diabetes Reports, 2*(2), 135–140.

Herz, M. I. (1984). Recognizing and preventing relapse in patients with schizophrenia. *Hospital and Community Psychiatry, 35*, 344–349.

Hogarty, G. E., McEvoy, J. P., Munetz, M., DiBarry, A. L., Bartone, P., Cather, R., et al. (1988). Dose of fluphenazine, familial expressed emotion, and outcome in schizophrenia. *Archives of General Psychiatry, 45*, 797–805.

Horan, W. P., Subotnik, K. L., Snyder, K. S., & Nuechterlein, K. H. (2006). Do recent onset schizophrenia patients experience a "social network crisis"? *Psychiatry-Interpersonal and Biological Processes, 69*, 115–129.

Isaac, R. J., & Armat, V. C. (1990). *Madness in the streets: How psychiatry and the law abandoned the mentally ill*. New York: Free.

Jablensky, A. (2000). Epidemiology of schizophrenia: The global burden of disease and disability. *European Archives of Psychiatry & Clinical Neuroscience, 250*, 274–285.

Jobe, T. H., & Harrow, M. (2005). Long-term outcome of patients with schizophrenia: A review. *Canadian Journal of Psychiatry, 50*, 892–900.

Kane, J. M., Woerner, M., & Sarantakos, S. (1986). Depot neuroleptics: A comparative review of standard, intermediate, and low-dose regimens. *Journal of Clinical Psychiatry, 47*(Suppl. 5), 30–33.

Kessler, R. C., Berglund, P., Demler, O., Jin, R., Merikangas, K. R., & Walters, E. E. (2005a). Lifetime prevalence and age-of-onset distributions of DSM-IV disorders in the national comorbidity survey replication. *Archives of General Psychiatry, 62*, 593–602.

Kessler, R. C., Demler, O., Frank, R. G., Olfson, M., Pincus, H. A., Walters, E. E., et al. (2005b). Prevalence and treatment of mental disorders, 1990 to 2003. *New England Journal of Medicine, 352*, 2515–2523.

Kessler, R. C., DuPont, R. L., Berglund, P., & Wittchen, H.-U. (1999). Impairment in pure and comorbid generalized anxiety disorder and major depression at 12 months in two national surveys. *American Journal of Psychiatry, 156*, 1915–1923.

Kessler, R. C., McGonagle, K. A., Zhao, S., Nelson, C. B., Hughes, M., Eshleman, S., et al. (1994). Lifetime and 12-month prevalence of DSM-III-R psychiatric disorders in the United States. Results from the National Comorbidity Survey. *Archives of General Psychiatry, 51*, 8–19.

Kopelowicz, A., Liberman, R. P., & Zarate, R. (2006). Recent advances in social skills training for schizophrenia. *Schizophrenia Bulletin, 32*, S12–S23.

Kring, A. M., Davidson, G. C., Neale, J. M., & Johnson, S. L. (2007). *Abnormal psychology* (10th ed.). Hoboken, NJ: John Wiley.

Kuyken, W., Byford, S., Taylor, R. S., Watkins, E., Holden, E., White, K., et al. (2008). Mindfulness-based cognitive therapy to prevent relapse in recurrent depression. *Journal of Consulting and Clinical Psychology, 76*, 966–978.

Lacro, J. P., Dunn, L. B., Dolder, C. R., Leckband, S. G., & Jeste, D. V. (2002). Prevalence of and risk factors for medication nonadherence in patients with schizophrenia: A comprehensive review of recent literature. *Journal of Clinical Psychiatry, 63*, 892–909.

Lamb, H. R., & Bachrach, L. L. (2001). Some perspectives on deinstitutionalization. *Psychiatric Services, 52*, 1039–1045.

Lehman, A. F., & Steinwachs, D. M. (1998). Patterns of usual care for schizophrenia: Initial results from the Schizophrenia Patient Outcomes Research Team (PORT) Client Survey. *Schizophrenia Bulletin, 24*, 11–20.

Lickey, M. E., & Gordon, B. (1991). *Medicine and mental illness*. New York: W. H. Freeman.

Lieberman, J. A., Stroup, T. S., McEvoy, J. P., Swartz, M. S., Rosenheck, R. A., Perkins, D. O., et al. (2005). Effectiveness of antipsychotic drugs in patients with chronic schizophrenia. *New England Journal of Medicine, 353*, 1209–1223.

Linehan, M., & Armstrong, H. (1991). Cognitive-behavioral treatment of chronically parasuicidal borderline patients. *Archives of General Psychiatry, 48*, 1060–1064.

Linehan, M., Comtois, C. A., Murray, A. M., Brown, M. Z., Gallop, R. J., Heard, H. L., et al. (2006). Two-year randomized controlled trial and follow-up of dialectical behavior therapy vs therapy by experts for suicidal behaviors and borderline personality disorder. *Archives of General Psychiatry, 63,* 757–766.

Lingam, R., & Scott, J. (2002). Treatment nonadherence in affective disorders. *Acta Psychiatrica Scandinavia, 105,* 164–172.

Lipsey, M. W., & Wilson, D. B. (1993). The efficacy of psychological, educational, and behavioral treatment: Confirmation from meta-analysis. *American Psychologist, 48,* 1181–1209.

Macias, C., Jackson, R., Schroeder, C., & Wang, Q. (1999). What is a clubhouse? Report on the ICCD 1996 survey of USA clubhouses. *Community Mental Health Journal, 35,* 181–190.

Mann, J. J. (2005). The medical management of depression. *New England Journal of Medicine, 353,* 1819–1834.

McEvoy, J. P., Lieberman, J. A., Stroup, S., Davis, S. M., Meltzer, H. Y., Rosenheck, R. A., et al. (2006). Effectiveness of clozapine versus olanzapine, quetiapine, and risperidone in patients with chronic schizophrenia who did not respond to prior atypical antipsychotic treatment. *American Journal of Psychiatry, 163,* 600–610.

McGlashan, T. H. (1988). A selective review of recent North American long-term followup studies of schizophrenia. *Schizophrenia Bulletin, 14,* 515–542.

McGrath, J., Saha, S., Welham, J., Saadi, O. E., MacCauley, C., & Chant, D. (2004). A systematic review of the incidence of schizophrenia: The distribution of rates and the influence of sex, urbanicity, migrant status, and methodology. *BMC Medicine, 2,* 13.

McGrew, J. H., Wilson, R., & Bond, G. R. (1996). Client perspectives on helpful ingredients of assertive community treatment. *Psychiatric Rehabilitation Journal, 19*(3), 13–21.

McGurk, S. R., & Mueser, K. T. (2004). Cognitive functioning, symptoms, and work in supported employment: A review and heuristic model. *Schizophrenia Research, 70,* 147–173.

McHugo, G. J., Drake, R. E., Whitley, R., Bond, G. R., Campbell, K., Rapp, C. A., et al. (2007). Fidelity outcomes in the National Implementing Evidence-Based Practices Project. *Psychiatric Services, 58,* 1279–1284.

McNeil, D. E., Binder, R. L., & Robinson, J. O. (2005). Incarceration associated with homelessness, mental disorder, and co-occurring substance abuse. *Psychiatric Services, 56,* 840–846.

McQuilken, M., Zahniser, J. H., Novak, J., Starks, R. D., Olmos, A., & Bond, G. R. (2003). The Work Project Survey: Consumer perspectives on work. *Journal of Vocational Rehabilitation, 18,* 59–68.

Mellman, T. A., Miller, A. L., Weissman, E. M., Crismon, M. L., Essock, S. M., & Marder, S. R. (2001). Evidence-based pharmacologic treatment for people with severe mental illness: A focus on guidelines and algorithms. *Psychiatric Services, 52,* 619–625.

Miller, A. L., Chiles, J. A., Chiles, J. K., Crismon, M. L., Rush, A. J., & Shon, S. P. (1999). The Texas Medication Algorithm Project (TMAP) schizophrenia algorithms. *Journal of Clinical Psychiatry, 60,* 649–657.

Miller, W. R., & Rollnick, S. (2002). *Motivational interviewing: Preparing people for change* (2nd ed.). New York: Guilford.

Minkoff, K. (1978). A map of chronic mental patients. In J. A. Talbott (Ed.), *The chronic mental patient* (pp. 11–37). Washington, DC: American Psychiatric Association.

Mitchell, A. J., & Subramaniam, H. (2005). Prognosis of depression in old age compared to middle age: A systematic review of comparative studies. *American Journal of Psychiatry, 162,* 1588–1601.

Möller, H., & Volz, H. (1996). Drug treatment of depression in the 1990s: An overview of achievements and future possibilities. *Drugs, 52,* 625–638.

Mowbray, C. T., Chamberlain, P., Jennings, M., & Reed, C. (1988). Consumer-run mental health services: Results from five demonstration projects. *Community Mental Health Journal, 2,* 151–156.

Moxley, D. P., Mowbray, C. T., & Brown, K. S. (1993). Supported education. In R. W. Flexer & P. L. Solomon (Eds.), *Psychiatric rehabilitation in practice* (pp. 137–153). Boston: Andover Medical.

Mueser, K. T., Bellack, A. S., & Brady, E. U. (1990). Hallucinations in schizophrenia. *Acta Psychiatrica Scandinavica, 82,* 26–29.

Mueser, K. T., Corrigan, P. W., Hilton, D. W., Tanzman, B., Schaub, A., Gingerich, S., et al. (2002). Illness management and recovery: A review of the research. *Psychiatric Services, 53,* 1272–1284.

Mueser, K. T., Drake, R. E., & Bond, G. R. (1997). Recent advances in psychiatric rehabilitation for patients with severe mental illness. *Harvard Review of Psychiatry, 5,* 123–137.

Mueser, K. T., & Gingerich, S. (1994). *Coping with schizophrenia: A guide for families.* Oakland, CA: New Harbinger.

Mueser, K. T., & Glynn, S. M. (1995). Families as members of the treatment team. In K. T. Mueser & S. Glynn (Eds.), *Behavioral family therapy for psychiatric disorder* (pp. 1–29). Needham Heights, MA: Allyn & Bacon.

Mueser, K. T., Goodman, L. B., Trumbetta, S. L., Rosenberg, S. D., Osher, F. C., Vidaver, R., et al. (1998). Trauma and posttraumatic stress disorder in severe mental illness. *Journal of Consulting and Clinical Psychology, 66,* 493–499.

Mueser, K. T., & Tarrier, N. (1998). *Handbook of social functioning in schizophrenia.* Boston: Allyn and Bacon.

Mueser, K. T., Torrey, W. C., Lynde, D., Singer, P., & Drake, R. E. (2003). Implementing evidence-based practices for people with severe mental illness. *Behavior Modification, 27,* 387–411.

National Alliance on Mental Illness. (2003). *NAMI mission & history.* Retrieved from http://www.nami.org/history.htm.

Nasar, S. (1998). *A beautiful mind.* New York: Simon & Schuster.

Nasrallah, H. A. (2002). Pharmacoeconomic implications of adverse effects during antipsychotic drug therapy. *American Journal of Health-System Pharmacy, 59*(Suppl. 8), S16–21.

Neugeboren, J. (2001). *Transforming madness: New lives for people living with mental illness.* Berkeley, CA: University of California Press.

New Freedom Commission on Mental Health. (2003). *Achieving the promise: Transforming mental health care in America. Final Report. DHHS Pub. No. SMA-03–3832.* Rockville, MD: Substance Abuse and Mental Health Services Administration.

Noll, K. M., Davis, J. M., & DeLeon-Jones, F. (1985). Medication and somatic therapies in the treatment of depression. In E. E. Beckham & W. R. Lebe (Eds.), *Handbook of depression: Treatment, assessment and research* (pp. 220–315). Homewood, IL: Dorsey.

Palmer, B. A., Pankratz, S., & Bostwick, J. M. (2005). The lifetime risk of suicide in schizophrenia. A reexamination. *Archives of General Psychiatry, 62,* 247–253.

Perese, E. F. (2007). Stigma, poverty, and victimization: Roadblocks to recovery for individuals with severe mental illness. *Journal of the American Psychiatric Nurses Association, 13,* 285–295.

Perkins, D. O., Gu, H., Boteva, K., & Lieberman, J. A. (2005). Relationship between duration of untreated psychosis and outcome in first-episode schizophrenia: A critical review and meta-analysis. *American Journal of Psychiatry, 162,* 1785–1804.

Pescosolido, B. A., Wright, E. R., & Lutfey, K. (1999). The changing hopes, worries, and community supports of individuals moving from a closing long-term care facility. *Journal of Behavioral Health Services & Research, 26,* 276–288.

Pfammatter, M., Junghan, U. M., & Brenner, H. D. (2006). Efficacy of psychological therapy in schizophrenia: Conclusions from meta-analyses. *Schizophrenia Bulletin, 32,* S64–S80.

Poutanen, O., Mattila, A., Seppala, N. H., Groth, L., Koivisto, A.-M., & Salokangas, R. K. R. (2007). Seven-year outcome of depression in primary and psychiatric outpatient care: Results of the TADEP (Tampere Depression) II study. *Nordic Journal of Psychiatry, 61,* 62–70.

Pratt, C. W., Gill, K. J., Barrett, N. M., & Roberts, M. M. (1999). *Psychiatric rehabilitation.* New York: Academic.

Ralph, R. O. (2000). *A synthesis of a sample of recovery literature 2000.* Alexandria, VA: National Technical Center for State Mental Health Planning, National Association for State Mental Health Program Directors.

Regier, D. A., Farmer, M. E., Rae, D. S., Locke, B. Z., Keith, S. J., Judd, L. L., et al. (1990). Comorbidity of mental disorders with alcohol and other drug abuse. Results from the Epidemiologic Catchment Area (ECA) Study. [comment]. *Journal of the American Medical Association, 264*(19), 2511–2518.

Regier, D. A., Rae, D. S., Narrow, W. E., Kaelber, C. T., & Schatzberg, A. F. (1998). Prevalence of anxiety disorders and their comorbidity with mood and addictive disorders. *British Journal of Psychiatry—Supplementum,* (34), 24–28.

Reichenberg, A., & Harvey, P. D. (2007). Neuropsychological impairments in schizophrenia: Integration of performance-based and brain imaging findings. *Psychological Bulletin, 133,* 833–858.

Robinson, D. G., Woerner, M. G., McMeniman, M., Mendelowitz, A., & Bilder, R. M. (2004). Symptomatic and functional recovery from a first episode of schizophrenia or schizoaffective disorder. *American Journal of Psychiatry, 161,* 473–479.

Rogers, E. S., Anthony, W. A., & Jansen, M. A. (1988). Psychiatric rehabilitation as the preferred response to the needs of individuals with severe psychiatric disability. *Rehabilitation Psychology, 33,* 5–14.

Rosenberg, S. D., Mueser, K. T., Friedman, M. J., Gorman, P. G., Drake, R. E., Vidaver, R. M., et al. (2001). Developing effective treatments for posttraumatic disorders among people with severe mental illness. *Psychiatric Services, 52,* 1453–1461.

Rosenheck, R. A., Leslie, D., Keefe, R., McEvoy, J., Swartz, M., Perkins, D., et al. (2006). Barriers to employment for people with schizophrenia. *American Journal of Psychiatry, 163,* 411–417.

Rubio, G., & Lopez-Ibor, J. J. (2007a). Generalized anxiety disorder: A 40-year follow-up study. *Acta Psychiatrica Scandinavia, 115,* 372–379.

Rubio, G., & Lopez-Ibor, J. J. (2007b). What can be learnt from the natural history of anxiety disorders? *European Psychiatry, 22,* 80–86.

Sartorius, N., Shapiro, R., & Jablonsky, A. (1974). The international pilot study of schizophrenia. *Schizophrenia Bulletin, 2,* 21–35.

Schinnar, A., Rothbard, A., Kanter, R., & Jung, Y. (1990). An empirical literature review of definitions of severe and persistent mental illness. *American Journal of Psychiatry, 147,* 1602–1608.

Segal, S. P., & Aviram, U. (1978). *The mentally ill in community-based sheltered care: A study of community care and social integration.* New York: Wiley-International.

Sharma, R. P., Dowd, S., & Janicak, P. G. (1999). Hallucinations in the acute schizophrenic-type psychosis: Effects of gender and age of illness onset. *Schizophrenia Research, 37,* 91–95.

Sheehan, S. (1982). *Is there no place on earth for me?* New York: Vintage Books.

Solomon, P. (2003). Case management and the forensic client. In W. Fischer (Ed.), *Community-based interventions for criminal offenders with severe mental illness* (pp. 53–71). Amsterdam: Elsevier.

Sorbara, F., Liraud, F., Assens, F., Abalan, F., & Verdoux, H. (2003). Substance use and the course of early psychosis: A 2-year follow-up of first-admitted subjects. *European Psychiatry, 18,* 133–136.

Stahl, S. M., & Buckley, P. F. (2007). Negative symptoms of schizophrenia: A problem that will not go away. *Acta Psychiatrica Scandinavica, 115,* 4–11.

Steadman, H. J., Mulvey, E. P., Monahan, J., Clark Robins, P., Appelbaum, P. S., Grisso, T. et al. (1998). Violence by people discharged from acute psychiatric inpatient facilities and by others in the same neighborhoods. *Archives of General Psychiatry, 55,* 393–401.

Stein, L. I., & Test, M. A. (1980). An alternative to mental health treatment. I: Conceptual model, treatment program, and clinical evaluation. *Archives of General Psychiatry, 37,* 392–397.

Substance Abuse and Mental Health Services Administration. (1997). *Just the facts: The prevalence of co-occurring mental and substance disorders in the criminal justice system.* Rockville, MD: National GAINS Center, Substance Abuse and Mental Health Services Administration.

Swanson, J. W., Holzer, C. E., 3rd, Ganju, V. K., & Jono, R. T. (1990). Violence and psychiatric disorder in the community: Evidence from the Epidemiologic Catchment Area surveys. *Hospital & Community Psychiatry, 41,* 761–770.

Swartz, M. S., Swanson, J. W., Hiday, V. A., Borum, R., Wagner, H. R., & Burns, B. J. (1998). Violence and severe mental illness: The effects of substance abuse and nonadherence to medication. *American Journal of Psychiatry, 155,* 226–231.

Switzer, G. E., Dew, M. A., Thompson, K., Goycoolea, J. M., Derricott, T., & Mullins, S. D. (1999). Posttraumatic stress disorder and service utilization among urban mental health center clients. *Journal of Traumatic Stress, 12,* 25–39.

Talbott, J. A. (Ed.). (1978). *The chronic mental patient.* Washington, DC: American Psychiatric Association.

Teplin, L. A., McClelland, G. M., Abram, K. M., & Weiner, D. A. (2005). Crime victimization in adults with severe mental illness. *Archives of General Psychiatry, 62,* 911–921.

Test, M. A. (1992). Training in community living. In R. P. Liberman (Ed.), *Handbook of psychiatric rehabilitation* (pp. 153–170). New York: Macmillan.

Thase, M. E. (2008). Selecting appropriate treatments for maintenance therapy for bipolar disorder. *Journal of Clinical Psychiatry, 69*(Suppl. 5), 28–35.

Thornicroft, G., & Sartorius, N. (1993). The course and outcome of depression in different cultures: 10-year follow-up of the WHO Collaborative Study on the Assessment of Depressive Disorders. *Psychological Medicine, 23,* 1023–1032.

Tondo, L., Isacsson, G., & Baldessarini, R. J. (2003). Suicidal behaviour in bipolar disorder: Risk and prevention. *CNS Drugs, 17,* 491–511.

Torrey, E. F. (2001). *Surviving schizophrenia: A manual for families, consumers, and providers* (4th ed.). New York: Harper-Collins.

Torrey, E. F., Erdman, K., Wolfe, S. M., & Flynn, L. M. (1990). *Care of the seriously mentally ill: A rating of state programs* (3rd ed.). Arlington, VA: National Alliance for the Mentally Ill.

Turkington, D., Kingdom, D., & Weiden, P. J. (2006). Cognitive behavior therapy for schizophrenia. *American Journal of Psychiatry, 163,* 365–373.

Turner, J. C., & TenHoor, W. J. (1978). The NIMH community support program: Pilot approach to a needed social reform. *Schizophrenia Bulletin, 4,* 319–348.

Twamley, E. W., Jeste, D. V., & Lehman, A. F. (2003). Vocational rehabilitation in schizophrenia and other psychotic disorders: A literature review and meta-analysis of randomized controlled trials. *Journal of Nervous and Mental Disease, 191,* 515–523.

U.S. Congress. (1963). *P. L. 88–164—Mental Retardation Facilities and Community Mental Health Centers Construction Act of 1963*, Washington, DC: U. S. Government Printing Office.

Verdoux, H., Tournier, M., & Cougnard, A. (2005). Impact of substance use on the onset and course of early psychosis. *Schizophrenia Research, 79,* 69–75.

Volkow, N. D. (2009). Substance use disorders in schizophrenia—clinical implications of comorbidity. *Schizophrenia Bulletin, 35,* 469–472

Wallace, C. J., Liberman, R. P., MacKain, S. J., Blackwell, G., & Eckman, T. A. (1992). Effectiveness and replicability of modules for teaching social and instrumental skills to the severely mentally ill. *American Journal of Psychiatry, 149,* 654–658.

Wang, P. S., West, J. C., Tanielian, T., & Pincus, H. A. (2000). Recent patterns and predictors of antipsychotic medication regimens used to treat schizophrenia and other psychotic disorders. *Schizophrenia Bulletin, 26,* 451–457.

Wehman, P., & Moon, M. S. (Eds.). (1988). *Vocational rehabilitation and supported employment.* Baltimore: Paul Brookes.

Weiden, P. J., & Olfson, M. (1993). The cost of relapse in schizophrenia. *Schizophrenia Bulletin, 21,* 419–428.

Weissman, M. M. (2006). A brief history of interpersonal therapy. *Psychiatric Annals, 36,* 553–557.

Whaley, A. L. (2004). A two-stage method for the study of cultural bias in the diagnosis of schizophrenia in African Americans. *Journal of Black Psychology, 30,* 167–186.

Wittlin, B. J. (1988). Practical psychopharmacology. In R. P. Liberman (Ed.), *Psychiatric rehabilitation of chronic mental patients* (pp. 117–145). Washington, DC: American Psychiatric Association.

Yulug, B., Ozan, E., Gönül, A. S., & Kilic, E. (2009). Brain-derived neurotrophic factor, stress, and depression: A mini review. *Brain Research Bulletin, 78,* 267–269.

Zygmunt, A., Olfson, M., Boyer, C. A., & Mechanic, D. (2002). Interventions to improve medication adherence in schizophrenia. *American Journal of Psychiatry, 159,* 1653–1664.

22

Pulmonary Disorders

Frederick A. Bevelaqua, MD, and Susan Garritan, PT, PhD, CCS

There are many pulmonary disorders that can cause disability. Probably the most common of these is chronic obstructive pulmonary disease (COPD). COPD is a term used to define a group of chronic lung conditions with a unifying characteristic of obstruction to airflow. The term encompasses a broad spectrum of disorders ranging from chronic bronchitis, which is primarily an airway disease, to emphysema, which is primarily a disease of the alveoli, the tiny air sacs in the lung where the exchange of oxygen for carbon dioxide occurs. COPD is extremely common and is a major cause of death, illness, and disability worldwide (Murray & Lopez, 1996). If current trends continue, it will become the third leading cause of death worldwide by 2020 (Murray & Lopez, 1997). It is generally acknowledged that cigarette smoking is by far the greatest risk factor for the development of COPD and that the risk for developing it in smokers is dose related (United States Department of Health and Human Services, 1984). However, not all smokers develop clinically significant COPD, which suggests that genetic factors play a role in determining susceptibility to the effects of cigarette smoke (Smith & Harrison, 1997). Once lung function is lost as a result of smoking, it is, for the most part, not regained after smoking cessation, although the rate of age-related decline in lung function in former smokers slows compared with that seen in nonsmokers (Camilli, Burrows, Knudson, Lyle, & Lebowitz, 1987). The economic impact of COPD can be measured in terms of the cost of treatment and reduced productivity due to morbidity and mortality. However, with proper treatment and rehabilitation, many individuals may achieve a greater degree of comfort and improved quality of life.

Initially, the symptoms of COPD may be relatively silent. The typical signs and symptoms of COPD such as persistent cough, increased sputum production, shortness of breath, wheezing, and chest tightness may not appear until there has been significant lung damage. Once symptoms appear, they typically worsen over time. Although bronchial asthma may be considered a separate disorder from COPD, it is also a disease of the airways and as such has many features similar to COPD. Other chronic pulmonary disorders including occupational lung diseases, interstitial lung diseases (ILDs), bronchiectasis, and cystic fibrosis (CF) share some clinical and pathophysiological characteristics with COPD and will be discussed later in this chapter. Therefore, an understanding of the clinical characteristics and pathophysiology of COPD will be helpful in understanding these other disorders as well.

BASIC PULMONARY ANATOMY, PHYSIOLOGY, AND PATHOPHYSIOLOGY

To understand COPD and pulmonary disease, it is helpful to understand the basic anatomy and physiology of the lungs. When you inhale, air travels down the trachea and into the bronchial passageways. These bronchial passageways branch into a myriad of smaller bronchial tubes called *bronchioles*. These bronchioles end in clusters of tiny air sacs called *alveoli*. These air sacs have very thin walls surrounded by tiny blood vessels known as "capillaries." It is through the alveoli and the capillaries that surround them that absorption of oxygen from the atmosphere and excretion of carbon dioxide produced by metabolism occurs. When one inhales, the muscles of the diaphragm and rib cage contract and in so doing expand the chest cavity, which draws air into the lungs. During normal unforced exhalation, the natural elasticity of the bronchial passageways and alveoli, known as elastic recoil pressure, causes the lungs to contract, thus expelling the air. However, there are many factors that combine to produce obstruction to airflow in COPD. Spasm of the smooth muscles of the respiratory tract, edema or swelling of the airways, excessive mucus production, and compression or collapse of the bronchial walls all contribute to airflow obstruction, particularly during expiration. The network of connective tissue and alveoli in the lung provides a supporting framework that helps to maintain the patency of the bronchioles, particularly during expiration. The loss of alveoli that occurs in emphysema causes diminished support for this framework, preventing the bronchioles from resisting the compressive forces that naturally occur during expiration. This in turn causes early collapse of the bronchioles during expiration, resulting in obstruction to airflow. Therefore, the reduction in expiratory airflow in COPD actually has two main causes. First, there is decreased expiratory airflow pressure that occurs from loss of elastic recoil of the lung. Second, there is increased resistance to airflow because of narrowing of the airways. This narrowing is due to a combination of factors that include hypertrophy of the smooth muscle lining the bronchial passageways, excess mucus production, edema of the airways occurring from inflammation, and premature collapse of the bronchioles on expiration that results from the loss of the supporting framework of the alveoli and connective tissue.

Clinically, COPD is often broken down into two subcategories, chronic bronchitis and emphysema, depending on which type of airflow obstruction predominates. In chronic bronchitis (sometimes called *Type B*), the obstruction to airflow is primarily due to inflammation of the airway that leads to increased airflow resistance. In chronic bronchitis, inflammation of the bronchial mucosa lining the bronchi is the primary pathological process. This inflammation may be caused by a variety of infections or irritants that result in damage to the lining of the respiratory tract. One result of this inflammation is mucus gland hypertrophy and the production of excess amounts of mucus that tend to clog the airways. The mucociliary clearance mechanism, which normally moves mucus upward and out of the respiratory tract, is also impaired (Isawa, Techima, Hirano, Ebina, & Kono, 1984). Therefore, the normal protective function of the mucus, which is to trap bacteria and irritants, is compromised. Hypertrophy of the smooth muscle lining the respiratory tract also plays an important role in causing airflow obstruction. In addition to damaging the mucosa lining the respiratory tract and causing excess mucus production, inflammation of the airways stimulates the parasympathetic nervous system, causing spasm of this hypertrophic smooth muscle lining the respiratory tract. Thus, there are primarily two types of airway obstruction in chronic bronchitis. One type involves direct mechanical blockage of the airway due to inflammation and swelling of the respiratory mucosa with mucus accumulation in the bronchial passageways. The other type involves smooth muscle hypertrophy and spasm triggered by inflammation and irritation. Both types of bronchial obstruction occur in asthma as well, but as mentioned previously, there tends to be a greater potential for reversibility of airflow obstruction caused by asthma. Patients with emphysema may also have some degree of airway disease similar to that described for COPD and asthma. However, in emphysema patients (sometimes called *Type A* patients), the decrease in expiratory airflow results primarily from loss of alveoli. Alveoli loss results in a decrease in bronchiole patency, causing obstruction to expiratory airflow and consequently to lung hyperinflation. It should be emphasized that most patients with COPD actually have elements of both chronic bronchitis and emphysema, although in any given patient, one form or the other may predominate.

The term *asthmatic bronchitis* is somewhat confusing and is used in two ways to describe two different clinical situations. It is sometimes used to refer to a variation of chronic bronchitis in which there is a more variable degree of airflow obstruction superimposed on a chronic, fixed degree of obstruction. The airflow obstruction in this situation is similar to asthma in that there is a potential for some reversal of the airflow obstruction that occurs from spasm of the smooth muscle lining the bronchial passageways. However, unlike asthma, there is only limited reversibility of airflow obstruction because of fixed airflow obstruction that is due to chronic airway inflammation and scaring characteristic of COPD. Therefore, the pathophysiology of asthmatic bronchitis in this situation is quite similar to that of chronic bronchitis with inflammation, edema, mucus plugging, and chronic scarring of the airways. However, it is characterized by some degree of reversible airflow obstruction that is caused by bronchial smooth muscle spasm. The other clinical situation in which the term asthmatic bronchitis is used refers to episodes of prolonged coughing, wheezing, and sputum production that occurs following episodes of acute bronchitis, which is usually triggered by respiratory tract infections.

The loss of alveoli associated with emphysema results in decreased surface area for the exchange of carbon dioxide and oxygen with the atmosphere. It also results in hyperinflation of the lung due to loss of elasticity. This hyperinflation is further compounded by the anatomical changes in the supporting structure of the small airways discussed previously that cause premature collapse of these airways on expiration, leading to air trapping in the lungs. Most patients with COPD have some degree of both airway and alveolar disease, although in any given patient, one form may be more dominant. The classic clinical definition of chronic bronchitis, namely, a chronic cough or mucus production for at least 3 months of the year for 2 consecutive years, is not really adequate to identify all patients with chronic bronchitis, although it useful in identifying most patients with this disorder. More useful is an understanding of the pathophysiology of these disease processes and what can be done to ameliorate symptoms, improve functional capacity, and prevent progression. Therefore, it is important to identify patients early in the course of their disease who have a potential for improvement with pharmacological therapy, physical therapy, exercise reconditioning, and the elimination of provocative factors such as cigarette smoking.

The bronchial obstruction that occurs in chronic bronchitis leads to a drop in arterial blood oxygen level (hypoxemia) and an increase in carbon dioxide retention (hypercapnia) because of a mismatch of ventilation of the lungs to blood perfusion of the lungs. Bronchial obstruction prevents inhaled air from effectively reaching alveoli, where the exchange of carbon dioxide for oxygen normally occurs. As a consequence, carbon dioxide builds up in the blood and oxygen levels fall. If the hypoxemia is chronic and severe enough, it may lead to pulmonary hypertension. Hypoxemia tends to cause constriction of blood vessels in the lung, resulting in pulmonary hypertension. This increases the strain on the right ventricle of the heart, causing right ventricular hypertrophy or enlargement (cor pulmonale), and ultimately right ventricular failure. Low blood oxygen may also induce a so-called syndrome referred to as *secondary polycythemia*, in which low blood oxygen levels stimulate the bone marrow to produce more red blood cells to carry oxygen to the tissues. This increase in red blood cell mass, if severe enough, can lead to increased risk of thrombosis and worsening pulmonary hypertension. Furthermore, the increased carbon dioxide retention (hypercapnia) seen in patients with severe COPD causes respiratory acidosis (a decrease in blood pH) that leads to worsening pulmonary vasoconstriction, pulmonary hypertension, and bronchoconstriction. As the disease progresses, respiratory failure eventually ensues.

EPIDEMIOLOGY OF COPD

Prevalence

Estimates regarding the prevalence of COPD in the United States and around the world are likely to be imprecise because of a number of factors. Varying definitions, underdiagnosis, underreporting, differences in survey techniques, and different criteria used to assess the severity of COPD make it very difficult to get an accurate assessment of the prevalence, severity, and morbidity of this disorder (Halbert, Isonaka, George, & Iqbal, 2003). However, COPD is generally recognized as a leading cause of morbidity and mortality throughout the world. The economic and social implications of this worldwide disorder are staggering and likely to worsen in the future because of air pollution, tobacco smoking, and the aging of the world's population. As individuals live longer with continued exposure to risk factors, the likelihood of developing COPD will increase. Although the estimates of the prevalence of COPD may vary, certain conclusions can be made based on the data that are available (Halbert et al., 2006): The prevalence of COPD is higher in smokers and ex-smokers than in those who have never smoked; the prevalence is greater in individuals older than 40 years compared to those younger than 40; and men are more likely to develop the disease than women (GOLD Report, 2008).

Morbidity and Mortality

Parameters used to measure morbidity usually include factors such as the number of doctor visits, emergency-room visits, and hospitalizations over a period of time. The data that are available based on these parameters indicate that the morbidity due to COPD increases with age and that it is greater in men than in women (National Heart, Lung and Blood Institute, 1998). COPD is generally regarded as being one of the leading causes of hospitalization of adults in the United States, particularly among the elderly (Sullivan, Strassels, & Smith, 1996). Moreover, deaths either directly related to or associated with COPD have been increasing steadily in the United States (Jemal, Ward, Hao, & Thun, 2005). Another indication of the importance of COPD as a disease entity is the years of life lost resulting from premature death as a consequence of this illness and the loss of functionality due to the disability it causes.

Etiology and Pathogenesis

The unifying factor in the development of COPD is the occurrence of inflammation in the respiratory tract and the response of the lung to this inflammation in terms of bronchoconstriction (spasm of the smooth muscle lining the airway), mucus production, edema of the airways, destruction of alveoli, and bronchial smooth muscle hypertrophy. Cigarette smoke and other inhalational toxins induce inflammation in the lungs as evidenced by increased numbers of white blood cells (neutrophils, lymphocytes, and macrophages) in the lumen of the airways (Barnes, 2004; Stockley, 2002). Both viral and bacterial infections contribute to the pathogenesis and progression of COPD (Sethi, Maloney, Grove, Wrona, & Berenson, 2001). The normal clearance mechanisms of the tracheobronchial tree are also impaired in COPD, leading to mucus plugging of the airways, which furthers the development of infection and inflammation (Burgel & Nadel, 2004). Although cigarette smoking is by far the most important etiological factor in the development of COPD, exposure to various dusts, vapors, and other airborne irritants, often on an occupational basis, can also lead to the development of airway inflammation, bronchospasm, edema, and mucus plugging of the airways. Epidemiological data suggest a close correlation between the severity of air pollution and the development of COPD (Abbey et al., 1998). However, genetic factors play an important role in any given individual's susceptibility to the development of COPD. The most well-known and best documented of these predisposing genetic factors is that of α1-antitrypsin deficiency. Although this disorder occurs in only a very small percentage of cases of COPD (Stoller & Aboussouan, 2005), its effects can be devastating. In this relatively rare genetic disorder, there is a deficiency of a proteolytic enzyme inhibitor in the blood known as α1-antitrypsin. In the presence of normal levels of this inhibitor, the enzymes that are normally released from blood leukocytes, alveolar macrophages, and bacteria during inflammation are prevented from causing excessive lung damage. However, when the levels of this proteolytic inhibitor are deficient, there is more extensive breakdown of lung tissue, with subsequent loss of alveoli and decreased elasticity of the lung. Without adequate levels of this proteolytic enzyme inhibitor, inflammation goes on unchecked for prolonged periods, leading to progressive alveolar destruction and loss of elastic lung tissue.

Clinical Characteristics of Chronic Bronchitis and Emphysema

Although the clinical and pathophysiological features of chronic bronchitis and emphysema frequently overlap, some patients with COPD have characteristics that more clearly place them in one category or the other. The reason why some patients develop a predominantly chronic bronchitis pattern and others a predominantly emphysematous pattern is unclear, but it may have to do with genetic factors that influence the response of the lung to inflammation. For the sake of simplicity, patients are often labeled as having one form of COPD or the other. The patients who have predominantly chronic bronchitis are characterized by a more chronic cough and sputum production and are more likely to be hypoxic and hypercapnia. Low blood oxygen level will cause these patients to look cyanotic, that is, to have a blue discoloration of the skin particularly in the nail beds and the lips. They are also more likely to develop cor pulmonale (enlargement of the right ventricle of the heart) secondary to the development of pulmonary hypertension. Furthermore, mucus gland hyperplasia, smooth muscle hypertrophy, and increased mucus production are likely to be more extensive in chronic bronchitis compared with emphysema leading to more pronounced cough and sputum production typically seen in the chronic bronchitis.

Patients who more predominantly have the emphysematous form of COPD tend to have less cough and sputum production. They also tend to be less hypoxic and hypercapnia until the disease is very far advanced. In emphysema, the loss of alveoli is more pronounced than in chronic bronchitis. This results in a decrease in elastic recoil of the lung that in turn results in greater hyperinflation. As a consequence, patients with emphysematous lungs tend to have a more flattened diaphragm that can be apparent on physical examination and X-ray. Flattening of the diaphragm also tends to impair the normal respiratory mechanics of breathing because the flattened diaphragm functions at a mechanical disadvantage. As discussed earlier, loss of lung elastic recoil also results in restricted airflow because it facilitates compression of the airways during expiration. In severe cases, airflow may be limited even when the individual is breathing at rest, causing an individual to appear to be short of breath (dyspneic) even when not engaged in any physical activity. The loss of alveoli in emphysematous lungs is also associated with the loss of alveolar capillaries. Therefore, emphysematous lungs contain many areas with a higher than normal ratio of ventilation to blood perfusion. This results in an increase of the so-called physiological dead spaces, which are areas of the lung that are ventilated with air but not well perfused by the blood so that gas exchange with the atmosphere is impaired. When this happens, the minute ventilation (liters per minute of air moved in and out of the lung) required to produce adequate levels of alveolar ventilation (liters of air actually involved with gas exchange in functioning alveoli) increases, thereby increasing the total work of breathing. As the disease progresses, the patient is less able to compensate even with the increased work required to breathe. A more severe impairment of gas exchange may occur in areas of the lung where there is underventilation in relation to perfusion. This results in so-called physiological shunting where blood passing through the lungs is exposed to poorly ventilated alveoli causing inadequate amounts of oxygen absorption, leading to hypoxemia and the clinical manifestation of cyanosis. This is a major cause of hypoxemia seen in COPD. Patients with emphysema may also have areas of low ventilation to perfusion similar to those with chronic bronchitis because inflammatory changes in the airways of emphysema patients may also contribute to airflow obstruction, resulting in decreased ventilation to perfusion. This is usually more striking in patients who present with acute bronchitis superimposed on pre-existing emphysema. Interestingly, patients who predominantly have emphysema usually maintain an arterial oxygen level remarkably close to normal despite a marked degree of airflow limitation until their disease is very far advanced. Such preservation of arterial oxygen level is unusual in patients who predominantly have severe chronic bronchitis. For an equivalent degree of airflow limitation, the patient with predominantly emphysema is less likely to develop low blood oxygen and high carbon dioxide compared with the patient with predominantly chronic bronchitis. This clinical characteristic also reflects the relatively well-preserved ventilatory response to carbon dioxide noted in the emphysema patient. In other words, the emphysema patient tends to maintain a greater degree of sensitivity to rising carbon dioxide levels as a stimulus to respiration compared with the patient with chronic bronchitis (Lane & Howell, 1970). The reason for this preservation of carbon dioxide responsiveness as a stimulus to respiration in emphysema patients and the apparently impaired responsiveness to increasing carbon dioxide levels in chronic bronchitis patients is not well understood. Although patients with emphysema tend to have less severe hypoxemia and hypercapnia than patients with chronic bronchitis, as emphysema progresses, both hypoxemia and hypercapnia are likely to develop once again, blurring the clinical distinctions between chronic bronchitis and emphysema.

When emphysema exists in relatively pure form, there is dyspnea on exertion, but the patient is relatively free from the productive cough or bronchospasm associated with chronic bronchitis. Cyanosis and clubbing (bulbous enlargement of the fingertips and toes) are usually absent, but use of accessory muscles of respiration and pursed-lip breathing occur. In so-called pursed lip breathing, the patient tends to breathe out against partially closed lips, similar to whistling. This maneuver tends to maintain pressure within the smaller airways during expiration helping to prevent their premature closure that is characteristic of emphysema. In the classic chronic bronchitis patient, there is also dyspnea with minimal exertion, but the patient usually has a more productive cough frequently associated with bronchospasm. In such patients, cyanosis is also more common. Use of accessory muscles of respiration and pursed lip breathing may also occur, but this is usually less pronounced than in the more emphysematous type patient.

On physical examination, the emphysematous patient tends to be more barrel chested than the patient with predominantly chronic bronchitis because of the hyperinflation of the lung. Hyperinflation of the lung in emphysema also makes the lung of the emphysema patient more hyperresonant or drum-like when the chest wall is percussed or tapped during the physical examination. Diaphragmatic excursion in the emphysema patient is also diminished because the hyperinflation of the lung impairs movement of the diaphragm. On auscultation (listening to chest sounds with a stethoscope), wheezes and rhonchi are less pronounced in patients with emphysema because these abnormal breath sounds are due to the type of airflow turbulence more likely caused by the pathophysiological changes in the airways associated with chronic bronchitis.

Chest X-rays of a patient with emphysema usually demonstrate an increased front-to-back diameter of the chest, low lying or flat diaphragms, increased air space behind the sternum, prominent or enlarged pulmonary arteries, and an elongated mediastinum (central compartment of the chest in which the heart, blood vessels, and other structures lie). So-called bullae may also be noted, which are areas of the lung that have undergone degenerative change because of loss of alveoli resulting in thin-walled cystic areas filled with air. Computed tomography (CT) scanning gives an even more precise picture of the anatomical changes in the lung associated with both chronic bronchitis and emphysema. However, it must be remembered that the diagnostic evaluation of the patient with COPD, be it primarily emphysema or chronic bronchitis, relies on a combination of factors including patient history, physical examination, pulmonary function studies, and radiological findings.

Other Types of Chronic Obstructive Lung Disease

Asthma, CF, and bronchiectasis are examples of other lung diseases in which the major pathophysiological processes involve the airways. Asthma and CF will be discussed in more detail later in this chapter. Bronchiectasis is characterized pathologically by chronic, irreversible dilatation and distortion of the bronchi. These abnormalities often develop following some sort of inflammatory injury to the respiratory tract (e.g., tuberculosis, severe pneumonia, or other respiratory tract infection). Anatomical bronchial abnormalities that are congenital in nature may also lead to the development of bronchiectasis. The clinical manifestations of bronchiectasis depend on the severity of the pathology and the degree of vascularity associated with the anatomical distortion of the bronchi. Patients with bronchiectasis usually have a chronic cough that is productive of excessive amounts of mucus that is often infected, although some patients may have minimal cough and sputum production. Hemoptysis (expectoration of blood) that at times may be severe and life threatening can also occur. Chronic sinusitis and clubbing of the fingers are common clinical characteristics often associated with bronchiectasis.

Functional Disabilities

The earliest clinical manifestations of COPD may be relatively mild. However, as time goes on, dyspnea becomes a predominant limiting factor. Years may pass before the degree of dyspnea is severe enough to limit routine daily activities such as stair climbing or walking. Until the disease is very far advanced, relatively sedentary activities may be accomplished without too much difficulty. Driving may be possible, but walking even limited distances may not be possible if an incline or stairs are involved. Nonetheless, there are some patients with severe obstructive lung disease who maintain a good level of physical activity despite reduced oxygen saturation of the blood and elevated carbon dioxide levels. Such individuals may be able to remain at work if the work is sedentary in nature and transportation is not a problem. Therefore, assessment of a given patient's functional capability as it relates to occupational activities may be difficult to determine based on pulmonary function studies and blood gases alone. In addition, depression, fear, and anxiety are potent ancillary factors that may further exacerbate the patient's physical limitations from a psychological standpoint. Recurrent respiratory tract infections and continued smoking greatly enhance the progression of the underlying disease process. Once a diagnosis of obstructive lung disease is made, preparation for a more sedentary occupation would be wise even at the onset of relatively mild disease since the rate of progression can be variable.

Medical Evaluation and Disability Assessment

In general, patients with symptomatic respiratory disease should be examined and evaluated by a specialist in internal medicine or pulmonary disease. A complete medical history should be taken including information regarding symptom severity and duration. Factors that precipitate the onset of symptoms need to be identified as well as the occupational and environmental factors that might be involved in the pathogenesis of the patient's illness. A history of smoking should be noted as well as any family history of pulmonary disease, followed by a detailed physical examination. A chest X-ray should be obtained to rule out other associated medical problems such as cancer and infection. However, while a chest X-ray often shows changes characteristic of emphysema and chronic bronchitis, there is frequently a poor correlation between X-ray findings, a patient's functional capacity, and rehabilitation potential. Although dyspnea (a sensation of uncomfortable shortness of breath) is often the most prominent symptom in a patient with pulmonary disease, it is not useful in determining level of impairment. Dyspnea can be attributed to both pulmonary and nonpulmonary causes such as cardiac disease or anxiety. Additionally, there are limitations in both the specificity and sensitivity of scales used to rate levels of self-reported dyspnea (Balmes & Barnhart, 2005).

The impact of pulmonary impairment on functional abilities and the ability to perform activities of daily living or maintain employment determines the degree of disability. Activity limitation and participation restriction are not as easy to quantify as impairment since they are affected by factors unique to each individual. These factors include age, gender, body mass index, educational level, economic status, social environment, and the physical or energy requirements of one's occupation (American Thoracic Society [ATS], 1986). The determination of activity limitation and participation restriction requires consideration of medical and nonmedical variables; therefore, individuals with similar levels of impairment may experience different levels of disability (ATS, 1993). Other tests such as blood studies and electrocardiogram may help identify nonpulmonary disorders that may be contributory to the patient's pulmonary symptoms.

Pulmonary function tests (PFTs) are particularly important in evaluating a patient's functional capacity. Two important parameters that are followed in patients with obstructive lung disease are the forced vital capacity (FVC) and the forced expiratory volume in 1 second (FEV_1). The FVC is the maximum amount of air that can be exhaled after a full inspiration. The FEV_1 is the volume of air expired during the first second of the forced expiratory maneuver after a full inhalation. Table 22.1, taken from the Global Initiative for Chronic Obstructive Lung Disease (GOLD Report, 2008), lists commonly used criteria for determining level of severity of COPD based on the FVC and FEV_1.

Global Initiative for Chronic Obstructive Lung Disease (GOLD)

Classification of COPD Severity

The volume exhaled with a forced expiratory maneuver during the second (FEV_2) and third (FEV_3) seconds are also often measured during simple spirometry testing. The FVC, FEV_1, FEV_2, FEV_3 are all reduced in obstructive lung diseases, but restrictive lung diseases (see "Interstitial Lung Diseases") can also reduce these parameters. However, in obstructive lung disease, the ratios of FEV_1, FEV_2, and FEV_3 to FVC are reduced, whereas in restrictive lung diseases, these ratios tend to be normal or at times above normal. Each agency that provides disability compensation will utilize its own specific rating scales for determining disability. Other scales that are often utilized include: the American Medical Association (AMA) *Guides to the Evaluation of Permanent Impairment*; Social Security (Disability Programs, Medical/Professional Relations, Disability Evaluation under Social Security, U.S. Department of Health and Human Resources); Workers Compensation Insurance; and the Department of Veterans Affairs (Balmes & Barnhart, 2005).

It should be noted that PFTs are useful in evaluating a patient's performance only when patient cooperation is complete and a competent technician is performing the study. Arterial blood gas determinations, lung volume measurements using various

TABLE 22.1 *Global Initiative for Chronic Obstructive Lung Disease (GOLD) Classification of COPD Severity*

| Stage | Lung Function[a] | | Symptoms |
	FEV_1 (%)	FEV_1/FVC	
I (Mild)	>80	<0.7	With or without cough, sputum
II (Moderate)	50–80	<0.7	With or without cough, sputum, dyspnea
III (Severe)	30–50	<0.7	With or without cough, sputum, dyspnea
IV (Very severe)	<30[b]	<0.7	Respiratory or right heart failure

[a]Based on postbronchodilator function.
[b]A postbronchodilator FEV_1 < 30% predicted or FEV_1 < 50% with respiratory failure.
Source: From GOLD Report, Global Initiative for Chronic Obstructive Lung Disease. Global strategy for the diagnosis, management, and prevention of chronic obstructive pulmonary disease (update 2008). GOLD website: www.goldcopd.org.

methodologies, and determination of airflow resistance are other types of PFTs that can be helpful in evaluating a patient's pulmonary limitations.

Cardiopulmonary stress testing is a further extension of pulmonary function testing during which the patient is actively exercised while ventilatory and cardiac monitoring is done to see if certain levels of exercise uncover pulmonary and/or cardiac limitations. Although exercise testing is not always necessary in the investigation of pulmonary impairment, it may be useful when the cause of shortness of breath cannot be determined by conventional PFTs done at rest or when the patient's complaints are out of proportion to lung function abnormalities found on conventional PFTs (AMA, 2008). Exercise testing provides more information about an individual's physiological responses to exercise and the maximal oxygen consumption (VO_2 max) attained during performance of a graded exercised protocol. Determining a person's VO_2 max can be helpful in estimating both exercise intensity and the general level of physical activity that can be safely performed. Such testing also provides a clearer picture of the patient's physical work capabilities.

Although PFTs and cardiopulmonary stress testing are helpful in assessing physical capabilities, it should be remembered that highly motivated, well-trained, and well-conditioned patients are likely to be more capable of performing physical activity compared with poorly motivated and deconditioned patients even though their pulmonary function studies may be comparable. After reviewing the medical history, physical examination, laboratory studies, radiological findings, PFTs, and, as needed, cardiopulmonary exercise testing, the physician is better able to categorize level of impairment regarding an individual's pulmonary disorder.

Treatment

Many patients with chronic pulmonary disease have potential for some reversibility or improvement that can be achieved with proper medical management. Periodical exacerbations caused by a variety of factors including infection may also occur. Such exacerbations may cause an acute deterioration in function that will improve as the acute process is treated. A wide variety of antibiotics are available to treat respiratory infections. There are also a number of medications that can help alleviate the bronchospasm found in many patients with COPD. Theophylline type drugs were commonly used in the past to alleviate bronchospasm, but they have been largely replaced by other more effective medications including inhaled β-adrenergic type drugs such as albuterol, salbutamol, and femoterol. Ipatropium bromide and titotropium bromide are atropine type derivatives that are also used as inhaled medications to alleviate bronchospasm. Oral, intravenous, and intramuscular corticosteroid drugs have marked antiinflammatory properties that can be extremely helpful in managing acute, severe bronchospasm. However, use of these drugs on a long-term basis can be associated with severe side effects such as osteoporosis, weight gain, muscle weakness, elevated blood sugar, cataract formation, and peptic ulcer disease. Inhaled corticosteroids type drugs such as beclomethasone, budesonide, fluticasone, mometasone, ciclesonide, and others may be particularly helpful for long-term management of steroid responsive bronchospasm because of their minimal systemic side effects. However, inhaled steroids are usually not very useful for acute, severe bronchospasm. Antileukotriene type drugs, which were primarily developed to reduce airway inflammation in asthma patients, may also be useful in reducing the inflammatory response in patients who have COPD with a bronchospastic component (Riccioni, DiIlio, Theoharides, & D'Orazio, 2004). Preventing dehydration in patients with COPD is also an important factor in treatment since it tends to thicken respiratory tract secretions, making it much more difficult for patients to clear their airways.

Chest physical therapy and pulmonary rehabilitation (PR) programs can be very useful to patients with chronic pulmonary disease. Postural drainage (use of gravity assisted positioning) and percussion techniques (manual tapping on the thorax over different lung segments) can assist the patient with clearance of respiratory tract secretions. Breathing exercises, relaxation techniques, and occupational therapy may help the patient more efficiently perform activities of daily living. Exercise reconditioning programs can be very useful in increasing a patient's physical endurance and work capacity. The benefits of exercise reconditioning include increased muscle strength and exercise tolerance, as well as decreased exertional dyspnea and fatigue (Nici et al., 2006; Troosters, Gosselink, Burtin, & DeCramer, 2008). In graded exercise programs, patients should be monitored closely for cardiac arrhythmias, myocardial ischemia, and oxygen desaturation that may occur during exercise. Supplemental oxygen may be useful and necessary during such programs. Monitoring nocturnal blood oxygen saturation is also helpful in patients who have underlying chronic pulmonary disease because they are at risk for developing hypoxemia as they sleep, which predisposes to other complications including pulmonary hypertension and cardiac arrhythmias. Improvement in oxygen saturation may have beneficial effects on a patient's pulmonary circulation, cardiac function, and sense of general well-being. Continuous oxygen therapy may be needed in patients who are chronically hypoxic. The careful use of oxygen therapy may be very useful in helping the patient with chronic pulmonary disease and hypoxemia maintain a more active lifestyle. However, oxygen supplementation requires careful monitoring and supervision. Transcutaneous oxygen saturation should be monitored periodically to ensure that the desired level of oxygen saturation is being achieved. Also, arterial blood gas determinations may periodically be needed to make sure that the patient's carbon dioxide level is not too high and that the acid–base balance in the blood remains satisfactory.

Vocational Implications

Although COPD is often considered a disease of the elderly, it also affects the working-age population (Sin, Stafinsk, Ng, Bell, & Jacobs, 2002). In a 2002 epidemiological survey, Eisner, Yelin, Trupin, and Blanc (2002) found that individuals with COPD were both more likely to report a perceived inability to work and less likely to be currently employed compared with individuals with nonrespiratory chronic health conditions. Most studies indicate that individuals with COPD who stop working have greater airflow limitation, as demonstrated by a lower FEV1, than those who continue to work (Kremer, Pal, & van Keimpema, 2006; Sin et al., 2002). Sin and colleagues, in 2002, found that COPD was associated with decreased participation in the work force: 3.4% for those with mild COPD, 3.9% for those with moderate COPD, and 14.4% for those with severe COPD. One study found that airflow limitation of equal severity was present in working and nonworking individuals with COPD; however, quality of life was reported to be less satisfactory in those unable to work (Orbon et al., 2005).

To increase the likelihood of remaining in the work force, it is imperative that individuals with COPD stop smoking and obtain optimal medical treatment for their lung disease including appropriate medications, exercise reconditioning, and secretion clearance techniques when needed. Once lung function is optimized, it is important to consider the energy requirements of different types of work. Individuals with COPD must be able to meet the energy demands of a job and work in an environment free of substances that pose a further risk of respiratory injury (ATS, 1986).

To estimate whether the energy demands of a particular job can be met, it is helpful to know the worker's VO$_2$ max. Oxygen consumption in the resting state is 3.5 ml/kg/minute (McArdle, Katch, & Katch, 1994). *To sustain activity at increasing levels of intensity, more oxygen would be required.* Generally, an individual can sustain a work level that is equal to 40% of his or her VO$_2$ max for an 8-hour time period (ATS, 1986; Gallagher, 1994), and for shorter periods of time, an individual can sustain a work level that is equal to 50% of his or her maximal oxygen consumption (ATS, 1986). Table 22.2 includes estimates of the energy requirements needed for the performance of different intensities of work (ATS, 1986).

TABLE 22.2   *Estimates of Energy Requirements for Work*

Type of Work	Required Oxygen Consumption
Office work	5–7 ml/kg/min
Moderate labor	15 ml/kg/min
Strenuous heavy labor	20–30 ml/kg/min

Source: American Thoracic Society (1986). Evaluation of impairment/disability secondary to respiratory disorders. *American Review of Respiratory Disease, 133,* 1205–1209.

Estimates of Energy Requirements for Work

If energy requirements of a particular job are unable to be met, individuals with COPD may need workplace accommodations, a change in employment setting, or possibly retirement. Workplace accommodations may be as simple as having access to supplemental oxygen to allow chronically hypoxic individuals or those who desaturate with exertion to remain employed in a sedentary occupation.

Other features of COPD may preclude working in certain occupations. If frequent coughing and expectoration are present, an individual may be unable to work in occupations that involve close personal interaction. If a protective mask is required in certain work environments, an individual with chronic bronchitis may be unable to wear it continuously because of the need to expectorate (Balmes & Barnhart, 2005). Finally, for individuals with COPD, the mode of travel to and from work must be considered, as this may pose a level of exertion that is beyond the individual's capacity. It is also extremely important that patients and their families develop a good understanding of the illness so that they can deal with it effectively. Frequently, proper use of medications results in significant symptom relief permitting resumption of some, if not all, routine activities. Smoking cessation is crucial in helping to delay disease progression. Proper nutrition, exercise reconditioning as part of a PR program, and chest physical therapy can sometimes provide great help to the patient trying to resume a more normal, active life. Psychological counseling can also help the patient deal with the anxiety and stress associated with chronic pulmonary disease. Anxiety and stress can symptomatically worsen the sense of shortness of breath associated with chronic pulmonary disease, thereby further compromising the patient's level of activity. However, learning to deal effectively with these symptoms and make satisfactory adaptations in lifestyle may make the difference between a productive life and a desperate one. In some cases, patients may have to change their employment goals. For patients who are severely compromised (e.g., FEV_1 of 1 or less), slow walking on a level surface may be possible, but stair climbing is likely to be very difficult. Likewise, resting hypoxemia (arterial oxygen level of 60 mmHg or lower) may be adequate for sedentary jobs, but even minimally strenuous activity may cause a significant drop in the oxygen level, which might preclude continued employment. Access to supplemental oxygen can often allow the chronically hypoxemia patient, or the patient who becomes hypoxemic with minimal exertion, to remain employed at a sedentary occupation. However, even sedentary activities may periodically require greater levels of activity that are not feasible. For example, traveling to and from work sometimes poses a level of exertion beyond the patient's capability.

PFTs are particularly important in evaluating pulmonary impairment, and criteria for impairment based on PFTs have been established by the Social Security Administration, other government agencies, and medical societies. Usually the degree of impairment based on PFTs is divided into mild, moderate, and severe, although the criteria for establishing these categories vary somewhat depending on which guidelines are selected. Mild impairment is usually not correlated with diminished ability to perform most jobs. Moderate impairment is correlated with a decreased ability to meet the demand of many jobs, particularly those that involve strenuous activity. Severe impairment prevents the patient from fulfilling the demands of most jobs. Formal exercise testing may be very helpful in more accurately estimating a patient's physical capacity to do work and as such may be very important in the evaluation of the patient's degree of disability.

ASTHMA

Etiology, Pathogenesis, and Clinical Characteristics

Asthma is an inflammatory airway disease that is characterized by a marked reversibility of airflow obstruction and bronchial hyperreactivity. It is often divided into allergic (extrinsic asthma) and nonallergic (intrinsic) asthma. The allergic or "extrinsic" type of asthma commonly has its onset in childhood, whereas intrinsic or nonallergic asthma usually has its onset in adulthood. In extrinsic asthma, exposure to an allergen such as pollen, dust, animal dander, mold, and certain foods may precipitate an attack. On the other hand, intrinsic asthma is more often precipitated by respiratory tract infection or by nonspecific airway irritation such as exposure to cold air. However, there is considerable overlap between the two groups, with many patients demonstrating clinical features of both. Because bronchial hyperreactivity or hyperresponsiveness is present in all asthmatics, attacks may be precipitated by many types of stimuli including extremes of temperature and humidity, inhaled chemicals, airborne particulate material, cigarette smoke, ozone, certain odors, aspirin, certain food additives (e.g., sulfites), and even exercise in many susceptible patients. When an asthma attack occurs, there is constriction of the bronchial smooth muscle lining the respiratory tract, which in conjunction with excessive mucus production leads to plugging of small airways. The end result of these processes is obstruction to airflow. The frequency, duration, and severity of asthmatic attacks vary markedly from patient to patient. An attack is typically characterized by shortness of breath and wheezing, which is often accompanied by cough and mucus production. In some individuals, cough may be the only symptom of asthma. During an acute attack, the patient breathes abnormally fast, often using accessory muscles of respiration in the neck and chest areas. Severe attacks may lead to exhaustion, with slowing of the respiratory rate causing hypoxemia, hypercapnia, and respiratory acidosis leading to respiratory arrest.

Reactive airways dysfunction syndrome (RADS) (Brooks, Weiss, & Bernstein, 1985) and irritant-induced asthma (IIA) (Brooks, Hammad, Richards, Giovinco-Barbas, & Jenkins, 1998) are similar clinical entities caused by exposure to toxic irritants and characterized by the absence of asthma symptoms for at least 2 years prior to exposure, persistence of asthma symptoms for at least 3 months after exposure, and objective evidence of nonspecific bronchial hyper-responsiveness on PFTs. Perhaps the most noteworthy outbreak of RADS/IIA yet described is that reported in individuals exposed to the irritants associated with the World Trade Center disaster of 9/11. Although these disorders are in many ways similar to asthma, current scientific evidence appears to support the conclusion that RADS and IIA are distinct clinical entities whose pathogenesis is different than that of asthma.

Functional Disability

During a severe asthmatic attack, the patient may be totally disabled. Even talking may be compromised because of severe breathlessness. The patient may be very restless and unable to lie flat. Eating and drinking may be difficult. Severe cough may ensue resulting in musculoskeletal pain of the chest wall. Depending on the severity of the patient's underlying asthma, the attack may be totally or partially reversible. Between acute attacks, the patient is typically able to resume normal activity. However, patients with severe, unremitting asthma may remain chronically symptomatic, resembling people with chronic bronchitis and emphysema in terms of disability.

Medical Evaluation

The standard evaluation of the asthmatic patient is similar to that of those with COPD. Essential components to the evaluation include obtaining a history of occupational and environmental exposure to irritants and toxins, in addition to a thorough allergy assessment. Laboratory evaluation should assess for the presence of CF especially in children and young adults since the diagnosis of CF is associated with prognostic and management issues that are different from those of COPD and asthma. Psychological evaluation may be very important because emotional factors can precipitate asthmatic attacks. In children and young adults, a social service evaluation may be helpful in identifying developmental and environmental factors that contribute to asthma, such as the presence of dust mites, cats, dogs, or mold in the home.

As with COPD, PFTs are used in the diagnosis and management of asthma patients. An improvement of greater than 12% or 200 ml in FEV_1 and FVC following inhalation of a bronchodilator medication is indicative of reversible or partially reversible airflow obstruction (AMA, 2008). When reversibility of airway obstruction is present, asthma or an asthmatic component exists in the pulmonary impairment (ATS, 2000–1999 official statement). In some cases, when an asthmatic component is suspected but reversible airflow limitation has not been demonstrated, a methacholine or histamine challenge may be administered to document airway hyperresponsiveness. Cardiopulmonary stress tests are not routinely performed in the investigation of asthma (ATS, 1993) but may be useful in investigating complaints of dyspnea by comparing spirometry measures before and after exercise (ATS, 1993). In most individuals, exercise-induced bronchospasm can be controlled with appropriate medications (ATS, 1986).

Impairment or disability related to asthma may be temporary or permanent (ATS, 1993). Temporary impairment is used to describe an individual's status when improvement is expected in the future through avoidance of trigger factors, use of optimal therapy, or both. Permanent impairment describes an individual's status when optimal medical management has maximized improvement, but airflow limitations persist (Balmes & Barnhart, 2005). Therefore, an individual with asthma must be clinically stable with maximal and optimal medical therapy in place prior to performing spirometry testing for the purpose of impairment evaluation.

The AMA *Guides to the Evaluation of Permanent Impairment* 2008 uses three separate criteria reflecting airway function to determine impairment classification in asthma. The criteria for impairment take into consideration the type and amount of medication required to control asthmatic symptoms; spirometric evidence of airway obstruction following administration of bronchodilator; and the degree of airway hyper-responsiveness present. Each of the three criteria is divided into five classes, with class 0 representing no disease and class 4 representing severe disease.

For disability compensation related to asthma, many agencies have established their own criteria for determining the presence of disability in asthmatic individuals. They include the following: Social Security (Disability Programs, Medical/Professional Relations, Disability Evaluation Under Social Security, U.S. Department of Health and Human Resources); Workers Compensation Insurance; and the Department of Veterans Affairs (for military personnel with illnesses attributed to military service) (Balmes & Bernhardt, 2005). Further information regarding the disability criteria of specific agencies can be obtained from their Web sites.

Treatment

Therapy is focused on the treatment and prevention of an asthmatic attack. The emphasis on prevention stems from the view that asthma is an inflammatory disease and that by controlling inflammation in the lung asthma can be controlled. Medical management of asthma has been greatly aided by the development of antiinflammatory agents. Asthma medications are typically divided into "controller medications" and "reliever medications." The controller medications are primarily antiinflammatory agents or long-acting bronchodilators that are taken on a regular basis. The reliever medications are used as needed to alleviate acute bronchospasm. Patients with very mild, intermittent asthma may be treated with rapid acting bronchodilators taken infrequently. However, patients with more frequent or chronic symptoms are usually treated with antiinflammatory agents such as inhaled corticosteroids sprays, antileukotriene drugs, and long-acting β-agonist type drug (so-called LABA drugs). Patients with severe asthma may require oral or parenteral corticosteroid type drugs given either intermittently or in the most severe cases on a more chronic basis. Self-monitoring with a home peak flow meter (a device that can measure airflow rates) can be helpful in determining the degree of airflow obstruction. Doing so can be useful to the patient and physician in recognizing the severity of an attack, adjusting treatment plans, and determining permitted levels of activity.

Careful monitoring of the asthmatic patient's status and making appropriate adjustments in outpatient management may oftentimes avoid emergency-room treatment and/or hospitalization. However, severe asthmatic attacks often require hospitalization despite appropriate outpatient treatment. Some patients with allergic (extrinsic) asthma may be helped by desensitization treatments in which the patient is exposed to very small amounts of the specific allergens to which he or she is sensitive, usually accomplished by subcutaneous injection. This treatment is designed to build up so-called blocking antibodies in the patient's body that attach themselves to the specific inhaled allergens to which the patient is sensitive. This inactivates the allergens before they can attach themselves to the antibodies that would otherwise trigger an allergic response. Careful avoidance of environmental allergens to which a patient is sensitive should be practiced at home and at work, thereby limiting the occurrences of asthmatic attacks. More recently, treatment for allergic asthma has centered on the use of omalizumab, a synthesized monoclonal antibody (IgG) that selectively binds to human immunoglobulin E antibody (IgE), thereby inactivating it and preventing it from attaching to an allergen that would trigger an allergic response.

Vocational Implications

The degree of disability in individuals with asthma can vary depending on the severity of the disease and on the effectiveness of prescribed treatment regimens in controlling attacks. Since asthma is characterized by variable airflow obstruction, a given individual's clinical status may change over time (Balmes & Barnhart, 2005). Individuals with asthma should avoid work situations where potential environmental irritants exist, including outdoor work and exposure to extremes of temperature, humidity, fumes, or cigarette smoke. Clinicians need to counsel individuals with asthma regarding the selection of appropriate work settings, which should include discussions pertaining to preventive, environmental, and behavioral factors that minimize risk and maximize function (ATS, 2004). In some instances, a worker with asthma may be able to continue employment with accommodations such as modification of the work required or changes in the worksite (ATS, 2004).

Occupational asthma results from sensitization to agents found only in the workplace. Once diagnosed, occupational asthma is managed by removing the worker from further exposure and considering him or her unable to return to that job or any other job where exposure to the same causative agent could occur (ATS, 1993). Early diagnosis and immediate removal from exposure are the most important factors in improving long-term outcomes in individuals with occupational asthma (Venables & Chan-Yeung, 1997).

In general, the asthmatic patient is younger than the patient with COPD and therefore has more potential for pursuing career changes through job retraining or additional education. Vocational rehabilitation interventions that train workers with chronic diseases, including

COPD and asthma, help develop feelings of self-confidence in dealing with work-related problems and are effective in maintaining employment (Varekamp, Verbeek, & Dijk, 2006).

CYSTIC FIBROSIS

Etiology, Pathogenesis, and Clinical Characteristics

Cystic Fibrosis (CF) is a genetic deficiency disease characterized by recurrent respiratory tract infections and progressive respiratory insufficiency. A specific gene responsible for CF was first discovered in 1989, although scientists have recently discovered that there are numerous gene mutations associated with CF (O'Sullivan & Freedman, 2009). Because of these varied gene mutations, the severity of CF may vary from person-to-person. It has been estimated that 1 out of every 20 people is a carrier of a defective gene associated with CF. It occurs more often in Caucasians (1 in 2,500 births) than in other racial groups (Tsui & Buchwald, 1991). Because of advances in treatment, median survival now exceeds 37.4 years (Cystic Fibrosis Foundation, 2007). However, even more prolonged survival is increasingly common with better medical management and lung transplantation. Increased survival has created a need for increased social and psychological support for these patients.

The primary genetic defect in CF affects the mechanism by which sodium and chloride pass out of cells. In CF, the epithelial cells that line the surface passageways of many organs such as the lung and pancreas retain increased amounts of sodium and chloride. The high concentration of these electrolytes draws water from the airways of the lung, pancreatic ducts, and the secretory ducts of other organs producing thicker, dehydrated mucus secretions. This highly viscous mucus obstructs and plugs the passageways leading to infection and destruction of tissue. Although pulmonary involvement is the most striking manifestation of CF, multiple organs may be affected including the pancreas, liver, intestines, and reproductive organs.

Functional Disability

Recurrent respiratory tract infection is characteristic of CF. The patient has a chronic cough with wheezing, dyspnea, recurrent bronchitis, pneumonia, and sinusitis. Hemoptysis (coughing up blood or bloody sputum) and bronchiectasis also occur. Pancreatic and intestinal involvement leads to nutrition malabsorption, poor growth, and abdominal discomfort. Liver involvement can lead to jaundice and cirrhosis while sodium loss in sweat may lead to circulatory compromise. Genitourinary tract abnormalities often cause reproductive failure and renal difficulties. There is considerable variation in the time of presentation of these symptoms. Although approximately 75% of patients with CF are diagnosed before age 6, some individuals may not exhibit serious symptoms until adolescence or later in life (Fitzsimmons, 1998).

Medical Evaluation

The diagnosis of CF is usually made clinically by the presence of pancreatic insufficiency and recurrent respiratory tract infections. The sweat test, demonstrating an elevated sodium concentration in sweat, continues to be the most readily available and clinically useful way of making the diagnosis for CF. In general, a diagnosis of CF can be made in an individual with clinical features of the disease if the concentration of chloride in sweat is greater than 60 mmol/L and two disease-causing CF transmembrane conductance regulator mutations are identified (O'Sullivan & Freedman, 2009). Chest X-ray findings depend on the stage of CF and show varying degrees of bronchiectasis, fibrosis, mucus plugging, and hyperinflation. PFTs are useful in documenting the progress and severity of the disease. As in patients with COPD and asthma, there is evidence of airway obstruction and ultimately "air trapping," which results in hyperinflation. Blood gases often reveal a decrease in oxygen levels early in the disease with elevation of carbon dioxide being noted later on. Progressive pulmonary disease may ultimately lead to cardiac failure as well.

Treatment

Advances in antibiotic therapy, nutritional support, airway clearance techniques, and having treatments coordinated at centers specializing in the care of individuals with CF have markedly increased survival into adulthood (O'Sullivan & Freedman, 2009). Heart–lung transplants are also being more commonly used with increasing success (Yankasas & Mallory, 1998). Genetic engineering may provide another approach that will ultimately increase survival, but this has been difficult to accomplish because of the large number of different genetic mutations that have been identified in individuals with CF. Patients with CF usually require daily chest physiotherapy to loosen secretions and prevent stagnation of mucus and subsequent infection. Antibiotics are essential in treating infections and usually must be given intravenously for prolonged periods. Inhalational antibiotic therapy has also been successfully used. Often intravenous and inhalational antibiotic therapy can be used at home, thereby decreasing hospitalization time. Because of the malabsorption problems inherent in this illness, nutritional support is critical in managing these patients.

Regular aerobic exercise has been shown to attenuate the decline in pulmonary function over a 3-year period in a randomized clinical trial (Schneiderman-Walker et al., 2000). In addition, appropriate vigorous physical activity enhances cardiovascular fitness, increases functional capacity, and improves quality of life. For these reasons, all adults with CF should be encouraged to exercise, unless their clinical condition prevents it (Yankaskas, Marshall, Sufian, Simon, & Rodman, 2004).

Vocational Implications

Patients with CF often have excellent educational abilities and can be very productive individuals. The patient's vocational counselor has to work with employers to provide needed support mechanisms that will allow the patient to remain in his or her workplace for as long as possible. This might include time for airway clearance techniques or antibiotic therapy during the workday. Also, the work environment must be reviewed to ensure the absence of inhaled irritants that might exacerbate the pulmonary aspect of this disease. Supplemental oxygen may sometimes be necessary to allow the patient to remain productive and ambulatory. Psychological problems often revolve around factors involving the patient's altered physical appearance, chronic cough, chronic dyspnea, loneliness, and family issues that normally arise in the course of any chronic illness. Faced with these numerous problems and additional concerns over sexual function, individuals with CF may develop anxiety and/or depression. Therefore, psychological evaluation and treatment will often be necessary. The counselor may also have to work with the patient's family to improve support at home that will allow the patient to increase his or her social and vocational activities.

INTERSTITIAL LUNG DISEASES

Etiology, Pathophysiology, and Clinical Features

ILDs are a group of pulmonary disorders that involve inflammation, scarring, and fibrosis of the alveoli, the gas exchanging units of the lung, and the supporting structure or interstitium of the lung in which the alveoli are located. Although ILD represents a heterogeneous group of diseases in which there is inflammation, fibrosis, and scarring of the alveolar walls (alveolitis), blood vessels, and small airways, there are many features common to this group of disorders. One major characteristic of ILD in general is the loss of lung volume, which causes what is described as a restrictive pattern on pulmonary function testing. In other words, the lungs are restricted in terms of their ability to expand on inhalation. This is in contrast to the obstructive pattern of COPD, asthma, and other similar diseases that are primarily airway diseases that result in obstruction to airflow.

The etiologies of the ILD and ensuing pulmonary fibrosis are often unknown. Inhalation of certain organic or inorganic dusts and chemicals may result in a hypersensitivity pneumonitis. This is an inflammatory disease of the lung in which inflammatory cells infiltrate into the lung tissue as a response to this exposure, causing the lung tissue to become thickened and fibrotic. These inhaled organic and inorganic particles, dusts, and chemicals may originate from a variety of sources including animal proteins, agricultural byproducts, and industrial byproducts. These illnesses are often named after the occupation with which they are associated. For example, *farmer's lung*, results from exposure to fungal particles found in moldy hay. *Bird breeder's lung* results from the inhalation of avian proteins such as those found in pigeon coops and birdcages. Sometimes the ILD caused by the inhalation of inorganic dusts and chemicals is termed "pneumoconiosis." Silica and asbestos are examples of inorganic dusts that may produce ILD and pulmonary fibrosis. Other potential causes of industrial dust pneumoconiosis are aluminum, beryllium, and cobalt. In pneumoconiosis, the duration and intensity of exposure to the offending material as well as the smoking history are important factors in determining etiology and severity. It should also be noted that the development of pulmonary fibrosis in pneumoconiosis can often occur years after the initial exposure and that symptoms frequently occur after the patient has left the occupation in which he or she was initially exposed (Muir et al., 1989).

Idiopathic pulmonary fibrosis (IPF) is a type of ILD in which the cause of the fibrosis is unknown. At times, pulmonary fibrosis will exist in conjunction with systemic diseases such as rheumatoid arthritis (rheumatoid lung). Sarcoidosis is another illness of unknown etiology, which can result in ILD and ultimately pulmonary fibrosis. Although sarcoidosis is often a benign disease of young adults that may present with eye or skin lesions, pulmonary involvement may result in severe fibrosis and disability.

A common clinical feature of patients with ILD is dyspnea or shortness of breath, particularly on exertion. With mild disease, the patient may be relatively asymptomatic. Difficulty in stair climbing may be noted first, but as the disease progresses, the patient may become quite symptomatic with marked shortness of breath and cough on minimal activity. Simple daily activities such as eating, dressing, and bathing may become progressively more difficult. Patients with severe disease demonstrate striking air hunger with rapid respiratory rates and obvious respiratory distress. Cough can also be a predominant feature. Patients with ILD, particularly those caused by hypersensitivity pneumonitis, may present with other constitutional symptoms such as fever. Patients with rheumatoid arthritis and pulmonary fibrosis will typically have severe joint disease, and patients with other connective tissue diseases such as systemic lupus erythematosus may have ILD associated with the typical symptoms of systemic lupus. Likewise, patients with pulmonary sarcoidosis may have extrapulmonary manifestations of their disease with involvement of skin, eyes, bones, and internal organs. The pulmonary fibrosis associated with progressive ILD can lead not only to the destruction of alveoli but also to the obliteration of the pulmonary capillary bed, resulting in pulmonary hypertension, right ventricular enlargement, and ultimately right ventricular failure.

Medical Evaluation

The medical evaluation of the patient with ILD will resemble that of the COPD and asthma patient as detailed earlier. A thorough and detailed occupational history will be necessary and is essential to the diagnosis of hypersensitivity pneumonitis and pneumoconiosis. Diagnosis will also depend on chest X-ray findings in many of these disease entities. In pneumoconiosis, the chest X-ray is often used as a means to grade severity and intensity of exposure. X-ray findings are particularly useful in establishing the diagnosis and severity of disease in silicosis and asbestosis. Oftentimes, the X-ray findings of pulmonary fibrosis may be nonspecific in terms of etiology, but they may be useful in helping to evaluate the severity of disease. High-resolution CT scanning may be helpful in providing a clearer picture of the anatomical abnormalities of ILD (AMA, 2008). In view of the large number of disease entities that comprise the category of ILD, a lung biopsy is often necessary to establish a more definitive diagnosis.

As with COPD and asthma patients, pulmonary function testing is essential in determining disability in patients with pulmonary fibrosis or ILD. The characteristic pulmonary function pattern in patients with ILD is restrictive, with loss of vital capacity (which is the maximum amount of air that can be expelled from the lungs by a forceful effort following a maximal inspiration), functional residual capacity (which is the additional amount of air that can be expelled forcefully following a normal exhalation), residual volume (which is the amount of air remaining in the lung following a maximal exhalation), and total lung capacity (which is the total amount of air in the lungs at maximal inspiration; see Figure 22.1)

In the early stages of inflammation and fibrosis, and occasionally in patients with more advanced disease, little change in lung volume may be noted, but more significant reduction will be seen in diffusion capacity and blood gases. Measurement of diffusion capacity for carbon monoxide may also be useful in detecting significant abnormalities in oxygen absorption across the alveolar-capillary membrane of the lung due to ILD. However, abnormalities in oxygenation and gas exchange at rest may not accurately predict the magnitude of the abnormality that may be seen during exercise (ATS, 2000). Therefore, exercise studies may be very useful in demonstrating deterioration in gas exchange during physical activity (Epler, Saber, & Gaensler, 1980), playing a greater role in the evaluation of impairment in ILD than in COPD or asthma (Balmes & Barnhart, 2005). Individuals with IPF demonstrate a marked decline in arterial oxygen saturation during mild to moderate exercise (Hsai, 1999). To increase their minute ventilation (volume of air breathed in and out in 1 minute) during exercise, individuals with IPF, unlike normal individuals, must increase their respiratory rate rather than tidal volume breath because of the restricted expansion capability of the lung (ATS, 2000). Therefore, individuals with restrictive lung disease develop a higher

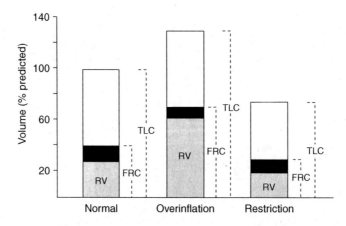

FIGURE 22.1 Lung volumes and capacities.

Source: From *Textbook of Pulmonary Diseases*, by E. L. Baum (Ed.), 1983, Boston: Little Brown. Copyright 1983 by Little Brown. Reprinted with permission from Lippincott Williams & Wilkins.

ventilatory requirement, a greater work of breathing, and a greater respiratory muscle oxygen requirement compared with normal individuals because of decreased lung compliance (Hsai, 1999).

Pulmonary impairment due to ILD is currently based on the same criteria as that used to evaluate impairment in COPD (AMA, *Guides to the Evaluation of Permanent Impairment*, 6th edition, 2008). For disability compensation related to ILD, specific agencies have rating scales for the determination of disability in ILD. These include: Social Security; Workers Compensation Insurance; Department of Veterans Affairs; U.S. Department of Labor and the Department of Energy.

Treatment

Knowledge of the natural history of each type of ILD is essential in regard to management. In this heterogeneous group of diseases, the ability to reverse the disease process will vary considerably according to the nature of the illness and the stage at which the diseases is first detected. In hypersensitivity pneumonitis, for example, withdrawal of the offending material from the patient's environment is necessary and may have dramatic results in terms of improvement. In pneumoconiosis, reduction of intensity and duration of exposure will help to reduce the severity of the disease. For a disease that may be reversible, introduction of drug therapy during the earliest stages of disease is essential. Because immunologically mediated inflammation is characteristic of many of these ILDs, corticosteroids are often the first drug of choice. Other immunosuppressive agents are also used in combination with corticosteroids or alone. In general, the decision to treat is often based on the severity of the symptoms, for example, cough and dyspnea.

Vocational Implications

In regard to occupational lung diseases, the counselor should work with the physician and employer in determining the offending substances that must be avoided. Retraining, relocation, and extension of education may be necessary for those with occupationally induced diseases. A counselor may have to work with employers to make adjustments in the workplace to achieve an environment that will allow the patient continued employment. Supplemental oxygen and rehabilitation programs may increase a patient's functional abilities. As in COPD, significant psychosocial disabilities may result from severe breathlessness in patients with ILDs. Anxiety and depression are very common not only as a result of the air hunger but also from a drastic change in lifestyle activities associated with respiratory compromise. Family members are also often affected by the patient's deteriorating health and concerns regarding the social and financial issues relating to the patient's inability to function normally. Social service evaluation in connection with the patient's family status may be helpful in determining the extent of the patient's support mechanisms at home.

ROLE OF PR IN CHRONIC LUNG DISEASE

Definition

Pulmonary rehabilitation is an evidence-based, multidisciplinary, and comprehensive intervention for patients with chronic respiratory diseases who are symptomatic and often have decreased daily life activities. Integrated into the individualized treatment of the patient, pulmonary rehabilitation is designed to reduce symptoms, optimize functional status, increase participation, and reduce health care costs through stabilizing or reversing systemic manifestations of the disease. (Nici et al., 2006)

PR has become an important part of the standard of care for individuals with lung disease and appears to benefit those with chronic lung diseases other than COPD (Ries et al., 2007).

Goals and Rationale

PR attempts to reverse the systemic consequences of lung disease, not to improve lung function (Casaburi & ZuWallach, 2009; Troosters et al., 2008). Systemic consequences contributing to exercise intolerance in pulmonary disorders include limitations in ventilation and gas exchange, as well as cardiac, skeletal muscle, and respiratory muscle dysfunction (Nici et al., 2006).

The goal of PR is to improve the functional abilities of those with chronic lung disease by addressing muscle weakness, exercise intolerance, exertional dyspnea, fatigue, nutritional deprivation, and psychological issues (Nici et al., 2006; Troosters et al., 2008). Target areas for improvement through PR include desensitization to dyspnea, decreased anxiety/depression, reduction in dynamic hyperinflation (air trapping during exercise), and improved skeletal muscle function (Casaburi & Zu Wallach, 2009).

PR Team Members and Areas of Focus

A comprehensive PR program is multidisciplinary and may include physicians, physical therapists, occupational therapists, nurses, exercise physiologists, psychologists, nutritionists, respiratory therapists, pharmacists, and social workers (British Thoracic Society, 2001). The multidisciplinary team will address the following areas to help optimize the individual's clinical status:

- Smoking cessation
- Disease education
- Proper use of hand-held nebulizers and inhalers for medication administration
- Secretion clearance techniques
- Controlled breathing techniques—pursed lip, paced and diaphragmatic breathing
- Recovery from shortness of breath positions and coping strategies
- Exercise training and strength training
- Nutritional counseling
- Energy conservation during activities of daily living
- Social support and psychological counseling

Exercise Training

The exercise portion is considered the cornerstone of a PR program and has the potential to reverse the effects of deconditioning (Troosters et al., 2008). Deconditioning occurs when individuals with lung disease experience dyspnea on exertion, and gradually limit their activity over time, which result in further muscle weakness. Pulmonary status should be maximized prior to initiating an exercise program. Optimal bronchodilator therapy is recommended for individuals with airflow limitations (Nici et al., 2006; Ries et al., 2007). Oxygen supplementation during PR, regardless of whether or not oxygen desaturation occurs, often allows higher training intensities and/or reduced symptoms in the research setting; however, it is still unclear whether this improves clinical outcomes (Nici et al., 2006; Ries et al., 2007).

Measures of baseline functional status are usually documented prior to initiation of an exercise program. The functional measure may be an established treadmill exercise testing protocol, a 6-minute walk test (ATS, 2002), or a bicycle ergometer test protocol. Following completion of the exercise program, the functional measure is repeated to determine whether improvement in functional status has been achieved.

Physiological monitoring to ensure patient safety during exercise training includes continuous heart rate and oxygen saturation monitoring, with blood pressure monitored at frequent intervals. Visual scales for rating level of exertion or dyspnea are also utilized to record symptoms, such as the Borg Scale of Perceived Exertion, which asks patients to rate their level of exertion by examining a number scale with word descriptions of exercise intensities. The numbers on the Borg Scale correlate roughly to the patient's pulse rate (Borg, 1982).

Principles of exercise training used in the healthy elderly population are utilized for those with COPD. Exercise is preceded by a warm-up session of stretching and warm-up exercises, a core exercise program, 30 minutes of continuous or intermittent active exercise, followed by a cool-down period (Troosters et al., 2008). Improvement in muscle function will be seen in the muscles that have actively participated in exercise training (specificity of training). Therefore, programs that emphasize endurance activities (treadmill walking and cycling) yield muscle changes that improve endurance, whereas training programs that emphasize tasks requiring strength (machine weights, free weight, elastic resistance, and lifting the body against gravity) yield muscle changes improving strength (Ries et al., 2007).

PR programs have traditionally focused on lower extremity training to improve ambulation (Nici et al., 2006; Ries et al., 2007). Currently, greater emphasis is being placed on the inclusion of upper extremity exercise as well, since the upper extremities, used in unsupported positions are crucial to the performance of many activities of daily living (Ries et al., 2007). When continuous exercise is difficult for those with severe lung disease, severe symptoms, or those just beginning to exercise, interval training can be helpful. Interval training involves performing several shorter exercise sessions separated by rest periods or by intervals of lower intensity exercise (Vogiatzis, Nanas, & Roussos, 2002).

Exercise Training Interventions Included in PR

Endurance exercise involves using large muscle groups in continuous repetitive motions, with emphasis on the muscles of ambulation (Ries et al., 2007). This includes cycling, walking/treadmill walking, and exercise stepping machines. Emphasis is also placed on training the smaller muscles of the upper extremities, which are needed for activities of daily living (Ries et al., 2007). This includes the use of upper body ergometry, ball tossing, and rowing machines. Cross-county ski machines, stationary bicycles with arm resistance, or swimming can exercise arms and legs simultaneously. Strength training can increase muscle strength and muscle mass (Ries et al., 2007). Strength training is particularly indicated for individuals with significant muscle atrophy (Nici et al., 2006). Exercise modalities used in strength training include machine or free weights, elastic resistance, and lifting the body against gravity (Ries et al., 2007). Respiratory muscle training provides resistance to the inspiratory muscles through the use of inspiratory muscle trainers (IMT) and is included in many PR programs. However, scientific evidence does not support the routine use of IMT as an essential component of PR programs (Ries et al., 2007).

Length of PR Programs and Outcome Measures

PR programs lasting 6–12 weeks have been recommended by the American College of Chest Physicians and the American Association of Cardiovascular and Pulmonary Rehabilitation to achieve physiological benefits. However, PR programs lasting longer than 12 weeks are noted to produce greater sustained benefits than shorter programs (Ries et al., 2007). PR programs are an important component in the management programs for individuals with chronic lung disease, particularly COPD, with statistically and clinically significant improvements seen in four important quality of life issues: dyspnea, fatigue, emotional state, and sense of control over the disease (Lacasse, Goldstein, Lasserson, & Martin, 2009). Significant improvements for the exercise measures of maximum exercise capacity, endurance time, and walking distance following PR for COPD were reported in a meta-analysis of outcome measures, with maximum exercise capacity and walking distance improvements sustained for up to 9 months after PR (Cambach, Wagenaar, Koelman, Ton van Keimpema, & Kemper, 1999).

Individuals with ILD may also achieve gains in functional status following PR by virtue of improved skills for coping with symptoms of their illness and better energy conservation with activity. Future research is needed to clarify the benefits and outcome measures for individuals with other chronic lung diseases following PR programs.

CONCLUSION

Chronic pulmonary diseases encompass a wide variety of disorders including COPD, asthma, CF, ILD, and others. The economic impact of these disorders is enormous and can only be estimated in terms of the cost of treatment, reduced work productivity, morbidity, and mortality. Understanding the etiology, pathogenesis, and pathophysiology of these diseases is crucial to the development of methods to prevent and treat these disorders. With proper medical treatment programs including PR, many individuals with pulmonary disease may achieve enough improvement in their physical capability to be able to return to useful work, thereby lessening the financial burden on society and improving their quality of life.

REFERENCES

Abbey, D. E., Burchette, R. J., Knutson, S. F., McDonnell, W. F., Lebowitz, M. D., & Enright, P. L. (1998). Long term particulate and other air pollutants and lung function in nonsmokers. *American Journal of Respiratory and Critical Care Medicine, 158,* 289–298.

American Medical Association (2008). The pulmonary system. In R. D. Rondinelli (Ed.), *Guides to the evaluation of permanent impairment* (6th ed., pp. 77–99). Chicago: American Medical Association.

American Thoracic Society (1986). Evaluation of impairment/disability secondary to respiratory disorders. *American Review of Respiratory Disease, 133,* 1205–1209.

American Thoracic Society (1993). Guidelines for the evaluation of impairment/disability in patients with asthma. *American Review of Respiratory Disease, 147,* 1056–1061.

American Thoracic Society (2000). Guidelines for methacholine and exercise challenge testing—1999. The official statement of the American Thoracic Society. *American Journal of Respiratory and Critical Care Medicine, 161,* 309–329.

American Thoracic Society (2000). Idiopathic pulmonary fibrosis: Diagnosis and treatment: International consensus statement. *American Journal of Respiratory and Critical Care Medicine, 161,* 646–664.

American Thoracic Society Statement (2002). Guidelines for the six-minute walk test. *American Journal of Respiratory and Critical Care Medicine, 166,* 111–117.

American Thoracic Society (2004). Guidelines for assessing and managing asthma risk at work, school and recreation. *American Journal of Respiratory and Critical Care Medicine, 169,* 873–887.

Balmes, J. R., & Barnhart, S. (2005). Evaluation of respiratory impairment/disability. In R. J. Mason, V. C. Broaddus, J. F. Murray, J. A. Nadel (Eds.), *Textbook of respiratory medicine* (4th ed., pp. 795–812). Philadelphia: Elsevier Saunders.

Barnes, P. J. (2004). Macrophages as orchestrators of COPD. *Journal of COPD, 1,* 59–70.

Borg, G. A. (1982). Psychophysical bases of perceived exertion. *Medicine and Science in Sports and Exercise, 14,* 337–381.

British Thoracic Society Standards of Care Subcommittee on Pulmonary Rehabilitation. (2001). Pulmonary rehabilitation. *Thorax, 56,* 827–834.

Brooks, S. M., Weiss, M. A., & Bernstein, I. L. (1985). Reactive airways dysfunction syndrome (RADS) after high level irritant exposures. *Chest, 88,* 376–384.

Brooks, S. M., Hammad, Y., Richards, I., Giovinco-Barbas, J., & Jenkins, K. (1998). The spectrum of irritant-induced asthma: Sudden and not-so-sudden onset and the role of allergy. *Chest, 113,* 42–49.

Burgel, P. R., & Nadel, J. A. (2004). Roles of epidermal growth factor receptor activation in epithelial cell repair and mucin production in airway epithelium. *Thorax, 59,* 992–996.

Cambach, W., Wagenaar, R. C., Koelman, T. W., Ton van Keimpema, A. R., & Kemper, H. C. (1999). The long-term effects of pulmonary rehabilitation in patients with asthma and chronic obstructive pulmonary disease: A research synthesis. *Archives of Physical Medicine and Rehabilitation, 80,* 103–111.

Camilli, A. E., Burrows, B., Knudson, R. J., Lyle, S. K., & Lebowitz, M. D. (1987). Longitudinal changes in forced expiratory volume in one second in adults. *American Review of Respiratory Disease 135,* 794–799.

Casaburi, R., & ZuWallach, R. (2009). Pulmonary rehabilitation for management of chronic obstructive pulmonary disease. *The New England Journal of Medicine, 360,* 1329–1335.

Cystic Fibrosis Foundation (CFF). 2007. *Patient Registry, 2007 Annual Data Report,* Bethesda, MD. Retrieved from www.cff.org

Eisner, M. D., Yelin, E. H., Trupin, L., & Blanc, P. D. (2002). The influence of chronic respiratory conditions on health status and work disability. *American Journal of Public Heath, 92,* 1506–1513.

Epler, G., Saber, F., & Gaensler, E. (1980). Determination of severe impairment (disability) in interstitial lung disease. *American Review of Respiratory Disease, 121,* 647–659.

Fitzsimmons, S. C. (1998). CFF Patient Registry, 1997 Annual Data Report, Bethesda, MD.

Gallagher, C. G. (1994). Exercise limitations and clinical exercise testing in chronic obstructive lung disease. *Clinics in Chest Medicine, 15,* 305–326.

GOLD Report, Global Initiative for Chronic Obstructive Lung Disease (2008). *Global strategy for the diagnosis, management, and prevention of chronic obstructive pulmonary disease.* Retrieved from www.goldcopd.org.

Halbert, R. J., Isonaka, S., George, D., & Iqbal, A. (2003). Interpreting COPD prevalence estimates: What is the true burden of disease? *Chest, 123,* 1684–1692.

Halbert, R. J., Natoli, J. L., Gano, A., Badamgarav, E., Buist, A. S., & Mannino, D. M. (2006). Global burden of COPD: Systematic review and meta-analysis. *European Respiratory Journal, 28,* 523–532.

Hsai, C. C. W. (1999). Cardiopulmonary limitations to exercise in restrictive lung disease. *Medicine and Science in Sports and Exercise, 31,* S28–S32.

Isawa, T., Techima, T., Hirano, T., Ebina, A., & Kono, K. (1984). Mucociliary clearance in smoking and non-smoking subjects. *Journal Nuclear Medicine, 25,* 352–359.

Jemal, A., Ward, E., Hao, Y., & Thun, M. (2005). Trends in the leading causes of death in the United States. 1970–2002. *Journal of the American Medical Association, 294,* 1255–1259.

Kremer, A. M., Pal, T. M., & van Keimpema, A. R. J. (2006). Employment and disability for work in patients with COPD: A cross-sectional study among Dutch patients. *Internal Archives of Occupational and Environmental Health, 80,* 78–86.

Lacasse, Y., Goldstein, R., Lasserson, T. J., & Martin, S. (2009). Pulmonary rehabilitation for chronic obstructive pulmonary disease (Review). *Cochrane Database Systems Review.* Retrieved from http://www.thecochranelibrary.com

Lane, D. J., & Howell, J. B. L. (1970). Relationship between sensitivity to carbon dioxide and clinical features in patients with chronic airways obstruction. *Thorax, 25,* 150–159.

McArdle, W. D., Katch, V. L., & Katch, F. I. (Eds.) (1994). Energy expenditure at rest and during exercise. In *Essentials of Exercise Physiology* (pp. 78—113). Philadelphia: Lea & Febinger.

Muir, D. C., Julian, J. A., Shannon, H. S., Verma, D. K., Sebestyen, A., & Bernholz, C. D. (1989). Silica exposure and silicosis among Ontario hardrock miners: III. Analysis and risk estimates. *The American Journal of Industrial Medicine, 16,* 29–43.

Murray, C. J. L., & Lopez, A. D. (Eds.). (1996). *The global burden of disease: A comprehensive assessment of mortality and disability from disease, injuries and risk factors in 1990 and projected to 2020.* Cambridge, MA: Harvard University Press.

Murray, C. J. L., & Lopez, A. D. (1997). Alternative projections of mortality and disability by cause 1990–2020: Global Burden of Disease Study. *Lancet, 349,* 1498–1504.

National Heart, Lung and Blood Institute, Morbidity & Mortality: Chartbook on Cardiovascular, Lung and Blood Diseases (1998). United States Department of Health and Human Services, Public Health Service. Bethesda, MD.

Nici, L., Donner, C., Woutres, E., Zu Wallack, R., Ambrosin, N., Bourbeau, J., et al. (2006). American thoracic society/European respiratory society statement on pulmonary rehabilitation. *American Journal of Respiratory and Critical Care Medicine, 173,* 1390–1413.

Orbon, K. H., Schermer, T. R., van der Gulden, J. W., Chavannes, N. H., Akkermans, R. P., van Schayck, O. P., et al. (2005). Employment status and quality of life in patients with chronic obstructive pulmonary disease. *International Archives of Occupational and Environmental Health, 78,* 467–474.

O'Sullivan, B. P., & Freedman, S. D. (2009). Cystic fibrosis. *Lancet, 373,* 1891–1904.

Riccioni, G., DiIlio, C., Theoharides, T., & D'Orazio, N. (2004). Advances in therapy with antileukotriene drugs. *Annals of Clinical Laboratory Science, 34,* 379–387.

Ries, A. L., Bauldoff, G. S., Carlin, B. W., Casaburi, R., Emery, C. F., Mahler, D., et al. (2007). Pulmonary rehabilitation: Joint ACCP/AACVPR evidenced based clinical practice guidelines. *Chest, 131,* 4S–42S.

Sethi, S., Maloney, J., Grove, L., Wrona, C., & Berenson, C. S. (2001). Airway inflammation and bronchial bacterial colonization in chronic obstructive pulmonary disease. *American Journal of Respiratory and Critical Care Medicine, 164,* 469–473.

Schneiderman-Walker, J., Pollack, S. L., Corey, M., Wilkes, D. D., Canny, G. J., Pedder, L., et al. (2000). A randomized controlled trial of a 3-year home exercise program in cystic fibrosis. *Journal of Pediatrics, 136,* 304–310.

Sin, D. D., Stafinsk, T., Ng, Y. C., Bell, N. R., & Jacobs, P. (2002). The impact of chronic obstructive pulmonary disease on work loss in the United States. *American Journal of Respiratory and Critical Care Medicine, 165,* 704–707.

Smith, C. A., & Harrison, D. J. (1997). Association between polymorphism in gene for microsomal epoxide hydrolase and susceptibility to emphysema. *Lancet, 350,* 630–633.

Stockley, R. A. (2002). Neutrophils and the pathogenesis of COPD. *Chest, 121*(Suppl. 5), 151S–155S.

Stoller, J. K., & Aboussouan, L. S. (2005). Alpha 1-antitrypsin deficiency. *Lancet, 365,* 2225–2236.

Sullivan, S. D., Strassels, S., & Smith, D. H. (1996). Characterization of the incidence and cost of COPD in the US. *European Respiratory Journal, 9*(Suppl. 23), S421.

Tsui, L. C., & Buchwald, M. (1991). Biochemical and molecular genetics of cystic fibrosis. *Advanced Human Genetics, 20,* 153–266, 311–312.

Troosters, T., Gosselink, R., Burtin, C., & DeCramer, M., (2008). Exercise training in COPD in clinical management of chronic obstructive pulmonary disease. In S. I. Rennard, R. Rodriguez-Rosin, G. Huchon, & N. Roche (Eds.), *Lung biology in health and disease* (2nd ed., pp. 371–384). New York: Informa Health Care.

United States Department of Health and Human Services. (1984). The health consequences of smoking: Chronic obstructive lung disease. (DHHS Publication No. [PHS] 84-50205). Rockville, MD: Author.

Varekamp, I., Verbeek, J. H. A. M., & Dijk, F. J. H. (2006). How can we help employees with chronic diseases to stay at work? A review of interventions aimed at job retention and based on an empowerment perspective. *International Archives of Occupational and Environmental Health, 80,* 87–97.

Venables, K. M., & Chan-Yeung, M. (1997). Occupational asthma. *Lancet, 349,* 1465–1469.

Vogiatzis, I., Nanas, S., & Roussos, C. (2002). Interval training as an alternative modality to continuous exercise in patients with COPD. *European Respiratory Journal, 20,* 12–19.

Yankasas, J. R., & Mallory, G. B. (1998). Lung transplantation in cystic fibrosis: Consensus Conference Statement. *Chest, 113,* 217–226.

Yankaskas, J. R., Marshall, B. C., Sufian, B., Simon, R. H., & Rodman, D. (2004). Cystic fibrosis adult care consensus conference report. *Chest, 125*(Suppl. 1), 1S–39S.

23

Chronic Kidney Disease

Kotresha Neelakantappa, MD, and Jerome Lowenstein, MD

Chronic renal failure poses a singular challenge for health professionals who deal with illness-related disability and rehabilitation. The course of progressive chronic kidney disease (CKD) leading to renal failure often spans many years; during the period before dialysis or renal transplantation is undertaken, the patient may experience disabilities related to cardiovascular disease, anemia, malnutrition, metabolic bone disease, neuropathy, muscle wasting, and acid–base and electrolyte disturbances. Dialysis treatment and transplantation significantly prolong the lives of patients with renal failure, but often allow some of the most disabling features of renal disease to persist or progress. Better understanding of the pathophysiological basis for many of the disabling aspects of chronic renal failure has led to therapies that may reduce the frequency and/or severity of these aspects of the disease. Prevention of disability and rehabilitation has become increasingly important as the number of patients treated with dialysis therapy and renal transplantation has become more common. U.S. Renal Data System's (USRDS, 2009) Annual Data Report (ADR) shows that the prevalence rate of end-stage renal disease (ESRD) was 527,282 in 2008, affecting 1,750 per million of population. This number has increased to more than six and a half times since 1980. The annual incidence rate (the number of new patients entering the program) fell 2.1%, for the first time since 1995, to 354 per million population.

ANATOMY OF THE NEPHRON

Each functioning unit of the kidney is called a nephron, and there are a million nephrons in each kidney. The nephron is comprised of the glomerulus, which is a tuft of capillaries invaginated in the Bowman's capsule. The glomerular tuft arises from the afferent arteriole. The glomerular capillaries reunite to form the efferent arteriole, which divides a second time to form peritubular capillaries which ultimately drain into the renal vein. The Bowman's capsule, which forms the urinary space, opens into the renal tubule.

The glomerular tuft contains the capillary network, an epithelial cell layer which arises from the Bowman's capsule and surrounds each of the capillaries and the mesangial cellular matrix forming the stalk. The barrier to glomerular plasma filtration is formed by the fenestrated capillary endothelium, the visceral epithelial layer of the Bowman's capsule, and the common basement membrane between these two. The visceral epithelial cell is a large specialized cell called podocyte, which forms long interdigitating foot processes that rest on the basement membrane, completely covering the outside of the basement membrane. The adjacent foot processes are separated by the slit diaphragm. Much is being learned about the biology of the podocyte, its foot processes, and the slit diaphragm as they relate to their important role as a barrier to protein filtration during health and alterations in their structure and function during disease. The ultrastructure of the filtration barrier is shown in Figure 23.1.

CKD AND CARDIOVASCULAR DISEASE

Although the kidney serves multiple functions, including regulation of red blood cell production and vitamin D synthesis, its main function is to excrete the daily generation of nitrogenous waste products, acid, and ingested water and electrolytes. To excrete the metabolic waste products, such as urea, in a reasonably small volume of fluid, at a concentration, much higher than in the plasma, the kidney filters 180 liters of plasma water a day (with all the dissolved solutes at the same concentration as that in the plasma) at the glomerulus and reabsorbs all of the filtrate with the essential components, such as water and electrolytes at the tubule, excreting only 1–2 liters of urine with a high concentration of waste products. Renal function is traditionally expressed in terms of glomerular filtration rate (GFR) per minute.

The National Kidney Foundation (Table 23.1) has proposed to consider CKD as a continuum, based largely on the presence of persistently increased protein excretion in the urine (proteinuria) and or impaired GFR (NKF-KDOQI, 2002).

The prevalence of CKD of stages 1–4 by the definitions in Table 23.1 was estimated to have increased from 11% to 13% between National Health and Nutrition Examination Surveys (NHANES) of 1988–1994 and 1999–2004. This may in part be secondary to increased identification. CKD classification carries the implicit message that renal disease (defined simply as reduced GFR) may be expected to progress, albeit at a variable rate, to renal failure and the need for renal replacement (either dialysis or renal transplantation.) This may not be the case.

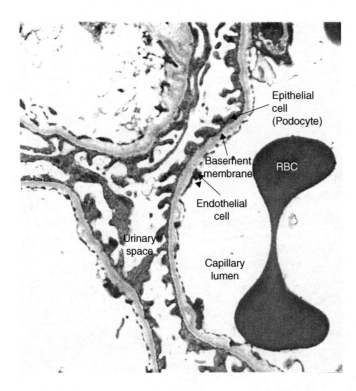

FIGURE 23.1   Electron micrograph of glomerular filtration barrier.

TABLE 23.1   *National Kidney Foundation Kidney Disease Outcome Quality Initiative (KDOQI) Classification of Chronic Kidney Disease*

Stage	Description	GFR (ml/min/1.73 m²)	Prevalence in the United States (NHANES 1999–2004)
1	Kidney damage with normal or ↑ in GFR	> 90	1.8%
2	Kidney damage with mild ↓ in GFR	60–89	3.2%
3	Moderate ↓ in GFR	30–59	7.7%
4	Severe ↓ in GFR	15–29	0.35%
5	Kidney failure	< 15 (or dialysis)	2.4%

Chronic kidney disease is defined as either evidence of kidney damage or impaired glomerular filtration rate (GFR) of < 60 ml/min/1.73 m² for ≥ 3 months. *Source:* Coresh, J., Selvin, E., Stevens, L. A., Manzi, J., Kusek, J. W., Eggers, P., et al. (2007). Prevalence of chronic kidney disease in the United States. *Journal of the American Medical Association, 298,* 2038–2047.

It is now well recognized that many patients classed as CKD 2 or 3 may not have intrinsic renal disease. Couser (2007) stated:

> Identification of stages of CKD implies, perhaps unintentionally, that CKD is a progressive process with those afflicted moving eventually from earlier to more advanced stages of disease. Although this clearly happens in many patients with *defined* [italics ours] forms of kidney disease like diabetes and glomerulonephritis, there is a paucity of data documenting such progression in patients with CKD defined *only* as GFR < 60 ml/min or with microalbuminuria. Indeed, it is clear from several studies that many such patients do not progress over several years of follow-up.

More recently, Hallan et al. (2009) have shown that combining GFR and albuminuria to classify CKD improves prediction of progression to ESRD. In a study of 65,589 adults, these authors showed that adding presence of albuminuria to impaired GFR would reduce the identified individuals who are predicted to progress to ESRD from 4.7% to 1.4% of the population and still identify 65.6% versus 69.4% of all individuals progressing to ESRD.

While reduced GFR in CKD classes 2, 3, and even 4 does not often progress to ESRD and the need for renal replacement therapy, there is abundant evidence that impaired GFR is associated with increased risk of cardiovascular morbidity and mortality. Several large multicenter studies (Khan et al., 2006; Tokmakova et al., 2004) reported that even mild reductions in GFR in patients with coronary artery disease and impaired left ventricular function is associated with higher mortality and morbidity. The relationship between impaired glomerular filtration and outcomes in cardiovascular disease is confounded by the fact that many important risk factors are common to both conditions. Diabetes mellitus, hypertension, and hyperlipidemia are risk factors common to both renal disease and coronary artery disease. Risk factor assessment using the scores developed in the Framingham studies appears to underestimate cardiovascular outcomes in the presence of reduced GFR (Henry et al., 2002). Analysis of cardiovascular and renal outcomes in the VALIANT study (Anavekar et al., 2004) composed of more than 14,000 patients with acute myocardial infarction and heart failure or left ventricular dysfunction demonstrated a significant and graded increase in mortality and cardiovascular events over a range of GFR that spanned the CKD categories 2 through 4. Patients presenting with greater reduction in GFR (CKD 5) were excluded from the study. Although the rate of renal events increased with declining estimated GFRs, the adverse outcomes were predominantly cardiovascular. Below 81.0 ml/min/1.73 m², each reduction of the estimated GFR by 10 ml/min/1.73 m² was associated with a hazard ratio for death and nonfatal cardiovascular outcomes of 1.10.

Although there is evidence of an association between renal disease with reduced GFR and accelerated atherosclerosis, it is not clear whether this can be ascribed to risk factors (e.g., hypertension, diabetes, hyperlipidemia), to factors unique to renal disease (e.g., profibrotic or proinflammatory mediators), or to an adverse effect of cardiac performance on renal function.

FUNCTIONAL ADAPTATION TO NEPHRON LOSS

As various kidney diseases destroy nephrons one at a time, a concept referred to as single nephron hypothesis, adaptive changes in residual nephrons permit the kidney to retain much of its function despite marked reduction in the number of nephrons. Systemic and intrarenal hemodynamic changes, hormonal stimuli, and possibly structural changes along the nephron lead to increase in single nephron GFR and to changes in tubular reabsorption and tubular secretion of various metabolites in the surviving nephrons. With further nephron loss, compensatory changes in the residual nephrons fail to maintain normal total renal function and abnormalities in blood composition become evident.

Minute changes in the body composition resulting from retention of some substances trigger mechanisms, which result in compensatory increase in their excretion with little change in the internal milieu. These mechanisms themselves are associated with varying degrees of untoward effects, but these are considered to be less harmful effects than those of retention of the substance in question. This is referred to as the *tradeoff hypothesis*. It is well illustrated by the compensatory responses that maintain external balance of sodium, potassium, hydrogen ion, calcium, and phosphate.

Sodium

Under normal circumstances, approximately 25,000 mEq of sodium (Na^+) are filtered daily. All except about 150 mEq (average daily intake) are reabsorbed. As the GFR and the filtered load of sodium decline with progressive renal disease, there is a reciprocal increase in the fraction of filtered sodium that escapes reabsorption. Despite marked reduction in filtered sodium in advanced renal failure, overt sodium retention and edema are not seen until the most advanced stage with decreased urine output, unless complicated by other problems such as heart disease. The mechanism responsible for rejection of an increased fraction of the filtered sodium may directly or indirectly be related to an increased systemic blood pressure. Hypertension may be the price to be paid for maintaining sodium balance in the face of declining GFR.

Potassium

Filtered potassium is completely reabsorbed before the glomerular filtrate reaches the distal convoluted tubule. Potassium balance is maintained mainly by secretion by the principal cells in the late distal convoluted tubule and cortical-collecting duct. Hyperkalemia (increased blood level of potassium) is usually not seen until GFR declines to less than 10–15% of normal. Tubular secretion of potassium depends on the negative electrical charge in the lumen created by sodium reabsorption and sodium conductance across the epithelium of the collecting duct, which in turn depend on the adrenal hormone aldosterone. Although plasma aldosterone concentration is not usually elevated in chronic renal disease, patients with moderately advanced renal failure are prone to develop hyperkalemia if drugs such spironolactone, eplerenone, angiotensin-converting enzyme inhibitors (ACEIs), angiotensin receptor blockers (ARBs), renin antagonists, or nonsteroidal anti-inflammatory agents are given.

Hydrogen Ion

Daily metabolism leads to generation of fixed acids (predominantly sulfuric acid), which dissociate into their respective anions (e.g., sulfate) and the cation, H^+ (proton). Daily metabolic production averages about 1 mEq/kg/day. The protons titrate the body buffers, predominantly bicarbonate. The kidney excretes the anions of the acids and regenerates the bicarbonate (and other body buffers). The regeneration of bicarbonate stores and the "back titration" of other body buffers (predominantly proteins) are accomplished by the excretion of H^+ with filtered urinary buffers such as phosphates and with ammonia (NH_3) synthesized in the proximal tubular cell, as NH_4^+. Renal acid excretion is reduced only modestly despite marked reduction in nephron number as renal disease progresses. This is the result of an increase in the filtered amount of titratable urinary buffers such as phosphates and enhanced ammonia production per residual nephron.

Calcium and Phosphorus

Calcium and phosphorus metabolism are markedly altered in progressive renal disease. The concentration of 1,25-D3, the active form of vitamin D, is governed by the enzymatic hydroxylation of 25-D3 by the kidneys. Because 1,25-D3 is reduced in renal failure the calcium absorption by the intestine decreases, resulting in hypocalcemia (reduced blood level of calcium).

Normally 80–90% of the filtered phosphorus is reabsorbed. In renal failure, even though the filtered load of phosphorus declines steadily, the serum phosphorus level does not rise, since the daily intake can be excreted by reduction in reabsorption down to nearly 50%. Beyond this point, steady state is achieved by a combination of further reduction in reabsorption and a relative increase in the filtered load achieved by a rise in the plasma level. Phosphate retention also contributes to hypocalcemia both by deposition of calcium phosphate in tissues and by reduced synthesis of 1,25-D3. Despite these perturbations in calcium and phosphorus balance, serum calcium and phosphorus concentrations are maintained within the normal range until GFR is markedly reduced. In large part this is attributable to increased parathyroid hormone (PTH) secretion. PTH not only reduces tubular reabsorption of phosphate, but also mobilizes calcium from the skeletal system. The pathogenesis of this "secondary hyperparathyroidism" involves several mechanisms. Hypocalcemia stimulates PTH release from parathyroid cells. Reduced vitamin D concentration leads to parathyroid hyperplasia by removing a normal suppressive effect it exerts on the parathyroid and a concomitant downregulation of vitamin D receptors on parathyroid cells. The "trade-off" for maintenance of calcium and phosphorus concentrations is the development of bone disease secondary to hyperparathyroidism characterized by osteomalacia and osteitis fibrosa cystica.

More recently, secretion of another regulatory hormone, fibroblast growth factor (FGF23) by the bone cells called osteocytes, has been discovered. Secretion of FGF23 also increases progressively in renal failure. FGF23 plays an important role in mitigating hyperphosphatemia in renal failure. Similar to PTH, it also decreases tubular phosphate reabsorption, leading to increased excretion; however, unlike PTH, it inhibits renal conversion of 25-D3 to the bioactive 1,25-D3, thereby decreasing intestinal phosphate absorption.

CKD AND ITS PROGRESSION

Most renal parenchymal diseases, regardless of the etiology of the underlying disease, exhibit progressive scarring and loss of function over a period of many years (see Table 23.1). In some instances, progression occurs because of persistent disease or repeated recurrences of the primary disease, but more frequently progression occurs without evidence of residual activity of the primary disease. Studies of the mechanisms underlying "nonimmunological" progression have provided therapeutical strategies for delaying the onset of renal failure.

The proposed mechanisms for progression fall into two categories—hemodynamic and signal-mediated fibrosis.

Many of the studies directed at understanding the hemodynamic mechanisms have been carried out in the "remnant kidney" model in rats subjected to removal of five-sixths of their kidneys. The animals go on to develop progressive renal failure. Studies have shown that after ablation of a critical mass of renal tissue, single nephron plasma flow and glomerular capillary hydrostatic pressure are increased in the remaining nephrons. The factors responsible for glomerular hemodynamic alterations and glomerular hypertrophy are not well understood. Increased levels of growth hormone, certain dietary amino acids, vasodilator renal prostaglandins, increased local concentrations of angiotensin II, endothelins (vasoconstrictor proteins produced by the endothelial cells), and autoregulation of glomerular blood flow leading to glomerular hypertension have all been implicated. The increase in glomerular hydrostatic pressure may occur in the absence of systemic hypertension. Increased surface area of the glomerular filtering bed and glomerular hypertension, while maintaining overall GFR close to normal, appear to lead to accelerated glomerular injury and fibrosis of the remaining nephrons. Treatment with antihypertensive agents is beneficial in slowing the rate of progression in various renal diseases in both experimental animals and humans. ACEIs and ARBs appear to exert a protective effect in CKD, which may be independent of the reduction in systemic blood pressure. More recently, the endothelin A receptor antagonist, avosentan, has been shown to reduce albumin excretion in patients with diabetic nephropathy (Wenzel et al., 2009).

Studies directed at identifying specific cellular mechanisms responsible for glomerular or interstitial fibrosis have usually been performed in experimental models of renal disease such as the unilateral obstructive nephropathy and forms of glomerular injury in which inflammation is absent (puromycin nephrotoxicity or experimental models characterized by the nephritic syndrome). Attention has been focused on the role of transforming growth factor β (Bottinger & Bitzer, 2002) and other profibrotic or proinflammatory molecules such as endothelin-1, monocyte attractant protein-1, and RANTES (Benigni & Remuzzi, 2001) in the progression of glomerular and tubulointerstitial renal diseases. While it is attractive to seek profibrotic factors in progressive renal diseases characterized by tissue fibrosis, other cellular mechanisms including apoptosis, proliferation, and endothelial–mesangial transdifferentiation may be important components in slowly progressive renal diseases.

TREATMENT OF CHRONIC RENAL FAILURE

Delaying Progression of Renal Disease

Although hypertension is almost always a result rather than a cause of renal disease, it leads to accelerated progression of the underlying disease, creating a vicious circle. Control of hypertension in renal disease is directed at both a reduction in cardiovascular morbidity and the slowing of progression of the underlying renal disease. Antihypertensive drugs have selective actions on afferent or efferent arterioles and differ in their ability to reduce glomerular hypertension. ACEIs (Lewis, Hunsicker, Bain, & Rohde, 1993) and ARBs (Brenner et al., 2001; Lewis et al., 2001), which lower glomerular capillary pressure (P_{GC}), have been shown to reduce proteinuria and delay progression in both diabetic and nondiabetic renal diseases (The GISEN Group, 1997). Although some studies have shown beneficial effect of the combination of ACEI and ARB in reducing proteinuria and delaying progression of renal disease, a randomized-controlled trial (Mann et al., 2008) of combination therapy of the ACEI, ramipril and ARB, telmisartan showed that there was no improvement in proteinuria or reduction in the rate of decline in renal function with either therapy alone or in combination. However, the increase in proteinuria during the study period was the least with combination therapy with ACEI and ARB. Calcium channel blockers differ in their effect on the kidney. Dihydropyridines, which are potent vasodilators, lead to an increase in proteinuria, perhaps because afferent arteriolar dilatation leaves P_{GC} unchanged or increased. Nondihydropyridines have been shown to reduce proteinuria, which is additive to that brought about by ACEI.

Other strategies to delay the progression have included antifibrotic agents such as tranilast, supplementation of glycosaminoglycans to restore glomerular integrity and function, counteracting advanced glycation end-products (AGEs) in diabetics with agents such as aminoguanidine, antagonists for the receptor for AGE, inhibitors of protein kinase C, preventing its oxidant injury, and so on. Unconventional effects of statins, erythropoiesis-stimulating agents, and vitamin D in delaying progression of renal disease have also been observed and are being explored. But, so far, either the benefit of these therapies has been marginal or the side effects have been significant, and therefore none of these has been advised.

Correcting the Metabolic Abnormalities

Metabolic acidosis in chronic renal disease is generally well tolerated and is usually not treated unless it is severe. The arguments against treatment have included the risk of sodium overload associated with sodium bicarbonate therapy, reduction in ionized calcium concentration resulting in tetany (sustained painful contraction of a group of muscles), and seizures and perhaps diminished oxygen (O_2) delivery to tissues due to reversal of an adaptive change in the O_2 dissociation curve. More recent evidence suggests that the benefits of treatment outweigh these objections. Treatment of metabolic acidosis with bicarbonate or with a metabolizable anion, which can act as a substitute for bicarbonate (e.g., citrate or lactate), has been shown to prevent growth retardation in children with renal tubular acidosis. It has been shown that correction of metabolic acidosis, by increasing dialysate bicarbonate concentration in patients with ESRD, improves bone mineralization, diminishes bone resorption, and reduces the severity of secondary hyperparathyroidism.

Chronic metabolic acidosis is associated with muscle weakness and decreased lean body mass. Forearm muscle studies in patients with chronic renal disease have demonstrated that the rate of protein degradation is directly related to the degree of acidosis and to plasma cortisol levels; plasma cortisol levels, in turn, are directly related to the degree of acidosis. Further, albumin synthesis is diminished and negative nitrogen balance increased in patients with chronic renal disease made acidotic by the administration of ammonium chloride. The downregulation of protein degradation seen in patients with chronic renal disease placed on a protein-restricted diet is impaired in those who also have metabolic acidosis; this can be corrected by treatment of acidosis with bicarbonate.

Anemia
Although there are many causes of anemia in chronic renal disease, reduced erythropoietin (EPO) production by the kidney seems to be the most important factor. Reduced oxygen delivery to the kidney, acting through hypoxia inducible factor (HIF-1), normally results in increased production of EPO, which increases the production of red blood cells (Semenza, 2000). However, EPO levels are markedly reduced in patients with anemia of chronic renal disease. Administration of recombinant human EPO (rHuEPO) corrects the anemia of renal disease in a dose-dependent manner. Ninety percent of patients on dialysis in the United States and many patients with chronic renal disease who are not yet on dialysis receive rHuEPO therapy. A longer acting preparation, darbepoetin alfa (Aranesp), has made administration and compliance more convenient for patients not yet receiving dialysis. The most common cause of resistance to rHuEPO is iron deficiency. Lack of response to oral iron administration is common among patients with ESRD and is attributed to the effects of hepcidin, which is produced by the liver, on the iron channel, ferroportin, preventing intestinal iron absorption

(Ganz, 2007). Patients with superimposed iron deficiency are treated with intravenous iron preparations quite safely. Other causes of resistance to EPO include bone marrow fibrosis, inflammatory conditions, poor nutrition, and underdialysis.

Anemia has been found to be an independent predictor of the de novo occurrence of congestive heart failure and increased mortality in ESRD. Left ventricular hypertrophy has also been found to be associated with increased mortality in ESRD. Successful treatment of anemia with rHuEPO has been shown to reverse cardiovascular and hemodynamic abnormalities such as left ventricular hypertrophy, increased cardiac output, and decreased peripheral vascular resistance. Patients report improved vitality and exercise tolerance; amelioration of angina, congestive heart failure, and fatigue have been observed. Other beneficial effects of EPO therapy include improvement in platelet dysfunction of uremia, uremic pruritus (itching), impaired carbohydrate and cortisol metabolism, and sexual function in male patients.

Despite such positive effects of treatment of anemia, attempts at complete correction of anemia with higher doses of epoetin are associated with increased cardiovascular risk and mortality (Drueke et al., 2006; Singh et al., 2006). The 2007 update by NKF-KDOQI (2007) is to maintain hemoglobin levels between 11 and 12 g/dl and not to exceed 13 g/dl. A recent placebo-controlled study (Pfeffer et al., 2009) showed that treatment of type 2 diabetes and CKD with darbepoetin alfa did not show a significant difference in death or cardiovascular events and death or ESRD, but that there was a significantly higher rate of fatal and nonfatal strokes in the darbepoetin group! There was only a modest improvement in the patient-reported fatigue in the darbepoetin group. Target hemoglobin was 13 g/dl and rescue darbepoetin was used even in the placebo group for hemoglobin of less than 9 g/dl. Subset analysis and finer details of the trial are still being studied.

Hepcidin is an inflammatory mediator produced by the liver as an acute phase reactant. The levels of hepcidin are elevated in CKD and ESRD as well as chronic inflammatory states. Elevated levels of hepcidin are associated with increased cardiovascular risk as well as decreased intestinal iron absorption and release from certain type of white cells (macrophages) and liver cells that store iron (Ganz, 2007). HIF-1 normally inhibits hepcidin. It has been suggested that higher doses of rHuEPO rather than the higher hemoglobin levels are responsible for the increased cardiovascular risk. It is thought that rHuEPO might lead to decreased HIF-1 levels in a feedback fashion, thus releasing the inhibitory effect on hepcidin. Newer classes of agents that stabilize HIF-1 and hence stimulate endogenous EPO production and at the same time have a suppressive effect on hepcidin are under investigation.

Vitamin D

Vitamin D plays a major role in bone metabolism and intestinal absorption of calcium and phosphorus. Sources of vitamin D include the following: (1) endogenous production by the skin from 7-dehydrocholesterol when exposed to UV radiation from the sun; (2) ingestion of preformed vitamin D from animal sources; and (3) from plants. Vitamin D derived from animals, including endogenously produced product, is named cholecalciferol or vitamin D_3 and the one derived from plants is named ergocalciferol or vitamin D_2.

Vitamin D, once produced or ingested, needs to have a hydroxyl ion (OH^-) attached both by the liver and the kidney before it is biologically active. Hydroxylation at the 25th carbon position occurs in the liver and at the 1st or 24th position in the kidney. Vitamin D deficiency (< 20–25 ng/ml) is defined by 25 hydroxy vitamin D levels. Patients with liver disease require supplementation of 25 hydroxy vitamin D (1–25 OH vitamin D is used in the United States since 25 OH vitamin D is not available) and those with kidney disease need either 1α-hydroxy D or 1–25 dihydroxy D. The role of 24–25 dihydroxy D is less well understood and is being investigated. Since hydroxylation at the 1 and 24 position occurs in the kidney, it is not surprising that the levels of 1–25 and 24–25 OH D are diminished in patients with kidney disease. The levels of 24–25 OH D are decreased early in the course of CKD and those of 1–25 OH D later in the course. However, 25 OH D deficiency is also known to exist in CKD and ESRD throughout the United States (LaClair et al., 2005) and is associated with decreased bone mineral density and increase in the risk of fractures (Elder & Mackun, 2006). Vitamin D supplementation has been shown to prevent the risk of fractures in elderly patients with low levels of vitamin D and a history of falling (Prince et al., 2008).

Treating the Symptoms of Renal Failure

Traditionally, treatment of patients with chronic renal disease has been directed at reducing uremic symptoms such as nausea, vomiting, pruritus, seizures, coma, and death. Most of these symptoms are effectively ameliorated by hemodialysis or peritoneal dialysis but other metabolic abnormalities and symptoms persist during renal replacement therapy.

CKD Mineral and Bone Disorder

This is the clinical syndrome that develops as a systemic disorder of mineral and bone metabolism due to CKD, manifested by abnormalities in bone and mineral metabolism and/ or extra-skeletal calcification.

Although symptomatic renal osteodystrophy, for example, bone pain and fractures, seldom occurs before the onset of ESRD, altered mineral metabolism is present early in the course of renal failure. The two classic forms of renal osteodystrophy are osteitis fibrosa, characterized by an increased rate of bone turnover secondary to hyperparathyroidism, and osteomalacia in which bone turnover is diminished and there is an increased volume of unmineralized bone (osteoid). Osteomalacia may result from vitamin D deficiency and aluminum toxicity in patients with ESRD. The incidence of aluminum toxicity has markedly diminished since the use of aluminum-containing phosphate binders has been discontinued and the aluminum content of the water used for dialysate is regularly monitored and kept below the recommended level. More recently, a third entity called adynamic bone disease or aplastic bone disease has been described. Low levels of PTH, diminished skeletal turnover, and reduced rate of osteoid formation characterize this condition. In some cases, it may result from excessive suppression of PTH or parathyroidectomy.

The management of renal osteodystrophy involves both suppression of hyperparathyroidism and control of hyperphosphatemia. Although the administration of 1–25 $(OH)_2$ vitamin D_3 has been extremely useful in the suppression of hyperparathyroidism, hypercalcemia (elevated calcium level) has been a limiting factor. This has led to the development of other vitamin D analogs, such as doxercalciferol and paricalcitol, which preferentially stimulate vitamin D receptors on the parathyroid gland and have less of an effect on intestinal calcium and phosphate absorption. These agents have better ability to suppress PTH for a given calcium level. Relative risk of death increases progressively with increasing levels of calcium, phosphorus, and calcium phosphorus product in the dialysis population (Block et al., 2004). Most recently, the first of a new generation of products, cinacalcet HCl (Sensipar), referred to as calcimimetic agents, has been available for use in the United States. These drugs increase the sensitivity of the calcium-sensing receptor to calcium and are devoid of the potential for hypercalcemia or hyperphosphatemia. The level of the calcium phosphorus product, which increases the risk of soft tissue calcification including vascular calcification and coronary artery disease, is not elevated with the use of cinacalcet. The key clinical event rates from the post hoc analysis of phase 3 studies show that parathyroidectomies were 0.3 per 100 patient years in the cinacalcet group versus 4.1 in the control group. Fractures were half as frequent, but mortality was not significantly different (NKF-KDOQI, 2003). Evaluation of Cinacalcet Therapy to Lower Cardiovascular Events (EVOLVE) is a global, phase 3, double-blind, randomized, placebo-controlled trial evaluating the effects of cinacalcet on mortality and cardiovascular events in hemodialysis patients with secondary hyperparathyroidism. Results are expected to be available in 2011 or 2012 (Chertow et al., 2007).

Most patients with stages 4 and 5 CKD need phosphate binders, even if they are on dialysis. Aluminum-containing antacids have been replaced by calcium carbonate and calcium acetate as dietary phosphate binders, to avoid the risk of aluminum toxicity. Even calcium-containing compounds have come under scrutiny because of the positive calcium balance and soft tissue calcification such as coronary and other vascular calcification in dialysis patients. Examples of calcium-free phosphate binders available in the United States include and sevelamer chloride (Renagel), recently replaced by sevelamer carbonate (Renvela) to avoid metabolic acidosis and lanthanum carbonate (Fosrenol). The ability to control hyperparathyroidism and hyperphosphatemia has resulted in a marked reduction in the incidence of renal osteodystrophy.

In certain instances, the nodular parathyroid hyperplasia is so severe that it is not possible to suppress it medically, a condition referred to as *tertiary hyperparathyroidism* in the past; this may necessitate surgical parathyroidectomy.

One interesting finding recently has been the discovery that higher vitamin D levels and treatment with vitamin D analogs are associated with a survival advantage and lower cardiovascular mortality (Wolf et al., 2007). The pathophysiological basis for this is not clear and needs to be studied further. Receptors for vitamin D have been identified in more than 30 tissues in the body. Vitamin D may favorably influence renin–angiotensin system, vascular smooth muscle cells, and cardiomyocytes. Ultrasound Doppler studies of the aortic pulse wave velocity and brachial artery distensibility indicate a correlation between low vitamin D levels and increased atherosclerosis (London et al., 2007).

Uremic Neuropathy

Uremic neuropathy can present as either a polyneuropathy or a mononeuropathy involving both sensory and motor fibers. It generally occurs in advanced renal failure and is an indication to start dialysis for ESRD. When it occurs in patients who are already on dialysis, one needs to consider inadequate dialysis as a cause. Pathologically, uremic polyneuropathy is associated with demyelination (loss of insulation surrounding nerve fibers) and axonal degeneration and the involvement is directly proportional to the length of the nerve, affecting longer axons first. It is usually symmetrical. The metabolic and chemical defects leading to these changes are not well understood. Clinically, it first presents as paresthesias (numbness), burning sensation, and pain in distal areas such as feet. Sensory symptoms usually precede motor symptoms. The onset of motor symptoms reflects advanced disease, which unlike the sensory neuropathy may not reverse with the institution of dialysis. Electrophysiological studies are very useful in detecting subclinical neuropathy. Uremic mononeuropathy usually involves median and ulnar nerves. Other nerves involved include seventh and eighth cranial nerves and peroneal nerves. Carpal tunnel syndrome is common in ESRD. It results from compression of median nerve at the wrist between carpal bones and transverse carpal ligament. Deposition of β-2-microglobulin-related amyloid fibrils in the carpal tunnel plays an important role in the pathogenesis of the syndrome. Early initiations of dialysis, the use of better dialysis membranes with higher clearance for β-2-microglobulin, and close attention to the adequacy of dialysis have reduced the incidence of uremic neuropathy. The extent of recovery is inversely related to the degree of dysfunction before initiation of dialysis. Restoration of renal function with renal transplantation results in remarkable recovery from even the most severe sensory and motor neuropathy.

Sexual Dysfunction

Erectile dysfunction and a decrease in both libido and frequency of intercourse are present in more than half the men with uremia. This is organic in nature as evidenced by a decline in nocturnal penile tumescence. The decline in nocturnal penile tumescence is more marked as compared with normal controls and in patients with other chronic illness, suggesting that it is the effect of uremia and yet does not improve with hemodialysis. Factors other than uremia that contribute to erectile dysfunction include peripheral neuropathy, autonomic nervous system dysfunction, and peripheral vascular disease. Psychological and physical stress may also play a role.

Lack of ovulation and scant menstruation are common in women with chronic renal failure. Some women may have menorrhagia (excessive menstrual bleeding) leading to worsening of anemia. Pregnancy can rarely occur with chronic renal failure but fetal loss is almost universal. Elevated prolactin levels are also seen in women with chronic renal disease. Although suppression of very high prolactin levels with bromocriptine in women with normal renal function improves the clinical syndrome of amenorrhea (loss of menstruation) and galactorrhea (abnormal milky discharge from the nipple), it fails to restore normal menstruation or correct galactorrhea in uremic women. Successful renal transplantation, however, leads to restoration of fertility and sexual function in most patients.

TREATMENT OF END-STAGE RENAL FAILURE

When Willem Johan Kolff (1912–2009) introduced his rotating drum artificial kidney in 1943, it was described as an effective treatment of patients with acute reversible renal failure. Today, hemodialysis and peritoneal dialysis serve to support and rehabilitate a growing number of patients with end stage irreversible renal failure. The incident hemodialysis population is now nearly eight times larger than what it was in 1978, and in 2006 it topped 100,000 patients for the first time. The number of new peritoneal dialysis patients peaked at 9,407 in 1995, and has since fallen to 6,725; this population now accounts for 6.2% of new dialysis patients, a ratio that continues to decline from its peak of 15% during 1982–1985.

As of December 31, 2006, the last year for which such data are available, nearly 328,000 patients were receiving hemodialysis therapy, 26,082 were on peritoneal dialysis (8.2% of the dialysis population), and 151,502 had a functioning renal transplant. The annual rate of growth has slowed in the prevalent hemodialysis population, from 8.5% in 1996 to 3.9% in 2006, whereas the peritoneal dialysis population has remained quite stable. The greatest growth has occurred in the renal transplant population, which has increased 5.5–6.0% each year since 2001. The number of patients who receive a kidney transplant as their first ESRD therapy reached 2,635 in 2006, with a growth rate of 7.3% each year since 1996. In 2006, 69,000 patients were waiting to receive a transplant. The total cost of ESRD to Medicare was $ 20.3 billion for 2006.

The National Kidney Foundation Disease Outcomes Quality Initiative (NKF-KDOQI) has provided evidence-based clinical practice guidelines for all stages of CKD and related complications (NKF–KDOQI, 1997) since 1997. Recognized throughout the world for improving the diagnosis and treatment of kidney disease, the NKF-KDOQI Guidelines have changed the practices of numerous specialties and disciplines and improved the lives of thousands of kidney patients.

Hemodialysis

Hemodialysis is typically performed three times a week. The procedure involves diffusion of solutes between the plasma and the dialysis bath (dialysate) across the semipermeable dialyzer membrane down a concentration gradient. Fluid (usually equal to the volume retained from one dialysis to the next) is removed by ultrafiltration by regulating the dialyzer transmembrane hydrostatic pressure. Blood flow rates through the dialyzers in the range of 350–450 ml/min are necessary to obtain sufficient clearance of solutes over a reasonably short period of time. Since the normal blood flow rates in peripheral veins are insufficient for this purpose, it is necessary to have some form of access to circulation where the blood flow rate is well in excess of this range. Simple catheters placed in a central vein and an arteriovenous fistula/ shunt, with or without the interposition of a synthetic vascular graft, serve as the most common forms of hemodialysis access. Although, tunneled central vein catheters are very useful to provide dialysis when a vascular access such as an AV fistula or AV graft is not available, continued use of these catheters is associated with the risk of serious infections, including bacterial endocarditis and decreased survival on dialysis and is greatly discouraged. Since 6–8 weeks is required for full maturation of an AV fistula, preemptive AV fistula creation in patients who anticipate going on hemodialysis leads to better outcome.

Peritoneal Dialysis

In this technique, the patient's peritoneum substitutes for the dialyzer membrane. When the peritoneal cavity is filled with dialysate solution, diffusion of solutes occurs between the plasma flowing in the capillaries supplying the peritoneum and the dialysate until concentration equilibrium is reached. In 1976 (Papovich, Moncrief, Decherd, Bomar, & Pyle, 1976), the basic concept of continuous ambulatory peritoneal dialysis (CAPD) was described. The authors made use of the fact that some solute transfer continued to occur for as long as 4–5 hours and one could achieve sufficient solute clearance with four to five 2-liter exchanges of dialysis fluid on a daily basis. This led the way to the use of peritoneal dialysis as a treatment option for patients with ESRD. The incidence of peritonitis as a complication of this procedure has been markedly reduced by improvements in techniques and the design of catheters, connections, and the use of automated cyclers, which can be used at night when the patients are asleep.

Newer Regimens of Hemodialysis

Despite advances in medical care, mortality in the ESRD population has remained relatively high (20% annually). Newer forms of dialysis techniques to improve this outcome have included short daily hemodialysis (SDHD), daily nocturnal hemodialysis (DNHD), and long overnight hemodialysis three times a week. SDHD is performed for 1.5–2.5 hours 5–6 days a week and has the advantage of removing the most solute in the shortest time (when the concentration gradient is highest) and avoiding symptoms such as muscle cramps and hypotension in the latter part of a conventional 3.5- to 4.5-hour dialysis. DNHD is performed at home while the patient is asleep at slower blood and dialysate flow rates than conventional hemodialysis. Patients are monitored remotely during treatment. It has been considered to be the best form of dialysis by some (Pierratos, 2004). A weekly dose of dialysis is high compared to conventional dialysis and it is particularly well suited for obese patients. Blood pressure control has been observed to be distinctly better on both SDHD and DNHD. Phosphate removal is twice as effective as in conventional hemodialysis. For the first time, patients with ESRD who are treated with DNHD do not need to take oral phosphate binders. They might even need phosphate supplementation to prevent hypophosphatemia. Removal of β-2-microglobulin (deposition of which leads to dialysis related amyloidosis) is increased fourfold compared to conventional hemodialysis. Other reported improvements include reduced severity of anemia associated with decreased requirement for rEPO, and improved cardiac function in those with decreased left ventricular ejection fraction. Because of increased direct cost involved with daily dialysis, long overnight dialysis three times a week is being explored. The most important difference between conventional dialysis and any of these may be a significantly increased dose of dialysis, improving removal of phosphate and larger molecular weight substances such as β-2-microglobulin. The effect on blood pressure control may be a reflection of the ease with which proper salt and fluid balance can be achieved and perhaps other factors as yet not well understood. Direct comparison between these modalities and proof of improved survival are lacking so far.

Survival of ESRD Patients

Although maintenance dialysis prevents death from uremia, patient survival is still limited. USRDS's 2008 ADR data show a mean expected remaining lifespan of 8.3 years for patients beginning dialysis between the ages of 40 and 44 and 4.6 years for those beginning between the ages of 60 and 64 years, for the year 2006. These are roughly one-fifth the expected lifespan for the general U.S. population of comparable age groups. In comparison, the remaining lifespan for patient with successful renal transplantation was 23.7 years for the 40–44 years age group and 12.7 years for those between 60 and 64 years. Understandably, survival depends on comorbid conditions. Probability of survival for 5 years after starting dialysis for incident diabetic patients during 1997–2001 was 27% for those on hemodialysis and 24% for those on peritoneal dialysis compared to 33% for all patients.

Although all-cause mortality has declined steadily since 1988, cardiovascular events (strokes and heart attack) account for about 50% of deaths in ESRD. The other important causes of death in ESRD are infections, most often stemming from hemodialysis access sites or peritonitis in those on peritoneal dialysis. The number of patients withdrawing from dialysis has increased from 21% in 2000–2001 to 24% in 2005–2006. Most of this increase has been in patients 75 years and older.

Adequacy of Dialysis

The National Cooperative Dialysis Study, a prospectively randomized and controlled study, demonstrated that the *dose of dialysis* as measured by urea clearance correlated with morbidity (Lowrie, Laird, Parker, & Sargent, 1981). The dose of dialysis therapy can be expressed as the virtual volume of plasma completely cleared of urea during dialysis, relative to the volume of distribution. The formula Kt/V expresses this, where K is urea clearance, t is duration of dialysis, and V is volume of distribution. The urea reduction ratio (URR) is also a correlate of Kt/V. Several studies (Hakim, Breyer, Ismail, & Schulman, 1994; Held et al., 1996; Parker, Husni, Huang, Lew, & Lowrie, 1994) have shown that increasing the dose of dialysis reduces mortality, which in one study (Held et al., 1996) was 7% for each 0.1 unit increment in Kt/V. However, increasing URR and Kt/V to higher levels (75% and 1.7) does not seem to be associated with further reduction in morbidity and mortality (Eknoyan et al., 2002). A target URR of more than 65% set by NKF-KDOQI was met by 96% of patients on hemodialysis in 2007.

Similar observations have been made regarding adequacy of dialysis and mortality and morbidity for patients on maintenance peritoneal dialysis. The Canada-USA (CANUSA) Peritoneal Dialysis Study Group (1996), in a prospective cohort study, found that a decrease in 0.1 unit Kt/V was associated with a 5% increase in the relative risk of death. Randomized controlled studies have supported lowering the minimum dose of weekly Kt/V to 1.7 (Moran & Correa-Rotter, 2006). As per USRDS data, 92.2% of patients in the United States met this goal as of 2006.

Survival on hemodialysis has been lower in the United States than in Japan and Europe. The reasons for regional variations in survival may be multiple, such as genetics, underlying comorbid conditions, different etiologies of ESRD, and relative prevalence of diabetes and atherosclerosis, as well as differences in criteria for accepting a patient for maintenance hemodialysis. One particular group from Tassin, France, has reported particularly excellent outcome in the control of blood pressure and anemia as well as survival and has drawn attention to their practice pattern (Charra et al., 1992). Patients are dialyzed for longer periods (24 hours compared to 9–12 hours per week) than any other place. A study of 22,000 patients from seven countries participating in the Dialysis Outcomes and Practice Patterns Study (DOPPS) found that longer treatment times and slower ultrafiltration rates are associated with better survival even after adjusting for comorbidities, dose of dialysis as determined by Kt/V and body size (Saran et al., 2006).

Nutrition

Malnutrition is common in chronic renal disease. It results not only from protein restriction in an attempt to slow the progression of renal disease, but also as a function of advancing renal disease. Analysis of the data from the modification of diet in renal disease study showed that body mass index, anthropometric measurements, and urinary creatinine excretion (an index of muscle mass) were lower than expected in patients with moderately advanced renal disease entering the study (Klahr et al., 1994). Several indices of nutrition, such as dietary protein intake, serum cholesterol, transferrin, insulin-like growth factor-1 (IGF-1), percent body weight, and urinary creatinine excretion decline as renal function deteriorates (Ikizler, Greene, Wingard, Parker, & Hakim, 1995).

Mild to moderate protein–calorie malnutrition is present in one-third of the patients on maintenance dialysis. Concentrations of plasma proteins such as albumin, prealbumin, transferrin, and IGF-1 as well as markers of tissue protein stores are already reduced in patients when dialysis is instituted. Factors contributing to malnutrition in the dialysis population include poor nutrient intake, intercurrent illness, and dialysis itself. Although several markers of malnutrition, such as low blood urea, serum cholesterol, creatinine, potassium, and phosphorus, have been associated with increased risk of mortality, low serum albumin concentration seems to be the strongest predictor of mortality. The odds ratio for the risk of death is inversely related, exponentially, to serum albumin concentration in patients maintained on either hemo- or peritoneal dialysis. Nearly half the patients with ESRD starting dialysis have serum albumin concentration below the normal range. Even though peritoneal losses contribute to hypoalbuminemia in CAPD patients (Lowrie, Huang, & Lew, 1995), the relative risk of death was the same for hemodialysis and CAPD patients with hypoalbuminemia, suggesting that regardless of the mechanism, hypoalbuminemia carried the same risk. Various interventions ranging from simple nutritional supplements to administration of intradialytic parenteral nutrition may be of value in correcting malnutrition in patients with ESRD. Experimentally, recombinant human growth hormone and recombinant human IGF-1 (rhIGF-1) have been shown to lead to positive nitrogen balance.

PHYSICAL REHABILITATION

As in any other chronic illness, rehabilitation is extremely important if patients with ESRD are to live as normal a life as possible. Even though hemodialysis and peritoneal dialysis provide means to sustain life in the absence of kidney function, patients are generally weak and disabled to a variable extent. The trend in favor of institution of dialysis before severe debility is incurred has made rehabilitation more effective.

Frailty is common among dialysis patients as the median age and comorbid conditions of these patients have increased in the recent years. A study of more than 2,000 patients in the Dialysis Morbidity and Mortality Wave 2 study (Johansen, Chertow, Jin, & Kutner, 2007) revealed that two-thirds met the definition of frailty, which comprised of self-reported poor physical functioning, exhaustion/fatigue, low physical activity, and undernutrition. Older age, female gender, and hemodialysis, rather than peritoneal dialysis, were independently associated with frailty. The hazard ratio for death was 2.24 among patients with frailty.

The 2008 ADR from USRDS show that the prevalence of walking disability in the CKD population is about twice that of the non-CKD population, and is much more likely to lead to death. Early identification of CKD patients with walking disabilities, and recognition that they are at high risk for falls, could lead to increased use of exercise interventions and rehabilitation to maintain or restore balance and function.

One of the most serious problems that patients with advanced renal disease experience is falling. Patients with renal disease have multiple risk factors for falls and "fragility fractures." Muscle weakness, low blood pressure, particularly when upright (orthostatic hypotension) either caused by fluid removal during hemodialysis or antihypertensive medications, peripheral neuropathy, and vitamin D deficiency all contribute to the risk of serious falls in patients with renal disease. Desmet, Beguin, Swine, and Jadoul (2005) identified older age, diabetes, increased number of prescription drugs, use of antidepressants, and inability to walk more than 10 m without assistance as risk factors associated with falls. A third of the falls required medical attention and 3.9% of patients with a history of falling during an 8-week period of the study sustained a fall fracture during that year. Falls have been shown to be an independent risk factor of increased mortality, even after adjusting for age, dialysis vintage, comorbidity, and laboratory variables in the dialysis population (Li, Tomlinson, Naglie, Cook, & Jassal, 2008).

Physical therapy aimed at improving flexibility, balance, and range of movement will help improve patients' abilities to perform activities of daily living, such as stooping, bending, and reaching. Although strengthening (isometric) exercises such as weight lifting have been shown to increase blood pressure, well-selected exercises such as lifting and carrying objects, in moderation, help maintain muscle strength, which is also important for activities of daily living.

Preliminary studies in patients with CKD indicate that resistance training reduces markers of inflammation such as C-reactive protein and interleukin-6 as well as leads to skeletal muscle hypertrophy (Castaneda et al., 2004).

Maximal aerobic capacity as measured by peak oxygen uptake (VO_2 max) is reduced in patients with ESRD to roughly half of what is seen in normal sedentary individuals. Correction of anemia with rHuEPO results in an increase in the arterial oxygen content and improves VO_2 max by an average of 28%, but the change in VO_2 max is much smaller than that expected for the change in hemoglobin and arterial oxygen content. Painter and Moore (1994) have determined that normal subjects get nearly twice the VO_2 change per change in hemoglobin as compared to dialysis patients. Exercise training alone has been shown to improve VO_2 max by 25%.

As is well appreciated in the general population, exercise training offers other health benefits in dialysis patients. Endurance exercise training in hemodialysis patients offers cardiovascular risk benefits, including lowering of both systolic and diastolic blood pressure sufficient to decrease or withdraw antihypertensive therapy in a number of patients, and a decline in plasma triglycerides and VLDL levels while increasing high-level lipoprotein level (Hagberg et al., 1983; Harter & Goldberg, 1985; Miller, Cress, Johnson, Nichols, Schnitzler, 2002).

Although the best time for exercise in relation to hemodialysis is not clear, exercising training during dialysis sessions has the advantages of supervision and encouragement by the staff as well as a productive use of dialysis time. One can expect an improved compliance to exercise program. Flexibility, strengthening, and aerobic exercises can all be performed effectively during dialysis. Because of the likelihood of hypotension and muscle cramps during the latter part of dialysis, exercise is best performed in the first hour of dialysis. It has been suggested that exercise during dialysis might improve efficiency of the latter. Although there are some risks of musculoskeletal injury associated with participation in an exercise program for a patient with ESRD, proper patient selection makes this risk negligible.

Although traditionally vitamin D has been viewed in relation to its effects on bone and mineral metabolism and much emphasis has been placed on the bioactive form, 1–25 dihydroxy D3 (1–25 OH D3), there has been renewed interest in its precursor 25 hydroxy D3 (25 OH D3) and its effects on muscle strength, pain, cognitive function, autoimmune disease, heart disease, cancer, and mortality (Kovesdy & Kalantar-Zadeh, 2008; Stechschulte, Kirsner, & Federman, 2009; Taskapan, Wei, & Oreopoulos, 2006; Wolf et al., 2007). 25 OH D3 levels are found to be low in most patients with CKD and are associated with muscle weakness and musculoskeletal pain. Supplementation with 25 OH D3 has been shown to result in improvement in muscle strength and decrease the incidence of falls (Prince et al., 2008). The need for supplementation of 25 OH D3 in addition to optimum management of secondary hyperparathyroidism with active form of vitamin D (1–25 OH D3) or its analogs in patients with kidney disease has not been well studied.

PSYCHOLOGICAL AND VOCATIONAL REHABILITATION

In addition to the appropriate management of the gamut of abnormalities resulting from chronic renal failure outlined earlier, one must also address the issue of the patient returning to living a full life. For some, this may not mean returning to work, but feeling well enough to enjoy one's family and surroundings. The goal should be to help the patient to resume all the duties, responsibilities, and benefits he/she enjoyed before the illness. Psychological problems stemming from chronic illness, dependence on dialysis, sexual dysfunction, and change in status from an earning and supporting member of the family to a dependent person need to be identified and addressed. Gainful employment is extremely important for an adult in the earning period of his/her life to regain self-esteem and to interact with the society he/she lives in with confidence. However, the fear of losing financial benefits such as Social Security disability insurance and Social Security income may deter some patients from seeking employment, even if they are able to return to work. In several states, there are work-incentive programs whereby the state agencies waive the termination of financial benefits to persons with disabilities if they seek employment (Renal Rehabilitation Report, 1997). Assistance by a knowledgeable social worker in the field is extremely helpful in this regard. The USRDS Dialysis Morbidity and Mortality Study: Wave 2 conducted in 1996 (USRDS 2003 ADR) found that 37% of younger (18–54 years) and 16% of older (55+ years) patients reported that they were able to work at the start of therapy for ESRD. Of these, only 60% of the younger and 40% of the older group were actually employed. Patients' educational levels correlated with reported ability to work and with employment status. Consistent with the association of lower educational level and increased risk of chronic disease in the general population, dialysis patients with lower educational status were more likely to be diabetic. Rasgon et al. (1993, 1996) have shown that multidisciplinary predialysis intervention leads to maintenance of employment in a larger number of patients starting dialysis, both in the in-center setting as well as in the home hemodialysis and ambulatory peritoneal dialysis population. The quality of life is significantly better after a successful transplantation. A long-term study (Matas et al., 1996) showed that more than 40% of transplant recipients were employed part time or full time 8 years after transplantation.

The Life Options Rehabilitation Advisory Council, which was formed in 1993 by a group of patients, health care providers, researchers, government representatives and private business persons, has played a major role in bringing the rehabilitation and quality-of-life issues into focus. Through its website, www.lifeoptions.org, it acts as a resource guide for important issues related to encouragement, education, exercise, employment, and evaluation—the 5 Es— described as the bridges to rehabilitation for people with kidney failure. There are free publications on these issues directed not only toward patients, but also for health care professionals and social workers.

REFERENCES

Anavekar, N. S., McMurray, J. J. V., Velazquez, E. J., Solomon, S. D., Kober, L., Rouleau, J. L., et al. (2004). Relation between renal dysfunction and cardiovascular outcomes after myocardial infarction. *New England Journal of Medicine, 351,* 1285–1295.

Benigni, A., & Remuzzi, G. (2001). How renal cytokines and growth factors contribute to renal disease progression. *American Journal of Kidney Disease, 37*(Suppl. 2), S21–S24.

Block, G. A., Klassen, P. S., Lazarus, J. M., Ofsthun, N., Lowerie, E. G., & Chertow, G. M. (2004). Mineral metabolism, mortality, and morbidity in maintenance hemodialysis. *Journal of the American Society of Nephrology, 15,* 2208–2218.

Bottinger, E. P., & Bitzer, M. (2002). TGF-ß signaling in renal disease. *Journal of the American Society of Nephrology, 13,* 2600–2610.

Brenner, B. M., Cooper, M. E., Zeeuw, D., Keane, W. F., Mitch, W. E., Parving, H. H., et al. (2001). Effects of losartan on renal and cardiovascular outcomes in patients with type 2 diabetes and nephropathy. *New England Journal of Medicine, 345,* 861–869.

Canada-USA (CANUSA) Peritoneal Dialysis Study Group. (1996). Adequacy of dialysis and nutrition in continuous peritoneal dialysis: Association with clinical outcomes. *Journal of the American Society of Nephrology, 7,* 198–207.

Castaneda, C., Gordon, P., Parker, R., Uhlin, K. L., Rubenoff, R., & Levy, A. S. (2004). Resistance training to reduce the malnutrition-inflammation complex syndrome of chronic kidney disease. *American Journal of Kidney Disease, 43*, 607–616.

Charra, B., Calemard, E., Ruffet, M., Chazot, C., Terrat, J.-C., Vanel, T., et al. (1992). Survival as an index of adequacy of dialysis. *Kidney International, 41*, 1286–1291.

Chertow, G. M., Pupim, L. B., Block, G. A., Correa-Rotter, R., Tilman, B., Drueke, T. B., et al. (2007). Evaluation of cinacalcet therapy to lower cardiovascular events (EVOLVE): Rationale and design overview. *Clinical Journal of the American Society of Nephrology, 2*, 898–905.

Coresh, J., Selvin, E., Stevens, L. A., Manzi, J., Kusek, J. W., Eggers, P., et al. (2007). Prevalence of chronic kidney disease in the United States. *Journal of the American Medical Association, 298*, 2038–2047.

Couser, W. G. (2007). Chronic kidney disease—The promise and the perils. *Journal of the American Society of Nephrology, 18*, 2803–2805.

Desmet, C., Beguin, C., Swine, C., & Jadoul, M. (2005). Falls in hemodialysis patients: Prospective study of incidence, risk factors and complications. *American Journal of Kidney Disease, 45*, 148–153.

Drueke, T. B., Locatelli, F., Clyne, N., Eckardt, K. U., Macdougall, I. C., Tsakiris, D., et al. (2006). Normalization of hemoglobin level in patients with chronic kidney disease and anemia. *New England Journal of Medicine, 355*, 2071–2084.

Eknoyan, G., Beck, G. J., Cheung, A. K., Dougirdas, J. T., Greene, T., Kusek, J. W., et al. (2002). Effect of dialysis dose and membrane flux in maintenance hemodialysis. *New England Journal of Medicine, 347*, 2010–2019.

Elder, G. J., & Mackun, K. (2006). 25-Hydroxyvitamin D deficiency and diabetes predict reduced BMD in patients with chronic kidney disease. *Journal of Bone and Mineral Research, 21*, 1778–1784.

Ganz, T. (2007). Molecular control of iron transport. *Journal of the American Society of Nephrology, 18*, 394–400.

The GISEN Group. (1997). Randomised placebo-controlled trial of effect of ramipril on decline in glomerular filtration rate and risk of terminal renal failure in proteinuric, non-diabetic nephropathy. *The Lancet, 349*, 1857–1863.

Hagberg, J. M., Goldberg, A. P., Ehsani, A. A., Heath, G. W., Delmez, J. A., & Harter, H. R. (1983). Exercise training improves hypertension in hemodialysis patients. *American Journal of Nephrology, 3*, 209–212.

Hakim, R. M., Breyer, J., Ismail, N., & Schulman, G. (1994). Effect of dose of dialysis on mortality and morbidity. *American Journal of Kidney Diseases, 2*, 661–669.

Hallan, S. I., Ritz, E., Lydersen, S., Romundstad, S., Kvenild, K., & Orth, S. R. (2009). Combining GFR and albuminuria to classify CKD improves prediction of ESRD. *Journal of the American Society of Nephrology, 18*, 1069–1077.

Harter, H. R., & Goldberg, A. P. (1985). Endurance exercise training: An effective therapeutic modality for hemodialysis patients. *Medical Clinics of North America, 69*, 159–175.

Held, P. J., Port, F. K., Wolfe, R. A., Stannard, D. C., Carroll, C. E., Daugirdas, J. T., et al. (1996). The dose of hemodialysis and patient mortality. *Kidney International, 50*, 550–556.

Henry, R. M. A., Kostense, P. J., Bos, G., Dekker, J. M., Nijpels, G., Heine, R. J., et al. (2002). Mild renal insufficiency is associated with increased cardiovascular mortality: The Hoorn Study. *Kidney International, 62*, 1402–1407.

Ikizler, T. A., Greene, J., Wingard, R. L., Parker, R. A., & Hakim, R. M. (1995). Spontaneous dietary protein intake during progression of chronic renal failure. *Journal of the American Society of Nephrology, 6*, 1386–1391.

Johansen, K. L., Chertow, G. M., Jin, C., & Kutner, N. G. (2007). Significance of frailty among dialysis patients. *Journal of the American Society of Nephrology, 18*, 2960–2967.

Khan, N. A., Ma, I., Thompson, C. R., Humphries, K., Salem, D. N., Sarnak, M. J., et al. (2006). Kidney function and mortality among patients with left ventricular systolic dysfunction. *Journal of the American Society of Nephrology, 17*, 244–253.

Klahr, S., Levy, A. S., Beck, G. J., Caggiula, A. W., Hunsicker, L., Kusek, J. W., et al. (1994). The effects of dietary protein restriction and blood pressure control on the progression of chronic renal disease. Modification of diet in renal disease study group. *New England Journal of Medicine, 330*, 877–884.

Kovesdy, C. P., & Kalantar–Zadeh, K. (2008). Vitamin D receptor activation and survival in chronic kidney disease VDRA and CKD survival. *Kidney International, 73*, 1355–1363.

LaClair, R. E., Hellman, R. N., Karp, S. L., Kraus, M., Ofner, S., Li, Q., et al. (2005). Prevalence of calcitriol deficiency in CKD: A cross-sectional study across latitudes in the United States. *American Journal of Kidney Diseases, 45*, 1026–1033.

Lewis, E. J., Hunsicker, L. G., Bain, R. P., & Rohde, R. D., for The Collaborative Study Group. (1993). The effect of angiotensin-converting-enzyme inhibition on diabetic nephropathy. *New England Journal of Medicine, 329,* 1456–1462.

Lewis, E. J., Hunsicker, L. G., Clarke, W. R., Berl, T., Pohl, M. A., Lewis, J. B., et al. (2001). Renoprotective effect of the angiotensin-receptor antagonist irbesartan in patients with nephropathy due to type 2 diabetes. *New England Journal of Medicine, 345,* 851–860.

Li, M., Tomlinson, G., Naglie, G., Cook, W. L., & Jassal, S. V. (2008). Geriatric comorbidities, such as falls, confer an independent mortality risk to elderly dialysis patients. *Nephrology Dialysis Transplantation, 23,* 1396–1400.

London, G. M., Guérin, A. P., Verbeke, F. H., Pannier, B., Boutouyrie, P., Sylvain, J., et al. (2007). Mineral metabolism and arterial function in end-stage renal disease: Potential role of 25-hydroxyvitamin D deficiency. *Journal of the American Society of Nephrology, 18,* 613–620.

Lowrie, E. G., Huang, W. H., & Lew, N. L. (1995). Death risk predictors among peritoneal dialysis and hemodialysis patients: A preliminary comparison. *American Journal of Kidney Diseases, 26,* 220–228.

Lowrie, E. G., Laird, N. M., Parker, T. F., & Sargent, J. A. (1981). Effect of the hemodialysis prescription on patient morbidity. *New England Journal of Medicine, 305,* 1176–1180.

Mann, J. F. E., Schmieder, R. E., McQueen, M., Dyal, L., Schumacher, H., Pogue, J., et al. (2008). Renal outcomes with telmisartan, ramipril, or both, in people at high vascular risk (the ONTARGET study): A multicentre, randomised, double-blind, controlled trial. *The Lancet, 372,* 547–553.

Matas, A. J., Lawson, W., McHugh, L., Gilligham, K., Payne, W. D., Dunn, D. L., et al. (1996). Employment patterns after successful kidney transplantation. *Transplantation, 61,* 729–733.

Miller, B. W., Cress, C. L., Johnson, M. E., Nichols, D. H., & Schnitzler, M. A. (2002). Exercise during hemodialysis decreases the use of antihypertensive medications. *American Journal of Kidney Diseases, 39,* 828–833.

Moran, J., & Correa-Rotter, R. (2006). Revisiting the peritoneal dialysis dose. *Seminars in Dialysis, 19,* 102–104.

NKF-KDOQI (National Kidney Foundation-Kidney Disease Outcomes Quality Initiative). (2002). Clinical practice guidelines for chronic kidney disease: Evaluation, classification, and stratification. *American Journal of Kidney Disease, 39,* S46–S75.

NKF-KDOQI (National Kidney Foundation-Kidney Disease Outcomes Quality Initiative). (2003). Clinical practice guidelines for bone metabolism and disease in chronic kidney disease. *American Journal of Kidney Diseases, 42*(Suppl. 3), S1–S201.

NKF-DOQI (National Kidney Foundation-Dialysis Outcomes Quality Initiative). (1997). Clinical practice guidelines for hemodialysis adequacy. *American Journal of Kidney Diseases, 30*(Suppl. 2), S32–S37.

NKF-KDOQI (National Kidney Foundation-Kidney Disease Outcomes Quality Initiative). (2007). Clinical practice guidelines and clinical practice recommendations for anemia in chronic kidney disease. 2007 update of hemoglobin target. *American Journal of Kidney Diseases, 50,* 474–529.

Painter, P. L., & Moore, G. E. (1994). The impact of recombinant human erythropoietin on exercise capacity in hemodialysis patients. *Advances in Renal Replacement Therapy, 1,* 55–65.

Papovich, R. P., Moncrief, J. W., Decherd, J. F., Bomar, J. B., & Pyle, W. K. (1976). The definition of a novel portable-wearable equilibrium peritoneal dialysis technique [Abstract]. *Transactions of American Society of Artificial Internal Organs, 5,* 64.

Parker, T. F., III, Husni, L., Huang, W., Lew, N., & Lowrie, E. G. (1994). Survival of hemodialysis patients in the United States is improved with a greater quantity of dialysis. *American Journal of Kidney Diseases, 23,* 670–680.

Pfeffer, M. A., Burdmann, E. A., Chen, C. Y., Cooper, M. E., Zeeuw, D., Eckardt, K. U., et al. (2009). A trial of darbepoetin alfa in type 2 diabetes and chronic kidney disease. *New England Journal of Medicine, 361,* 2019–2032. Available from www.nejm.org

Pierratos, A. (2004). Daily nocturnal home hemodialysis. *Kidney International, 65,* 1975–1986.

Prince, R. L., Austin, N., Devine, A., Dick, I. M., Bruce, D., & Zhu, K. (2008). Effects of ergocalciferol added to calcium on the risk of falls in elderly high-risk women. *Archives of Internal Medicine, 168,* 103–108.

Rasgon, S., Schwankovsky, L., James-Rogers, A., Widrow, L., Glick, J., & Butts, E. (1993). An intervention for employment maintenance among blue-collar workers with end-stage renal disease. *American Journal of Kidney Diseases, 22,* 403–412.

Rasgon, S. A., Chemleski, B. L., Ho, S., Widrow, L., Yeoh, H. H., Schwankovsky, L., et al. (1996). Benefits of a multidisciplinary predialysis program in maintaining employment among patients on home dialysis. *Advances in Peritoneal Dialysis, 12,* 132–135.

Saran, R., Bragg-Gresham, J. L., Levin, N. W., Twardowski, Z. J., Wizemann, V., Saito, A., et al. (2006). Longer treatment time and slower ultrafiltration in hemodialysis: Associations with reduced mortality in the DOPPS. *Kidney International, 69,* 1222–1228.

Semenza, G. L. (2000). Surviving ischemia: Adaptive responses mediated by hypoxia-inducible factor 1. *Journal of Clinical Investigation, 106,* 809–812.

Singh, A. K., Szczech, L., Tang, K. L., Barnhart, H., Sapp, S., Wolfson, M., et al. (2006). Correction of anemia with epoetin alfa in chronic kidney disease. *New England Journal of Medicine, 355,* 2085–2098.

Stechschulte, S. A., Kirsner, R. S., & Federman, D. G. (2009). Vitamin D: Bone and beyond, rationale and recommendations for supplementation. *The American Journal of Medicine, 122,* 793–802.

Taskapan, H., Wei, M., & Oreopoulos, D. G. (2006). 25(OH) Vitamin D3 in patients with chronic kidney disease and those on dialysis: Rediscovering its importance. *International Urology Nephrology, 38,* 323–329.

Tokmakova, M. T., Skali, H., Kenchaiah, S., Braunwald, E., Rouleau, J. L., Packer, M., et al. (2004). Chronic kidney disease, cardiovascular risk, and response to angiotensin-converting enzyme inhibition after myocardial infarction: The survival and ventricular enlargement (SAVE) study. *Circulation, 110,* 3667–3673.

United States Renal Data System 2008 Annual Data Report. (2009). Available from http://www.usrds.org

Wenzel, R. R., Littke, T., Kuranoff, S., Jurgens, C., Bruck, H., Ritz, E., et al. (2009). Avosentan reduces albumin excretion in diabetics with macroalbuminuria. *Journal of the American Society of Nephrology, 20,* 655–664.

Work incentives: Thoughts from an expert. (1997). *Renal Rehabilitation Report, 5,* 3.

Wolf, M., Shah, A., Gutierrez, O., Ankers, E., Monroy, M., Tamez, H., et al. (2007). *Kidney International, 72,* 1004–1013.

24

Rheumatic Diseases

Sicy H. Lee, MD, and Steven B. Abramson, MD

Rheumatic diseases encompass all disorders in which some portion of the musculoskeletal system, including synovial joints, periarticular structures, or muscles, is involved. Arthritis is the general term used when the joint disease predominates in the patient's illness. Examples of some inflammatory arthritides include rheumatoid arthritis (RA), Reiter's syndrome, and psoriatic arthritis. In other conditions, the periarticular soft tissue or muscle disease is the primary concern, and the joint complaints are only a minor component. Some examples of these diseases include fibromyalgia, polymyositis, polymyalgia rheumatica, and scleroderma.

The classification of rheumatic diseases established by the American College of Rheumatology (ACR), the professional medical organization of the subspecialty of rheumatology, lists 116 rheumatic diseases under 10 major general classes of disorders. The current classification is based on known pathological changes induced in affected tissues, clinical patterns, and/or causative agents of each disease. The classification of the rheumatic diseases is a dynamic process that undergoes periodic review as important new information and concepts concerning pathophysiological mechanisms of these diseases are discovered.

According to the latest estimates derived from numerous surveys, there are more than 43 million persons suffering from some form of arthritis or related diseases in the United States. This number will reach 60 million by year 2020 (Centers for Disease Control and Prevention [CDC], 1990, 1994, 1998; Lawrence, Helmick, & Arnett, 1998). Among these individuals, at least 26% are partially disabled and about 10% are totally disabled. Arthritis and related diseases resulted in at least 45 million lost workdays yearly. These figures underscore the magnitude and the problems in diagnosis and management of these diseases. Furthermore, because most rheumatic diseases are chronic disabling conditions, these diseases as a group have significant social and economic ramifications. The rheumatic diseases detailed in this chapter, RA, spondyloarthropathies, and degenerative joint disease, are important because they are chronic disabling diseases that occur with relative frequency among individuals within the working population.

RHEUMATOID ARTHRITIS

The prevalence of RA in most White populations approaches 1% among adults aged 18 and older and increases with age, approaching 2% and 5% in men and women, respectively, by 65 years. The incidence also increases with age, peaking between the fourth and sixth decades. The annual incidence for all adults has been estimated at 67/100,000. Both prevalence and incidence are two and three times greater in women than in men (Hochberg, 1981).

Racial factors appear to be important in RA. American Blacks, native Japanese, and Chinese may have a lower prevalence of RA than do Whites, whereas several North American Indian tribes (the Yakima of central Washington State and the Mille-Lac Band of Chippewa in Minnesota) have a high prevalence of RA (Cunningham & Kelsey, 1984). Reasons for these differences are unknown but may relate to both genetic and environmental factors.

Genetic factors have an important role in the susceptibility to RA. The concordance among monozygotic twins is 25–50%, whereas the concordance among dizygotic twins is only 10%. Studies have demonstrated a strong association between the major histocompatibility complex (MHC) Class II antigen HLA-DR4 and RA across several racial groups. Furthermore, a region of the β-1 chain in the DR molecule, amino acid positions 67 to 74, is common among DR4 and non-DR4 individuals with RA, suggesting that this amino acid sequence may be integral to presenting autoimmunological peptides and thus confers the susceptibility to RA more specifically than the entire DR4 molecule (Gregersen, Lee, Silver, & Winchester, 1987).

The role of environmental factors, particularly infectious agents, as a causal factor in RA remains under active investigation.

Etiology and Pathogenesis

RA is an autoimmune disease in which the normal immune response is directed against an individual's own tissue, including the joints, tendons, and bones, resulting in inflammation and destruction of these tissues. The cause of RA is not known, but current evidence suggests that the initiating event is an immune reaction to a foreign antigen such as a virus or bacteria. In an individual with the genetic susceptibility for RA, this normal immune response is unchecked, perpetuating the inflammatory response. This theory is supported by the existence of an antibody called the rheumatoid factor (RF), which is initially formed in the synovial fluid and can be found in the serum of about 80% of patients who have had RA for several months. This antibody is unique in that it interacts with normal immunoglobulin G, which itself is an antibody. An experimental arthritis in animals similar to RA can be induced following inoculation of protein substances similar to these antibodies, supporting this hypothesis in part (Holmdahl, Nordling, Rubin, Tarkowski, & Klareskog, 1986).

During this process of inflammation, cells of the immune system, including monocytes, T lymphocytes, B lymphocytes, and neutrophils, are activated to secrete a variety of chemical substances. These chemicals further stimulate proliferation of the synovial cells that normally line the joints, causing fluid accumulation in the joints (effusion), destruction of cartilage, and erosion of bone. The erosions in the bone can be observed radiographically and are characteristic of RA. Pathologically, the typical feature is the invasion of the cartilage and bone by the pannus, a vascular granulation tissue composed of various numbers of inflammatory cells, synovial cells, and new blood vessels. The tendons and ligaments can be similarly affected.

Clinical Manifestations

RA is a systemic disease manifested primarily as polyarthritis. Although the diagnosis is made on clinical grounds, the most recent criteria, established by the ACR in 1987, afford a sensitivity of 91.2% and a specificity of 89.3% for diagnosing RA (Arnett et al., 1988). These include the following: (a) morning stiffness lasting at least 1 hour before maximal improvement; (b) arthritis of three or more joints or joint areas simultaneously for more than 6 weeks; (c) at least one of the joints involved should be the wrist, metacarpophalangeal joints (MCPs), or proximal interphalangeal joints (PIPs); (d) symmetrical pattern of joint involvement; (e) subcutaneous nodules over bony prominence, or extensor surfaces; (f) positive RF tested by any method that has been positive in less than 5% of normal control subjects; (g) radiographic changes that are typical of RA on posteroanterior views of the hands and wrists, including periarticular osteopenia or erosions.

RA usually has an insidious, slow onset over weeks to months. About 15–20% of individuals have a more rapid onset that develops over days to weeks. About 8–15% of individuals actually have acute onset of symptoms that develop over days. The initial symptoms may be systemic or articular. In some patients, fatigue, malaise, low-grade fever, or diffuse musculoskeletal pain may be the first nonspecific complaints. Morning stiffness is frequently the first presenting symptom prior to onset of joint pain. Although symmetrical pattern is common, asymmetric presentation is not unusual. The usual involvement is oligoarthritis progressing to polyarthritis in an additive but not migratory pattern. The most common joints involved in RA are MCPs (87%), PIPs (82%), and wrists (63%). Among larger joints, knees are most commonly involved (56%), followed by the shoulders (47%) and the hips. Medium-sized joints are the least commonly involved, with the ankles (53%) affected more frequently than the elbows (21%) (Harris, 1997).

The natural history of RA is varied. In a minority of patients, the intermittent course is marked by partial to complete remission without need for continuous therapy. This pattern of disease is usually mild. Initially, only a few joints are involved. Insidious return of the disease is often marked by progressive joint involvement. The majority of patients develop persistent disease requiring chronic therapy. At least 50% of patients will develop erosive disease of cartilage in bone, which in a significant minority of patients is progressive and debilitating. Recent studies by Pincus and Callahan (1992) and others underscore the increased mortality and morbidity among patients with RA.

Functional Presentation and Disability

In the initial stages of each joint involvement, there is warmth, pain, and redness, with corresponding decrease of range of motion of the affected joint. In the hand, soft-tissue swelling occurs as an early finding in RA and usually appears as fusiform enlargement of the PIPs. Patients describe difficulty in activity requiring motion of these joints, particularly in the morning. Progression of the disease results in reducible and later fixed deformities, including ulnar deviation, swan-neck, or boutonnière deformities (Figures 24.1 and 24.2). The distal

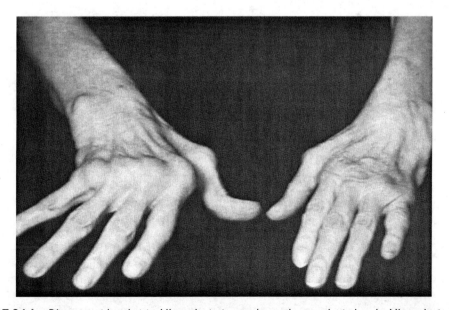

FIGURE 24.1   Rheumatoid arthritis: Ulnar deviation and muscle atrophy in hands. Ulnar deviation and subluxation of metacarpophalangeal joints are present in the hand on the left. The joints also appear swollen. Muscle atrophy has developed in the dorsal musculature of both hands. Reprinted with permission from American College of Rheumatology, 2009. From http://images.rheumatology.org

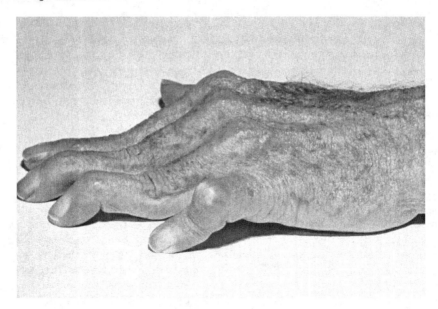

FIGURE 24.2   Rheumatoid arthritis: Swan-neck and boutonnière deformity in hand. Swan-neck deformities are seen in the second, third, and fourth digits of a patient with chronic rheumatoid arthritis. A boutonnière deformity of the fifth digit is present. Reprinted with permission from American College of Rheumatology, 2009. From http://images.rheumatology.org

interphalangeal joints (DIPs) are seldom involved in RA. Many patients are able to continue performing activities of daily living as well as various nondexterous vocational tasks. The most severe form is arthritis mutilans, in which there is complete bone and joint destruction and all movement is severely limited. At the wrist, there is decreased ability to extend or flex, with progression toward eventual fusion. An exaggerated flexion with near dislocation (subluxation) can occur in severe disease.

Deformities also occur at other joints. At the neck, there can be limitation in extension/flexion as well as rotation. The more serious deformities are those that result in neurological problems such as weakness and paralysis. The transverse ligaments that stabilize C-1 and C-2 vertebrae can become eroded. This results in C-1–C-2 (atlantoaxial) subluxation and can cause instability, with possible compression of the spinal cord or upward migration of the cervical spine and impingement of the medulla (brain). Such neurological involvement requires surgical intervention. The knees can decrease in flexion and can also develop flexion contracture. The hip may become limited in rotation or flexion extension. The ankle can be affected, with decreased ability to invert/overt or flex/extend. With inflammation or rupture of certain tendons, the foot can become flat. The toes mirror what occurs in the hands with involvement of the metatarsal phalangeal joints (MTPs) and PIPs. The most common deformities are hammer or cock-up toes with MTP subluxation and callus formation of the planter surface.

Muscle weakness and atrophy develop early in the course of the disease in many patients. The exact cause of these problems is not clear. One observation is that perhaps the patients are unable to move because of pain, and this lack of movement can cause further muscle atrophy and weakness. The combination of pain and muscle atrophy further diminishes the patient's ability to perform activities requiring both strength and dexterity. Therefore, the vocational and functional skills of the patient may be impaired early by pain, inflammation, and weakness. If the inflammation clears after several weeks and no damage has been done to the bone or cartilage, there will be usually no residual impairment. If the inflammation persists, permanent deformities can develop such that the mechanics of the joint are altered and the joint cannot function well, even though pain and inflammation may subside eventually.

Complications

There are a number of complications in RA. These include carpal tunnel syndrome, Baker's cyst, vasculitis, subcutaneous nodules, Sjögren's syndrome, peripheral neuropathy, cardiac and pulmonary involvement, Felty's syndrome, and anemia (Hurd, 1984). With the exception of carpal tunnel syndrome and Baker's cyst, these complications usually occur in the presence of seropositive, progressive, and destructive disease.

Carpal tunnel syndrome occurs when the proliferating synovial tissue compresses on the median nerve as it travels through the narrow space in the flexor surface of the wrist. It is characterized by numbness, tingling, and eventual loss of feeling in the thumb, second, and third fingers. The small muscles of the thumb may weaken and atrophy when the compression is not relieved.

Baker's cyst occurs when the synovial fluid escapes from the knee and collects in the space behind the knee, with extension into the calf. Rupture of the Baker's cyst can occur abruptly and cause sudden pain and swelling in the calf. These symptoms must be distinguished from venous thrombophlebitis by ultrasound studies.

Vasculitis is the inflammation of blood vessel, affecting capillaries and small- and medium-sized blood vessels. It can lead to skin lesions such as ulcers and subcutaneous nodules and to more severe problems, such as mononeuritis multiplex.

Subcutaneous nodules may develop in approximately 20–25% of patients. They typically occur in areas subject to pressure, such as the elbows, occiput, or sacrum. They may occasionally break down or become infected but generally are asymptomatic.

In Sjögren's syndrome, lymphocytes invade the glandular tissue of the mouth, nose, eyes, throat, and lungs, resulting in dry eyes (keratoconjunctivitis sicca) and dry mouth (xerostomia). The loss of glandular function may cause ulcers of the eye tissue, dental caries, and an inability to chew food normally. When dry eyes and dry mouth occur alone, the sicca syndrome is said to be present. When sicca syndrome is accompanied by RA, the condition is termed Sjögren's syndrome. The lymphocytes can also invade the kidneys, liver, lungs, and other internal organs, resulting in their dysfunction.

Many patients with RA can develop peripheral neuropathy and complain of mild numbness and tingling in their fingers and toes. Rarely, they can develop mononeuritis and lose complete function of a major nerve. This loss of nerve function is due to inflammation of the blood vessels that supply the nerve. When more than one nerve is involved, it is termed mononeuritis multiplex.

The most common cardiac involvement in RA is pericardial effusion or accumulation of fluid around the heart, which is reported in about 40% of patients at autopsy but is usually clinically asymptomatic. When symptomatic pericarditis occurs, it will rarely proceed to pericardial tamponade where emergency surgical intervention to relieve the pressure around the heart is necessary. Sometimes, a focal myocarditis may be recognized. Lesions similar to rheumatoid nodules may be found involving the myocardium and the valves. Valvular insufficiency, conduction abnormalities, and myocardial infarction secondary to these inflammatory lesions may occasionally be seen as clinical manifestations of rheumatoid heart disease.

There is an increased risk of premature death in patients with RA. Recently, it has become clear that this is largely due to cardiovascular disease, particularly coronary artery disease (CAD). A meta-analysis of 24 observational studies comprising 111,758 patients concluded that the risk of CAD mortality was higher by 59% in patients with RA (Avina-Zubieta et al., 2008).

Several forms of pulmonary disease can occur in patients with RA. Rheumatoid pleural disease, though frequently found at autopsy, is most commonly asymptomatic. Pleural effusions or fluid in the pleural cavity can develop, but rarely will they accumulate to significant size and cause respiratory distress. Multiple pulmonary nodules may occur bilaterally. Another more serious pulmonary manifestation of RA is interstitial fibrosis with pneumonitis. This may progress to a honeycomb appearance on X-rays, with bronchiectasis, chronic cough, and progressive dyspnea. Lung biopsy can show chronic inflammatory cell infiltration accompanied by neutrophils and eosinophils. Laryngeal obstruction can also be caused by arthritis of the cricoarytenoid joint.

Felty's syndrome is characterized by splenomegaly, lymphadenopathy, anemia, thrombocytopenia, and neutropenia in association with chronic active RA. Systemic manifestations such as fever, fatigue, anorexia, and weight loss are common. Hyperpigmentation and leg ulcers may accompany Felty's syndrome.

The anemia of RA can be due to either chronic inflammation that primarily affects the production of red blood cells in the bone marrow or to iron deficiency secondary to occult blood loss in individuals treated with medications that can cause gastritis or peptic ulcer disease. Frequently, a combination of both factors can be present.

Laboratory Diagnosis

RF, antibodies to cyclic citrullinated peptides (CCPs), increased levels of the erythrocyte sedimentation rate (ESR), and C-reactive protein (CRP) are often found in patients with RA. RFs and anti-CCP antibodies are useful in diagnosis and may be helpful in monitoring the activity of disease (Visser, le Cessie, Vos, Breedveld, & Hazes, 2002). RFs, which are antibodies to the constant region of immunoglobulins, occur in 70–80% of patients with RA. They are not specific for RA, as they are also found in patients with mixed cryoglobulinemia, Sjögren's syndrome, 20–30% of those with *systemic lupus erythematosus*, and 5–10% of healthy individuals. In contrast, anti-CCP antibodies are found in 60–70% of patients with RA but less often in other diseases. Both RF and anti-CCP antibodies predict erosive disease among patients with RA.

Treatment and Prognosis

A variety of medications are available in the treatment of RA (Harris, 1997). The approach to the individual patient with RA is determined by a careful analysis of the severity of the patient's disease and rate of progression of the disease, as well as an assessment of the patient's other comorbid conditions. Clinical assessment is supplemented by laboratory and radiographic assessment. Because articular cartilage or bone in humans cannot be replaced, the goal of the therapy must be to arrest the synovitis prior to any irreversible damage (American College of Rheumatology, 2002). The drugs available to treat RA can be divided into several broad categories (Table 24.1).

Analgesics
These drugs include topical (e.g., capsaicin or diclofenac) and oral agents (e.g., acetaminophen [paracetamol], propoxyphene, tramadol), and more potent opioids (e.g., oxycodone, hydrocodone). Nonsteroidal anti-inflammatory drugs (NSAIDs), which include cyclooxygenase 2 (COX-2) selective agents, have both analgesic and anti-inflammatory properties but do not alter disease outcomes. Selective inhibitors are preferred for patients at higher risk for adverse gastroduodenal effects (Desai et al., 2008).

Glucocorticoids
In patients with extensive synovitis who do not obtain relief from NSAIDs, low-dose steroids can be given for temporary relief. Prednisone in doses up to 7.5 mg daily is used in RA for symptomatic control. Even at low doses, oral corticosteroids may promote osteoporosis, and therefore concomitant treatment with antiresorptive agents should be considered. Moreover, patients who require treatment with corticosteroids should be considered for disease-modifying antirheumatic drug (DMARD) treatment, and once the disease is controlled or improved on DMARDs, steroid therapy should be tapered and discontinued. Steroids alone should never be the mainstay of medical therapy because they do not appear to prevent cartilage damage and because of their side effects. Long-term steroid use can result in early cataract

TABLE 24.1 *Agents Used to Treat RA*

Agent (Brand Name)	Dose
Analgesics/anti-inflammatories	
Salicylates	1,000–5,000 mg/day (adjusted based on serum salicylate levels)
Aspirin	
Sodium salicylate	
Salicylic acid (Trilisate)	
Diflunisal (Dolobid)	
NSAIDs	
Ibuprofen (Motrin/Advil)	400–800 mg t.i.d.-q.i.d.
Sulindac (Clinoril)	150–200 mg b.i.d.
Piroxicam (Feldene)	10–20 mg q.d.
Indomethacin (Indocin)	25–50 mg b.i.d.-q.i.d., 75 mg SR
Meclofenamate (Meclomen)	50–100 mg b.i.d.-q.i.d.
Naproxen (Naprosyn/Aleve)	250–500 mg b.i.d.
Ketoprofen (Orudis/Oruvail)	50–75 mg b.i.d.-q.i.d., 200 mg q.d.
Oxaprozin (Daypro)	1,200–1,800 mg q.d.
Tolmetin (Toextin)	200–400 mg b.i.d.-q.i.d.
Diclofenac (Voltaren/Arthrotec)	25–75 mg b.i.d.
Flurbiprofen (Ansaid)	50–100 mg b.i.d.
Corticosteroids	5.0–15 mg q.d. for arthritis
Oral prednisone	Higher doses for extra-articular disease
Intra-articular	Varies with joint size
Disease-modifying agents (slow-acting agents)	
Gold	
Oral (Ridaura)	3 mg q.i.d.-b.i.d.
Parenteral (Solganal)	50 mg q month IM
D-penicillamine (Depen)	125–1,000 mg q.d.
Hydroxychloroquine (Plaquenil)	200–600 mg q.d.
Sulfasalazine (Entab)	1,000–1,500 mg b.i.d.
Immunosuppressive agents	
Methotrexate (PO, IM, IV)	5.0–30 mg/week
Azathioprine (Imuran)	25–150 mg q.d.
Leflunomide (Arava)	10–20 mg q.d.
Cyclophosphamide (Cytoxan)	25–150 mg q.d.
Mycophenolate acid (Cellcept)	1 gm b.i.d.
Cyclosporin (Neoral)	2–4 mg/kg/day
Biologic agents	
TNF receptor antagonist	
Etanercept (Enbrel)	SQ 50 mg q week
Adalimumab (Humira)	SQ 40 mg q 2 weeks
Infliximab (Remicaide)	IV 3–10 mg/kg q 2 months
Golimumab (Samponi)	SQ 50 mg q month
Certulizumab (Cimzia)	SQ 200 mg q 2 weeks
IL-1 receptor antagonist (Kineret)	SQ 10 µg q.d.
IL-6 monoclonal antibody	
Tocilizumab (Actemra)	IV 8 mg/kg q month
Anti-CTLA-4 monoclonal antibody	
Abatacept (Orencia)	IV 500–1,000 mg q month

formation, osteoporosis, peptic ulcer disease, augmentation or initiation of hypertension and diabetes, increased skin and vascular fragility, delayed wound healing, muscle weakness, unsightly weight gain and fat accumulation on the face and the trunk, and poor resistance to bacterial and other opportunistic (e.g., fungal) infections.

DMARDs

DMARDs may be either traditional or biological drugs, which are produced by recombinant DNA technology. DMARDs have the potential to reduce or prevent joint damage and preserve joint integrity and function. In individuals who have persistent disease, DMARDs should be initiated as soon as possible.

There is now an increasing tendency to begin DMARDs earlier and more aggressively in the course of the patient's illness. This tendency resulted from the emerging view that there is a brief window of opportunity early in the patient's illness to halt the inflammatory process. Once articular damage occurs, the destructive process appears to self-perpetuate and cannot be reversed with medications. There is evidence that radiographic damage can occur within 2 years of onset of disease. Therefore, individuals who have evidence of disease activity as measured by swollen and tender joints, elevated CRP or sedimentation rate, elevated RF and/ or anti-CCP, and constitutional symptoms including morning stiffness, fever, and weight loss should be aggressively treated with DMARDs so that remission is achieved as soon as possible. The traditional DMARDs include hydroxychloroquine, sulfasalazine, methotrexate, leflunomide, and minocycline. The ACR 2008 recommendations, based upon a systematic literature review and expert consensus, differentiate among these agents: methotrexate and leflunomide are preferred to sulfasalazine in patients with high disease activity and features associated with a poor prognosis (Saag et al., 2008; Smolen, Kalden, & Scott, 1999).

Parenteral gold and D-penicillamine are rarely used and have potential major side effects, including nephrosis (protein in the urine), anemia, leukopenia, thrombocytopenia, stomatitis, skin rash, and interstitial pulmonary fibrosis. Therefore, close laboratory and clinical monitoring is required while patients are on these medications. For the patient to accept these potentially toxic medications, the physician must adequately explain the necessity for their use. Oral gold and antimalarials have less toxic side effects but are also less likely to be effective. Because of the potential damage to the retina, regular ophthalmological examination is necessary while the patient is on antimalarials. Methotrexate has gained widespread use and is relatively easy to administer as it is given once a week. The drug is effective, but there are concerns about its long-term toxicity, particularly pulmonary and hepatic fibrosis (Tugwell, Bennett, & Gent, 1987). Sulfasalazine has gained popularity in Europe as an effective DMARD (Pinals, Kaplan, Lawson, & Hepburn, 1986). The adverse effects associated with the use of this drug include blood dyscrasias, drug fever, hepatitis, allergic pneumonitis, drug-induced lupus, vasculitis, and significant cutaneous reaction including exfoliative dermatitis. Very few serious reactions have been reported in RA patients, and the adverse events appear to occur more commonly among slow acetylators. Leflunomide (Arava) is a reversible pyramidine inhibitor and appears similar to methotrexate and sulfalazine in efficacy; its major potential adverse effect is hepatotoxicity, and monitoring is required monthly (Strand, Cohen, & Schiff, 1999). Other cytotoxic drugs (azathioprine, cyclosporine, cyclophosphamide) appear effective but also have many potential side effects, particularly hepatic, renal, and hematological toxicities, and require careful monitoring (Yocum, Klippel, & Wilder, 1988).

The newest group of DMARDs in the treatment of RA is the biological agents (Siddiqui, 2007). These agents are unique in that they target a specific arm or subpopulation of cells within the immune system so that the inflammatory response in RA is abrogated. The majority of the approved agents target tumor necrosis factor (TNF). Etanercept (Enbrel) is a soluble TNF-receptor antagonist and is a recombinant receptor fusion protein (Bathon, Martin, & Fleishmann, 1967). Infliximab (Remicaide) is a chimeric anti-TNF monoclonal antibody (approximately 25% mouse protein) and approved for the treatment of RA in combination with methotrexate (Maini, Clair, & Breedveld, 1999). Adalimumab (Humira) is a fully humanized anti-TNF monoclonal antibody (Weinblatt, Keystone, & Furt, 2003). Anikinra (Kineret) is an IL-1 receptor antagonist and the only approved IL-1 antagonist; it has not proven to be among the more efficacious of the available RA biological treatments (Bresnihan, Alvaro-Gracia, & Cobby, 1998; Dayer, 1990). More recently approved biological therapies for RA include rituximab (Ritxuan, anti-CD20) and abatacept (Orencia, cytotoxic T-lymphocyte antigen 4 immunoglobulin), and tocilizumab (Actemra), an anti-interleukin (IL)-6 receptor.

Another growing trend in the medical management of RA is the early use of combination drug therapy in aggressive disease. Smaller doses of multiple drugs with synergistic effects are used, in effect lowering the level of toxicity of individual drugs and enhancing the efficacy of treatment. Multiple studies have demonstrated that giving all the biological agents in combination with methotrexate is more effective in preventing radiographic progression than when methotrexate or any of the biological agents are given as monotherapy. The ultimate challenge for the future is to devise safe and effective therapies that can be administered in early stages of the disease.

Surgical treatment in RA should be used in combination with medical therapy. In patients with severe synovitis and in whom the slow-acting agents have not yet taken effect, early synovectomy (removal of the synovial tissue to as great a degree as possible) can be considered for the elbows and knees. When permanent deformities have developed despite medical therapy, surgery can be performed to correct these deformities to decrease pain and improve the patient's functional status. These procedures include joint fusions (e.g., wrist fusion to provide a stable and painless wrist), resections (e.g., resection of the distal ends of the metatarsal heads to reduce foot pain and improve comfort and walking), and joint prostheses. The most successful total joint replacements are the hips and knees; joint replacements for the shoulder, elbow, and ankle are available but are less successful.

Rehabilitation therapy is an integral part of treatment in RA. In early disease, the goal is to reduce pain and inflammation and to prevent deformities and muscle atrophy. As the disease progresses, it is an important modality to correct deformities and increase strength. The major goal at each stage is to improve functional skills in the patient. Modalities that are used to reduce pain and inflammation include moist heat, paraffin baths, and cold packs that allow more activities to be performed with less discomfort. Acupuncture sometimes can be used as an adjunct to decrease swelling or pain. The choice of treatment depends largely on patient's preference because there are few data upon which one can base the choice. The pain relief is temporary, lasting perhaps 2 hours. It is important, therefore, that the patient be taught how to perform these treatments at home. Placing a joint in plastic, fiberglass, or plaster splints will protect the joint and diminish the inflammation. There must be a balance between exercise and rest, however, to prevent deterioration of motion and muscle atrophy. Splints are most conveniently placed on the wrists or hands. For some, night use alone may be sufficient.

Exercise is important to help prevent contractures as well as preserve and improve muscle strength. Nonweight-bearing and isometric exercises will allow improvement in strength without joint inflammation. Passive range-of-motion exercises will help preserve motion without stress on the joints. Physical and occupational therapists should also evaluate the patient's functional limitations in activities of daily living and ambulation. Patients should be taught ambulation and transfer techniques. Devices such as reachers, hooks, and built-up utensil handles can be provided. The occupational therapist may also make energy- or labor-saving recommendations for the home, such as the raising or lowering of tabletops or changing to more easily activated faucet handles. All of these measures aim to allow the patient to be more functional and independent.

The majority of patients with RA respond partially to some form of therapy, but few go into true remission, defined as absence of radiographic progression and clinical symptoms. The general course of RA, then, is gradual diminution of inflammation but progression of deformities (Pincus & Callahan, 1992). The speed with which the deformities occur varies from patient to patient. Factors associated with poor prognosis include persistent inflammation despite aggressive medical therapy of more than 1 year's duration; onset of disease below age 30; presence of extra-articular manifestation of RA, including subcutaneous nodules, vasculitis, Sjögren's syndrome, and neuropathy; and high-titer RF.

Psychological and Vocational Implications

Patients with RA undergo several stages of psychological adjustments. In the early stages of disease, it is common for patients with RA to be frightened because of the uncertainty of the prognosis of the disease and the degree of disability. Many patients also tend to blame themselves or a particular incident for the onset of the disease. Along with this feeling of guilt, there is also denial. Many patients do not give up hope that one day the disease and pain will miraculously vanish. This type of denial may lead to unrealistic expectations and resistance to medical treatment. As the disease progresses, the patient may express various degrees of anger, frustration, resentment, and depression. Some patients adapt to their disease and disability, and function well with limited abilities, whereas other patients seem incapacitated by fairly minimal involvement. Adaptation to RA requires the patient to have self-confidence and willingness to adjust certain aspects of his or her lifestyle without sacrificing independence. This adaptation is difficult and may be thwarted by pain denial, anger, and depression. Another reaction to the disease is hopelessness and increased dependency. Faced with the prospect of progressive deformities and apparent deterioration, the patient may give up trying to remain active by increasingly depending on others for care.

Not all individuals with RA progress unremittingly to disability. In the minority of patients with mild disease, fewer adjustments are required and vocational goals can be easily met. However, in individuals in whom the disease is an evolving and dynamic process, the vocational counselor should make frequent assessment of the patient's functional ability as the disease progresses and provide realistic goals and support through the more difficult periods so that employment can be sustained.

In general, motor coordination, finger and hand dexterity, and eye–hand–foot coordination are adversely affected by RA. Vocational goals dependent upon fine, dextrous, or coordinated movements of the hand are therefore not ideal for patients with RA. Loss of motion and pain on motion slow the patient's movements and diminish coordination. Therefore, the operation of machines requiring repetitive, dexterous, and rapid movements is also not a desirable choice. However, if the force required is quite low, dexterous tasks such as the use of an electric typewriter or computer are quite possible.

Most jobs requiring medium to heavy physical activity are also not desirable. Although most patients may be able to perform moderate manual labor (i.e., lift 25–30 lb), such level of activity will not be sustainable as the disease progresses. In addition, such a workload may be harmful to the joints. Activities such as climbing, balancing, stooping, kneeling, standing, or walking are all hampered by pain on weight bearing or with motion. Although these activities can be accomplished by most individuals with milder forms of RA, jobs requiring such activities repetitively and without periods of rest cannot be sustained and indeed may damage joints.

It is usual for patients with RA to detect changes in humidity, temperature, or barometric pressure. Therefore, extremes of weather or abrupt changes in temperature should be avoided, and an indoor climate in which the environment is relatively controlled is recommended. Excessive noise, vibration, fumes, gases, dust, and poor ventilation have no specific effects on patients with RA except for those individuals with appreciable pulmonary involvement.

Advanced or additional educational goals such as vocational training and/or college courses of 2–4 years should be strongly considered for individuals with recent-onset RA and those with long-standing disease despite increased mortality and morbidity among the latter. Educational goals should be guided by the patient's interest and aptitude. It is important to realize that the individual with RA does not have a permanent invariant disability but rather a changing disability with chronic pain (which can vary from day to day) that generally results in a progressive and unfavorable outcome. Such individuals require ongoing coordinated counseling that provides a combination of empathy, encouragement, and adequate evaluation and treatment.

SERONEGATIVE SPONDYLOARTHROPATHIES

The seronegative spondyloarthropathies consist of a group of related disorders that include Reiter's syndrome, ankylosing spondylitis, psoriatic arthritis, and arthritis in association with inflammatory bowel disease. This group of diseases occurs more commonly among young men, with a mean age at diagnosis in the third decade and a peak incidence between ages 25 and 34. The prevalence appears to be approximately 1%. The male-to-female ratio approaches 4 to 1 among adult Caucasians (Hochberg, 1992).

Genetic factors play an important role in the susceptibility to each disease. Among Caucasians, more than 90% of patients with ankylosing spondylitis are HLA-B27, and approximately 20% of individuals with the HLA-B27 antigen will develop some form of spondyloarthritis. In addition, disease concordance for ankylosing spondylitis among monozygotic twins exceeds 50%. Linkage to other MHC Class I antigens that are cross-reactive with B27 (B7, B22, B40, B42) has also been observed, particularly among Blacks, in whom the association between ankylosing spondylitis and HLA-B27 (40–50%) is not as striking as that in Caucasians (Arnett, 1984).

Etiology and Pathogenesis

The cause of spondyloarthritis is unclear, but there is strong evidence that the initial event involves interaction between genetic factors determined by Class I MHC genes and environmental factors, particularly bacterial infections. The onset of musculoskeletal symptoms following exposure to infections suggests an immunologically mediated process, as does the finding of lymphocytes at the sites of inflammation.

Reiter's syndrome may follow a wide range of gastrointestinal infections, including species of *Salmonella, Shigella, Yersinia, Campylobacter,* and *Escherichia coli* (Arnett, 1984). Recent work by Schumacher has identified chlamydial organisms in the synovial tissue. *Giardia, Brucella,* and *Streptococcus* organisms have also been implicated, as well as amoebas and episodes of diarrhea in which no specific pathogen can be identified have been reported (Callin & Fries, 1976; Voltonen, Leirisalo, & Pentikainen, 1985). Arthritis also occurs in association with inflammatory bowel disease in patients who have undergone intestinal bypass operations for obesity and in Whipple's disease. Bowel inflammation has been implicated in the pathogenesis of endemic Reiter's syndrome, psoriatic arthritis, and ankylosing spondylitis. A putative link between these diverse conditions is the ability of enteric organisms to gain access to the systemic circulation and to initiate an immune response in a genetically susceptible individual. The observation that some bacterial antigens share certain amino acid sequences with the HLA-B27 molecule suggests molecular mimicry as a plausible mechanism to explain the link between infection and arthritis in the presence of HLA-B27 (Inman, Chiu, Johnston, & Falk, 1992). This association, however, does not explain why only 20% of HLA-B27 individuals develop arthritis in the face of appropriate enteric infection. Whether there are fewer evident genetic differences between healthy and diseased HLA-B27-positive individuals remain under investigation.

Clinical Manifestations

The spondyloarthropathies share certain common features, including the absence of serum RF, an oligoarthritis commonly involving large joints in the lower extremities, frequent involvement of the axial skeleton, familial clustering, and linkage to HLA-B27. Unlike RA, in which the predominant site of inflammation is the synovium, these disorders are characterized by inflammation at sites of attachment of ligament, tendon, fascia, or joint capsule to bone (enthesopathy).

Because the musculoskeletal presentation in each of the seronegative disorders is indistinguishable, current classification schemes are based on the presence of extra-articular features such as psoriasis, colitis, urethritis, aphthous stomatitis, inflammatory eye disease, nail changes, and keratoderma blenorrhagicum. Unfortunately, none of these features is unique to any particular disease. Psoriasis may occur in the setting of inflammatory bowel disease, aphthous stomatitis may occur in any of the seronegative disorders, keratoderma may be indistinguishable from pustular psoriasis, and axial changes in psoriatic or colitic arthritis can be indistinguishable from primary ankylosing spondylitis. Overlap syndromes are common. Finally, there are patients with oligoarthritis and enthesopathy who lack sufficient extra-articular features to allow a specific diagnosis by existing criteria. HLA typing may provide a means of establishing that these patients have a disorder that falls within the spectrum of spondyloarthropathy. Given these pitfalls, the most accurate way of classifying a given patient may be to delineate fully the clinical features of the disease as well as the immunogenetic background in which it occurs.

Ankylosing spondylitis is the prototype disease among this group of disorders. The diagnosis is confirmed by clinical and radiographic findings. Existing criteria include the Rome and the New York criteria (Table 24.2) (Bennett & Burch, 1967). Ankylosing spondylitis is considered primary if no other rheumatological disorder is present and secondary if the patient has evidence of Reiter's syndrome, psoriasis, or colitis.

Reiter's syndrome was first described by Reiter in 1916 and consists of the triad of arthritis, urethritis, and conjunctivitis. Paronen (1948) subsequently pointed out the association of antecedent infectious urethritis or dysentery with the clinical triad. Arnett introduced the concept of incomplete Reiter's syndrome to describe those individuals who had only two of the features of the triad and underscored the association of the incomplete syndrome with HLA-B27 (Arnett, McClusky, & Schacter, 1976). The most current ACR criteria are much broader; they define Reiter's syndrome as a seronegative arthritis that follows urethritis, cervicitis, or dysentery. Possible associated features include balanitis, inflammatory eye disease, oral ulcers, and keratoderma. Callin has proposed a broader definition (Table 24.3) that gives added weight to these extra-articular features (Fox, Callin, Gerber, & Gibson, 1979).

Psoriatic arthritis is not a single disease entity but consists of many different patterns of musculoskeletal disorders occurring in individuals with psoriasis. Patients may present with disease that is clinically indistinguishable from RA, ankylosing spondylitis, or Reiter's syndrome. The most widely used criteria are those of Moil and Wright (Table 24.4) (Bennett,

---

TABLE 24.2 *New York Criteria for Ankylosing Spondylitis (AS) (1966)*

Diagnosis:
  Limitation of the lumbar spine in all three planes—anterior flexion, lateral flexion, and extension
  History of or presence of pain in the dorsolumbar junction or in the lumbar spine
  Limitation of chest expansion to 1 inch (2.5 cm) or less measured at the level of the fourth intercostal space

Grading (requires radiographs of sacroiliac joints):
  Definite AS
    Grade 3–4 bilateral sacroiliitis with at least one clinical criterion
    Grade 3–4 unilateral or grade 2 bilateral sacroiliitis with clinical criterion 1 or with clinical criteria 2 and 3
  Probable AS
    Grade 3–4 bilateral sacroiliitis with no clinical criteria

From Bennett, P. H., & Burch, T. A. (1967). New York symposium on population studies in the rheumatic diseases: New diagnostic criteria. *Bulletin on the Rheumatic Diseases, 17*, 453–469. Reprinted with permission.

TABLE 24.3   *Clinical Criteria for Reiter's Syndrome*

Seronegative asymmetric arthropathy (predominately lower extremity) plus one or more of the following:
  Urethritis
  Cervicitis
  Inflammatory eye disease
  Mucocutaneous disease: balanitis, oral ulceration, or keratoderma
Exclusions:
  Primary ankylosing spondylitis
  Psoriatic arthropathy
  Other rheumatic disease

From Fox, R., Callin, A., Gerber, R. C., & Gibson, D. (1979). The chronicity of symptoms and disability in Reiter's syndrome: An analysis of 131 consecutive patients. *Annals of Internal Medicine, 91*, 190–207. Reprinted with permission.

1979). Complicating this classification scheme is the observation that in up to 20% of patients, the musculoskeletal disease antedates the onset of psoriasis. Therefore, an individual with dactylitis and radiographic evidence of pencil-in-cup deformities may be considered to have psoriatic arthritis even if the patient lacks skin disease. A family history of psoriasis or the presence of psoriasis-associated HLA alleles would further support this diagnosis (Mielants, Veys, & Cuvelier, 1985).

There are no distinct criteria for the enteropathic arthritis accompanying ulcerative colitis or Crohn's disease. A clinical spectrum of diseases similar to those seen in association with psoriasis may be observed. In an individual patient, axial disease, peripheral arthritis, or enthesopathy may predominate. Peripheral arthritis tends to parallel activity of bowel disease, whereas axial disease may progress independent of bowel activity. Complicating the

TABLE 24.4   *Diagnosis of Psoriatic Arthritis*

Established inflammatory musculoskeletal disease (joint, spine or entheseal) with three or more of the following:

1. Psoriasis	
(a) Current*	Psoriatic skin or scalp disease present today as judged by a qualified health professional
(b) History	A history of psoriasis that may be obtained from patient or qualified health professional
(c) Family history	A history of psoriasis in a first- or second-degree relative according to patient report
2. Nail changes	Typical psoriatic nail dystrophy including onycholysis, pitting, and hyperkeratosis observed on current physical examination
3. Negative test for RF	By any method except latex but preferably by enzyme-linked immunosorbent assay or nephelometry, according to the local laboratory reference range
4. Dactylitis	
(a) Current	Swelling of an entire digit
(b) History	A history of dactylitis recorded by a qualified health professional
5. Radiological evidence of juxta-articular new bone formation	Ill-defined ossification near joint margins (but excluding osteophyte formation) on plain X-rays of hand or foot

* Current psoriasis awarded 2 points. Criteria yield specificity 98.7%, sensitivity 91.4%
From Taylor, W. J., Gladman, D., Helliwell, P., Marchesoni, A., Mease, P., Mielants, H., et al. (2006). Classification criteria for psoriatic arthritis: Development of new criteria from a large international study. *Arthritis and Rheumatism, 54*, 2665–2673. Reprinted with permission.

concept of enteropathic arthritis as a distinct disease is the observation that low-grade bowel inflammation may be found on colonic or ileal biopsy in all of the seronegative disorders.

Patients with spondyloarthropathy may also develop inflammation of the aorta (aortitis) and the aortic valve, resulting in aortic insufficiency. Pulmonary fibrosis may also occur, resulting in diminished diffusion capacity and restrictive lung disease.

Functional Presentation and Disability

When the axial skeleton is involved, the initial symptom is morning stiffness and lower-back pain. As the disease worsens, there is progressive diminution of motion of the spine. Eventually, the sacroiliac joints and lumbar, thoracic, and cervical spine become fused, although the process may skip over parts. At this stage, the spine is no longer painful, but the patient has lost all ability to flex or rotate the spine and generally develops a hunched-over posture with fused flexion of the cervical spine and flexion contracture of the hips to compensate for the loss of the lordosis curvature in the lumbar spine. The joints where the ribs attach to the vertebrae are also affected, and chest expansion and lung volume are decreased. Frequently, peripheral joints are involved, and the pattern is usually asymmetric oligoarthritis involving primarily the large or medium joints, including the hips, knees, and ankles. Rarely are smaller joints or the joints in the upper extremities involved. Enthesopathy can occur at multiple sites but more commonly presents as planter fasciitis, Achilles tendonitis, and medial or lateral epicondylitis.

Loss of motion of the spine or pain in the spine with motion generally affects a patient's mobility, making certain chores difficult. Walking, however, remains unimpaired unless the hips and knees are affected. Frequent stooping and bending becomes impossible. Toilet activities and dressing may be difficult, but rarely does the patient become dependent. In fact, a patient with ankylosing spondylitis is typically able to continue vocational activity despite progressive stiffness, unless it requires significant back mobility or physical labor.

Treatment and Prognosis

NSAIDs are the initial primary agents in the treatment of seronegative spondyloarthritis. Indomethacin is commonly regarded as being the most effective. Other NSAIDs, including naproxen, piroxicam, meclofenamate, and flurbiprofen, are also efficacious. Salicylates are generally not effective treatment. Corticosteroids, when given at significantly higher doses than that used in RA, can also be quite effective. If the inflammation does not completely resolve with NSAIDs alone or erosive disease is present at the initial evaluation, DMARDs should be given to prevent joint destruction and fusion. Just as in RA, the initiation of DMARDs in early disease is recommended to prevent progression of disease. The more common DMARDs used in the treatment of spondyloarthritis include sulfasalazine and methotrexate (Nissila, Lehtinen, & Leirisalo-Repo, 1988). Parenteral gold has been found to be effective therapy in patients with the form of psoriatic arthritis that mimics RA. Anti-TNF biological agents are currently approved by the FDA in the treatment of psoriatic arthritis and ankylosing spondylitis. Surgical intervention includes either early synovectomy or total joint replacement in the later stages of disease. Physical therapy is also an integral part of treatment in this disease. Exercises should be done daily and should include those that enable the patient to maintain maximum chest expansion and erect posture as well as maximal axial flexibility.

Spondyloarthritis follows at least three different courses. The majority of the patients experience recurrent episodes of arthritis. A minority have only one self-limiting episode of the disease. A smaller minority of patients suffer a continuous and unremitting aggressive course. Although most patients can continue to work, most are affected and become disabled as the disease progresses (Fox et al., 1979).

Vocational Implications

The patient with spondylitis should be considered for vocational or professional education as resources and interests dictate. Although motor coordination, eye–hand coordination, and eye–hand–foot coordination will not be impaired among individuals with minimum peripheral arthritis, a stiff back will limit the patient's rotation and flexion so that overall dexterity may be affected. Tasks that require reaching or bending will be difficult. Work requiring lifting of more than 10–15 lb may cause increased back pain. Climbing and balancing skills, stooping, and kneeling may be tolerated initially but become difficult as the disease worsens. Even with sedentary tasks, the patient must be allowed the opportunity to stretch the spine frequently. Although many individuals describe joint pain in relation to weather changes, patients with spondylitis should not necessarily require an indoor environment. Some noise, vibration, fumes, gas, dust, and poor ventilation should not be more intolerable than they are to an individual without spondyloarthritis unless significant pulmonary involvement is present. In general, patients with advanced education or clerical skills will frequently be able to continue meaningful employment, whereas those with only manual skills will become disabled.

DEGENERATIVE JOINT DISEASE

Degenerative joint disease (osteoarthritis [OA]) is the most common rheumatic disease and is characterized by progressive loss of cartilage and reactive changes at the margins of the joint and in the subchondral bone. The disease usually begins in the fourth decade; prevalence increases with age, and the disease becomes almost universal in individuals aged 65 and older (Scott & Hochberg, 1984). It primarily affects weight-bearing joints such as the knees, hips, and lumbosacral spine. Frequently, the DIPs and PIPs are involved. Rarely, the shoulder can also be affected.

Etiology and Pathogenesis

OA involves three tissues—bone, articular cartilage, and the synovium. Mechanical stress, trauma, joint misalignment, meniscal surgery, and genetic predisposition can all contribute to the development of OA. Obesity is frequently associated with degenerative joint disease in the weight-bearing joints (Hartz, Fischer, & Bril, 1986). Genetic factors play a role in the development of OA of the PIPs and DIPs and appear to involve a single autosomal gene that is sex-influenced and dominant in females, resulting in an incidence 10 times greater than in men.

Degenerative changes begin as focal erosion of cartilage at various points of stress. There follows an increase in water content of the cartilage and quantitative and qualitative changes in the cartilage proteoglycans. Enzymes capable of degrading proteoglycans and collagen are increased in the OA cartilage. As disease progresses, cartilage erosions become confluent and lead to large areas of denuded surface. The final outcome is full-thickness loss of cartilage down to bone. In contrast with this structural ulcerative breakdown, there is a proliferative cartilage and bone response leading to thickening of the subchondral bone and increased bony formation (osteophyte). Low-grade synovitis is common, particularly in advanced disease, and is due to release of inflammatory mediators or humoral and cell-mediated immune responses to damaged joint components (Samuels, Krasnokutsky, & Abramson, 2008).

Abnormal mechanical stress can result in production of inflammatory cytokines including TNF-α and interleukins (ILs)-1β, -6, and -8 and proteases (e.g., matrix metalloproteinase) that can degrade cartilage (Samuels et al., 2008). It is important to note that inflammatory events also contribute to the pain characteristic of OA. Inflammatory molecules, including prostaglandin E_1 and leukotriene B_4, can sensitize nerve fibers in joints so that their responses are increased to both painful and nonpainful stimuli. Other inflammatory molecules (e.g., bradykinin, histamine, serotonin, prostacyclin) released in joints can cause fibers to signal pain even when the joint is still (Bonnet & Walsh, 2005).

Clinical Manifestations

In early disease, pain occurs only after joint use and is relieved by rest. As disease progresses, pain occurs with minimal motion or even at rest. Nocturnal pain is commonly associated with severe disease. Acute inflammatory flares may be precipitated by trauma or, in some patients, by crystal-induced synovitis in response to crystals of calcium pyrophosphate or apatite. Stiffness usually occurs only in affected joints. Local tenderness, pain on passive motion, and crepitus are prominent findings. Joint enlargement results from synovitis, synovial effusion, or proliferative changes in cartilage and bone (osteophyte formation). Clinical symptoms usually show positive correlation with radiological abnormalities. In a given patient, however, the lack of correlation between joint symptoms and radiographic findings may be striking.

Osteophytes formed at the DIPs are termed Heberden's nodes, and similar changes at the PIPs are called Bouchard's nodes. Flexor and lateral deviations of the DIPs are common. In most patients, Heberden's nodes develop slowly over months or years. These deformities are generally asymptomatic and primarily concern the patient for cosmetic reasons. In other patients, onset is rapid and associated with moderately severe inflammatory changes. This pattern of OA is termed erosive OA and frequently occurs during the fourth decade in women with a strong familial history. The first metacarpal (MP) joints are frequently involved, leading to tenderness at the base of the first MP bone and a squared appearance of the hand.

OA of the knee is characterized by localized tenderness over various components of the joint and pain on passive or active motion. Crepitus is usually present, and muscle atrophy is seen secondary to disuse. Disproportionate losses of cartilage localized to the medial or lateral compartments of the knee lead to secondary genu varum or valgum deformity. Chondromalacia patellae are commonly detected and is associated with softening and erosion of the patellar articular cartilage. Pain, localized around the patella, is aggravated by activity such as climbing stairs.

Osteoarthritic changes in the hip present with an insidious onset of pain. Pain is usually localized to the groin or along the inner aspect of the thigh, although patients often complain of pain in the buttocks, sciatic region, or the knee due to pain referral along contiguous nerves. Physical examination shows loss of hip motion, initially most marked on internal rotation or extension.

OA of the MTPs can lead to MTP subluxation with corresponding hammer toe deformities. In the first MTP, the most common change is hallux valgus deformities. The severity of these deformities is usually aggravated by inappropriate footwear such as high heels and narrow, pointed, tight shoes.

OA of the spine results from involvement of the intervertebral disks, vertebral bodies, or posterior apophyseal articulations. Associated symptoms include local pain and stiffness and radicular pain due to compression of contiguous nerve roots. Lumbar stenosis is the term used when compression of the spinal cord occurs at multiple levels. The presenting symptom can be pain on walking and must be differentiated from claudication secondary to vascular incompetence. The presence of nocturnal pain can be a differentiating symptom for lumbar disease. In severe cases, myelopathy can develop, leading to muscle atrophy and disability. Surgical intervention is recommended when there are signs of neuropathy or myelopathy.

Functional Disabilities

OA affects the patient's performance by impeding use of the involved joint. Because the hips, knees, and lower back are common sites of degenerative joint disease, walking and transfer activities may be impaired. At first, the patient will be able to function well in a limited area, but as the disease progresses, the patient's functional capability decreases. Generally, however, activities of daily living, including dressing and eating, will not be significantly impaired.

Treatment and Prognosis

Major guidelines for the treatment of OA are all quite similar in that all of them recommend a combination of nonpharmacological and pharmacological treatments (Zhang et al., 2008). All guidelines also recommend a stepped approach to pharmacotherapy for pain management in OA patients. The primary goal in the treatment of OA is pain control and improvement of function in the affected joint. NSAIDs should be used in patients who show signs of inflammatory response in the affected joint. Analgesic agents such as acetaminophen may be used on a continuous basis, in combination with NSAIDs, to enhance pain control. Oral or parenteral therapy with corticosteroids is contraindicated in the treatment of OA. Intra-articular injections of corticosteroids, however, may be beneficial when used judiciously in the management of acute flares, when inflammatory response appears to be a major component. Injections should be infrequent because joint deterioration may be accelerated by masking of pain and subsequent joint overuse or by a direct deleterious effect of these drugs on cartilage.

Newer therapies are on the horizon aimed at preserving the joint function and preventing further damage. These potential treatments can be divided into disease- or structure-modifying drugs and those that improve functional status only. The disease-modifying agents include tetracyclines, gene therapy, and use of growth factors and cytokines (Howell & Altman, 1993). The mode of action is through inhibition of collagenase activity, increase in the level of tissue inhibitor of metalloproteinases (TIMPs), or manipulation of these factors via cytokines or gene therapy. Increased understanding of molecular events involved in the pathobiology of OA has prompted development of disease-modifying OA drugs. Many of these agents (e.g., matrix metalloproteinase inhibitors, TNF-α inhibitors, IL-1β inhibitors) are aimed at blocking the actions of the inflammatory cytokines and degradative enzymes described in the preceding paragraphs, and they may also decrease the pain experienced by OA patients (Hunter & Hellio Le Graverand-Gastineau, 2009). However, pain should also be a primary focus in the overall management of OA patients because it has been repeatedly shown that the achievement of significant pain relief is associated with significant improvements in quality of life for this population (Rabenda et al., 2005). Potential agents that are used only for symptomatic treatment of OA include glucosamine sulfate, chondroitin sulfate, and intra-articular administration of hyaluronic acid derivatives. Glucosamine sulfate and chondroitin sulfate are available in the United States as nutritional supplements. Some evidence exists from Europe that these drugs may modify symptoms in selected patients, but no adequate controlled trial has been conducted to establish their effect in structural modification. Although hyaluronic acid derivatives are often mentioned as potential structure-modifying drugs, these products are currently considered to be long-acting symptom-modifying drugs only (Peyron, 1993).

The goal in early rehabilitation is to improve the functional status and prevent further deterioration of the affected joint. Patients should be instructed in daily non-weight-bearing exercise to strengthen muscles and thus protect joints from overuse. In addition, they should be taught weight-bearing techniques. Appliances such as canes are also beneficial.

Surgical procedures in the treatment of OA include arthroplasty, osteotomy, and total prosthetic replacement. Hip and knee replacement procedures produce striking symptomatic relief and improved range of motion. Advances in arthroscopic techniques have led to increased surgical management such as debridement to remove loose bodies and abrasion chondroplasty earlier in the disease.

OA is a slowly progressive disease. Although medical and rehabilitative treatment can lead to improvement of function and diminution of pain in most patients, the effect is generally temporary. There is currently no established disease-modifying drug in the treatment of OA.

The eventual outcome is complete destruction of the joint, and ultimately surgical intervention is required.

Vocational Implications

Because OA is not always a systemic disease, successful treatment of a single involved joint may result in continued employment in the patient's current job unless it requires dexterous or heavy use of the involved joint. Even if surgical or medical treatment results in an increased range of motion, diminished pain, and increased functional ability of the affected joint, the use of that joint should be limited. Heavy lifting, which repeatedly places stress on the hips, knees, or lumbosacral spine, should be avoided by those who have OA in these areas. Light to medium work should be possible. Climbing, balancing skills, stooping, and kneeling will be impaired in many patients with OA. The environment has no significant effect on patients with OA even though changes in relative humidity and barometric pressures may cause transient joint discomfort.

Returning to work after undergoing successful surgery requires intensive postoperative rehabilitation and continued exercise to maintain muscle strength. As the patient's endurance and tolerance for activity normalize, work can be resumed. However, heavy manual work should be avoided, as the durability of the prosthetic implants is still limited. Stooping and kneeling may be accomplished without pain following surgery but should be limited. Certain motions involved with stooping and kneeling may cause dislocation of a prosthetic hip. Climbing and balancing can be accomplished, but such repetitive motions are hazardous and should also be limited. Most individuals with OA are able to sustain gainful employment and a normal level of activity following successful medical and surgical therapy.

REFERENCES

American College of Rheumatology. Subcommittee on Rheumatoid Arthritis Guidelines. (2002). Guidelines for the management of rheumatoid arthritis. 2002 update. *Arthritis and Rheumatism, 46,* 328–346.

Arnett, F. C. (1984). HLA and the spondyloarthropathies. In A. Callin (Ed.), *Spondyloarthropathies* (pp. 297–321). Orlando, FL: Grune & Stratton.

Arnett, F. C., Edworthy, S. M., Bloch, D. A., McShane, D. J., Fries, J. F., Cooper, N. S., et al. (1988). The American Rheumatism Association 1987 revised criteria for the classification of rheumatoid arthritis. *Arthritis and Rheumatism, 31,* 315–324.

Arnett, F., McClusky, O. E., & Schacter, B. Z. (1976). Incomplete Reiter's syndrome: Discriminating features and HLAB w27 in diagnosis. *Annals of Internal Medicine, 84,* 8–13.

Avina-Zubieta, J. A., Choi, H. K., Sadatsafavi, M., Etminan, M., Esdaile, J. M., & Lacaille, D. (2008). Risk of cardiovascular mortality in patients with rheumatoid arthritis: A meta-analysis of observational studies. *Arthritis and Rheumatism, 59,* 1690–1697.

Bathon, J. M., Martin, R. W., & Fleishmann, R. M. (2000). A comparison of etanercept and methotrexate in patients with early rheumatoid arthritis. *New England Journal of Medicine, 343,* 1586–1593.

Bennett, P. H., & Burch, T. A. (1967). New York symposium on population studies in the rheumatic diseases: New diagnostic criteria. *Bulletin on the Rheumatic Diseases, 17,* 453–469.

Bennett, R. M. (1979). Psoriatic arthritis. In D. J. McCarty (Ed.), *Arthritis and allied conditions* (9th ed., pp. 453–466). Philadelphia, PA: Lea & Febiger.

Bonnet, C. S., & Walsh, D. A. (2005). Osteoarthritis, angiogenesis, and inflammation. *Rheumatology (Oxford), 44,* 7–16.

Bresnihan, B., Alvaro-Gracia, J. M., & Cobby, M. (1998). Treatment of rheumatoid arthritis with recombinant human interleukin-1 receptor antagonist. *Arthritis and Rheumatism, 41,* 2196–2204.

Callin, A., & Fries, J. F. (1976). An "experimental" epidemic of Reiter's syndrome, revisited: Follow-up evidence on genetic and environmental factors. *Annals of Internal Medicine, 84,* 564–574.

Centers for Disease Control and Prevention. (1990). Prevalence of arthritic conditions in the United States. *Morbidity and Mortality Weekly Report, 39,* 99–102.

Centers for Disease Control and Prevention. (1994). Arthritis prevalence and activity limitations—United States, 1990. *Morbidity and Mortality Weekly Report, 43*, 433–438.

Centers for Disease Control and Prevention. (1998). Prevalence and impact of chronic joint symptoms—Seven states, 1996. *Morbidity and Mortality Weekly Report, 47*, 345–351.

Cunningham, L. S., & Kelsey, J. L. (1984). Epidemiology of musculoskeletal impairments and associated disability. *American Journal of Public Health, 74*, 574–579.

Dayer, J. M. (1990). Use of an IL-1 inhibitor in inflammation. In V. Strand (Ed.), *Proceedings: Early decisions in DMARD development: 2. Biologic agents in autoimmune disease* (pp. 44–46). Atlanta, GA: Arthritis Foundation.

Desai, S. P., Solomon, D. H., Abramson, S. B., Buckley, L., Crofford, L. J., Cush, J. C., et al. (2008). American College of Rheumatology Ad Hoc Group on use of selective and nonselective nonsteroidal antiinflammatory drugs. *Arthritis and Rheumatism, 59*, 1058–1073.

Emery, P., Szczepaanski, L., & Szechinski, J. (2003). Sustained efficacy at 48 weeks after single treatment course of rituximab in patients with rheumatoid arthritis [Abstract 1095]. *Arthritis and Rheumatism, 48* (Suppl.), S439.

Fox, R., Callin, A., Gerber, R. C., & Gibson, D. (1979). The chronicity of symptoms and disability in Reiter's syndrome: An analysis of 131 consecutive patients. *Annals of Internal Medicine, 91*, 190–207.

Gorman, J. D., Sack, K. E., & Davis, J. C., Jr. (2002). Treatment of ankylosing spondylitis by inhibition of tumor necrosis factor. *New England Journal of Medicine, 346*, 1349–1356.

Gregersen, P. K., Lee, S., Silver, J., & Winchester, R. (1987). The shared epitope hypothesis: An approach to understanding the molecular genetics of rheumatoid arthritis susceptibility. *Arthritis and Rheumatism, 30*, 1205–1213.

Harris, H. D., Jr. (1997). The clinical features of rheumatoid arthritis & treatment of rheumatoid arthritis. In W. N. Kelly, E. D. Harris, S. Ruddy, & C. Sledge (Eds.), *Textbook of rheumatology* (pp. 898–950). Philadelphia, PA: W. B. Saunders.

Hartz, A. J., Fischer, M. E., & Bril, G. (1986). The association of obesity with joint pain and osteoarthritis. *Journal of Chronic Diseases, 39*, 311–319.

Hochberg, M. C. (1981). Adult and juvenile rheumatoid arthritis: Current epidemiologic concepts. *Epidemiology Review, 3*, 27–41.

Hochberg, M. C. (1992). Epidemiology. In A. Callin (Ed.), *Spondyloarthropathies*. Orlando, FL: Grune & Walton.

Holmdahl, R., Nordling, C., Rubin, K., Tarkowski, A., & Klareskog, L. (1986). Generation of monoclonal rheumatoid factors after immunization with collagen II-anti-collagen II immune complexes: An anti-idiotype antibody to anti-collagen II is also a rheumatoid factor. *Scandinavian Journal of Immunology, 24*, 197–212.

Howell, D. S., & Altman, R. D. (1993). Cartilage repair and conservation in osteoarthritis. *Rheumatic Diseases Clinics of North America, 19*, 713–724.

Hunter, D. J., & Hellio Le Graverand-Gastineau, M. P. (2009). How close are we to having structure-modifying drugs available? *Medical Clinics of North America, 93*, 223–234, xiii.

Hurd, E. R. (1984). Extra-articular manifestations of rheumatoid arthritis. *Seminars in Rheumatic Diseases, 8*, 151–163.

Inman, R. D., Chiu, B., Johnston, M. E. A., & Falk, J. (1992). Molecular mimicry in Reiter's Syndrome: Cytotoxicity and ELISA studies of HLA-microbial relationships. *Immunology, 58*, 501–512.

Lawrence, R. C., Helmick, C. G., & Arnett, F. C. (1998). Estimates of the prevalence of arthritis and selected musculoskeletal disorders in the United States. *Arthritis and Rheumatism, 41*, 778–799.

Maini, R., St. Clair, E. W., & Breedveld, F. (1999). Infliximab versus placebo in rheumatoid arthritis patients receiving concomitant methotrexate, a randomized phase III trial: ATTRACT Study Group. *Lancet, 354*, 1932–1939.

Mielants, H., Veys, E. M., & Cuvelier, C. (1985). HLA B27 related arthritis and bowel inflammation: Part 2. Ileocolonoscopy and bowel histology in patients with HLA B27 related arthritis. *Journal of Rheumatology, 12*, 294–299.

Nissila, M., Lehtinen, K., & Leirisalo-Repo, M. (1988). Sulfasalazine in the treatment of ankylosing spondylitis: A 26-week placebo-controlled clinical trial. *Arthritis and Rheumatism, 31*, 1111–1117.

Paronen, A. (1948). Reiter's disease: A study of 344 cases observed in Finland. *Acta Medica Scandinavica, 131*, 1–143.

Peyron, J. G. (1993). Intraarticular hyaluronan injection in the treatment of osteoarthritis: State-of-the-art review. *Journal of Rheumatology, 20*, 10–15.

Pinals, R. S., Kaplan, S. B., Lawson, J. G., & Hepburn, B. (1986). Sulfasalazine in rheumatoid arthritis. *Arthritis and Rheumatism, 29,* 1427–1434.

Pincus, T., & Callahan, L. F. (1992). Taking mortality in rheumatoid arthritis seriously: Predictive markers, socio-economic status and co-morbidity. *Journal of Rheumatology, 13,* 841–845.

Rabenda, V., Burlet, N., Ethgen, O., Raeman, F., Belaiche, J., & Reginster, J. Y. (2005). A naturalistic study of the determinants of health related quality of life improvement in osteoarthritic patients treated with non-specific non-steroidal anti-inflammatory drugs. *Annals of the Rheumatic Diseases, 64,* 688–693.

Reiter, H. (1916). Über eine bisher unbekannte Spirochaeten Infektion (Spirochaetosis arthritica). *Deutsche Medicin Wochenschrift, 42,* 1535–1536.

Saag, K. G., Teng, G. G., Patkar, N. M., Anuntiyo, J., Finney, C., Curtis, J. R., et al. (2008). Recommendations for the use of nonbiologic and biologic disease-modifying antirheumatic drugs in rheumatoid arthritis. *Arthritis and Rheumatism, 59,* 762–784.

Samuels, J., Krasnokutsky, S., & Abramson, S. B. (2008). Osteoarthritis: A tale of three tissues. *Bulletin of the NYU Hospital for Joint Diseases, 66,* 244–250.

Scott, J. C., & Hochberg, M. C. (1984). Osteoarthritis. *Maryland Medical Journal, 33,* 712–716.

Siddiqui, M. A. (2007) The efficacy and tolerability of newer biologics in rheumatoid arthritis: Best current evidence. *Current Opinion in Rheumatology, 19,* 308–313.

Smolen, J. S., Kalden, J. R., & Scott, D. L. (1999). Efficacy and safety of leflunomide compared with placebo and sulphasalazine in active rheumatoid arthritis: A double-blind, randomized, multicentre trial. European Leflunomide Study Group. *Lancet, 353,* 259–266.

Strand, V., Cohen, S., & Schiff, M. (1999). Treatment of active rheumatoid arthritis with leflunomide compared with placebo and methotrexate. European Leflunomide Study Group. *Archives of Internal Medicine, 159,* 2542–2550.

Taylor, W. J., Gladman, D., Helliwell, P., Marchesoni, A., Mease, P., Mielants, H., et al. (2006). Classification criteria for psoriatic arthritis: Development of new criteria from a large international study. *Arthritis and Rheumatism, 54,* 2665–2673

Tugwell, P., Bennett, K., & Gent, M. (1987). Methotrexate in rheumatoid arthritis: Indications, contraindications, efficacy, and safety. *Annals of Internal Medicine, 107,* 358–366.

Visser, H., le Cessie, S., Vos, K., Breedveld, F. C., & Hazes, J. M. (2002). How to diagnose rheumatoid arthritis early: A prediction model for persistent (erosive) arthritis. *Arthritis and Rheumatism, 46,* 357–365.

Voltonen, V. V., Leirisalo, M., & Pentikainen, P. J. (1985). Triggering infections in reactive arthritis. *Annals of Rheumatic Diseases, 44,* 399–412.

Weinblatt, M. E., Keystone, E. C., & Furt, D. E. (2003). Adalimumab, a fully human anti-tumor necrosis factor a monoclonal antibody, for the treatment of rheumatoid arthritis in patients taking concomitant methotrexate: The ARMADA trial. *Arthritis and Rheumatism, 48,* 35–45.

Yocum, D. E., Klippel, J. H., & Wilder, R. L. (1988). Cyclosporin: A treatment of refractory rheumatoid arthritis. *Annals of Internal Medicine, 1,* 863–873.

Zhang, W., Moskowitz, R. W., Nuki, G., Abramson, S., Altman, R. D., Arden, N., et al. (2008). OARSI recommendations for the management of hip and knee osteoarthritis, Part II: OARSI evidence-based, expert consensus guidelines. *Osteoarthritis Cartilage, 16,* 137–162.

25

Spinal Cord Injury

Jung Ahn, MD, and Jeffrey Berliner, DO

Sir Ludwig Guttmann, a physician who was a pioneer in the care and treatment of patients with spinal cord injury (SCI), put it succinctly when he said, "Of the many forms of disability which can beset mankind, a severe injury or disease of the spinal cord undoubtedly constitutes one of the most devastating calamities in human life." Given that we do not have a cure as of now, the best treatment continues to be prevention.

Since World War I, great strides have been made in understanding the pathophysiology of SCI.

Physicians who work with patients with SCI deal not only with spinal stability and physical disability but also with secondary medical complications. These secondary medical complications involve the dysregulation of the nerve supply to the cardiopulmonary, digestive, integumentary, and urological systems.

Over the past three decades we have witnessed great progress in the management of SCI-related complications, significant changes in SCI epidemiology, new diagnostic modalities used to assess the status of spinal trauma, and tremendous strides in research aimed at alleviating secondary functional deficits resulting from SCI.

Researchers strive to restore function in both acute and chronic SCI patients. Hope has never been higher that we are now on the road to finding a cure for paralysis. Although progress has been slow, and no magic bullet has yet been discovered, this hard work and dedication continues to increase our knowledge and understanding of how injuries affect the spine. The complexity of the spinal cord leaves many unknown variables that play key roles in the functioning spinal cord. When an injury occurs, it triggers a cascade of events that all play a role in the effects seen afterward. We are just beginning to understand the role of the mediators of damage caused by the cascade and their effects. Research is now focused on interrupting the pathological processes at different points and on helping foster an environment to regrow healthy nerve tissue.

This chapter addresses the medical, physical, neurological, psychological, social, and vocational aspects of SCI medicine.

HISTORY

The first recorded account describing SCI was discovered in the Edwin Smith papyrus and dates back to 3000 B.C. (Donovan, 2007). It was described as an "ailment not to be treated." Centuries later in Greece, treatment for SCIs had changed little. According to the Greek physician Hippocrates (460–377 B.C.), "there were no treatment options for spinal cord injuries that resulted in paralysis; unfortunately, those patients were destined to die" (Hughes, 1988). Hippocrates did, however, create a traction machine to help realign the spinal column. Revolutionary gains in treatment of SCI were not made until centuries later when Paul of Aegina (625–690 A.D.) recommended surgical intervention for vertebral fractures. Surgical treatments were discussed in further detail and refined in India in the Sushrutu Samhita during the sixth century and the Royal Book written in Baghdad during the tenth century (Belen & Aciduman, 2006; Delisa & Hammond, 2002; Donovan, 2007; Eltorai, 2002; Hughes, 1988).

Through modern times, advances in the care of SCI patients have come through prevention of injury and secondary complications. Today, there is hope that with better understanding of the inner workings of the spinal cord and the neuronal damage caused by SCI, in conjunction with new technology, a cure appears to be on the horizon.

TERMINOLOGY

SCI is defined as an insult to the spinal cord resulting in a change, either temporary or permanent, in normal motor, sensory, or autonomic function. The term paraplegia refers to the lower extremities, whereas tetraplegia (formally referred to as quadraplegia) refers to all extremities (Dawodu, 2008). SCI does not only affect one's ability to walk or the usage of the hands, but also alters one's interaction with people and the environment. The injury can affect any or all of the following: the ability to earn income and to obtain or hold a job, relationships with loved ones and friends, sexuality, bowel and bladder functioning, dynamics of marriages, health, and emotion. Although the initial injury often provides a bleak picture, persons with SCI can enjoy fruitful and fulfilling lives.

FACTS AND FIGURES

These data were obtained from the National Spinal Cord Injury Database. The database has been in existence since 1973 and is a culmination of the efforts of Model Spinal Cord Injury Systems. In 2009, there were 14 model system centers across the United States which worked in a collaborative effort, with the goal of improving care for persons affected by SCI. The model systems are sponsored by the National Institute on Disability and Rehabilitation Research (National SCI Statistical Center, 2008).

The incidence of SCI in the United States is approximately 12,000 new cases per year and the prevalence or number of people alive with SCI in the United States is estimated to be approximately 250,000. The majority of SCIs occur from motor vehicle accidents (42%), whereas falls account for 23% and violence 15%. The average age of onset of injury is 39 with a bimodal peak. The highest incidence of SCI occurs during the teenage years through the mid-20s and then another increase is seen after the age of 70. The mechanism of injury between these two subgroups is different; the former occurs from motor vehicle accidents and sport-related injuries, whereas the latter is predominantly caused by falls and degenerative spinal stenosis (a narrowing of the spinal canal due to ligamentous and bony overgrowth). SCI affects males roughly four to one over females with a causal relationship to high-risk behaviors (DeVivo, Krause, & Lammertse, 1999; National SCI Statistical Center, 2008).

Figures Affecting Monetary and Psychosocial Aspects

The cost of care for a patient with SCI is colossal. In 2008, the average hospitalization cost was $150,000, and the average first-year expense for a ventilator-dependent tetraplegic was estimated at $700,000. The lifetime-associated medical cost for an injury occurring at the age of 25 for a paraplegic is >$1 million and the estimated lifetime cost for a tetraplegic is >$3 million. The cost of the injury is augmented by the fact that only 52% of patients are covered by insurance at the time of injury and that income is generally lost during hospitalization and recovery. Unemployment among those with SCI is extremely high and estimated to be approximately 63% at 8 years after injury. Only 51% of persons who sustained injury at an early age were employed by the age of 25 (National SCI Statistical Center, 2008).

Life expectancy for a person with SCI has dramatically risen over the past 50 years. A paraplegic injured at the age of 20 can be expected to live for 45 years after the injury. Life expectancy for the able-bodied counterpart is 78.8 years. A patient who becomes tetraplegic and ventilator dependent at the age of 20 has an average life expectancy of 18 years after injury, although if the patient has a C1–C4 injury and is able to be weaned from the ventilator, the life expectancy rises to 35 years. This underscores the importance of ventilator weaning (DeVivo & Ivie, 1995).

PSYCHOSOCIAL STATISTICS

People with SCI undergo a dramatic change in lifestyle. This change in lifestyle not only affects the injured person but also the family members, friends, and loved ones. This may put a strain on relationships as persons now attempt to redefine their roles as caregiver and patient. Among those married at the time of injury (52%), there is a slightly increased divorce rate when compared with the general population (El Ghatit & Hanson, 1975; National SCI Statistical Center, 2008). Among those who remain married, a limited number of studies showed a better quality of marriage and life-satisfaction rating for both the injured person and his/her spouse.

SCI is often associated with risk-taking behavior. The prevalence of alcohol abuse is high when compared with that of the general population. Mckinley, Kolakowsky, and Kreutzer (1999) found that at the time of initial injury, 53% of patients had positive toxicology screens and among those, 75% were over the state legal limit for intoxication. About 25% of positive toxicology screens were positive for both drugs and alcohol (Allen & Darlene, 1998). Heinemann and colleagues also found that "persons with spinal cord injury have a greater lifetime exposure to and use of substances" as compared to their able-bodied counterparts in the age group of 18–25 year olds (Charles & Carl, 1998).

ANATOMY AND PHYSIOLOGY OF THE SPINAL CORD

Armed with a basic understanding of spinal cord anatomy and physiology, location of the injury, and extent of the spinal cord insult, it becomes possible to predict and anticipate the functions that may be lost, impaired, and regained.

The Spinal Cord

The spinal cord is composed of a bundle of tracts and neurons that are responsible for modulating and transmitting information between the outside environment and the brain and vice versa. The brain and the spinal cord comprise the central nervous system; the spinal cord contains lower motor neurons (LMNs) as well. Upper motor neurons (UMNs) have their origins in the brain or brain stem and transmit information to the spinal cord level, whereas LMNs connect the information from the UMNs to the muscle. Both UMNs and LMNs aid in the movement of muscles. The peripheral nervous system has its origin outside the central nervous system and connects the central nervous system to various muscles and organs (Hammond & Burns; Kalat, 1998).

An adult spinal cord contains more than 1 billion neurons, some of which extend roughly 45 cm in length (American Spinal Injury Association, 2002). These neurons form two specific regions of the spinal cord referred to as gray and white matter. To understand this concept better, it helps to think of the brain and the spinal cord as two computers gathering information and sharing it with one another. The white matter functions to connect the two computers. The gray matter, located in the center of the spinal cord, is made of neuronal cell bodies and processes information. After the information is processed, it is then passed to connector neurons, termed inter-neurons, and then to the white matter. The white matter is composed of axons and is organized into long tracts. Separate tracts relay sensory, motor, and autonomic information to and from the brain.

To gain a better understanding of how the spinal cord works, let us follow the pathway of the sensation of vibration. The feeling of vibration is sensed by receptors, underneath the skin termed Pacinian corpuscles. The information is transmitted to the back of the spinal cord via peripheral nerves. This information is relayed to the posterior gray matter in the back of the spinal cord, processed and transferred to the ascending long tracts (fasciculus gracilis and fasciculus cuneatus) of the white matter, and then transferred to the brain. These ascending tracts are situated in the back of the spinal cord, and are known as the posterior column. The information is processed within the brain and delivered to the sensory cortex of the parietal lobe.

The Vertebrae

The spinal cord is encased and protected by the vertebrae, numbering about 33 at birth. Taken together, the 33 vertebrae make up the vertebral (spinal) column. This column is typically divided into four levels, referred from top to bottom as the cervical, thoracic, lumbar, and sacral spine. The cervical spine contains seven bones located in the neck region. The thoracic spine contains 12 vertebrae. The next three levels, caudal to the thoracic spine, are the lumbar spine, sacrum, and coccyx. The spinal cord terminates around the inferior border of the first lumbar vertebra, forming the conus medullaris (Figure 25.1).

Sequelae of SCI

SCIs are classified using the American Spinal Injury Association (ASIA) Impairment Scale. Using a standard classification scale allows clinicians to communicate the location and the extent of injury accurately. The scale also allows clinicians to predict the potential for recovery and monitor the effects of particular interventions on outcome more accurately.

Neurological examination for SCI involves 10 key muscle groups (myotomes) and 28 key sensory levels (dermatomes) on each side of the body. After testing all myotomes and dermatomes, a score of A through E is given. The scale below is truncated for improved ease of understanding (Oleson, Burns, Ditunno, Geisler, & Coleman, 2005).

A complete injury is the most severe injury and is graded as an ASIA A. This infers that there is no sensory perception or motor strength in the sacral segments. An injury that has sensation in the most caudal sacral dermatome is termed incomplete and confers a better prognosis for recovery (Figure 25.2).

Prognosis

"Will I walk again?" This is one of the first questions asked just after a person becomes paraplegic or tetraplegic, and the answer is very complicated. Different mechanisms of injury are known to have different prognoses. Tumors convey a different prognosis as compared to traumatic SCI, and falls have a different prognosis for return of function than bullet injuries. This section will focus on the return of function in traumatic SCI. Even with accurate research, however, there is still a dearth of literature on return of function and many questions remain unanswered.

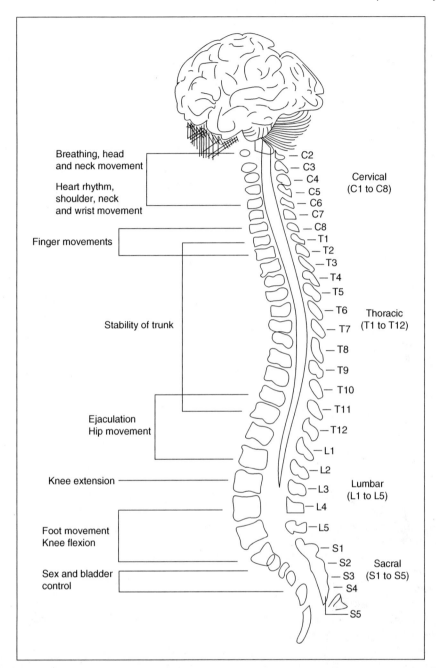

Breathing, head
and neck movement

Heart rhythm,
shoulder, neck
and wrist movement

Finger movements

Stability of trunk

Ejaculation
Hip movement

Knee extension

Foot movement
Knee flexion

Sex and bladder
control

— C2
— C3
— C4
— C5
— C6
— C7
— C8

Cervical
(C1 to C8)

— T1
— T2
— T3
— T4
— T5
— T6
— T7
— T8
— T9
— T10
— T11
— T12

Thoracic
(T1 to T12)

— L1
— L2
— L3
— L4
— L5

Lumbar
(L1 to L5)

— S1
— S2
— S3
— S4
— S5

Sacral
(S1 to S5)

FIGURE 25.1   The spine, spinal cord, and associated functions. Courtesy of ASIA and ISCOS.

Functional recovery is predicted using the ASIA Impairment Scale (Figure 25.3). Improvements in predicting functional recovery has been demonstrated by Curt, Keck, & Dietz, 1999. when combining the ASIA Impairment Scale with electrodiagnostic testing. In tetraplegics, most of the recovery of arm function is believed to occur over the first 6 months after injury. Studies by Ditunno and colleagues (1994) found that if subjects had a complete injury with no motor function at the level of injury by 1 week, only 45% of patients

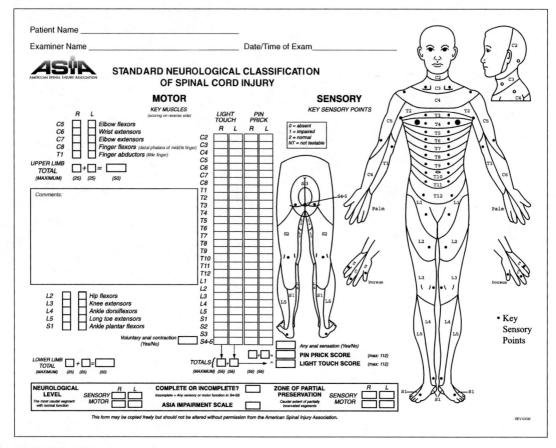

FIGURE 25.2 Standard neurological classification of spinal cord injury. Courtesy of ASIA and ISCOS.

demonstrated antigravity strength in that same muscle by 9–12 months. However, if subjects had some motor power, more than 90% gained antigravity strength over the same period (Kirshblum & O'Connor, 1998). This is important because antigravity strength helps make muscles functional on their own. The quicker the recovery begins, the quicker the progress is made, and often the recovery is more complete. For patients who have incomplete injuries, recovery is often faster and more complete.

Walking in the tetraplegic and paraplegic is accomplished through return of lower extremity motor strength (Crozier et al., 1992; Waters, Yakura, & Adkins, 1993). Prediction of walking in complete and incomplete SCI, studied by Burns and colleagues (1997) and most recently by Scivoletto and coworkers (2004), has yielded interesting results. A person with a complete SCI (ASIA A) has a 5% chance of recovering to an ASIA C and a 3% chance of recovering to an ASIA D by 1 year's time. How this correlates into walking with or without assistive device remains largely unknown. With the development of new technology, such as tractography, an MRI technology that is able to look at individual tracts of the spinal cord, and advances in electrodiagnostic testing, it may be possible that in the future physicians will be better able to predict recovery for the individual patient.

Secondary Complications
When asked to visualize a patient with an SCI, people typically envision a person in a wheelchair. The inability to walk is only one of many alterations of function that affects the quality

```
┌─────────────────────────────────────────┐
│                                           │
│        ASIA Impairment Scale              │
│                                           │
│  □  A = Complete: No motor or sensory     │
│     function is preserved in the          │
│     segments S4–S5.                       │
│                                           │
│  □  B = Incomplete: Sensory but not       │
│     motor function is preserved below     │
│     the neurological level and            │
│     includes the sacral segments S4–S5    │
│                                           │
│  □  C = Incomplete: Motor function is     │
│     preserved below the neurological      │
│     level, and more than half of key      │
│     muscles below the neurological        │
│     level have a muscle grade less        │
│     than 3.                               │
│                                           │
│  □  D = Incomplete: Motor function is     │
│     preserved below the neurological      │
│     level, and at least half of key       │
│     muscles below the neurological        │
│     level have a muscle grade of 3 or     │
│     more                                  │
│                                           │
│  □  E = Normal: Motor and sensory         │
│     function is normal                    │
│                                           │
├─────────────────────────────────────────┤
│                                           │
│        Clinical Syndromes                 │
│                                           │
│     □  Central cord                       │
│     □  Brown-Sequard                      │
│     □  Anterior cord                      │
│     □  Conus medullaris                   │
│     □  Cauda equina                       │
│                                           │
└─────────────────────────────────────────┘
```

FIGURE 25.3 American Spinal Injury Association Impairment Scale. Courtesy of Wings for Life.

of life for a person living with an SCI. Understanding the repercussions that an SCI has on daily life offers a window into the injury's psychosocial ramifications.

RESPIRATORY SYSTEM. Injuries involving the cervical and thoracic spinal cord have a deleterious effect on the respiratory system. The more cephalad (closer to the head) the cord injury, the more affected the respiratory system becomes by virtue of decreasing the number of muscles involved in respiration. The levels of cervical nerve 3, 4, and 5 are of particular importance. These nerves join to form the phrenic nerve, which innervates the primary muscle of respiration known as the diaphragm. Weakness or paralysis of the diaphragm may result in respiratory failure, requiring the assistance of mechanical ventilation, which may be temporary or permanent depending upon ensuing recovery.

Physicians specializing in Spinal Cord Injury Medicine and pulmonologists are gaining a better understanding of how to help people with SCI gain independence from ventilators. When medically feasible, avoiding mechanical ventilation improves quality of life and extends the life span. Although lifelong ventilator support may appear to paint a bleak picture, studies have demonstrated that patients on a ventilator can enjoy a high quality of life.[44]

Prevention of respiratory complications is of the utmost importance. In general, tetraplegics with loss of the diaphragm and accessory respiratory muscle function are unable to remove phlegm by themselves because of their inability to cough effectively. This can cause pneumonia, the leading cause of death in both the acute and chronic phases of SCI. Other complications include atelectasis, mucus plugging, pleural effusion, empyema, pneumothorax, and pulmonary embolism.

Measures to prevent respiratory complications in the acute phase of high-level SCI require a team approach. Secretion management, cough assist techniques, proper pulmonary toileting, chest physical therapy, in-line ventilator equipment, and proper oral hygiene are just a few of the many techniques that help reduce pulmonary complications. Long-term pulmonary management includes yearly influenza vaccination and pneumococcal vaccination every 5 years.

Phrenic nerve pacing provides an exciting alternative to long-term ventilator support. This involves pulsatile electrical stimulation applied to the phrenic nerves, provided by a diaphragmatic pacemaker, resulting in stimulation of the diaphragm and thus ventilator-free breathing. To qualify for the procedure, the patient must have at least partially preserved function of the phrenic nerve in addition to an intact diaphragm. The procedure is not without complications, such as electrical failure and electrode migration (Berliner & Ahn, 2006; Onders et al., 2007). The diaphragmatic pacemaker is a device in which the electrodes are implanted directly into and provide stimulation to the diaphragm. Research on the practicality and efficacy of the diaphragmatic pacemaker is underway but preliminary results demonstrated by Onders and colleagues are encouraging (Smith, Gangitano, Munoz, & Salas, 2008). With advances in respiratory care for high-level tetraplegics as well as advances in technology, it is hopeful that quality of life of high-level cervical SCI patients can be improved.

GENITOURINARY SYSTEM. The importance of proper urinary management for SCI patients cannot be overstated. Before World War II, the leading cause of death among patients with SCI was related to urinary complications (Boone, 2000). Over the past three decades we have learned to reduce urinary tract complications including infection, stone formation, and hydronephrosis (kidney damage).

The urinary system is made up of the kidneys, ureters, urinary bladder, bladder neck (internal sphincter), external urethral sphincter, and urethra. Storage and excretion of urine works in a coordinated manner that is under the control of the brain, brainstem, spinal cord, and peripheral nervous system. Following SCI, there is a disruption in the signals being sent between the brain and the genitourinary system. The effects seen on the bladder depends on whether UMNs or LMNs have been affected.

UMN injuries cause a reflexogenic bladder; as the bladder fills, an uncontrollable contraction of the bladder occurs. This contraction occurs against a closed outlet (external sphincter). This can cause one of two problems: incontinence or a backflow of urine to the kidneys. Long-standing backflow of urine to the kidneys causes kidney damage (hydronephrosis). LMN lesions cause flaccidity of the detrusor (muscles of the bladder), resulting in areflexia of the bladder with urinary retention. An areflexic bladder has no nervous control of the bladder or urinary sphincters. The lack of muscle tone in the bladder and the external sphincter causes urinary retention and occasionally overflow incontinence.

Treatment of a neurogenic bladder is tailored to individual needs and may consist of catheter care, pharmacological intervention, and surgery. Two common forms of initial management for the neurogenic bladder are intermittent catheterization or indwelling urinary catheterization. These two approaches are performed in an effort to eliminate residual urine from the bladder and to protect the kidneys from backflow. To perform intermittent catheterization, a catheter is inserted through the urethra and into the urinary bladder to drain the urine. This is usually performed every 4–6 hours depending on daily fluid intake and urine output. This means that every 4–6 hours a person will need to find an appropriate place to perform catheterization. An indwelling catheterization is an alternative procedure and, in this treatment, a catheter is placed in the bladder to drain the urine constantly into a bag. Both of these methods have advantages and disadvantages.

Pharmacological treatment has also provided an increased quality of life for SCI patients by increasing urine flow, preventing incontinence, and decreasing urinary tract infections (Berliner & Ahn, 2006; Raghavan & Shenot, 2009).

Surgical intervention may be considered to increase the size of the urinary bladder, reduce the tone of the external sphincter, and increase independence with self-care with bladder management. One of examples is the Monti Procedure. This procedure allows a patient with poor hand function to catheterize through a small opening, usually placed in the umbilicus, which is connected to the bladder by a piece of the small intestine (ileum). Other procedures include suprapubic tube placement, external sphincterotomy, bladder augmentation, ileal conduit surgery and artificial sphincter placement.

The use of botulinum toxin has also evolved for the management of a spastic bladder. In this procedure, botulinum toxin is injected directly into the bladder wall. This allows for increased storage capacity and decreased incontinence episodes. This procedure is usually effective for 3–6 months, and needs to be repeated to maintain efficacy (Darouiche, 2001; Raghavan & Shenot, 2009).

Bladder care research offers hope for improved quality of life for patients with neurogenic bladder. Spastic (overactive) bladders often become small and contracted, and may require augmentation surgery to increase the size of the bladder. A new augmentation surgery is currently being investigated using an autologous neo-bladder construct. In this study, a patient's own bladder cells are isolated and grown in a medium and placed in a scaffold in the shape of the bladder. The neo-bladder is then surgically placed to augment the patient's own bladder (Spinal Cord Injury Bowel Management, 2009).

In the past, renal failure was the leading cause of death in the SCI population. Subsequent research, antibiotics, and proper urinary management have decreased the number and severity of urinary tract complications. A new novel approach to prevent urinary tract infections involves inoculating the bladder with noninvasive forms of bacteria. The idea is to have the nonvirulent forms of bacteria colonize the bladder in an effort to keep out the pathological strains (Randell et al., 2001).

GASTROINTESTINAL SYSTEM. In SCI, the normal physiology of defecation is impaired. The gastrointestinal system relies on coordinated neural function between the central nervous system and the autonomic nervous system to function properly. When interrupted, there is a disruption of normal stool transit time and defecation. In general, "if the spinal cord injury is above the twelfth thoracic vertebrae, the ability to feel when the rectum is full may be lost. The anal sphincter muscle may remain tight, and bowel movements will occur on a reflex basis" (Rosito, Nino-Murcia, Wolfe, Kiratli, & Perkash, 2002). The injury to the bowel is termed an UMN-type bowel. "A spinal cord injury below the twelfth thoracic vertebrae may damage the defecation reflex and cause paralysis of the anal sphincter muscle. Fluid absorption in the transverse colon is also partially impaired. This is known as a lower motor neuron or flaccid bowel." The two bowel problems mentioned earlier, the UMN and LMN bowels, must be treated differently (Rosito et al., 2002).

The UMN reflexic bowel may be treated with diet modification, gentle digital stretching to the anal sphincter, digital disimpaction, and medications in the form of stool softeners, bulking agents, colonic stimulants, suppositories and enemas. Taken together, the bowel regimen is termed a "bowel care program," which is typically performed daily or every other day. In preparation of bowel movements, the patient or care provider checks the rectal vault for stool. If no stool is present in the rectum, an enema or suppository may be inserted. If no result is noted 15 minutes of insertion, digital anal stretching or digital rectal stimulation may be necessary. Digital stimulation is performed by inserting a lubricated, gloved finger inside the anus maintaining contact with the rectal mucosa. The patient or care provider then rotates the finger in a circular motion until the wall relaxes. This usually takes 15–60 seconds. Digital stimulation takes advantage of an intact reflex which causes peristalsis (reflex contraction of the intestines) to occur, which in turn pushes the stool along (Kalat, 1998).

The LMN bowel routine is different from that of the UMN bowel program because there are no reflexes. This renders digital stimulation and many medications such as suppositories and laxatives useless. There is also a flaccid anal sphincter, which allows stool to pass uninhibited. The LMN bowel treatment program may consist of a high-fiber diet and bulking agents such as fiber-based medicines. It may also require high colonic enemas to empty the distal colon and rectum for prevention of fecal incontinence.

In some cases, the bowel care program may take >3 hours, greatly compromising quality of life. One alternative is the Malone Procedure (appendicostomy). The Malone Procedure involves connecting the appendix to the abdominal wall creating a stoma with a one-way valve. The person can then place an enema into the intestines through this opening using a catheter. The one-way valve when working properly ensures that no fecal matter passes to the abdomen. Another alternative to the bowel treatment program is a colostomy. This procedure involves connecting the colon to the anterior abdominal wall, creating a stoma. The feces then evacuate through the stoma and into a collecting bag. High satisfaction with this procedure for both the caregiver and patient has been reported (Priebe, Martin, Wuermser, Castillo, & McFarlin, 2002; Susan Garber et al., 2005).

INTEGUMENTARY SYSTEM. Patients with SCI are at high risk of developing pressure ulcers over the bony prominences below the level of injury due to loss of sensation. The skin is truly one of areas where "an ounce of prevention is worth a pound of cure" (Benjamin Franklin). "Now let us look at a means of preventing bedsores. Daily care must be devoted to keep integrity of the skin for once they appear, it is often difficult to get rid of them" (Paget, 1873).

Normal skin is resistant to the development of a pressure sore by means of sensory feedback to the brain from the peripheral nervous system. This feedback alerts our body that it is time to move. Changing positions or performing "weight shifts" will allow the arterial blood supply to reach the skin and underlying soft tissue to provide oxygen as well as to wash out noxious waste (Regan et al., 2007). It is estimated that 50–80% of all SCI patients experience pressure ulcers within their lifetime. The cost of pressure ulcers remains high and a single pressure ulcer can cost between $2,000 and $7,000 per year (Regan et al., 2007). This cost is enormous, but the emotional cost to the affected person may be even higher. A patient with an ischial pressure ulcer will need to avoid sitting for prolonged periods of time. Since sitting in and pushing a wheelchair is the primary means of locomotion, stopping this activity may cause time missed at work and school, in addition to social isolation and financial hardship.

A pressure ulcer is defined by the National Pressure Ulcer Advisory Panel (NPUAP), as a "localized injury to the skin and/or underlying tissue usually over a bony prominence, as a result of pressure, or pressure in combination with shear, moisture and/or friction. A number of contributing or confounding factors are associated with pressure ulcers" (Figure 25.4).

Proper lying and sitting surfaces reduce pressure on vulnerable areas. Cushioned mattresses and wheelchair seating systems effectively disperse pressure over the entire region rather than over a bony prominence (Regan et al., 2007). Educating patients and families on ways to relieve pressure and to perform daily skin inspection is an imperative means of preventing pressure ulcers (O'Connor & Salcido, 2002); Brown, Hill, & Baker, 2006). Pressure relief while lying in bed entail changing position every 2 hours. To perform pressure relief when sitting, tetraplegics with active tricep function (C7) and strength can lift the upper body from the wheelchair for either 15 seconds every 15 minutes or 30 seconds every 30 minutes, termed the 15/15 or 30/30 rule (Kalat, 1998; Sipski & Arenas, 2006). Patients who do not possess enough upper extremity strength to lift themselves can modify local pressure using an electric wheelchair that tilts or reclines the upper body posteriorly. This will take pressure off the sitting surface. Pressure mapping is a way to evaluate the safety of a sitting surface further. It involves using sensors to quantify the pressure between the person and the seat cushion. Other means of improving skin care include good nutritional support, maintaining proper body weight, smoking cessation, and avoiding moist and caustic substances, such as urine or stool to remain on the skin for prolonged periods of time (Brown et al., 2006).

The treatment of a pressure ulcer depends on many variables including its appearance, cleanliness, degree of penetration through the skin and underlying structures, location, and

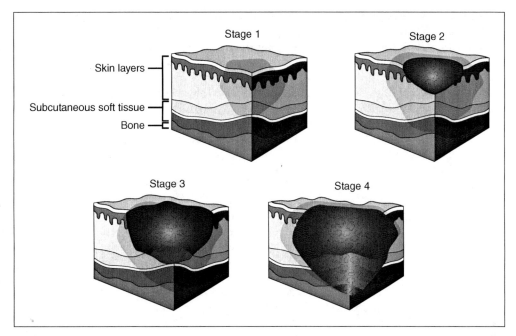

FIGURE 25.4 Pressure ulcer staging. Courtesy of the Wound Care Information Network.

drainage. The general principles of pressure ulcer treatment are to eliminate predisposing conditions, avoid friction, shear stress and tissue maceration, and debride devitalized tissue (Sipski & Arenas, 2006). There are multiple pharmacological agents that aid in pressure ulcer healing. Treatments that may be used in conjunction with pharmacological management include whirlpool therapy, electrical stimulation, hyperbaric oxygen, and vacuum-assisted dressings. Eating a nutritious diet high in protein and cessation of smoking are encouraged to provide a proper medium for wound healing.

If a wound is large, deep, and complex, a surgical closure may be a viable alternative. Surgical techniques include sharp debridement and rotational myocutaneous flap closure. After the operation, an air-fluidized bed is frequently used for surgical site care. Typically, a patient is kept on bed rest for 3 weeks. Afterward, a slowly progressive sitting program under close observation by a treating physician and rehabilitation nurse is implemented as long as the surgical site remains intact.

SEXUALITY AND FERTILITY. Sexuality and intimacy are important ingredients to psychological health and emotional well-being. Sexuality encompasses much more than just the act of sex but involves closeness and interpersonal relationship between people. Persons with SCI may continue to express sexual desire and remain sexually active but often face many barriers to a return to intimacy. Often these embarrassing topics remain largely unaddressed by health-care providers, leaving persons with SCI and their partners in the dark. They are left without answers to questions regarding sexuality and childbearing.

SCI affects sexuality in both males and females and may affect interest, arousal, ejaculation, and orgasm. Interest in performing sexual activity remains high in the SCI community but there are logistical considerations and hurdles. Before sexual activity, bowel and bladder care may need to be performed to prevent incontinence during the sexual act (Kalat, 1998). Males may need to premedicate to achieve erection, and females may need added lubrication. Sexual positioning may also need to be planned. In the right environment and with open dialogue, many of the aforementioned obstacles are incorporated into, as opposed to being a deterrent from, the sexual act.

The effect of SCI on sexual response is generally discussed based upon the degree of completeness or incompleteness of the patient's injury, and whether the neurological damage caused an upper or LMN injury. In males, SCI may affect the ability to achieve or maintain an erection. Erections if achieved are often incomplete or unsustainable for the purpose of intercourse (Westgren & Levi, 1995). A multitude of treatment options are available for men with erectile dysfunction. These include vacuum tumescence devices (vacuum-assisted erections), oral medications, placement of medication into the urethral opening, injection of medication into the penile shaft (intracavernous injections), and penile implantation surgery.

The effects of SCI on sexuality and fertility of females is less evident and has been less well studied. The arousal stage for females is affected, manifested by a decrease in vaginal lubrication.

Ejaculation is defined as the expulsion of seminal fluid from the urethra. This is greatly diminished in the male with SCI and may occur in up to 4% of persons. If the goal of ejaculation is for siring a child, then assistive reproductive technology may be tried. Methods of semen retrieval include vibroejaculation, electroejaculation, and removal of semen directly from the testicles or seminal tract (Bors & Commar, 1960; Kirshblum et al., 2002; Kreuter, Siösteen, & Biering-Sørensen, 2008; Linsenmeyer, 2002; Outcomes Following Traumatic Spinal Cord Injury, 1999; Ricciardi, Szabo, & Poullos, 2007; Westgren & Levi, 1995; Wirz, van Hedel, Rupp, Curt, & Dietz, 2006).

Female reproductive capability does not appear to be affected by SCI. It is important for an obstetrician to be familiar with SCI as secondary complications during pregnancy occur at a substantially higher rate than their able-bodied counterparts.

Parenting after SCI has been studied by Westgren and Levi (1995), and there appears to be no negative consequences for the child or parents. Children stated that mothers with SCI were no different than other mothers, and the partner did not feel that extra burden of care shifted toward them. "We found an overall favorable outcome as regards to the parameters evaluated. The families seem to live a rich and complete family life with very little demand for external help. They report a well functioning social network and seem socially integrated both as individuals and as families" (Crozier et al., 1992).

REHABILITATION

The Rehabilitation Team

Rehabilitation begins in the early acute phase of the SCI and continues as a lifelong process. The rehabilitation team may consist of many or all of the following disciplines: a physiatrist (physicians specializing in Physical Medicine and Rehabilitation), rehabilitation nurse, physical therapist, occupational therapist, speech pathologist, swallow therapist, psychologist, nutritionist, recreational therapist, respiratory therapist vocational counselor, and social worker.

The team, led by the physiatrist, provides medical care, therapies, and psychosocial support to foster medical stability, improve function, and assist with community return. The acute period is always an intense and rough period for the person with a newly acquired SCI. Many SCI patients feel that a piece of them has been taken away, and that they are not whole anymore. The goal of the team is to support and encourage the patient to overcome many difficulties the patient will face in activities of daily living and to come out as a strong, independent, and confident individual. The interdisciplinary team communicates with one another to ensure that the patient, patient's family, and caregivers receive the support they need.

The ultimate goal of rehabilitation after SCI is to maximize function, minimize dysfunction, and facilitate a smooth return to life activities. The rehabilitation process begins once the patient enters the emergency room and is a lifelong process thereafter. Just as no two patients are the same, no two rehabilitation programs can be the same. It must be tailored to each patient. In the acute phase of SCI, rehabilitation focuses on patient and family/caregiver education and prevention of secondary complications.

Such initial rehabilitation program includes prevention of joint contractures, pneumonia, pressure ulcers, urinary tract infections, ileus, autonomic dysreflexia, orthostatic hypotension, and thromboembolic disease. This helps provide optimal patient care and alleviates physical suffering (Waters, Adkins, Yakura, & Vigil, 1994). The information provided in the acute phase will be reinforced throughout the entire rehabilitation process. Once the patient with SCI is medically and surgically stabilized, he or she is transferred to an inpatient rehabilitation hospital for acute SCI inpatient rehabilitation

Attainable goals for patients with SCI are based on level of injury, ASIA Impairment Scale, comorbidities, previous function, precautions, and psychosocial status. These interdisciplinary goals are reassessed weekly, as function, endurance, and task achievement may change over the inpatient stay.

Injury levels have been correlated with functional outcome, and individuals may attain or often exceed expectations. Adaptive technology can also allow the injured to become more independent in activities of daily living. Patients with high complete injury at cervical levels 1 through 4 have no hand function but can obtain independence in wheelchair mobility, weight shifts, and directing transfers. Environmental controls units allow persons to open and close doors, turn on and off lights, use computers, and control the television. Persons with high SCIs have learned to hunt and fish with mouth units termed sip and puff even without arm or hand movement. The more caudal (toward the feet) the injury and the more key muscles a patient recovers for usage, the more functional and independent an individual can become (Albin, White, Yashon, & Harris, 1969).

Walking and Standing

It is the goal of every patient with an SCI to "walk again." Walking after SCI is often divided into three different categories: walking for exercise only, walking for household distances, and walking in the community. As of now it is possible for paraplegics with injury as high as the second thoracic level to ambulate short distances using a walking aid with bilateral long leg braces. Most patients without motor strength in their legs walk for exercise only as the energy requirement for walking is too great, and the quality of the gait is poor and inefficient. Walking for exercise is not without merit as walking and standing even for short periods of time has been shown to be beneficial for the psychosocial aspect of the patient. Walking is also good for cardiovascular health. However, it is true that the lower the level of injury and the greater the strength in the lower extremities, the higher the predictive value for functional gait (Chen, 2000; Freund et al., 2007; Kwon et al., 2008).

A multitude of research studies are being conducted to evaluate the effects of interventions on walking and return of function in patients with SCI. Some equipment and therapies currently under investigation are examining the effects of functional electrical stimulation on muscle recovery and body weight-supported treadmill training on functional recovery.

SCI: AN AILMENT TO BE CURED

The cure for SCI has been elusive, but current research is paving the way for a future cure.

Acute Injury

In an ideal world, clinicians would be able to stop the cascade of damaging events triggered by an SCI. One attempt at stopping the cascade is spinal cord hypothermia. This procedure was originally invented by Dr. Alfred Reginald Allen in 1911 and was used to treat SCI by

Dr. Maurice Albin, but in 1969 it was deemed to have no medical value (Belen & Aciduman, 2006). Spinal cooling has recently been repopularized after use on a professional football player who was injured during a game. Although a cogent biological rationale may exist for the use of local or systemic hypothermia in acute traumatic SCI, little scientific literature is currently available to substantiate the clinical use of either in human patients (Festoff et al., 2006). Experiments are currently underway using different methods of cooling in an attempt to prove efficacy.

Other attempts to stop neural tissue inflammation have included activated macrophage trials, antibodies against NOGO-A, a molecule that destroys the protective covering of nerve cells, and inhibitors of nitrous oxide synthetase. No single agent has yet been successful to alter outcome of SCI (Yick, So, Cheung, & Wu, 2004).

Immunosuppressive therapy has recently gained ground in SCI research as a means of blocking the entire inflammatory cascade. Tacrolimus and Cyclosporine are primarily used to inhibit autoimmune reactions in transplanted organs or tissue. It has been hypothesized that, through the same mechanism, the body would be unable to mount an immune and inflammatory response after SCI (Sayer, Kronvall, & Nilsson, 2006).

Other attempts have also been made to stop programmed cell death (apoptosis) after injury in the form of inhibitors of caspase and calpain, and with the use of minocycline (Hurlbert, 2001). Lithium, a drug long known to alter sodium transport and inhibit the body's immune reaction, is currently being trialed as well (Early Acute Management in Adults with Spinal Cord Injury, 2008).

Neuroprotection After SCI

The use of steroids for treating SCI is noted as early as the 1970s; during this time, steroids were thought to have no efficacy in treating cervical SCI sustained from trauma. After results of the Second National Acute Spinal Cord Injury Study were reported in 1990, administration of high-dose steroids within 8 hours of SCI appeared to be standard of care. However, the use of steroids is still a debated topic, and only time and additional research will determine its usefulness (Fouad et al., 2005; Keirstead, 2005; Nistor, 2004).

Neural Regeneration

Cajal and Golgi, two neuroscientists in the late 1800s, laid the framework for the modern view of neuroanatomy and are believed to be the founders of modern neuroscience. Since that time, many efforts have been made to assess and promote neural reconnections in the spinal cord. As early as 1980, it was shown that neural regrowth is possible after SCI in a rodent model (Fawcett, 2009). Attempts to translate that experiment and many subsequent experiments have not been able to provide a functional recovery in humans.

Cell Transplantation and Replacement

Stem cell research offers hope for recovery of SCI and has provided evidence of efficacy in animal models. Stem cells have been isolated from the bone marrow, olfactory cells, umbilical cord blood, placenta, and embryo. When placed in an appropriate medium, these cells undergo division and regenerate a line of cells, which produce a desired function.

In the case of SCI, the goal of stem cell research is to generate viable neurons within a damaged lesion. One successful experiment produced oligodendrocytes, cells that produce a sheath covering over the nerve, called myelin. An experiment by McDonald and colleagues. (1999) provided evidence that transplanted mouse embryonic stem cells into the damaged spinal cord could not only survive up to 5 weeks but could also differentiate into oligodendrocytes.

Improvement in motor function was also reported. Keirstead (2005) showed that embryonic cells taken from human fetal tissue, when transplanted into a rat, could also grow, survive, and produce cells that helped replace the myelin. Current stem cell research offers hope for a cure for paralysis (Eltorai, 2002).

CONCLUSION

SCI is a devastating disease, which affects almost all aspects of a person's life. Through proper medical management, psychosocial support, and rehabilitation therapies as well as the patient's motivation and family/caregiver's participation, it is possible for a person with SCI to pursue a productive and satisfying life.

REFERENCES

Albin, M. S., White, R. J., Yashon, D., & Harris, L. S. (1969). Effects of localized cooling on spinal cord trauma. *The Journal of Trauma, 9,* 1000–1008.

Allen W. H. & Darlene, H. (1998). Substance abuse and medical complication following spinal cord injury. *Rehabilitation Psychology, 43,* 219–231

American Spinal Injury Association. (2002). *International Standards for Neurological Classification of SCI.* Chicago: Author.

Belen, D., & Aciduman, A. (2006). A pioneer from the Islamic Golden Age: Haly Abbas and spinal traumas in his principal work, The Royal Book. *Journal of Neurosurgery. Spine, 5,* 381–383.

Berliner, J. C., & Ahn, J. H. (2006). Pharmacological management of urological dysfunction. *Journal of Korean American Medical Association, 12,* 85–93.

Boone, T. B. (2000). Recent advances in the management of neurogenic bladder. *Urology, 56,* 76–81.

Bors, E., & Commar, A. E. (1960). Neurological disturbances of sexual function with special reference to 529 patients with spinal cord injury. *Urological Survey, 10,* 191–222.

Brown, D. J., Hill, S. T., & Baker, H. W. (2006). Male fertility and sexual function after spinal cord injury. *Progress in Brain Research, 152,* 427–439.

Burns, S. P., Golding, D. G., Rolle, W. A., Jr., Graziani, V., & Ditunno, J. F. (1997). Recovery of ambulation in motor incomplete tetraplegia. *Archives of Physical Medicine and Rehabilitation, 78,* 1169–1172.

Charles, H. B., & Carl, T. R. Alcohol use and readiness to change after spinal cord injury. (1998). *Archives of Physical Medicine and Rehabilitation, 79,* 1110–1115.

Chen, M. S. (2000). Nogo-A is a myelin-associated neurite outgrowth inhibitor and an antigen for monoclonal antibody IN-1. *Nature, 403,* 434–439.

Crozier, K. S., Cheng, L. L., Graziani, V., Zorn, G., Herbison, G., & Ditunno, J. F., Jr. (1992). Spinal cord injury: Prognosis for ambulation based on quadriceps recovery. *Paraplegia, 30,* 762–767.

Curt, A., Keck, M. E., & Dietz, V. (1999). Functional outcome following spinal cord injury: Significance of motor-evoked potentials and ASIA scores. *Archives of Physical Medicine and Rehabilitation, 79,* 81–86.

Darouiche, R. (2001). Pilot trial of bacterial interference for preventing urinary tract infection. *Urology, 58,* 339–344.

Dawodu, S. T. (2008). Spinal Cord Injury Definition, Epidemiology, Pathophysiology. *Emedicine,* http://emedicine.medscape.com/article/322480-overview

Delisa, J., & Hammond, M. (2002). The history of the subspecialty of spinal cord injury medicine. In S. Kirshblum, D. Campagnolo, & J. Delisa (Eds.), *Spinal Cord Medicine* (pp. 1–4). Philadelphia, PA: Lippincott, Williams and Wilkins.

DeVivo, M. J., & Ivie, C. S. III. (1995). Life expectancy of ventilator-dependent persons with spinal cord injuries. *Chest, 108,* 236–232.

DeVivo, M. J., Krause, J. S., & Lammertse, D. P. (1999). Recent trends in mortality and causes of death among persons with spinal cord injury. *Archives of Physical Medicine and Rehabilitation, 80,* 1411–1419.

Ditunno, J., Flanders, A., Kirshblum, S., Graziani, V., & Tessler, A. (1994). Predicting outcomes in traumatic spinal cord injuries. In S. Kirshblum, D. Campagnolo, & J. Delisa (Eds.), *Spinal cord medicine* (pp. 108–120). Philadelphia, PA: Lippincott, Williams and Wilkins.

Donovan, W. H. (2007). Spinal cord injury—Past, present, and future. *Journal of Spinal Cord Medicine, 30,* 85–100.

Early Acute Management in Adults with Spinal Cord Injury. (2008). A Clinical Practice Guideline for Health Care Professionals, consortium for Spinal Cord Injury Medicine, Paralyzed Veterans Association.

El Ghatit, A. Z., & Hanson, R. W. (1975). Outcome of marriages existing at the time of a male's spinal cord injury. *Journal of Chronic Diseases, 28,* 383–388.

Eltorai, I. M. (2002). History of spinal cord medicine. In V. Lin (Ed.), *Spinal cord medicine, principles and practice* (pp. 3–14). New York: Demos Medical Publishing.

Fawcett, J. W. (2009). Recovery from spinal cord injury: Regeneration, plasticity and rehabilitation. *Brain, 132,* 1417–1418.

Festoff, B. W., Ameenuddin, S., Arnold, P. M., Wong, A., Santacruz, K. S., & Citron, B. A. (2006). Minocycline neuroprotects, reduces microgliosis, and inhibits caspase protease expression early after spinal cord injury. *Journal of Neurochemistry, 97,* 1314–1326.

Fouad, K., Schnell, L., Bunge, M. B., Schwab, M. E., Liebscher, T., & Pearse, D. D. (2005). Combining Schwann cell bridges and olfactory-ensheathing glia grafts with chondroitinase promotes locomotor recovery after complete transection of the spinal cord. *Journal of Neuroscience, 25,* 1169–1178.

Freund, P., Wannier, T., Schmidlin, E., Bloch, J., Mir, A., Schwab, M. E., et al. (2007). Anti-Nogo-A antibody treatment enhances sprouting of corticospinal axons rostral to a unilateral cervical spinal cord lesion in adult macaque monkey. *Journal of Comparative Neurology, 502,* 644–659.

Garber, S., et al. (2005). *Pressure ulcer prevention and treatment following spinal cord injury: A clinical practice guideline for health care professionals.* Consortium for Spinal Cord Injury Medicine, Paralyzed Veterans Association.

Hammond, M. C., & Burns, S. C. *Yes, you can! A guide to self-care for persons with spinal cord injury.* Paralyzed Veterans of America 3rd edition.

Hughes, J. T. (1988). The Edwin Smith Papyrus: An analysis of the first case reports of spinal cord injuries. *Paraplegia, 26,* 71–82.

Hurlbert, R. J. (2001). Methylprednisolone for acute spinal cord injury. An inappropriate standard of care. *Journal of Spinal Disorders, 13,* 185–199.

Kalat, J. W. (1998). *Biological Psychology* (6th ed.). Pacific Grove, CA: Brooks/Cole. p. 24.

Keirstead, H. S. (2005). Human embryonic stem cell-derived oligodendrocyte progenitor cell transplants remyelinate and restore locomotion after spinal cord injury. *Journal of Neuroscience, 25,* 4694–4705.

Kirshblum et al., Rehabilitation of spinal cord injury. (2002). In S. Kirshblum, D. Campagnolo, & J. Delisa (Eds.), *Spinal cord medicine* (pp. 275–298). Philadelphia, PA: Lippincott, Williams and Wilkins.

Kirshblum, S. C., & O'Connor, K. C. (1998). Bowel care practices in chronic spinal cord injury. *Archives of Physical Medicine and Rehabilitation, 79,* 1456–1466.

Kreuter, M., Siösteen, A., & Biering-Sørensen, F. (2008). Sexuality and sexual life in women with spinal cord injury: A controlled study. *Journal of Rehabilitation Medicine, 40,* 61–69.

Kwon, B. K., Mann, C., Sohn, H. M., Hilibrand, A. S., Phillips, F. M., Wang, J. C., et al. (2008). Hypothermia for spinal cord injury. *The Spine Journal, 8,* 859–874.

Linsenmeyer, T. (2002). Sexual function and fertility following spinal cord injury. In S. Kirshblum, D. Campagnolo, & J. Delisa (Eds.), *Spinal cord medicine* (pp. 322–328). Philadelphia, PA: Lippincott, Williams and Wilkins.

McDonald, J. W., Liu, X. Z., Qu, Y., Liu, S., Mickey, S. K., Turetsky, D., et al. (1999). Transplanted embryonic stem cells, survive, differentiate and promote recovery in injured rat spinal cord. *Nature Medicine, 5,* 1410–1412.

McKinley, W. O., Kolakowsky, S. A., & Kreutzer, J. S. (1999). Substance abuse, violence, and outcome after traumatic spinal cord injury. *American Journal of Physical Medicine & Rehabilitation, 78,* 306–312.

National SCI Statistical Center. (2008). *Spinal cord injury: Facts and figures at a glance.* Birmingham, AL: University of Alabama at Birmingham National Spinal Cord Injury Center.

Nistor, G. I. (2004). Human embryonic stem cells differentiate into oligodendrocytes in high purity and myelinate after spinal cord transplantation. *Glia, 49,* 385–396.

O'Connor, K. & Salcido, R. (2002). Pressure ulcer management and spinal cord injury. In S. Kirshblum, D. Campagnolo, & J. Delisa (Eds.), *Spinal cord medicine.* Philadelphia, PA: Lippincott, Williams and Wilkins.

Oleson, C. V., Burns, A. S., Ditunno, J. F., Geisler, F. H., & Coleman, W. P. (2005). Prognostic value of pinprick preservation in motor complete, sensory incomplete spinal cord injury. *Archives of Physical Medicine and Rehabilitation, 86,*988–992.

Onders, R., McGee, M. F., Marks, J., Chak, A., Schilz, R., Rosen, M. J., et al. (2007). Diaphragm pacing with natural orifice transluminal endoscopic surgery: Potential for difficult-to-wean intensive care unit patients, *Surgical Endoscopy, 21,* 471–479.

Outcomes Following Traumatic Spinal Cord Injury. (1999). Clinical Practice Guideline for Health Care Professionals, Consortium for Spinal Cord Injury Medicine, Paralyzed Veterans Association.

Priebe, M. M., Martin, M., Wuermser, L. A., Castillo, T., & McFarlin, J. (2002). The medical management of pressure ulcers. In V. Lin (Ed.), *Spinal cord medicine, principles and practice* (pp. 567–587). New York: Demos Medical Publishing.

Raghavan, A. M., & Shenot, P. J. (2009). Bladder augmentation using an autologous neo-bladder construct. *Kidney International, 76,* 236.

Randell, N., Lynch, A. C., Anthony. A, Dobbs, B. R., Roake, J. A., & Frizelle, F. A. (2001). Does a colostomy alter quality of life in patients with spinal cord injury? A controlled study. *Spinal cord, 39,* 279–282.

Regan, M., et al. (2007). Pressure Ulcers following Spinal Cord Injury, Spinal Cord Injury Rehabilitation Evidence, ICORD (http://www.icord.org/scire)

Ricciardi, R., Szabo, C., & Poullos, A. (2007). Sexuality and spinal cord injury. *Nursing Clinics of North America, 42,* 675–684.

Rosito, O., Nino-Murcia, M., Wolfe, V. A., Kiratli, B. J., & Perkash, I. (2002). The effects of colostomy on the quality of life in patients with spinal cord injury: A retrospective analysis. *Journal of Spinal Cord Medicine, 25,* 174–183.

Sayer, F., Kronvall, E., & Nilsson, O. (2006). Methylprednisolone treatment in acute spinal cord injury: The myth challenged through a structured analysis of published literature. *The Spine Journal, 6,* 335–343.

Scivoletto, G., Di Donna, V., Kim, C. M., Eng, J. J., & Whittaker, M. W. (2004). Level walking and ambulatory capacity in persons with incomplete spinal cord injury: Relationship with muscle strength *Spinal Cord, 42,* 156–162.

Sipski, M. L., & Arenas, A. (2006). Female sexual function after spinal cord injury. *Progress in Brain Research, 152,* 441–447.

Smith, C. P., Gangitano, D. A., Munoz, A., & Salas, N. A. (2008). Botulinum toxin type A normalizes alterations in urothelial ATP and NO release induced by chronic spinal cord injury. *Neurochemistry International, 5,* 1068–1075.

Spinal cord injury bowel management. (2009). http://www.sci-info-pages.com/bowel.html

Waters, R. L., Adkins, R., Yakura, J., & Vigil, D. (1994). Prediction of ambulatory performance based on motor scores, derived from standards of the American Spinal Injury Association. *Archives of Physical Medicine and Rehabilitation, 75,* 756–760.

Westgren, N., & Levi, R. (1995). Motherhood after traumatic spinal cord injury. *Obstetrics and Gynecology, 50,* 260–261.

Wirz, M., van Hedel, H. J., Rupp, R., Curt, A., & Dietz, V. (2006). Muscle force and gait performance: Relationships after spinal cord injury. *Archives of Physical Medicine and Rehabilitation, 87,* 1218–1222.

Yick, L. W., So, K. F., Cheung, P. T., & Wu, W. T. (2004). Lithium chloride reinforces the regeneration-promoting effect of chondroitinase ABC on rubrospinal neurons after spinal cord injury. *Journal of Neurotrauma, 21,* 932–943.

26

Stroke

Michal Eisenberg, MD, and Ira Rashbaum, MD

Stroke is the second leading cause of death worldwide, with 15 million strokes occurring annually. Of these, 5 million people die and another 5 million are left permanently disabled, placing an immense burden on family and community (Grysiewicz, Thomas, & Pandey, 2008). In the United States, according to data from the National Stroke Association and the American Heart Association, stroke continues to be the third leading cause of death after cardiac disease and cancer, killing about 150,000 people each year and accounting for the leading cause of long-term disability in adults.

In the United States, death due to stroke fell to 14% from 1995 to 2005, with the total deaths from stroke falling by 30%. According to the American Heart Association, in 2005, the incidence of new stroke was approximately 600,000 with another 185,000 recurrent strokes, totaling 785,000 cerebral infarcts. At younger ages, men have a higher incidence of stroke compared with women, whereas at older ages there is no gender difference in incidence. Nonetheless, according to the American Heart Association 2009 update, given that women live longer than men and that stroke more commonly occurs in the older population, more women than men die yearly of stroke. Women accounted for 60.6% of death due to stroke in the United States in 2004. In patients aged 45–64, death occurs within 30 days of stroke, in 8–12% of ischemic strokes and 37–38% of hemorrhagic strokes (Rosamond et al., 1999). African Americans have almost double the risk of first-ever stroke compared with White Americans. The most common type of stroke is ischemic, accounting for approximately 87% of all strokes (Conroy, DeJong, & Horn, 2009).

Whereas intracerebral hemorrhages account for only 13% of all strokes, they are responsible for more than 30% of all stroke deaths. Intracerebral hemorrhage has an annual incidence of 10–30 per 100,000 population, representing 2 million (10–15%) of the 15 million strokes reported yearly worldwide. Hospital admissions for cerebral hemorrhages have increased by 18% in the past 10 years. This increase in hospitalizations may be attributable to the aging population, in many cases associated with suboptimal blood pressure management and the increased use of anticoagulants, thrombolytics, and antiplatelet medication. Populations vary in the incidences of intracranial hemorrhage, with deep intracranial hemorrhage more common in the young and middle-aged populations. White Americans show a lower incidence of hemorrhagic stroke than Mexicans, Latinos, Native Americans, African Americans, Japanese, and Chinese populations (Qureshi, Mendelow, & Hanley, 2009).

According to the American Heart Association 2009 update, the median number of years of survival after a first stroke declines with age of onset, such that survival is 6.8 years for men and 7.4 years for women aged 60–69, 5.4 years for men and 6.4 years for women aged 70–79, and 1.8 years for men and 3.1 years for women aged 80 and older.

Although the life-altering cost to the individual who suffers a stroke is immeasurable, the burden overall to society including health care costs in 2008 has been estimated to be $65.5 billion in the United States (Grysiewicz et al., 2008).

STROKE ETIOLOGY AND RISK FACTORS

According to the National Stroke Association, "a stroke occurs when a blood clot blocks an artery or a blood vessel breaks, interrupting blood flow to an area of the brain," leading to brain cell death and resultant brain damage (National Stroke Association, 2009). When brain cells die during a stroke, abilities controlled by that area of the brain are lost, which may include speech, movement, and memory (National Stroke Association, 2009). In contrast to a permanent stroke, a transient ischemic attack (TIA), is a focal neurological deficit lasting less than 24 hours (Grysiewicz et al., 2008). Stroke is not limited to adults and may occur in children and adolescents.

Age is one of the main risk factors for stroke (Garrison, Rolak, Dodaro, & O'Callaghan, 1988). For each consecutive decade after 55 years of age, the risk for stroke approximately doubles (Grysiewicz et al., 2008). Hypertension is the greatest treatable risk factor for ischemic and hemorrhagic stroke (Garrison et al., 1988). The relationship between high blood pressure and stroke risk is continuous, consistent, and independent of other risk factors (Garrison et al., 1988). Hypertension accelerates the development of atherosclerosis that ultimately leads to an increased number of atherosclerotic events (Sacco et al., 2006). The incidence of stroke rises as blood pressure rises (Kannel, Wolf, Verter, & McNamara, 1970). Data consistently show higher incidence of stroke among Blacks than Whites (Garrison et al., 1988).

Cardiac disease is the third most important risk factor for stroke after age and hypertension. Cardiac disease predisposing to stroke includes coronary artery disease, atrial fibrillation, valvular heart disease, congestive heart failure, patent foramen ovale (PFO), and atrial septal aneurysm. Coronary artery disease is a process where the arteries supplying the heart with oxygen-rich blood become clogged. Atrial fibrillation is an irregular heart rhythm when multiple impulses originate and spread within the smaller two heart chambers. Atrial fibrillation causes stagnation of blood flow within the left atrium of the heart that may lead to thrombus formation and embolism (Grysiewicz et al., 2008). Valvular heart disease is a disease process involving any of the heart's four valves, the aortic, mitral, tricuspid, or pulmonic. Congestive heart failure is a process when the heart cannot pump blood sufficiently. A PFO is a flap-like opening between two heart chambers that can lead to turbulent blood flow. An atrial septal defect is a hole between two heart walls that may also lead to turbulent blood flow.

Diabetes is another important risk factor for stroke development. It is estimated that nearly 40% of all ischemic strokes are attributed to the effects of diabetes either alone or in combination with hypertension (Kissela et al., 2005). This risk may be due to the accelerated development of atherosclerosis over time and the increase of other risk factors including central obesity, accumulation of belly fat, elevated cholesterol, and hypertension associated with diabetes (Goldstein et al., 2006).

Hyperlipidemia, or elevated blood cholesterol levels, is a clear risk factor for cerebrovascular disease. Cholesterol-lowering medication decreases the primary risk of stroke by 25% (Straus, Majumdar, & McAlister, 2002). Clinical studies have indicated that the use of statins, a type of cholesterol-lowering medication, can significantly lower the risk of stroke as a primary prevention measure in patients with known high-risk vascular disease, including those with hypertension and diabetes (Reddy et al., 2009). Data presented in 2009 by the Stroke Prevention by Aggressive Reduction in Cholesterol Levels (SPARCL) group suggest that stroke victims who achieve optimal levels of low-density lipoprotein cholesterol, high-density lipoprotein cholesterol, triglycerides, and blood pressure were 65% less likely to have another stroke compared with people who did not reach an optimal level of any risk factor (Sacco, 2009).

A stroke is itself a risk factor for another stroke (Garrison et al., 1988). A patient with prior stroke has an approximately 7% annual risk of recurrent stroke (Hankey & Warlow, 1999). In general, stroke is more prevalent in men than in women (Brown, Whisnant, Sicks, O'Fallon, & Wiebers, 1996), although this is reversed in the 35–44 age group. Parental history of stroke is associated with 1/4- to 1/3-fold increased stroke risk (Kiely, Wolf, Cupples, Beiser, & Myers, 1993).

Smoking has been identified as an independent risk factor for stroke with a relative risk of 1.5 (Grysiewicz et al., 2008). Relative risk is the ratio of the risk of a disease among the exposed (smoking, in this example) versus the unexposed. Exposure to environmental or second-hand, tobacco smoke also increases the risk for stroke (Bonita, Duncan, Truelsen, Jackson, & Beaglehole, 1999).

Other risk factors for stroke include obesity, irregular and heavy alcohol use, elevated homocysteine levels, hypercoagulability syndromes, dialysis for chronic renal failure, cancer, illicit use of drugs such as cocaine or amphetamines, and cerebral amyloid angiopathy. Elevated serum cholesterol has not been clearly identified as a stroke risk factor (Grysiewicz et al., 2008).

Thrombotic stroke is the most common kind of stroke, accounting for about 40% of all ischemic cerebrovascular disease (Mohr et al., 1978). They are usually due to atherosclerotic stenosis or occlusion of a large blood vessel, especially the carotid or middle cerebral artery (Garrison et al., 1988). Embolic strokes comprise about 30% of all strokes. They arise from platelets, cholesterol, or fibrin, breaking off an arterial wall or from the heart, that travel to the brain, causing occlusion of a cerebral artery. Lacunar strokes comprise approximately 20% of all strokes (Mohr, 1982). These are very small strokes that occur where small perforating arterioles that branch directly off large vessels become blocked.

Hemorrhagic strokes account for approximately 10% of all strokes. They tend to occur in the basal ganglia, internal capsule, cerebellum, thalamus, or pons. Hypertension can rupture the penetrating arteries. Prognosis for hemorrhagic stroke is generally worse than ischemic stroke in terms of both mortality and functional recovery; however, if the patient recovers, the blood in the brain may be reabsorbed leaving relatively milder deficits (Garrison et al., 1988).

STROKE SIGNS AND SYMPTOMS

The signs and symptoms of stroke depend upon whether the left or right side of the brain is affected, and whether the patient is right-hand dominant (left brain dominant) or left-hand dominant (right brain dominant). For our discussion, we will presume a left cerebral dominant person, who typically is right handed.

An individual with a dominant left hemisphere stroke may have difficulty with moving the right side of the body, and have communication difficulty such as reading, speaking, writing, understanding, or judgment. An individual with a nondominant right hemisphere stroke often has difficulty with judgment, vision, and perception as well as left-sided weakness.

In the United States, it has been found that the middle cerebral artery is the most common artery affected by stroke. When this occurs, there is weakness on the body opposite the side of the stroke location. The upper limb is often weaker than the lower limb. Sensation may also be affected. When the anterior cerebral artery is involved in stroke, sensory deficits are usually absent and motor impairment often involves the lower limb more than the upper limb. In strokes involving the posterior cerebral artery, sensation and motor ability may be affected minimally, if at all, but impairment involving balance and vision may be marked.

In strokes involving the brain stem, sensory and motor abnormalities may be bilateral. They may produce cranial nerve abnormalities and adversely affect eye movement, tongue movement, and/or swallow function.

Strokes involving the occipital lobe typically cause visual deficits. Apraxia is the inability to execute a voluntary motor movement despite being able to demonstrate normal muscle function. Aphasia is the inability to use or understand language. Hemianopia is blindness in one half of the visual field of one or both eyes. Agnosia is the inability to recognize, interpret, or identify objects or people despite having prior knowledge of them. Aprosodia is the impaired ability to comprehend the emotion conveyed.

Anosognosia is decreased awareness of one's impairment and/or disability. Prosopagnosia is the decreased recognition of objects, faces in particular. Abulia is the impaired ability to make decisions or act independently.

COURSE AND PROGNOSIS

After the initial identification of a stroke and presentation to an emergency department, the course of treatment and prognosis vary depending on the type of stroke, either ischemic or hemorrhagic, as well as time of symptom onset, severity, and other comorbid medical conditions. A lower score on the Glasgow coma scale is an early indicator of poor prognosis.

Initially, the differentiation of hemorrhagic versus ischemic stroke or other brain pathology is determined by brain imaging such as computed tomography (CT) or magnetic resonance imaging (MRI). In some instances, an endotracheal tube is inserted if the airway is threatened to support breathing and adequate oxygenation. Patients are initially stabilized in the emergency department, with attention to and management of blood pressure, glucose control, intravenous or intraarterial blood clot treatments, antiplatelet therapy with aspirin or other drugs, and various surgical and endovascular interventions. The use of blood-thinning agents, that is, anticoagulation with heparin or similar agents, was a common practice in the past, but is no longer a recommended treatment modality for ischemic stroke (Adams et al., 2007).

For a hemorrhagic stroke, poorer prognostic factors include a larger volume of blood at presentation, enlargement of the hematoma volume, blood in the ventricles, and patients previously on oral blood thinners (Nassisi, 2008).

For an ischemic stroke, the treating emergency physician determines whether the patient is a candidate for blood clot removal therapy, that is, thrombolytic therapy. As of May 2009, the American Heart Association and the American Stroke Association provided guidelines for the administration of the blood-thinning agent recombinant tissue-type plasminogen activator (rt-PA) in a treatment window of 3–4.5 hours from stroke onset (Del Zoppo, Saver, Jauch, Adams, & American Heart Association Stroke Council, 2009). The 2007 American Heart Association guidelines highlight that for ischemic stroke, time of symptom onset is the single most crucial part of the history for determining the treatment course.

Patients are generally hospitalized for further management and observation after the initial emergency room course. Within the first 24–48 hours, neurological worsening occurs in approximately 25% of patients. Unfortunately, predicting which patients will deteriorate is difficult (Adams et al., 2007). The course of treatment during the hospitalization phase is designed to reduce the incidence of secondary complications, plan for secondary prevention treatments, and initiate rehabilitation and supportive services (Adams et al., 2007). Mobilization of patients generally begins as soon as their medical condition is considered stable, noting any changes in their neurological condition and acclimation to movement and sitting upright (Adams et al., 2007). Advantages of early mobilization include reducing risks for pneumonia, deep vein thrombosis, pulmonary embolism, joint contracture, and nerve palsies. The average length of hospitalization following stroke on an acute medical service is 4.9 days (2006 National Hospital Discharge Survey, National Health Statistics Reports, No. 5).

ACUTE STROKE MANAGEMENT

In the not so distant past, care of the patient with acute stroke emphasized supportive measures. Acute stroke care in recent years has been transformed by diagnostic and therapeutic advances and by the creation of stroke care centers as will be described below. Stroke must be treated in a timely manner (Gorelick, Gorelick, & Sloan, 2008). The adage is "time is brain," as delays in diagnosis and treatment may render the patient neurologically impaired and disabled (Gorelick et al., 2008). The American Heart Association describes stroke-warning signs including sudden numbness or weakness of the face, arm, or leg, especially on one side of the body; sudden confusion, trouble speaking, or understanding; sudden trouble seeing in one or both eyes; sudden trouble walking, dizziness, or loss of balance or coordination; and sudden, severe headache with no known cause (American Heart Association, 2009). Emergency preparedness is also strongly encouraged. Several states have enacted legislation for emergency medical services to preferentially triage patients suspected of having acute stroke to stroke care centers capable of rapid assessment and treatment (Gorelick et al., 2008).

Acute stroke recognition and intervention in the emergency department is crucial to improving stroke outcomes (Gorelick et al., 2008). Once the patient has arrived, a focused history and physical examination is efficiently performed followed by timely procurement of appropriate laboratory data. The National Institutes of Health Stroke Scale (NIHSS), a key neurological scale often utilized by emergency medicine and neurology personnel, assesses the patient's level of consciousness, motor, sensory, speech, and language skills. The NIHSS helps to localize what part of the brain was affected by the stroke, quantify the deficit(s), and guide treatment (Gorelick et al., 2008).

After a history and the initial physical examination have been completed and appropriate laboratory tests have been drawn, suspected stroke patients are sent immediately for a brain neuroimaging study (Gorelick et al., 2008). The most practical and widely available study to diagnose acute stroke is noncontrast brain CT that can be obtained within minutes. CT identifies brain hemorrhage and subdural hematoma nearly 100% of the time and subarachnoid hemorrhage 85–97% of the time (Gorelick et al., 2008).

Brain MRI has been shown to be better than CT for detecting acute ischemia or hemorrhage, with diffuse-weighted imaging (DWI) being particularly sensitive in detecting acute ischemic stroke (Gorelick et al., 2008). CT offers certain advantages in terms of availability and ease of use but MRI is likely the preferred test for accurate diagnosis in acute suspected stroke (Gorelick et al., 2008). MRI may not be readily available at all centers and it may take longer to complete; therefore, CT is an accepted initial imaging modality in acute stroke.

In the hospital, appropriate medical care is provided while the medical team is trying to determine if an acute stroke has occurred. Management of blood pressure, cardiac disease, blood sugar, and body temperature is essential. Arguably, the most important development in acute stroke treatment is intravenous thrombolytic therapy. Approved by the Food and Drug Administration after a milestone report in 1995 (The National Institute of Neurological Disorders and Stroke rt-PA Stroke Study Group, 1995), rt-PA can be administered intravenously within the first 3 hours after ischemic stroke sign or symptom onset with clinical improvement noted compared with placebo. For every 18 patients treated with intravenous rt-PA, two will achieve as good an outcome as they would have without the treatment, and one will have significant hemorrhage related to treatment (Gorelick et al., 2008).

Many patients being screened for rt-PA administration do not qualify for therapy based on their presentation time. They are either outside the 3-hour time window or meet other exclusion criteria, such as stroke or serious head injury within 3 months, major surgery within 14 days, history of intracranial hemorrhage, rapidly improving or minor symptoms, gastrointestinal or genitourinary hemorrhage within 21 days, arterial puncture within 7 days at a noncompressible site, seizure at stroke onset, systolic blood pressure above 185 mmHg, diastolic blood pressure above 110 mmHg, prothrombin time greater than 15 seconds, international normalized ratio greater than 1.4, platelet count less than 100,000, and glucose less than

50 mg/dl or greater than 400 mg/dl (Gorelick et al., 2008). Historically, there appeared to be no significant clinical benefit when administering intravenous rt-PA after 3 hours, with an increased risk of internal bleeding; however, emerging evidence suggests it could be beneficial to give rt-PA up to 4.5 hours after stroke in selected cases (Hacke et al., 2008).

Intraarterial thrombolysis, when a clot-dissolving medication is delivered to a stroke patient through the artery instead of a vein for up to 6 hours after demonstrating stroke signs and or symptoms, has been investigated and may prove to be an effective tool in acute ischemic stroke treatment (Gorelick et al., 2008). It has not been approved in the United States for routine clinical use as it requires specialized catheter labs and skilled clinicians for administration.

Clot retrieval devices attempt to literally retrieve blood clots lodged in brain blood vessels. Interventional neuroradiologists thread catheters into a patient's body, as is done during cardiac catheterization, and reach the vascular system of the brain where this type of device can remove a clot partially or completely. One such device is approved for clot retrieval within the first 8 hours after acute ischemic stroke; however, debate has ensued over its efficacy (Gorelick et al., 2008). A study is ongoing to investigate the efficacy of the MERCI clot retrieval device in the United States utilizing the 50 most active medical centers.

Combined intravenous and intraarterial thrombolytic approaches are being studied as is the development of new agents that may be safer and used concomitantly with clot retrieval devices (Gorelick et al., 2008).

Regardless of the use of newer agents and/or technologies in patients with acute stroke, good general medical management remains of paramount importance (Khaja, 2008).

MEDICAL COMPLICATIONS OF STROKE

Bowel and Bladder Dysfunction

Urinary incontinence occurs in about 30% to 80% of stroke patients, making it fairly common during the early stages, yet it continues in only about 10% of patients 2 years after stroke onset (O'Neill, Geis, Bogey, Moroz, & Bryant, 2004). Incontinence may result in urinary tract infection, skin breakdown, and social embarrassment (Roth, 1991). Stroke-related incontinence typically results from injury to the central descending pathways that control urination. This causes loss of voluntary inhibition of bladder muscle (detrusor) contraction, resulting in a hyperactive bladder (Roth, 1991). Patients describe the sensation of a full bladder but cannot prevent the bladder from contracting, resulting in uncontrolled voiding. Overflow incontinence may be due to weakness of the detrusor. In this situation, patients are incapable of completely emptying their bladder when voiding, causing an "overflow" incontinence. Incontinence may be related to weakness, cognitive-perceptual impairment, and/or lack of mobility (Roth, 1991). Transferring onto a toilet and adjusting one's clothing are often difficult tasks for stroke patients (Roth, 1991).

Various other conditions that many stroke patients have, such as diabetes mellitus, peripheral vascular disease, and coronary artery disease, may negatively affect bladder control as well (O'Neill et al., 2004).

Urodynamic testing, generally performed by a urologist, assesses the filling pressures of the bladder and sphincter muscle activity. In many cases, though, assessment of bladder volumes after urinating, known as the postvoid residual volume, obtained by either ultrasound bladder scans or catheterizing the bladder immediately after voiding is sufficient to determine the cause of incontinence.

Managing bladder dysfunction includes fluid intake regulation, scheduled toileting, and, in selected cases, medication. Medications need to be used with some caution in stroke patients, particularly the elderly, as the common classes of medications used to treat bladder dysfunction have anticholinergic properties (drowsiness and dry mouth, for example) and/or sympathomimetic properties (such as drowsiness and adverse cardiac effects).

Bowel dysfunction is common in stroke patients and is often considered an indicator of limited functional prognosis (Roth, 1991). The most common complications are constipation and impaction, but incontinence and diarrhea can also be frustrating and embarrassing (Roth, 1991). Diarrhea and incontinence often indicate bowel impaction as the fluid flows around the obstructing stool (Roth, 1991). Improper diagnosis can lead to treatment with constipating agents that only worsens the problem (Roth, 1991). One should always exclude bowel infection, medication effects, or other causes.

Often, bowel dysfunction is an indirect consequence of common problems caused by stroke, such as difficulty in transferring to the toilet or cognitive dysfunction (Roth, 1991). Often, once an effective bowel regimen is established, bowel dysfunction may be improved, which can significantly enhance quality of life by minimizing bowel accidents that may lead to embarrassment and/or skin moisture, the latter a risk factor for skin ulcers.

Cardiac Complications

One of the most frequent conditions accompanying, and potentially complicating, stroke rehabilitation is heart disease (Roth, 1991). According to the Framingham study, the most common heart disease forms included hypertensive heart disease, coronary artery disease, and heart failure (Roth, 1991). Heart disease is the second largest cause of death within the first 30 days among stroke patients (Roth, 1991). Heart disease can adversely affect the clinical and functional course of stroke rehabilitation by, among other things, limiting therapy participation, decreasing endurance, and impairing function (Roth, 1991). Recognition of heart disease manifestations in stroke patients before and during rehabilitation is the first step toward initiating appropriate intervention (Roth, 1991). Stroke patients often present a unique challenge to rehabilitation professionals, particularly when there are impairments of cognition and/or communication. Therefore, one has to have a high index of suspicion in considering the possible presence of life-altering heart disease, especially when patients may not be able to give a complete or succinct history.

Central Pain/Complex Regional Pain Syndrome

Central pain may be one of the most enigmatic complications of stroke. Although once associated with thalamic stroke, we know now that most thalamic strokes are not associated with central pain, and that most stroke patients with central pain do not have thalamic strokes.

The pain may be deep, superficial, localized, or diffuse, often with a burning, aching, or tingling quality (Roth, 1991). The onset is usually weeks to months after the stroke occurs.

It is treated often with a multidisciplinary approach including nursing care, medication, psychological therapy, and physical/occupational therapy. Surgery generally appears to have little or no role in managing this; however, deep brain stimulation, where electrodes are implanted in the brain to stimulate pain regions with the goal of reducing or eliminating pain, is an option.

Joint Contractures

Joints are at risk of becoming stiff and contracted following stroke. Surrounding muscles, tendons, ligaments, and joint capsules may tighten and shorten if a joint is not moved through its full range of motion (ROM) multiple times a day, leading to contractures, occurring most commonly at the shoulder, hip, and ankle. Contractures may develop more readily in the presence of spasticity (Anderson, 1981). The topic of spasticity is discussed in greater detail later in this chapter.

Depression

Depression has been the most frequently discussed psychological complication of stroke (Roth, 1991). Several studies have found the rate of clinically significant depression in stroke populations to be between 20% and 60% (O'Neill et al., 2004; Roth, 1991). It is a serious problem deserving prompt attention because it not only impedes participation in rehabilitation but is also linked with higher 12- and 24-month mortality after adjustment for factors associated with stroke severity (O'Neill et al., 2004). A combination of judicious antidepressant medication linked with talk therapy when indicated is an appropriate course of action.

Dysphagia

Dysphagia, or disorder of swallowing function, remains the most significant dietary concern after stroke (Reddy et al., 2009). Stroke may cause dysphagia by leading to impairment in oral-motor control, pharyngeal peristalsis, and/or swallow initiation and coordination. Untreated dysphagia can lead to pneumonia and malnutrition (Reddy et al., 2009).

A bedside clinical swallowing evaluation is often useful to identify patients at risk. These at-risk patients should be considered candidates for a more objective swallowing examination called a modified barium videofluoroscopic swallow study, or MBVFSS, which is performed by a swallowing therapist. The MBVFSS is performed in a radiology suite and assesses the patient's ability to swallow various consistencies of solids and liquids. If a patient does not pass a swallowing study, that is, if she/he does not demonstrate the ability to swallow safely solids and/or liquids, even soft or pureed solids and/or thickened liquids, the safest approach to ensure adequate nutrition is by feeding through a tube. If a patient passes a swallowing study, a diet modified to maximize patient safety is ordered.

Selected stroke patients with dysphagia may be able to eat and/or drink a modified diet while receiving a certain portion of their nutrition by a tube inserted into their stomach. When a tube for feeding is anticipated to be needed for more than several days, a gastroenterologist may place the tube directly through the abdominal wall into the stomach, known as a percutaneous enteral gastrostomy (PEG). This is often preferable to a nasogastric tube that passes through the nose and into the stomach. Swallowing therapists may also apply exercise and/or electric stimulation to specific muscles to restore swallow function more quickly and completely.

Falls

Falls are a potentially serious occurrence after stroke. Although many patients with stroke are susceptible to falls, those with nondominant hemisphere strokes manifesting decreased safety awareness, impaired attention to their environment opposite to the side of the lesion, and cognitive/perceptual impairments are particularly at risk. Interestingly, another risk for falls is increased mobility, essentially enabling patients to try to mobilize and/or ambulate themselves when they should not. Management centers on environmental modifications, such as the use of bedside commodes, may decrease the need for bathroom trips at night. In inpatient centers, frequent or continuous direct observation of patients at risk may be necessary. Bed or chair alarms that sound and alert staff when a patient attempts to stand have also been advocated as a way of decreasing falls in stroke and nonstroke patients. Our center has developed a falls committee that identifies at-risk patients and works on prevention and treatment strategies in a multidisciplinary way (Dunbar, September 9, 2008).

Pneumonia

Pneumonia, or lung infection, may occur due to a patient's overall illness; however, aspiration pneumonia occurs commonly in stroke patients. Aspiration pneumonia occurs when food and/or liquid may pass into the lung instead of the stomach.

Pneumonia is the third largest cause of death within the first month after stroke (Roth, 1991). Treatment includes antibiotic therapy, chest physical therapy including tracheobronchial hygiene, and proper mobilization (Roth, 1991).

Pressure Sores

Pressure sores and skin irritation can develop after stroke when immobility and increased physical pressure lead to ischemia overlying specific areas of the body.

Roth (1991) noted that pressure sores may be seen on weight-bearing surfaces of stroke patients, including the occiput (back of the head), scapula (shoulder blade), sacrum (lower part of the spine), buttocks, and heels. These sores are mainly preventable and are the direct result of immobility and skin insensitivity. Other factors such as shear forces, moisture, infection, and inadequate nutrition also play a role.

Prevention is key. Skin inspection, good nutrition, appropriate bladder and bowel regimens, and body position changes are extremely important. Position changes can allow blood circulation flow more freely as weight is shifted. When a pressure sore exists, wound care, and, when indicated, surgical management are required (Roth, 1991).

Seizures

Seizures are fairly uncommon after stroke, occurring in about 5% of cases. Strokes caused by emboli have the highest risk followed by hemorrhagic strokes. Neurological consultation for judicious use of antiseizure medication is suggested. However, one would prefer not to place a patient on continued medication, if possible, as this class of medications can cause lethargy and other mental status changes (Roth, 1991).

Shoulder Pain

Another common occurrence after stroke is hemiplegic shoulder pain. It is thought to occur in about 23% of stroke patients at 6 months. It can limit functional participation and lead to poorer outcomes and decreased quality of life (Reddy et al., 2009). Adhesive capsulitis, or shoulder ROM limitation due to tightness of the surrounding fibrous joint capsule, is the most common cause of poststroke shoulder pain. Primary adhesive capsulitis is essentially idiopathic (of unknown cause); however, stroke patients tend to be immobile, increasing the likelihood of limited motion at the shoulder. Rotator cuff tendon pain and/or tears can cause shoulder pain in this population and even contribute to secondary adhesive capsulitis. Complex regional pain syndrome and spasticity, both covered elsewhere in this chapter, are also causes of shoulder pain in this patient population. Management of hemiplegic shoulder pain starts with primary prevention. Limb positioning with acrylic wheelchair lap trays and/or slings may be utilized. Electrical stimulation of the supraspinatus, trapezius, and posterior deltoid muscles along with therapeutic exercise to these muscles may decrease pain and increase function (Reddy et al., 2009).

Thromboembolism

Deep venous thrombosis (blood clots in deep veins) and pulmonary embolism (blood clots in the pulmonary blood vessels) are potentially serious, even life-threatening, events that commonly occur in stroke patients. Incidence of deep venous thrombosis in stroke patients has been described as being between about 25% and 75% (Roth, 1991). The incidence of pulmonary embolism in stroke patients is lower but still significant at about 10–15%, and is the fourth most common cause of death in the first 30 days after stroke (Roth, 1991). Pulmonary embolism occurs less frequently in all patient populations than deep venous thrombosis.

Stroke patients may be more susceptible to thromboembolic disease due to immobility, leading to decreased overall physical functioning, such as limited ambulatory distances, and, occasionally, hypercoagulability of the blood (i.e., the blood is somewhat thicker than normal). Hypercoagulable state of the blood is a risk factor for stroke in itself.

All stroke rehabilitation professionals should be vigilant in checking for signs of deep venous thrombosis, which include limb swelling, tenderness, warmth, and color changes. When a deep venous thrombosis and/or pulmonary embolism are suspected, diagnostic evaluation should occur immediately, including venous duplex studies and/or spiral CT of the chest, respectively.

When a deep venous thrombosis is identified, a distal and/or nonocclusive thrombosis is theoretically less concerning than a proximal or occlusive one; however, in our experience, treatment is almost always embarked upon with anticoagulation using oral warfarin with or without heparin, either administered intravenously or under the skin when no medical or surgical contraindication exists. Oral warfarin generally is taken for 3 months for deep venous thrombosis and 6 months for pulmonary embolism. When contraindication exists, an inferior vena cava (IVC) filter is introduced by an interventional radiologist as soon as possible. An IVC filter is a device that is placed in the IVC, one of the major veins returning blood from the body back to the heart, to prevent blood clots, which could possibly dislodge from a vein, from entering the general blood circulation so as to not occlude an artery such as to the lungs. This is not used as often as blood-thinning medication, but is used when blood-thinning medication cannot be used or is deemed unsuccessful. Medical and/or surgical professionals are consulted before making therapeutic decisions such as these.

Generally, patients with deep venous thrombosis stay on the rehabilitation medicine service as long as they are deemed medically stable and generally resume full therapy activities after a day or less of bed rest. However, many stroke patients with newly diagnosed pulmonary embolism require transfer to an acute care hospital setting for closer observation and further care.

Urinary Tract Infections

Urinary tract infections may occur in stroke patients due to bladder dysfunction (as described previously) or poor hygiene. Indwelling bladder catheters increase the risk of developing a urinary tract infection and are therefore avoided whenever possible in favor of intermittent bladder catheterization if mechanical bladder emptying is required. Intermittent bladder catheterization may be performed by a nurse, by the patient, whenever possible, or by a caregiver trained in proper clean technique.

REHABILITATION MANAGEMENT

Rehabilitation after stroke is designed to regain function through a combination of recovery of abilities and adaptation to deficits. Comprehensive management of stroke rehabilitation requires attention to multiple aspects of human functioning. The team approach utilized in rehabilitation facilities provides a framework to address patients' needs in a thorough and systematic way. Another approach suggests dividing patients' needs into three domains: physical, psychological, and social (Vanhook, 2009). Either approach is appropriate, provided attention is given to all aspects of human functioning.

Initiation of rehabilitation begins during acute hospitalization with consultation from a rehabilitation physician, a.k.a physiatrist, and assessments by occupational, physical, and speech therapists. The patient's cognitive and physical abilities during this initial period are key determinants regarding both the need and level of intensity for continued inpatient hospitalization in a rehabilitation facility or for a discharge home.

Using the rehabilitation team approach, a physician, generally a physiatrist, leads a team of rehabilitation nurses, therapists, psychologists, and social workers. Whether a patient is discharged home directly from acute medical care or is transferred to an inpatient rehabilitation unit, these services should evaluate and treat patients to address their functional needs. After the initial evaluation, goals are set on a weekly basis, addressing the patient's deficits and needs. The rehabilitation team meets weekly to evaluate progress and determine next steps of care in a comprehensive and an interdisciplinary manner. A partial list of functions that need to be considered and managed in the rehabilitation program include pain control, bladder and bowel needs, bed mobility, sitting, standing, walking, activities of daily living, cognitive training, speech, language, swallowing, mood, and transition to home and the community.

Using the three domains approach, the medical caregiver should address the physical domain of cognition and function, psychological domain of self-concept and health perception, and social domain of relationships and role change. These needs demand the interdisciplinary skills of a variety of trained medical professionals for complete poststroke rehabilitation management (Vanhook, 2009).

After the acute inpatient rehabilitation phase, patients are either medically and physically well-enough to return home or continue to have a need for ongoing nursing and caregiver care that is best provided in an inpatient rehabilitation facility. In either case, it is crucial to emphasize the importance of continued medical follow-up to adequately address both ongoing medical problems and continued therapy to further functional recovery. When patients are discharged to the community, the process of rehabilitation often continues with home therapy services followed by outpatient physical, occupational, and speech therapy services as needed. Following the completion of acute rehabilitation, many patients remain incapable of returning to their community yet retain the capacity to improve functionally, albeit over longer periods of time. In this scenario, patients are typically transferred to a subacute facility, where rehabilitation, medical, and nursing services continue but generally at a less intense level than in acute rehabilitation centers, facilitating recovery with additional therapy while providing necessary custodial and physical needs.

For patients who have returned home, the efforts to maximize recovery and return to desired societal roles continue. Managing activities of daily living in addition to handling new challenges in home and community environments are often daunting tasks. For this reason, patients should be guided by continued outpatient rehabilitation services to initiate new tasks in stepwise patterns that build on small successful steps.

SPASTICITY

Spasticity can be described as muscle overactivity, defined as a velocity-dependent increase in muscle tone. It is part of the upper motor neuron syndrome that occurs following injuries to the spinal cord, brain stem, or brain, including stroke. Spasticity is manifested by hyperreflexia, spread of reflexes beyond stimulated muscles, hypertonicity, simultaneous contraction of agonist and antagonist muscles (e.g., triceps and biceps), clonus, and rigidity (Elovic, Eisenberg, & Jasey, 2009). When present, spasticity is problematic for most patients causing pain, difficulty with proper position of limbs and hygiene, and interference with normal motor function. In some situations, spasticity can be useful to achieve functional goals in the absence of motor strength.

Management of spasticity is often one of the greatest challenges after stroke for the patient and the treating rehabilitation team. It is best managed by a cohesive rehabilitation team, using multiple interventions in an integrated treatment plan. There are various interventions for spasticity treatment, with the goal of reducing muscle overactivity with the smallest side effect profile.

Spasticity management generally addresses both passive and active aspects of motor control. Passive functions include pain, positioning, hygiene, splint wearing, and prevention of contracture. Active functions include reducing the interference of spasticity on antagonistic muscle activity, thereby improving volitional movement.

The first step in spasticity management is preventing a wide variety of conditions that stimulate increased muscle tone, such as a pressure ulcer, ingrown toenail, contracture, kinked urinary drainage catheter, renal and bladder stones, urinary tract infection, blood clots in the leg, heterotopic ossification (abnormal bone growth across a joint or within muscle tissue), fecal impaction, infection, and fracture. Proper positioning is part of this first step, for poor positioning can cause increased spasticity, decreased ROM, contractures, and pain, which can exacerbate and potentiate a vicious cycle of worsening spasticity (Elovic et al., 2009). Various postures to avoid include leg crossing (scissoring), windswept position, and frog-leg position, which can worsen spasticity.

Stretching of the limbs is crucial to implement early in the treatment of both spasticity and stroke in general, serving as a focal treatment to prevent development of muscle shortening and contracture and to maintain ROM (Elovic et al., 2009; Gracies, 2001). Stretch needs to be applied for a prolonged period of time to achieve functional benefit. Applications of braces or casts made of plaster or fiberglass on spastic limbs are a means of achieving prolonged stretch. Serial casting uses a series of casts to increase joint ROM by progressively changing the angle of joint positioning with each new cast applied every 1–7 days (Pohl et al., 2002). Casting can be an important adjunct to other spasticity interventions, but caution must be taken to avoid skin breakdown or irritation from poorly fitted casts. Splints can also provide sustained stretch, with a reduced risk of skin problems as they are easily removed by patients or caregivers.

Physical modalities, such as cooling or heating, similar to stretching, are localized treatments with no significant systemic or major side effects, other than local skin irritation. Cooling modalities include quick icing, prolonged cooling, or an evaporating spray, such as ethyl chloride. Forms of heating include ultrasound, paraffin, fluidotherapy, superficial heat, and whirlpool. These modalities should be followed immediately by stretching and exercise (Elovic et al., 2009; Pohl et al., 2002).

Electrical stimulation in the form of transcutaneous electrical nerve stimulation units is a modality used in reducing pain, and through its nociceptive action it may reduce spasticity. No strong evidence exists regarding the effectiveness of massage therapy; however, it is often requested by patients and families (Elovic et al., 2009; Pohl et al., 2002).

Medications for spasticity management can be administered via four means: enteral system (oral or via gastrostomy tube), transdermal system, cerebrospinal fluid space (intrathecal) administration, and local injection into nerves and muscles.

Oral agents, including baclofen, tizanidine, dantrolene, and benzodiazepines, have systemic absorption and may therefore have widespread effects throughout the body, including the desired effect of reducing spasticity. Catapres-TTS is a transdermal medication, that is absorbed through the skin from a patch and also achieves its effects with systemic absorption. Given that these medications are absorbed systemically, their side effect profiles need to be taken into account and each patient treated individually given the risks of sedation, impaired cognition, fatigue, weakness, nausea, dizziness, paresthesias, blood pressure changes, and liver and kidney damage in patients at risk.

Intrathecal delivery of medications, such as baclofen, morphine, or clonidine, places the drug in close proximity to the spinal cord, where it acts to decrease spasticity by directly affecting structures involved in its generation. A pump filled with the medication is implanted surgically and is connected via a tube to the intrathecal space that surrounds the spinal cord. The pump is programmed to deliver precise amounts of drug to the intrathecal space, permitting effective management of spasticity in selected cases. Local intramuscular injections with phenol, ethanol, or botulinum toxin can treat focal spasticity. Both these methods involve more invasive procedures but offer the benefit of delivering the drug to its site of action, thereby reducing the incidence of side effects throughout the body associated with oral and transdermal methods of drug administration.

Optimal management of spasticity involves multiple and simultaneous application of these treatment modalities, interventions, and medications, and is best provided by a comprehensive rehabilitation team that includes therapists, nurses, and physicians in addition to providing patient and caregiver education.

MECHANISMS AND PATTERNS OF RECOVERY

It is known that stroke causes areas of cell death and scarring, yet patients have varying degrees of sensory, motor, and other functional recovery poststroke. The degree of recovery depends on various factors including severity of injury, location, size, and type of stroke, and premorbid dementia. Overall outcomes of stroke recovery are also dependent on other factors such as social support, emotional well-being, and coexisting medical conditions.

The mechanisms of recovery from stroke at the brain level can be attributed to some degree to blood resorption after hemorrhagic stroke and resolving edema. The degree and timing of recanalization and reperfusion therapies that restore blood flow following an acute ischemic stroke also play a role in the recovery process (Molina & Alvarez-Sabín, 2009). The stroke treatments and interventions described in previous sections are extrinsic and are designed to limit injury, assist in the recovery process, and improve specific functional skills. An emerging body of research is also investigating intrinsic cerebral factors that may help the healing process from within the brain itself. Neuronal factors contributing to recovery are thought to be attributable to axonal sprouting and new nerve growth. Animal studies have shown that there is axonal sprouting in areas connected to or near stroke lesions. Sprouting axons have been demonstrated in animal studies to arise from intact areas on the opposite side or nonaffected brain areas (Carmichael, 2008). Similarly, animal studies have demonstrated that axonal sprouting occurring in response to motor cortex injury extended from the premotor cortex in the frontal lobe into the somatosensory cortex in the parietal lobe (Dancause et al., 2005). Although this information is encouraging, it has not yet been able to demonstrate a promotion in functional recovery. New nerve regeneration has been shown to continue in the adult mammalian brain, and recent evidence supports new neuron growth in human adults (Dancause et al., 2005; Lichtenwalner & Parent, 2006). Self-repair of injured brain may be possible with endogenous neural stem cells and persistent neuronal production, which was thought impossible in the past.

Motor recovery generally occurs in a proximal-to-distal pattern, whereby muscles more proximally regain strength before more distal muscles. For example, elbow motor control is likely to return before wrist or finger control, and similarly hip and upper leg movement before the ankle. As more is learned about neuronal recovery, therapies will be developed in the future to restore neurological function at the level of brain cells (Dancause et al., 2005; Lichtenwalner & Parent, 2006; Zhang, Zhang, & Chopp, 2005).

EMERGING STROKE TREATMENTS

Stroke rehabilitation, as with all rehabilitation, has embraced both the "high-tech" and "high-touch" therapeutic modalities. Some of the emerging treatments will be described further.

Constraint-Induced Movement Therapy

Constraint-induced movement therapy (CIMT), in its purest form, is an intensive therapeutic regimen provided over the course of 10 consecutive treatment days, 6 hours each day, that restricts the use of the uninvolved upper limb, forcing individuals to use their weaker upper limb to perform activities of daily living. It is based on the theory of nonuse that says a limb weakened by stroke will not improve if it is not actively rehabilitated. The patient uses a mitt, sling, and/or splint to the unimpaired upper extremity for up to 90% of waking hours (Taub et al., 1993) The Extremity Constraint Induced Therapy Evaluation (EXCITE) trial is the largest trial known to date that demonstrated clinical and functional improvement compared with traditional therapy (Wolf et al., 2006).

Because of the logistics of providing such intense treatment for those 10 days, modifications in the treatment protocol have evolved. Modified constraint-induced movement therapy (mCIMT) provides treatment 5 hours daily for 5 days, followed by 3 hours a day, three times weekly over approximately 10 additional weeks (Page, Sisto, Johnston, Levine, & Hughes, 2002). Other modifications have used online computer sessions or combined CIMT with robot therapy (Page & Levine, 2007). Other factors potentially limiting the efficacy and application of CIMT include the considerable effort and motivation required, the frequently low mitt-wearing compliance rate, and the minimally required strength and ROM at the distal upper limb, the latter markedly limiting the number of total individuals who can benefit from CIMT.

Virtual Reality

Computer technological development has led to virtual reality programs where individuals can interact in computer-generated "environments" simulating real-world settings (Chute, 2002; Rizzo & Buckwalter, 1997). Theoretically, specific therapeutic modalities can be safely provided that otherwise would be too dangerous or complex. The technology is flexible, reproducible, and capable of meeting clinical, research, and assessment needs. Virtual reality may be combined in research settings relatively easily with functional magnetic resonance imaging (fMRI) to assess virtual reality's effect on neuroplasticity.

Transcranial Magnetic Stimulation

Transcranial magnetic stimulation (TMS) is essentially brain stimulation with magnetic energy designed to induce neuroplasticity, or purposeful brain rewiring, to enhance functional recovery after stroke. TMS uses short magnetic pulses generated by passing a very brief current held to the scalp's surface. The primary risk of TMS is the induction of seizures. This can generally be avoided by adhering to strict technical protocol (Wasserman, Pascual-Leone, Davey, Rothwell, & Puri, 2002). Repetitive TMS was shown in one study to be associated with improvement in disability scales after a 10-day treatment course compared with sham rTMS (Khedr, Ahmed, Fathy, & Rothwell, 2005).

Electric Stimulation

Electric stimulation can be provided in various ways in an attempt to improve both motor and functional skills following a central nervous system injury such as stroke. It can be applied to muscles and/or nerves in the form of neuromuscular electric stimulation or at the brain via electrodes. Electric stimulation, either applied to muscles and nerves or to the motor cortex of the brain, provides a means to enhance motor relearning and, theoretically, improve the functional use of the weak limb.

Electric stimulation may also be incorporated into braces shown to improve both upper and lower limb function. Electric stimulation may also reduce shoulder subluxation after stroke. Shoulder subluxation occurs when the head of the humerus bone depresses in the shoulder socket due to surrounding muscle weakness caused by stroke.

Robot Therapy

Clinicians and biomedical engineers have collaborated to develop various robotic devices with the goal of improving both motor and functional recovery poststroke. Robotics takes advantage of evidence suggesting that intensive, highly repetitive, functionally relevant, and challenging therapies are critical factors contributing to motor and functional recovery (Butefisch,

Hummelsheim, Denzler, & Mauritz, 1995). Rehabilitation robots have been designed to provide intensive and highly repetitive therapies providing a means to improve motor and functional recovery in ways not feasible or practical using traditional rehabilitation approaches. Robots use computer programs that constrain inaccurate limb movement during specific tasks that can be modified as patients progress in their recovery, promoting more functionally appropriate motor skills. The intensity and automated components of robot therapies specifically address the time and labor constraints associated with traditional therapies, as they can be used with less involvement of trained professionals. Robot therapy can also enhance patient compliance by combining games with treatment, which provide immediate feedback on performance that serve to increase motivation. Changes in motor skills can be readily tracked and documented to help guide therapy, evaluate the efficacy of treatment interventions, and provide an additional means to monitor progress. However, some robotic devices are labor intensive, and most require considerable start-up costs. Although they hold great promise, there is currently a lack of validation from clinical trials. However, the initial labor intensiveness arising from staff training plus the cost of equipment may be offset by the long-term cost effectiveness derived from decreasing the amount of direct contact time therapists must spend with patients. Robot therapy has also been combined with CIMT and virtual reality. Future studies will need to address the functional implications of robot devices as well as their economic feasibility and advantage over conventional treatments (Rashbaum & Flanagan, in press).

Body Weight-Supported Treadmill Training

Body weight-supported treadmill training (BWSTT) uses a harness system that supports a percentage of a patient's body weight that unloads the lower extremities while training to walk on a treadmill. Evidence suggests that this may be an effective method of improving gait quality, walking speed, and trunk stability after stroke. It may also be an effective means to encourage a symmetrical gait pattern early in the rehabilitation process as well as a more appropriate method to facilitate sensory input and maximize much-needed repetition during the critical recovery period (Rashbaum & Flanagan, in press).

BWSTT attempts to facilitate automatic walking movements within the context of task-specific training. The patient is placed on a treadmill moving at the maximal comfortable walking speed with a portion of the weight being supported at the trunk by an overhead harness. The combination of the therapist(s) and the physical apparatus of the system controls leg movement, patient posture, and balance that aids in mimicking the normal rhythmic nature of gait. The system offers patients the support to maintain the standing position, which is useful for those who do not have the muscle strength or postural control to begin over-the-ground gait training. Furthermore, it may decrease the fear of falling. It may avoid the development of gait deviations often associated with traditional ambulation training (Rashbaum & Flanagan, in press). Gait improvement following BWSTT has been associated with changes in brain activation patterns in the cerebellum and midbrain suggesting its ability to enhance cerebral plasticity (Luft et al., 2008).

BWSTT is receiving widespread clinical acceptance. A primary drawback has been the time and physical demands placed on therapy staff (Bogey & Hornby, 2007), which, with emerging improvements in technique, should decrease.

COMMUNITY REINTEGRATION

The transition from the hospital to the community requires overcoming many potential obstacles for people with stroke because of the associated difficulties in physical, cognitive, and psychological skills combined with varying degrees of social support. An important role of the rehabilitation team prior to discharge is to prepare patients and their caregivers for their new roles at home. The continuum of care, including follow-up for medical care, rehabilitation needs, therapy, and social services, is crucial to a successful return to the community.

Patients and their caregivers need clear instructions and direction on how to follow-up with many of the physicians, such as neurosurgeons, neurologists, and endovascular interventionalists, who managed their stroke while hospitalized, particularly when patients are being discharged home from rehabilitation facilities and access to physicians may be challenging. Both nursing and attendant care are often required at home to ensure safety and maximal independence, and therefore need to be arranged prior to hospital discharge. Attention to psychological states can also affect successful resumption of everyday activities, as depression has been shown to be common in stroke survivors and can have an impact on activities of daily living and longevity in this population (Cameron, Tsoi, & Marsella, 2008; Dancause et al., 2005; Lichtenwalner & Parent, 2006; Zhang et al., 2005).

VOCATIONAL RETURN

Given that 15–20% of stroke survivors are of working age (Vestling, Tufvesson, & Iwarsson, 2003), the issues relating to vocational rehabilitation for return to work are crucial to this population. Vocational rehabilitation can be defined as a process by which patients with disabilities or illness can be assisted to achieve, maintain, or return to prior employment or seek out new useful occupation (Chamberlain et al., 2009). Current advancements in United States' law as determined by the Americans with Disabilities Act (ADA) Amendment of 2008 establishes the rights of persons with disabilities to have employers provide reasonable accommodations, without regard to ameliorating factors that would mitigate the disability to disqualify the person as qualifying for accommodations (Petrila, 2009). The ADA empowers persons with disabilities to seek rights for adaptations in the workplace.

Percentages of stroke survivors returning to work ranges from 19% to 73% (Treger, Shames, Giaquinto, & Ring, 2007). Those who have returned to work have shown subjectively rated higher levels of well-being and life satisfaction, yet approximately 75% of patients do not resume their prior work role poststroke. Various barriers to return to work after stroke include hemiplegia and physical factors, lack of transportation, poor local economy with high unemployment, and stereotypes against persons with disabilities. For stroke survivors who return to work, this is usually accomplished within the first 3–6 months, with minimal return to work at 1 year. Predictors for return to work include younger age, stroke severity, cognitive and behavioral impairments, and functional disability as measured by the Barthel Index or Glasgow Outcome Scale (Treger et al., 2007). A study from New Zealand found that psychiatric and physical morbidities are determinants of the outcome to return to work (Glozier, Hackett, Parag, & Anderson, 2008). Overall, return to work after stroke is an important outcome factor in stroke recovery and remains a challenge both to quantify and to achieve in many stroke survivors (Treger et al., 2007).

CONCLUSION

Stroke is a sudden life-changing event with lifelong implications, often with chronic disability, decreased independence, and increased need for medical, social, and caregiver support. This disease of the brain is common throughout the world and the United States, rendering it one of the greatest dangers to health and well-being, particularly in the older population. The process to recovery can be long and arduous for patients and caregivers. Access to follow-up medical and rehabilitation care, adequate social support and services, and psychological disposition and motivation are factors that play key roles in helping patients progress day to day toward their maximal recovery and return to improved functioning.

Stroke survivors are heros of the brain, and overcoming devastating damage to this critical body organ depends on rapid response of emergency systems and experienced initial treatment in acute care hospitals, followed by the expertise of experienced and well-trained rehabilitation teams to guide survivors and their caregivers. Well-orchestrated treatment protocols and teams continue to improve survival and reduce disability after stroke.

Patients with a history of stroke should be encouraged to follow up with a rehabilitation physician, physiatrist, or other medical stroke specialist to ensure prompt access to post-stroke medical care, rehabilitation, and social services, and thereby improve quality of life and maximize functioning. In the hands of well-trained stroke physicians and rehabilitation teams, stroke survivors can improve their quality of life and improve functioning of mind and body.

REFERENCES

Adams, H. P., Jr., del Zoppo, G., Alberts, M. J., Bhatt, D. L., Brass, L., Furlan, A., et al. (2007). Guidelines for the early management of adults with ischemic stroke: A guideline from the American Heart Association/American Stroke Association Stroke Council, Clinical Cardiology Council, Cardiovascular Radiology and Intervention Council, and the Atherosclerotic Peripheral Vascular Disease and Quality of Care Outcomes in Research Interdisciplinary Working Groups: The American Academy of Neurology affirms the value of this guideline as an educational tool for neurologists. *Circulation, 115,* e478–e534.

American Heart Association. *Stroke warning signs.* Retrieved May 23, 2009 from www.americanheart.org/presenter

Anderson, T. P. (1981). Stroke and cerebral trauma: Medical aspects. In W. C. Stolov & M. R. Clowers (Eds.), *Handbook of severe disability* (p. 121). Washington, DC: US Department of Education.

Bogey, R., & Hornby, G. T. (2007). Gait training strategies utilized in poststroke rehabilitation: Are we really making a difference? *Topics in Stroke Rehabilitation, 14,* 1–8.

Bonita, R., Duncan, J., Truelsen, T., Jackson, R. T., & Beaglehole, R. (1999). Passive smoking as well as active smoking increases the risk of acute stroke. *Tobacco Control, 8,* 156–160.

Brown, R. D., Whisnant, J. P., Sicks, J. D., O'Fallon, W. M., & Wiebers, D. O. (1996). Stroke incidence, prevalence, and survival: Secular trends in Rochester, Minnesota, through 1989. *Stroke; a Journal of Cerebral Circulation, 27,* 373–380.

Butefisch, C., Hummelsheim, H., Denzler, P., & Mauritz, K. H. (1995). Repetitive training of isolated movements improves the outcome of motor rehabilitation of the centrally paretic hand. *Journal of the Neurological Sciences, 130,* 59–68.

Cameron, J. I., Tsoi, C., & Marsella, A. (2008). Optimizing stroke systems of care by enhancing transitions across care environments. *Stroke; a Journal of Cerebral Circulation, 39,* 2637–2643.

Carmichael, S. T. (2008). Themes and strategies for studying the biology of stroke recovery in the post-stroke epoch. *Stroke, 39,* 1380–1388.

Chamberlain, M. A., Moser, V., Ekholm, K., O'Connor, R., Herceg, M., & Ekholm, J. (2009). Vocational rehabilitation: An educational review. *Journal of Rehabilitation Medicine. Supplement, 41,* 856.

Chute, D. L. (2002). Neuropsychological technologies in rehabilitation. *Journal of Head Trauma Rehabilitation, 17,* 369–377.

Conroy, B., DeJong, G., & Horn, S. (2009). Hospital-based stroke rehabilitation in the United States. *Topics in Stroke Rehabilitation, 16,* 34.

Dancause, N., Barbay, S., Frost, S. B., Plautz, E. J., Chen, D., Zoubina, E. V., et al. (2005). Extensive cortical rewiring after brain injury. *Journal of Neuroscience: The Official Journal of the Society for Neuroscience, 25,* 10167–10179.

Del Zoppo, G. J., Saver, J. L., Jauch, E. C., Adams, H. P., Jr., & American Heart Association Stroke Council. (2009). Expansion of the time window for treatment of acute ischemic stroke with intravenous tissue plasminogen activator: A science advisory from the American Heart Association/American Stroke Association. *Stroke; a Journal of Cerebral Circulation, 40,* 2945–2948.

Dunbar, S. D. (September 9, 2008). Safety huddles. Advance for Nurses. Retrieved March 26, 2010, from http://nursing.advanceweb.com/Editorial/Content/Editorial.aspx?CC=121501

Elovic, E. P., Eisenberg, M. E., & Jasey, N. N. (Eds.). (2009). *Physical medicine and rehabilitation: Principles and practice* (5th ed.). Philadelphia: Lippincott Williams & Wilkins.

Garrison, S. J., Rolak, L. S., Dodaro, R. R., & O'Callaghan, A. J. (1988). Rehabilitation of the stroke patient. In J. A. Delisa (Ed.), *Rehabilitation medicine: Principles and practice* (pp. 565–583). Philadelphia: Lippincott.

Glozier, N., Hackett, M., Parag, V., & Anderson, C. (2008). The influence of psychiatric morbidity on return to paid work after stroke in younger adults: The Auckland Regional Community Stroke (ARCOS) study, 2002 to 2003. *Stroke, 39*, 1526.

Goldstein, L. B., Adams, R., Alberts, M. J., Appel, L. J., Brass, L. M., Bushnell, C. D., et al. (2006). Primary prevention of ischemic stroke: A guideline from the American Heart Association/American Stroke Association Stroke Council: Cosponsored by the Atherosclerotic Peripheral Vascular Disease Interdisciplinary Working Group; Cardiovascular Nursing Council; Clinical Cardiology Council; Nutrition, Physical Activity, and Metabolism Council; and the Quality of Care and Outcomes Research Interdisciplinary Working Group. *Circulation, 113*(24), e873–923.

Gorelick, A. R., Gorelick, P. B., & Sloan, E. P. (2008). Emergency department evaluation and management of stroke: Acute assessment, stroke teams and care pathways. *Neurologic Clinics, 26*, 923–942, viii.

Gracies, J. M. (2001). Pathophysiology of impairment in patients with spasticity and use of stretch as a treatment of spastic hypertonia. *Physical Medicine and Rehabilitation Clinics of North America, 12*, 747–768, vi.

Grysiewicz, R. A., Thomas, K., & Pandey, D. K. (2008). Epidemiology of ischemic and hemorrhagic stroke: Incidence, prevalence, mortality, and risk factors. *Neurologic Clinics, 26*, 871–895, vii.

Hacke, W., Kaste, M., Bluhmki, E., Brozman, M., Davalos, A., Guidetti, D., et al. (2008). Thrombolysis with alteplase 3 to 4.5 hours after acute ischemic stroke. *New England Journal of Medicine, 359*, 1317–1329.

Hankey, G. J., & Warlow, C. P. (1999). Treatment and secondary prevention of stroke: Evidence, costs, and effects on individuals and populations. *Lancet, 354*, 1457–1463.

Kannel, W. B., Wolf, P. A., Verter, J., & McNamara, P. M. (1970).Epidemiologic assessment of the role of blood pressure in stroke: The Framingham study. *Journal of American Medical Association, 214*, 301–310.

Khaja, A. M. (2008). Acute ischemic stroke management: Administration of thrombolytics, neuroprotectants, and general principles of medical management. *Neurologic Clinics, 26*, 943–961, viii.

Khedr, E. M., Ahmed, M. A., Fathy, N., & Rothwell, J. C. (2005). Therapeutic trial of repetitive transcranial magnetic stimulation after acute ischemic stroke. *Neurology, 65*, 466–468.

Kiely, D. K., Wolf, P. A., Cupples, L. A., Beiser, A. S., & Myers, R. H. (1993). Familial aggregation of stroke. the Framingham study. *Stroke; a Journal of Cerebral Circulation, 24*, 1366–1371.

Kissela, B. M., Khoury, J., Kleindorfer, D., Woo, D., Schneider, A., Alwell, K., et al. (2005). Epidemiology of ischemic stroke in patients with diabetes: The greater Cincinnati/Northern Kentucky stroke study. *Diabetes Care, 28*, 355–359.

Lichtenwalner, R. J., & Parent, J. M. (2006). Adult neurogenesis and the ischemic forebrain. *Journal of Cerebral Blood Flow & Metabolism, 26*, 1.

Luft, A. R., Macko, R. F., Forrester, L. W., Villagra, F., Ivey, F., Sorkin, J. D., et al. (2008). Treadmill exercise activates subcortical neural networks and improves walking after stroke: A randomized controlled trial. *Stroke; a Journal of Cerebral Circulation, 39*, 3341–3350.

Mohr, J. P. (1982). Lacunes. *Stroke; a Journal of Cerebral Circulation, 13*, 3–11.

Mohr, J. P., Caplan, L. R., Melski, J. W., Goldstein, R. J., Duncan, G. W., Kistler, J. P., et al. (1978). The Harvard cooperative stroke registry: A prospective registry. *Neurology, 28*, 754–762.

Molina, C. A., & Alvarez-Sabín, J. (2009). Recanalization and reperfusion therapies for acute ischemic stroke. *Cerebrovascular Diseases, 27*, 162–167.

Nassisi, D. (2008). *Stroke, hemorrhagic*. Available from http://emedicine.medscape.com/article/793821-overview

National Stroke Association. *What is stroke?* Retrieved May 23, 2009 from www.stroke.org

O'Neill, B. J., Geis, C. C., Bogey, R. A., Moroz, A., & Bryant, P. R. (2004). Stroke and neurodegenerative disorders acute stroke evaluation, management, risks, prevention, and prognosis. *Archives of Physical Medicine and Rehabilitation, 85*, S3–S10.

Page, S. J., & Levine, P. (2007). Modified constraint-induced therapy extension: Using remote technologies to improve function. *Archives of Physical Medicine and Rehabilitation, 88*, 922–927.

Page, S. J., Sisto, S., Johnston, M. V., Levine, P., & Hughes, M. (2002). Modified constraint-induced therapy in subacute stroke: A case report. *Archives of Physical Medicine and Rehabilitation, 83*, 286–290.

Petrila, J. (2009). Congress restores the Americans with disabilities act to its original intent. *Psychiatric Services, 60*, 878.

Pohl, M., Ruckriem, S., Mehrholz, J., Ritschel, C., Strik, H., & Pause, M. R. (2002). Effectiveness of serial casting in patients with severe cerebral spasticity: A comparison study. *Archives of Physical Medicine and Rehabilitation, 83*, 784–790.

Qureshi, A., Mendelow, D. A., & Hanley, D. F. (2009). Intracerebral haemorrhage. *The Lancet, 373*, 1632–1644.

Reddy, C., Chae, J., Lew, H., Lombard, L., Edgley, S., & Moroz, A. (2009). Stroke management in the acute care setting. *PM & R: The Journal of Injury, Function, and Rehabilitation, 1*, S4–S12.

Rizzo, A. A., & Buckwalter, J. G. (1997). Virtual reality and cognitive assessment and rehabilitation: The state of the art. In G. Riva (Ed.), *Virtual reality in neuro-psycho-physiology*. Amsterdam, Netherlands: IOS Press.

Rosamond, W. D., Folsom, A. R., Chambless, L. E., Wang, C. H., McGovern, P. G., Howard, G., et al. (1999). Stroke incidence and survival among middle-aged adults: 9-year follow-up of the atherosclerosis risk in communities (ARIC) cohort. *Stroke; a Journal of Cerebral Circulation, 30*, 736–743.

Roth, E. J. (1991). Medical complications encountered in stroke rehabilitation. *Physical Medicine and Rehabilitation Clinics of North America, 2*, 563.

Sacco, R. (2009, July). Breakthroughs in stroke prevention and treatment. *Bottom Line Personal, 1*, 9.

Sacco, R. L., Adams, R., Albers, G., Alberts, M. J., Benavente, O., Furie, K., et al. (2006). Guidelines for prevention of stroke in patients with ischemic stroke or transient ischemic attack: A statement for healthcare professionals from the American Heart Association/American Stroke Association Council on Stroke: Co-sponsored by the Council on Cardiovascular Radiology and Intervention: The American Academy of Neurology affirms the value of this guideline. *Stroke; a Journal of Cerebral Circulation, 37*, 577–617.

Straus, S. E., Majumdar, S. R., & McAlister, F. A. (2002). New evidence for stroke prevention: Scientific review. *Journal of the American Medical Association, 288*, 1388–1395.

Taub, E., Miller, N. E., Novack, T. A., Cook, E. W., 3rd, Fleming, W. C., Nepomuceno, C. S., et al. (1993). Technique to improve chronic motor deficit after stroke. *Archives of Physical Medicine and Rehabilitation, 74*, 347–354.

The National Institute of Neurological Disorders and Stroke rt-PA Stroke Study Group. (1995). Tissue plasminogen activator for acute ischemic stroke. The National Institute of Neurological Disorders and Stroke rt-PA Stroke Study Group. *New England Journal of Medicine, 333*, 1581–1587.

Treger, I., Shames, J., Giaquinto, S., & Ring, H. (2007). Return to work in stroke patients. *Disability and Rehabilitation, 29*, 1397–1403.

Vanhook, P. (2009). The domains of stroke recovery: A synopsis of the literature. *Journal of Neuroscience Nursing: Journal of the American Association of Neuroscience Nurses, 41*, 6–17.

Vestling, M., Tufvesson, B., & Iwarsson, S. (2003). Indicators for return to work after stroke and the importance of work for subjective well-being and life satisfaction. *Journal of Rehabilitation Medicine: Official Journal of the UEMS European Board of Physical and Rehabilitation Medicine, 35*, 127–131.

Wasserman, E. M., Pascual-Leone, A., Davey, N. J., Rothwell, J., & Puri, B. K. (Eds.). (2002). *Handbook of transcranial magnetic stimulation*. New York: Oxford University Press.

Wolf, S. L., Winstein, C. J., Miller, J. P., Taub, E., Uswatte, G., Morris, D., et al. (2006). Effect of constraint-induced movement therapy on upper extremity function 3 to 9 months after stroke: The EXCITE randomized clinical trial. *JAMA: The Journal of the American Medical Association, 296*, 2095–2104.

Zhang, R. L., Zhang, Z. G., & Chopp, M. (2005). Neurogenesis in the adult ischemic brain: Generation, migration, survival, and restorative therapy. *The Neuroscientist: A Review Journal Bringing Neurobiology, Neurology and Psychiatry, 11*, 408–416.

27

Visual Impairments

Bruce P. Rosenthal, OD, FAAO, and Roy Gordon Cole, OD, FAAO

The world population clock stood at 67,945,803,019 on November 3, 2009, and will add 2 billion plus people by the year 2040 (U.S. Census Bureau, n.d.). The marked increase in the numbers of older persons will translate into millions and millions of visually impaired persons worldwide from age-related eye conditions such as macular degeneration, diabetic retinopathy, cataract, and glaucoma. In the United States, there are currently 1.8 million persons with age-related macular degeneration (AMD), 2.2 million with glaucoma, 4.1 million with diabetic retinopathy, and 20.5 million with cataract. These numbers will increase to 2.9 million for AMD, 3.3 for glaucoma, 7.2 for diabetic retinopathy, and 30.1 for cataract in 2020 (Eye Disease Prevalence Research Group, 2004).

In the United States, there will be a significant increase in the number of aging citizens, especially in the 60–85+ categories. In 2009, the baby-boomers demographic ranged in age from 45 to 63 years and had their first member sign up for Medicare. In 2025, the age range will be 61–79 years, and by 2050, this group will range in age from 86 to 104 years.

The increase is especially significant, as Congdon and colleagues (2004) have noted, because Americans aged 80 and older have the highest rates of blindness as well as being in the fastest growing segment of the population. It was also noted that although those aged 80 and older make up only 8% of the population, they accounted for 69% of the cases of blindness. There will also be a concomitant increase in the life expectancy in the United States from 75.8 in males and 80.9 in females in 2010 to 80.8 in males and 85.3 in females in 2050 (Figure 27.1; U.S. Census Bureau, n.d.).

The marked increase in the numbers of older persons will translate into millions and millions of additional visually impaired persons worldwide. These individuals will in turn require access to vision rehabilitation and particularly low-vision services.

DEFINITIONS AND STATISTICS

Vision Impairment

Vision impairment can be described as reduced vision that interferes with an individual's ability to do their normal daily activities. It can be defined as having a visual acuity of 20/70 or worse in the better eye, even with eyeglasses, or as the presence of a significant visual field loss (ICD-9, 2009). A broader definition of vision impairment, according to the Prevent Blindness America (2008), is having a visual acuity of 20/40 or worse in the better eye even with eyeglasses. Visual impairment may be categorized as moderate, severe, profound,

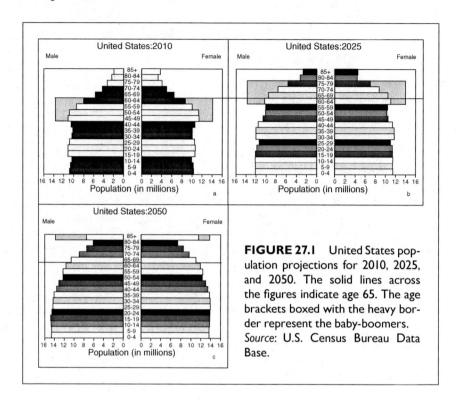

FIGURE 27.1 United States population projections for 2010, 2025, and 2050. The solid lines across the figures indicate age 65. The age brackets boxed with the heavy border represent the baby-boomers. *Source*: U.S. Census Bureau Data Base.

near-total, or total vision loss depending on the degree of loss of visual acuity or visual field (ICD-9, 2009). (There are also categories of vision called normal and near normal that are not considered to be impaired vision.) There is no official definition of impairment based on reduced contrast sensitivity, but clinicians recognize the important effect this can have on function and provide compensatory devices and techniques to patients. This is becoming more important with the newer medical treatments that often leave patients with relatively good acuity and minimal visual field loss but with significant contrast loss, which can be debilitating.

Vision impairment affects a significant proportion of middle-aged and older Americans but can be present from birth. It also has an effect on the national economy and has been estimated to cost $4 billion in benefits and lost taxable income (Vision Problems in the United States, 2002). In less than 5 years, the estimate of the annual cost of adult vision problems in the United States, including those with vision impairment, escalated to $51.4 billion (Prevent Blindness America, 2007). Visual impairment is also correlated with a risk of mortality, and McCarty, Nanjan, and Taylor (2001) noted that even those persons with mild visual impairment have a twice higher risk of dying over a 5-year period.

According to the National Eye Institute (2004), the estimated prevalence rates of visual impairment and blindness in the United States at age 75 years is 2% in the White population and 4% in the Hispanic and Black populations (Figure 27.2). By age 80 years, the prevalence markedly increases to 14% in the Hispanic population, 9% in Blacks, and 8% in Whites. Congdon and colleagues. (2004) estimated that there are 2.4 million Americans older than 40 years who are categorized as having low vision. In another study, one in six adults (17%) aged 45 years and older, representing 13.5 million Americans, reported some form of vision impairment even when wearing glasses or contact lenses (The Lighthouse, National Survey on Vision Loss, 1995). The Eye Disease Prevalence Group (2004) estimated that 38 million Americans aged 40 and older experience blindness, low vision, or an age-related eye disease.

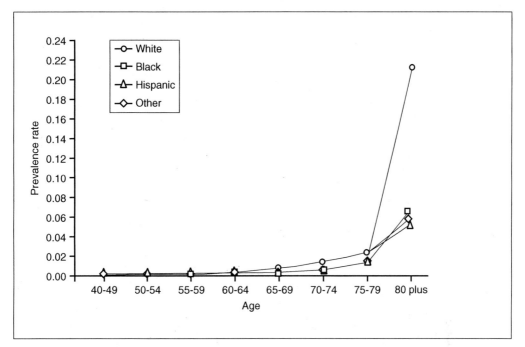

FIGURE 27.2 Estimated specific prevalence rates for vision impairment and blindness in the United States. *Source*: Friedman, D., Congdon, N., Kempen, J., & Tielsch, J. (2002). *Vision problems in the U.S.: Prevalence of adult vision impairment and age-related eye disease in America.* Chicago, IL: Prevent Blindness America.

As one can see, there is some discrepancy among the various statistics regarding blindness and vision impairment (Figure 27.3).

According to a Gallup poll, blindness is only second to cancer when it comes to health conditions that people fear most. It has also been reported that 71% of Americans, aged 45 years and older, fear being blind more than being deaf, and 76% fear being blind more than having to use a wheelchair (The Lighthouse, 1995). Fortunately, the blindness that people often think of (cannot see light, needs a guide dog, and has to learn Braille) rarely occurs. However, it is not uncommon to have a loss of vision to the point that one has a significant problem in maintaining a satisfactory quality of life. What this means can vary from individual to individual; therefore, a careful evaluation of the patient's abilities and needs is required before attempting to implement a rehabilitation program.

Legal Blindness

Probably the most common definition of blindness is that used by the Social Security Department to determine disability. It states that an individual is legally (statutorily) blind (according to the National Eye Institute, the leading causes of new cases of legal blindness are macular degeneration, glaucoma, and diabetic retinopathy) if either the best-corrected visual acuity (with standard lenses) is 20/200 (6/60) or worse in the better eye or if the remaining central visual field is restricted to 20° or less in the widest meridian of the better eye. To take into account the visual acuity charts that are often used in clinical low-vision care (e.g., the Early Treatment of Diabetic Retinopathy Study chart) the visual acuity criteria were recently clarified by the Social Security Department to be a visual acuity of less than 20/100 (Social Security Online, n.d.).

Age, years	Blindness[1]		Low vision[1]		All vision impaired	
	Persons	(%)	Persons	(%)	Persons	(%)
40–49	51,000	0.1	80,000	0.2	131,000	0.3
50–59	45,000	0.1	102,000	0.3	147,000	0.4
60–69	59,000	0.3	176,000	0.9	235,000	1.2
70–79	134,000	0.8	471,000	3.0	605,000	3.8
>80	648,000	7.0	1,532,000	16.7	2,180,000	23.7
Total	937,000	0.8	2,361,000	2.0	3,298,000	2.7

FIGURE 27.3 Prevalence of blindness and low vision among adults aged 40 years and older in the United States. [1]Blindness as defined by the U.S. definition is the best-corrected visual acuity of 6/60 or worse (=20/200) in the better-seeing eye; low vision is defined as the best-corrected visual acuity of less than 6/12 (<20/40) in the better-seeing eye (excluding those who were categorized as being blind by the U.S. definition). *Source:* National Eye Institute. Eye disease prevalence and projections (Number of adults 40 years and older in the U.S.). *Archives of Ophthalmology, 122,* **444,** 477–485.

The acuity part of this definition dates back to 1935, when the Social Security Act, with its benefits to the blind, was passed. The visual field part was added as an amendment the following year (Simons, 1991). This definition has been adopted widely by federal, state, and local agencies throughout the United States to determine eligibility and benefits. It is even used by the Internal Revenue Service to determine tax benefits.

The problem with this definition of legal blindness is that it has little or no validated experimental basis. Anyone working in the field has had patients with relatively poor visual acuity or visual field (considered legally blind) who functioned well and other patients with relatively good visual acuity and fields (not legally blind) who could barely do anything for themselves. It also does not address reduced contrast sensitivity, field loss as result of stroke (e.g., hemianopia), and central scotomas that interfere with functional capability but do not necessarily impact acuity significantly. Thus, from a rehabilitation point of view, it makes more sense to talk in terms of visual disability.

MODELS OF DISABILITY

Two models of disability are generally discussed in the literature:

- The medical model that views disability as a problem (loss of function) caused by a medical problem (disease, trauma, or other health conditions).
- The social model that views disability to be caused by social or environmental factors.

The International Classification of Disease (ICD) is the international standard classification of diseases and other health problems adopted by the World Health Organization (WHO). The current revision is ICD-10, but the United States is still using ICD-9, with plans to adopt ICD-10 in 2013. ICD-11 is currently being prepared.

In 1980, WHO published the International Classification of Impairments, Disabilities and Handicaps, a system that expanded the coverage of the ICD by looking at the medical origin of handicaps and loss of function. It has been used to define vision impairment and its effect on disabilities and handicaps from the medical perspective and has been referred to as a medical model of disability.

In May 2001, WHO revised the International Classification of Impairments, Disabilities and Handicaps into the International Classification of Functioning, Disability and Health (ICF), a classification of health and health-related domains. "These domains are classified from body, individual, and societal perspectives by means of two lists: a list of body functions and structure and a list of domains of activity and participation. Because an individual's functioning and disability occurs in a context, the ICF also includes a list of environmental factors. ... ICF takes into account the social aspects of disability and does not see disability only as a 'medical' or 'biological' dysfunction" (WHO, n.d.). The ICF can be thought of as bringing together the medical and social models of disability. It should be noted that the WHO has adopted new terms for "disability" and "handicap," namely, "activity" and "participation," respectively. Thus, an impairment leads to an inability to do an activity (the disability), which can lead to an inability of participation in society (the handicap) (WHO, n.d.).

There is a continuum in the classification of visual performance. Individuals classified with low vision may have visual acuity ranging from 20/70 to 20/1000, with the term *blindness* applied to all categories with performance worse than this (including counting fingers at 1 m or less, seeing hand motion at 5 m or less, some light perception, and no light perception). Another continuum includes peripheral visual field loss down to 5° (ICD-9-CM, 2009).

Colenbrander (1977) described how *impairment* relates to *disorder* and *disability*. A disorder may be defined as "any deviation from normal structure and or function of the body or parts thereof" (e.g., a cataract). A disorder can lead to an impairment, which is "a disorder interfering with an organ function" (e.g., reduced visual acuity, reduced visual field, and reduced contrast sensitivity). An impairment can lead to a disability, which is "the lack, loss, or reduction of an individual's ability to perform certain tasks" (e.g., cannot read a newspaper). It should be noted that impairment refers to the basic functions performed by a part of the body, whereas disability refers to tasks performed by a person.

A handicap is "a disadvantage for a given individual, resulting from an impairment or a disability that limits or prevents the fulfillment of a role that is normal (depending on age, sex, and social-cultural factors) for that individual" (Visio, 1993). A patient could be considered *handicapped* if reading the newspaper is an activity that is important in this person's life and the activity cannot be done. Individuals who do not need to read the newspaper and do not want to should not be considered handicapped by this disability.

The ICF promotes the "social model of disability," emphasizing functioning and participation in a social context, instead of function loss and handicap due to an individual medical condition (A. Colenbrander, personal communication, July 22, 2008). Although these classification systems would be helpful in sharing information, defining function, and doing research, they have not been adopted for use in the United States. Doctors and rehabilitation professionals generally code with a medical diagnosis code (ICD-9) combined with a procedure code. It should be noted that there are some vision impairment codes in the ICD-9 that are used by rehabilitation professionals and some low-vision doctors, but most doctors still use only the medical diagnosis codes.

Arditi and Rosenthal (1996) included contrast sensitivity and defined visual impairment as a significant limitation of visual capability resulting from disease, trauma, or congenital condition that cannot be fully ameliorated by standard refractive correction, medication, or surgery. Impairment is manifested by one or more of the following:

1. Insufficient visual resolution (worse than 20/60 in the better eye with best correction of ametropia).
2. Inadequate field of vision (worse than 20° along the widest meridian in the eye, with the more intact central field, or homonymous hemianopia).
3. Reduced peak contrast sensitivity (<1.7 log CS binocularly).

Unfortunately, this definition has not been adopted for use, and the problem with a lack of accepted criteria for reduced contrast sensitivity continues.

In addition to reduced contrast sensitivity, two other problems can cause functional performance issues in individuals: lighting and glare problems and visual skills problems.

Although recognized and addressed in low-vision rehabilitation care, these have not been defined to an extent that will allow them to be included in a classification system.

WHERE WE HAVE COME FROM AND WHERE WE ARE

Vision rehabilitation got its start after World War II (as did medical rehabilitation) when the blinded veterans who came back from the war recovered from their wounds but were still blind. Attention was paid more to psychosocial and vocational issues, and care was provided by an interdisciplinary team. The two rehabilitation programs (vision and medical) split apart, and the first civilian Low Vision Rehabilitation Center was opened at the VA Hospital in Hines, Illinois, in 1948. Initially, this system (vision rehabilitation) worked mainly with healthy, blind veterans, but in 1978, there was an amendment to the Rehabilitation Act of 1973 designating funds for independent living skills training for older adults. Because older adults develop many other health problems, it would make sense for these two systems to come back together, and that is what seems to be happening now (Wainapel, 2001).

Currently, there are two parallel systems in the United States that provide services to older adults, but they have not really collaborated: the Blindness System (sometimes referred to as an educational model) and the Health Care System (sometimes referred to as a medical model). There is also a third system, the Aging System, that works with aging and sick adults but not really with the visually impaired or blind. Aging visually impaired people sometimes fall through the cracks, each group (vision and aging) feeling that the other should be taking care of this person. Again, this seems to be being addressed somewhat at present (Warren, 2000).

Occupational therapists have been getting more involved in providing vision rehabilitation care, thus bringing together the health and vision issues of the patient. In addition, there have been changes in Medicare and also legislative attempts to provide more care and coverage for these visually impaired or blind adults. This will be discussed at the end of this chapter.

FACTORS AFFECTING VISUAL FUNCTION AND ITS TREATMENT

The main impairments affecting visual function are reduced visual acuity, visual field loss (central or peripheral), poor contrast sensitivity, lighting and glare problems, and visual skills problems (scanning, tracking, fixating, etc.).

Visual Acuity

There are more than 38 million Americans aged 40 and older who are classified as either "blind" and have low vision or an age-related eye disease (Eye Disease Prevalence Research Group, 2004). These estimates are based on only two parameters in the United States: visual acuity or visual field loss.

In 1861, Franciscus Donders coined the term *visual acuity* to describe the "sharpness of vision" and defined it as the ratio between a subject's VA and a standard VA. Hermann Snellen, who worked with Donders, published his famous letter chart in 1862 with newly designed targets called optotypes and changed from using feet to meters (e.g., 20/20 to 6/6). Eye doctors in the United States, other than low-vision specialists, continue to use feet notation, whereas most of the rest of the world uses the metric system (Figure 27.4).

Measured visual acuity gives us an indication of the patient's ability to resolve detail. "Normal" acuity (i.e., 20/20) is based on the assumption that an individual should be able to separate objects that are 1 minute apart in visual angle. People can have even better vision (20/15 and even 20/10). The limitation on acuity is generally determined by the spacing of the retinal cells.

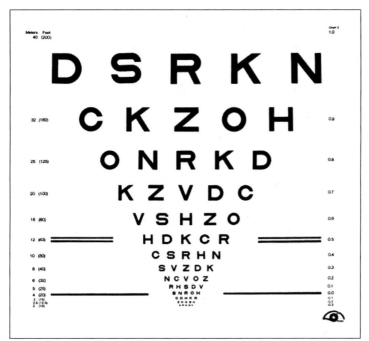

FIGURE 27.4 Visual acuity chart. *Source:* National Eye Institute, National Institutes of Health, Ref#: EC06. Accessed October 21, 2009, from http://www.nei.nih.gov/photo/keyword.asp?conditions=Eye+Charts&match=all.

Visual acuity is usually written as a fraction, the numerator represents the test distance, and the denominator represents the letter size.

$$\text{Visual acuity} = \frac{\text{Testing distance}}{\text{Letter size}}$$

The letter size is actually a distance measurement: the distance at which the letter must be held to subtend a visual angle of 5 minutes at the eye, that is, look like a 20/20 letter. When test distances in feet are used, we see acuities such as 20/20 or 20/200. When metric distances are used, these acuities become 6/6 and 6/60. All acuities can be represented as decimal acuities, and this is done by "dividing out the fraction"; that is, 20/20 becomes 1.0 and 20/200 becomes 0.1. Another way of defining visual acuity is as follows:

$$\text{Visual acuity} = \frac{\text{Distance at which letter was used}}{\text{Distance at which letter subtends 5' of arc}}$$

For example, a 20-foot letter size read at 10 feet would be equivalent to 10/20 or 20/40 acuity. When working with people whose vision is significantly reduced, the acuity can still be measured accurately. One technique simply involves walking the patient up to the test chart, thus reducing the test distance and increasing the sensitivity of the chart. Another technique is to use a test chart with larger letters or numbers and a larger selection of intermediate sizes. In this case, low levels of vision can still be measured, even worse than 20/2000. Legal (statutory) blindness in the United States is based on a best-corrected (with standard glasses or contact lenses) visual acuity of 20/200 or less.

A patient with reduced visual acuity is unable to resolve detail. In some cases, all that is needed is an up-to-date refraction, resulting in a new pair of glasses for general wear. When glasses by themselves are not adequate, additional interventions must be initiated. This is generally accomplished by making the image on the retina larger, that is, using some form of magnification. Magnification can be provided in one of the three ways: making the object larger (e.g., large-print books), moving the object closer (e.g., sitting closer to the television or bringing the reading material closer to the eyes when using stronger reading glasses), or using some optical device to make the object look bigger (e.g., a telescope to see distant objects better or a magnifier for reading). One of the goals of the low-vision examination is to determine and prescribe the appropriate level and type of magnification.

Visual Field

Visual acuity gives us an indication of the patient's ability to resolve detail, whereas the visual field gives us information regarding the patency of the whole retina (the central and peripheral areas of the retina). When we test the visual field, we are generally, but not exclusively, evaluating peripheral field (side vision). This is important for the patient to be able to detect objects around him. Once the individual detects an object, he or she can look at it and identify it (using visual acuity and central field). The visual field becomes an especially important factor when discussing and considering training for mobility problems. Peripheral visual field is the other way someone can be certified as legally blind. The criteria used in the United States is that the peripheral field is constricted resulting in a central field of vision subtending an angle of 20° or less at the eye.

Perimetry, which is the technique of measuring the visual field, uses a variety of techniques. These may include manual and automated evaluation of the entire visual field with kinetic or static stimuli. The automated perimeter has paved the way for more standardized and accurate visual field testing in all types of patients, including those with low vision (Bass & Sherman, 1996).

There are different ways that the visual field can be affected. A loss of vision in a specific area is referred to as a scotoma (scotomas can range from "black holes" in vision to areas that are "hazy" to see through). It should be noted that scotomas in the visual field can have almost any size and shape, and the number of scotomas a patient has can also vary significantly. Scotomas can be located in the center of the macula (referred to as a central scotoma), affecting straight-ahead vision with a concurrent reduction in visual acuity. The magnification principles discussed above would apply. Scotomas can also be located adjacent to the central area (paracentral scotoma). In this case, acuity is usually not affected; interference comes from the closeness of scotoma to what is being viewed. Central and paracentral scotomas can be plotted using a microperimetry technique such as scanning laser ophthalmoscopy. Central scotomas can also be plotted with a handheld laser as described by Fletcher and Cole (Cole, 2008). Sometimes, central scotomas or distortions can be identified with a diagnostic test known as the Amsler grid (a grid of 20×20 squares that is equivalent to 20° of the visual field when held 13 in. from the eye).

An overall peripheral field defect, which may be caused by glaucoma or retinitis pigmentosa (RP), can interfere with mobility. This is the situation when only a small central part of the visual field remains. Mobility problems generally occur when the overall remaining central field subtends an angle of about 5° or less (the normal field of vision with both eyes open is 180° and with one eye is 140°), but some patients are bothered even earlier. Scotomas usually caused by stroke or head trauma can be limited to one side of the visual field (hemianopia). These can be detrimental to patient function because the patient cannot see objects to that side. This can interfere significantly with general mobility and with near tasks such as reading and writing, and laser photocoagulation for diabetic retinopathy results in scotomas as well.

The treatment of a visual field defect will vary depending on the size, location, number, and severity of the scotomas. Generally, there is no good optical treatment available for significant loss of the visual field. However, optical remediation with prisms, mirrors, or reversed telescopes has been used in training and maximizing the residual visual field. Usually, the patient must learn to live with and compensate for the defect. Orientation and mobility training (especially cane travel), and visual scanning training, will often be helpful in the case of peripheral field loss and sometimes in the case of severe central field loss. For patients who have central field loss (central and paracentral scotomas), eccentric viewing training, which teaches the patient to look off-center, that is, away from the fovea (the area of the retina that gives us the greatest detail when looking at an object), can help with tasks such as reading and even with seeing in general.

Contrast

Visual acuity charts measure high-contrast vision (the ability to resolve black letters on a light background). Most of the world, however, is not high contrast, and this can explain some situations in which patients feel that their vision has worsened, although the measured visual acuity on the eye chart is the same. Contrast sensitivity charts are specially designed charts that can measure any decrement in this visual function and would account for the patient's perception in the vision.

Contrast sensitivity is increasingly recognized as an important factor influencing the quality of vision. There is an increase in the risk for accidents, because of a loss of spatial awareness, when there is a decrease in the contrast sensitivity function. Reduced contrast sensitivity may also affect the ability to walk down steps, recognize faces, drive at night or in the rain, find a telephone number in a directory, read instructions on a medicine container, or navigate safely through unfamiliar environments.

The benefit of contrast sensitivity testing is that it often gives us an indication of who will respond poorly to standard magnification levels (sometimes needing significantly higher magnification) or who will need higher levels of lighting or glare control to perform their desired tasks. In fact, it is not unusual to see patients with contrast sensitivity problems function with significantly weaker lenses when bright lighting is incorporated into the task (along with appropriate glare-control techniques).

Lighting and Glare

It is often impossible to predict how much light a patient needs. Too much can be as detrimental as not enough. The best way to determine the appropriate lighting level is to see how the patient responds to different light levels and note the effect of the light levels on patient performance. The easiest way to change the intensity of light on a page is to change the distance of the light from the page. Intensity follows the inverse-square law: if you move the light, the intensity (I) changes by an amount inversely proportional to the square of the change in the distance (d) from the page: $I = I_o/(d^2)$. For example, if you move a light to one half the original distance from the page, the intensity on the page increases by 4 times:

$$(1/0.5)^2 = 4\times$$

Patients also complain about glare. One broad definition of glare is "light that does not contribute to retinal imagery but has an adverse effect on visual efficiency, visual comfort, or resolution" (Waiss & Cohen, 1991). Intraocular glare problems can sometimes be solved by removing the source of glare (e.g., cataracts). If the glare source is external, one can either modify the environment or filter out the distracting wavelengths causing the glare problem by using special filters, such as yellow or amber lenses, or visors. One very handy device is a typoscope (also called a reading guide). This is simply a matte-black card with a slot cut in it that, when placed on printed material, exposes two to three lines of print. The surrounding black material reduces the reflected light from the page, thus reducing the total amount of light entering the eye. Concurrently, the intensity of light on the exposed printed material can be increased, thus increasing the perceived contrast of the print.

Visual Skills Problems

Some people have problems moving their eyes (scanning), locating objects, fixating (aiming the eyes at the object), and maintaining this fixation when following the object (tracking). They might also have trouble moving the eyes accurately across a printed line or jumping from the end of one line to the next when reading. When this happens, skills training can be done. This consists of a series of exercises that are designed to improve these skills and are generally done over a period of some weeks. Optometrists, occupational therapists, and vision rehabilitation therapists generally provide this type of training.

OVERVIEW OF VISION REHABILITATION

Vision rehabilitation addresses functional deficits resulting from a medical condition (congenital or acquired). Before any type of visual rehabilitation is considered, the patient must have a thorough medical eye evaluation, along with the initiation of any medical and/or surgical interventions. The patient should also have standard refractive eye care to be certain that the cause of reduced vision is not uncorrected or undercorrected refractive error or presbyopia. The ultimate goal in the rehabilitation of a visually impaired person is to maximize the use of any residual vision and compensate for vision loss by using either vision enhancement or vision substitution techniques and devices. Vision rehabilitation can be thought of as having two components:

1. Clinical low-vision care results in the prescription of and training with vision assistive devices and the development of a treatment plan for vision rehabilitation training. These services are provided by optometrists or ophthalmologists.
2. Vision rehabilitation training to instruct and train the patient in the use of techniques and devices to allow for greater independence and the achievement of the patient's goals and objectives to the greatest extent possible. These services are provided by occupational therapists and other nonmedically licensed professionals such as vision rehabilitation trainers, orientation and mobility specialists, and low-vision instructors.

Maximizing the Use of Residual Vision With Clinical Low-Vision Care

Before vision rehabilitation training is recommended and implemented, it is important to perform a low-vision examination. The low-vision examination will identify the patient's functional goals (visual), assess the patient's current level of visual functioning, and determine whether any modifications can be made to attain these goals. These modifications (or interventions) can include the provision of magnification, lighting, glare control, visual field loss compensation, and visual skills training. As mentioned, the objective of the low-vision examination is to maximize the use of the residual vision. On the basis of the results of this examination, the patient will be categorized as either "sighted" or "blind" and will be guided into the rehabilitation model with the appropriate emphasis. Thus, the low-vision examination is the key component tying together medical care and rehabilitative care, making certain that patients are channeled into the correct programs. It is this service that mostly responds to the chief complaint of older persons with vision loss (The Lighthouse, 1990b, p. 3). The chief complaint of a majority of older persons was previously identified (in this same reference) as "I want to see well."

Compensating for Vision Loss With Vision Rehabilitation Training

Once the clinical low-vision care has been completed or has progressed to the point that current functional levels and desired goals have been determined, the vision rehabilitation training of the patient can be initiated. Sometimes the entry point for the patient into rehabilitation services occurs in the settings providing vision rehabilitation training. A low-vision examination must be an essential and early component of any rehabilitation services. Rehabilitation can include but is not necessarily limited to the following:

ADL training and IADL training, the activities of which are described as follows:

> ADLs refer to Activities of Daily Living, which are basic but important general tasks required for day to day living, such as bathing, dressing, grooming, eating, mobility and help in the bathroom.... IADLs are Instrumental Activities of Daily Living [which] consist of activities that are less basic then ADLs....[and] need to be done but on a less time sensitive schedule. For example, IADLs include paying bills, cleaning, laundry and meal preparation. (Lake Shore Assisted Living Facility, 2008).

Sometimes, these activities are grouped together and loosely referred to as ADL training, providing instruction in the use of special devices or techniques to compensate for visual impairment.

Communications skills training is designed to develop the ability of the patient to handle common interactions with other individuals. This includes both direct verbal communication between individuals, writing techniques, and use of the telephone, and special hearing-amplifying devices. Some examples would be bold-lined pens to make writing more visible, talking books, or Braille books.

Orientation and mobility training is designed to enable the patient to navigate safely both indoors and outdoors. Orientation training refers to knowing where one is, where one wants to go, and how to go there. Mobility training stresses safe travel and teaches techniques that can be used when traveling alone or with someone else (sighted guide technique), including detecting obstacles ahead, crossing the street, locating the destination, and using public transportation.

Educational and vocational training is designed to provide the patient with the educational background (possibly including college and graduate school) and training to achieve a specific goal. At a minimum, this would be the educational experience needed to attain a basic level of competency, followed with the vocational training so that the patient can learn the work skills necessary to be employed and maintain a certain degree of independence. Included in this is the provision of any special optical or adaptive devices needed for the specific task being performed, including any special equipment (e.g., special computer systems) needed by the patient.

Psychological and social counseling is designed to help the patient deal with problems in acknowledging and accepting the loss of vision and interacting with other people. Support groups may also provide help for adjusting to vision loss. Depression is a major problem with vision loss, and Javit, Zhou, and Wilke (2007) found that a progression of vision loss from normal to blind is associated with more than 1.5-fold increased odds of depression and injury and 2.5- to 3-fold increased odds of utilization of skilled nursing facilities and long-term care. Horowitz, Reinhardt, and Kennedy (2005) note in a study of new applicants for rehabilitative services who had recent vision loss that 7% had current major depression and 26.9% met the criteria for subthreshold depression.

Family and peer counseling is designed to help family and friends understand and deal with the problems that both they and the patient are having because of the vision impairment.

Other needed services are required by some patients with specific and unusual needs. It is important that these are identified and addressed and the patient is referred to receive the necessary services.

THE ROLE OF PATHOLOGY IN VISUAL IMPAIRMENT

One of the ways to understand the various pathologies that cause a visual impairment is to understand how light travels through the eye (Figure 27.5).

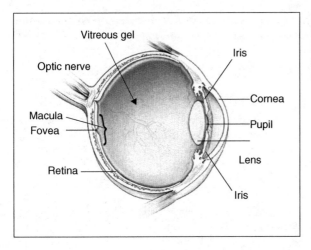

Vitreous gel

Optic nerve

Macula
Fovea

Retina

Iris

Cornea

Pupil

Lens

Iris

FIGURE 27.5 The eye. *Source*: National Eye Institute. (n.d.). National Institutes of Health. Retrieved June 14, 2010, http:// www. nationaleyeinstitute.net/photo/keyword.asp? conditions=Normal+Eye+Images&match=all

The cornea (the transparent window in the front) and the lens, which are the primary refracting structures of the eye, are the main systems that focus images onto the retina, which is located at the back of the eye. After passing through the lens, the light must travel through the vitreous, which is a clear, jellylike material that fills the interior of the eye. Problems such as cataracts and corneal disease affect these systems and generally result in the person experiencing an overall blurred image (reduced visual acuity), decreased contrast, and glare.

Eventually, the light will fall on the retina, a structure that is, in effect, a dual image-processing system. The central portion of the retina (macular area) is associated with straight-ahead vision, including detail discrimination and color. The macular area plays a major role in reading, facial discrimination, and object identification. Problems in the macular area can cause a reduction in visual acuity or a loss of central visual field (a central scotoma or blind spot). Some of the common conditions in which the macular region is affected include macular degeneration, diabetic retinopathy, and albinism.

The second portion of the retina, the peripheral retina, is associated with object awareness and motion detection. Its function is to allow one to become aware of objects to the side (peripherally; i.e., up, down, right, left, etc.), and it plays a major role in mobility (one's ability to navigate around objects and people without bumping into them). Conditions that affect the peripheral retina result in a loss of side vision, with or without a concurrent reduction in visual acuity. Some of these conditions are glaucoma, RP, strokes, and tumors.

The retina changes light into electrical impulses, which leave the eye through the optic nerve and travel a route through the brain (the visual pathways) to the occipital region, in particular, areas 17, 18, and 19, as well as other areas in the brain, where the interpretation and interaction with other body systems take place.

Cataract

Description of Medical Condition
The lens is composed of three layers: the nucleus (center), the cortex, and the capsule. It is clear at birth, but throughout life, the lens continues to produce cells that become increasingly yellow with age. Cataracts develop as a result of aging, trauma, hereditary factors, birth defects, or a systemic condition such as diabetes.

Cataracts (opacity or clouding of the lens) may appear in all parts of the lens and are classified into four main anatomical types: the nuclear, cortical, posterior subcapsular, and mixed.

Cataracts become significantly more prevalent after 40 years of age, with nearly 20.5 million Americans having some type of cataract. This number is expected to markedly increase to 30.1 million by 2020. It has also been found that in the United States, women have a higher prevalence of cataracts than men (Congdon et al., 2004) and that Caucasians are three times as likely as Blacks to develop cataracts, and women smoking at least 35 cigarettes a day increased the risk by about 50% (Lindblad, Håkansson, Svensson, Philipson, & Wolk, 2005).

Functional Presentation of Medical Condition
The greater the progression of the cataract, the greater the visual impairment from the effects of decreased visual acuity, loss of contrast, and glare.

Treatment and Prognosis
Cataract is the fourth major eye disease in the United States, and surgery is considered to be a routine outpatient procedure. The most common procedure involves a "stitchless" incision and replacement of the cataractous lens with an intraocular lens. Cataract extraction is considered to be one of the safest and cost-effective surgical procedures. Assuming a healthy retina, the prognosis for functional cure and restoration of normal vision is high. However, there may be complications when an underlying ocular pathology, such as macular degeneration, prevents visualization of the retina. Cataract surgery is indicated when (a) visual function is impaired and it becomes difficult to pursue normal activities such as reading or independent travel, or (b) there are medical complications occurring from advanced cataracts.

Two types of cataract surgery are generally performed. Extracapsular extraction involves the removal of the lens nucleus in one piece from the capsular bag. An intraocular lens is then inserted in the posterior chamber of the eye (behind the iris) during surgery to replace the lens that has been removed. A second procedure, more commonly used in developing countries (but changing to extracapsular even in those countries), is intracapsular extraction which involves removal of the entire contents (lens and capsule) during surgery. The surgical removal of the lens is then followed by an optical correction with an aphakic (to make up for the lack of the lens) spectacle correction or contact lenses.

In some cases, the capsule that is left in the eye after the initial surgery is done can become opaque over time. This is referred to as a secondary cataract or secondary membrane. This can usually be simply treated in the office with a yttrium aluminum garnet laser, which opens a hole in the membrane. Patients who go in with poor vision generally leave with good vision (assuming there are no problems elsewhere in the eye).

The patient should be referred for a low-vision examination if cataract surgery cannot be done or complications occur during or following the surgery. Although magnification itself might not be as successful as in other eye conditions, approaches using lighting, glare control, and contrast enhancement can often go a long way in helping the patient.

Psychological and Vocational Implications
Assuming no complications, there should be no psychological or vocational implications after cataract surgery. In fact, many individuals are amazed that the visual acuity and color vision is so improved with surgery and that the glare disability has disappeared. In general, there is a significant improvement in the quality of life with cataract surgery.

Corneal Disease

Description of Medical Condition
Composed of three layers and two membranes, the cornea is normally clear, but changes in any of the corneal layers or membranes can cause the retinal image to be blurred. The cornea is a structure that is prone to degenerations, dystrophies, deposition, edema, neovascularization, scarring, pigmentation, ulcers, cysts, noninflammatory progressive thinning (keratoconus), infection, viral diseases, and trauma. Visual function can sometimes be restored with medical treatment, such as require laser treatment, a corneal transplant, or a keratoprosthesis.

Functional Presentation of Medical Condition

Interference with corneal integrity can result in a blurred or distorted image on the retina. A totally opaque cornea can prevent light from reaching the retina altogether. Patients with corneal disease may experience severe glare, cloudy vision, and problems with reduced visual acuity.

Phototherapeutic keratectomy may be used to replace irregularities in the corneas. However, more severe damage to the cornea may require a replacement of the cornea. Keratoplasty is the primary method of restoring vision for an individual with a diseased, irregular, or scarred cornea. The procedure involves transplanting a healthy cornea from a compatible donor. It is done to improve the visual acuity, preserve the anatomy and physiology of the cornea, remove active disease tissue, and improve the cosmetic appearance of the eye. Lasers are also used to treat some corneal problems. When surgery is contraindicated, a scarred or disfigured cornea can be cosmetically "corrected" with a contact lens to match the fellow eye. New treatments involve high-speed lasers, endothelial keratoplasty, stem cell transplants, and artificial corneas (Hicks et al., 2006). The latter include synthetic corneal keratoprosthesis (also known as K-Pro) that can dramatically return vision to an individual who has been totally blind with no useable vision (Chew et al., 2009). A person with a scarred and opaque cornea resulting from chlorine splashing back into the eye would be an example of an individual who may be a candidate for this new and radical treatment.

If the treatment is not totally successful in restoring vision, the patient should be referred for a low-vision examination. Although magnification itself might not be as successful as in other eye conditions, approaches using lighting, glare control, and contrast enhancement can often go a long way in helping the patient.

Psychological and Vocational Implications

In addition to improving visual function with corneal surgery, a cosmetic contact lens or prosthetic shell should be considered when the cosmetic appearance will enhance professional or personal goals. Consultations with a prosthetic specialist should be considered as early as possible. Vocational goals will be dependent on the degree to which the retinal image is compromised.

Macular Degeneration

Description of Medical Condition

Macular degeneration is considered one of the leading causes of visual impairment in older adults. There is an estimated increase in people aged 40 years and older with advanced AMD from 1.7 million to 2.95 million in 2020, with another 7.3 million at risk for vision loss (Friedman et al., 2004). Age is also a significant risk factor in developing macular degeneration, increasing from 2% for those aged 50–59 years to nearly 30% for those older than 75 years (National Eye Institute, 2004).

The retina, the lens-sensitive tissue of the eye, is 0.5 mm thick and composed of a central and a peripheral area of receptors. The macula is centrally located in the retina and is the area in which most of the color photoreceptors (the cones) are concentrated and tightly packed. The macula specializes in object identification (visual acuity/resolution tasks such as facial recognition and letter reading), daylight vision, and color perception. The peripheral retina contains the majority of the rods that are specialized for night vision as well as object detection and motion detection.

The macula has the highest resolution as well as the best visual acuity in the retina. It is composed of the fovea, 1.5 mm in diameter, as well as a rod-free 0.5-mm area. These areas are surrounded by the parafoveal and perifoveal areas. This region, which is most frequently affected by the aging process, may develop "dry" (atrophic) or "wet" (exudative) changes. The degenerative changes can result in atrophy, hemorrhage, exudates, fibrovascular scars, or cyst formation of the macular and the surrounding paramacular areas.

There are many risk factors (Clemons, Milton, Klein, Seddon, & Ferris, 2005) associated with macular degeneration, which include ethnicity (Caucasian), family history, high blood pressure, obesity (Seddon, Cote, Davis, & Rosner, 2003), or a history of hypertension (Klein, Klein, Tomany, & Cruickshanks, 2003), and light iris color (Maguire, 1997). Another risk factor associated with macular degeneration is smoking. The incidence of macular degeneration in smokers (Congdon, 2004) seems to be two to four times higher than that in nonsmokers, and genes are also playing an ever-increasing role in the development of AMD. Individuals having the CFH gene variant were found to have an increased risk for developing macular degeneration by about 2.5–5.5 times (Haines et al., 2005).

The Age-Related Eye Disease Study (Clemons et al., 2005) showed that supplementing the diet with antioxidant vitamins, including C and E, zinc, and copper, along with the beta-carotenoid has been shown to be effective in reducing the severity of AMD. The Age-Related Eye Disease Study II being run by the National Eye Institute (2004) is studying the effect of dietary xanthophylls (lutein and zeaxanthin) along with omega-3 long-chain polyunsaturated fatty acids docosahexaenoic acid and eicosapentaenoic acid on the development, reduction, and stabilization of AMD.

Functional Presentation of Medical Condition
The effect of structural changes on the macula may be visually manifested when viewing objects as distortions, decreased visual acuity, decreased color recognition, loss of contrast, or as a "black hole" (area of no vision [scotoma]). Reading may become progressively more difficult as the disease progresses, driving may have to be discontinued, and employment may be impossible without special low-vision intervention. In addition, macular degeneration has been linked with depression.

Treatment and Prognosis
Optical coherence tomography is becoming the gold standard in imaging the retina and in treating retinal disorders (Wolfgang et al., 2003). The new imaging tests allow the ultrahigh resolution and imaging of precise pathological lesions. The images are similar to viewing a histological section of the retina and capture up to 40,000 scans of the eye per second. Fluorescein angiography and indocyanine green angiography (Yannuzzi, Slakter, Sorenson, Guyer, & Orlock, 1992) are two of the diagnostic procedures used, along with optical coherence tomography, to evaluate the proliferative angiogenic (porous blood vessels that form in response to vascular endothelial growth factor [VEGF]) blood vessels in macular degeneration. It is used to determine whether anti-VEGF (intravitreal injections of ranibizumab or bevacizumab into the eye) treatment might be indicated to slow the progression of the disease. Laser photocoagulation has been replaced in slowing down the exudative or hemorrhagic (wet) type of macular disease if detected in the early stages by anti-VEGF therapy.

Patients are also able to monitor the course of the disease with the Amsler grid (a grid of 20 × 20 squares that subtend 20° overall of the visual field when held at 13 in. from the eye) to determine whether there is a change in the macular function from disease processes (Figure 27.6).

Any sudden change of the grid (such as waviness, black areas [scotomas], or distortion) may be indicative of a leaking retina that might be amenable to anti-VEGF treatment, especially if done early. Additional treatments that have been under investigation are combination therapies, including anti-VEGF treatment (ranibizumab) with photodynamic therapy (cold laser) and dexamethasone. The rationale for the combination therapies is the targeting of different processes in the development of new blood vessels (Figure 27.7).

Fortunately, patients with macular degeneration can often be helped with low-vision interventions. A low-vision examination is recommended to determine which lenses are of value for distant, intermediate, and near tasks. The power and type of magnification is determined by the extent of the visual loss. Except in a minority of cases, functional ability is generally retained to the end, with the use of low-vision devices such as microscopic and telescopic lens systems and absorptive lenses. Electronic closed-circuit televisions (CCTVs) allow the ability

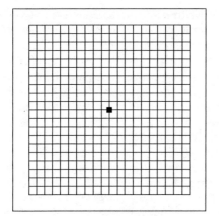

FIGURE 27.6   Amsler grid. *Source:* National Eye Institute, National Institutes of Health.

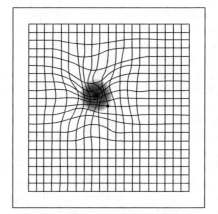

FIGURE 27.7   Amsler grid as it might appear to someone with age-related macular degeneration. *Source:* National Eye Institute, National Institutes of Health.

to magnify as well as enhance the contrast of the letters from black letter on a white background to white letters on a black background. A new generation of portable CCTVs allows for greater freedom such as reading menus under poor lighting conditions.

Talking books are available, free of charge, from the local library system through the federal government. Bold felt-tip pens, talking clocks, and checkbook stencils are some other nonoptical devices that are available for the person with macular disease and low vision. Through the use of low-vision devices, individuals are often able to function with visual acuity as low as 20/1000. However, a new generation of portable optical character recognition devices enables individuals with little or no vision to access newspapers, magazines, or books. Other types of rehabilitation, as discussed in this chapter, are also generally beneficial to the patient.

Psychological and Vocational Implications

As with most visual losses, individuals are most concerned that the condition will progress to complete blindness. Where possible, the eye care provider and low-vision specialist must reassure the patient that low-vision devices will generally permit the patient to return to normal activities of daily living, such as reading, maintaining a checkbook, or going to museums and the theater. If necessary, other rehabilitation services, such as training in orientation and mobility and activities of daily living, should be advised.

Diabetic Retinopathy

Description of Medical Condition

It is estimated that 4.1 million Americans aged 40 years and older have diabetic retinopathy (Kempen et al., 2004) and that 5% of the population aged 74 years and older (824,000 Americans) have diabetic retinopathy (Friedman, Congdon, & Tielsch, 2002). Nearly, all persons with type I diabetes will develop diabetic retinopathy, and 60% of patients with type 2 will develop retinopathy within two decades of the diseases (Fong et al., 2004). In the National Eye Institute Los Angeles Latino Eye Study, the Latino population has been shown to have a significant prevalence of diabetic retinopathy. It was found that approximately 50% of the participants who had diabetes had diabetic retinopathy (Varma, Torres, Peña, Klein, & Azen, 2004). In the United States, diabetic retinopathy causes vision loss during the working years. This translates into more disability and person-years of vision lost than any other eye disease (Kempen et al., 2004).

The early, or background, stage manifests itself with small hemorrhages in the eye. This eventually may lead to the more serious proliferative type, which can cause retinal scarring, hemorrhaging into the vitreous, and even retinal detachment.

Functional Presentation of Medical Condition
Diabetic individuals often experience fluctuating or severely decreased visual acuity, which in turn may cause difficulty in reading and seeing the markings on a syringe. They are at a higher risk for cataracts, which may be manifested by glare and reduced contrast sensitivity (e.g., how black a letter needs to be seen), and various types of visual field problems. In addition, diabetic individuals can even have transient episodes of diplopia.

Treatment and Prognosis
The Diabetes Control and Complications Trial study showed that strict control of blood sugar is required to reduce the incidence of complications once considered an inevitable result of diabetes (Diabetes Control and Complications Trial Research Group, 1995;Fuchs, 1996). Intensive blood glucose control was shown to reduce the risk for eye disease by 76%, kidney disease by 50%, and nerve disease by 60%. Study results also showed that intensive therapy reduced the risk for developing retinopathy by 76%.

Despite regulation of the condition with diet, oral medication, or insulin, many individuals still continue to have progressive visual loss. Photocoagulation may be indicated when there is leaking of the blood vessels. In addition, panretinal photocoagulation of the peripheral retina may be indicated to preserve remaining vision, as well as the possibility of having cataracts removed.

Despite continued vision loss, low-vision devices, including prisms for transitory diplopia, will often be of value in enabling an individual to maintain everyday activities.

Psychological and Vocational Implications
Individuals are often depressed and should be directed to a social worker, psychiatrist, psychologist, or discussion group for support. Rehabilitation considerations must include not only vision but also the effect of this debilitating disease on other systems.

Glaucoma

Description and Demographics of Medical Condition
An estimated 2.2 million Americans aged 40 and older have glaucoma. Of these, 711,000 Americans aged 80 and older (7.7% of the population) have the condition (Friedman, 2004). Glaucoma is more prevalent in the Hispanic and Black population and accounts for 28.6% cases of blindness (Congdon et al., 2004).

Glaucoma is a disease in which the optic nerve is damaged when the intraocular pressure (IOP) of the eye is increased. Generally, "normal" eye pressure ranges between 10 and 20 mm Hg, but it has been found that thin corneas may be a significant risk factor in damaging the optic nerve. If left untreated, glaucoma will result in the destruction of the peripheral retina as well as affect night vision.

The causes of glaucoma are varied and generally result from a blockage in the drainage canal in the eye known as the canal of Schlemm. The blockage takes place in an area known as the trabecular meshwork; the causes may be congenital, hereditary, systemic, traumatic, secondary, drug induced, neoplastic, or surgically induced. There is new gene research that has revealed a defect in the chromosome-1 open-angle gene (GLCI). It is believed that the defective gene will block the drainage of the aqueous fluid (Fingert, Stone, Sheffield, & Alward, 2002) (Figure 27.8).

The philosophy of the cause of glaucoma has been changing. There are basically three types of glaucoma that affect the eye: (1) chronic (open-angle) glaucoma, in which increased pressure over time eventually affects the optic nerve and visual field; (2) acute (closed-angle) glaucoma, in which there is a rapid increase or spiking of the IOP that may be accompanied

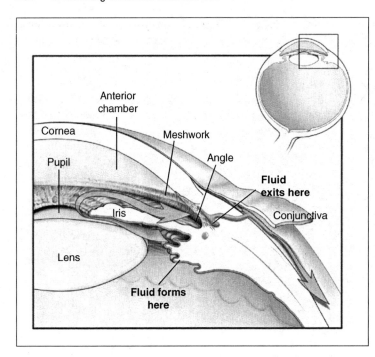

FIGURE 27.8 The aqueous fluid. A clear fluid flows continuously in and out of the anterior chamber and nourishes nearby tissues. The fluid leaves the chamber at the open angle where the cornea and iris meet. When the fluid reaches the angle, it flows through a spongy meshwork and leaves the eye. *Source*: National Eye Institute, National Institutes of Health.

by intense pain and even nausea or vomiting; and (3) low-tension glaucoma, which may be caused by a decrease in blood flow to the optic nerve.

Risk factors have been found to include thin corneas (Gordon et al., 2002) and optineurin (defect in the gene directing the production of the protein found in the trabecular meshwork) (Sarfarazi & Rezaie, 2004).

Functional Presentation of Medical Condition

Over a period of time, especially if left untreated, irreversible optic nerve and visual field damage will occur, impairing night vision, visual acuity, mobility, and even the reading skills of the patient. In addition, glare and light sensitivity are also prevalent in individuals with glaucoma.

Treatment and Prognosis

Medications that decrease production of aqueous humor or facilitate outflow of fluid through the trabecular meshwork are generally the first treatments instituted with the glaucoma patient (Figure 27.9). Some of the drugs used to reduce the IOP are the anticholinergic drugs, beta-adrenergic receptor antagonists, alpha-2 adrenergic agonists, sympathomimetics (epifrin), carbonic anhydrase inhibitors, prostaglandin analogs, and miotic agents (parasympathomimetics such as pilocarpine).

Argon laser trabeculoplasty, in use since 1979, relieves buildup of pressure by creating drainage holes. Another procedure is a trabeculectomy, which is designed to lower pressure by cutting out a small section of the drainage system (Parc, Johnson, Oliver, Hattenhauer, & Hodge, 2001).

Low-vision devices, including spectacles, hand and stand magnifiers, CCTV, lighting, and nonoptical devices, are used to return an individual with glaucoma to normal, or at least improved, visual function. Absorptive lenses, especially those that transmit in the yellow visible portion of the spectrum, seem to enhance the contrast and seem to be especially beneficial for outdoor and indoor wear. These lenses also may enhance the apparent brightness of the scene and often aid in mobility.

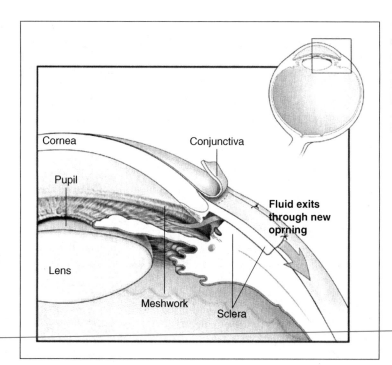

FIGURE 27.9 Conventional surgery to treat glaucoma makes a new opening in the meshwork. This new opening helps fluid to leave the eye and lowers intraocular pressure. *Source*: National Eye Institute, National Institutes of Health.

Psychological and Vocational Implications

Progressive loss of vision, even with the most rigid compliance, may result in difficulty in performing one's job or pursuing normal activities. Modifications in the work space may be required, with high technology including voice-input and speech-output devices. Intervention and support groups should also be considered, along with orientation and mobility training for independent travel.

Albinism

Description of Medical Condition/Disability Condition

Albinism is a trait that is inherited through autosomal recessive or sex-linked transmission and results in characteristics that affect the pigmentation of the skin and hair as well as the iris and retina. In addition, nystagmus and a significant refractive error are also generally associated with albinism. There is a lack of the pigment in the body and the eye in the tyrosinase-negative (ty-neg oculocutaneous) form of albinism. The "typical" individual with albinism has white or platinum hair and irises that appear to be pink. In the tyrosinase-positive (ty-positive oculocutaneous) type of albinism, there is some degree of pigmentation in the eye and skin. The ocular albino, however, is distinctive in that the lack of pigmentation is restricted to the eyes only. This person has a normal (and often dark) skin and hair coloring.

Functional Presentation of Medical Condition/Disability Condition

Photophobia varies with the type of albinism. For example, the ty-negative albino is characteristically more sensitive to light than the ty-positive or ocular albino. Nystagmus is also more noticeable in the ty-neg albino than in the ocular albino.

Persons with albinism have a decrease in visual acuity because of macular aplasia, but, as mentioned, the severity of the loss of vision varies with the type of albinism. With regard to visual acuity, the ty-neg albino has the severest visual impairment, and the ocular albino has the least.

Treatment and Prognosis

Because refractive errors are generally significant, persons with albinism should be evaluated for corrective spectacle lenses, as well as for absorptive lenses, as early as possible to reduce light sensitivity. The individual with albinism also responds favorably to low-vision devices, including strong microscopic reading lenses, magnifiers, absorptive lenses, and telescopic lenses, and should be referred to a low-vision specialist before entry into school. The presence of nystagmus is in no way a contraindication to the use of low-vision devices, and people with albinism are often our best low-vision patients.

Psychological and Vocational Implications

The individual with albinism is generally singled out early in life by his or her peers as being different because of physical appearance. Parents and children should have family counseling by an individual familiar with visual disabilities. Vocational implications have changed dramatically with the acceptance of persons having albinism into most occupations, including medicine.

Retinitis Pigmentosa

Description of Medical Condition/Disability Condition

RP, which is a progressive eye disease that affects the pigmentary layer of the retina, is the most common cause of inherited blindness (National Eye Institute, 1993). In addition, approximately 30% of people with RP report some degree of hearing loss (National Retinitis Pigmentosa Foundation, 1995). Although there are many variants of RP, it most commonly affects the periphery or midperiphery of the retina. The speed of the progression of visual field loss varies with each individual; some progress to a significant loss of functional visual field. Multiple genes, when mutated, can cause the RP phenotype.

The electroretinogram is essential in the differential diagnosis of RP. The electroretinogram will typically reveal a decreased or absent scotopic response and a reduction in the photopic response as the condition progresses. The visual field is also diagnostically significant in recording the progression of the visual field loss. It is impossible, however, to predict whether an individual diagnosed in the early stages will rapidly progress to a loss of functional vision.

Functional Presentation of Medical Condition/Disability Condition

Night vision and peripheral vision loss go hand in hand. The more advanced the RP, the greater the loss of peripheral vision and the more difficult it is to travel. Legal blindness, as previously noted, is a field restricted to 20° or less in the better eye. Mobility, however, does not generally become a significant problem until the remaining visual field is 5° or less. Reading also becomes progressively more difficult as the visual field becomes small.

Glare or light sensitivity is frequently associated with RP, especially when a small posterior subcapsular cataract is associated with the condition. The need for good lighting, however, is an important factor in providing optimal visual function.

Treatment and Prognosis

Currently, no medical or surgical treatments are known to stop or decrease the progression of RP. Periodic eye examinations are essential in monitoring the progression of the condition. Refractive corrections are necessary, along with absorptive lenses, to cut down on glare or light sensitivity. In addition, contrast-enhancing lenses such as the NOIR or Corning CPF series may be beneficial in enhancing performance and reducing adaptation times between outdoors and indoors.

The CCTV is also indicated when reading becomes too difficult with optical devices. The CCTV provides the ability to reverse polarity so that white letters can be seen on a black background, and it enables one to regulate the brightness and contrast of the image viewed. Special prism lenses have been used in the later stages of RP to increase the awareness of the periphery. The Nightscope, which was intended to be used for mobility under dim illumination by individuals with RP, has been found to have limited use.

As the progression of the RP continues, so will the loss in mobility. A traveling cane, long cane, sensory device, or seeing-eye dog may be indicated to assist in independent travel.

Psychological and Vocational Implications

The fear of total blindness and loss of independence are uppermost in the minds of most individuals with RP. Psychological and family counseling, as well as genetic counseling, are indicated for persons contemplating having children.

In accordance with motor vehicle laws, individuals with serious progressive visual field loss should not contemplate occupations that will necessitate driving. They also might have trouble driving because of the field loss even though their acuity is still relatively good.

Peripheral Visual Field Loss From Strokes or Tumors

Description of Medical Condition

Peripheral visual field loss can be the result of inflammatory, vascular, congenital, toxic, or degenerative changes that can occur anywhere in the visual pathway as well as the eye itself. A person who has a stroke or tumor can be left with a resultant visual field loss that may be partial, bilateral, unilateral, homonymous, eccentric, bitemporal, superior, inferior, or nasal. This problem may be compounded by the cognitive, motor, and language disorders that may result from stroke or head trauma (Cohen & Waiss, 1994). In addition, there are more complex aspects of the visual process that can be affected. These include perception of visual form, color, object meaning, recognition, and attention. There may also be disorders of the visual system such as hallucinations (Brown & Murphy, 1992).

Functional Presentation of Medical Condition

A complete bilateral loss of the left or right side of vision (homonymous hemianopia) is often the result of a vascular accident in the head. Reading disability is greater when the defect falls in the right visual field. The strategy behind the treatment of hemianopia is to take the visual information present in the nonseeing portion of the field and transfer it for processing into the functioning area of the field (Cohen & Waiss, 1996). Optical treatment generally involves the use of prisms and mirrors. Mobility and night vision may be impaired, and losing one's place while reading is often the result if there is a loss in either the left visual field (finding the beginning of the next line to be read) or the right visual field (reading to the end of the line being read).

Treatment and Prognosis

Generally, visual field loss is accompanied by "spatial neglect" in the area of the field loss. Prisms have been used to enhance rather than expand spatial awareness when there is a loss in the peripheral visual field. Furthermore, mirrors have been placed on glasses, with less success than prisms, to facilitate peripheral field awareness. Low-vision devices, including the CCTV, have also been of value in reading and vocational pursuits.

Psychological and Vocational Implications

Individuals with peripheral field loss may need counseling to understand the extent of the loss. Driving, although legal, may be dangerous when there is a significant peripheral loss, especially to one side. Individuals with this condition should therefore be discouraged from driving.

MEDICARE, THIRD-PARTY COVERAGE, AND LEGISLATION

The problem with Medicare coverage in the past was that there was no distinct national policy. Local medical review policies were inconsistent and/or nonexistent. Vision-impaired patients were denied full and consistent access to rehabilitation services. This started to change with statements in two appropriations bills in two consecutive years (2001 and 2002):

> The committee is concerned that although one in six people older than 65 years has a vision impairment, the Medicare program has not been responsive to the needs of visually impaired older adults, and coverage of low-vision services is inconsistent and inadequate. *The committee urges HCFA to study the impact of vision loss on beneficiary health status and health care costs* [emphasis by author]. (Appropriations Bill, 2001)

> Medicare beneficiaries who are blind or visually impaired are eligible for physician-prescribed rehabilitation services from approved health care professionals on the same basis as beneficiaries with other medical conditions that result in reduced physical functioning. *The committee urges Centers for Medicare & Medicaid Services (CMS) to direct its carriers to inform physicians and other providers about the availability of medically necessary rehabilitation services for these beneficiaries* [emphasis by author]. (Appropriations Bill, 2002)

Program Memorandum—2002

These statements resulted in the issuing of a Program Memorandum by Medicare (AB-02–78) on May 29, 2002. It clarified equal access and coverage of necessary rehabilitation services, and it directed the local carriers to publish the Memorandum in provider newsletters/bulletins. It stated that Medicare-covered therapeutic services could include mobility, activities of daily living, and other rehabilitation goals that are medically necessary. It discussed coverage and limitations and listed the applicable HCPCS Therapeutic Procedures and the ICD-9 Codes for Vision Impairment that support medical necessity. One major change that this Memorandum brought was the fact that visually impaired people who are *not* legally blind can get coverage. It raised the acuity level requirement from 20/200 (severely impaired—legally blind) to 20/70 (moderately impaired) and added a number of visual field conditions that could also now be covered (Program Memorandum, 2003).

Medicare Vision Rehabilitation Services Act of 2003

In 2003, Congress encouraged CMS to recognize the additional component of in-home care:

> The committee commends CMS for issuing a program memorandum...and believes that vision rehabilitation services provided in a clinical setting may be enhanced by a brief course of additional vision rehabilitation in the home. *The committee encourages CMS to direct carriers and intermediaries to recognize the delivery of additional vision rehabilitation in the home that are included in a clinical care plan* [emphasis by author]. (Appropriations Bill, 2003)

Medicare Prescription Drug, Improvement, and Modernization Act of 2003

There had been legislative attempts at coverage since 1999, but none had passed either House as of late 2009. The latest language coming out of Congress was in the Medicare Drug Bill, Section 645, which was signed into law in December, 2003. When the compromise bill finally came out, it directed the secretary to study the feasibility and advisability of Medicare payment for services of vision rehabilitation professionals (orientation and mobility specialists, rehabilitation teachers, or low-vision therapists) (CMS Legislative Summary, 2004).

Two other provider proposals came out in 2003 in the Conference Report on H.R. 2673, Consolidated Appropriations Act, 2004—(House of Representatives—November 25, 2003):

> Page H12580 directed the Secretary to report on the provision of services by vision rehabilitation professionals (including in the home) under "general" supervision. Retrieved April 22, 2004, from http://thomas.loc.gov/cgi-bin/query/F?r108:11:./temp/~r108PAbkWk:e2549639
>
> Page H12745 requested a nationwide outpatient vision rehabilitation services demonstration project to examine the effect of "standardized" national vision rehabilitation provided in the home by physicians, occupational therapists, and vision rehabilitation teachers. Retrieved April 22, 2004, from http://thomas.loc.gov/cgi-bin/query/F?r108:11:./temp/~r108PAbkWk:e3813207

Because other third-party coverage generally follows Medicare, it is expected that other policies will ultimately cover vision rehabilitation, if they are not already doing so. It should be noted that Medicare does not cover the low-vision examination done by optometrists and ophthalmologists. The medical part of the examination would be covered, but there is generally a charge to the patient for the noncovered part ("refractive" or "optical"). Currently, Medicare also does not cover the provision of low-vision devices that are so beneficial to most of these patients. The American Academy of Ophthalmology and the American Optometric Association are currently trying to address these issues. In the current climate of downsizing and budget limitations, this is not an easy task.

Demonstration Project Gets Underway

The Demonstration Project, described in the Medicare Prescription Drug, Improvement, and Modernization Act of 2003, began on April 1, 2006, and will run through March 31, 2011. It will be run in six demonstration sites—New Hampshire, North Carolina, Kansas, Washington state, the New York City Area, and the Atlanta area. Additional areas were added to the Atlanta as well as the New York City region to capture more patients. The Demonstration Project extends the provider list for the rehabilitation training component to include certified low-vision therapists, orientation and mobility specialists, and rehabilitation teachers. The Demonstration Project also allows these individuals to provide services in the patient's home without the physician being present, that is, under general supervision.

At the conclusion, the Department of Health and Human Services and the CMS will produce a report based on the data collected during the study to determine whether low-vision rehabilitation services should be covered for the additional providers for all Medicare recipients across the country.

It should be noted that concerns about the Demonstration Project have been expressed: "...there are intrinsic flaws in the scope and design of the project that preclude its successful implementation and may even undermine the services that have been expended by Medicare to beneficiaries with visual impairments in the last decade" (Mogk, Watson, & Williams, 2008). The article concludes that the Demonstration Project should be either completely restructured or terminated. No changes have occurred as of the close of 2009.

ADA Amendments Act of 2008

The American with Disabilities Act of 2008 was passed by Congress and signed by the president on September 25, 2008. Its purpose is to restore the intent and protections of the

Americans with Disabilities Act of 1990. It includes two important features of particular interest to the vision loss community:

- If an individual has a visual disability that impacts a major life activity such as reading and is using low-vision devices to compensate for that disability, their disability status is evaluated based on the person's normal visual abilities with ordinary eye glasses or contact lenses, but not with low-vision devices.
- It makes the important distinction between glasses/contact lenses (lenses that are intended to correct refractive error) and low-vision devices (optical systems that magnify, enhance, or otherwise augment a visual image). (http://www.govtrack.us/congress/billtext.xpd?bill=h110–3195; accessed 2/17/09)

SUMMARY

The prevalence of vision loss markedly increases with the aging U.S. and worldwide populations. The leading conditions resulting in serious vision loss in the aging population will continue to be AMD, glaucoma, diabetic retinopathy, and cataracts.

Advances in the treatment and understanding of the mechanisms in the "dry" and "wet" forms of AMD, as well as new treatments for diabetic retinopathy and glaucoma, will ultimately have long-term effects in preserving visual function. This is of great importance, especially because the annual cost of adult vision problems in the United States was around $51.4 billion in 2007 (Prevent Blindness America, 2007).

It is estimated that visual impairment and blindness accounted for $8 billion in lost productivity in 2006 (Rein et al., 2006). Screening and early detection, along with new therapies and treatments, will result not only in great cost savings to society but also in increased quality of life for persons affected with age-related eye disease.

REFERENCES

Arditi, A., & Rosenthal, B. (1996, July). *Developing an objective definition of visual impairment*. Paper presented at the VISION 96 International Conference on Low-Vision Proceedings, Book 1, Madrid, Spain.

Bass, S. J., & Sherman, J. (1996). Visual field testing in the low vision patient. In B. P. Rosenthal & R. G. Cole (Eds.), *Functional assessment of low vision*. St. Louis, MO: C. V. Mosby.

Brown, G. C., & Murphy, R. P. (1992). Visual symptoms associated with choroidal neovascularization: Photopsias and the Charles Bonnet Syndrome. *Archives of Ophthalmology, 110*, 1251.

Chew, H. F., Ayres, B. D., Hammersmith, K. M., Rapuano, C. J., Laibson, P. R., Myers, J. S., et al. (2009). Boston keratoprosthesis outcomes and complications. *Cornea, 28*, 989–996.

Clemons, T. E., Milton, R. C., Klein, R., Seddon, J. M., & Ferris, F. L. 3rd. (2005). Age-related eye disease study research group: Risk factors for the incidence of advanced age-related macular degeneration in the age-related eye disease study (AREDS) AREDS report No. 19. *Ophthalmology, 112*, 533–539.

CMS Legislative Summary. (2004). Retrieved October 19, 2009, from http://www.cms.hhs.gov/MMAUpdate/downloads/PL108–173summary.pdf

Cohen, J. M., & Waiss, B. M. (1994). An overview of visual rehabilitation for stroke and head trauma patients. *Aging and Vision News, 6*, 3, 11.

Cole, R. J. (2008). Modifications to the Fletcher central field test for patients with low vision. *Journal of Visual Impairment & Blindness, 102*, 659.

Colenbrander, A. (1977). Dimensions of visual performance. *Transactions of the American Academy of Ophthalmology and Otolaryngology, 83*, 322.

Cong, R., Zhou, B., Sun, Q., Gu, H., Tang, N., & Wang, B. (2008). Smoking and the risk of age-related macular degeneration: A meta analysis. *Annals of Epidemiology, 18*, 647–656.

Congdon, N., Vingerling, J. R., Klein, B. E., West, S., Friedman, D. S., Kempen, J., et al. (2004). Prevalence of cataract and pseudophakia/aphakia among adults in the United States. *Archives of Ophthalmology, 122,* 487–494.

Congdon, N., O'Colmain, B., Klaver, C., Klein, R., et al. (2004). For the Eye Disease Prevalence Research Group. Prevalence of open-angle glaucoma among adults in the United States. *Archives of Ophthalmology, 122,* 532–538.

2004. Eye disease prevalence and projections (Number of adults 40 Years and Older in the U.S.). *Archives of Ophthalmology, 122,* 444, 477–485.

Eye Disease Prevalence Research Group. (2004). Blindness. *Archives of Ophthalmology, 122,* 437–676.

Fingert, J., Stone, E., Sheffield, V., & Alward, W. (2002). Myocilin glaucoma 1. *Survey of Ophthalmology, 47,* 547–561.

Fong, D. S., Aiello, L., Gardner, T. W., King, G. L., Blankenship, F., Cavallereno, J. D., et al. (2004). Retinopathy in diabetes. *Diabetes Care, 27,* S99–S102.

Friedman, D. S., Congdon, J., & Tielsch, J. (2002). *Vision problems in the U.S.: Prevalence of adult vision impairment and age-related eye disease in America.* Chicago, IL: Prevent Blindness America.

Friedman, D. S., O'Colmain, B. J., Munoz, B, Tomany, S. C., McCarty, C., de Jong, P. T., et al. For the Eye Disease Prevalence Research Group. (2004). Prevalence of age-related macular degeneration in the United States. *Archives of Ophthalmology, 122,* 564–573.

Fuchs, W. (1996). Preventing diabetic vision loss. *Aging and Vision News, 8,* 6–7.

Gallup poll. (n.d.). Retrieved November 20, 2009, from http://www.mmf.umn.edu/initiatives/insight/2009/spring/research.cfm

Gordon, M. O., Beiser, J. A., Brandt, J. D., Heuer, D. K., Higginbotham, E. J., Johnson, C. A., et al. (2002). The ocular hypertension treatment study: Baselines factors that predict the onset of primary open-angle glaucoma. *Archives of Ophthalmology, 120,* 714–720.

Haines, J. L., Hauser, M. A., Schmidt, S., Scott, W. K., Olson, L. M., Gallins, P., et al. (2005). Complement factor H variant increases the risk of age-related macular degeneration. *Science, 308,* 419–421.

Horowitz, A., Reinhardt, J. P., & Kennedy, G. J. (2005). Major and subthreshold depression among older adults seeking vision rehabilitation services. *American Journal of Geriatric Psychiatry, 13,* 180–187.

Hicks, C. R., Crawford, G. J., Dart, J. K., Grabner, G., Holland, E. J., Stulting, R. D., et al. (2006). AlphaCor: Clinical outcomes. *Cornea, 25,* 1034–1042.

ICD-9-CM. (2009). Published by PMIC. 331.

Javitt, J. C., Zhou, Z., & Wilke, R. J. (2007). Association between vision loss and higher medical care costs in medicare beneficiaries: Costs are greater for those with progressive vision loss. *Ophthalmology, 114,* 238–245.

Kempen, J. H., O'Colmain, B. J., Leske, M. C., Haffner, S. M., Klein, R., Moss, S. E., et al. For the Eye Disease Prevalence Research Group. (2004). The prevalence of diabetic retinopathy among adults in the United States. *Archives of Ophthalmology, 122,* 552–563.

Klein, R., Klein, B. E. K., Tomany, S. C., & Cruickshanks, K. J. (2003). The association of cardiovascular disease with the long-term incidence of age-related maculopathy: The Beaver Dam eye study. *Ophthalmology, 110,* 636–643.

Krachmer, J., & Palay, D. (1991). Corneal disease. *New England Journal of Medicine, 325,* 1805–1806.

Lake Shore Assisted Living Facility (2008). What are ADLs and IADLs? Retrieved February 6, 2008, from http://lakeshoreli.com/assisted-living-faq/what-are-adls-and-iadls.htm.

Lindblad, B., Håkansson, N., Svensson, H., Philipson, B., & Wolk, A. (2005). Intensity of smoking and smoking cessation in relation to risk of cataract extraction: A prospective study of women. *American Journal of Epidemiology, 162,* 73–79.

Maguire, M. (1997). Who is at risk? *Aging and Vision News, 9,* 5.

McCarty, C., Nanjan, M., & Taylor, H. (2001). Vision impairment predicts 5 year mortality. *British Journal of Ophthalmology, 85,* 322–326.

Mogk, L., Watson, G., & Williams, M. (2008). A Commentary on the Medicare Low Vision Rehabilitation Demonstration Project. *Journal of Visual Impairment & Blindness, 102,* 69–75.

National Eye Institute. (1993). *Vision research: A National plan 1994–1998* (NIH Publication No. 95–3186). Bethesda, MD: Author.

National Eye Institute. (2004). Statistics. Retrieved http://www.nei.nih.gov/eye-data/tables.asp

National Retinitis Pigmentosa Foundation. (1995). *Fact sheets: Information about retinitis pigmentosa.*

Parc, C. E., Johnson, D. H., Oliver, J. E., Hattenhauer, M. G., & Hodge, D. O. (2001). The long-term outcome of glaucoma filtration surgery. *American Journal of Ophthalmology, 132,* 27–35.

Prevent Blindness America. (2007). *The economic impact of vision problems. The toll of major adult eye disorders, visual impairment and blindness in the U.S. economy.* Chicago, IL: Prevent Blindness America.

Prevent Blindness America. (2008). http://www.preventblindness.org/vpus/2008_update/VPUS_2008_update.pdf

Program Memorandum. (2003). Retrieved February 13, 2009, from http://www.cms.hhs.gov/Transmittals/downloads/AB03050.pdf

Rein, D. B., Zhang, P., Wirth, K. E., Lee, P. P., Hoerger, T. J., McCall, N., et al. (2006). The economic burden of major adult visual disorders in the United States. *Archives of Ophthalmology, 124,* 1754–1760.

Sarfarazi, M., & Rezaie, T. (2004). Optineurin in primary open angle glaucoma. *Ophthalmology Clinics of North America, 16,* 529–541.

Seddon, J. M., Cote, J., Davis, N., & Rosner, B. (2003). Progression of age-related macular degeneration: Association with body mass index, waist circumference, and waist-hip ratio. *Archives of Ophthalmology, 121,* 785–792.

Simons, K. (1991). Visual acuity and the functional definition of blindness. In W. Tasman & E. A. Jaeger (Eds.), *Duane's clinical ophthalmology* (Vol. 5, pp. 1–21). Philadelphia, PA: J. B. Lippincott.

Social Security Online. (n.d.). Retrieved February 18, 2009, http://www.ssa.gov/disability/professionals/bluebook/2.00SpecialSensesandSpeechAdult.htm

The Lighthouse. (1990b). *Statistics on blindness and vision impairment: A resource manual.* New York: Author.

The Lighthouse. (1995). *The Lighthouse National Survey on Vision Loss: The experience, attitudes, and knowledge of middle-aged and older Americans.* New York: Author.

U.S. Census Bureau. (n.d.). Retrieved November 11, 2009, from http://www.census.gov

U.S. Census Bureau. (n.d.). Retrieved November 6, 2009, http://www.census.gov/popest/estimates.php

Varma, R., Torres, M., Peña, F., Klein, R., & Azen, S. P. (2004). Prevalence of diabetic retinopathy in adult Latinos: The Los Angeles Latino Eye Study. *Ophthalmology, 111,* 1298–1306.

Visio. (1993, June). *Interdisciplinary model for the rehabilitation of visually impaired and blind people.* Visio Report No 93–2, English version. Huizen, The Netherlands: Author.

Vision Problems in the U.S. (2002). Prevalence of Adult Eye Disease and Vision Impairment in America, Prevent Blindness America. Retrieved from http:// www.preventblindness.org/resources/vision_data.html

Wainapel, S. F. (2001). Low vision rehabilitation and rehabilitation medicine: A parable of parallels. In R. W. Massof & L. Lidoff (Eds.), *Issues in low vision rehabilitation—Service delivery, policy, and funding* (pp. 55–59). New York: AFB Press.

Waiss, B., & Cohen, J. (1991). Glare and contrast sensitivity for low vision practitioners. *Problems in Optometry, 3,* 436.

Warren, M. (2000). An overview of low vision rehabilitation and the role of occupational therapy. In M. Warren (Ed.), *Low vision: Occupational therapy with the older adult* (pp. 11–14). Bethesda, MD: American Occupational Therapy Association.

Wolfgang, D., Sattmann, H., Hermann, B., Ko, T., Stur, M., Unterhuber, A., et al. (2003). Enhanced visualization of macular pathology with the use of ultrahigh-resolution optical coherence tomography. *Archives of Ophthalmology, 121,* 695–706.

World Health Organization. (n.d.). Retrieved October 15, 2009, from http://www.who.int/classifications/icf/en

Yannuzzi, L. A., Slakter, J. S., Sorenson, J. A., Guyer, D. R., & Orlock, D. A. (1992). Digital indocyanine green videoangiography and choroidal neovascularization. *Retina, 12,* 191–223.

28

Complementary and Alternative Medicine

Alex Moroz, MD, FACP, and Robert A. Schulman, MD

According to a 2007 government survey (Nahin, Barnes, Stussman, & Bloom, 2009; National Center for Health Statistics, 2009), Americans spent $33.9 billion out of pocket on complementary and alternative medicine (CAM) over the past 12 months. To put these figures in context, the $14.8 billion spent on nonvitamin, nonmineral, natural products is equivalent to approximately one-third of total out-of-pocket spending on prescription drugs, and the $11.9 billion spent on CAM practitioner visits is equivalent to approximately one-quarter of total out-of-pocket spending on physician visits.

CAM is a group of diverse medical and health care systems, practices, and products that are not generally considered to be part of conventional medicine. Although scientific evidence exists for some CAM therapies, for most there are key questions that are yet to be answered through well-designed scientific studies—questions such as whether these therapies are safe and whether they work for the purposes for which they are used (National Center for Complementary and Alternative Medicine [NCCAM], 2009).

Integrative medicine, also called integrated medicine, combines treatments from conventional medicine and CAM for which there is evidence of safety and effectiveness. The NCCAM groups CAM practices into four domains (mind–body medicine, biologically based practices, manipulative and body-based practices, and energy medicine), recognizing that there can be some overlap. In addition, NCCAM studies CAM whole medical systems, which cut across all domains. Although it is not practical to present a comprehensive overview of all CAM practices in this chapter, we will review representative therapies for each NCCAM domain.

MIND–BODY MEDICINE DOMAIN

Mind–body medicine uses various techniques designed to enhance the mind's capacity to affect bodily function and symptoms. Some techniques that were considered CAM in the past have become conventional (e.g., patient support groups and cognitive-behavioral therapy). Other mind–body techniques are still considered CAM, which include meditation (a conscious mental process using certain techniques—such as focusing attention or maintaining a specific posture—to suspend the stream of thoughts and relax the body and mind), prayer, mental healing, and therapies that use creative outlets such as art, music, or dance.

Example: Meditation

The term *meditation* (from the Latin *meditari*: to measure, to study) refers to a group of techniques, such as mantra meditation, relaxation response, mindfulness meditation, and Zen Buddhist meditation. Most meditative techniques started in Eastern religious or spiritual traditions. These techniques have been used by different cultures throughout the world for thousands of years. Today, many people use meditation outside of its traditional religious or cultural settings for health and wellness purposes.

In meditation, a person learns to focus attention. Some forms of meditation instruct the practitioner to become mindful of thoughts, feelings, and sensations and to observe them in a nonjudgmental way. This practice is believed to result in a state of greater calmness and physical relaxation, and psychological balance. Practicing meditation can change the way in which a person relates to the flow of emotions and thoughts in the mind.

Most types of meditation have four elements in common:

- *A quiet location.* Meditation is usually practiced in a quiet place with as few distractions as possible. This can be particularly helpful for beginners.
- *A specific, comfortable posture.* Depending on the type being practiced, meditation can be done while sitting, lying down, standing, walking, or in other positions.
- *A focus of attention.* Focusing one's attention is usually a part of meditation. For example, the meditator may focus on a mantra (a specially chosen word or set of words), an object, or the sensations of the breath. Some forms of meditation involve paying attention to whatever is the dominant content of consciousness.
- *An open attitude.* Having an open attitude during meditation means letting distractions come and go naturally without judging them. When the attention goes to distracting or wandering thoughts, they are not suppressed; instead, the meditator gently brings attention back to the focus. In some types of meditation, the meditator learns to "observe" thoughts and emotions while meditating (NCCAM, 2009).

A 2007 national Government survey (Barnes, Bloom, & Nahin, 2008) that asked about CAM use in a sample of 23,393 U.S. adults found that 9.4% of respondents (representing more than 20 million people) had used meditation in the past 12 months—compared with 7.6% of respondents (representing more than 15 million people) in a similar survey conducted in 2002. The 2007 survey also asked about CAM use in a sample of 9,417 children: 1% (representing 725,000 children) had used meditation in the past 12 months.

People use meditation for various health problems (Bonadonna, 2003), such as anxiety, pain, depression, stress, insomnia, and physical or emotional symptoms that may be associated with chronic illnesses (such as heart disease, human immunodeficiency virus/acquired immune deficiency syndrome, and cancer) and their treatment. Meditation is also used for overall wellness.

Practicing meditation has been shown to induce changes in the body (Newberg & Iversen, 2003). Some types of meditation might work by affecting the autonomic nervous system. This system regulates many organs and muscles, controlling functions such as the heartbeat, sweating, breathing, and digestion. It has two major parts:

- The *sympathetic nervous system* helps mobilize the body for action. When a person is under stress, it produces the "fight-or-flight response": the heart rate and breathing rate go up and blood vessels narrow (restricting the flow of blood).
- The *parasympathetic nervous system* causes the heart rate and breathing rate to slow down, the blood vessels to dilate (improving blood flow), and digestive juices to increase.

It is thought that some types of meditation might work by reducing activity in the sympathetic nervous system and increasing activity in the parasympathetic nervous system.

In one area of research, scientists use sophisticated tools to determine whether meditation is associated with significant changes in brain function (Davidson & Lutz, 2007). These changes include alterations in patterns of brain function assessed with functional magnetic resonance imaging (fMRI), changes in the cortical evoked response to visual stimuli that reflect the effect of meditation on attention, and alterations in amplitude and synchrony of high-frequency oscillations that may play an important role in connectivity among widespread circuitry in the brain. A number of researchers believe that these changes account for many of meditation's effects.

It is also possible that practicing meditation may work by improving the mind's ability to pay attention (Jha, Krompinger, & Baime, 2007; Lutz, Slagter, Dunne, & Davidson, 2008). Since attention is involved in performing everyday tasks and regulating mood, meditation might lead to other benefits.

A 2007 NCCAM-funded review of the scientific literature found evidence suggesting that meditation is associated with potentially beneficial health effects (Ospina et al., 2007). However, the overall evidence was inconclusive. The reviewers concluded that future research needs to be more rigorous before firm conclusions can be drawn.

BIOLOGICALLY BASED PRACTICES DOMAIN

Biologically based practices in CAM use substances found in nature, such as herbs, foods, and vitamins. Some examples include dietary supplements, herbal products, and the use of other so-called natural but as yet scientifically unproven therapies (e.g., using shark cartilage to treat cancer).

Acupuncture (a family of procedures involving the stimulation of anatomical points on the body using various techniques [NCCAM, 2009]) is a commonly used biologically based practice and also part of the traditional Chinese medicine whole medical system (see below). Acupuncture will not be covered in detail here because the evidence accumulated to date is extensive and a comprehensive review requires at least a separate chapter and probably a dedicated manuscript.

Example: Prolotherapy

Prolotherapy is a technique that involves the injection of various fluids into joints, ligaments, tendons, and muscles (Reeves, 2000). The goal is stimulation of endogenous growth factors thereby initiating tissue repair and healing. The proliferants are thought to strengthen and "reorganize" injured tissue and decrease pain by creating an irritation that alters the inflammatory process (Jensen, Rabago, Best, Patterson, & Vanderby, 2008). Materials used for injections may include dextrose, glycerin, phenol, and lidocaine. George S. Hackett, MD, is reported to have developed the technique, which was subsequently popularized by Gustav Anders Hemwall, MD.

Prolotherapy is used to treat tendonopathies such as lateral epicondylitis and Achilles tendonitis, general musculoskeletal conditions, coccygodynia, osteoarthritis (OA) of the hand, sacroiliac disorders, various types of neck pain, temporomandibular joint (TMJ) dysfunction, cervicogenic headaches, chronic headaches, and foot problems.

A Cochrane review of prolotherapy injections for chronic low-back pain (LBP) found that when combined with spinal manipulation, exercise, and other cointerventions, it may improve chronic LBP and disability (Dagenais, Yelland, Del Mar, & Schoene, 2004). Conclusions were confounded by clinical heterogeneity among studies and by the presence of cointerventions.

Another interesting retrospective study of patients with TMJ pain found that prolotherapy can be an effective therapeutic modality that reduces TMJ pain and joint noise in most patients who have reached a plateau using an intraoral appliance, physical therapy, or home care (Hakala, 2005).

In an analysis of evidence of using prolotherapy in musculoskeletal disorders, data from 34 case reports and case series and two nonrandomized controlled trials suggested that prolotherapy is efficacious for many musculoskeletal conditions (Rabago, Best, Beamsley, & Patterson, 2005). However, results from six randomized controlled trials (RCTs) were conflicting. Two RCTs on OA reported decreased pain, increased range of motion, and increased patellofemoral cartilage thickness after prolotherapy. Two RCTs on LBP reported significant improvements in pain and disability compared with control subjects, whereas two did not. All studies had significant methodological limitations. Another group of authors concluded that on the basis of the scarce body of literature critically reviewed to date (Kim, Stitik, Foye, Greenwald, & Campagnolo, 2004), the clinical efficacy of prolotherapy in treating OA remains inconclusive.

Several placebo-controlled studies, together with uncontrolled studies, suggest that regenerative injection therapy is effective in treating painful cervical ligament and tendon pathology (Linetsky, Miguel, & Torres, 2004).

MANIPULATIVE AND BODY-BASED PRACTICES DOMAIN

Manipulative and body-based practices in CAM are based on manipulation (the application of controlled force to a joint, moving it in an effort of restoring health). Manipulation may be performed as a part of other therapies or whole medical systems (see following text), including chiropractic medicine, massage, and naturopathy. Some examples include chiropractic or osteopathic manipulation (a type of manipulation practiced by osteopathic physicians that is combined with physical therapy and instruction in proper posture), and massage (pressing, rubbing, and moving muscles and other soft tissues of the body, primarily using the hands and fingers, aiming to increase the flow of blood and oxygen to the massaged area).

Example: Massage

Massage is the stimulation of soft tissue by applying pressure on them for therapeutic purposes, and is one of the oldest forms of medical treatment in the world, with origins in various societies. Chinese writings dating back to 2700 B.C. and 2598 B.C. mention massage in religious documents and a medical work, respectively. The depiction of massages were found on the wall of an Egyptian physician's tomb in Saqqara, ca. 2330 B.C. Massage was also mentioned and approved in the Indian medical work, *Ayurveda*, written around 1800 B.C as well as the book *On Articulations* by Hippocrates in 400 B.C.

Since its origins, the popularity of massage as a form of medical treatment has fluctuated, particularly in Western civilizations. In Western civilizations, the acceptance and use of massage declined from the fifth century to the Renaissance. This was largely due to the influence of the Church; it condemned massage for bringing pleasure to the body. However, in 1819, massage became more acceptable in Western medicine when Piorry analyzed its physiological effects.

Modern massage came into effect when the practice became more systematic. In 1863, the French publication of Estradere's *Du Massage*, "systematically classified each massage technique according to the bodily system affected." This influenced the rise of scientific massage techniques (Tan, 2002). Such techniques include the Swedish massage developed by Per Henrik Ling in the early 19th century. In the United States, modern scientific massage therapy was introduced in the mid-1800s, where physicians utilized it until the early 20th century. After the pharmaceutical revolution occurred in the 1940s, massage therapy became less acceptable and was categorized as an alternative form of health care. In the 1960s, physical therapy began to use massage for treating musculoskeletal impairments and other physical impairments. During the same era, the growth in the movement toward emphasizing human psychology and spirituality greatly increased massage therapy's popularity. Following the 1960s, massage therapy eventually became incorporated into the "normal," healthy lifestyle. Nursing and physical therapy have come to reincorporate massage techniques including simple backrubs, reflexology, therapeutic touch, and aromatherapy massage. Presently, surveys in the United States have indicated the growing popularity of massage; it is one of the most commonly used therapies for both the general population as well as individuals with disabilities, and it is one of the top physician referrals for alternative therapies (Tan, 2002). Several common stroke techniques can be found among the myriad of massage techniques. These include effleurage, friction, pressure, petrissage, vibration, and percussion. Effleurage involves rhythmic and gentle skin contact. Generally, the palm is used for larger body surfaces while the fingers are used for smaller body surfaces. In the friction stroke technique, moderate pressure is applied to one area with the thumbs or fingers. The pressure stroke is, "similar to the friction stroke, except that pressure strokes are made with the hands." Petrissage, also known as kneading, involves lifting and holding skin and the underlying muscle. The tissues are pushed against the bone. Tissues are supported by one hand while kneading is performed using the other hand. Kneading is generally limited to areas of the body with large muscles mass. Vibration strokes involve the use of continuous motion. For percussion strokes, the wrist is used for tapping areas of the body (Snyder, 2006).

Ernst evaluated systematic reviews of massage therapy (MT) and chiropractic effects on reduction of any type of pain (Ernst, 2004). Two systematic reviews were found, and there was equivocal evidence for effectiveness of MT in controlling musculoskeletal or other pain. However, a meta-analysis of 37 studies that used random assignment concluded that single applications of MT did not reduce immediate assessment of pain, whereas multiple applications reduced delayed assessment of pain (Moyer, Rounds, & Hannum, 2004).

Back and colleagues described a pilot program to evaluate the efficacy of employer-funded on-site MT on job satisfaction, workplace stress, pain, and discomfort (Back, Tam, Lee, & Haraldsson, 2009). Twenty-minute massage therapy sessions were provided. Evaluation demonstrated possible improvements in job satisfaction, with initial benefits in pain severity, and the greatest benefit for individuals with preexisting symptoms. A long-term effect was not demonstrated.

A number of authors addressed the prevalence of use of MT, with results ranging from 6.9% to 61% depending on the population studied. Wells studied the use of complementary and alternative therapies in 189 women with nonsmall cell lung cancer (Wells et al., 2007). MT was used by 6.9% of participants, most commonly for pain (54.8%). Women who were younger, experienced more symptoms, and who lived on the West coast or the South (vs. the Northeast) were more likely to use complementary and alternative therapies. In a nationally representative survey that sampled 2,055 adults, Wolsko and colleagues discovered that 54% of those reporting back or neck pain in the past 12 months used complementary and alternative therapies, including 14% that used MT (Wolsko, Eisenberg, Davis, Kessler, & Phillips, 2003). Fifteen percent of midlife U.S. women used massage and chiropractic medicine, most commonly for pain (Brett & Keenan, 2007).

Palinkas and Kabongo (2000) surveyed 542 patients attending 16 family practice clinics belonging to a community-based research network in San Diego, California, and found that 17.2% used MT. The results of a survey and interviews of older adults showed that the most prevalent motivation for using complementary and alternative therapies was pain relief (54.8%), and that MT was used by 35.7% (Williamson, Fletcher, & Dawson, 2003). Prevalence of MT use in a large military family practice clinic was found to be 36%, most commonly used for back or other musculoskeletal pain (Drivdahl & Miser, 1998). In a telephone interview survey of Chicago adults aged 45 years and above, Feinglass and colleagues (2007) discovered that more than half of the respondents used complementary and alternative therapies, most commonly MT and relaxation techniques. Similarly, more than half of traumatically injured spinal cord patients with shoulder pain received MT or physical therapy (McCasland, Budiman-Mak, Weaver, Adams, & Miskevics, 2006).

Use of MT with neck, back, and other musculoskeletal pain has been studied extensively. A review by Trinh and others concluded that there is limited evidence suggesting that MT is less effective than acupuncture in chronic mechanical neck pain (Trinh et al., 2007). Ezzo et al. (2007) analyzed 19 trials of MT in neck pain and found that 12 were not designed well. Descriptions of the massage intervention, massage professional's credentials, or experience were frequently missing, while six of the trials examined massage as a stand-alone treatment. Not surprisingly, the results were inconclusive (Ezzo et al., 2007). Results were also inconclusive in 14 trials that used massage as part of a multimodal intervention because none were designed such that the relative contribution of MT could be ascertained.

Sherman and others surveyed randomly selected acupuncturists, chiropractors, and massage therapists in two states (Sherman et al., 2006). Back pain was the most common reason for visits to each of these providers, with chronic back pain representing about 12% of visits to massage therapists.

Cherkin, Sherman, Deyo, and Shekelle (2003) reviewed MEDLINE, Embase, and the Cochrane Controlled Trials Register, and included three RCTs that evaluated massage and reported that it is effective for subacute and chronic back pain.

Similarly, Furlan, Brosseau, Imamura, and Irvin (2002) conducted a systematic review of MEDLINE, Embase, Cochrane Controlled Trials Register, HealthSTAR, Cumulative Index to Nursing and Allied Health Literature (CINAHL), and dissertation abstracts describing use of MT for lower back pain. Nine publications reporting on eight randomized trials were included. Three had low and five had high methodological quality scores. Massage was compared with an inert treatment (sham laser) in one study that showed that massage was superior, particularly if given in combination with exercises and education. In the other seven studies, massage was compared with different active treatments. They showed that massage was inferior to manipulation and transcutaneous electrical nerve stimulation; equal to corsets and exercises; and superior to relaxation therapy, acupuncture, and self-care education. The beneficial effects of massage in patients with chronic LBP lasted at least 1 year after the end of the treatment. One study comparing two different techniques of massage concluded in favor of acupuncture massage over classic (Swedish) massage.

Wright and Sluka (2001) reviewed the use of several modalities including MT in the management of painful musculoskeletal disorders, and concluded that although evidence from basic scientific research suggests that many of the therapies could have potential therapeutic effects, there is a paucity of high-quality evidence from RCTs to support the therapeutic effectiveness of these therapies.

Best, Hunter, Wilcox, and Haq (2008) reviewed evidence for using massage for muscle and soft-tissue pain and weakness after intense exercise. Analysis of 27 studies that met inclusion criteria led authors to conclude that while case series provide little support for the use of massage to aid muscle recovery or performance after intense exercise, RCTs provide moderate data supporting its use to facilitate recovery from repetitive muscular contractions. It also appears that the experience of the massage therapist may be directly related to effectiveness of MT in relieving muscle soreness after a 10-km race (Moraska, 2007).

Dryden, Baskwill, and Preyde (2004) reviewed evidence of MT's utility for orthopedic problems and concluded that it may be effective for patients with low-back problems and potentially beneficial for other orthopedic problems. MT appears to be safe and effective in reducing both pain and dysfunction with high patient satisfaction.

In a randomized, double-blind, placebo-controlled trial of 140 subjects with knee OA, physiotherapy including MT appeared no more effective in reducing pain at 12 and 24 weeks than regular contact with a therapist (Bennell et al., 2005).

Several investigators studied use of massage in cancer pain. Ferrell-Torry and Glick (1993) administered 30 minutes of therapeutic massage on two consecutive evenings to nine hospitalized males diagnosed with cancer who were experiencing cancer pain. Massage therapy significantly reduced the subjects' level of pain perception and anxiety. In addition to these subjective measures, all physiological measures (heart rate, respiratory rate, and blood pressure) tended to decrease from baseline, providing further indication of relaxation. Building on the work of these authors, Grealish, Lomasney, and Whiteman (2000) administered 10-minute foot massage (5 minutes per foot) to 87 subjects hospitalized with cancer and found a significant immediate effect on the perceptions of pain, nausea, and relaxation when measured with a visual analog scale.

In a larger study, Currin and Meister (2008) assessed the effect of a Swedish massage intervention on 251 oncology patients' perceived level of distress. The analysis found a statistically significant reduction in patient-reported distress for both pain and physical discomfort, regardless of gender, age, ethnicity, or cancer type.

Jane, Wilkie, Gallucci, and Beaton (2008) reviewed 15 studies published in English between 1986 and 2006 for study design, methods, and massage efficacy in adult patients with cancer. Methodological issues identified included less rigorous inclusion criteria, failure to consider potential confounding variables, less than rigorous research designs, inconsistent massage doses and protocols, measurement errors related to sensitivity of instruments and timing of measurements, and inadequate statistical power.

Use of massage for postoperative pain control has been addressed by several authors.

Forchuk and colleagues (2004) evaluated the usefulness of arm massage from a significant other following lymph node dissection surgery in a randomized clinical trial that included 59 women. Participants reported a reduction in pain in the immediate postoperative period and better shoulder function.

Anderson and Cutshall (2007) reviewed benefits of massage in the reduction of pain, anxiety, and tension in cardiac surgical patients, and described a clinical case example of a patient who has experienced cardiac surgery and received massage therapy.

In a study attempting to test the effectiveness of physiotherapy-based rehabilitation starting 1 week after lumbar disc surgery, Erdogmus and coworkers (2007) compared "comprehensive" physiotherapy, "sham" neck massage, and no therapy. LBP at 12 weeks was equally improved in both the "comprehensive" and the "sham" massage groups, compared to controls.

Finally, in a randomized trial of MT in 605 veterans with acute postoperative pain after major surgery, Mitchinson and colleagues (2007) found that compared with the control group, patients in the massage group experienced very significant short-term decreases in pain (intensity $p = 0.001$), pain unpleasantness, and anxiety. In addition, patients in the massage group experienced a significantly faster rate of decrease in pain intensity and unpleasantness during the first 4 postoperative days compared with the control group.

Another area that deserves discussion is use of massage in patients with pain related to burn injuries. Field and coworkers (1998) randomly assigned 28 adult patients with burns before debridement to either a massage therapy group or a standard treatment control group. The massage therapy group demonstrated decreased pain on the McGill Pain Questionnaire, Present Pain Intensity Scale, and Visual Analogue Scale compared to the control group. In their review, Gallagher, Rae, and Kinsella (2000) described massage as one of nonpharmacological modalities routinely used in treating patients with burns.

Hernandez-Reif and coworkers (2001) studied 24 young children (mean age = 2.5 years) hospitalized for severe burns who received standard dressing care or massage therapy in addition to standard dressing care before dressing changes. The massage therapy was conducted to body parts that were not burned. During the dressing change, the children who received massage therapy showed minimal distress behaviors and no increase in movement other than at the torso. In contrast, the children who did not receive MT responded to the dressing change procedure with increased facial grimacing, torso movement, crying, leg movement, and reaching out. Nurses also reported greater ease in completing the dressing change procedure for the children in the MT group. MT has also been described by Schneider and coworkers (2006) as a common alleviating factor in their review of neuropathic-like pain after burn injury.

ENERGY MEDICINE DOMAIN

Energy therapies involve the use of energy fields. They are of two types:

1. *Biofield therapies* are intended to affect energy fields that purportedly surround and penetrate the human body. The existence of such fields has not yet been scientifically proven. Some forms of energy therapy manipulate biofields by applying pressure and/or manipulating the body by placing the hands in, or through, these fields. Examples include tai chi (a component of traditional Chinese medicine and martial arts that combines movement, meditation, and controlled breathing), Reiki (a therapy in which practitioners seek to transmit a universal energy to a person, either from a distance or by placing their hands on or near that person; the intent is to heal the spirit and thus the body), and therapeutic touch (a therapy in which practitioners pass their hands over another person's body with the intent to use their own perceived healing energy to identify energy imbalances and promote health).
2. *Bioelectromagnetic-based therapies* involve the unconventional use of electromagnetic fields, such as pulsed fields, magnetic fields, or alternating-current or direct-current fields.

Example: Tai Chi Chuan

Tai chi chuan is a martial art rooted in the philosophy of Daoism that emphasizes fluid, continuous movement. Literally translated as the "supreme ultimate fist" (Chen, 2006), tai chi chuan strives for balance and harmony in the practitioners' movements vis-à-vis chi or qi, the metaphysical life force that Daoism believes to run through all living beings. Through the correct positioning of the body, the gracefully proper transitions between positions, as well as mental concentration, tai chi chuan aims for harmony within the practitioner and between the practitioner and the way of nature. Since the emphasis of tai chi chuan is precise and fluid motion, it can be practiced by a wide range of age groups (Wolf, O'Grady, & Xu, 2002).

The way of nature is a fundamental aspect of both Daoism and tai chi chuan. The quintessential book of Daoism, the *Dao De Jing*, states that the Dao has no set form but can be understood through the cyclical movement of nature as well as through the opposite, yet complementary forces in nature (Morton, 2004). The Dao has been described as being, "like empty space, but emptiness has been undervalued, since the hollow in the center of a bowl, the space in a wheel between rim and hub, or the empty space of a window or door in a room are the very things which give these objects their point and usefulness." In essence, the passiveness of the Dao helps the flow of Chi in the body (Morton, 2004).

The recorded history of tai chi chuan began in the 17th century, a transition period between the Ming and Qing dynasties. The art of tai chi chuan was a secret and closely protected heirloom of the Chen family. This pattern was broken around the 19th century when Yang Luchan, the first notably nonmember of the Chen family, learned the art from Chen Changxing. Eventually Yang made his own contributions to the art, leading to the creation of the Yang style. Proliferation of tai chi chuan continued and as a result, multiple variations of tai chi chuan exist today, with the Chen, Yang, Sun, Wu and alternative Wu, as the more popular of the variations (Wolf et al., 2002).

Tai chi chuan practice is based on 10 principles created by Grand Master Yang Chen-Fu in the late 1920s:

1. Keep the head and neck straight (as if suspended from above).
2. Upper and lower back is kept in a straight line with the pelvis tucked in.
3. Waist is relaxed and rotates easily, including the muscles of the hips and groin.
4. Shoulders and elbows are relaxed and sinking down.
5. Upper and lower parts of the body always move as one coordinated unit.

6. Always differentiate between a full (solid) and an empty leg when moving (i.e., be aware to which leg a weight shifting is occurring).
7. Move using only the intention of the mind and no external muscle force.
8. Make each movement flow into the next in a smooth, continuous manner.
9. Ensure a sense of harmony between the internal and external body feeling.
10. Experience a tranquil, meditative state. (Wolf et al., 2002).

From these principles, the actual practice of tai chi chuan begins with warm-up exercises such as foot massages and gentle patting of the face, neck and arms; this is done to stimulate the movement of chi. The final part of the warm-up involves the "waiving arms" exercise; the exercise involves shifting the body weight among the legs and other parts of the body, as well as free swinging of the arms in a backward motion. After the warm-up, the exercises begin. Common to all the variations of tai chi chuan is the review. At the beginning of each session, previous motions are reviewed to ensure they have been practiced adequately and that the motions are correct. Typically, a session lasts between 60 and 90 minutes (Wolf et al., 2002).

Comprehensive benefits of tai chi were reviewed by Klein and Adams (2004). Of the more than 200 published reports examined, 17 controlled clinical trials were judged to meet a high standard of methodological rigor. Controlled research evidence was found to confirm therapeutic benefits of tai chi practice with regard to pain management.

Use of tai chi among other mind–body interventions in neurology patients was reviewed by Wahbeh, Elsas, and Oken (2008). Authors discussed applications of mind–body therapy to general pain, back and neck pain, carpal tunnel syndrome, headaches, and fibromyalgia, and concluded that the evidence for the efficacy of mind–body therapies is quite strong in some conditions, such as migraine headache.

Research-based use of tai chi for reducing pain and stress as a potential nursing intervention was summarized by Chen and Snyder (1999). Authors critically evaluated existing literature and suggested that additional studies on the effects of tai chi from a nursing perspective are needed to make clear when it is beneficial as a nursing intervention.

On the other hand, Siu, Chan, Poon, Chui, and Chan (2007) used tai chi as a control intervention in a study evaluating a 6-week Chronic Disease Self-Management Program (CDSMP) in 148 subjects with chronic illness. CDSMP subjects used more cognitive methods to manage pain and had a tendency to adopt the cognitive methods of diverting attention, reinterpreting pain, ignoring sensations, and making positive self-statements, as opposed to subjects assigned to the tai chi (control) group.

In a survey of Boston and Seattle patients with chronic LBP, Sherman and colleagues (2004) found that knowledge about complementary alternative therapies was low, except for chiropractic.

Yocum, Castro, and Cornett (2000) reviewed the role of exercise, education, and behavioral modification as alternative therapy for pain and stress in rheumatic disease. Their analysis indicated that programs using alternative therapies such as tai chi in combination with traditional medications appear to be beneficial for patients with arthritis, and that these individuals appear to live better lives and have better long-term outcomes.

A number of investigators studied the effectiveness of tai chi in patients with OA pain. Lee, Pitler, and Ernst (2008) conducted a systematic review of use of tai chi for OA on MEDLINE, AMED, British Nursing Index, CINAHL, Embase, PsycINFO, The Cochrane Library 2007, Issue 2, the UK National Research Register and ClinicalTrials.gov, Korean Medical Databases, the Qigong and Energy database, and Chinese Medical Databases (until June 2007). Hand searches included conference proceedings and author's own files. Five RCTs assessed the effectiveness of tai chi on pain of OA. Two RCTs suggested significant pain reduction on visual analog scale and the Western Ontario and McMaster Universities Osteoarthritis Index (WOMAC) as compared with routine treatment and an attention control program in knee OA. Three RCTs did not report significant pain reduction on multiple sites pain.

In a prospective, pretest–posttest clinical trial, Shen and colleagues (2008) examined the effects of tai chi exercise on gait kinematics, physical function, pain, and pain self-efficacy in elderly with knee OA. After 6 weeks of tai chi exercise, knee pain was significantly decreased, whereas no change was observed in pain self-efficacy.

Lee et al. (2008) studied effects of tai chi exercise on pain and stiffness of knee joint in 46 community-dwelling elderly subjects with OA. The experimental group had significantly less pain and stiffness than the control group.

Wang and colleagues (2008) discuss the challenges of designing an RCT with long-term follow-up. Their RCT examines the effects of a 12-week tai chi program compared with an attention control (wellness, education, and stretching) on pain, functional capacity, psychosocial variables, joint proprioception, and health status in elderly people with knee OA. The challenges encountered by the authors included strategies for recruitment, avoidance of selection bias, the actual practice of tai chi, and the maximization of adherence and follow-up while conducting the clinical trial for the evaluation of the effectiveness of tai chi on knee OA.

Two studies examined comparative efficacy of hydrotherapy and tai chi in patients with OA. Lee (2006) compared the effects of tai chi, aquatic exercise, and a self-help program in 50 patients. There were significant differences in joint pain and stiffness for both the tai chi and the aquatic exercise groups compared with the self-help group. In a larger RCT, Fransen, Nairn, Winstanley, Lam, and Edmonds (2007) randomly allocated 152 older persons with chronic symptomatic hip or knee OA for 12 weeks to hydrotherapy classes, tai chi classes, or a waiting list control group. Outcomes were assessed 12 and 24 weeks after randomization and included pain and physical function (WOMAC). At 12 weeks, compared with controls, participants allocated to hydrotherapy classes and tai chi classes demonstrated significant improvements for pain scores. All significant improvements were sustained at 24 weeks. Interestingly, class attendance was higher for hydrotherapy, with 81% attending at least half of the available 24 classes, compared with 61% for tai chi. Similarly, while demonstrating significant pain reduction in the tai chi group, the drop-out rate in the study by Song, Lee, Lam, and Bae (2007) was 41%.

In contrast to these findings, Brismee et al. (2007) found that although 6 weeks of group tai chi followed by another 6 weeks of home tai chi training resulted in significant improvements in mean overall knee pain and maximum knee pain compared with controls, all improvements disappeared after stopping practice for 18 weeks.

Several studies investigated the use of tai chi in pain associated with rheumatoid arthritis. Han and coworkers (2004) attempted to assess the effectiveness and safety of tai chi as a treatment for people with rheumatoid arthritis. Cochrane Controlled Trials Register, MEDLINE, PEDro, and CINAHL databases, the Chinese Biomedical Database, and the Beijing Chinese Academy of Traditional Medicine were searched. RCTs and controlled clinical trials examining the benefits and harms of exercise programs with tai chi instruction or incorporating principles of tai chi philosophy were selected for review and included four trials encompassing 206 participants. Although the included studies did not assess the effects on patient-reported pain, the results suggest that tai chi does not exacerbate symptoms of rheumatoid arthritis.

A systematic review of MEDLINE, PubMed, AMED, British Nursing Index, CINAHL, Embase, PsycINFO, The Cochrane Library, the UK National Research Register and ClinicalTrials.gov, Korean Medical Databases, Qigong and Energy Medicine Database, and Chinese databases identified two RCTs that assessed pain outcomes and did not demonstrate effectiveness on pain reduction compared with education plus stretching exercise and usual activity control (Lee, Pittler, & Ernst, 2007).

In a controlled trial of 61 subjects with rheumatoid arthritis, Lee and Jeong (2006) found that pain and fatigue significantly decreased in the experimental group. Koh (1982) describes his personal experience with using tai chi for symptoms of ankylosing spondylitis unresponsive to conventional therapies. After 2.5 years of daily practice the author felt less pain in addition to other positive results. However, pain returned if practice was neglected for as little as 1 week.

There were also several studies that examined the effects of tai chi on pain in college students and the elderly.

Wang, Taylor, Pearl, and Chang (2004) administered a 3-month intervention of tai chi exercise to college students, and multidimensional physical and mental health scores including bodily pain were assessed using the SF-36 health survey questionnaire before and after the intervention. Bodily pain improved significantly after tai chi exercise intervention.

Reid and colleagues (2008) reviewed the evidence regarding self-management interventions for pain due to musculoskeletal disorders among older adults. After searching the MEDLINE and CINAHL databases, the authors identified 27 articles that evaluated programs including yoga, massage therapy, tai chi, and music therapy. Positive outcomes were found in 96% of the studies. Proportionate change in pain scores ranged from an increase of 18% to a reduction of 85% (median = 23% reduction). Identified issues with the generalization of subjects included limited enrollment of ethnic minority elders, as well as nonethnic elders aged 80 and above.

Another review conducted by Morone and Greco (2007) found limited support for meditation and tai chi for improving function or coping in older adults with LBP or OA. Several studies included older adults, but did not analyze benefits by age. Tai chi, yoga, hypnosis, and progressive muscle relaxation were significantly associated with pain reduction in these studies. Ross, Bohannon, Davis, and Gurchiek (1999) evaluated effects of tai chi exercise on 11 elderly women. Findings included significant improvement ($p = 0.05$) in pain perception as measured by the visual analog scale. Ho and coauthors compared health-related quality of life in 140 elderly practicing tai chi and 560 age- and sex-matched control subjects taken from the general population (Ho et al., 2007). The authors found no significant difference in the bodily pain scales between tai chi and control groups.

Despite these findings, in a larger study using similar design, Kin, Toba, and Orimo (2007) found that when the 804 elderly participants who participated were further subdivided in age cohorts, the 70- to 80-year-old subjects practicing tai chi had significantly better bodily pain scores ($p < 0.05$) than the age- and sex-matched national average.

Finally, in a fascinating study involving 112 healthy older adults aged 59–86 years, Irwin, Olmstead, and Oxman (2007) set out to evaluate the effects of tai chi on resting and vaccine-stimulated levels of cell-mediated immunity (CMI) to varicella zoster virus (VZV) and on health functioning. In this prospective RCT, the subjects were vaccinated with the live attenuated VZV vaccine licensed to prevent varicella. The tai chi group showed significant improvements in SF-36 scores for bodily pain, vitality, and mental health.

WHOLE MEDICAL SYSTEMS

Whole medical systems are built upon complete systems of theory and practice. Often, these systems have evolved apart from and earlier than the conventional medical approach used in the United States (NCCAM, 2009). Examples of whole medical systems that have developed in Western cultures include

1. Homeopathic medicine: A whole medical system that originated in Europe, homeopathy seeks to stimulate the body's ability to heal itself by giving very small doses of highly diluted substances that in larger doses would produce illness.
2. Naturopathic medicine: A whole medical system that originated in Europe, naturopathy aims to support the body's ability to heal itself through the use of dietary and lifestyle changes together with CAM therapies such as herbs, massage, acupuncture, and so on.

Examples of systems that have developed in non-Western cultures include

1. Traditional Chinese Medicine, which is a whole medical system that originated in China, based on the concept that disease results from disruption in the flow of qi and imbalance

in the forces of yin and yang. Practices such as herbs, meditation, acupuncture, and Qi Gong comprise an elegant system of preventing, diagnosing, and treating somatic and emotional illness.

2. Ayurveda, which is a whole medical system that originated in India that aims to integrate the body, mind, and spirit to prevent and treat disease. Therapies used include herbs, massage, and yoga.

CONCLUSION

Complementary and alternative practices are well established in our society and may be able to address various health-related issues.

Only by holding CAM modalities to the highest standards of evidence will we best facilitate the creation of an integrated health care delivery system in which conventional physicians and CAM practitioners work as an interdisciplinary team. As the Prince of Wales commented in 1998, "This isn't a question of orthodox medicine taking over, or of CAM diluting the intellectual rigor of orthodoxy. It is about reaching across the disciplines to help and to learn from one another for the ultimate benefit of the patients you all serve" (Prince of Wales, 1998).

REFERENCES

Anderson, P. G., & Cutshall, S. M. (2007). Massage therapy: A comfort intervention for cardiac surgery patients. *Clinical Nurse Specialist, 21*, 161–165.

Back, C., Tam, H., Lee, E., & Haraldsson, B. (2009).The effects of employer-provided massage therapy on job satisfaction, workplace stress, and pain and discomfort. *Holistic Nursing Practice, 23*(1), 19–31.

Barnes, P. M., Bloom, B., & Nahin, R. (2008). *Complementary and alternative medicine use among adults and children: United States, 2007* (CDC National Health Statistics Report No. 12). Hyattsville, MD: National Center for Health Statistics.

Bennell, K. L., Hinman, R. S., Metcalf, B. R., Buchbinder, R., McConnell, J., McColl, G., et al. (2005). Efficacy of physiotherapy management of knee joint osteoarthritis: A randomized, double blind, placebo controlled trial. *Annals of the Rheumatic Diseases, 64*, 906–912.

Best, T. M., Hunter, R., Wilcox, A., & Haq, F. (2008). Effectiveness of sports massage for recovery of skeletal muscle from strenuous exercise. *Clinical Journal of Sport Medicine, 18*, 446–460.

Bonadonna, R. (2003). Meditation's impact on chronic illness. *Holistic Nursing Practice, 17*, 309–319.

Brett, K. M., & Keenan, N. L. (2007). Complementary and alternative medicine use among midlife women for reasons including menopause in the United States: 2002. *Menopause, 14*, 300–307

Brismee, J. M., Paige, R. L., Chyu, M. C., Boatright, J. D., Hagar, J. M., McCaleb, J. A., et al. (2007). Group and home-based tai chi in elderly subjects with knee osteoarthritis: A randomized controlled trial. *Clinical Rehabilitation, 21*(2), 99–111.

Chen, K. M., & Snyder, M. (1999). A research-based use of Tai Chi/movement therapy as a nursing intervention. *Journal of Holistic Nursing, 17*, 267–279.

Chen, K. M. (2006). Tai Chi. In M. Snyder (Ed.), *Complementary/alternative therapies in nursing* (5th ed., p. 313). New York: Springer. http://site.ebrary.com/lib/nyulibrary/Doc?id=10171392&ppg=316

Cherkin, D. C., Sherman, K. J., Deyo, R. A., & Shekelle, P. G. (2003). A review of the evidence for the effectiveness, safety, and cost of acupuncture, massage therapy, and spinal manipulation for back pain. *Annals of Internal Medicine, 138*, 898–906.

Currin, J., & Meister, E. A. (2008). A hospital-based intervention using massage to reduce distress among oncology patients. *Cancer Nursing, 31*, 214–221

Dagenais, S., Yelland, M. J., Del Mar, C., & Schoene, M. L. (2004). Prolotherapy injections for chronic low-back pain. *Cochrane Database of Systematic Reviews.* Retrieved March 19, 2010, from http://www2.cochrane.org/reviews/en/ab004059.html

Davidson, R. J., & Lutz, A. (2007). Buddha's brain: Neuroplasticity and meditation. *IEEE Signal Processing, 25*, 171–174.

Drivdahl, C. E., & Miser, W. F. (1998). The use of alternative health care by a family practice population. *Journal of the American Board of Family Practice, 11*, 193–199.

Dryden, T., Baskwill, A., & Preyde, M. (2004). Massage therapy for the orthopaedic patient: A review. *Orthopaedic Nursing, 23*, 327–332.

Erdogmus, C. B., Resch, K. L., Sabitzer, R., Müller, H., Nuhr, M., Schöggl, A., et al. (2007). Physiotherapy-based rehabilitation following disc herniation operation: Results of a randomized clinical trial. *Spine, 32*, 2041–2049.

Ernst, E. (2004). Manual therapies for pain control: Chiropractic and massage. *Clinical Journal of Pain, 20*(1), 8–12.

Ezzo, J., Haraldsson, B. G., Gross, A. R., Myers, C. D., Morien, A., Goldsmith, C. H., et al. (2007). Massage for mechanical neck disorders: A systematic review. *Spine, 32*, 353–362.

Feinglass, J., Lee, C., Rogers, M., Temple, L. M., Nelson, C., & Chang, R. W. (2007). Complementary and alternative medicine use for arthritis pain in 2 Chicago community areas. *Clinical Journal of Pain, 23*, 744–749.

Ferrell-Torry, A. T., & Glick, O. J. (1993). The use of therapeutic massage as a nursing intervention to modify anxiety and the perception of cancer pain. *Cancer Nursing, 16*(2), 93–101.

Field, T., Peck, M., Krugman, S., Tuchel, T., Schanberg, S., Kuhn, C., et al. (1998). Burn injuries benefit from massage therapy. *Journal of Burn Care and Rehabilitation, 19*, 241–244.

Forchuk, C., Baruth, P., Prendergast, M., Holliday, R., Bareham, R., Brimner, S., et al. (2004). Postoperative arm massage: A support for women with lymph node dissection. *Cancer Nursing, 27*(1), 25–33.

Fransen, M., Nairn, L., Winstanley, J., Lam, P., & Edmonds, J. (2007). Physical activity for osteoarthritis management: A randomized controlled clinical trial evaluating hydrotherapy or Tai Chi classes. *Arthritis and Rheumatism, 57*, 407–414.

Furlan, A. D., Brosseau, L., Imamura, M., & Irvin, E. (2002). Massage for low-back pain: A systematic review within the framework of the Cochrane Collaboration Back Review Group. *Spine, 27*, 1896–1910.

Gallagher, G., Rae, C. P., & Kinsella, J. (2000). Treatment of pain in severe burns. *American Journal of Clinical Dermatology, 1*, 329–335.

Grealish, L., Lomasney, A., & Whiteman, B. (2000). Foot massage: A nursing intervention to modify the distressing symptoms of pain and nausea in patients hospitalized with cancer. *Cancer Nursing, 23*, 237–243.

Hakala, R. V. (2005). Prolotherapy (proliferation therapy) in the treatment of TMD. *Cranio, 23*, 283–288.

Han, A., Robinson, V., Judd, M., Taixiang, W., Wells, G., & Tugwell, P. (2004). Tai chi for treating rheumatoid arthritis. *Cochrane Database of Systematic Reviews*, (3):CD004849.

Hernandez-Reif, M., Field, T., Largie, S., Hart, S., Redzepi, M., Nierenberg, B., et al. (2001). Childrens' distress during burn treatment is reduced by massage therapy. *Journal of Burn Care and Rehabilitation, 22*, 191–195.

Ho, T. J., Liang, W. M., Lien, C. H., Ma, T. C., Kuo, H. W., Chu, B. C., et al. (2007). Health-related quality of life in the elderly practicing Tai Chi Chuan. *Journal of Alternative and Complementary Medicine, 13*, 1077–1083.

http://nccam.nih.gov/health/acupuncture/introduction.htm, retrieved December 9, 2009.

http://nccam.nih.gov/health/meditation/overview.htm, retrieved December 6, 2009.

http://nccam.nih.gov/health/whatiscam/overview.htm, retrieved November 8, 2009.

http://nccam.nih.gov/health/whatiscam/overview.htm, retrieved December 6, 2009.

Irwin, M. R., Olmstead, R., & Oxman, M. N. (2007). Augmenting immune responses to varicella zoster virus in older adults: A randomized, controlled trial of Tai Chi. *Journal of the American Geriatrics Society, 55*, 511–517.

Jane, S. W., Wilkie, D. J., Gallucci, B. B., & Beaton, R. D. (2008). Systematic review of massage intervention for adult patients with cancer: A methodological perspective. *Cancer Nursing, 31*(6), E24–35.

Jensen, K. T., Rabago, D. P., Best, T. M., Patterson, J. J., & Vanderby, R., Jr. (2008). Early inflammatory response of knee ligaments to prolotherapy in a rat model. *Journal of Orthopaedic Research, 26*, 816–823.

Jha, A. P., Krompinger, J., & Baime, M. J. (2007). Mindfulness training modifies subsystems of attention. *Cognitive, Affective and Behavioral Neuroscience, 7*(2), 109–119.

Kim, S. R., Stitik, T. P., Foye, P. M., Greenwald, B. D., & Campagnolo, D. I. (2004). Critical review of prolotherapy for osteoarthritis, low back pain, and other musculoskeletal conditions: A physiatric perspective. *American Journal of Physical Medicine and Rehabilitation, 83*, 379–389.

Kin, S., Toba, K., & Orimo, H. (2007). Health-related quality of life (HRQOL) in older people practicing Tai Chi—Comparison of the HRQOL with the national standards for age-matched controls. *Nippon Ronen Igakkai Zasshi. Japanese Journal of Geriatrics, 44*, 339–344.

Klein, P. J., & Adams, W. D. (2004). Comprehensive therapeutic benefits of Taiji: A critical review. *American Journal of Physical Medicine and Rehabilitation, 83*, 735–745.

Koh, T. C. (1982). Tai Chi and ankylosing spondylitis—a personal experience. *American Journal of Chinese Medicine, 10*(1–4), 59–61.

Lee, H. Y. (2006). Comparison of effects among Tai-Chi exercise, aquatic exercise, and a self-help program for patients with knee osteoarthritis. *Daehan Ganho Haghoeji, 36*, 571–580.

Lee, H. Y., & Lee, K. J. (2008). Effects of Tai Chi exercise in elderly with knee osteoarthritis. *Daehan Ganho Haghoeji, 38*(1), 11–18.

Lee, K. Y., & Jeong, O. Y. (2006). The effect of Tai Chi movement in patients with rheumatoid arthritis. *Daehan Ganho Haghoeji, 36*(2), 278–285.

Lee, M. S., Pittler, M. H., & Ernst, E. (2007). Tai chi for rheumatoid arthritis: Systematic review. *Rheumatology, 46*, 1648–1651.

Lee, M. S., Pittler, M. H., & Ernst, E. (2008). Tai chi for osteoarthritis: A systematic review. *Clinical Rheumatology, 27*, 211–218.

Linetsky, F. S., Miguel, R., & Torres, F. (2004). Treatment of cervicothoracic pain and cervicogenic headaches with regenerative injection therapy. *Current Pain and Headache Reports, 8*(1), 41–48.

Lutz, A., Slagter, H. A., Dunne, J., & Davidson, R. J. (2008). Attention regulation and monitoring in meditation. *Trends in Cognitive Sciences, 12*, 163–169.

McCasland, L. D., Budiman-Mak, E., Weaver, F. M., Adams, E., & Miskevics, S. (2006). Shoulder pain in the traumatically injured spinal cord patient: Evaluation of risk factors and function. *Journal of Clinical Rheumatology, 12*, 179–186.

Mitchinson, A. R., Kim, H. M., Rosenberg, J. M., Geisser, M., Kirsh, M., Cikrit, D., et al. (2007). Acute postoperative pain management using massage as an adjuvant therapy: A randomized trial. *Archives of Surgery, 142*, 1158–1167.

Moraska, A. (2007). Therapist education impacts the massage effect on postrace muscle recovery. *Medicine and Science in Sports and Exercise, 39*(1), 34–37.

Morone, N. E., & Greco, C. M. (2007). Mind-body interventions for chronic pain in older adults: A structured review. *Pain Medicine, 8*, 359–375.

Morton, W. S. (2004). *China: Its history and culture.* Blacklick, OH: McGraw-Hill. p. 39.

Moyer, C. A., Rounds, J., & Hannum, J. W. (2004). A meta-analysis of massage therapy research. *Psychological Bulletin, 130*(1), 3–18.

Nahin, R. L., Barnes, P. M., Stussman, B. J., & Bloom, B. (2009). *Costs of Complementary and Alternative Medicine (CAM) and frequency of visits to CAM practitioners: United States, 2007* (National health statistics reports; No 18). Hyattsville, MD: National Center for Health Statistics.

Newberg, A. B., & Iversen, J.(2003) The neural basis of the complex mental task of meditation. *Medical Hypotheses, 61*, 282–291.

Ospina, M. B., Bond, T. K., Karkhaneh, M., Tjosvold, L., Vandermeer, B., Liang, Y., et al. (2007). *Meditation practices for health: State of the research.* Evidence Report/Technology Assessment no. 155. Rockville, MD: Agency for Healthcare Research and Quality; AHRQ publication no. 07–E010. p. 288.http://site.ebrary.com/lib/nyulibrary/Doc?id=10171392&ppg=291

Palinkas, L. A., & Kabongo, M. L. (2000). The use of complementary and alternative medicine by primary care patients. *Journal of Family Practice, 49*, 1121–1130.

Rabago, D., Best, T. M., Beamsley, M., & Patterson, J. (2005). A systematic review of prolotherapy for chronic musculoskeletal pain. *Clinical Journal of Sport Medicine, 15*, 376–380.

Reeves, K. D. (2000). Prolotherapy: Basic science, clinical studies, and technique, In T. A. Lennard (Ed.), *Pain procedures in clinical practice* (2nd ed., pp. 172–190.). Philadelphia: Hanley and Belfus.

Reid, M. C., Papaleontiou, M., Ong, A., Breckman, R., Wethington, E., & Pillemer, K. (2008). Self-management strategies to reduce pain and improve function among older adults in community settings: A review of the evidence. *Pain Medicine, 9*, 409–424.

Ross, M. C., Bohannon, A. S., Davis, D. C., & Gurchiek, L. (1999). The effects of a short-term exercise program on movement, pain, and mood in the elderly: Results of a pilot study. *Journal of Holistic Nursing, 17*(2), 139–147.

Schneider, J. C., Harris, N. L., El Shami, A., Sheridan, R. L., Schulz, J. T., III, Bilodeau, M. L., et al. (2006). A descriptive review of neuropathic-like pain after burn injury. *Journal of Burn Care and Research, 27*, 524–528.

Shen, C. L., James, C. R., Chyu, M. C., Bixby, W. R., Brismée, J.-M, Zumwalt, M. A., et al. (2008). Effects of Tai Chi on gait kinematics, physical function, and pain in elderly with knee osteoarthritis—a pilot study. *American Journal of Chinese Medicine, 36*, 219–232.

Sherman, K. J., Cherkin, D. C., Connelly, M. T., Erro, J., Savetsky, J. B., Davis, R. B., et al. (2004). Complementary and alternative medical therapies for chronic low back pain: What treatments are patients willing to try? *BMC Complementary and Alternative Medicine, 4*, 9.

Sherman, K. J., Cherkin, D. C., Deyo, R. A., Erro, J. H., Hrbek, A., Davis, R. B., et al. (2006). The diagnosis and treatment of chronic back pain by acupuncturists, chiropractors, and massage therapists. *Clinical Journal of Pain, 22*, 227–234.

Siu, A. M., Chan, C. C., Poon, P. K., Chui, D. Y., & Chan, S. C. (2007). Evaluation of the chronic disease self-management program in a Chinese population. *Patient Education and Counseling, 65*(1), 42–50.

Snyder, M. (2006). *Complementary/alternative therapies in nursing* (5th ed.). New York: Springer Publishing Company.

Song, R., Lee, E. O., Lam, P., & Bae, S. C. (2007). Effects of a Sun-style Tai Chi exercise on arthritic symptoms, motivation, and the performance of health behaviors in women with osteoarthritis. *Daehan Ganho Haghoeji, 37*, 249–256.

Tan, J. C. (2002). Massage as a form of complementary and alternative healing modality for physical manipulation. In S. F. Wainapel (Ed.), *Alternative medicine and rehabilitation: A guide for practitioners* (pp. 77–98). New York: Demos Medical Publishing.

The Prince of Wales. (1998, May 28). *Speech before the Integrated Healthcare Conference, London.* Retrieved March 19, 2010, from http://news.bbc.co.uk/2/hi/health/102246.stm

Trinh, K., Graham, N., Gross, A., Goldsmith, C., Wang, E., Cameron, I., et al. (2007). Acupuncture for neck disorders. *Spine, 32*, 236–243.

Wahbeh, H., Elsas, S. M., & Oken, B. S. (2008). Mind-body interventions: Applications in neurology. *Neurology, 70*, 2321–2328.

Wang, C., Schmid, C. H., Hibberd, P. L., Kalish, R., Roubenoff, R., Rones, R., et al. (2008). Tai Chi for treating knee osteoarthritis: Designing a long-term follow up randomized controlled trial. *BMC Musculoskeletal Disorders, 9*, 108.

Wang, Y. T., Taylor, L., Pearl, M., & Chang, L. S. (2004). Effects of Tai Chi exercise on physical and mental health of college students. *American Journal of Chinese Medicine, 32*, 453–459.

Wells, M., Sarna, L., Cooley, M. E., Brown, J. K., Chernecky, C., Williams, R. D., et al. (2007). Use of complementary and alternative medicine therapies to control symptoms in women living with lung cancer. *Cancer Nursing, 30*(1), 45–55.

Williamson, A. T., Fletcher, P. C., & Dawson, K. A. (2003). Complementary and alternative medicine: Use in an older population. *Journal of Gerontological Nursing, 29*(5), 20–28.

Wolf, S. L., O'Grady, M. J., & Xu, T. (2002). Tai chi chuan. In S. F. Wainapel (Ed.), *Alternative medicine and rehabilitation: A guide for practitioners* (pp. 99–138). New York: Demos Medical Publishing.

Wolsko, P. M., Eisenberg, D. M., Davis, R. B., Kessler, R., & Phillips, R. S. (2003). Patterns and perceptions of care for treatment of back and neck pain: Results of a national survey. *Spine, 28*, 292–297.

Wright, A., & Sluka, K. A. (2001). Nonpharmacological treatments for musculoskeletal pain [see comment]. *Clinical Journal of Pain, 17*(1), 33–46.

Yocum, D. E., Castro, W. L., & Cornett, M. (2000). Exercise, education, and behavioral modification as alternative therapy for pain and stress in rheumatic disease. *Rheumatic Diseases Clinics of North America, 26*, 145–159, x–xi.

29

Rehabilitation Nursing: Educating Patients Toward Independence

Jeanne Dzurenko, BSN, MPH, RN

Health care is rapidly changing the face of traditional rehabilitative services, with many implications for patient education as a result. Patients now transfer to rehabilitation facilities sooner and with many acute medical processes. The rehabilitation team treats these sicker patients and begins restoration to optimal functioning in less time. Seven-days-a-week therapy services while being sought by managed care companies in an effort to minimize inpatient days has been cost prohibitive to most inpatient facilities.

Home care and outpatient rehabilitative services have expanded in an effort to continue patient therapies in lower cost environments. Thus, patients are required to learn without the round-the-clock presence of professionals. The family becomes an essential member of the rehabilitative team to support and reinforce those self-care techniques taught by the professional staff.

The goals of any rehabilitation program are to maximize independence and minimize the effects of a chronic illness or acute traumatic injury. In addition to treating the physical disability, the therapeutic philosophy of rehabilitation addresses the emotional, social, and psychological problems of patients. Existing rehabilitation programs are based on the pioneering efforts of Dr. Howard A. Rusk, which began to develop in 1942 to assist injured World War II personnel.

Rehabilitation encompasses caring for a variety of disabilities. The case mix may be composed of individuals who have had amputations, or other neurological impairments, strokes, and spinal cord injuries (SCI). Whether adult or pediatric, inpatient or outpatient, education is a key component of any comprehensive rehabilitation program.

Following traumatic injury or chronic illness, restorative therapy teaches patients to bathe, dress, and feed themselves. The ultimate goal is to enable the individual to perform activities of daily living (ADL) independently. Measuring functional ability after setting realistic, attainable goals will foster success. Self-efficacy is measured as patients change behaviors that foster independence. As they transition back into the community, it is essential for them to have resources necessary to continue to do what is important to them to achieve the quality of life. For patient education, it has been demonstrated that the use of computerized information has improved patient education outcomes when used with printed materials (Yeh, Chen, & Liu, 2005).

The approach to rehabilitation is interdisciplinary as well as multidisciplinary. Physical therapy, occupational therapy, speech, vocational rehabilitation, therapeutic recreation, psychology, social services, and nursing are the key disciplines involved. This approach allows each specialty to focus on the individual's affected function, which its profession aims to maximize. Depending on the person's age, the goals of the rehabilitation program may vary. In the elderly, vocational training may not be relevant, as retirement may have occurred prior to the onset of disability; therefore, functional independence is the highest achievable goal. On the other hand, a young adult may require functional retraining as well as educational and vocational programs to develop skills necessary to reintegrate into the workforce.

The ability of the health care professional to understand educational techniques that are individualized to the patient maximize success of any rehabilitation program. Technology has changed not only how therapy is provided but also how patient education is delivered. Health care providers now incorporate computer-assisted technology into many aspects of rehabilitation. For example, the use of the Sony Wii has been used in rehabilitation settings.

There are countless resources on the Web and access in most instances is free for the public. Most health care institutions enter into licensing agreements with software providers and/ or produce their own patient education materials. Here are a few of the many sites available. The National Library of Medicine has MEDLINE Plus, which provides many interactive tools on the Web. This Web site offers a catalog of interactive patient education tools on a variety of topics. For stroke and cardiac rehabilitation, there are two offerings. At New York University Langone Medical Center, the Patient Family Resource Center Web site offers links to many health education resources. In this example, the patient education video on rehabilitation hospital discharge is available and can be viewed on the Web.

Many nonprofit organizations also offer pod casts, downloads of patient information, and videos for patients and families from their Web sites. Discussion of some of the disability-specific Web sites is in the following conditions.

The education component is at the core of every rehabilitation program. The sections that follow describe prevalent diagnoses found in dedicated rehabilitation hospitals and the roles of the health care professional in educating individuals with these disabilities.

WHAT IS A STROKE?

Stroke affects 795,000 people each year and accounted for over 140,000 deaths in the United States in 2005, according to the American Heart Association (2009). Although the majority of stroke victims are elderly, stroke can affect individuals of all ages. Some patients may recover from this event with little residual dysfunction; however, many demonstrate physical, cognitive, and behavioral changes. An educational program about stroke should include the following:

- Definition of stroke
- Risk factors
- Functional changes
- Behavioral changes
- Visual changes
- Cognitive changes
- Communication deficits
- Sensory changes
- Complications of stroke

Because of the varying levels of injury, poststroke education should include both group and individual teaching. Group sessions can be utilized to cover the definition of stroke, associated risk factors, and prevention; individual sessions will help patients and their caregivers to better understand specifically what has happened to them. Combining both methods with frequent reinforcement and clear, concise audiovisual aids and handouts will improve the patient's ability to cope with the changes associated with stroke. Patients with aphasia and their family members benefit from direct interaction with each other (Simmons-Mackie, Kearns, & Potechin, 2005).

A stroke results from a blockage (cerebral thrombosis) or a ruptured blood vessel (cerebral hemorrhage). The severity of this event, which occurs in the brain, determines how bodily functions are affected. Depending on which side of the brain the stroke occurs in, stroke patients will present with different disabilities. Audiovisual aids describing blood flow to the brain and pictorials demonstrating a thrombosis versus a hemorrhage should be available. Risk factors can be grouped into two categories; those that can be controlled and those that cannot. Discussing risk factors according to these categories is essential for patients and families to better understand why strokes occur. High blood pressure, heart disease, and transient ischemic attacks are medical problems that increase a person's risk for a stroke. Cigarette smoking also has been demonstrated to be a cause of stroke. Medical management of the first three and abstinence from the fourth risk factor should be reinforced.

The noncontrollable risk factors include advancing age, being male, being of African American heritage, having a history of a prior stroke, and having a family history of stroke.

THE EFFECTS OF STROKE

A left cerebrovascular accident (CVA) typically results in right hemiparesis. Nursing care objectives for patients in this group are an understanding of right-sided paralysis, speech–language deficits such as aphasia and dysarthria, behavioral changes manifested by slow, disorganized movements, and memory deficits. For a right CVA, paralysis on the left side of the body, spatial-perceptual deficits, impulsive behavior, and memory deficits should be the topics of learning. Descriptive examples of behavioral changes and expected responses will assist patients and families to adjust to the cognitive changes associated with stroke.

After the general explanation of the two types of strokes, patient education must be centered on routine care and management. Prevention of blood clots and pressure ulcers due to immobility are important aspects of care.

Safe transfers and mobility to prevent falls and related injuries should be addressed. Toileting routines can be difficult and frustrating for both patient and family. Incontinence, although usually temporary in stroke patients, must be controlled to maintain personal hygiene and the dignity of the patient. Teaching the family to use external or indwelling catheters, incontinence briefs, and enemas routinely facilitates coping with this sequelae. To achieve a return to self-management, stroke rehabilitation often involves repetitive therapy. Because the patient may present with cognitive and perceptual deficits, this retraining may seem nonpurposeful. Maintaining quality of life for both the patient and caregiver is essential to the educational process.

Bugge, Alexander, and Hagen (1999) found that 37% of caregivers of patients with stroke experience strain as a result of providing that care. Because the average age of a caregiver is in the 60s to 70s, it is essential to thoroughly assess the ability of the caregiver to participate in training. The changes in roles, functional ability, and overall quality of life are impacted by a stroke. Health care professionals must address these elements during the education.

SPINAL CORD INJURY

SCIs occur from falls, sports, or motor vehicle-related trauma. Impairments result in varying degrees of disability, depending on the location of the injury. SCI rehabilitation can be grouped into four general categories, which can be addressed by nursing care and include the injury's effect on:

- Mobility
- Bladder function
- Bowel function
- Sexuality.

In order for patients to better understand the nature of their disability, a discussion about the anatomy and physiology of the nervous system, types of injuries, and levels of impairments should be the introductory phase of the program. Paraplegia versus tetraplegia, complete versus incomplete injuries, and functional levels will demonstrate to patients the variation within spinal cord impairment.

Utilization of audiovisual aids to define the central nervous system function and differentiate between the types of injuries is essential. Reinforcement of learning through pictorials will foster a better understanding of what has happened. There are various videos currently available that will assist the nurse in explaining spinal cord function and the effects of injuries.

Bladder Management

Bladder management is an important focus of SCI care. Proper urinary management can positively influence self-esteem, dignity, and autonomy. Patients must have an understanding of catheter care, whether suprapubic or transurethral. If the patient requires intermittent catheterization, the procedure for clean intermittent catheterization (CIC) using soap and water are the most popular cleansing agents for home use. Bladder management should focus on preventing urinary tract infections; therefore, CIC is an integral part of the program.

Patients should be taught to recognize the signs and symptoms of complications related to altered bladder function, such as reflux of urine into the kidney, bladder or kidney stones, and infections. The use of the Internet education on bladder function and management has been demonstrated to facilitate the provision of user-friendly and culturally sensitive information (Brillhart, 2007).

Bowel Management

Bowel management is another area that requires attention in SCI patients. A successful bowel routine should be completed within 45 minutes to minimize complications and avoid accidents. Components of a bowel management education program may vary depending on whether the bowel is spastic or flaccid. Medications for the neurogenic bowel include laxatives, stool softeners, and suppositories. Proper dosing and scheduling enhance the development of a routine.

Potential problems associated with an inadequately managed neurogenic bowel include constipation and impaction, diarrhea, and autonomic dysreflexia, the later being a potentially dangerous condition associated with a rapid rise in blood pressure. Maximizing independence with a bowel routine is achieved through detection of these complications and early intervention. Coping with bowel incontinence is attainable through education.

A spastic bowel results from upper motor neuron disease. It is demonstrated by the presence of increased anal muscle tone on examination. Diet, stool softeners, laxatives, and a suppository inserted on a regularly timed basis will help to regulate a spastic bowel. Other components of a bowel routine might include medications, digital stimulation, and the Valsalva maneuver. In patients with a history of autonomic dysreflexia, overstimulation should be minimized with the use of a topical anesthetic jelly when performing digital stimulation or inserting a suppository. In a flaccid bowel with absent anal tone, bulk formation of stool using a high-fiber dietary supplement rather than stool softening is indicated.

The nurse should facilitate an understanding of the need for a bowel routine and hopefully foster compliance. Individuals with SCI may take weeks or even months to establish a routine. In any case, the combination of one-to-one instruction and attendance at SCI group sessions should be encouraged. While individual instruction addresses each person's own situation, group instruction for SCI has the advantages of motivation, sharing of experience, and peer support.

Sexuality

Sexuality is a topic that should be raised with all SCI patients and their partners. Whether they are young or old, this population requires assistance in expressing their fears about sexuality as well as in learning alternatives to intercourse.

Depending on the level of SCI, a patient may experience altered physical sensation. The SCI patient should be made to realize that sexuality is not merely physical but rather part of the emotional being of the individual.

In both cases, the nurse must have competence about the topic and feel comfortable discussing issues of sex and sexuality. Comfort with the topic is equally important. Many health care professionals have difficulty discussing sexuality issues because of the sensitivity of the content. As with any other education program, repetition will increase comfort because each session will build on previous knowledge and experience.

Sexuality covers a broad range of issues. The concerns of women are different from those of men. The focus of sex education programs should be on addressing sexual behavior, desire, orgasms, erection, and infertility. Volumes have been written on these topics. Whatever an individual's education need, it is essential that the learning process preserve his or her dignity.

Personal expectations must be a focus of education. For example, the nurse should not minimize a man's need to experience an erection if that is what is important to him. For that person, therapeutic rehabilitation may include review of technical and pharmacological aids or penile implants.

In any case, persons with SCI should have the opportunity to discuss and learn about options. Focusing on receiving pleasure as well as giving it will boost confidence. Adapting to SCI will include taking responsibility for one's own sexual pleasure. Often the focus lies in pleasing the partner or "performing." Effective education in this area will redirect the individual to explore his or her own sexuality and discover that the only difference between SCI patients and others is the interrupted connection between the higher centers of the brain and the lower body. Intimacy is still possible. Rehabilitation nurses must provide culturally sensitive and developmentally appropriate coaching and hope for this patient population (Kautz, 2007).

Coping Strategies

Patients with SCI must develop effective coping strategies to adjust to their disability as well as to the social aspect of living with a disability. Patient education in this population should center on developing appropriate coping strategies. Effective strategies have a positive influence on social adjustment and physical function in people with SCI. Coping skills training should be integrated into the comprehensive rehabilitation program to facilitate the transition into the community (Song & Nam, 2010).

AMPUTEES

Amputees require a comprehensive rehabilitation program. Limb loss can be devastating to both patient and family. In addition to being disabled, the patient has to cope with an altered body image. The nursing care plan should include psychological support and education focusing on residual limb care, phantom pain, use of a prostheses, and mobility.

Nursing interventions will include skin care of the residual limb, such as assessment of the suture line for signs of infection and methods to prevent skin breakdown. Limb wrapping is generally taught early in the postoperative phase to minimize edema and prepare the residual limb for prosthesis. Safe transfer training and mobility must be taught. Adaptive equipment needs also should be assessed and education about safe use implemented.

Advanced prosthetics technology has allowed for lighter and more comfortably fitting artificial limbs. The Amputation Coalition of America has comprehensive resources on their Web site. From their quarterly newsletter, cornerstone to their list of patient education materials, and links to other Web sites, this organization provides various tools for the individual with a limb loss and their families.

Finally, the need for psychological support should not go untended. The grieving process should be encouraged as a normal reaction for both patient and family members. Learning to verbalize the feelings associated with limb loss may be difficult; therefore, nurses must teach the involved parties what to expect and how to cope. Depending on the existing coping skills, support groups or individualized psychotherapy may be appropriate. The involvement of a social worker and psychologist will help the patient to adjust to the anticipated lifestyle changes.

OTHER NURSING CARE ISSUES

Although nursing care can be disability focused, general plans of care are common to all rehabilitation patients. Pressure ulcer prevention for any patient with limited mobility should be incorporated into patient education. Frequent position change, skin care, and adequate nutritional intake should be addressed. Proper wheelchair positioning to minimize pressure over bony prominences through the use of cushions and other devices can be beneficial to any disabled person with limited mobility. Keeping skin clean and the inclusion of moisturizers and barrier creams for patients with incontinence may be added to this daily routine. Finally, adequate nutrition intake, particularly for a patient susceptible to skin breakdown, will minimize the adverse effects to the skin.

Foot care is another focus of education for rehabilitation candidates. Self-assessment of toes and feet, cleansing, and gentle care will minimize the complications that can develop.

Discharge planning can never be discussed too much. Although patients are interviewed about the discharge plan early in the hospitalization and the discussion continues until the actual discharge, there should be a formal class in which to discuss options and have a question-and-answer period. Opening the class to all patients and families at any point in their rehabilitation stay can reflect positively on the outcome of the class. By listening to other people's fears and concerns, patients and families are able to encourage and support one another. A camaraderie develops as each patient sees that he or she really is not alone when planning to reenter the community. Common topics included in the program are equipment and its uses, community referrals, follow-up visits, and medication regimens.

This type of program also allows family members who may have missed some of the one-to-one meetings with the social workers or discharge planner to seek answers and reassurance from the rehabilitative staff.

SELF-CARE DAYS AND INDEPENDENT LIVING EXPERIENCE

After the individual disciplines have completed their therapeutic regimens, patients should participate in self-care days accompanied by a family member. With the assistance of the interdisciplinary team, the patient progresses toward a higher level of independence, and family members observe the patient as he or she completes the tasks of self-care. The interdisciplinary team also evaluates the patient's readiness for an independent living experience (ILE). Once the patient has mastered self-care, the ILE is arranged.

The ILE is the final step in the rehabilitation continuum prior to discharge. Its objectives are fourfold:

1. Promote a realistic experience
2. Provide an opportunity to apply newly learned ADL skills

3. Develop confidence
4. Develop abilities to manage community living.

The patient and caregiver are invited to this "day at home" simulation in an apartment-like setting. A team member will observe and supervise the patient through all of the activities learned during the hospitalization. Proper transfer techniques, bathing, showering, dressing, and meal preparation will be performed. This program facilitates the experience of a post-discharge routine for patient and caregiver while they are still in the supportive environment of the hospital. Patients and their families are offered this "trial and error day" to experience their anticipated challenges of living at home and to allay their fears.

Often, patients are able to perform ADLs in the rehabilitation setting, but the techniques learned are forgotten because of the stress of being home alone or because of the changed environment. For example, a patient may have mastered bathing independently in the roll-in shower at the rehabilitation facility; however, once home, showering requires the additional step of transferring to a tub chair. Because of the extra energy and step involved, the patient may become discouraged and never attempt to shower. The ILE will occur in a similar home environment and permit the patient to practice the activity. This process can be individualized to mimic the barriers of the permanent home. Through a thorough home assessment, the nurse or therapist can re-create the setting and foster independence within the home constraints.

Families are encouraged to participate, share their concerns, discuss fears, and ask questions. Their involvement in the ILE will offer insight to the future patient living at home. The goal and plan that have been set for admission can be demonstrated with confidence. Depending on individual needs, patient and family may grocery-shop, prepare a meal, or launder clothes. The choice of activities is left to patient and family, but patients are encouraged to select the tasks they feel most unsure performing. Ultimately, the ILE will restore the patient's ability to function within the community.

COMMUNITY REFERRALS

The transition from hospital to home requires additional support to patients and their families. An efficient discharge plan from a rehabilitation setting includes referrals to community agencies. Various disease-related organizations offer comprehensive services to their members. Support groups for both patients and family members can be found for diseases such as stroke, SCI, and multiple sclerosis. Community support varies from state to state and even county to county. In New York City, for example, the Center for Independent Living of the Disabled in New York offers counseling, equipment loan, entitlement advice, and housing information. Other agencies may offer transportation, recreational activities, and respite care. Early assessment of individual patients' communities will enable the interdisciplinary team to incorporate the services of community agencies into the discharge plan.

SUMMARY

As health care provisions change and lengths of hospitalizations continue to shorten, the ways in which rehabilitative services are provided will evolve. As lengths of stay shorten, it will become even more imperative that health care professionals perform accurate evaluation and begin therapy immediately.

Patient and family education is the backbone of every rehabilitation plan of care and helps to facilitate a smooth transition from hospital to home. Individual and group classes reinforce the accomplishments achieved in physical, occupational, and speech therapy. Motivation and progress are fostered through an interdisciplinary approach that includes the patient and family as integral participants in the process. To do this effectively, goals must be individualized, mutual, and realistic. No matter how small the gains may seem to others, it is these achievements that produce the larger and ultimate goals of independence. Finally, the use of the computerized assistive technology and the Internet to supplement all individual and group education has become routine. It is the responsibility of rehabilitation providers to help patients find reputable resources that will provide them accurate information at home. In some instances, development of a handout is necessary to meet the individual's educational needs of a particular population. This requires the health care professional to create culturally sensitive health information that is understandable. Health literacy is essential for the development process and to achieve this the average grade level (AGL) minus 4 grades should be utilized when developing the patient education material. Currently, in the United States, the AGL is tenth grade so the recommended reading level should be sixth grade.

REFERENCES

American Heart Association. (2009). *Heart disease and stroke statistics—2009 update at a glance.* Dallas, TX: Author.

Brillhart, B. (2007). Internet education for spinal cord injury patients: Focus on urinary management. *Rehabilitation Nursing, 32,* 214–219.

Bugge, C., Alexander, H., & Hagen, S. (1999). Stroke patients' informal caregivers: Patient, caregiver, and service factors that affect caregiver strain. *Stroke, 30,* 1517–1523.

Kautz, D. (2007). Hope for love: Practical advice for intimacy and sex after stroke. *Rehabilitation Nursing, 32,* 95–103.

Simmons-Mackie, N. N., Kearns, K. P., & Potechin, G. (2005). Treatment of aphasia through family member training. *Aphasiology, 19,* 583–593.

Song, H. & Nam, K. (2010). Coping strategies, physical function, and social adjustment in people with spinal cord injury. *Rehabilitation Nursing, 35,* 8–15.

Yeh, M. L., Chen, H. H., & Liu, P. (2005). Effects of multimedia with printed nursing guide in education on self efficacy and functional activity in patients with hip replacement. *Patient Education and Counseling, 57,* 217–224.

30

Social Work in Physical Medicine and Rehabilitation

Patrick Inniss, PhD

This chapter provides an overview of the role of social work in the field of physical medicine. The chapter will explain the scope of the rehabilitation social workers' involvement with the newly defined disabled and demonstrate that their ongoing collaboration and assessment of patient/families needs are key to helping promote independence within the parameters of realistic expectations.

The chapter will begin with a historical review of the beginning of social work in the health care field in the early part of the 20th century, followed by highlighting the current educational requirements for social work practice within hospital settings. With this background information, the chapter proceeds to detail, via case examples, the components that formulate specifically the rehabilitation social worker's evaluation of disabled patients during their hospitalization. The factors in the evaluation/assessment that influence the discharge process such as the patient's emotional reactions, family relationships, and support systems will be addressed as relevant to the social workers' interventions. Disability-specific issues follow the evaluation/assessment section to emphasize how individualized discharge plans vary and are directly related to the nature of the disability. Finally, a review of concrete services and entitlements is included to provide information related to current resources available. The chapter concludes with thoughtful considerations for the future in respect to ongoing work with the disabled population.

BRIEF HISTORY OF SOCIAL WORK IN HEALTH CARE

Social work has had a long association with the health care field and owes its introduction in hospitals to Dr. Richard Cabot, a physician who practiced medicine at Massachusetts General Hospital in the early 1900s. It was Dr. Cabot's belief that "the individual's health and social environment were intertwined: disease, social circumstance and even religious beliefs could not be easily separated" (Dodds, 1993). In 1905, tired of what he described as "medicine's blindness to the social context of illness," Dr. Cabot conceived and then implemented what may be his most enduring achievement: hospital social work. Dr. Cabot hired Ida B. Cannon, a former visiting nurse who had experienced firsthand the plight of the disadvantaged in their homes and community settings. In her new role as social worker in the hospital, Ms. Cannon seized the opportunity to help and treat patients in what she viewed to be a more meaningful way. This innovative approach to health care not only helped lay the foundation for comprehensive intervention with hospitalized and clinic patients but also gave rise to a more formalized practice in the emerging field of medical social work.

In 1914, Ms. Cannon was named Chief of the Massachusetts General Hospital Social Work Department, the first of its kind to be developed within a hospital setting. Although the initial focus of social work services was aimed at patients seen and treated in the outpatient clinics, the services were later expanded to the inpatient setting. From its inception, the Department of Social Work was an interdisciplinary unit, with a staff that included nurses, physicians, teachers, and volunteers. Dr. Cabot and Ms. Cannon implemented systems and procedures to document interventions in medical charts. In addition, they established ongoing collaboration with medical professionals and promoted social work's input in the overall patient treatment plan. Their efforts firmly established the importance of the role of social workers within the hospital and recognized the value of having designate hospital staff to represent the "patient's point of view." This collaborative work between the Massachusetts General Hospital's medical staff and the interdisciplinary treatment team placed social work in the forefront of standards of care. The collaboration led to the investigation and systematic study of patients suffering from tuberculosis, identification of the needs of pregnant teenagers, documentation of the incidence of orthopedic problems in children, and numerous other ills that affected the community at large at that time (Massachusetts General Hospital Department of Social Services, 1958). Not only were thorough records kept of the incidence of these ills, but the education and directives shared with the patients and families helped to promote a more informed and better-served patient population.

The concept of team collaboration, which is today very much a part of the physical rehabilitation model, is rooted in a philosophy and approach that considers psycho/social issues as one of the factors having a direct relationship to the success of medical outcomes in the overall treatment plan (Rosenberg & Rehr, 1982). In the early 20th century, in response to economic pressures on the health care system by immigration and poverty, hospital social work spread throughout the country (Otis-Green, 2008). Since then, social work in health care has not only grown in general hospitals, but has evolved into a variety of subspecialties that include social work services in areas such as transplant programs, dialysis treatment, oncology treatment programs, substance abuse, physical rehabilitation, mental illness, and so on.

As the practice of social work became more ingrained within hospital settings, the need to establish the role of the social worker within the professional hierarchy became more important. Schools of social work were established with the intent to formalize education to apply principles and theories to practice. In essence, the curriculum of social work education integrated psychodynamic theory of human behavior with application of the same to on-site supervision and instruction in a variety of settings. In 1952, the Council of Social Work Education was subsequently established as the sole accrediting body in social work and has since recognized programs for bachelor's, master's, and doctorate degrees. The master's degree program, which entails 2 years postgraduate studies, is the accepted level of education for individuals employed in the medical and mental health field. Social workers with a master's degree are required to be licensed in the state to perform clinical work within a hospital/rehabilitation and mental health setting (Hoffman et al., 2008).

SOCIAL WORK WITHIN THE FIELD OF REHABILITATION

Although the field of social work in the 20th century has broadened in levels of formal education, specialized training, and practice, it has remained essentially focused on the person and his or her environment. This perspective enables rehabilitation social workers to advance the vision that "individuals with disabilities can be viewed as fully capable of health and well being within the context of their chronic condition or disability" (Stuifbergen & Roberts, 1997). In keeping with this approach, the social worker's role in physical rehabilitation is to assess the bio/psycho/social aspects of a patient's reaction to chronic illness or disability.

This assessment includes taking a social history, determining the patient's ability to cope with a new diagnosis, exploring the family dynamics impacting on the patient's adjustment to illness or disability, and identifying the strengths and weaknesses within the patient/family system.

Generally, patients with newly acquired disabilities will experience a range of emotions and reactions in attempting to incorporate what has occurred. Based on theory and practice, five adjustment patterns among the disabled or people facing end-of-life issues have been identified as fairly common. These reactions, which will be described in detail later in this section, include the following: (1) shock and anger, (2) bargaining and denial, (3) realization or recognition, (4) retaliation and reintegration, and (5) adjustment or adaptation (Kubler-Ross, 1969/1997; Power & Dell Orto, 2004). The ultimate goal for the social worker is to establish a discharge plan that meets the needs identified by the patient and the family and, at the same time, remains sensitive to their emotional well-being. Although the theoretical approaches in this specialization and other areas of social work have undergone various transformations, the principles of practice essentially remain the same: identify the problems, strategize interventions, and work toward helping individuals regain control over their life situation and their home environment.

Although social work practice in the field of rehabilitation has a specific approach, the ongoing need to evaluate effectiveness is encouraged. For example, a study conducted with disabled individuals and social workers looked at how they perceived their interactions with each other. The study identified that what the social worker perceived as his or her mission and what the patient perceived as his or her need were not always in sync. The study suggested that ongoing formal training in understanding disability is needed so that professionals can be more attuned to the fact that a patient does not want to be treated in the context of the recent disability but rather in the context of the person he or she has always been (Kim & Canda, 2007). Rather than defining the disability in terms of illness and disease, the rehabilitation social worker should define the disability by the meaning the disability carries for the patient. People with disabilities are people for whom a disability is a *part* of their lives—not the definition of their lives (Mackelprang & Salsgiver, 1999).

The independent living movement of the 1970s–1980s gave impetus to promoting health care workers among others to view the disabled in a more interactive way, and this view continues to be the emphasis in discharge planning. With help from others, advocacy groups succeeded in having their conceptualizations of self-determination, consumer control, and nondiscrimination codified in a variety of federal laws. The most important of these laws are the Rehabilitation Act of 1973, its amendments (1978), the Individuals with Disability Education Act (1997), and the American Disability Act of 1990. These Acts contain mandates for the inclusion of people with disabilities into mainstream American life to the maximum extent possible (Beaulaurier & Taylor, 2001). The rehabilitation social worker is therefore challenged to incorporate general principles of practice and, at the same time, appreciate the uniqueness of each patient/family situation to provide a balanced approach in the delivery of service.

DISCHARGE PLANNING ASSESSMENT AND INTERVENTION

The primary focus of discharge planning is to facilitate the promotion of independence and rehabilitation and to prevent readmission or further unwarranted treatment (Blumenfield & Rosenberg, 1988). This section will review the components of the bio/psycho/social assessment and is aimed specifically at the major areas of exploration which the social worker is expected to examine to formulate a discharge plan. At the same time, the process of the assessment provides a focal point from which to examine issues that have an impact on the disabled person and the family system. Case examples are referenced to highlight the psycho/social dynamics occurring in the overall process. Family system for the purposes of this chapter will be defined as any significant individual or individuals who are a part of the patient's immediate environment and play a role in the process of rehabilitation. The connotation "family system" will not necessarily imply a biological relationship except in the instances where an actual family member is identified such as a wife or husband.

The rehabilitation social worker is the provider of information reporting the patient's premorbid functioning, current coping abilities, perceptions regarding posthospital care needs, and the impact of the patient's disability within the family system. Although the focus may vary according to the medical issues addressed, the basic tasks remain in the realm of assessment, communication, counseling, coordination, and referral (Holliman, Dziegielewski, & Priyadarshi, 2001). Because rehabilitation occurs in a multidisciplinary milieu, it is not uncommon for information gathering to overlap among the assessments of other team members. In the process of identifying the discharge needs, the planning is individualized depending on the patient's diagnosis. For example, the discharge planning for a stroke patient will have different implications than the discharge planning involved for a patient with a spinal cord injury (SCI).

Gathering information to determine an appropriate plan is dependent on a good psycho/social assessment. The importance of a good assessment cannot be understated as the discharge planning will rest on information that is accurate and useful to other team members. For example, accessibility in the home environment for a wheelchair-dependent patient would be a major factor in exploring discharge planning needs. The social worker and the rehabilitation team as a whole will place particular emphasis in determining accessibility because of its impact not only on the patient but the family system as a whole. The patient's and/or family's input along with their concerns will contribute to projecting a plan and strategy for intervention. However, the assessment can be viewed in different ways depending on who is asking the questions.

It has been observed that when "persons with disabilities do not adopt the views of professionals, they are at risk of being labeled as 'problematic' in denial" or resistant. When everyone around them views their situation as a tragedy, it is difficult to view their situation differently (Mackelprang & Salsgiver, 1999). The following case highlights an environmental issue and the significance of the perceptions between patient and staff in addressing the problem in the discharge planning process.

Several years ago while working with an elderly female patient who had a below-the-knee amputation, the social worker was approached by the physical therapist who was concerned that the patient was being discharged to a one flight walk-up apartment. The therapist had spoken several times to the patient and her husband about moving to an apartment that would be more accessible for her. The couple refused to consider relocating as an option. The therapist felt that they were not dealing with the reality of their situation and that the social worker should attempt to convince the couple that a move to another apartment would be in the patient's best interest. Although the couple's living situation had been discussed during the initial psycho/social evaluation, the social worker revisited the concerns of the therapist with the patient and her husband. Although the couple was touched by the concerns of the staff, they were adamant that relocation was not an immediate consideration. Their primary concern was financial. They had lived in their rent-controlled apartment for more than 30 years, and living on a fixed income prevented them from considering any other option. They also pointed out that because of their longevity at their residence, they had many friends and neighbors who could be of help when needed. If an apartment on the ground floor became available at some point, they acknowledged that they might consider moving but expressed that financial considerations were their primary concern.

This example has several considerations in the context of assessment and discharge planning. While the patient had initially acknowledged feeling overwhelmed in the initial assessment, she also had to consider her overall living situation. One might argue that the therapist was correct in her perception that returning to a walk-up apartment was directly related to the patient's denial and refusal to appreciate her changed circumstance, "reactions; not atypical of someone dealing with a new disability" (Bhuvaneswar, Epstein, & Stun,

2007). To the therapist, the obvious was simple: move to another place. In reality, it would be unlikely that an apartment in the same complex would be so readily available so that even if the patient and her husband had wanted to move, it would not happen within the time frame of her hospitalization. Second, having the support of neighbors and being around people she knew at a critical time of her life was very important to her well-being. Finally, living on a fixed income had limited her choices. In reassessing the situation, it became clear that denial was not as much at play as financial concerns and the availability of neighbors in the overall decision process. Sharing feedback with the team after further discussion with the patient and her husband enabled the staff to gain a different perspective on the couple's decision making. With current emphasis on shorter term hospitalizations, what may ultimately be viewed as the best plan for the patient may not always be accomplished prior to discharge.

The ability of the rehabilitation social worker to be flexible and willing to appreciate the patient's preferences may override what we view as the optimal in discharge planning. It is expected that the patient may have a range of reactions to the catastrophic change in a life situation, so it is the rehabilitation social worker's ongoing assessment that will determine not only what stage of adjustment the patient is experiencing, but whether the patient's decision is influenced by his or her emotional state or by other factors such as financial concerns in the case cited. It has been suggested in the literature that among the number of principles in making an adequate assessment, the social work practitioner must ascertain the person's perception of the disability. The individual's understanding of the facts and issues related to a new diagnosis is of foremost importance (Cowger, 1994). Furthermore, the rehabilitation social worker as well as other members of the health care team must listen to each person's personal perceptions of the emotional impact of his or her disability rather than anticipating the patient will or should react in preconceived ways. The social worker's ongoing feedback to the team is therefore vital in helping the patient stay where she is while at the same time appreciating the staff's "take" on the patient's situation.

In the initial psycho/social assessment, the collection of demographics such as where and with whom the patient lives, the current and future income, level of education, work history, and religious affiliations/beliefs are essential to creating a description of the person and his or her environment. Although this information is concrete in nature, it is the action of gathering these data in conjunction with the psycho/social information assembled that, when bound together, formulates a discharge plan.

In the overall evaluation or impression section of an assessment, the social worker provides initial impressions regarding the patient's coping skills. This process requires thoughtful consideration so that one does not misinterpret someone's own reactions in the context of expected responses as occurred in the case previously described. The individualized responses may vary and the patient may remain "emotionally immobilized" in any one stage of adjustment for long periods of time, preventing the individual from progressing in the rehabilitation process. Roberta Treischman, in her study of SCI patients, felt that there was not enough consistent evidence to validate that everyone experiences the same adjustment patterns and/or that they occur in any fixed order. Nonetheless, there is general consensus that these patterns of adjustment are likely to occur in some form and with varying degrees of intensity (Treischman, 1979). As mentioned earlier, the most common stages of adjustment are as following: (1) shock and anger, (2) bargaining and denial, (3) realization or recognition, (4) retaliation, and (5) reintegration or adjustment/adaptation (Kubler-Ross, 1969/1997; Marinelli & Dell Orto, 1984).

Shock, the first stage, is associated with the patient's inability to come to terms with a diagnosis. This reaction is likely to be observed during the initial stages of an acquired disability. Therefore, the social worker should expect that the ability to establish sound discharge plans will be minimal at best while the patient is going through this particular period.

Bargaining, the second stage, is the period where the patient hopes for full recovery and may tap into spiritual beliefs as a resource for bringing about change to his or her situation.

The fulfillment of this request for help may occur in the form of a promise to be more devoted to one's faith in the future or a commitment to give back in some way to society.

The patient progresses at a certain point from the second stage of bargaining to the third stage of denial. This next stage emerges prior to the beginning of facing the permanency of the disability. It is likely that patients may not be able to move on at this point as they attempt to make sense of their physical disability. The denial stage typically presents a challenge to the social worker and interdisciplinary team. The importance of team collaboration is therefore critical not only in helping the patient progress through this particular stage, but also in providing supportive intervention throughout the rehabilitation process.

The additional stages of realization/recognition, anger, and finally acknowledgment or acceptance are the most common progressions of the adjustment continuum. As mentioned earlier, not everyone will progress through these stages in the same order, and some individuals may linger longer than expected in a particular stage without necessarily experiencing a negative outcome (Gunther, 1969; Linveh, 1991). Therefore, the social worker should expect that there will be periodic downtimes when the patient is going through a particular episode of emotional turmoil that impedes the ability to think or plan ahead. Support and intervention have to be carefully staged utilizing clinical judgment as to when the patient is able to discuss long-range plans. Setting short-term goals is more practical during these phases. Identifying the patient's emotional state and providing appropriate support are critical. The following case scenario typifies the identification of one stage of adjustment, recognition, and the appropriate intervention that was utilized to help the patient.

A 16-year-old teenager who became a C5 tetraplegic because of an accident at his high school was initially very confidant and resistant to talking about his disability when first entering the rehabilitation program. He attended his daily therapy sessions and minimized any discussions about future goals or planning. He preferred to charm the therapists and made it known that he did not believe in discussing his problems with the social worker or the psychologist. After a period of time, the therapists noted that they were having more difficulty engaging the patient in discussing equipment needs for discharge and that he more or less had refused to discuss plans any further. He eventually stopped going to therapy or showed up late to a therapy session. It was obvious that the patient was going through a period of mourning and depression as he began to recognize the reality of his situation. Attempts to have the patient refocus were unsuccessful.

A joint discussion with the team resulted in the decision to invite a former patient to meet with the young man to offer support. The former patient was a man in his 20s who had the same level of injury and had experienced the injury when he was in his teens as well. The two young men met one evening in the hospital where they had a one-to-one talk. The following day, the former patient reported to the team that the younger man was at first reluctant to speak and had scrutinized him very carefully (Interview with social worker, 1987). After a time, the younger patient began to ask questions and became more open with his feelings and his fears about the future. The former patient reassured him that he would go through many changes but that ultimately he would not only get through this but would have a life that would be fulfilling. At the end of their session, they proceeded to leave when they both realized that the door to the room they were in had been closed behind them and they would have difficulty exiting. The young patient panicked, and looking at his new-found friend asked, "What do we do now?" The former patient managed to position his chair so that he was able to lift his hands and turn the knob so they could leave the room. On leaving, the former patient counseled the younger one that this is how it will be from here on, saying, "There won't always be someone to open a door for you, you have to learn to do it yourself."

This one session had a major influence on the patient and demonstrates the vulnerability of patients' emotional functioning throughout the rehabilitation process. The social workers' ongoing collaboration with the team along with their reassessments is therefore essential. When this special session was scheduled, the patient had begun to realize the severity of his disability, which led to depression and a period of mourning for his loss. Depression in and of itself is healthy, "but it is only when the depressed behavior interferes with the individual's participation in the therapy program and is reflected in social withdrawal that the depression may be considered maladaptive" (Rosenthal, 1989). Recognizing not only the patient's difficulties at this point but also the limited impact of the staff on his depression necessitated drawing on other resources. Once the patient was able to identify with someone who was in the same situation, he not only had a role model but began to feel more hopeful. "It seems critical that at some point during the framing process people with newly-defined disabilities have an opportunity to interact with others who actually live with similar conditions" (Braschler, 2006). It is also important that in the ongoing reassessment one is able to not only identify the stage of adjustment but also apply the appropriate strategy of intervention. This is to say, the intervention may be other than the worker's own expectation to resolve the problem and bring about change. Sometimes, being effective requires recognition of our own limitations in our role as social workers in reaching a patient and calling on someone who may be more effective at that moment in time. In essence, the social worker is expected to use clinical judgment as to the effectiveness of the intervention. In this instance, the use of peer counseling helped lift the patient out of his depression, motivating him to attend therapy sessions regularly and providing the incentive to learn more skills toward achieving independent functioning.

The road to adjustment can be different for each individual and as mentioned may occur at any time. Major adjustment reactions to disability may occur after the patient has been discharged back into the community. The final stage identified in the recovery process, adjustment and/or adaptation, cannot be defined in terms of weeks or years. The stage may ebb and flow throughout the person's lifetime (Braschler, 2006). If a patient experiences any of the behavioral reactions as mentioned while in the hospital setting, the professional staff is available to provide support and intervention. Quite often, patients experience major reactions following discharge when the support of the rehabilitation team is no longer readily available. It has been noted, for example, that one-third of stroke patients experience depression up to 2–3 years following the initial onset (Flick, 1999). Others have noted that adjustment is a continuous struggle (Cohen & Napolitano, 2007). In either case, the ability to get through these fragile periods will depend not only on the patient's strengths but also on the patient's support systems outside the hospital setting.

BIO/PSYCHO/SOCIAL ASSESSMENT OF THE PATIENT IN THE FAMILY SYSTEM

The rehabilitation social worker's overall assessment must include information on how the patient fits into the family system. Is the patient a son, daughter, father, mother, grandparent? This information may not initially come from the patient, particularly during the acute care stage of diagnosis and treatment, for example, while the patient is in a hospital intensive care unit. Obtaining this information may not even occur while patients are in the initial stages of rehabilitation as they may be caught up with the medical issues that render them unwilling to share information. The patient may feel so helpless that a family member may be assigned to be the spokesperson. In the instance of someone with a traumatic brain injury or stroke, the inability to provide information may not be a matter of choice but rather a result of cognitive deficits and inability to provide reliable information.

The input of family members or significant others is therefore essential in respect to defining the patient's place within the family system. Determining how strong the family support systems are and who is going to be the major player in joining the patient in the discharge planning process has to be identified. In addition, during the course of information gathering, there is opportunity to observe and interpret the reactions of family members to the patient's trauma. The following case illustrates the importance of understanding family involvement.

A psychiatrist who sustained a severe stroke and suffered a loss of speech among his deficits was unable to communicate during his initial and subsequent psychosocial evaluations. His wife, therefore, became the patient's spokesperson. She described him as an intelligent man who had written numerous professional articles and books in his field. His wife was saddened by her husband's losses and worried that he would not be able to return to his work. She therefore hoped that he would be restored to full functioning not only for his own well-being but for hers as well. As time progressed, the patient made minimal progress and his wife became more despondent. She began to express that she would not know what to do if her husband did not regain full functioning. Although options were discussed regarding hiring private home care services, the wife did not seem to be worried about financial considerations, but there remained an element of hesitation in her ability to plan. When the wife was confronted about this, she confessed that bills were mounting up and that she had not paid any of them. When this was pursued further, she indicated that the funds to pay the bills were not the concern. She was embarrassed to admit that she did not know how to write a check or balance a check book. She revealed that her husband had always handled the finances and that she did not know how to go about paying her bills. The social worker reassured the wife that she could learn to manage this task and began the process of teaching her how to write checks and maintain a record.

In this case, the patient who had become severely disabled would not likely be able to resume all the responsibilities he carried prior to his illness. His family support system, his wife, was rendered helpless by her inability to assume his tasks in the home. The appropriate intervention to help the patient required that the social worker provide education, guidance, and emotional support to the wife as the reversal of roles met with challenges on its most basic levels.

Role reversal, whether it is short term or long term, is just one of a number of stressors that can occur within the patient and family system. The nature of the disability, as well as the patient's age, economic status, and marital status, can present varying degrees of stress and may continue long after the patient has been discharged from the rehabilitation setting. In a study of caregivers for stroke survivors, it was found that 1 month after discharge, family members complained of three common problems: the safety of the patient; difficulty in managing activities of daily living and managing cognitive; and behavioral and emotional changes (e.g., mood swings, lack of motivation, forgetfulness, memory loss, depression, and calling the caregiver often) (Grant, Glandon, Elliot, Giger, & Weaver, 2004).

The reactions of the family or significant others are therefore equally important in determining the coping abilities and expectations during and after the rehabilitation process. Some of the same responses experienced by the patient previously cited—shock, anger, depression, mourning, and adjustment—are likely to be felt by the family member, as well. If the family's coping skills during a crisis have met with success in the past, the same coping skills will usually be adopted in the new crisis. However, if previous illness or crisis incited major dysfunction within the family system, it is very likely that previous stressors will resurface again. Anxiety, blame, and a reluctance to communicate openly can impede pulling the family together to plan for aftercare. An inability to confront or avoidance can impede adjustment for all concerned, whereas the family who are able to be open and honest with each other are likely to have better outcomes (Power & Dell Orto, 2004). In addition, patients who have a history of dysfunction within the family, for example, substance abuse or risk taking behavior, are likely to be forced to confront these same issues as they become dependent on the family to assist in their care. The following case illustrates this situation.

A young man, intoxicated at a high school graduation party, dove into a shallow pool and suffered injuries that resulted in his becoming a tetraplegic. On his admission to the rehabilitation unit, the mother announced to the team that her son was not allowed to return home because he had been directly responsible for his injury, and she could not take on another tragedy within the family. A subsequent family meeting with the social worker revealed that the patient had come from a family where all the men in the household, father and siblings, were alcoholics. One son had previously died in an accident as a result of driving while intoxicated. The patient's mother was an active member of a family support group called AL-Anon (Statement of Purpose)[1] and was committed to setting limits and boundaries to any of the family members who continued to cause problems in the home because of drinking. The mother had now taken the lead in holding the family together with set boundaries and conditions.

None of the other family members had challenged her insistence that the patient had to make his own way. They would remain supportive, but he could not come home. Their affirmation of the mother was intensified by the patient's refusal to admit he had a drinking problem. The patient's mother remained an active participant in planning by helping the patient apply for benefits and remaining supportive services. However, he had to find his own place to live. With the help of the rehabilitation team, physical therapists, occupational therapists, psychologist, social worker, and vocational counselor, the patient ultimately moved to a college campus that included student housing for the disabled. Arrangements were made with able-bodied students to assist with his care. Environmental equipment was prescribed and ordered to allow the patient to record class lectures and submit assignments.

This case, however, points to a number of issues within the family system that had an impact on the direction of discharge planning. The premorbid dysfunctional issues gave rise to renewed confrontations for the family as a whole. Despite the problems inherent within the family system, there was still opportunity, nonetheless, to set expectations and negotiate with the patient and his family in setting reasonable goals. The major players in planning his after-care would have to be identified. In this instance, the mother was clearly the strong person in the family who while setting boundaries was also able to mobilize around the things she felt she could reasonably assist with, namely, helping her son obtain entitlements, securing documents, and so on. The patient, on the other hand, had to make choices as to the best possible options for himself. Fortunately, the patient possessed sufficient intellectual ability and skills that enabled him to pursue his goal of a college education. With the support of the team, he was able to map out a plan to move beyond the hospital setting. The issue of substance abuse was put on hold although follow-up counseling was recommended. Most often, patients are unable to focus on other issues while in the process of physical rehabilitation.

DISABILITY-SPECIFIC ISSUES

The previous section has looked at the components of a social work assessment of the patient and family system to develop a discharge plan. In this process, the psychosocial issues that potentially arise have been highlighted to demonstrate that the relationships between the patient/family and their reactions to the newly acquired disability will have an impact on the nature of the social worker's intervention.

Essentially, the strategies for intervention are geared toward providing concrete services, emotional support in the form of individual and/or family counseling, and the coordination of services with the rehabilitation team. The social worker's ongoing reassessment of how the patient and family are coping and the sharing of this information with staff are critical so that the team is made aware of any changes in plans and can tailor their interventions to meet the patient's and family's needs. In addition, although social workers contribute to the rehabilitation process through assessment, education, and planning, it is also important that patients and families are encouraged to engage in the earliest stages of treatment and rehabilitation (Keleher, Dixon, Holliman, & Vodde, 2003). Although specific indicators have been cited as common reactions to disability, each individual adjusts in his or her own way, and the timing and length of adjustment are difficult to gauge. The disability in and of itself may dictate what issues play a major role.

SCIs, which tend to occur in a younger population, can result in permanent impairment. The ability to regain independent functioning will depend on the level of injury and whether the injury is complete, that is, with little chance of neurological recovery. Loss of independence for this group often affects the ability to return to work or school. Although the ability to resume previous activities is achievable, it does present a number of challenges for the patient and the discharge planner. As pointed out in the previous case example, planning involved a major effort of the rehabilitation team to achieve a safe and adequate discharge arrangement. The shorter length of hospital stay may not allow the time for working out all the details in community readjustment. Most often, the plans for reintegration into the community occur after the patient is discharged and may take a very long time before one's life is normalized. Major structural changes to the home for accessibility and/or obtaining accessible housing may also be foremost in discharge planning but usually do not occur until long after discharge.

In the previous case of the 16-year-old tetraplegic, his concerns focused around life beyond the hospital setting in respect to living arrangements and mapping out a future. The role model session helped the young man see someone with the same disability living positively and emphasizing independence. Issues regarding housing, education, and securing entitlements were most important to him. Numerous studies with SCI patients, including my study of SCI women, point to the desire of this population to resume premorbid activities after a period of adjustment (Inniss, 1996).

The cognitive deficits of a stroke or traumatic brain injured patient have different implications regarding the development of an aftercare plan. Memory loss and impairment in thought processes may impede the ability to reach a level of independence that consequently places the family in the caregiving role for an indefinite period of time. This raises a number of issues in respect to family ability, willingness, and stamina to provide the support over a long period of time (DeJong, Batavia, & Williams, 1991). Role reversal and the need for a spouse to assume new tasks are challenging. This was clearly evident, for example, with the stroke victim's wife, who had to assume the financial responsibilities for the household.

When a patient suffers a traumatic brain injury, the family system must contend with personality changes and cognitive impairments, as well as management of the medical and social service needs. The levels of emotional and personality disturbances that are evidenced in the patient's behavior are more strongly associated with levels of family disturbances than the patient who presents a physical disability (Albert, Im, Brenner, Smith, & Waxman, 2002). A follow-up study of caregivers 5 years after their family member sustained a traumatic brain injury found that the more severe the injury the more likely the family member reported high levels of stress (Brooks, Campsie, Symington, Beatric, & Mokinlay, 1986).

Although each disability presents its special challenges, there are common threads among the disabled population as a whole. Financial concerns, insurance limitations, inadequate family support, and issues of sexual dysfunction can complicate the discharge planning. In instances where the family is required to provide the major caregiving role, the stress and strain incurred can lead to deeper family dysfunction, in some instances resulting in divorce and/or ongoing marital discord.

It is the uniqueness of each situation that requires the social worker to be creative, supportive, and proactive in helping the patient and family make the transition from hospital to home. In the process of providing information, directing clients to aftercare services and connecting them to organizations specifically geared toward addressing disability-specific issues are essential. Discharge from the hospital can cause rapid deterioration within the home setting as the patient/family begin to settle in and live with the disability in absence of the support they have received thus far. Aligning with support groups, maintaining peer counseling relationships can be significant in sustaining coping abilities for both patient and family.

AFTERCARE SERVICES

Discharge options following acute rehabilitation may include returning to the rehabilitation center for outpatient therapy or receiving in-home therapy if recommended. Most fee-for-service insurance carriers will cover both venues of therapy, although the extent and approval will depend on the range of available benefits. Managed care insurance carriers may be more limited in the number of hours of therapy allowed. In addition, home care may be a very limited benefit and cannot be factored in as fulfilling the need for providing assistance to the patient in the home. The family will therefore be expected to provide assistance to the discharged patient in performing activities of daily living. Application to Medicaid for more comprehensive supportive service care may be appropriate if the discharged patient meets income requirements. Patients who have cognitive deficits are likely to have difficulty obtaining coverage for outpatient services as some managed care companies do not always view this as a therapeutic need.

Some patients who do not meet criteria for continued acute rehabilitation because of limited progress may move on to continued rehabilitation at a subacute level. Most skilled nursing facilities now provide units that offer rehabilitation for an extended period. There are a limited number of facilities that have subacute units specifically geared to work with the brain-injured patient. The payment for these subacute programs can be time limited, and justification for payment is based on documented evidence of progress by the therapy staff from the host facility. Although managed care is attractive because of its potential to improve delivery and coordination of services, the inherent financial incentives to provide fewer services under capitated rates may cause people with chronic conditions to be underserved (Regenstein, Schroer, & Meyer, 1998).

Transitional living facilities provide extended care for disabled patients beyond acute rehabilitation settings. These programs are geared toward teaching independent living skills and are aimed at transitioning the patient to community living. These facilities are limited in number and may require individuals to be placed out of state because their needs cannot be met locally. New York State Medicaid, for example, will approve out-of-state placements provided a well-documented history of placement attempts within the patient's home area has been demonstrated. Insurers are likely to be hesitant to provide coverage unless a cost containment analysis can be demonstrated in respect to saving on aftercare services. The availability of services may also be limited in respect to the person's age as skilled nursing facilities generally serve the elderly population. In sum, although the goal is to promote independent living for the patient, the limitations with insurance coverage and the family availability to take on care of the patient can be impediments to a patient's transitioning to the community.

The independent living movement that emerged in the 1970s was a direct result of the disabled population's frustration with limited services and society's insensitivity toward their expectation of being fully integrated into community living. It became the mission of disabled individuals to collectively set up their own network of services that would guide, direct, and demand services so that living independently would be seen as a right and not as a privilege. The independent living movement was a political concept with a clearly defined social model for the integration of people with disabilities in their communities. The basic characteristics of the movement have been to promote self-determination, self-image, public education, peer support, and advocacy (Roberts, 1989). This effort is supported by the concept that when individuals redefine their role from that of patient, client, or recipient of goods and services to that of consumer of services with specific demands and standards, their sense of control over their own lives is elevated (Tower, 2003).

FINANCIAL ISSUES

In 2004, the U.S. Bureau of Statistics revealed that 45 million American citizens had no health insurance coverage. Clearly, this dearth of coverage has created a strain on the U.S. health care system in trying to provide care for the uninsured. In the instance of someone accessing services for rehabilitation, the extended care and cost beyond an acute care hospital is daunting (Center on Budget and Policy Priorities, 2006). Because of cost containment issues, the federal government has encouraged and supported managed care programs that began with private insurances in the 1980s. Essentially, costs are held down by the provision of services deemed necessary by the insurance overseeing how dollars are spent. These programs may only have limited contracts with homecare agencies, skilled nursing facilities that consequently limit choice. A disabled person may therefore not be able to obtain necessary homecare services if the insurance only allows for a limited number of hours per day.

For those who are uninsured or needing coverage beyond their insurance benefits, the federal and state governments fund the Medicaid program that provides reimbursement for medical care services for those individuals who meet specific state-defined income criteria. The elderly and the disabled make up 25% of Medicaid beneficiaries, but they account for 70% of the program's costs. Each state maintains its own formula for eligibility. For individuals with a disability, Medicaid covers a range of services, including homecare, medical equipment, transportation to medical appointments, and medications. For people with chronic conditions, it is likely that at some point they will apply and receive Medicaid when they have exhausted benefits of their insurance carriers (Gold, White, Justin, & Fries, 2006). The SCI patients described in this chapter are examples of individuals who became Medicaid recipients.

During the 1990s, states began to view managed care as a way to control cost for Medicaid beneficiaries. Most of the plans were initially developed for low-income families and were not targeted specifically for the disabled (Regenstein et al., 1998). Because persons with disabilities are a costly population, state Medicaid programs began incorporating younger persons with disabilities into managed care insurance plans. Forty-eight states and Washington D.C. now either require or allow some or all of their Medicaid population to enroll in some form of managed care (Vladek, 2003). States vary on their mandates for disabled in respect to managed Medicaid enrollment, and the impact of its ability to meet the needs of this population continue to be evaluated.

Individuals who are aged 65 and have paid into the Social Security system are eligible to apply to and receive insurance coverage under the Medicare program. In 1972, 7 years after the Medicare Act was enacted, a provision was added to enable individuals who have been disabled for 2 years and have worked a number of quarters to qualify for Medicare benefits at a younger age. This change to the Medicare benefit was a significant addition in assisting the disabled to apply for the benefit before retirement age. Medicare benefits, however, are more time-focused than Medicaid. Medicare, Part A, covers inpatient hospital care, skilled nursing facility care, home health care, and hospice care. There are deductibles and coinsurance that a patient is responsible for paying during each benefit period. A benefit period begins when you are admitted to the hospital or skilled nursing facility and ends when you are discharged from the hospital or skilled nursing facility after 60 consecutive days. Currently, the initial deductible is $1,028. After 60 days, the coinsurance cost is $267 per day for days 61–90, then $534 per day for days 91–150 of a hospital stay. Medicare covers the first 20 days of a skilled nursing facility at 100%, with a subsequent co-pay if the individual remains beyond 20 days (U.S. Department of Health and Human Services, 2009). Medicare also implemented assistance with medications under the Medicare D program, enacted in 2003; however, this is also administered by a formula that calculates out-of-pocket expenses with assistance after yearly costs go beyond predetermined limits (Center on Budget and Policy Priorities, 2006). In the case example of the female amputee, when the patient considered finances, the limits of Medicare were factored in as well. The cost for private help can be high, and elderly patients are particularly concerned about depleting their resources. When this patient referred to the importance of relying on friends to assist her, clearly the limitations of Medicare and financial issues as mentioned earlier influenced their decision making for postdischarge and aftercare planning.

Many of the Medicare recipients have signed on to managed care programs. These programs tend to be economically beneficial for doctor visits, reduced medications cost, and coverage for examinations that would otherwise be expensive. Managed care, however, presents challenges for the consumer and the health care provider who must work within the boundaries of the coverage. Case managers assigned to insurance companies and/or employed within hospital settings generally provide direction to health care personnel as to the parameters of someone's coverage and how to be cost effective in the application of service needs.

There are numerous other insurance plans that may be available to the disabled person depending on eligibility. These would include worker's compensation, which is provided in the instance of on-the-job injuries and covers the services directly related to the disability. No-fault insurance, which covers injuries related to auto accidents, however, varies according to state in respect to the amount of coverage. Spinal cord-injured and traumatic brain injury patients are often the victim of auto accidents; consequently, other insurance coverage is needed to supplement payment for services.

Veterans are in a special category and generally must be enrolled with a Department of Veterans Affairs (VA) health care facility to receive benefits. Eligibility for most VA benefits is based on active military service under other than dishonorable conditions. Veterans can be treated in the VA system for those injuries related to active duty. In the absence of other insurance, veterans may receive rehabilitation in a VA hospital for a non-war-related injury, if they meet other criteria to be treated within the VA system.

Financial assistance in the form of income is available via disability through one's employer. This benefit is time limited, usually lasting 6 months. If the individual has paid into the Social Security system, an application can be made for benefits only after the disability has lasted for 6 months and is likely to remain permanent or end in death. This benefit is known as Social Security Disability or Social Security Disability Income. The counterpart to SSD, Social Security Income is paid to those individuals who meet criteria as permanently disabled and have not paid into Social Security. The above cover most of the basic plans although individuals may have coverage under long-term insurance plans.

SUMMARY

The rehabilitation social worker must recognize that as the numbers of individuals with impairments in body structures or body functions escalate, the nature of the interventions must expand in scope to include referrals to support groups and organizations that actively advocate for entitlements.

There is growing awareness within the social work arena to view the disabled in a different way. That is, there is more emphasis to promote self-determination and provide the skills to allow the person to act on his or her own behalf. This same approach is recommended for families who often flounder following the hospitalizations of loved ones without ongoing support (Patchner, 2005). Studies have shown that the aftercare support can make a critical difference in the healthy survival of patients and the family members. It is important also that health care providers become more sophisticated in advocating and promoting the needs of the disabled through professional interventions. The number of individuals needing personal assistance whether it is from family members or from paid caregivers will also increase. Health insurances and its related issues will continue to be the focus for changes and discussion in the future. The direction of changes will be dependent on what factors are at play that influence options considered. Issues of cost containment will continue to be a major factor, but there needs to be some compromise in respect to ensuring that the disabled population is not left with minimal benefits that render them dependent on others when there could be a wider range of choices for independence. I refer to the disincentives inherent in government entitlements. Essentially, someone who works and makes an income that is beyond the limits for Medicaid/Medicare coverage will likely opt to remain unemployed to receive the benefit of home attendant services. If the system has built in allowances for the disabled to contribute to their benefit to maintain home attendant service, it might allow an individual to remain gainfully employed (Institute of Medicine of the National Academies, 2007).

Government and the private sector need to confront the demands of the disabled population. Research, both in the medical arena and in the social sciences, is important to demonstrate the needs and proposed solutions. The thrust of this chapter has been not only to explain the social workers' involvement with the disabled but also to demonstrate that their ongoing collaboration and assessment of patient/families needs are key to helping promote independence and make it a realistic expectation.

NOTE

1. Statement of Purpose: Al-Anon Family Groups are a fellowship of relatives and friends of alcoholics who share their experience, strength and hope in order to solve their common problems. We believe alcoholism is a family illness and that changed attitudes can aid recovery." www.al-anon-alateen.org.

REFERENCES

Albert, S., Im, A., Brenner, L., Smith, M., & Waxman, R. (2002). Effect of a social work liaison program on family caregivers to people with traumatic brain injury. *Journal of Head Injury Rehabilitation, 20,* 175–189.

Beaulaurier, R., & Taylor, S. (2001). Social work practice with people with disabilities in the era of disability rights. *Social Work in Health Care, 32,* 67–91.

Bhuvaneswar, C., Epstein, L., & Stun, T. (2007). Reactions to amputation-recognition and treatment. *Journal of Clinical Psychiatry, 9,* 303–308.

Blumenfield, S., & Rosenberg, G. (1988). Towards a network of social health services: Redefining discharge planning and expanding the social work domain. *Social Work in Health Care, 13,* 31–48.

Braschler, R. (2006). Social work practice and disability issues. In S. Gehlert & T. Browne (Eds.), *Handbook of health social work.* Hoboken, NJ: John Wiley and Sons.

Brooks, N., Campsie, L. Symington, C., Beatric, A., & Mokinlay, W. (1986). The five year outcome of severe blunt injury: A relative's view. *Journal of Neurology, Neurosurgery and Psychiatry, 49,* 704–770.

Center on Budget and Policy Priorities. (2006). *The number of uninsured Americans is at an all-time high.* Washington, DC: Staff Report.

Cohen, C., & Napolitano, D. (2007). Adjustment to disability. *Journal of Social Work in Disability and Rehabilitation, 6,* 135–155.

Cowger, C. (1994). Assessing client's strengths: Clinical assessments for client empowerment. *Social Work, 39,* 262–268.

DeJong, G., Batavia, A., & Williams, J. (1991). Who is responsible for the lifelong well being of a person with a head injury. *Journal of Head Trauma, 3,* 9–22.

Dodds, T. (1993). Richard Cabot: Medical reformer during the progressive era (1890–1920). *Annals of Internal Medicine, 38,* 417–422.

Flick, C. (1999). Stroke rehabilitation, stroke outcome and psychosocial consequences. *Archives of Physical Medicine Rehabilitation, 80,* S21–S26.

Gold, R. M., White, S., Justin, T., & Fries, E. (2006). The Medicaid managed care program. In S. L. Isaacs & J. Knickman (Eds.), *The Robert Wood Johnson Foundation Anthology* (Vol. 9). New Jersey: Robert Wood Johnson Foundation.

Grant, J. S., Glandon, G. L., Elliott, T. R., Giger, J. N., & Weaver, M. (2004). Care giving problems and feelings experienced by family caregivers after discharge. *International Journal of Rehabilitation Research, 27,* 105–111.

Gunther, M. S. (1969). Depressed mood during rehabilitation of persons with spinal injury. In D. Ruge (Ed.), *Spinal cord injuries.* Springfield, IL: Charles C. Thomas Hohmann.

Hoffman, K., et al. (2008). Social work education. In T. Mizrahi & L. Davis (Eds.), *The encyclopedia of social work* (20th ed., Vol. 4). National Association of Social Workers and Oxford University Press.

Holliman, D., Dziegielewski, S., & Priyadarshi, D. (2001). Discharge planning and social work practice. *Social Work in Health Care, 32,* 1–19.

Inniss, P. (1996). *Daily living activities of spinal cord injured women.* Unpublished doctoral dissertation, School of Social Work, New York University.

Institute of Medicine of the National Academies. (2007). Committee on Disability in America Board on Health Sciences Policy. In M. J. Field & A. M. Jette (Eds.), *The future of disability in America.* Washington, DC: The National Academies Press.

Keleher, C., Dixon, D., Holliman, D., & Vodde, R. (2003). Biopsychosocial perspectives and primer for social workers. *Journal of Social Work in Disability and Rehabilitation, 2,* 57–77.

Kim, K., & Canda E. (2007). Supporting the well being of people with mobility disabilities through social work practice. *Journal of Social Work in Disability and Rehabilitation, 6,* 31–51.

Kubler-Ross, E. (1997). *On death and dying—what the dying have to teach doctors, nurses, clergy, and their own families.* New York: Simon and Shuster, Touchstone. (Original work published by New York, Macmillan, 1969)

Linveh, H. (1991). A unified approach to existing models of adaptation to disability: A model of adaptation In R. Marinelli & A. D. Orto (Eds.), *The psychological and social impact of disability.* New York: Springer Publishing Company.

Mackelprang, R., & Salsgiver, R. (1999). *A diversity model approach in human services practice.* California: Brooks/Cole.

Marinelli, R., & Dell Orto, A. D. (1984). *The psychological and social impact of disability.* New York: Springer Publishing Company.

Massachusetts General Hospital Department of Social Services. (1958). *Selected papers and reports: Fiftieth anniversary celebration of the social service.* Retrieved April 4, 2009, from www.mghsocialwork.org/history.html

Otis-Green, S. (2008). Health care social work. In T. Mizrahi & L. Davis (Eds.), *The encyclopedia of social work* (20th ed., Vol. 2). New York: Oxford University Press.

Patchner, L. (2005). Social work practice and people with disabilities: Our future selves. *Advances in Social Work, 6,* 109–120.

Power, P. W., & Dell Orto, A. E. (2004). *Families living with chronic illness and disability: Interventions, challenges, and opportunities.* New York: Springer Publishing Company.

Regenstein, M., Schroer, C., & Meyer, J. A. (1998). *Medicaid managed care for persons with disabilities: Case studies of programs in Florida, Kentucky, Michigan and New Mexico.* Washington, DC: Kaiser Commission on Medicaid and the Uninsured.

Roberts, E. (1989). A history of the independent living movement: A founder's perspective. In B. W. Heller, L. S. Zegans, & L. M. Flohr (Eds.), *Psychosocial interventions with physically disabled persons.* Piscataway, NJ: Rutgers University Press.

Rosenberg, G., & Rehr, H. (1982). *Advancing social work practice in the health care field: Emerging issues and new perspectives.* New York: Haworth Press.

Rosenthal, M. (1989). Psychosocial evaluation of physically disabled persons. In B. W. Heller, L. S. Zegans, & L. M. Flohr (Eds.), *Psychosocial interventions with physically disabled persons.* Piscataway, NJ: Rutgers University Press.

Stuifbergen, A. K., & Roberts, G. J. (1997). Health promotion practices of women with multiple sclerosis. *Archives of Physical Medicine and Rehabilitation, 98,* S3–S9.

Tower, K. (2003). Disability through the lends of culture. *Journal of Social Work in Disability and Rehabilitation, 12,* 5–22.

Treischman, R. (1979). *Spinal cord injuries: Psychological social and vocational adjustment.* New York: Pergamon Press.

U.S. Department of Health and Human Services. (2009). *Medicare & you.* Baltimore, MD: Centers for Medicare and Medicaid Services.

Vladek, B. (2003). Where the action really is: Medicaid and the disabled. *Health Affairs, 22,* 1–10.

31

The Computer Revolution, Disability, and Assistive Technology

Mark A. Young, MD, and Bryan O'Young, MD

Accessible technology (AT) can be employed as a powerful tool to modify disablement and enable participation in activities of daily living and in recreational and vocational pursuits (Stiens, 1998). This chapter, intended as an introduction to AT for Physical Medicine and Rehabilitation (PM&R) physicians, therapists, and others in allied disciplines, provides an overview of available AT solutions to address four common categories of physical impairments: hearing, visual, hearing and visual (combined hearing and visual), and motor and dexterity. These broad categories represent the major groups of impairments that are likely to be encountered in rehabilitation practice. The chapter addresses each of the four common categories in separate modules. Although computer-associated and software-based AT solutions are emphasized, AT modalities that are not specifically computer related are also discussed. The final section of this chapter discusses emerging AT.

BACKGROUND TO ACCESSIBLE TECHNOLOGY

Accessible Technology is a general term used to describe "any item, piece of equipment or system, whether acquired commercially, modified or customized, that is utilized to increase, maintain or improve functional capabilities of individuals with disability" (Assistive Technology Act of 1998, 1998). With more than 54 million Americans with a disability (U.S. Department of Health & Human Services, 2009), AT has emerged as an essential tool in the rehabilitation and functional self-sufficiency of this growing and often neglected population. AT is used as an abbreviation for accessible technology, which was recently introduced by the disability community as an alternative to *assistive technology* to emphasize a person's abilities.

AT can enable disabled people to carry out activities of daily living, and it can help them communicate, further their education, and pursue vocational or recreational activities (Gerard, 2001). Also, AT tools can improve cognitive, mental, and physical functioning by helping disabled people compensate for impairments. For example, an electronic "prosthesis" can aid a patient impaired by a foot drop, and a low-tech memory-reminder board can help a stroke patient remember the time and date. AT has become one of the most powerful tools in helping disabled people achieve social equality (Santiago-Pintor, Hernández-Maldonado, Correa-Colón, & Méndez-Fernández, 2009).

AT solutions can take on many different forms and can dramatically influence all aspects of a person's life. However, AT need not be a sophisticated, high-cost solution such as an

Ibot wheelchair designed to ascend stairs (www.ibotnow.com; demonstrated at www.you-tube.com/watch?v=z1RhmvxcpfI). Instead, AT can be a simple, low-tech solution designed to address a particular impairment, such as a sticky note which a patient with a traumatic brain injury can use to compensate for memory deficits. AT can help disabled people achieve a sense of heightened independence, improve their quality of life, and in some cases promote accomplishing educational goals (Guyer & Uzeta, 2009) and workplace re-entry.

It is estimated that more than 216 million Americans (72%) currently use the Internet (Internet World Stats, 2009) and that 210 billion e-mails are sent worldwide every day (The Radicati Group, 2009). The computer revolution resulted in a growing commitment of rehabilitation providers and their patients to successfully deploy technology to creatively accommodate impairments (Young, Tumanon, & Sokal, 2000). The global proliferation of desktops, laptops, notebooks, and PDAs has been met with a simultaneous increase in the number of disabled people who use these devices for various purposes, including social (establishing friendships and relationships), medical (providing information about conditions and treatment options), personal and house-hold (accomplishing daily activities, such as shopping and ordering meals), psychological (com-pensating for cognitive deficits), and vocational (optimizing employment outcomes) purposes (National Council on Disability, 1993).

The world of PM&R and neurorehabilitation has seen a proliferation of academic attention and scientific activities devoted to technological means of promoting equality among persons with disability via AT provision and innovation. Recent regional and international confer-ences have focused on the expanding role of AT solutions. To advance the role of AT for the aging workforce, one historical forum was conducted at the Rusk Institute of Rehabilitation Medicine. This forum served as a "learning lab" and informational session on how health care providers can successfully incorporate AT into their treatment arsenal to enable peo-ple with disabilities or age-related impairments to re-enter or competitively remain in the workforce (Zaretsky, Young, Lee, Crounse, & Stiens, 2005). On an international level, there have also been several seminal meetings focused on emerging technologies and the critically important role of technology-assisted neurorehabilitation (International Neurorehabilitation Symposium, 2009).

Although there are an increasing number of commercial technology and fee-based "add-on" programs available to meet the needs of disabled people, this chapter emphasizes emerging technologies and basic complementary computer-based commercial applications, which are commonly found as part of standard operating systems. With computer technology, includ-ing Internet applications, serving as an indispensable tool to enhance vocational re-entry and personal satisfaction, the chapter has a major emphasis on profiling specific AT solutions that enhance prognostic efficacy of vocational rehabilitation programs. Often, the process is simple and may involve the clinician suggesting a specific "tweak and adjustment" made to standard operating systems that enable the activation of disability access utilities freely avail-able on all computers. Disabled people are thought to benefit from AT in many ways: within their own bodies, such as through cochlear transplantation to enhance hearing; within their immediate environment, such as with a scooter to improve mobility; and within an extended environment, such as a wheelchair-adapted van (Boninger et al., 2008).

Because enhancing quality of life for people with disabilities is an overarching goal of rehabilitation, health care providers treating people with disabilities must be well versed in AT solutions to better serve patients. When physical limitations and impairments hamper basic activities of daily living and functional skills, health care providers must serve as a vital intermediary to suggest solutions.

Module I: AT for Hearing-Impaired and Deaf Patients

Auditory and hearing impairments are commonly encountered in rehabilitation settings and have the potential to impact vocational involvement. Hearing impairments, represented by a wide range of conditions including mild hearing loss to deafness, are often coincidentally discovered on the rehabilitation unit or in the outpatient PM&R setting. Although the incidence of hearing impairments is higher among older individuals, auditory problems emerge among younger persons as well. The incidence and prevalence of hearing impairment rises dramatically with age and its presence frequently thwarts the rehabilitation process. Hearing impairments within the occupational setting that go unaddressed can lead to reduced work productivity and decreased efficiency.

Deafness is broadly defined as "a hearing impairment that impairs the processing of linguistic information through hearing, with or without amplification." Therefore, deafness can be viewed as a sensory state that prevents an individual from receiving sound in all or most of its forms. In contrast, "hearing loss" generally includes some level of responsiveness to auditory stimuli, including speech.

Amplification devices, such as hearing aids and amplification telephones, have long been the mainstay for hearing-impaired people (Ross, 2008b). However, it is important for the clinician to remember that hearing aids are often incapable of providing adequate assistance in many situations, such as in noisy environments. In such situations, hearing impairment might be remedied instead by use of directional microphones or devices based on induction loops, infrared, or frequency modulation. These devices make obtrusive movies, meetings, and seminars more accessible to hearing-impaired people. An alternative AT solution is TV monitor closed captioning.

There are many technological devices to aid deaf people in common daily activities. Some of these technologies include flashing lights and vibrating signals to alert them to ringing phones, doorbells, smoke detectors, and alarm clocks. Vibrational watch alarms and pagers are other valuable assistive technologies for those with hearing impairments. One consideration that must be taken into account when developing AT for deaf people is that some might be able to hear sounds but not spoken words.

With the prevalence of technology in modern society, it is important to understand the various challenges computers present for people with hearing impairments and what physicians and caregivers can do to overcome these challenges. It is estimated that one in five adult computer users in the United States has a hearing difficulty. Add-on software, in which it is possible for the user to adjust volume and other sound options, enables hearing-impaired or deaf computer users to receive information visually. The maturation and development of cell phone technology and instrumentation have created new challenges for deaf persons, such as noisy feedback that occurs when hearing aids interfere with cell phone frequencies (Experience No Interference by Using Hearing Aid Compatible Cell Phones, August 8, 2008. Retrieved June 8, 2009, from Articlesbase Free Online Articles Directory Web site: http://www.articlesbase.com/diseases-and-conditions-articles/experience-no-interference-by-using-hearing-aid-compatible-cell-phones-514101.html; Ross, 2008a). However, there are many assistive technologies that allow deaf people to communicate using standard telephones without encountering the issues that arise on cell phones.

One such example is text telephone (TTY), a standard communications protocol for people who are deaf or hearing impaired. When used in conjunction with a relay service, TTY serves an important role for these people by providing telephone service that enables deaf people to access others with normal hearing. A deaf person wishing to speak over the phone can use a "Voice Carry Over Relay Service," which are telephones that operate by vocalizing outgoing messages while simultaneously displaying incoming messages. Currently, "Video Relay Technology" enables deaf people who communicate in sign language to place a call through a signing intermediary to those who do not communicate by sign language (Video Relay Service, Corliss Community. Retrieved June 8, 2009, from The Corliss Institute, Inc., Web site: http://www.corliss.org/).

Those hearing-impaired and deaf people who cannot speak benefit from using synthetic speech software, which generates speech produced by an electronic synthesizer activated by a keyboard.

Various software companies (www.microsoft.com/enable/guides/hearing.aspx, last updated: May 20, 2009, accessed June 3, 2009; www.apple.com/accessibility/macosx/hearing. html, accessed June 3, 2009) manufacture products that enhance computer accessibility for hearing-impaired and deaf people. For example, audio alerts can be replaced by visual alerts. Physicians can suggest some of these features for their hearing-impaired patients to facilitate smoother use of various computer operating systems.

Increasingly, deaf and hearing-impaired people are searching for technological solutions to adapt emerging technology, including wired and wireless telephones, for their use. A growing body of literature describes the ways in which deaf consumers are advocating to the wireless industry about issues such as wireless emergency communications, touch screen usability, iPhone applications, and hearing-aid compatibility of mobile phones (Wireless RERC, 2009).

With the expansion of technological applications to address hearing loss, there has been a national emphasis placed on drafting legislation designed to ensure equal access to technology for people with sensory impairments, including impairments in hearing and vision. Furthermore, the proposed Twenty-First Century Communications and Video Accessibility Act and the Americans with Disabilities Restoration Act provide regulatory goals and safeguards for people with disabilities of all types (Hamlin, 2008). This includes the next major category of disability: AT for vision-impaired and blind patients.

Module 2: AT for Vision-Impaired and Blind Patients

Vision-impaired and blind people can benefit by listening to books on tapes and to radio stations that broadcast readings. Various read-aloud devices, including watches, clocks, thermostats, thermometers, scales, calculators, microwave ovens, money identifiers, compasses, sphygmomanometers, toys, dictionaries, talking signs, and a recently introduced device, the *talking glucometer*, are valuable tools for this population.

Failing or completely absent vision or blindness is frequently encountered in diabetic patients. A talking glucometer "speaks out" blood glucose concentrations, time, date, and historical blood glucose levels. Use of this device has revolutionized the lives of diabetic patients with vision impairments and other disabilities. Vision-impaired diabetic patients often experience difficulty in monitoring and managing blood glucose concentrations. For a vision-impaired diabetic patient who does not have access to help from others such as nurses, caregivers, relatives, or volunteers to monitor blood glucose, a talking glucometer can provide essential assistance. The talking glucometer is one type of AT that should be introduced as part of comprehensive management of diabetes-related vision impairment.

For people with low vision, many magnification options, including handheld optics and monocular glasses, are available. For greater magnification, closed circuit television (CCTV) may be used to magnify and enhance images. CCTVs are readily available in a variety of formats, including handheld cameras, self-contained units, and virtual-reality helmets.

Braille technology applications have been used to promote self-sufficiency in activities of daily living, such as walking and wayfinding. A new AT system was designed to aid vision-impaired people in wayfinding through the use of a camera cell phone, which is held by the user to find and read aloud specially designed signs in the environment. These signs are wayfinding barcodes marked with simple color patterns (targets) that can be quickly and reliably identified using image-processing algorithms running on the camera cell phone (Coughlan & Manduchi, 2007). Another approach to aid blind people is the application of Braille or other tactile markings on items such as thermostats, telephones, rulers, clocks, calendars, ATM machines, and keyboards.

Blind people using a computer with a QWERTY keyboard layout can obtain output through the use of screen-reader software, which provides computer-synthesized voice output. For those who prefer to obtain Braille output, refreshable Braille displays are available. This display, which is hardware that is attached to a computer, receives messages from the computer through screen translator software and presents these messages to the user in Braille. The message the Braille displays is refreshable, that is, it keeps updating as the user moves the cursor on the computer screen. Screen color configurations can be altered to match the requirements of vision-impaired computer users. These users may also benefit from using screen magnification software and cursor enhancement features. Several screen magnification programs offer a connected speech component that supplements the visible text with voice interpretation. Vision-impaired and blind people also often benefit from using text-to-speech software, which reads aloud the text that is on a computer screen. A host of solutions are available to make the keyboard and mouse easier to use. A user can dispense with mouse and keyboard altogether by typing on screen and by using speech recognition software. A growing number of Certified Vocational Rehabilitation Programs throughout the United States, including the Workforce & Technology Center in Baltimore, MD, have pioneered technology programs for blind diabetic patients seeking to mainstream back into the workplace (Young, Desai, & Young, 2009).

In the acute rehabilitation setting and in the subacute and outpatient arena, these diabetes-related visual impairments often become obvious to the clinician. For those diabetic patients identified in the rehabilitation setting who do not have visual disturbances or other forms of secondary diabetic complications, the rehabilitation team can play an essential preventive and educational role in averting the long-term consequences of the disease.

However, if the disease has progressed such that a diabetic patient experiences serious visual impairment, the job of the physicians becomes much more challenging, and disease management becomes more complicated. The blind diabetic patient poses a special rehabilitation challenge because of the critically important goals of balancing optimal management of glycemic control (maintaining sugars at a normal level) while increasing the ability to perform essential activities of daily living, thus improving overall functional status.

Blind diabetic patients who live alone often encounter problems reading their standard glucose meters and drawing up insulin. This may lead to worsening of complications of many diabetes-related conditions. It is important to understand the relevance of vision-related problems in diabetic patients and the respective challenges they pose for physicians and caregivers alike. A better understanding on the part of physicians can enhance their ability to provide better care and more thorough chronic disease management to the blind diabetic patients.

TECHNOLOGICAL SOLUTIONS TO ENABLE BLIND AND VISION-IMPAIRED PATIENTS TO USE COMPUTERS

Speech Technology

The most recent version of Mac OS X includes a text-to-speech (TTS) system (known as Alex), which is helpful to blind persons, enabling natural intonation even when set at quick speaking rates. This program works with all applications that support Apple speech synthesis. One of the advantages of the Mac OS X TTS system is that it analyzes text one paragraph at a time and is thought to interpret the context more accurately. The Alex program will speak a sentence differently depending on its precise location in the text and based on concepts found in prior sentences. This is in contrast to most TTS systems that analyze and synthesize text one sentence at a time and are not context sensitive.

Another advantage of Alex is that it is easier to understand the flow and nuance of human speech, since its voice more closely resembles human speech rather than computerized speech. There is a breath capability built inside the speech synthesizer so that when Alex recites a long passage it sounds more natural. The synthesizer inserts a breath based on a variety of factors, including appropriateness, time duration since last breath, syntax of the given text, and the time required for Alex to finish speaking.

In addition to the speech synthesizer, developers have found ways of improving the ease of functionality of the keyboard and mouse for vision-impaired patients. In terms of making the keyboard easier to use, the patient can press keyboard shortcuts one key at a time (sticky keys), hear a tone when they press Caps Lock, Num Lock, or Scroll Lock (toggle keys), ignore or slow down brief or repeated keystrokes (filter keys), turn on bounce keys or repeat keys and slow keys, underline keyboard shortcuts and access keys, choose a Dvorak Simplified Keyboard layout, adjust cursor blink rate and character repeat rate, and find keyboard short-cuts. The mouse may be made easier to use by changing the color and size of mouse pointers, controlling the mouse pointer with the keyboard (mouse keys), activating a window by hovering over it with the mouse, changing what the mouse pointer looks like, and altering mouse button settings. Further, patients can type without using the keyboard (on-screen keyboard) and start speech recognition if they prefer to use the computer without either a mouse or a keyboard. These examples illustrate the myriad of ATs that help vision-impaired patients use the computer independently on a daily basis.

Module 3: AT for People With Hearing and Vision Impairments

People with both hearing and vision impairments are sometimes referred to as being deaf–blind. Many of the technologies helpful to people with individual sensory impairments also apply to the deaf–blind population. However, adaptations are often necessary. For example, telephone access can be optimized through the use of TTYs with large print capability. People with even partial residual hearing can use amplification phones equipped with Braille markings; these ATs are a necessity for people who are deaf–blind (Fellbaum & Koroupetroglou, 2008).

Devices in the home and the workplace can attract the attention of deaf–blind people to inform them of particular environmental circumstances. In the home, alarm clocks equipped with crystal and tactile markings and pillow alarms are available. At the workplace, devices can use vibration, scents, or fan-driven air to alert that a telephone is ringing or that a smoke-detector is sounding.

Given the prevalence of visual and hearing impairments in the PM&R field, it is critical for physicians to understand the impact these disabilities have on the long-term care of their patients. With the goal of promoting better case management, physicians can use AT to improve the quality of life in a deaf–blind patient. Two mainstream operating systems, Windows Vista and Mac OS v10.5 Leopard, can be adapted to enable those with visual or auditory impairments to enjoy unconstrained computer usage. The following section describes examples of how each operating system can be employed to help those with hearing impairments.

Solutions for Persons With Hearing Impairments: The Windows Environment (Windows Vista)
To enable people with hearing impairments to receive notifications for system sounds *visually* rather than *audibly*, the clinician can select "Turn on visual notifications for sounds (Sound Sentry)" and then choose the visual warnings needed. (Make Windows XP More Accessible for Everyone. Retrieved June 8, 2009, from Microsoft Web site: http://www.microsoft.com/windowsxp/using/accessibility/default.mspx) Table 31.1 outlines more detailed instructions for activating visual warnings in the Windows Vista operating system.

Apple has also made provisions in its operating system that cater to hearing and visually impaired persons. Since Mac computers tend to be most prevalent in educational institutions, this section is especially important for physicians who encounter children and college students with the aforementioned disabilities. It is important to stress the importance of both operating systems and the intricacies of each so that physicians can choose the right match for a particular person. For example, someone who is deaf–blind will need different provisions than someone who is only deaf and can benefit from visual notifications as described below.

TABLE 31.1 *Solutions for Persons With Hearing Impairments: The Windows Environment (Windows Vista)*

	Mouse Actions	Keyboard Actions
1.	To open the **Ease of Access Center**, select: **Start.** **Control Panel.** **Ease of Access.** **Ease of Access Center.**	To open the **Ease of Access Center**, press: Windows logo key+U.
2.	Under **Explore all settings**, select: **Use text or visual alternatives for sounds.**	Under **Explore all settings**, select: **Use text or visual alternatives for sounds** by pressing TAB, and then ENTER.
3.	Under **Use visual cues instead of sounds**, select: **Turn on visual notifications for sounds (Sound Sentry).**	Under **Use visual cues instead of sounds**, select: **Turn on visual notifications for sounds (Sound Sentry)** by pressing ALT+R.
4.	Under **Choose visual warning**, select one of the following options: **None.** **Flash active caption bar.** **Flash active window.** **Flash desktop.** Select **Save.**	Under **Choose visual warning**, select one of the following options: **None** by pressing ALT+N. **Flash active caption bar** by pressing ALT+B. **Flash active window** by pressing ALT+W. **Flash desktop** by pressing ALT+K. Select **Save** by pressing ALT+S.

Make Windows XP More Accessible for Everyone. Retrieved June 8, 2009, Web site: http://www.microsoft.com/windowsxp/using/accessibility/default.mspx

Solutions for Persons With Hearing Impairments: The Apple OS (Leopard) Environment

Mac OS X v10.5 Leopard provides a variety of features designed to assist those who have difficulty hearing computer speech or discerning sounds. Within the employment setting, this is an important accessibility feature, enabling a deaf or hearing-impaired employee to accomplish occupational tasks such as hearing an incoming e-mail alert.

VISUAL ALERT FEATURES. This application within Apple OS (Leopard) enables the computer user to see a flashing screen cue when an alert sound is heard. Growl is a notification system for Mac OS X which enables applications that support Growl to send the deaf user notifications via e-mail or visual prompt. Notifications are a way for Apple applications to provide the deaf or hearing-impaired user with new information, in written hearing impairment–friendly format, without the hearing-impaired user having to switch applications. Growl notifications can be configured to appear as spoken notifications (useful to blind users) and e-mail messages or can be viewed on the screen with or without accompanying sound effects (the most common configuration; Buchanan, 2008).

iCHAT. For deaf employees in the workplace, several AT solutions address the need for multiple means of communication. For example, iChat is an Internet-based text, audio, and video chat application that enables employees to communicate with each other. iChat can be used with existing chat programs such as AIM (the largest instant messaging community in the United States), MobileMe, Google Talk, and Jabber. Utilizing iChat, employees can communicate with fellow employees on either Mac or Windows PC through text, audio, or video chats.

Although iChat has been available on earlier versions of Mac OS, the Mac OS X Leopard version includes a number of enhanced text messaging features including the ability to log into multiple services simultaneously, manage multiple chats using tabs in a single window, forward short messaging service (SMS) messages, and transfer files to a buddy during a chat session.

iChat incorporates a high-quality video frame rate, which optimizes communication for employees using sign language. It is also a helpful utility for hands-on video relay service at HOVRS.com. The finger and hand movements of others taking part in the chat can be readily seen.

CLOSED CAPTIONING. Within the Apple OS, deaf or hearing-impaired persons can set QuickTime player and DVD player to display open and closed captioning. The clinician can help his/her patient by activating the captions feature in the system preferences or the application preferences, then have them displayed onscreen.

Module 4: AT for Motor- and Dexterity-Impaired Patients

Although voice-recognition technology is often useful in helping motor- and dexterity-impaired patients meet their needs, many of these patients prefer to use whatever residual dexterity and motor functioning they have. Patients with quadriplegia, stroke, amyotrophic lateral sclerosis, amputations, or cerebral palsy can benefit from using environmental control units (ECUs), which can be defined as "various apparatus for disabled persons that control devices such as lamps, television, radio, telephone, and alarm systems. Similar to television remote control devices, they are typically switches manipulated by the lips, chin, or other body movements" (The Free Dictionary by Farlex. Retrieved June 8, 2009, from The Free Dictionary by Farlex Web site: http://medical-dictionary.thefreedictionary.com/environmental+control+units). Examples of such ECUs include doors equipped with electronic openers, electronic locks, coffee makers, lights, call buttons, and TV sets controlled by switch control. While most of these ECUs are typically used in the home setting, workplaces can also be ergonomically configured to optimize access by motor- and dexterity-impaired people (Guide for Individuals with Dexterity and Mobility Impairments, June 4, 2009. Retrieved June 8, 2009, from Microsoft Web site: http://www.microsoft.com/enable/guides/dexterity.aspx).

An estimated one in four adult computer users in the United States has impairment in dexterity. Dexterity impairment and difficulty with coordination are caused by a number of neurological and musculoskeletal conditions, including stroke, carpal tunnel syndrome, arthritis, cerebral palsy, Parkinson's disease, multiple sclerosis, loss of limbs or digits, spinal cord injuries, and repetitive stress injury, among others. The textbook by Sears and Young (2003) comprehensively surveys health conditions that induce impairments affecting computer use.

A new and evolving generation of AT has facilitated the use of computers by people with motor or dexterity impairments. A Microsoft Web site (www.microsoft.com/enable/guides/dexterity.aspx) summarizes resources available to dexterity-impaired people. Computer access can be optimized by simple switch access or by using an on-screen keyboard. For people without any use of the hands, hands-free devices, such as a chin mouse, a headset that generates a radio signal, an eye-gaze unit, or a mouth stick are viable alternatives to a single switch.

People with motor or dexterity impairments often encounter difficulty using standard "hands-on" input items such as the keyboard, mouse, or track pad. Several hardware and software alternatives or enhancements are available. Word prediction software improves typing accuracy and limits keystroke errors by guessing the next word and presenting a list of alternatives. Input items are available in different sizes. Speech recognition systems have users issue commands and enter data by voice instead of using an input device. On-screen keyboard programs provide an image of a standard or modified keyboard on the computer screen. The user selects the keys with a mouse, touch screen, trackball, joystick, switch, or electronic pointing device that allows the user to control their computer entirely with a keyboard. Keyboard filters include typing aids such as word prediction utilities and add-on spelling checkers. This technology reduces the minimum number of keystrokes and enables users to quickly access letters and to avoid selecting the wrong keys.

Touch screens are devices placed on the computer monitor (or built into it) that allow direct selection or activation of the computer by touching the screen and completely eliminate the need for a mouse (for a comparison of hands-on vs. hands-free modes of computer-related AT for people with motor problems, see Table 31.2).

Software-Based (Operating System) Adaptations

In addition to input devices, there are various software-based adaptations to help people with motor impairments operate computers more easily. For instance, the Microsoft filter key feature blocks repeated keystrokes, ignores rapid or extraneous keystrokes, and slows down repeated key rates. This enables quick access to letters and helps users avoid inadvertently selecting the wrong keys. The filter key feature can help patients suffering from chronic neurological disorders such as Parkinsonism or other condition that manifest symptoms such as tremors, stiffness, and poor coordination. For many with poor motor coordination, there is a frame that fits over the keyboard and helps reduce errant keystrokes.

Spelling-Prediction Software

In spelling-prediction software, as each key is typed, the list changes accordingly and predicts the current word (word completion) the user is trying to enter. The software also predicts the next word (word prediction) and offers abbreviation expansion and speech output. Spell check is another feature of spelling prediction software, reducing the number of keys typed and improving word accuracy.

Researchers are developing and testing a system that provides computer cursor control for individuals who are unable to use their hands. The system inputs consisted of electromyogram (EMG) signals from muscles in the face and point-of-gaze coordinates produced by an eye-gaze tracking (EGT) system. Each input is processed by an algorithm that produces its own cursor update information. These algorithm outputs were fused to produce an effective and efficient cursor control. Experiments were conducted to compare the performance of EMG/EGT, EGT-only, and mouse cursor controls. Results revealed that although EMG/EGT control was slower than EGT-only and mouse control, it effectively controlled the cursor without a spatial accuracy limitation. The system also facilitated a reliable click operation (Chin, Barreto, Cremades, & Adjouadi, 2008).

TABLE 31.2 *Hands-On vs. Hands-Free AT Input Modes*

Hands-On AT	Hands-Free AT
Keyboard	Sips and puffs
Mouse	Head movement
Joystick	Eye movement
Trackball	Touch screen
Touch pads	Foot movement
Touch screen	

NEW FRONTIERS IN AT: THE COMPUTER AND INTERNET REVOLUTION

This chapter would not be complete without a brief discussion of new frontiers and novel horizons in the field of AT. Undoubtedly, the emergence of new and unique computer, Internet, cyberspace technology, and program applications has revolutionized accessibility for people with all types of disabilities. For example, the role of Internet-based cognitive retraining programs designed to assist persons with brain injury has helped to streamline the rehabilitation process utilizing Internet messaging technology (Bergquist, Gehl, Lepore, Holzworth, & Beaulieu, 2008).

The use of computers and the Internet by persons with traumatic spinal cord injury is the subject of a large study involving 2,926 patients. Results revealed that 69% of participants with spinal cord injury used a computer and 94% of computer users accessed the Internet. Of the computer users, 19% used assistive devices for computer access. Among the Internet users, 69% went online 5–7 days/week. The most frequent use for Internet was e-mail (91%), followed by shopping sites (66%) and health sites (61%). There was no statistically significant difference in computer use by sex or by extent of neurological injury, and there was no difference in Internet use by extent of neurological injury. The highest computer and Internet access rates were seen among participants injured before the age of 18 (Goodman, Jette, Houlihan, & Williams, 2008).

With the maturation of cyberspace, cell phone technology, and the introduction of new services and innovative applications, many new programs and imaginative products originally intended for the general public have been serendipitously discovered by the disabled community and have proven to serve as a viable means of accommodation.

Recent notable examples include freely available programs such as Pinger, which allows voice-based text messaging from a cell phone. Composing a text message by voice may be of benefit for a person with a motor impairment involving the upper extremities; here, the text message is automatically transcribed and sent to a voice-selected e-mail recipient. Along with the text message, an option also exists for sending a voice file.

Cutting-edge research developments recently spawned the growth of a new generation of AT that successfully deploys robotics controlled by a neural-computer interface. Currently, neural interface systems (NISs), which are in an early stage of development, are emerging medical devices that enable people with paralysis and other motor disorders to deploy AT to reanimate muscles based on command signals directly from the brain (Donoghue, Black, Nurmikko, & Hochberg, 2007).

NISs represent a unique approach to restoring function and to managing nervous system disorders. They work by coupling the nervous system to a device that stimulates tissue in a closed loop (Donoghue, 2002). Examples of currently used NISs include cochlear implants for restoration of hearing and deep brain stimulators to attenuate tremor in patients with Parkinson's and other movement disorders. Motor cortex–based NISs that produce robotic motor movements in patients with tetraplegia and other paralytic states are in the early stages of development, which show tremendous promise as a new neurotechnology (Donoghue et al., 2006).

Twitter

Twitter is a freely available Internet-based social networking and microblogging service (text posts of fewer than 140 characters) that allows users to send and receive messages known as tweets. Like text messaging or SMS, Twitter enables people to stay in contact. Recent technological developments by researchers at the University of Wisconsin–Madison has extended the capabilities of Twitter and text messaging even further by the creation of a new Twitter interface device designed for people with disabilities who are unable to communicate or type (e.g., locked in syndrome). This enables such users to input information to a computer via a brain-monitoring cap, which receives brain messages (letters concentrated on or actions focused on) that in turn instructs the computer [for reference and demo, see Heasley (2009)]. Physiatrists can play an important role in caring for people with disabilities by identifying particular disabilities likely to benefit from AT. They can also forge collaborative partnerships with patients by assisting them in integrating AT into their lives.

CONCLUSION

The coming of the computer age and the marvelous and revolutionary array of Internet technologies have enabled persons with disabilities to optimize their quality of life through creative accommodation of disability (Young et al., 2000). While the practice of medicine and the domain of PM&R have traditionally emphasized healing and rehabilitation through physical modalities, exercise, pharmacological modulation, and psychological intervention, the rehabilitation process often requires another critical yet overlooked component—evaluation for and provision of assistive technology. Assistive technology has been aptly dubbed a "magical bridge" (NYU-Rusk Seminar on AT and the Ageing Workforce 2005) because it allows people with disabilities to traverse the barriers that separate them from their family, home environment, and workplace.

This chapter has attempted to provide a comprehensive overview of available and emerging technologies that provide persons with disabilities the opportunity to further their rehabilitation process through accessibility and accommodation. By focusing on four fundamental categories of impairment likely to benefit from AT (hearing, visual, hearing and visual, and motor and dexterity), this chapter provides a broad framework for understanding the barriers faced by persons with disabilities and the proposed technological solutions. In addition, specific software, hardware, and Internet-based solutions are proposed to provide the practitioner and patient with specific "fixes." As Sigmund Freud proclaimed, "The two most important tasks in life are to love and to work." AT has the potential to help disabled people do both by providing an important framework for enablement.

ACKNOWLEDGMENT

The authors acknowledge the help and support of Michael J. Young of the University of Maryland Baltimore County, who assisted by providing valuable information relating to emerging computer and Internet technologies for people with disabilities.

The authors also wish to acknowledge the editing contributions of Amy Morgan, a History of Science, Medicine and Technology major and Theater Arts and Studies minor at The Johns Hopkins University in Baltimore, Maryland.

REFERENCES

Assistive Technology Act of 1998. (1998). Retrieved March 15, 2009 from http://www.section508.gov/docs/AT1998.html

Bergquist, T., Gehl, C., Lepore, S., Holzworth, N., & Beaulieu, W. (2008). Internet-based cognitive rehabilitation in individuals with acquired brain injury: A pilot feasibility study. *Brain Injury, 22,* 891–897.

Boninger, M. L., Choi, H., Johnson, K., Young, M. A., Steins, S. A., & Sears, A. (2008). Assistive technologies: Catalysts for adaptive function. In B. O'Young, M. Young, & S. Stiens (Eds.), *Physical medicine & rehabilitation secrets* (3rd ed., pp. 201–206). Philadelphia, PA: Mosby Elsevier.

Buchanan, R. (2008). *Growl—Useful notifications that you control.* Retrieved April 27, 2009, from http://atmac.org/growl-useful-notifications-that-you-control/

Chin, C. A., Barreto, A., Cremades, J. G., & Adjouadi, M. (2008). Integrated electromyogram and eye-gaze tracking cursor control system for computer users with motor disabilities. *Journal of Rehabilitation Research and Development, 45,* 161–174.

Coughlan, J., & Manduchi, R. (2007, April). Functional assessment of a camera phone-based wayfinding system operated by blind users. In *Conference of IEEE Computer Society and the Biological and Artificial Intelligence Society (IEEE-BAIS)*. Research on Assistive Technologies Symposium (RAT '07), Dayton, Ohio, USA.

Donoghue, J. P. (2002). Connecting cortex to machines: Recent advances in brain interfaces. *Nature Neuroscience, 5*, 1085–1088.

Donoghue, J. P., Black, M., Nurmikko, A., & Hochberg, L. R. (2007). Assistive technology and robotic control using MI ensemble-based neural interface systems in humans with tetraplegia. *Journal of Physiology, 569*, 603–611.

Donoghue, J. P., Friehs, G. M., Caplan, A. H., Stein, J., Mukand, J. A., Chen, D., et al. (2006). BrainGate neuromotor prosthesis: First experience by a person with brainstem stroke. *Society for Neuroscience Abstracts,* 256.10.

Fellbaum, K., & Koroupetroglou, G. (2008). Principles of electronic speech processing with applications for people with disabilities. *Technology and Disability, 20*, 55–85.

Gerard, D. (2001). *What is assistive technology*. Retrieved March 13, 2009, from http://www.rehabtool.com/forum/discussions/1.html

Goodman, N., Jette, A. M., Houlihan, B., & Williams, S. (2008). Computer and Internet use by persons after traumatic spinal cord injury. *Archives of Physical Medicine and Rehabilitation, 89*, 1492–1498.

Guyer, C., & Uzeta, M. (2009). Assistive technology obligations for postsecondary education institutions. *Journal of Access Services, 6*, 12–35. Retrieved May 14, 2009, from http://www.informaworld.com/10.1080/15367960802286120

Hamlin, L. (2008). National update: Equal access to technology for people with hearing and vision loss. *Hearing Loss, 29*, 24–26.

Heasley, S. (2009). *Disability scoop: Twittering for those who can't talk or type*. Retrieved May 15, 2009, from http://www.disabilityscoop.com/2009/04/23/brain-twitter/2989/

International Neurorehabilitation Symposium 2009. (2009). Retrieved April 20, 2009, from http://www.inrs2009.com/

Internet World Stats. (2009). Retrieved March 4, 2009, from http://www.internetworldstats.com/am/us.htm

National Council on Disability. (1993). *Study on the financing of assistive technology devices and services for individuals with disabilities: Report to the President and the Congress of the United States,* Washington, DC.

Ross, M. (2008a). Bluetooth and hearing aids: Ready for prime time? *Hearing Loss Magazine, 29*, 28–30.

Ross, M. (2008b). What did you expect? Hearing aids—expectation and aural rehabilitation. *Hearing Loss, 29*, 20–24.

Santiago-Pintor, J., Hernández-Maldonado, M., Correa-Colón, A., & Méndez-Fernández, H. L. (2009). Assistive technology: A health care reform for people with disabilities. *Puerto Rico Health Sciences Journal, 28*, 44–47.

Sears, A., & Young, M. (2003). *Physical disabilities and computing technologies: An analysis of impairments.* Hillsdale, NJ: L. Erlbaum Associates.

Stiens, S. A. (1998). Personhood, disablement, and mobility technology. In D. B. Gray, L. A. Quatrano, & M. Lieberman (Eds.), *Designing & using AT: The human perspective* (pp. 29–49). Towson, MD: Paul Brookes.

The Radicati Group, Inc. (2009). Retrieved March 5, 2009, from http://www.radicati.com/

U.S. Department of Health & Human Services. (2009). *Office on disability*. Retrieved March 20, 2009, from http://www.hhs.gov/od/

Wireless RERC. (2009). *Wireless RERC: Consumer advisor newsletter: First quarter, 2009*. Retrieved April 27, 2009, from http://www.wirelessrerc.org/publications/consumer-advisory-newsletter-can/consumer-advisory-network-newsletter-q1–2008-pdf/

Young, M. A., Desai, M., & Young, M. J. (2009, March). *ADVANCE for Directors in Rehabilitation.* pp. 29–31.

Young, M. A., Tumanon, R. C., & Sokal, J. O. (2000). Independence for people with disabilities: A physician's primer on assistive technology. *Maryland Medical Journal, 1*, 28–32.

Zaretsky, H., Young, M. A., Lee, M. H. M., Crounse, B., & Stiens, S. (2005, July). *Proceedings of "Technology & Innovations for a Healthy Workforce."* New York: *New York University/Rusk Institute.*

32

Trends in Medical Rehabilitation Delivery and Payment Systems

Mary C. Ellis, PT, and Kristofer J. Hagglund, PhD, ABPP

Over the past 20 years, the U.S. health care system has been buffeted by explosive growth in utilization and costs of health care services. Both private and public payers have implemented a variety of controls on service and payment systems to slow the growth of spending. The changes in reimbursement systems have not always succeeded in reducing spending, but they have contributed to changes in the delivery of health care. Medical rehabilitation was initially protected from cost-containment forces, but it has been undergoing significant transformation over the past 5 years. This chapter focuses on the current status and trends in the payment and delivery of medical rehabilitation services in the United States.

Rehabilitation care is evolving within the larger and complex health care system that continues to be shaped by changing demographics and economic forces. A principal characteristic of the changing health care landscape is the rapid rise in costs. The average annual per capita cost of health care in 1965 was $202, and total health costs consumed 5.7% of the U.S. gross domestic product (GDP). In 2002, the cost was $5,440, and total health costs consumed 14.9% of the GDP or nearly 15 cents of every dollar spent in the United States (Levit, Smith, Cowan, Sensenig, & Catlin, 2003). In 2009, health care expenditures approached 2.5 trillion dollars or 17.6% of the GDP. By 2018, the United States is on track to spend 4.4 trillion dollars on health care, which is more than double the spending in 2007. This growth in the proportion of the GDP consumed by health care has alarmed citizens, employers, providers, and government policy makers. Growth in overall health care expenditures has been reflected in the growth of the rehabilitation field. For example, the number of freestanding rehabilitation hospitals increased from 68 in 1965 (Frederickson & Cannon, 1995) to 216 in 2002 (U.S. Department of Health and Human Services [HHS], 2003). By 2006, there were 217 freestanding inpatient rehabilitation hospitals (MedPac, 2007). There were 936 rehabilitation units within health care facilities in 2003 (HHS, 2003), which grew to 1,010 units by 2006. The number of skilled nursing facilities (SNFs) increased from 8,200 in 1989 (Frederickson & Cannon, 1995) to 14,755 in 2001 (HHS) to 15,600 in 2006 (MedPac, 2007). In 2007, the number of SNFs and inpatient rehabilitation facilities (IRFs) decreased slightly (MedPac, 2008).

Various factors have contributed to the tremendous growth in rehabilitation services. Advances in medical care have allowed more people to survive disabling conditions, thus increasing demand for services over longer periods of time. Buchanan, Rumpel, and Hoenig (1996) described an additional dynamic. They found that among Medicare recipients, growth in outpatient services from 1987 to 1990 was related to the availability of reimbursable services.

Their analysis suggested that this growth was more highly attributable to good reimbursement to providers for their services and to provider decision making, than to changes in demographics. Findings such as these were largely responsible for prompting the federal government (through Medicare) and private insurers to implement the substantial changes in service and payment systems described in this chapter.

CONTINUUM OF REHABILITATION CARE

Inpatient Care

Medical rehabilitation services are delivered in a variety of settings, including intensive or critical care units, acute hospital units, inpatient rehabilitation programs, outpatient clinics, subacute rehabilitation, and home care. By far, the most common entry point for patients into the rehabilitation settings is from acute inpatient medical settings. A report to the assistant secretary of HHS for Planning and Evaluation documented that

> over a third (35.2 percent) of all beneficiaries discharged from acute hospitals go on to use other services. Of those who do, almost 80.0 percent are discharged to either skilled nursing facilities (SNF, 41.1 percent) or sent home with home health services (HHA, 37.4 percent). Another 9.0 percent are discharged to outpatient therapy services (OP). The remaining 10–12.0 percent are leaving the hospital for continued services at a specialized hospital, such as an acute-level inpatient rehabilitation facility (IRF, 10.3 percent) or long term care hospital (LTCH, 2.0 percent).

Patients sometimes receive rehabilitation services from part or all of the rehabilitation team when they are in an intensive care or acute medical unit. If they transfer to a comprehensive medical rehabilitation unit or facility, the services consume significant portions of the patients' days. In the case of Medicare and most other patients, this constitutes a minimum of 3 hours per day, because of insurer participation requirements. Typically, the interdisciplinary rehabilitation team will meet weekly in patient care conferences to discuss each patient's individualized plan of care and progress toward discharge goals and to address barriers to discharge, treatment strategies, and discharge plans, ensuring that services are delivered in a coordinated and efficient fashion.

In the summer and fall of 2009, regulatory changes in the form of the IRF Final Rule followed by Transmittal 112, Medicare Benefit Policy on Coverage of Inpatient Rehabilitation Services introduced much more specific regulations and instructions to IRFs. In the August 7, 2009, Federal Register, the IRF final rule for fiscal year (FY) 2010 was published. The final rule adopted substantial changes to the existing regulations on IRF admissions, patient screenings, and related criteria. Under the FY 2010 Final Rule, IRFs receive a market basket update of 2.5%, resulting in an overall increase of $145 million in Medicare payment in FY 2010. The Benefit Manual provides specific instructions that describe coverage for inpatient rehabilitation services provided in IRFs. Under the new coverage policy, the decision to admit the patient to the IRF is the key to determining whether the admission is reasonable and necessary. The revisions are extensive, particularly regarding documentation of the need for inpatient rehabilitation services as well as hours and types of therapy. Effective with IRF discharges on and after January 1, 2010, contractors must use these updated coverage policies in medical review of IRF claims.

Although the demand for inpatient rehabilitation services has remained strong, cost-containment efforts by the Centers for Medicare and Medicaid Services (CMS), Medicaid, and private insurers have put pressure on providers to reduce the length of rehabilitation hospitalization. This has created an increased need for rehabilitation services following hospital discharge and has been one reason for an increase in growth of subacute rehabilitation programs (Chan & Ciol, 2000) home-care services, and outpatient programs.

Subacute Rehabilitation, SNFs, and Residential Programs

Patients who can be safely discharged from the hospital but are not ready to return home may go to a subacute program, which is often a part of an SNF (CMS, 2002). Alternatively, they may go to a regular nursing unit at an SNF or be admitted to a residential treatment program (sometimes licensed as an adult foster-care facility). Medicare recipients were more than twice as likely to be admitted to an SNF in 1999 than in 1994 (CMS). Careful consideration of potential medical risks and patient safety in posthospital placement decisions is an important part of discharge planning (Wright, Rao, Smith, & Harvey, 1996).

The least restrictive types of residential care are supervised living situations, where a person may live in an apartment alone or with a roommate. These persons live in the community but require some assistance or supervision by a rehabilitation provider or other provider, who may have contact with them once or several times a day. A new and growing living option, especially for the elderly, is an assistive living facility (sometimes licensed as a home for the aged). Individuals usually live in apartment-like accommodations with assistance in homemaking chores and the availability of some supervision and personal assistance. These facilities are not regular venues for the delivery of rehabilitation services, but they constitute a major growth market in housing options for elderly persons with disabilities who do not have significant nursing care needs. In 1999, 1.5% of Medicare beneficiaries were living in an assisted living setting (CMS, 2002).

Home Care

In the continuum of care, another increasingly utilized component of postacute care (PAC) is living at home with services provided either in an outpatient clinic or by home-care providers. These community-based services may include personal assistance services, skilled nursing, and/or other services, such as occupational or physical therapy. From 2004 to 2007, acute care discharges to home health care increased from 21% to 29%. This reflects a change in the application of the 75% rule which decreased admission of total joint replacement patients to IRFs and increased the care of total joint patients in the home health and SNF settings. Personal assistance services are often a critical part of home care for persons with severe disabilities. These services usually include help with activities of daily living (ADLs), such as eating, bathing, grooming, and mobility. The availability of personal care assistance has been shown to have a positive relationship with physical and mental health for persons with stroke, spinal cord injury (SCI), or traumatic brain injury. These providers are typically not professionals, although a small percentage of them complete certification programs. Family members often provide services. When only family members provide personal assistance, the interpersonal relationships may become strained or "distorted." Combining the assistance of unrelated persons with that of family members seems to be associated with the best health outcomes (Nosek, 1993). The need to improve funding for such services to avoid unnecessary institutionalization has been a major goal of public policy activism by consumer groups of disabled persons. The Medicaid Home and Community-Based Waiver programs offer, at a state level, services not otherwise covered under Medicaid to persons who otherwise would live in a nursing home. Services available under the waiver programs include respite care, home modifications, nonmedical transport, case management, and personal care assistance. There are significant waiting lists in some states for the waiver applicants.

Outpatient Care

Outpatient rehabilitation clinics may be hospital based, or freestanding clinics that are privately owned by the providers working in the clinic (e.g., private practice clinic), or owned by a hospital, health system, or corporation that specializes in providing rehabilitative care. Some clinics may contain just one rehabilitation discipline, such as psychology or physical therapy. Other clinics may provide a range of rehabilitative services. The Medicare designation for the latter is a Comprehensive Outpatient Rehabilitation Facility. These settings are appropriate for patients who no longer require the same level of physician and/or skilled nursing support available in a hospital but need extensive therapy to improve functioning. Some outpatient facilities may contain programs where patients receive a specialized, highly interdisciplinary and integrated care, such as day treatment. These patients may include those with spinal cord injuries, chronic musculoskeletal pain, traumatic brain injuries, stroke, work-related injuries, or those in need of vocational rehabilitation services. For those with work-related injuries or chronic musculoskeletal pain, the treatment venue may be the workplace, where individuals receive therapy guided by the rehabilitation staff to resume their previous job duties. In other cases, a periodic appointment with a single provider may meet the patient's needs.

Telehealth

With many rehabilitation centers and specialty programs residing in large metropolitan areas, and few programs in smaller cities and rural areas, accessibility to services remains a problem. The transmission of voice, data, and images using telecommunications techniques has given rise to increased opportunities for rehabilitation providers to offer some specialized information and services to remote locations, such as the offices of less specialized rural providers or the homes of rehabilitation or patients with disabilities. Important services may include training and counseling, monitoring and assessment of rehabilitation progress, monitoring wound healing, and therapeutic interventions. Various challenges remain to be overcome, such as reimbursement, licensing requirements in different states, privacy, and confidentiality, as well as improvement in the technology of the telecommunication devices. Telecommunication has the potential to augment care, as opposed to the view of it being a poor substitution for traditional care (Lathan, Kinsella, Rosen, Winters, & Trepagnier, 1999). Telehealth has begun to be used as a method for providing some rehabilitation services and education to persons with disabilities living in rural areas (Schopp, Johnstone, & Merveille, 2000).

INTERDISCIPLINARY REHABILITATION CARE

Patients receive services from a variety of therapists to diagnose, evaluate, and treat cognitive, behavioral, and physical functioning. The core rehabilitation team in the IRF setting typically includes a physician (often a physiatrist, who is a physician practicing the specialty of physical medicine and rehabilitation), rehabilitation psychologist or neuropsychologist, social worker, nurse, physical therapist, occupational therapist, and speech/language pathologist. Other professionals, such as case managers, orthotists, prosthetists, therapeutic recreation specialists, dietitians, rehabilitation engineers, chaplains, vocational rehabilitation counselors, and teachers, may supplement the team.

In some rehabilitation programs, a team that specializes in a particular diagnosis, such as SCI or brain injury, may treat the patient. An accreditation model of programmatic approach to patient care is the Commission on Accreditation of Rehabilitation Facilities (CARF). CARF provides field-based standards for accreditation of specialized rehabilitation programs, focused on the persons served (patient), quality, and outcomes. Specialized programs and teams have been shown to reduce length of stay (e.g., Tator, Duncan, Edmonds, Lapczak, & Andrews, 1993) with equal or better outcomes, presumably through greater efficiencies in patient care. The goal of therapeutic intervention is maximal independence and discharge to the "least restrictive," and usually least costly, environment. Rehabilitation has been quite successful in this endeavor. Using SCI as an example, a review of data collected from 1973 to 1996 reveals that 95.3% of individuals reside in private residences in the community following discharge and only 4.3% of persons with SCI are transferred to nursing homes. Recently, there has been a rise in discharge of spinal cord injured patients to nursing homes, which may reflect both a change in case mix (older people or people on ventilators) and the trend for reducing the inpatient rehabilitation length of stay because of cost-containment considerations (DeVivo, 1999).

Technological aides that can assist persons with disability are a promising and increasingly important component of rehabilitative care (Symington, 1994). Rehabilitation engineers may be involved in the evaluation and consideration of more elaborate, specialized equipment, such as environmental control units, computer systems, power mobility devices, and seating/positioning devices that are customized to meet a particular patient's needs. Funding to purchase the more advanced assistive technology remains out of reach of many consumers. One frequently accessed resource is state vocational rehabilitation agencies, when assistive technology is part of the plan to return to work. Usage of more simple assistive technology, such as canes and walkers, results in fewer reported mobility difficulties in the disabled population (Agree, 1999). The Rehabilitation Engineering and Assistive Technology Society of North America (RESNA) is an association whose membership is multidisciplinary and international. As an organization, RESNA promotes research and development, education, advocacy, and the provision of assistive technology while at the same time supporting the individuals engaged in these activities. RESNA offers certification in the field of assistive technology as well as education and research opportunities in the field.

Over the past 20 years, rehabilitation case managers have become a more significant part of the rehabilitation team. The role of the case manager is often multifaceted and may be carried out by individuals with specific roles on the team, such as a physician, nurse, physical therapist, occupational therapist, psychologist, or social worker. In recent years, an individual who specializes in this activity and is not a direct treatment provider has often assumed this role. Most commonly, the rehabilitation provider and the patient's insurance company employ this person. These individuals, representing the provider and the insurance company, in partnership with the patient, clarify benefits and coordinate care provided by the team. Increasingly, case managers play a pivotal role in recommending, clarifying, and arranging for the provision of needed care for the patient through the rehabilitation continuum. Also, this person may provide the patient and team with information against the approval or payment of services. This decision may be based on lack of insurance coverage for benefits, lack of perceived need for the service, or the availability of a more cost-effective alternative. This role has sometimes led to friction between case managers and providers who see their professional judgment challenged, and with patients who resent being denied benefits to which they feel entitled.

Economic pressures have continued to mount for streamlining the rehabilitation team. Payers restrict the services and/or disciplines they will cover under benefits. Insurers restrict the number of days they will cover the inpatient rehabilitation setting. This effort is taking several forms. Because of lack of coverage by payers, for example, many rehabilitation hospitals no longer provide recreation therapy by a licensed recreation therapist.

Another form of severe economic pressure for Medicare providers is in the form of Recovery Audit Contractor (RAC) audits. Section 302 of the Tax Relief and Health Care Act of 2006 makes the RAC program permanent and requires the Secretary to expand the program to all 50 states by no later than 2010. By 2010, CMS plans to have four RACs in place. Each RAC will be responsible for identifying overpayment and underpayments in approximately one-fourth of the country. In the demonstration project, the RACs resulted in more than $900 million in overpayments being returned to the Medicare Trust Fund between 2005 and 2008 and nearly $38 million in underpayments returned to health care providers. The RACs will be paid on a contingency fee basis on both the overpayments and underpayments they find RAC audits are a significant expense for providers of rehabilitation services, including preparation time for the auditors and personnel, legal, and court fees. Many RAC findings for overpayments returned to Medicare have been overturned when providers take the case to the Administrative Law judge.

FUNDING SOURCES FOR MEDICAL REHABILITATION

Private Payers

Employers pay for or subsidize health care coverage for the majority of working Americans and their families. Over the last 2 decades, enrollment in managed care insurance plans has increased dramatically to approximately 95% of workers with health insurance (Henry J. Kaiser Family Foundation, 2004a). The most common types of managed care plans are health maintenance organizations (HMOs), preferred provider organizations (PPOs), and point-of-service plans (POSs). Although thorough descriptions of these types of managed care plans are beyond the scope of this chapter, the following summarizes the key differences between these plans.

HMOs are the oldest type of managed care plan, the most famous of which is Kaiser Permanente. This HMO began its public operation in 1945 and now has 24% of all managed care enrollees (Henry J. Kaiser Family Foundation, 2004a). Traditional HMOs accept a capitation payment from the employer (or other payer) to deliver all the care necessary for its employees and their covered dependents. In a capitated contract, the HMO is paid a fixed sum of dollars for each member or enrollee of a plan, usually on a "per person per month" basis. The plan must meet the medical needs of all covered persons using the aggregate of this fixed dollar amount. Typically, each enrollee in an HMO selects a primary care provider, who coordinates all care and who authorizes all care that he or she does not provide, including specialty care, hospitalization, and so on. The HMO may directly employ all, some, or none of the health care providers on its panel. If they are not employees of the HMO, the providers will usually have a contract with the HMO to provide care and share in the financial risks associated with the provision of care.

PPOs are plans where a managed care organization (MCO) develops and contracts with groups of providers who agree to accept the plan's payment rates. The enrollee has a financial incentive to seek out the "preferred providers" because there may be no or lower copayments. PPOs do not always have an assigned/selected primary care provider who authorizes services. POSs have both preferred (or "in-network") providers and "out-of-network" providers. Usually, enrollees select or are assigned a primary care provider who coordinates and authorizes care (often including out-of-network services). Again, the enrollee has a financial incentive to seek "in-network" services because the payment coverage is better.

Government Programs

Publicly financed health care programs accounted for nearly 46% of total national health care expenditures in 2002 ($713.4 billion; Levit et al., 2003). Medicare and Medicaid account for most of this spending, much of it directed to rehabilitation and other services for the elderly and people with disabilities. Patient populations at some rehabilitation facilities are composed primarily of Medicare and Medicaid recipients. Since their inception, both Medicare and Medicaid expenditures have consistently outpaced the rate of inflation and the rate of growth in expenditures of private funds. Federal and state legislative bodies have acted to slow this rapid growth rate through regulatory legislation and by encouraging experimentation in health care delivery models (Levit, Lazenby, & Braden, 1998). Health care delivery is being rapidly converted from fee-for-service (FFS) reimbursement to managed care, especially capitated contracts with commercial MCOs.

Medicare

Title XVIII of the Social Security Act of 1965, otherwise known as Medicare, is the largest public payer of health care (Levit et al., 2003). Medicare is a social insurance program for persons older than 65 years and for people with disabilities who have a sufficient work history to qualify for Social Security Disability Insurance for 24 consecutive months. In 2003, approximately 15% of Medicare beneficiaries (6 million) had a disability and were younger than 65 years (Henry J. Kaiser Family Foundation, 2004b).

Part A of Medicare covers inpatient hospitalization, SNF care, home health care, and hospice care. Supplemental Medical Insurance (Part B) of Medicare is optional coverage that pays for physician and psychological services and other services such as durable medical equipment (DME), laboratory tests, medical supplies, and therapies (Hoffman, Klees, & Curtis, 2000). Contrary to popular belief, Medicare Part A expenditures are derived from mandatory payroll deductions from current wage earners. As health care costs rise and the population ages, Medicare Part A increasingly grows closer to financial insolvency. Depending on legislative action, Medicare Part A could exhaust its funds within the next few years. To slow down Medicare's cost inflation, federal legislation has encouraged experimental health care delivery programs and use of voluntary enrollment in managed care programs. The Medicare Part A Hospital Insurance Trust Fund has faced projected funding shortfalls throughout its history. The latest Trustees report projects that the Part A trust fund will be exhausted by 2017, unless Congress acts to slow spending or increase revenues. Medicare eligibility status is projected to grow from 42.5% in 2005 to 46.6% in 2010 (Kaiser Family Foundation, 2001–2007).

Medicaid

In 2010, Medicare is projected to be 13% of the total federal outlay, with Medicaid and the State Health Insurance Assistance Program projected at 13% of the total federal outlay.

Medicaid (Title XIX of the Social Security Act) is a jointly sponsored program between the federal government and the states/territories. Within broad federal guidelines, each state establishes its own eligibility guidelines, determines the type and amount of services, sets provider payment rates, and administers its own program (Hoffman et al., 2000). States receive matching funds from the federal government to help offset the costs of care. The matching formula is based on the per capita income of each state/territory. Medicaid is the largest purchaser of health care services for the neediest and poorest people in the United States. The recession that began in December of 2007 put significant pressure on Medicaid. Unemployment escalated from 4.9% in December 2007 to 9.7% in August 2009. As in the past recession of 2002, this created a dramatically higher demand for Medicaid funding in the face of severe state budget shortfalls. In 2002, Medicaid covered approximately 47 million individuals, and in 2009, because of the recession Medicaid covered 60 million people, making it the most significant component of the "safety net." The American Recovery and Reinvestment Act of 2009 provides financial support to the states to alleviate their need to cut Medicaid payments to providers, reduce benefits, and tighten eligibility for coverage. Despite this federal infusion of dollars, there have been provider payment cuts in many states which may reduce access through reduced incentive for provider participation. Total Medicaid spending growth averaged 7.9% across all states in fiscal year (FY) 2009, the highest rate of growth in 6 years and higher than the original projections of 5.8% growth.

Medicaid directors overwhelmingly attributed the growth to higher than expected increases in caseload due to the recession. Enrollment growth averaged 5.4% in FY 2009, significantly higher than the 3.6% enrollment growth projected at the start of FY 2009. For FY 2010, states projected that Medicaid enrollment growth would continue to accelerate, increasing on average by 6.6% over 2009 growth.

A significant portion of Medicaid beneficiaries have multiple disabilities, further complicating health care service delivery. Furthermore, the elderly or disabled with low incomes who are eligible for Medicare are also eligible for supplemental Medicaid coverage. In 2002, there were approximately 7 million people who were dually enrolled in Medicaid and Medicare. In 2005, this figure grew to 8.8 million. In this era of cost containment and experimentation with health care delivery, it is important to remember that people younger than 65 years with disabilities comprise 18% of the enrollees in Medicaid, but spending for this group accounted for 46% of the costs in 2005 (Henry J. Kaiser Family Foundation, 2004c).

Limitations of the Medicare and Medicaid System for Persons With Disabilities

Overall, Medicare and Medicaid are critical and effective sources of health care for persons with disabilities. However, there are limitations of these programs that often exacerbate the health problems of persons with disabilities. Low reimbursement rates, limitations in coverage, and poor coordination of services place people with disabilities in a confusing and unfriendly health care maze. Furthermore, many people with disabilities have concomitant psychological and social problems, including affective and anxiety disorders, substance abuse/dependence, and social isolation (see, e.g., Heinemann, Keen, Donohue, & Schnoll, 1988). For many, behavioral difficulties, such as poor adherence to treatment regimens, result in costly complications and secondary disabilities. These problems are exacerbated by low incomes, unemployment, and difficulties meeting everyday basic living needs (Blendon et al., 1993). Primary care needs of persons with disabilities are often specialized. Internists and family care physicians may not be trained to meet these specialized needs. However, under the Medicare and Medicaid programs, the primary care physician is most often the internist. Another significant limitation is coverage for DME including wheelchairs, assistive devices, and ADL equipment. The coverage is often restrictive and not individualized to meet the needs of persons. When psychological, social, and daily living needs go unmet, quality of life and medical status are worsened and health care costs are significantly increased (Friedman, Sobel, Myers, Caudill, & Benson, 1995). In addition, problems in obtaining health care worsen the health status and quality of life for persons with disabilities (Neri & Kroll, 2003).

As with Medicare, basic medical services are covered by Medicaid. The states, however, have wide discretion in providing "optional services," such as outpatient clinic services, diagnostic services, optometry, psychological care, rehabilitation, and physical therapy. These services are subject to cuts in times of recession and budget cuts. Also, similar to Medicare, FFS reimbursement is the traditional payment system in Medicaid. Medicaid costs have been rising dramatically over the last decade. State legislatures and governors, working with the federal government, have been rapidly converting their Medicaid systems from FFS to managed care. Both reimbursement/payment methodologies have created problems for obtaining health care for people with disabilities. The health care needs of people with disabilities, combined with the low reimbursement to providers from Medicaid, contribute to many providers "not accepting Medicaid patients."

Catastrophic Insurance

Little is known about how health care changes will affect the delivery of rehabilitation services paid for by other forms of disability insurance, such as no-fault automobile catastrophic insurance, long-term disability insurance, and workers' compensation. Workers' compensation is different from most health programs because it provides for income replacement for injured workers as well as medical care. The significant costs associated with these benefits have led to tremendous efforts to rehabilitate workers and return them to the job. Workers' compensation carriers have used medical case management for many years in an attempt to control excessive costs secondary to overutilization of services. Prolonged disability is responsible for the greatest costs and involves medical, psychological, and socioecological issues that are best addressed from a multidisciplinary team. It is not clear, however, how often a rehabilitation model has been used effectively for temporarily or permanently disabled workers despite its proven efficacy with some groups of disabled persons.

Over the last 2 decades, workers' compensation costs rapidly rose to become a substantial business expense. Dembe, Himmelstein, Stevens, and Beachler (1997) reported that workers' compensation costs rose 64% from 1984 to 1993, after adjusting for inflation, and made up 2.4% of the private sector payroll in 1991. Medical care costs overtook income replacement in total workers' compensation costs, something that had not happened in many years. Also, market competition among workers' compensation carriers, workers' demand for improved care, and employers' efforts to reduce costs and streamline administration have contributed to reform efforts. With these concerns in mind, more than 25 states began to enact legislation to reform workers' compensation, most of them authorizing or mandating managed care health delivery (Dembe et al., 1997). Also, efforts have increased to link workers' compensation and general health care to reduce administrative costs, control cost shifting, and increase coordination of care, financing, and administration (Dembe et al., 1997).

Only a few studies have examined either the short-term or long-term outcomes among people with disabilities using payer source, such as workers' compensation, as a variable. Tate and colleagues (1994), for example, examined the effects of payer type (Medicaid, catastrophic insurance, and private payer), extent of benefits, and independent living resources on functional, psychological, and social outcomes among 111 individuals with SCI. All participants were at least 2 years postdischarge from acute rehabilitation. Among the most significant findings was that people who had private insurance reported greater work and school activities compared with those with Medicaid or catastrophic no-fault insurance. Transportation benefits also were positively related to participation in work and school activities. Surprisingly, there was an inverse relationship between the extent of benefits and psychological and social outcome. The authors caution that the type of payment system and rules may foster dependency and poorer psychosocial outcome. Persons receiving catastrophic insurance benefits continually are forced to dramatize their needs to the insurance carrier or case manager to obtain benefits, sometimes creating a disincentive to increase independence. They suggested that a voucher system that allows personal choice of health care benefits might facilitate less dependency, improve psychological and social outcomes, and increase participation in functional activities, including work and school. The voucher system could be accompanied by an educational program to help individuals make choices of benefits that would maximize their independence and fit their unique situation.

FUNDING OF HEALTH CARE FOR CHILDREN WITH DISABILITIES

Approximately 5% of U.S. children and adolescents have a chronic health condition that interferes with one or more major life activities. Less than 1% of children have three or more chronic conditions, but developmental delays, learning disabilities, and emotional and behavioral problems are much more prevalent among this group of children with multiple chronic conditions (Newacheck & Stoddard, 1994). In general, children with chronic disabling conditions require coordinated specialized services, including occupational therapy, physical therapy, psychological and social services, speech and language therapy, and home care. As with adults, children with chronic disabling conditions are a relatively small percentage of all children, but they utilize a large percentage of health care services (Newacheck & Taylor, 1992). Medicaid covered approximately 2.1 million children with physical or mental disabilities and spent more than $20 billion on health care for these children in 2000. This represented approximately 12% of the total Medicaid expenditures for 4% of the Medicaid population (Crowley & Elias, 2003). Also, children with special health care needs (CSHCN) such as those with chronic disabling conditions receive services funded by Title V programs (Social Security Act), through the Bureau of Maternal and Child Health, state health care programs, and school systems.

In addition to federal and state funded health care programs, approximately 60% of children with chronic disabling conditions receive services funded by private insurance. Often, these policies have restrictions on the type and scope of services, especially ancillary services and home care (Shonkoff et al., 1994). Also, many of these plans have annual or lifetime caps on benefits and/or cover only part of the costs of health care services. The children receiving health care through Medicaid and private insurance are rapidly being enrolled into managed care programs. The implications of these changes have yet to be fully realized, but health care advocates of many children have expressed concerns similar to those stated about the limitations of managed care for adults with disabilities.

Research has revealed mixed results on the effects of managed care on the outcomes of children with chronic disabling conditions. For example, Horwitz and Stein (1990) compared benefits for a sample of HMOs with traditional indemnity insurers in Connecticut paying for services with children on a FFS basis. HMOs were found to offer more preventive care and increased access to care. However, both plans tended to have restrictions on services most commonly used by these children (mental health services and DME). Case managers from both plans focused more on controlling costs than coordinating care. The study concluded that neither organization offered a comprehensive system of care to CSHCN. Fox and Wicks (1993) conducted a cross-sectional survey of almost 700,000 children with disabilities due to chronic conditions. HMOs typically approved specialty care only when significant improvement could be documented within a short period of time. Other identified problems included difficulty accessing specialists, along with an insufficient number of specialists to provide consumer choice. Another survey (Fox, Wicks, & Newacheck, 1993) of state Medicaid offices documented that some HMOs were resistant to providing necessary mental health, speech, and occupational therapy services to CSHCN. For example, coordination of services for children at risk for serious emotional disturbance was hampered by the move toward managed care in one study (Hocutt, McKinney, & Montague, 2002). In general, it was found that managed care plans for CSHCN who were Medicaid recipients referred the children to adult subspecialists more often than pediatric subspecialists. Also, long-standing provider relationships were disrupted in the transition to managed care. Furthermore, more parents of these children were dissatisfied with managed care than with FFS Medicaid (Stroul, Pires, Armstrong, & Zaro, 2002).

State Children's Health Insurance Program

The State Children's Health Insurance Program, now known as CHIP codified as Title XXI of the Social Security Act, was enacted as part of the Balanced Budget Act of 1997. The purpose of this law was to extend insurance/health care to approximately 40% of the uninsured children in the United States. As a federal "grant-in-aid" program, this law encourages states to extend health care coverage either through Medicaid or through an alternative program to low-income, uninsured children. In return, the states may receive matching funds from the federal government. These programs increased the income threshold of eligibility for subsidized coverage to 214% of the federal policy level and insured 5.3 million children during FY 2002. In a sample of states, CHIP enrolled a higher percentage of CSHCN, including children with a high level of unmet heath care needs, compared with the general child population (Szilagyi et al., 2003). These investigators suggest that CHIP may need to consider a variety of financing mechanisms, including risk-adjustment funding strategies, high-risk pools, reinsurance mechanisms, and improved compensation for primary care practitioners, for case management of the severe CSHCN population within CHIP. Access to care under CHIP is generally described as good for those enrolled in urban areas with managed care arrangements (Wooldridge et al., 2003). An important regulation of CHIP for children with disabilities is that states may not deny enrollment or coverage because of preexisting conditions (Rosenbaum, Johnson, Sonosky, Markus, & DeGraw, 1998).

The Children's Health Insurance Program Reauthorization Act of 2009 (CHIPRA), enacted in February 2009 by President Obama, extends and expands the CHIP. CHIPRA requires states to include dental services (equivalent to benchmark packages) in CHIP plans. In addition, CHIPRA would allow states the option to provide dental-only supplemental coverage for children who otherwise qualify for a state's CHIP program but have other health insurance without dental benefits. The Act includes provisions related to the development and dissemination of dental education materials, data reporting on dental access and quality, and state requirements to post lists of participating dental providers. The Act also requires mental health parity for states that chose to include mental health or substance abuse services in their CHIP plans. CHIPRA includes provisions to reduce barriers to providing premium assistance.

CHIPRA establishes the Medicaid and CHIP Payment and Access Commission to review Medicaid and CHIP access payment policies and then submit reports and recommendations to Congress. CHIPRA includes $225 million over 5 years, child health quality initiatives including the development of quality measures and electronic health records. The Act also establishes demonstration programs to improve quality, combat obesity, and develop information technology. CHIPRA includes $20 million for the Census Bureau to improve state-specific estimates of children and requires a federal evaluation of the program.

MANAGED CARE FOR PERSONS WITH DISABILITIES

Theoretically, managed care has the potential to improve care for medically complex, high-cost populations, such as people with disabilities (Reilly, Coburn, & Kilbreth, 1990), by employing organized delivery systems that emphasize timely, comprehensive, and community-based services. MCOs have traditionally avoided complex, high-cost populations and, therefore, have limited experience in implementing effective programs.

Evaluation studies of managed care performance in the general population have focused on utilization of services and costs. Rarely are these measures of performance paired with analyses of the health status of the population. The results of the performance of managed care on health outcomes have been mixed, and there are virtually no data on functional health-related quality of life (Miller & Luft, 1994). This is particularly true of those with disabilities or chronic illness where there is a need for better outcome measures and evaluations that estimate the program effects (Ireys, Thornton, & McKay, 2002). Beatty and colleagues (2003) found few differences in access to care or outcomes across FFS or managed care payment systems for persons with arthritis, SCI, multiple sclerosis, or cerebral palsy.

The ability of a publicly funded managed care system in Tennessee to serve blind and disabled persons who receive Supplemental Security Income was examined (Hill & Wooldridge, 2003). They found that this disabled population had worse access to care (specialists, medication, and equipment) and less satisfaction with care compared with other managed care enrollees. Elderly Medicare managed-care enrollees were also less satisfied with access to specialists, but they were more satisfied with costs compared with non-managed care enrollees (Iezzoni, Davis, Soukup, & O'Day, 2002).

In another study, Medicare beneficiaries in poorest health or most severely disabled perceived both access to care and cost difficulties irrespective of whether they were in managed care plans or had traditional FFS Medicare coverage (Beatty & Dhont, 2001). A qualitative study examining health care of people with cerebral palsy, multiple sclerosis, or SCI found that a lack of disability-specific knowledge, limited provider time, and poor communication among providers were obstacles to care coordination that were generally equally prevalent between persons in managed care and FFSs health plans (Kroll & Neri, 2003). Porell and Miltiades (2001) found that Medicare managed care resulted in no adverse risk of decline in functional status in a large general population of Medicare recipients compared with FFS Medicare.

MANAGED CARE MODELS IN GOVERNMENT-FUNDED PROGRAMS

Both Medicaid and Medicare have been experimenting with health care delivery models that provide an alternative to the FFSs system. Medicaid's conversion to managed care has been much more rapid than that of Medicare. Additionally, the Medicare program is exclusively administered through the federal government, whereas Medicaid is essentially 56 separate programs. This creates numerous obstacles to developing and implementing model managed care programs for Medicare recipients with disabilities compared with Medicaid, where each state government has some latitude in experimenting with alternative delivery systems.

Although most states began converting FFS Medicaid to managed care with the use of a primary-care case-management model, there has been rapid growth in risk-based managed care contracting since 1994. In this situation, a Medicaid agency contracts with an MCO to provide an agreed-upon set of services in exchange for a preset capitated payment for the entire health care needs of a patient. Payment is not contingent on the level of service provided, unless special services or programs (e.g., transplant services) are exempted from the contract and paid by Medicaid on an FFS basis.

In many Medicaid programs, mental health services are also "carved out," creating a separate subcapitation despite the fact that most policy analysts recommend complete integration of mental health services. For rehabilitation clients, this can result in a subcontract with a separate set of mental health providers, who may not be a part of the rehabilitation team and may lack specialized knowledge of the role of the person's disability. Savings incurred by this integration are also not available for use to fund non-mental health care. Until such services are integrated, the false distinction between mind and body will be perpetuated, and health care delivery will continue to be uncoordinated and ineffective. Also, Medicaid plans often do not include people who receive both Medicare and Medicaid. The regulations of the two programs are often incompatible, thereby complicating the coordination of health care services and financing. States can apply for waivers to combine the funding streams of these two programs to develop innovative health care delivery programs. A successful example of a public private partnership is the Community Medical Alliance in Boston, Massachusetts, which has adapted principles of prepaid managed care. The Alliance developed a contract with Medicaid to care for people with physical disabilities as well as late-stage *acquired* immune deficiency syndrome (AIDS). Experience to date suggests that the flexibility of capitation can be used to substantially shift care from its usual hospital focus to clinicians in home and community settings, especially nurse practitioners, with a high degree of patient satisfaction and without apparent compromise in quality. Instead of limiting access, managed care can use prepayment to support early interventions, coordination, and the development of services specifically designed to meet the needs of the target population. The Community Health Alliance coordinates care through the nurse practitioner for services including medical, rehabilitation, and mental health services.

FOR-PROFIT VERSUS NOT-FOR-PROFIT SECTORS IN THE DELIVERY OF REHABILITATION CARE

Many rehabilitation clinics and hospital services are for-profit taxpaying businesses with accountability to owners/stockholders for profitability. This means that the less the income that is paid out for patient care and administrative expenses, the more money there is to invest in the growth of the company or to pay owners/stockholders. A study of the impact of ownership arrangements and profitability in outpatient physical therapy clinics found that clinics jointly owned by physicians and physical therapists saw patients for 39–45% more visits than in nonphysician-owned comprehensive rehabilitation facilities providing services, and concomitantly their revenue per patient was 30–40% higher (Mitchell & Scott, 1992). Furthermore, it appeared that unlicensed personnel in the physician-owned practices delivered more care. Such findings have contributed to the regulations limiting the practice of physician referrals to rehabilitation facilities that they own. A study of home health agencies found that care was four times more expensive in for-profit proprietary agencies than in public agencies (Williams, 1994). When comparisons were made between for-profit and not-for-profit rehabilitation hospitals, for-profit hospitals showed higher net revenue and profits and employed fewer people than did nonprofit hospitals (McCue & Thompson, 1995). A large part of the growth in outpatient programs has been by for-profit corporations. Clearly, these companies have recognized the potential for profit and growth.

Using 100% of Medicare claims data for 2002, 2003, and 2004, the Office of the Inspector General analyzed physicians' billing patterns for outpatient physical therapy. They concluded that CMS should consider revisions, clarifications, and further study of the "incident to" rule to ensure that Medicare beneficiaries are receiving skilled therapy services from appropriately trained and licensed staff and that the services meet professionally recognized standards of care. The "incident to" rule allows physicians to bill, at the full physician fee schedule rate, for physical therapy performed by any nonphysician staff if certain Medicare rules are met. Beginning June 2005, CMS mandated that medical professionals rendering physical therapy services under the "incident to" rule meet the same Medicare requirements delineated for qualified physical therapists with the exception of licensure.

Nonprofit entities do not pay corporate profits and do not answer to shareholders, but they still face pressures to hold down costs and realize a positive financial margin to reinvest in the company's future. Some health care systems are owned and operated by local or state governments or the federal government. These include city, county, or state health facilities and agencies as well as most public university medical centers. In addition, the military and veterans administration are one of the largest providers of rehabilitation services (Wilson & Kizer, 1997). The Veterans Administration Medical Center (VAMC) rehabilitation departments are particularly well known for work with military service veterans with stroke, SCI, and those with amputations. VAMCs offer comprehensive care including some options for care in nursing homes, residential placements, and home care. Coverage and benefits are dependent on several factors, including whether the health problem was incurred during or related to service in the military (i.e., service connected), and financial resources. The VAMCs and the Department of Defense (DoD) Hospitals have been severely stressed by the Iraq War. Under scrutiny from the public, the military, and the federal government, the VAMCs and DoD programs have undergone significant restructuring while developing and coordinating with services to ensure quality care for injured warriors.

SPECIFIC COST-CONTAINMENT STRATEGIES

Prospective Payment and Case Mix Groups

As mentioned earlier, much of the expansion in the continuum of rehabilitation care can be credited to a stable source of funding through Medicare and Medicaid. A decade ago, Medicare and Medicaid recipients comprised approximately half of patients seeking rehabilitation services (Aitchison, 1993). More recent statistics estimate that roughly 70% of all patients treated at IRFs are Medicare beneficiaries (CMS, 2004b). A second funding boon was the adoption of the Tax Equity and Fiscal Responsibility Act (TEFRA) in 1982, which allowed many rehabilitation hospitals and units to be reimbursed by Medicare based on the hospital's cost per discharge, rather than on what was considered a less lucrative prospective payment system (PPS) where facilities are reimbursed a predetermined fee for hospitalization based on the patient's diagnosis or diagnosis-related groups (DRGs).

Exemption from prospective payment for rehabilitation facilities was done because DRGs did not account well for the high variability in hospital resource utilization for rehabilitation patients. An analysis by Schneider, Cromwell, and McGuire (1993) found that TEFRA limits were insufficient to account for increases in costs of providing care by rehabilitation facilities. However, the TEFRA payment system also provided a financial incentive for rehabilitation hospitals to discharge patients quickly (Chan et al., 1997). The hospital could collect incentive payments from Medicare for reducing its per-patient charge compared with a "base year." This could be accomplished by reducing length of patient stay, which did occur, but has caused the number of discharges from rehabilitation hospitals to SNFs to increase 48% from 1992 to 1994 (Wynn). It also caused facilities to try to admit less complex and less severely disabled patients. In response to these issues, Congress passed a provision in the Balanced Budget Act of 1997 that mandated a revision for the entire PAC reimbursement system as a means of controlling costs (Cotterill & Gage, 2002). In the case of rehabilitation facilities, this mandated a change to a PPS, which was originally scheduled for implementation on October 1, 2000. Subsequent modification of the Act by the Balanced Budget Refinement Act of 1999 and the Benefits Improvement Act of 2000 resulted in final adoption of an IRF PPS effective January 1, 2002.

When ultimately adopted, the PPS reflected a significant sea change from the previous retrospectively based TEFRA system. The new reimbursement system avoided per-diem charges, mandating instead a diagnostic-specific flat rate based on anticipated resources required for provision of patient rehabilitation services. Reimbursement rates were established for Case Mix Groups (CMGs) based on the patient's clinical characteristics as derived from the 21 defined Rehabilitation Impairment Categories, motor and cognitive level of function as defined by the Functional Independence Measure (FIM), and the patient's age. This classification scheme yielded 95 CMG categories with five additional categories for special situations. An additional important feature of the total reimbursement schedule is a three-tiered adjustment for comorbidities. Specific comorbidities have been defined by the CMS and can be classified as high cost (tier 1), medium cost (tier 2), or low cost (tier 3). The level of comorbidity provides a weighted adjustment to the overall prospective reimbursement rate. The only other adjustments to this rate are designed to address variations in cost due to geographic location, percentage of low-income patients, and rural location (CMS, 2004b). Concern has also been expressed regarding the capacity of the new system to compensate appropriately for medically complex cases with higher acuity (Hoffman et al., 2003; Stineman, 2002). In general, IRF providers greeted the PPS with initial uneasiness. Most have faired well financially under the system (Schmelling, 2003), and the PPS is widely considered to be more equitable (Fowler, 2003).

An additional important goal for the PPS was to gather more and better information for purposes of improved future decision making relative to rates and desired treatment locations. As part of the new PPS, patients are classified using a standard data collection instrument titled the Inpatient Rehabilitation Facility—Patient Assessment Instrument or IRF-PAI. Based on the FIM, the IRF-PAI provides a uniform set of patient data regarding admission and discharge levels of functional independence (Carter, Relles, Ridgeway, & Rimes, 2003). The IRF-PAI classification provides a reasonably uniform measure of time and resources required for inpatient rehabilitation. It has been described as one of the best CMS-designed PPSs (Morrison, 2002). Beyond its utility as a classification measure, it provides a growing and comprehensive information base of standardized data for use in future decision-making.

The 75% Rule Update to the 60% Rule

The change to a PPS has indeed been a fundamental sea change in the character of reimbursement for IRFs. Yet, the long-standing "75% rule" represented perhaps a significantly greater threat to the capacity to provide patients with rehabilitation services as well as to the financial viability and ultimate survival of many inpatient facilities. As noted earlier, IRFs were exempted from participation in the earlier acute care PPS (DRGs) because of the high variability in the resources needed for inpatient rehabilitation. A higher intensity of IRF services also resulted in generally higher reimbursement rates. However, as a condition for classification as an IRF, the provider was required to demonstrate that 75% of patients treated at the facility came from 10 diagnostic groups: stroke, SCI, congenital deformity, amputation, major multiple trauma, fracture of the femur (hip fracture), brain injury, polyarthritis (including rheumatoid arthritis), specified neurological disorders, and burns (CMS, 2004b).

For a variety of reasons, the 75% rule was never consistently enforced. In particular, there has been considerable confusion regarding clear diagnostic classification, particularly for patients who undergo prosthetic joint replacement for severe arthritis (most frequently hips and knees). At question is whether individuals who have undergone such surgery still can be classified as experiencing arthritis in that joint. Also at question has been the adequacy of documentation of polyarthritis. Interestingly, it has been the improved quality of standardized data available from the IRF-PAI that has helped illuminate the inconsistencies in enforcement of this rule. According to CMS (2004b) estimates, only 13.35% of facilities were meeting the 75% rule. Nationally, only 50% of patients being served in the IRF setting fell into one of the 10 categories.

If the 75% rule were enforced in the current environment, the financial consequences for patients and IRF providers could be described as severe (American Medical Rehabilitation Providers Association, 2004). Failure to meet the 75% rule would result in reclassification of the facility as an acute care facility with reimbursement at the substantially lower inpatient PPS rate (CMS, 2004a). Given the significantly higher costs for the more intensive patient rehabilitation services (IPPS) and the significantly lower reimbursement rates in the IPPS, the consequences of such reclassification would be financially disastrous for an IRF. Enforcement of the 75% rule was slated for initiation on July 1, 2004. There were minor revisions to diagnostic categories that could be included under the 75% rule, and the rule was to be progressively phased in over 3 years with full implementation on July 1, 2007 (CMS). However, provisions in the Medicare, Medicaid, and SCHIP Extension Act of 2007 required CMS to set the compliance rate no higher than the 60% compliance rate that became effective for cost-reporting periods beginning on or after July 1, 2006. Furthermore, the statutory provisions also required CMS to continue the use of comorbidities (i.e., patient-specific conditions that are secondary to the patient's principal diagnosis) in addition to the patient's primary reason for being in the IRF in determining the IRF's compliance percentage under this rule.

Bundling Payment for PAC

Bundling, especially bundling acute and PAC into one payment, is seen as a way to make acute care hospitals more accountable for preventable readmissions and as a way to bring greater efficiencies and costs savings to an entire episode of care. In the Conference on Bundling Post-Acute Payment hosted by the Center for Post-Acute Studies, National Rehabilitation Hospital, and the School of Nursing and Health Studies, Georgetown University, in 2009, the building blocks and policy infrastructure needed for bundling for PAC were identified. A "menu" of policy choices that lie ahead were identified and summarized in the conference report. Currently, the financial incentives in PAC and acute care are contained within each setting, with the primary incentive to discharge a patient so that a new patient with a new payment may be admitted into the bed. In a bundling model, the incentive changes. Payments that have been provided to Medicare beneficiaries through the silos of acute care, inpatient acute rehab, home health, and subacute settings will, through proposed bundling policy, be disseminated through one provider with the incentive to provide quality outcomes within the bundled payment. It is argued that incentives within the silos of PAC will go away in bundling. Various trade associations continue to work with Congress, HHS, and acute, postacute and other health care organizations to develop consensus regarding bundling.

CARE Tool

The Deficit Reduction Act of 2005 directed CMS to develop a PAC Payment Reform Demonstration. This demonstration was to be in place in early 2008, with a report submitted to Congress in 2011. The goal of this initiative is to standardize patient assessment information from PAC settings and to use these data to guide payment policy in the Medicare program. This demonstration will provide standardized information on patient health and functional status, independent of PAC site of care, and examine resources and outcomes associated with treatment in each type of setting. Consistent case-mix data are needed to determine whether similar patients are treated in different settings. Similarly, good information on resource use within each setting is needed to understand differences in patient treatment and outcomes.

CMS has contracted with RTI International to carry out this mandate through several initiatives, including the following:

1. *Development of a standardized patient assessment tool* for use at acute hospital discharge and at PAC admission and discharge. This tool, the Continuity Assessment Record and Evaluation (CARE), will measure the health and functional status of Medicare acute discharges and measure changes in severity and other outcomes for Medicare PAC patients.
2. *Conduct a PAC payment reform demonstration* to examine differences in costs and outcomes for PAC patients of similar case mix who use different types of PAC providers. CMS recognizes the variation in local practice patterns and available services across the United States and will examine how different service compositions affect PAC costs and outcomes, all else equal.

CMS has also contracted with Northrop Grumman to establish a web application at CMS for providers to submit the patient assessment data.

Decreased Hospitalization

With the increased penetration of managed care and the specter of additional cost-containment methodologies, traditional, institutionally based rehabilitation is undergoing significant changes in service delivery. Already, lengths of stay have been severely shortened. From 1986 to 1992, rehabilitation inpatient days declined by 3–4 days, or about 15% of the total rehabilitation stay (Wolk & Blair, 1994). This has resulted in a shorter time to reach rehabilitation goals. At the same time, occupancy rates have shown only slight changes, reflecting the increased number of patients admitted to most IRFs even in the face of an increase in the number of inpatient programs. Decreased length of hospitalization has resulted in improved efficiency in the average patient's gains in functional status per week, with little negative effect on the total level of functional gains achieved during the rehabilitation stay during the 3-year period from 1990 to 1992 (Granger & Hamilton, 1994).

It can be anticipated that health care intensity and services will be tied to the reimbursement system that supports it. Cotterill and Gage (2002) noted that location for service provision (acute vs. acute rehab vs. SNF, etc.) tends to shift in response to reimbursement policies. As such, it is reasonable to assume that providers in all postacute settings will seek to provide services in the most efficient and financially viable manner. If the CMS reform goals are to reduce costs and tie medical care to the realities of cost, it is reasonable to expect that services will adhere to the laws of the marketplace (Banja & DeJong, 2000). Ultimately, the challenge will be one of balancing the financial decisions with the needs for socially responsible medical care.

CONSUMER PROTECTION/RIGHTS

Pay for Performance, Reporting Quality Measures

In the past, consumers have generally viewed their health provider as an advocate for their obtaining the best care possible. It has been understood by consumers that most providers were paid under a FFS arrangement, where the more service that they delivered, the more money they were paid, and that they profited from caring for the patient. There was little reason to doubt that the provider would order everything that was medically necessary for the patient's care. Furthermore, because the provider made the decisions regarding care, they were legally liable for mistakes in decision-making or service delivery. At times, this led to the provision of excessive care and unnecessary health care costs for payers.

Now, the concern is the opposite. In a prepaid or capitated system, the provider of services may receive a fixed amount based on diagnosis, or have decisions regarding the kind or amount of treatment reviewed by payers or based on guidelines determined by others. In these managed health plans, the provider may be subject to strong financial incentives to limit care or provide less expensive care. In this case, the health care consumer can be less certain regarding the degree to which a treatment decision is motivated more by cost savings than by optimal care. In a poll commissioned by the American Psychological Association, 81% of adults sampled were very concerned about changes in the health care system. Thirty-six percent indicated that their main concern was quality of care, 25% indicated that their concern was access or availability of care, and 21% were most concerned about cost (Newman, 1997). Nonelderly sick persons with managed health plans are significantly more likely than those with traditional FFS insurance to complain of problems obtaining treatment, diagnostic tests, and uncaring physicians (Donelan, Blendon, Benson, Leitman, & Taylor, 1996).

These concerns have led to state and federal legislative and regulatory initiatives to safeguard consumer rights in key aspects of health care. In his 1998 State of the Union Address to Congress, President Clinton stated that physicians and not health plan "accountants" should make medical decisions. He called on Congress to pass a Patients' Bill of Rights that includes many patient protections. As the century turned, there was considerable interest in a Patients' Bill of Rights. In fact, separate, though rather similar, "Patient Protection Acts" were passed in both the House and Senate. Provisions included guidelines for access to services, choice of providers, continuity of care, appeal processes, and external review, among others. The largest differences between the bills involved definitions of liability for decision-making by insurance plans. However, in the tragedy and aftermath of the World Trade Center attack on September 11, 2001, the Acts languished, as did almost all other legislation of the session. Although patient rights and responsibilities are defined to some extent by accrediting bodies such as the Joint Commission on Accreditation of Healthcare Organizations and CARF, further federal legislation has not been forthcoming.

Coalitions representing business and insurance interests assert that such regulation is not needed since the consumer is able to change health plans or providers if they are not satisfied with the care that they receive. In a perfect market system, this may be true, but this assertion ignores several important points. First, consumers may not always be able to judge when they are receiving inferior care, or be in a position to change health plans or providers when they experience poor care. Second, consumers who receive their health benefits through an employer may be at the mercy of limited options that the employer offers. Third, many persons receiving rehabilitative care require services that are very costly to managed health plans. Such plans may not have a financial incentive to keep such patients as part of their plan and actually benefit if such a patient chooses another health plan.

There has been long-standing concern about the lack of consumer ability to influence factors that would allow marketplace forces to operate in an efficient manner in health care (Bingaman, Frank, & Billy, 1993). Kuttner (1997) indicates that consumers lack the "symmetrical" market power with providers of health care that would allow self-correcting for exploitative practices. Various solutions to rectifying this inequity have been proposed. These include publication of "report cards" on health plans and hospitals. Another suggestion is to establish consumer councils elected by consumers who work with the managers of health care plans to improve service (Rodwin, 1997).

In addition, there has been significant legislation affecting the privacy of medical information. In 1996, President Clinton signed into law the Health Insurance Portability and Accountability Act (HIPAA) as a measure to protect health insurance coverage for workers and their families when they lose or change jobs. To accomplish this, HIPAA also required the establishment of standards for electronic data transfer and management, as well as the security and privacy of health information (CMS, 2002). The regulations were in many ways complex and far-reaching (Parver, 2001). Confusion was common following their implementation, though HIPAA was described by some commentators as manageable with knowledge, planning, and common sense (Murer, 2004).

THE FUTURE: A CONSUMER-DRIVEN SYSTEM OF HEALTH CARE

People with disabilities require health delivery systems designed specifically for their complex health care needs. As DeJong (1997) points out, people with disabilities have a "thinner margin of health" and need unique programs to engage in preventive and health maintenance practices. Also, they are more likely to acquire secondary conditions and have greater needs for access to specialists and ancillary services, such as DME and assistive technologies (DeJong). The field of rehabilitation is uniquely suited to the needs of people with disabilities because of its focus on long-term outcomes.

However, traditional rehabilitation needs to be restructured. Rehabilitation providers and institutions are beginning to consider delivering comprehensive services under capitated, full-risk payment systems. The implications of these changes for people with disabilities and for the provision of rehabilitation services are profound and not yet fully understood. Initial evidence suggests that managed health care models designed specifically to meet the highly variable and complex health care needs of people with disabilities can successfully enhance long-term outcome and be cost-effective. This requires understanding the long-term needs and costs of people with disabilities, and delivering rehabilitation services in a cost-efficient but high-quality manner.

Community-based programs emphasizing preventive and health-promotion intervention will be integral to high-quality care that maximizes long-term outcomes and cost control. Additionally, the independent living movement has become more sophisticated and is making headway in convincing policy makers that a consumer-driven health care system is not only appropriate to promote independent living but is likely to be cost-effective. For example, consumer-driven personal assistance programs are gaining popularity. A voucher system in which consumers exert greater control over where health care dollars are spent may be the next shift in reimbursement systems. This would force providers and MCOs to compete for limited dollars by improving services and emphasizing outcomes. Information and marketing will be a major component of health delivery systems, but it will need to be supported by research on the long-term success of interventions and organized delivery systems.

REFERENCES

Agree, E. (1999). The influence of personal care and assistive devices on the measurement of disability. *Social Science & Medicine, 48*, 427–443.

Aitchison, K. W. (1993). Rehabilitation at the crossroads: Financial and other considerations. *American Journal of Physical Medicine and Rehabilitation, 72*, 405–407.

American Medical Rehabilitation Providers Association (AMRPA). (2004, April 30). Statement of AMRPA. Real-time outcomes reports (news release).

Banja, J. D., & DeJong, G. (2000). The rehabilitation marketplace: Economics, values, and proposals for reform. *Archives of Physical Medicine and Rehabilitation, 81*, 233–240.

Beatty, P. W., & Dhont, K. R. (2001). Medicare health maintenance organizations and traditional coverage: Perspectives of health care among beneficiaries with disabilities. *Archives of Physical Medicine and Rehabilitation, 82*, 1009–1017.

Beatty, P. W., Hagglund, K. J., Neri, M. T., Dhont, K. R., Clark, M. J., & Hilton, S. A. (2003). Access to health care services among people with chronic or disabling conditions: Patterns and predictors. *Archives of Physical Medicine and Rehabilitation, 84*, 1417–1425.

Bingaman, J., Frank, R. G., & Billy, C. L. (1993). Combining a global health budget with a market-driven delivery system. Can it be done? *American Psychologist, 48*, 270–276.

Blendon, R. J., Donelan, K., Hill, C., Scheck, A., Carter, W., Beatrice, D., et al. (1993). Medicaid beneficiaries and health reform. *Health Affairs, 12,* 132–143.

Buchanan, J. L., Rumpel, J. D., & Hoenig, H. (1996). Changes for outpatient rehabilitation: Growth and differences in provider types. *Archives of Physical Medicine and Rehabilitation, 77,* 320–328.

Carter, G. M., Relles, D. A., Ridgeway, G. K., & Rimes, C. M. (2003). Measuring function for Medicare inpatient rehabilitation payment. *Health Care Financing Review, 24,* 25–44.

Centers for Medicare and Medicaid Services. (2002). Overview of the Medicare program. Retrieved from http://www.cms.hhs.gov

Centers for Medicare and Medicaid Services. (2004a). CMS announces changes in criteria for classifying inpatient rehabilitation facilities. *CMS News* (Press Release). Retrieved April 30, 2004, from http://www.cms.hhs.gov/ media/press/release.asp

Centers for Medicare and Medicaid Services. (2004b). *Changes to the criteria for being classified as an inpatient rehabilitation facility: Final rule.* Washington, DC: Author.

Center for Post-acute Studies. (2009). *Bundling payment for post-acute care: building blocks and policy options.* Washington, DC: National Rehabilitation Hospital. Available at www.postacuteconference.org

Chan, L., & Ciol, M. (2000). Medicare's payment system: Its effect on discharges to skilled nursing facilities from rehabilitation hospitals. *Archives of Physical Medicine and Rehabilitation, 81,* 715–719.

Chan, L., Koepsell, T. D., Deyo, R. A., Esselman, P. C., Haselkorn, J. K., Lowery, J. K., et al. (1997).The effects of Medicare's payment system for rehabilitation hospitals on length of stay, charges, and total payments. *New England Journal of Medicine, 337,* 978–985.

Cotterill, P. G., & Gage, B. J. (2002). Overview: Medicare post-acute care since the Balanced Budget Act of 1007. *Health Care Financing Review, 24,* 25–44.

Crowley, J. S., & Elias, R. (2003). *Medicaid's role for people with disabilities.* A report of the Kaiser Commission on Medicaid and the Uninsured. Retrieved from http://www.kff.org/medicaid

DeJong, G. (1997). Primary care for persons with disabilities. *American Journal of Physical Medicine and Rehabilitation, 76*(Suppl. 3), S2–S8.

Dembe, A. E., Himmelstein, J. S., Stevens, B. A., & Beachler, M. P. (1997). Improving workers' compensation health care. *Health Affairs, 16,* 253–257.

DeVivo, M. J. (1999). Discharge disposition from model spinal cord injury care system rehabilitation programs. *Archives of Physical Medicine and Rehabilitation, 80,* 785–790.

Donelan, K., Blendon, R. J., Benson, J., Leitman, R., & Taylor, H. (1996). All payer, single payer, managed care, no payer: Patients' perspectives in three nations. *Health Affairs, 15,* 254–265.

Fowler, F. J. (2003, August/September). Straight talk. *Rehab Management.*

Fox, H. B., & Wicks, L. B. (1993). Health maintenance organizations and children with special health needs: A suitable match? *American Journal of Diseases of Children, 147,* 546–552.

Fox, H. B., Wicks, L. B., & Newacheck, P. W. (1993). State Medicaid health maintenance organization policies and special needs children. *Health Care Financing Review, 15,* 25–37.

Frederickson, M., & Cannon, N. L. (1995). The role of the rehabilitation physician in the postacute continuum. *Archives of Physical Medicine and Rehabilitation, 66*(Suppl. 12), S5–S9.

Friedman, R., Sobel, D., Myers, P., Caudill, M., & Benson, H. (1995). Behavioral medicine, clinical health psychology, and cost offset. *Health Psychology, 14,* 509–518.

Granger, C. V., & Hamilton, B. B. (1994). The uniform data system for medical rehabilitation report of first admissions for 1992. *American Journal of Physical Medicine and Rehabilitation, 73,* 51–55.

Heinemann, A., Keen, M., Donohue, R., & Schnoll, S. (1988). Alcohol use in persons with recent spinal cord injuries. *Archives of Physical Medicine and Rehabilitation, 69,* 619–624.

Henry J. Kaiser Family Foundation. (2004a). *Trends and indicators in the changing health care marketplace, 2004 update.* Retrieved June 10, 2004, from http://www.kff.org/insurance/7031/ti2004–2–3.cfm

Henry J. Kaiser Family Foundation. (2004b). *Fact sheet: Medicare at a glance.* Retrieved June 10, http:// www.kff.org/medicare/loader.cfm?url=/commonspot/security/getfile.cfm&PageID=33319

Henry J. Kaiser Family Foundation. (2004c). *Fact sheet: Medicaid Program at a glance.* Retrieved June 10, 2004, from http://www.kff.org/medicaid/loader.cfm?url=/commonspot/security/getfile.cfm&PageID=30463

Hill, S. C., & Wooldridge, J. (2003). SSI enrollees' health care in TennCare. *Journal of Health Care for the Poor and Underserved, 14,* 229–243.

Hocutt, A. M., McKinney, J. D., & Montague, M. (2002). The impact of managed care on efforts to prevent development of serious emotional disturbance in young children. *Journal of Disability Policy Studies, 13,* 51–60.

Hoffman, E. D., Klees, B. S., & Curtis, C.A. (2000). Overview of the Medicare and Medicaid program. *Health Care Financing Review, Medicare and Medicaid Supplement,* 1–19.

Hoffman, J. M., Doctor, J. N., Chan, L., Whyte, J., Jha, A., & Dikmen, S. (2003). Potential impact of the new Medicare prospective payment system on reimbursement for traumatic brain injury inpatient rehabilitation. *Archives of Physical Medicine and Rehabilitation, 84*, 1165–1172.

Horwitz, S. M., & Stein, R. E. (1990). Health maintenance organizations versus indemnity insurance for children with chronic illness: Trading gaps in coverage. *American Journal of Diseases of Children, 144*, 581–586.

Iezzoni, L. I., Davis, R. B., Soukup, J., & O'Day, B. (2003). Satisfaction with quality and access to health care among people with disabling conditions. *International Journal for Quality in Health Care, 14*, 369–381.

Ireys, H. T., Thornton, C., & McKay, H. (2002). Medicaid managed care and working-age beneficiaries with disabilities and chronic illnesses. *Health Care Financing Review, 24*, 27–42.

Kroll, T., & Neri, M. T. (2003). Experiences with care co-ordination among people with cerebral palsy, multiple sclerosis, or spinal cord injury. *Disability & Rehabilitation, 25*, 1106–1114.

Kuttner, R. (1997). *Everything for sale: The virtue and limits of markets.* New York: Alfred A. Knopf.

Lathan, C., Kinsella, M. A., Rosen, M. J., Winters, J., & Trepagnier, C. (1999). Aspects of human factors engineering in home telemedicine and telerehabilitation systems. *Telemedicine Journal, 5*, 169–175.

Levit, K. R., Lazenby, H. C., & Braden, B. R. (1998). National health spending trends in 1996. *Health Affairs, 17*, 35–51.

Levit, K., Smith, C., Cowan, C., Sensenig, A., Catlin, A., & the Health Accounts Team (2003). Health spending rebound continues in 2002. *Health Affairs, 23*, 147–159.

Master, R, Dreyfus, T., Connors, S., Tobias, C., Zhou, Z., & Kronick, R. (1996 Spring). Medicaid Working Group, Boston, MA 02116, USA. The Community Medical Alliance: An integrated system of care in Greater Boston for people with severe disability and AIDS. *Managed Care Quarterly, 4*, 26–37.

McCue, M. J., & Thompson, J. M. (1995). The ownership difference in relative performance of rehabilitation specialty hospitals. *Archives of Physical Medicine and Rehabilitation, 76*, 413–418.

Miller, R., & Luft, H. (1994). Managed care plan performance since 1980: A literature analysis. *Journal of the American Medical Association, 271*, 1512–1519.

Mitchell, J. M., & Scott, E. (1992). Physician ownership of physical therapy services. Effects on charges, utilization, profits, and service characteristics. *Journal of the American Medical Association, 268*, 2055–2059.

Morrision, M. H. (2002, April). The positive spin. *Rehab Management, 24*, 26.

Murer, C. G. (2004, March). Trends and issues. *Rehab Management*, 46–48.

Neri, M. T., & Kroll, T. (2003). Understanding the consequences of access barriers to health care: Experiences of adults with disabilities. *Disability and Rehabilitation, 25*, 85–96.

Newacheck, P. W., & Stoddard, J. J. (1994). Prevalence and impact of multiple childhood chronic illnesses. *Journal of Pediatrics, 124*, 40–48.

Newacheck, P. W., & Taylor, W. R. (1992). Childhood chronic illness: Prevalence, severity, and impact. *American Journal of Public Health, 82*, 364–371.

Newman, R. (1997, March). *Keynote Address.* Paper presented at the meeting of the American Psychological Association State Leadership Conference, Washington, DC.

Nosek, M. A. (1993). Personal assistance: Its effect on the long-term health of a rehabilitation hospital population. *Archives of Physical Medicine and Rehabilitation, 74*, 127–132.

Parver, C. (2001, November). Protecting your patients and practice. *Rehab Management, 82*, 74–75.

Porell, F. W., & Miltiades, H. B. (2001). Disability outcomes of older Medicare HMO enrollees and fee-for-service Medicare beneficiaries. *Journal of the American Geriatrics Society, 49*, 615–631.

Reilly, P., Coburn, A. F., & Kilbreth, E. H. (1990). *Medicaid managed care: The state of the art.* Portland, ME: National Academy for State Health Policy.

Rodwin, M. A. (1997). The neglected remedy: Strengthening consumer voice in managed care. *The American Prospect, 34*, 45–50.

Rosenbaum, S., Johnson, K., Sonosky, C., Markus, A., & DeGraw, C. (1998). The children's hour: The State Children's Health Insurance Program. *Health Affairs, 17*, 75–89.

Schmelling, S. (2003, August/September). Trends and issues: Interview with Cherilyn G. Murer, JD, CRA. *Rehab Management.*

Schneider, J. E., Cromwell, J., & McGuire, T. P. (1993). Excluded facility financial status and options for payment system modification. *Health Care Financing Review, 15*, 7–30.

Schopp, L. H., Johnstone, B. R., & Merveille, O. C. (2000). Multidimensional tele-care strategies for rural residents with brain injury. *Journal of Telemedicine and Telecare, 6*(Suppl. 1), S146–S149.

Shonkoff, J., Sweeney, M., McManus, M., Corro, D., Skubel, E., & McPherson, M. (1994). *Meeting the needs of chronically disabled children in a changing health care system* (Issue Brief No. 651). Washington, DC: National Health Policy Forum, George Washington University.

Stineman, M. G. (2002). Prospective payment, prospective challenge. *Archives of Physical Medicine and Rehabilitation, 83,* 1802–1805.

Stroul, B. A., Pires, S. A., Armstrong, M. I., & Zaro, S. (2002). The impact of managed care on systems of care that serve children with serious emotional disturbances and their families. *Children's Services: Social Policy, Research, & Practice, 5,* 21–36.

Symington, D. C. (1994). Megatrends in rehabilitation: A Canadian perspective. *International Journal of Rehabilitation Research, 17,* 1–14.

Szilagyi, P. G., Shenkman, E., Brach, C., LaClair, B. J., Swigonski, N., Dick, A., et al. (2003). Children with special health care needs enrolled in the State Children's Health Insurance Program (SCHIP): Patient characteristics and health care needs. *Pediatrics, 112,* e508–e520.

Tate, D. G., Stiers, W., Daugherty, J., Forchheimer, M., Cohen, E., & Hansen, N. (1994). The effects of insurance benefits coverage on functional and psychosocial outcomes after spinal cord injury. *Archives of Physical Medicine and Rehabilitation, 75,* 407–414.

Tator, C. H., Duncan, E. G., Edmonds, V. E., Lapczak, L. I., & Andrews, D. F. (1993). Neurological recovery, mortality and length of stay after acute spinal cord injury associated with changes in management. *Paraplegia, 33,* 254–262.

U.S. Department of Health and Human Services (2003). *2003 CMS statistics.* CMS Publication no. 03445. Washington, DC: Author.

Williams, B. (1994). Comparison of services among different types of home health agencies. *Medical Care, 32,* 1134–1152.

Wilson, N. J., & Kizer, K. W. (1997). The VA health care system: An unrecognized national safety net. *Health Affairs, 16,* 200–204.

Wolk, S., & Blair, T. (1994). *Trends in medical rehabilitation.* Reston, VA: American Rehabilitation Association.

Wooldridge, J., Hill, I., Harrington, M., Kenney, G., Hawkes, C., & Haley, J. (2003). *Interim evaluation report: Congressionally mandated evaluation of the State Children's Health Insurance Program.* Report submitted to the U.S. Department of Health and Human Services. Retrieved from http://aspe.hhs.gov/health/schip/interimrpt/index.htm

Wright, R. E., Rao, N., Smith, R. M., & Harvey, R. F. (1996). Risk factors for death and emergency transfer in acute and subacute inpatient rehabilitation. *Archives of Physical Medicine and Rehabilitation, 77,* 1049–1055.

33

Legislation and Rehabilitation Professionals

Susanne M. Bruyère, PhD, CRC, Sara A. Van Looy, BA,
and Thomas P. Golden, MS, CRC

Over the course of the past decades, the field of rehabilitation has seen sweeping changes, as laws have been enacted to support the rights of individuals with disabilities, and subsequently the efforts of the professionals who provide services to these people have also changed. These legislative mandates have granted rights to persons with disabilities in accessibility of goods and services, transportation, telecommunications, housing, and employment (U.S. Department of Justice, 2002).[1] Although each of these areas is vital for accessing a full life as an American citizen, it is the area of employment that is the center of attention in this chapter. Economic self-sufficiency and the ability to use one's talents and abilities in meaningful work are key to a person's financial independence and experience of personal well-being (Fujiura, Yamaki, & Czechowicz, 1998; Stapleton, O'Day, Livermore, & Imparato, 2006). To provide the broadest possible perspective on employment issues that may affect the functioning of rehabilitation professionals, we focus not only on rehabilitation legislation and legislation specifically targeted to persons with disabilities, but also on other pieces of employment legislation that provide protections for persons with disabilities. For the purposes of this discussion, the laws that will be focused on are presented as follows: Titles I (Vocational Rehabilitation Services) and V (Rights and Advocacy) of the Rehabilitation Act of 1973 as amended, the employment provisions of the Americans with Disabilities Act (ADA) of 1990, the Ticket to Work and Work Incentives Improvement Act of 1999 (TWWIIA), the Workforce Investment Act (WIA) of 1998, the Family Medical Leave Act (FMLA), the Occupational Safety and Health Act (OSHA), the National Labor Relations Act (NLRA), and state workers' compensation laws.

This chapter provides a brief overview of each law with an explanation of issues, concerns, or critical areas in service delivery that may arise from it. These are issues that have caused much consternation to employers who attempt to fulfill their responsibilities under several—at times seemingly conflicting—pieces of disability and employment legislation (Gault & Kinnane, 1996). They are therefore of concern to the individual with a disability who is trying to either gain or maintain employment, as well as to rehabilitation professionals who serve people with disabilities. The intent of this chapter is to contribute to the ability of rehabilitation professionals to assist employers and individuals with disabilities in navigating this maze. The authors offer a summary of some key strategies for operating effectively within this regulatory environment, which rehabilitation professionals can use either for coaching individuals about their rights or for providing consultation to employers about their responsibilities to persons with disabilities to lessen or eliminate discrimination in the employment process.

More broadly, an understanding of the legislative environment that affects an employer's receptivity in hiring and retaining individuals with disabilities is important to not only rehabilitation professionals who are providing direct services, but also to service administrators and those in state and national leadership positions contributing to public policy evolution. Since the initiation of many of these laws, significant changes have occurred in the U.S. economic, political, and social contexts. As two examples, U.S. involvement in wars abroad and the aftermath of returning veterans with disabilities, as well as the unprecedented weakening of the American economic infrastructure, necessitate an informed rehabilitation professional who can be vigilant in advocating for the inclusion of people with disabilities in all facets of new public policy initiatives. Knowledge of the legislative roots of specific public policy proposals, as well as of our country's response to contemporary challenges in the public policy arena, is imperative for the rehabilitation professional's maximal effectiveness.

EMPLOYMENT LEGISLATION AFFECTING REHABILITATION SERVICE DELIVERY

The Rehabilitation Act of 1973 as Amended

Two titles of the Rehabilitation Act will be discussed here: Title I, which deals with employment and related support services available to persons with disabilities as provided by the state-federal vocational rehabilitation (VR) system, and Title V, which prohibits discrimination on the basis of disability in programs conducted by federal agencies, in programs receiving federal financial assistance, in federal employment, and in the employment practices of federal contractors.

Title I of the Vocational Rehabilitation Act of 1973, as modified by the Rehabilitation Act amendments of 1992 and 1998, has the following as its purpose:

> To assist States in operating statewide comprehensive, coordinated, effective, efficient, and accountable programs of vocational rehabilitation, each of which is (A) an integral part of a statewide workforce investment system; and (B) designed to assess, plan, develop, and provide vocational rehabilitation services for individuals with disabilities, consistent with their strengths, resources, priorities, concerns, abilities, capabilities, interests, and informed choice, so that such individuals may prepare for and engage in gainful employment. (Sec. 100(a)(2))[2]

Some of the earliest legislative seeds for the VR service delivery system as we know it today were sown over 80 years ago with the 1920 Civilian Rehabilitation (Smith-Fess) Act, Public Law 66–236 (Wright, 1980). The Rehabilitation Act has provided funds to states on a formula basis since that time. In the years following the passage of this legislation, VR services have evolved and greatly expanded to provide an extensive array of both public- and private-sector services to address the employment and independent living needs of persons with disabilities.

The federal funding appropriation for the VR service delivery system during fiscal year 2009 was more than $2.8 billion (National Rehabilitation Association 2008). In addition, under the American Recovery and Reinvestment Act of 2009, an additional $540 million was appropriated for grants to state VR programs (U.S. Department of Education, 2009). The state VR system is made up of 80 agencies in 56 states and territories. Twenty-four states have two agencies: one designed for specific services to the blind and visually impaired, and the other providing VR services to all other individuals with disabilities. The remaining 32 agencies offer combined services.[3] Examples of the services that can be provided to persons with disabilities, as authorized under the legislation, are as follows: vocational assessment, career counseling, vocational training, job development and job placement, assistive technology, supported employment, and follow-along services. The legislative mandate requires that the order of selection for the provision of VR services shall be determined on the basis of first serving those individuals with the most significant disabilities. Individuals with disabilities, including individuals with the most significant disabilities, are generally presumed to be capable of engaging in gainful employment, and the provision of individualized rehabilitation services is designed to improve their ability to become gainfully employed. A successful outcome is considered to be placement in an integrated employment setting at a prevailing wage for a minimum of 90 days, although other vocational outcomes, such as homemaker and unpaid family worker, are accepted as legitimate closures for certain individuals who are deemed unable to seek competitive employment. The state and federal VR program serves approximately 1.2 million individuals with disabilities a year, placing close to a quarter of a million consumers into competitive employment (Council of State Administrators of Vocational Rehabilitation, n.d.).

The following are the provisions of Title V of the Rehabilitation Act, which prohibits discrimination against persons with disabilities. Section 501 requires affirmative action and nondiscrimination in employment by federal agencies of the executive branch.[4] Section 503 requires affirmative action and prohibits employment discrimination by federal government contractors and subcontractors with contracts of more than $10,000.[5] Section 504 states that "no qualified individual with a disability in the United States shall, solely by reason of her or his disability, be excluded from, denied the benefits of, or be subjected to discrimination under" any program or activity that either receives federal financial assistance or is conducted by any executive agency or the U.S. Postal Service. Requirements include reasonable accommodation for employees with disabilities, program accessibility, effective communication with people who have hearing or vision disabilities, and accessible new construction and alterations.[6] Although the ADA does not apply to workplaces with fewer than 15 employees, the Tenth Circuit has ruled that that limit does not apply to claims brought under the Rehabilitation Act against entities that receive federal funds (Hellwege, 2002).

Section 508 of the Rehabilitation Act applies to all federal agencies when they develop, procure, maintain, or use electronic and information technology. Section 508 was added to the Rehabilitation Act in 1986, but lacked teeth until 1998, when Congress amended the Rehabilitation Act to require federal agencies to make their electronic and information technology accessible to people with disabilities and pushed the Executive branch to develop accessibility standards. Those standards were developed by the Architectural and Transportation Barriers Compliance Board (Access Board),[7] and served to advance the development of new accessible technologies. Federal Web designers also have to make their sites accessible to users with disabilities, and anyone in government who develops or maintains technology products has to make sure that those technologies are accessible (Jaeger, 2006).

The standards for determining employment discrimination under the Rehabilitation Act are the same as those used in Title I of the ADA, and therefore the issues for rehabilitation professionals in dealing with how these rights play out in the workplace are similar. The implications for rehabilitation professionals are discussed in greater detail under the presentation of issues around implementation of Title I of the ADA, which follows.

The ADA of 1990

The ADA is a landmark piece of civil rights legislation that extends the prohibitions against discrimination on the basis of race, sex, religion, and national origin to persons with disabilities.[8] Individuals may have both rights and responsibilities under the law, depending on the roles they assume: as employers or consultants to employers, as practitioners providing health services to the public, or as individuals who today or in the future may be protected by the Act (O'Keeffe, 1994). Title I, the employment provisions of the ADA, applies to private employers with at least 15 employees and to state and local government employers. The ADA protects qualified individuals with disabilities from discrimination. A qualified individual with a disability is a person who meets the necessary prerequisites for a job and can perform the essential functions with or without reasonable accommodation. A reasonable accommodation is any modification or adjustment to a job, an employment practice, or the work environment that makes it possible for a qualified individual with a disability to participate in the job application process, perform the essential functions of a job, and/or enjoy benefits and privileges of employment equal to those enjoyed by employees without disabilities (U.S. Equal Employment Opportunity Commission, 1992).[9]

The ADA employment provisions make it unlawful to discriminate on the basis of disability in a wide range of employment-related actions, including recruitment, job application, hiring, advancement, compensation, benefits, training, and discharge. Title I prohibits both intentional discrimination and employment practices with discriminatory effect. Additionally, Title I limits the use of both pre-employment and postemployment medical examinations and inquiries. An individual with a disability may be subjected to a pre-employment medical examination and inquiry only after a conditional offer of employment has been made and only if all entering employees in the job category, regardless of disability, are subjected to such an examination. Postemployment medical examinations and inquiries must be job-related and consistent with business necessity. Employee medical information is to be maintained separately from other personnel information, treated in a confidential manner, and shared only with supervisors and managers who need to know about necessary restrictions on the work duties of the employee and necessary accommodations. First aid and safety personnel can also be given selected information if the disability might require emergency medical treatment, as can government officials investigating compliance with the ADA.

The reasonable accommodation requirement is central to the mandate of nondiscrimination against people with disabilities. Reasonable accommodation is not an entirely new concept. Reasonable accommodation is required under the Rehabilitation Act regarding the employment and participation of individuals with disabilities under federal contracts and programs, and under Title VII of the Civil Rights Act with respect to religious observances of employees. The ADA provides the following examples of reasonable accommodations: job restructuring; part-time or modified work hours; reassignment to a vacant position; acquisition or modification of equipment or services; appropriate adjustment or modifications of examinations, training materials, or policies; and provision of qualified readers or interpreters.

Employers are not, under the ADA, required to hire employees who may pose a "direct threat" to the workplace safety or health environment (U.S. Equal Employment Opportunity Commission [EEOC], 1992). The statutory definition of the term direct threat is "a significant risk to the health or safety of others that cannot be eliminated by reasonable accommodation." Employers may use the direct-threat defense only in cases where risk is significantly increased, and standards for determining how severe a risk is must be applied to all employees—both with and without disabilities (EEOC, 1997).

Despite these landmark civil rights employment protections for people with disabilities, enforcement of the law as originally intended has been problematic. The U.S. EEOC holds responsibility for receiving and investigating reports of disability-related employment discrimination. An ongoing concern is that the EEOC has had significant difficulty handling complaints that it receives in a timely fashion (Moss & Johnsen, 1997; Percy, 2001). In addition, the Supreme Court has issued a number of decisions that have dramatically changed the way the ADA is interpreted (National Council on Disability, 2004). Decisions on the definition of disability, who can be considered "disabled," and the applicability of the statute to state governments limited the application of the ADA in many cases (National Council on Disability, 2007).

In addition, questions and concerns about accommodations for persons with psychiatric disabilities have been voiced by employers and their legal representatives (Billitteri, 1997; Pechman, 1995), and employer surveys have found that the majority still hold patronizing or potentially discriminating attitudes (Scheid, 1998). In response to these concerns, the EEOC issued enforcement guidance on the ADA as it applies to persons with psychiatric disabilities (EEOC, 1997). This publication provides useful information to persons with disabilities as well as to rehabilitation practitioners who provide services to them, about the rights of persons with disabilities to accommodation and disclosure of disability under the ADA. However, this area continues to warrant further attention, as a study by Ullman, Johnson, Moss, and Burris (2001) of disability discrimination claims to the EEOC found that psychiatric illnesses were significantly less likely to be classified as Category A claims and fully investigated than were other disabilities, whereas a study by Goldberg, Killeen, and O'Day (2005) found lingering issues surrounding disclosure of disabled status on the part of people with psychiatric disabilities.

When the ADA employment provisions first became effective, some industries were predominantly concerned about their hiring practices and restraints than being able to ask questions about prior injuries (Setzer, 1992); other employers responded with concerns about additional facets of employment that would be affected, such as the implications for insurance benefits and compensation (Huss, 1993; Nobile, 1996; Zolkos, 1994). Over the 2 decades since the law's passage, employers also have become aware of the importance of examining how they treat job incumbents with disabilities. According to statistics kept by the U.S. Equal Employment Opportunity Commission, the federal agency that oversees compliance with the ADA employment provisions, more than half (55%) of charges filed from 1993 to 2007 were related to alleged unlawful discharge, twice as many as were filed for the next most common issue, reasonable accommodation (25%). (Bjelland, Bruyère, Houtenville, Ruiz-Quintanilla, & Webber, 2009). Thus, it appears that employers need assistance in navigating requirements for nondiscrimination across all phases of the employment process. Informed rehabilitation professionals can be of great assistance in this process both to these employers and to job applicants and job incumbents with disabilities.

The ADA Amendments Act of 2008

The ADA definition of disability, intended by legislators to be broad and open-ended, was so contentious and was so limited by subsequent court rulings that, in 2008, Congress passed the ADA Amendments Act of 2008 (ADAAA.) The intent of the ADAAA was to reject the increasingly narrow judicial constructions of the ADA in favor of the broad coverage that was the original intent of the Act (EEOC, 2008). The ADAA specifically overturned Supreme Court rulings on the definition of disability and the effect of mitigating measures such as medications or assistive devices. It retained the basic definition of disability, but provided clearer definitions of terms, expanding on the description of other terms, and providing nonexhaustive lists of examples. It also clarified that a condition that is episodic or in remission (such as bipolar disorder or depression) can still be a disability if it would be considered a disability when active (EEOC, 2008).

TWWIIA of 1999

The TWWIIA, signed into law on December 17, 1999, was intended to provide beneficiaries and recipients of either Supplemental Security Income (SSI), Social Security Disability Insurance (SSDI), or both, the incentives and supports needed to either prepare for, attach to, or advance in work.[10] TWWIIA attempted to reduce and remove certain barriers to employment for individuals who receive SSI and SSDI and to encourage beneficiaries and recipients to access the services and supports needed to assist them in their pursuit of employment. At the heart of the Act was a desire by Congress to increase options available to beneficiaries of the Social Security Administration's (SSA's) disability programs by expanding upon the existing network of service providers available and creating a more comprehensive set of supports for people with disabilities considering work.[11]

The TWWIIA includes three important titles: Ticket to Work and Self-Sufficiency, Expansion of Health Care, and Demonstration Projects/Studies. Title I expands vocational services options for persons with disabilities. The Ticket to Work and Self-Sufficiency Program is an important provision of Title I. This program replaces the Social Security Administration's (SSA's) existing VR program with an outcomes-based and market-driven program.

All SSI recipients and SSDI beneficiaries who have been determined to be disabled under SSA's adult definition of disability, are more than 18 years of age, and receive benefits will receive a Ticket to Work. The SSA administers the provisions of Title I.[12]

The Ticket Program permits the individual beneficiary or recipient to choose from an array of service providers (called Employment Networks [ENs]), placing control over provider selection in the hands of the consumer. The Ticket Program is purely voluntary and beneficiaries and recipients can choose whether to use their Ticket or not, decide who to deposit their Ticket with, and decide at any point to retract their Ticket from a provider if they feel the services they are receiving are inadequate.

The EN, an approved service provider under the Ticket Program, can be a private organization or public agency that agrees to work with SSA to provide vocational rehabilitation, employment, and/or other support services to assist a SSA beneficiary/recipient to prepare for, obtain, and remain at work. Under the Ticket Program, a service provider can elect to become an EN, become a service provider under another EN, or both. A state VR agency can be a part of multiple ENs across a given state, but each EN must have an agreement with VR before initiating a referral to the designated state VR agency. An EN that agrees to provide services can decide to receive either outcome payments for months in which a beneficiary does not receive benefits due to work activity (up to 60 months), or reduced outcome payments in addition to payments for assisting the beneficiary to achieve phased milestones connected with employment. In addition, state VR agencies can also elect to receive payment as they have in the past under the cost reimbursement option. This special status is in recognition of the fact that under the Rehabilitation Act of 1973 as amended, state VR agencies cannot deny services and supports to a consumer who is eligible. State VR agencies differ from other ENs in that the other ENs can make a decision to not accept someone's Ticket.

Despite SSA's efforts to promote the Ticket Program from its outset, initial studies have found that participation rates have remained low, and that most beneficiaries have remained in the traditional payment system. Thus, SSA has attempted to strengthen the Ticket with revisions to the regulations. These revisions took effect in late 2008, and their effects remain to be studied (Stapleton et al., 2008).

Title II of TWWIIA governs the provision of health care services to workers with disabilities. This section of the law attempted to reduce the disincentives to employment for people with disabilities posed by the threat of loss of health care benefits by encouraging states to improve access to health care coverage available under Medicaid (Goodman & Livermore, 2004). Under this provision, new optional eligibility groups are established, creating two new Medicaid Buy-In eligibility categories, and also extending the period of premium-free Medicare Part A eligibility and requiring protection for certain individuals with Medigap. The Department of Health and Human Services, through the Centers for Medicare and Medicaid Services, administers the health care provisions.[13]

WIA of 1998

The WIA of 1998[14] was intended to consolidate workforce preparation and employment services into a unified system of support that is responsive to the needs of job seekers, employers, and communities (Public Law 105–220). Title I of the Act developed a framework for the delivery of workforce investment activities at the state and local level to provide services in an effective and meaningful way to all customers, including persons with disabilities. The law is positioned not only to empower customers, but also to provide opportunities for business and human resource professionals to focus public programs on marketplace needs.

WIA created a workforce development system that encourages and facilitates One-Stop service delivery (WIA of 1998, August 7, 1998). This employment and training system was intended to serve every job seeker through a central location that provides access to numerous workforce development programs. Core services—including assessment, basic job readiness, and help with job searches—are open to a universal population. For those who require further assistance finding employment, intensive services and job training are also available. The One-Stop system is based on four principles: (1) Universal Access—making core services available to all people; (2) Customer Choice—allowing customers to select services based on their needs; (3) Service Integration—consolidation of all workforce development services into One-Stop centers; and (4) Accountability—Centers are evaluated on the basis of measurable outcomes with future funding linked to the results of services provided to customers (Imel, 1999).

Title IV of the WIA reauthorizes the VR program. The law specifically states that "linkages between the VR program and other components of the statewide workforce investment system are critical to ensure effective and meaningful participation by individuals with disabilities in workforce investment activities." Collaboration between the state units administering the VR program and generic workforce development services (Departments of Labor) is intended to produce better information, more comprehensive services, easier access to services, and improved long-term employment outcomes (WIA of 1998, Title IV, Section 403: 2).

To ensure such participation, WIA and the Department of Labor's (DOL's) Employment and Training Administration (ETA) stress the need for access and partnership when addressing the needs of people with disabilities. Universal access to one-stop services is a central component of WIA.[15] In a notice published in April 2000, the ETA stated: "the Department of Labor is committed to ensuring that the programs, services, and facilities of each One-Stop delivery system are accessible to all of America's workers, including individuals with disabilities" (U.S. DOL, 2000). Every job seeker should have access to the core services available at their local One-Stop Center. Federal law mandates that all WIA activities, from core to intensive services, must be accessible to individuals with disabilities. While physical access to the One-Stop Center is important, access to all tools and services offered by the center—including virtual and computer-based resources—is critical if job seekers with disabilities are to benefit fully from the One-Stop system.

WIA mandates a series of partnerships in the One-Stop system, including Vocational Rehabilitation. VR has a seat on state and local Workforce Investment Boards and, ideally, is involved in the design of the workforce development system. States and local areas also can bring other disability organizations into the system as partners. The U.S. DOL encourages state and local policy makers to develop partnerships with disability-specific organizations to create an effective and universal workforce investment system.

Although VR's involvement in the workforce investment system is critically important and the Rehabilitation Act of 1973 as amended was incorporated into Title IV of WIA, it does not appear that the two systems have become completely integrated. This is evidenced in the fact that both systems maintain separate administrations and in some states the systems are housed in entirely separate state agencies. The challenge of integrating a specialized field (vocational rehabilitation) into the broader workforce development system posed opportunity for development of articulation agreements established to provide clarity regarding who provides what types of services and supports within the One-Stop infrastructure (Golden, Zeitzer, & Bruyère, in press). Articulation of these roles and responsibilities was further reinforced by the 2002 launch of the Disability Program Navigator (DPN) position within the DOL, jointly sponsored by the SSA and the U.S. DOL's ETA. The DPN pilot was administered through the state DOL infrastructure and in some cases states actually expanded resources beyond the federal appropriation to ensure that individuals with disabilities who wanted to go to work have assistance accessing and maneuvering the One-Stop System.

FMLA of 1993

The FMLA (Public Law 103–3) went into effect on August 5, 1993.[16] It established, for employers with 50 or more employees, a minimum labor standard with regard to leaves of absence for family or medical reasons.

Under the FMLA, an eligible employee may take up to 12 work-weeks of leave during any 12-month period for one or more of the following reasons: the birth of a child and to care for the newborn child; the placement of a child with the employee through adoption or foster care and to care for the child; to care for the employee's spouse, son, daughter, or parent with a serious health condition; and a serious health condition of the employee that makes the employee unable to perform one or more of the essential functions of his or her job.[17] An FMLA serious health condition is an illness, injury, impairment, or physical or mental condition that involves inpatient care or continuing treatment by a health care provider. During the FMLA leave, the employer must maintain the employee's existing level of coverage under a group health plan. At the end of FMLA leave, an employer must take an employee back into the same or an equivalent job. The FMLA does not require an employer to let an employee who is medically unable to do his job return to work, nor does it require modification of the job or reassignment to a new position. In 2008, the FMLA was amended to clarify the rights of military personnel and their families to take and use FMLA leave (U.S. DOL, 2009c).

Some of the questions that arise in use of the FMLA that relate to the functioning of rehabilitation professionals arise from the interplay of FMLA leave with accommodation and return-to-work efforts (Geaney, 2004; Scott, 1996; Shalowitz, 1993). The interaction between FMLA, the ADA, and workers' compensation has been dubbed "the Bermuda Triangle of employment law" by some writers (Postol, 2002). In some cases, the FMLA leave itself can be an accommodation (FMLA Leave can be ADA Accommodation, 2002). In other situations, the FMLA may create difficulties for an employer attempting to get injured workers back to work and off benefits. Many employers have used "light duty" to bring an injured worker back to work within his or her medical restrictions. Light-duty jobs typically are very different from the job an employee was doing at the time of injury. Because the FMLA requires that a worker be restored to the same or an equivalent position on return from leave, an employer may not compel an injured worker to accept light-duty work in lieu of exercising his or her FMLA entitlement. Likewise, the DOL has taken the position that an employer may not require an FMLA-eligible employee to accept reasonable accommodation instead of FMLA leave.

An employer may offer accommodation or light duty but may not compel it. On the other hand, if an employee rejects an offer of employment that is within his or her medical restrictions, an employer may contest the employee's entitlement to workers' compensation indemnity benefits. In addition, if an employee voluntarily accepts light duty, an employer may not designate time on light duty as FMLA leave, as the employee is working. However, time spent on light duty does not lessen an employee's right to be restored to the same or an equivalent position held at the time leave commenced.

The issue of FMLA employee notice provisions and ADA prohibitions on medical inquiries has raised many questions for employers (Geaney, 2004). FMLA allows employers to ask for certification of a serious health condition, whereas the ADA places restrictions on disability-related inquiries by employees. The EEOC issued a fact sheet to address some of these most-often-asked questions about the ADA and FMLA interaction (EEOC answers, 1997).[18] This publication clarifies the point that when an employee requests leave under the FMLA for a serious health condition, employers will not violate the ADA by asking for the information specified in the FMLA certification form. The ADA allows medical inquiries that are "job-related" and consistent with business necessity. However, employers continue to note that differences between FMLA and the ADA cause difficulties when leave requests trigger obligations under each statute (Lipnic & DeCamp, 2007). After amendments to the FMLA in 2008 that clarified the definition of "serious health condition" and required that employees follow their employer's usual sick leave call-in requirements immediately upon the start of their health condition, the DOL published revised rules and guidance for employers and employees (U.S. DOL, 2009a).

The FMLA form requests only information relating to the particular serious health condition for which the person is seeking leave. An employer is entitled to know why an employee, who otherwise should be at work, is requesting time off under the FMLA. Medical inquiries that are strictly limited in this fashion are therefore not ADA violations (EEOC, 2000).

OSHA of 1970

The OSHA of 1970 represents the culmination of nearly a century of Congress's growing concern for workplace safety (Rothstein, 1990). Throughout the 20th century, laws were passed in response to specific workplace health issues, but no piece of legislation covered all safety and health issues in every workplace for every employee until the passage of OSHA in 1970. Unlike some other employment regulation, OSHA is applied universally to all employers, regardless of the volume of business they conduct or the number of people they employ (Rothstein, 1990).

At OSHA's core is the recognition that every worker has a right to a workplace that is free from recognized hazards. Therefore, when a potential hazard is identified, the OSH Administration, through the Labor Department, develops a standard against which workplace practices or conditions should be measured (Bureau of National Affairs, 1997).

After the implementation of a standard, the Labor Department can determine which workplaces will be inspected—either by the request of an employee in the particular workplace or at the OSH Administration's discretion. Inspections are conducted with the permission of the employer and according to OSHA guidelines. Violations of a standard are punishable by government-ordered abatement and monetary fines, set according to the size of the business, the seriousness of the violation, the good faith of the employer, and the record of prior violations. Violations that result in the death of an employee can be punished by criminal law (Bureau of National Affairs, 1997).

Section 18 of OSHA encourages states to develop and operate their own job safety and health programs. These state plans must be approved and monitored by the federal government. As of 2009, there were 22 states operating complete state plans, while an additional 4 states had OSH plans covering only public employees. States must set job safety and health standards that are at least as affective as comparable federal standards, but have the option of promulgating standards covering hazards not addressed by the federal regulations (U.S. DOL, 2009b).

A major way in which this law may affect the functioning of rehabilitation professionals is its interplay with ADA requirements regarding employment screening prohibitions, medical confidentiality of records, and required accommodations. The ADA's limitations on employee testing can be in conflict with OSHA's need for testing in furtherance of workplace safety goals.

The ADA places significant restrictions on an employer's right to require pre-employment physicals, to make medical inquiries of employees and applicants, and to require that employees submit to physical examinations, and it restricts access to such information in an effort to prevent potential discrimination. OSHA, in contrast, affirmatively requires employers to conduct testing in various situations to assure safety. For example, employees exposed to high noise levels are required to be included within an audiometric testing program, which includes among other things annual hearing tests (Taylor, 1995; U.S. DOL, 2001). The ADA requires strict confidentiality of medical records. OSHA, on the other hand, requires employers to provide employees, their representatives with signed authorizations, and OSHA personnel access to such records in the interest of exposing potential hazards and their causes. By having the employee sign an information release, the employer can better assure that the information being released stays in the appropriate hands and that the ADA confidentiality requirements are not violated. The EEOC has stated that the ADA does not override health and safety requirements established under other federal laws, such that if certain standards are required by another law, an employer does not have to show that it is job-related and consistent with business necessity (EEOC, 1992; Occupational Injury and Illness Recording and Reporting Requirements, 2001).

OSHA requires certain employers to develop and maintain a written emergency action plan. Although the ADA does not require emergency planning, it does require that any plan created in compliance with OSHA standards must include people with disabilities (U.S. DOL, 2005).

Although OSHA requirements can often take precedence over the ADA requirements to assure adherence to health and safety requirements, the reasonable accommodation element of the ADA can still be applied to OSHA-mandated policies and modifications. For example, an eyewash station, which may be required by OSHA for certain positions, must be installed in such a way that a wheelchair user would have access to it.

The lines are not always so clear, however, particularly in terms of the direct-threat defense to ADA claims. Take, for example, the case of an employee with epilepsy working on an assembly line. The way an employer handles the situation is largely contingent on which legislation he or she believes is more likely to be invoked. Removal of the employee, satisfying the general duty clause of OSHA, may violate the ADA. The direct-threat defense is so difficult to prove that employers are likely to avoid the ADA claim at all costs, often leaving themselves in violation of OSHA standards. The complications arise when OSHA doesn't explicitly call for an action such as removal of an employee who has seizures. As a general rule, OSHA standards "trump" the ADA's duty to accommodate, but employers cannot rely on using OSHA as a defense to ADA claims unless the employment action in question was specifically called for by OSHA (Skoning & McGlothlen, 1994).

NLRA of 1935

The NLRA, also called the Wagner Act, was passed in 1935. It stands as the established framework for labor relations in the United States, covering union-management relations in almost every private firm in operation. The law protects workers from the effects of unfair labor practices by employers, and requires employers to recognize and bargain collectively with a union that the workers elect to represent them (Gold, 1998).

Among the main principles of the NLRA are the idea of exclusivity of representation, a policy against direct dealing, and the duty to provide information. Seniority rights gained through collective bargaining are also among the most valued benefits of having a unionized workplace (Gold, 1998). All of these areas may yield conflict for individuals seeking to invoke protection from laws such as the ADA, FMLA, or the Rehabilitation Act. These laws rely on making exceptions to or changes in terms and conditions of employment on an individual basis, while collective bargaining agreements under the NLRA make the union the broker of employment rights for all its members (Schwab, 2009). Compliance with these laws may include dealing with the employer to discuss and secure those agreements that may fall outside the scope of the union's normal interactions, the unilateral implementation of an accommodation for an employee, and often the security of medical information, which the union may feel it has the right to access under the NLRA (Evans, 1992).

Reasonable accommodations for individuals with disabilities may present an especially problematic situation for employers and unions alike. Both parties are required by law to operate in a nondiscriminatory manner: the employer must accommodate a worker so that his or her essential job functions may be performed regardless of disability and must provide terms and conditions of employment that are free of discriminatory intent. The union must represent its constituency equally and consistently, as well as allow accommodations for people with disabilities to be implemented without unreasonable opposition (President's Committee, 1994).

Whenever a modification in the terms or conditions of employment is required, a review of the collective bargaining agreement would be advisable, as well as some kind of communication between the employer and the union concerning the accommodation and the potential effects it may have on the lives of other workers (President's Committee, 1994). An effective way to approach this is the use of joint labor-management teams (Bruyère, Gomez, & Handelmann, 1996).

In a unionized workplace, the rehabilitation professional can contribute to an injured worker's effective return to the workplace, taking into the account the interests of the employee, the employer, and the union to effect a successful reintegration. Organized labor has been an important part of the history of fighting for worker rights and against job discrimination, and these social issues are very important to workers with disabilities. Yet many employment professionals have little experience with unions and little knowledge of their purpose and structure (Bruyère, 1996). Adopting a position that favors both the person with a disability and the union will go a long way in the service delivery process to minimize conflict and maximize union support in the accommodation process.

A 2002 Supreme Court decision (U.S. Airways, Inc. v. Barnett) ruled that employees with disabilities are not always entitled to reassignment to a job intended for workers with more seniority. The Supreme Court held that, in situations involving a conflict between a requested accommodation and an employer-created seniority system, the "seniority system will prevail in the run of cases." However, the court left open the possibility of an employee showing that reassignment would be a reasonable accommodation in a particular case despite the existence of a seniority system (Ford & Harrison, 2002). Thus, questions remain about the legalities of accommodating workers with disabilities within a collective bargaining agreement (Flores, 2008).

Workers' Compensation

Workers' compensation programs are government-sponsored, employer-financed systems for compensating employees who incur an injury or illness in connection with their employment. They are designed to ensure that employees who are injured on the job receive timely compensation for their losses without proof of fault. Workers' compensation laws allow employees or their survivors to file claims for economic losses resulting from work-related injuries or occupational diseases. Benefits provided under workers' compensation laws include medical care, disability payments, rehabilitation services, survivor benefits, and funeral expenses. Employers who participate in workers' compensation programs usually are protected against tort actions that employees might otherwise pursue to redress their losses.

State workers' compensation statutes generally provide benefits to employees for job-related injuries, whether or not the injury is permanently disabling. In addition to medical care and treatment for job-related injuries, these statutes typically also provide benefits for temporary incapacity, scarring, and permanent impairment of specific parts of the body. Workers' compensation laws are maintained by all 50 states, the District of Columbia, American Samoa, Guam, the Virgin Islands, and Puerto Rico. In addition, the federal government administers workers' compensation programs authorized by the Federal Coal Mine Health and Safety Act, the Longshore and Harbor Workers' Compensation Act, and the Federal Employers' Liability Act. Rehabilitation professionals working in private-sector rehabilitation and in the return-to-work process for persons with disabilities must interact with this system and its regulations regularly.

Although much attention was paid immediately after the passage of the ADA to disability nondiscrimination and the hiring process, some employers were already focusing on its effect on job incumbents with disabilities (Walworth, Damon, & Wilder, 1993). Now, even more attention is being paid to the ADA's effect on job retention aspects of the employment process. Of the ADA charges filed with the EEOC between 1992 and 2007, 12.2% were cited as being related to a back impairment (Bjelland, Bruyère, von Schrader, Houtenville, Ruiz-Quintanilla, & Webber, 2009), which is a disability or injury often seen in the workers' compensation system. It is inevitable that the rehabilitation practitioner will deal with some persons for whom there will be an interplay of these two pieces of legislation.

Some authors have pointed out that disability nondiscrimination legislation such as the ADA appears to rest on very different principles than the workers' compensation system (Bell, 1994; Geaney, 2004). The ADA is predicated on the premise that disability does not necessarily mean inability to work, and focuses on how accommodation can assist in removing barriers to employment caused by the interaction between functional limitations and the workplace. Workers' compensation legislation, however, focuses on the apparently contrasting premise that impairments are the cause of work limitations, and employees must prove loss of earning capacity because of injury. For workers' compensation purposes it is often necessary for an employee to emphasize the limitations caused by a disability, but these statements can be detrimental to requests for reinstatement and accommodation under the ADA (Geaney, 2004).

Rehabilitation professionals in this area will need to concern themselves with clarifying for individuals with disabilities and for employers the significant aspects of workers' compensation legislation as they relate to protections provided by the ADA and FMLA. These include such issues as the injured worker as a protected person under the ADA, queries by an employer about a worker's prior workers' compensation claims, hiring persons with a prior history of an occupational injury and application of the direct threat standard, reasonable accommodation for persons with disability-related occupational injuries, light-duty issue, and exclusive remedy provisions in workers' compensation laws. In response to a need for clarification of these issues, the EEOC issued enforcement guidance concerning the interaction between Title I of the ADA and state workers' compensation laws that can greatly assist rehabilitation professionals in responding to many of these employer questions (EEOC, 1996; Welch, 1996).

IMPLICATIONS FOR REHABILITATION SERVICE DELIVERY

To prepare persons with disabilities appropriately for initial entry or re-entry into the workplace, and to provide effective consultation to employers on disability nondiscrimination and equal access in the workplace, rehabilitation professionals must be apprised of state and federal legislation that affects both safety and equity practices in the workplace. The issues presented here in the implementation of specific pieces of legislation, and more specifically as they interrelate with disability nondiscrimination legislation, such as the ADA, and workforce preparation and benefits support, such as the Ticket legislation and WIA, point to areas where rehabilitation professionals need more knowledge and expertise and also where they can provide effective service. A listing of specific skill and knowledge areas needed by rehabilitation professionals in implementing the ADA as consultants were identified by Pape and Tarvydas (1994) as cutting across the following three distinct areas: core rehabilitation principles, knowledge, and functions; disability concepts, functions, and knowledge; and ADA knowledge and functions. The implications of disability nondiscrimination legislation specifically for the role of psychologists were addressed by Crewe (1994), who encourages specialized pre- or postdoctoral preparation in disability and rehabilitation for psychologists who are planning to apply their clinical or counseling psychology training to services for people with disabilities. The implications of disability nondiscrimination legislation such as the ADA for preparation of rehabilitation undergraduate and graduate professionals are discussed by Stude (1994), who encourages rehabilitation educators to include this information in existing course-work rather than isolating it into a specialized course. The importance of examining the gap between existing employment and disability policy and desired employment outcomes for persons with disabilities was the focus of a recent conference and resulting publication sponsored by the American Psychological Association and the National Institute of Disability and Rehabilitation Research (Bruyère et al., 2003).

The ADA has afforded rehabilitation professionals who contribute to employment opportunities for persons with disabilities a tool to more effectively combat discrimination in the recruitment, hiring, retention, and termination processes. Under the ADA, a significant service that VR counselors might provide is assisting employers with job analyses, writing job descriptions, and helping develop or design the reasonable accommodations that will make initial hiring or return to work feasible for workers with disabilities (Walker & Heffner, 1992). Employers need assistance in the development of policies and procedures that do not discriminate against people with disabilities in the recruitment, hiring, health and other employment benefits, promotion and training, and termination processes.

The workers' compensation system is one that is cited as being difficult for both employees and employers, seemingly fanning the fires for a contentious and litigious relationship. One of the most important things rehabilitation professionals can do is to facilitate communication between the employer and the employee (Commerce Clearing House, 1997). Rehabilitation professionals can either themselves be that bridge with employers or serve as consultants to encourage supervisors and others in the workplace to address the employees' questions and provide supportive follow-up during disability leave. Rehabilitation professionals also can play a role in bringing human resource, safety, and health professionals within a given organization together to develop a unified approach to the ADA and workers' compensation (Walker & Heffner, 1992).

In all facets of this legislation, working both with individuals with disabilities and with employers and teaching them how to communicate their respective needs effectively is imperative. Often, when coached appropriately, both employees with disabilities and their supervisors or the human resources staff in a given organization can effectively address accommodation requests and resolve any conflicts that arise in negotiating final decisions on accommodations. Problems arise when there has been a prior history of poor performance, of poor relationship between supervisor and employee, or of general discord or conflict in a unit or workplace environment, creating a culture of mistrust in responding to employee needs.

SUMMARY

The purpose of this chapter has been to provide rehabilitation professionals with a basic overview of some of the pieces of disability and employment legislation that may affect their functioning in the rehabilitation and return-to-work process. Several of these laws, such as the NLRA and the OSHA, are designed to protect workers' rights before injury occurs, and to emphasize employer responsibilities in the safety and equitable treatment of workers in all terms and conditions of employment. Regulatory requirements such as the FMLA, short-term disability leave requirements as dictated by state regulations, and workers' compensation legislation are designed to deal with the rights of employees once an injury or illness has occurred. These laws protect the right to a medical leave that gives the worker the time needed for the rehabilitation process and they assure the security of benefits to cover part of the medical costs and salary lost to time off work due to illness or injury, as well as a job upon their return. Legislation such as the Rehabilitation Act of 1973 as amended and the ADA and ADAAA focuses more specifically on the rights of workers with disabilities. These laws require equal access in the seeking and securing of employment, as well as retention and equitable access to other terms and conditions of employment. Regulatory requirements such as confidentiality of medical information also serve a role here, in terms of providing requirements for employers to keep confidential any medical diagnostic information on employees that they may gain access to. Legislation such as the SSA's TWWIIA and the U.S. DOL's WIA provide needed supports and services to remove barriers to employment and provide needed supports in the employment-seeking process.

Assisting the individual through the rehabilitation process to return to productive functioning in the community and in the workplace is the core of the rehabilitation professional's job. When employment outcomes are part of the rehabilitation goal, knowledge of the regulatory requirements that surround the workplace and have an effect on employer and employee behavior is vital for the rehabilitation professional to function effectively. This chapter has pointed out some of the possible areas of conflict or concern that may influence both worker and employer behaviors, and has provided a basic introduction for practitioners to pursue further information, given the nature of their services and interventions for persons with disabilities.

ACKNOWLEDGMENTS

The authors' efforts in writing this material were supported by a grant from the U.S. Department of Education National Institute on Disability and Rehabilitation Research for a Rehabilitation Research and Training Center for Employment Policy for Persons with Disabilities (Grant #H113B040013). The authors thank the work of Rebecca DeMarinis, a coauthor on a prior version of this chapter published in 1999. Erin Sullivan, Fordham University Law Student, and Sara Furgusun, Cornell University ILR Student, assisted in the review of recent literature for this edition.

NOTES

1. A brief publication discussing these pieces of legislation, entitled *A Guide to Disability Rights Laws*, is available from the U.S. Department of Justice Civil Rights Division, Disability Rights Section, P. O. 66738, Washington, DC 20035–6738; (800) 514–0301 (voice), (800) 514–0383 (TTY), or go to http://www.usdoj. gov/crt/ada/cguide.pdf to download the full publication.
2. See http://www.rcep6.org/rehabilitation_act.htm for complete text of the Rehabilitation Act.
3. For further information, visit the Council for State Administrators in Vocational Rehabilitation (CSAVR) at http://www.rehabnetwork.org, or contact the Executive Office: 4733 Bethesda Avenue, Suite 330, Bethesda, MD 20814; phone (301) 654–8414; fax (301) 654–5542.
4. To obtain more information or to file a complaint, employees should contact their agency's Equal Employment Opportunity Office; call 1–800-669–4000 (voice), 1–800-669–6820 (TTY), or visit http://www.eeoc.gov.
5. For more information on section 503, contact Office of Federal Contract Compliance Programs, U.S. Department of Labor, 200 Constitution Ave., NW, Washington, DC 20210; (202) 693–0101. Visit http://www.dol.gov/esa/ofccp/ for a list of regional offices, section 503 information, and instructions for filing complaints.
6. For information on how to file complaints under section 504 with the appropriate agency, contact U.S. Department of Justice, 950 Pennsylvania Avenue, NW, Civil Rights Division, Disability Rights Section—NYAV, Washington, DC 20530; (800) 514–0301 (voice), (800) 514–0383 (TTY), or see http://www.ada.gov.
7. Information about these standards can be found at the Access Board web site at http://www.access-board.gov/news/508.htm.
8. Cornell University has developed an online guide to the ADA and reasonable accommodations for people with specific disabilities. See http://www.hrtips.org for more information.
9. A modification or adjustment is "reasonable" if it seems reasonable on its face, that is, ordinarily or in the run of cases; this means it is "reasonable" if it appears to be "feasible" or "plausible." A deeper discussion of what is "reasonable" accommodation can be found in U.S. Equal Employment Opportunity Commission (2002).
10. For more information on the Work Incentives Improvement Act, see the Social Security Administration (SSA) web site at http://www.ssa.gov/work/Ticket/ticket_info.html
11. Cornell University has developed a series of Policy and Practice Briefs on Social Security issues, including one on the Ticket program. They can be found at http://www.ilr.cornell.edu/ped/dep/pp.html

12. Further information about the Ticket Program is available through the SSA on their toll-free number at 1–800-772–1213, or on the Social Security Administration web site at http://www.ssa.gov/work
13. Further information about the Medicaid Buy-In program can be found at the Centers for Medicare and Medicaid Services (CMS) web site at http://www.cms.hhs.gov/twwiia/factsh01.asp
14. For further information about the Workforce Investment Act, see http://www.doleta.gov/usworkforce/asp/wialaw.txt
15. The U.S. Department of Labor has developed an online toolkit (http://www.onestoptoolkit.org/) for One-Stops to help grantees ensure access for people with disabilities.
16. See http://www.dol.gov/esa/regs/statutes/whd/fmla.htm for the complete text of this law.
17. For additional information about the FMLA, or to file an FMLA complaint, individuals should contact the nearest office of the Wage and Hour division, Employment Standards Administration, U.S. Department of Labor. The Wage and Hour division is listed in most directories under U.S. Government, Department of Labor, or you can visit their Web site at http://www. dol.gov/esa/whd/. For further information, contact the Office of Legal Counsel's Attorney of the Day at (202) 663–4691.
18. The EEOC fact sheet, the *Family and Medical Leave Act, the Americans with Disabilities Act, and Title VII of the Civil Rights Act* can be ordered by writing or calling the EEOC's Office of Communications and Legislative Affairs at 1801 L St., NW, Washington, DC 20507; telephone (202) 663–4900, TTY (202) 663–4494, or at http://www.eeoc.gov/policy/docs/fmlaada.html on the EEOC Web site.

REFERENCES

Bell, C. (1994). The Americans with Disabilities Act and injured workers: Implications for rehabilitation professionals and the workers' compensation system. In S. Bruyère & J. O'Keeffe (Eds.), *Implications of the Americans with Disabilities Act for psychology* (pp. 137–149). New York: Springer Publishing & Washington, DC: American Psychological Association.

Billitteri, T. (1997). Mental health policy: The issues. *CQ Researcher, Congressional Quarterly Inc., 7*, 795–797.

Bjelland, M., Bruyère, S., Houtenville, A., Ruiz-Quintanilla, A., & Webber, D. (2009). *Trends in disability employment discrimination claims: Implications for rehabilitation counseling practice, administration, training, and research.* Ithaca, NY: Cornell University Employment and Disability Institute.

Bjelland, M., Bruyère, S., von Schrader, S., Houtenville, A., Ruiz-Quintanilla, A., & Webber, D. (2009). Age and disability employment discrimination: Occupational rehabilitation implications. *Journal of Occupational Rehabilitation.* DOI: 10.1007/s10926–009-9194-z

Bruyère, S. (Ed.) (1996). *A job developer's guide to working with unions: Obtaining the support of organized labor for the hiring of employees with disabilities.* St. Augustine, FL: Training Resource Network.

Bruyère, S., Erickson, W., VanLooy, S., Sitaras, E., Cook, J., Burke, J., et al. (2003). Employment and disability policy: Recommendations for a social sciences research agenda. In F. E. Menz & D. F. Thomas (Eds.), *Bridging gaps: Refining the disability research agenda for rehabilitation and the social sciences—Conference proceedings.* Menomonie, WI: University of Wisconsin-Stout, Stout Vocational Rehabilitation Institute, Research and Training Centers.

Bruyère, S., Gomez, S., & Handelmann, G. (1996). The reasonable accommodation process in unionized environments. *Labor Law Journal, 48*, 629–647.

Bureau of National Affairs, Inc. (1997). Job safety and health (No. 228). In *The Laws in Brief: OSHA.* Washington, DC: Author.

Commerce Clearing House. (1997). Communication and concern help workers return to work. In *Workers' compensation business management guide* (pp. 299–301). Chicago: Author.

Council of State Administrators of Vocational Rehabilitation (n.d.). *Public Vocational Rehabilitation Program Fact Sheet.* Retrieved July 22, 2009, from http://www.rehabnetwork.org/press_room/vr_fact_sheet.htm

Crewe, N. (1994). Implications of the Americans with Disabilities Act for the training of psychologists. *Rehabilitation Education, 8*, 9–16.

Evans, B. (1992). Will employers and unions cooperate? *HR Magazine, 37*, 59–63.

FMLA Leave can be ADA Accommodation. (2002, September). *HR Focus, 79*, 2.

Flores, C. (2008). A disability is not a trump card: The Americans with Disabilities Act does not entitle disabled employees to automatic reassignment. *Valparaiso University Law Review, 43*, 195–260.

Ford & Harrison, L. L. P. (2002, July 19). *Potential violation of collective bargaining agreement does not make requested accommodation unreasonable.* News release. Retrieved February 9, 2004, from http://www.fordharrison. com/fh/news/articles/07192002collective.asp

Fujiura, G., Yamaki, K., & Czechowicz, S. (1998). Disability among ethnic and racial minorities in the United States. *Journal of Disability Policy Studies, 9,* 111–130.

Gault, R., & Kinnane, A. (1996). Navigating the maze of employment law. *Management Review, 85,* 9–11.

Geaney, J. (2004). The relationship of workers' compensation to the Americans with Disabilities Act and Family and Medical Leave Act. *Clinics in Occupational and Environmental Medicine, 4,* 273–293.

Gold, M. (1998). *An introduction to labor law.* Ithaca, NY: Cornell University, ILR Press.

Goldberg, S., Killeen, M., & O'Day, B. (2005). The disclosure conundrum: How people with psychiatric disabilities navigate employment. *Psychology, Public Policy, and Law, 11,* 463–500.

Golden, T., Zeitzer, I., & Bruyère, S. (in press). New approaches to disability in social policy: The case of the United States. In T. Guloglu (Ed.), *Social policy in a changing world.* Munster: MV Wissenschaft Publishing.

Goodman, N., & Livermore, G. (2004, July 28). *The effectiveness of Medicaid Buy-In programs in promoting the employment of people with disabilities.* Briefing paper prepared for the Ticket to Work and Work Incentives Advisory Panel of the Social Security Administration. Retrieved November 20, 2009, from http://www.ssa.gov/work/panel/panel_documents/pdf_versions/Buy-in%20paper%20Goodman_Livermore%20072804r.pdf

Hellwege, J. (2002). Tenth Circuit blocks attempt to narrow Rehabilitation Act in disability cases. *Trial, 38,* 88–90.

Huss, A. (1993). ADA, insurance, and employee benefits. *Journal of the American Society of CLU & ChFC, 47,* 82–89.

Imel, S. (1999). *One stop career centers* (ERIC Digest No. 208). Columbus, OH: ERIC Clearinghouse on Adult, Career, and Vocational Education. ERIC Document Reproduction Service NO. ED434244.

Jaeger, P. (2006). Assessing Section 508 compliance on federal e-government Web sites: A multi-method, user-centered evaluation of accessibility for persons with disabilities. *Government Information Quarterly 23,* 169–190.

Lipnic, S., & DeCamp, P. (2007). *Family and Medical Leave Act Regulations: A report on the Department of Labor's request for information.* Washington, DC: U.S. Department of Labor. Retrieved November 30, 2009, from http://digitalcommons.ilr.cornell.edu/key-workplace/315

Moss, K., & Johnsen, M. (1997). Employment discrimination and the ADA: A study of the administrative complaint process. *Psychiatric Rehabilitation Journal, 21,* 111–121.

National Council on Disability. (2004). *Righting the ADA.* Washington, DC: Author. Retrieved November 15, 2009, from http://www.ncd.gov/newsroom/publications/2004/pdf/righting_ada.pdf

National Council on Disability. (2007). *Implementation of the Americans with Disabilities Act: Challenges, best practices, and new opportunities for success.* Washington, DC: Author. Retrieved November 15, 2009, from http://www.ncd.gov/newsroom/publications/2007/pdf/implementation_07–26-07.pdf

National Rehabilitation Association (2008). The President's 2009 Federal Budget. Retrieved July 22, 2009, from http://nationalrehab.org/index.php?option=com_content&task=view&id=83&Itemid=2

Nobile, R. (1996). How discrimination laws affect compensation. *Compensation & Benefits Review, 28,* 38–42.

Occupational Injury and Illness Recording and Reporting Requirements, 66 Fed Reg 5916. (January 19, 2001) (to be codified at 29 CFR pts 1904 and 1952). Retrieved November 23, 2009, from http://www.osha.gov/pls/oshaweb/owadisp.show_document?p_table=FEDERAL_REGISTER&p_id=16312

O'Keeffe, J. (1994). Disability, discrimination, and the Americans with Disabilities Act. In S. Bruyère & J. O'Keeffe (Eds.), *Implications of the Americans with Disabilities Act for psychology* (pp. 1–14). New York: Springer Publishing & Washington, DC: American Psychological Association.

Pape, D., & Tarvydas, V. (1994). Responsible and responsive rehabilitation consultation on the ADA: The importance of training for psychologists. In S. Bruyère & J. O'Keeffe (Eds.), *Implications of the Americans with Disabilities Act for psychology* (pp. 169–186). New York: Springer Publishing & Washington, DC: American Psychological Association.

Pechman, L. (1995). Coping with mental disabilities in the workplace. *New York State Bar Journal, 67,* 22, 24–26, 49.

Percy, S. (2001). Challenges and dilemmas in implementing the Americans with Disabilities Act: Lessons from the first decade. *Policy Studies Journal, 29,* 633–640.

Postol, L. (2002). Sailing the employment law Bermuda Triangle. *The Labor Lawyer, 18,* 165–192.

President's Committee on Employment of People with Disabilities. (1994). *Seniority and collective bargaining issues and the Americans with Disabilities Act—A strategy for implementation.* Final Report of the Seniority/Collective Bargaining Agreement Work Group. Washington, DC: Author.

Rothstein, M. A. (1990). *Occupational safety and health law* (3rd ed.). St. Paul, MN: West Publishing Co.

Scheid, T. (1998). The Americans with Disabilities Act, mental disability, and employment practices. *Journal of Behavioral Health Sciences and Research, 25,* 312–324.

Schwab, S. (2009). *The union as broker of employment rights.* Cornell Law Faculty Working Papers. Retrieved December 3, 2009, from http://scholarship.law.cornell.edu/clsops_papers/55

Scott, M. (1996). Compliance with ADA, FMLA, workers' compensation, and other laws requires road map. *Employee Benefit Plan Review, 50,* 20–30.

Setzer, S. (1992, February 24). Hiring restraints loom in disability law. *ENR News,* pp. 8–9.

Shalowitz, D. (1993, December 6). Return to work obstacle. *Business Insurance, 53,* 2.

Skoning, G., & McGlothlen, C. (1994). Other laws shape ADA policies. *Personnel Journal, 73,* 116.

Stapleton, D., Livermore, G., Thornton, C., O'Day, B., Weathers, R., Harrison, K., et al. (2008, September). *Ticket to Work at the crossroads: A solid foundation with an uncertain future.* Report submitted to the Social Security Administration Office of Disability and Income Support Programs. Washington, DC: Mathematica Policy Research Institute. Retrieved November 30, 2009, from https://www.policyarchive.org/bitstream/handle/10207/15739/TTW_crossroads.pdf

Stapleton, D., O'Day, B., Livermore, G., & Imparato, A. (2006). Dismantling the poverty trap: Disability policy for the twenty-first century. *The Milbank Quarterly, 84,* 701–732.

Stude, E. (1994). Implications of the ADA for master's and bachelor's level rehabilitation counseling and rehabilitation services professionals. *Rehabilitation Education, 8,* 17–25.

Taylor, R. W. (1995). Medical examinations under the ADA and OSH Act: A dilemma for employers. *Employment in the Mainstream, 20,* 23–25.

Ullman, M., Johnson, M., Moss, K., & Burris, S. (2001). The EEOC charge priority policy and claimants with psychiatric disabilities. *Psychiatric Services, 52,* 642–649.

U.S. Department of Education. (2009). *American Recovery and Reinvestment Act of 2009: Vocational Rehabilitation Recovery Funds.* Retrieved July 15, 2009, from http://www.ed.gov/policy/gen/leg/recovery/factsheet/vr.html

U.S. Department of Justice. (2002). *A guide to disability rights laws.* Washington, DC: Author. Retrieved February 5, 2004, from http://www.usdoj.gov/crt/ada/cguide.pdf

U.S. Department of Labor. (2000, April 12). *Training and Employment Information Notice No. 16–99.* Retrieved February 17, 2004, from http://wdsc.doleta. gov/disability/htmldocs/tein_16_99.cfm

U.S. Department of Labor. (2001). *Frequently asked questions: Various Topics: What if an employee declines an audiometric test?* Retrieved November 30, 2009, from http://www.osha.gov/html/faq-various.html

U.S. Department of Labor. (2005). *Innovative workplace safety accommodations for hearing impaired workers* (Safety and Health Information Bulletin SHIB 07–22-2005). Retrieved December 1, 2009, from http://www.osha.gov/dts/shib/shib072205.html

U.S. Department of Labor. (2009a). *Frequently asked questions and answers about the revisions to the Family and Medical Leave Act.* Washington, DC: Author. Retrieved May 15, 2009, from http://www.dol.gov/whd/fmla/finalrule/NonMilitaryFAQs.pdf

U.S. Department of Labor. (2009b). *Frequently asked questions about State Occupational Safety and Health Plans.* Retrieved December 1, 2009, from http://www.osha.gov/dcsp/osp/faq.html

U.S. Department of Labor. (2009c). *Military family leave provisions of the FMLA (Family and Medical Leave Act): Frequently asked questions and answers.* Washington, DC: Author. Retrieved May 15, 2009, from http://www.dol.gov/whd/fmla/finalrule/MilitaryFAQs.pdf

U.S. EEOC answers biggest FMLA/ADA questions. (1997). *Disability Leave and Absence Reporter, 104,* 4.

U.S. Equal Employment Opportunity Commission [EEOC]. (1992). *A technical assistance manual on the employment provisions (Title I) of the Americans with Disabilities Act.* Washington, DC: Author.

U.S. Equal Employment Opportunity Commission [EEOC]. (1996). *EEOC enforcement guidance: Workers' compensation and the ADA.* Washington, DC: Author.

U.S. Equal Employment Opportunity Commission [EEOC]. (1997, March 25). *EEOC enforcement guidance on the Americans with Disabilities Act and psychiatric disabilities* (No. 915.002). Washington, DC: Author.

U.S. Equal Employment Opportunity Commission [EEOC]. (2000). *The Family and Medical Leave Act, the Americans with Disabilities Act, and Title VII of the Civil Rights Act of 1964.* Retrieved February 4, 2004, from http://www.eeoc.gov/pol-icy/docs/fmlaada.html

U.S. Equal Employment Opportunity Commission [EEOC]. (2003). *Annual Report, Fiscal Year 2002.* Retrieved February 5, 2004, from http://www.eeoc.gov/litigation/02annrpt.html

U.S. Equal Employment Opportunity Commission [EEOC]. (2008). *Notice Concerning the Americans with Disabilities Act (ADA) Amendments Act of 2008.* Retrieved May 15, 2009, from http://www.eeoc.gov/ada/amendments_notice.html

Walker, J., & Heffner, F. (1992). The Americans with Disabilities Act and workers compensation. *CPCU Journal, 45,* 151–152.

Walworth, C., Damon, L., &, Wilder, C. (1993). Walking a fine line: Managing the conflicting obligations of the Americans with Disabilities Act and workers' compensation laws. *Employee Relations, 19,* 221–232.

Welch, E. (1996). The EEOC, the ADA, and WC. *Ed Welch on Workers' Compensation, 6,* 178–179.

Wright, G. (1980). *Total rehabilitation.* Boston: Little Brown.

Zolkos, R. (1994, July 18). Avoiding charges of bias. *Business Insurance,* p. 85.

34

Accreditation—A Quality Framework in the Consumer-Centric Era

Brian J. Boon, PhD

Arguably, health care stands out as the most complex of service industries. As a sector within this industry, medical rehabilitation struggles with its many unique challenges. Downstream from acute care services, medical rehabilitation is now confronted with the task of demonstrating its value in a reimbursement environment that is directed toward more services for less money. Payment systems have not kept up to changes in service demand driven by patient's need and the rising requirement for specialized rehabilitation services.

In response to the many challenges in the rehabilitation industry, leadership is intensely focused on efforts to improve quality to demonstrate value to their many constituents. Although the use of formalized quality frameworks have been the norm in the manufacturing industry, such as total quality control or management, it is only in the past 20 years that the rehabilitation industry has employed with vigor the many quality frameworks available. Because practitioners in rehabilitation are key participants in quality improvement efforts conducted by organizations, it is a professional obligation that they critically understand features of the quality framework to be used, and where possible, influence decisions regarding which framework to embrace. Often an administrator or business leader in an organization will lean toward a quality framework employed in other industries, such as manufacturing, and extend it to health care because of their familiarity to quality programs or awards in terms of consumer products or services. For the rehabilitation industry, it is argued that a rehabilitation-focused accreditation quality model is the best fit as a quality framework for advancing the performance of organizations that provide medical rehabilitation services.

To be comparable with other quality management alternatives, an accreditation model must include quality standards that reflect sound business practices and address the systematization of continuous improvement efforts. However, to become a best-fit quality model in medical rehabilitation, quality standards must also include a prominent place for the person served and, by extension, specific quality standards directed to advancing service to unique rehabilitation populations, such as persons with brain injury, spinal cord injury, and chronic pain. It is these population-specific standards that differentiate accreditation as a quality framework from other frameworks as the best fit.

To understand and appreciate the value of accreditation for medical rehabilitation as a quality framework, it is important that accreditation be considered within its evolutionary context in relation to the dynamics of the broader health care industry. Accreditation as a quality framework was constructed by the rehabilitation industry in response to environmental pressures to demonstrate a commitment to quality. Since its inception in 1966, as the only rehabilitation-specific accreditor, the Commission on Accreditation of Rehabilitation Facilities (CARF) has been setting quality standards for the broad rehabilitation industry, including medical rehabilitation. As the primary rehabilitation accreditor, CARF's quality standards have changed to meet the demands of the broader health care environment. Since 1966, many new quality management approaches have been trialed by the industry. It is argued that a rehabilitation-specific quality framework will continue to serve both the rehabilitation industry and its patients in that industry well into the future of consumer-directed care. Further, the CARF quality model of accreditation will be compared and then differentiated through its unique focus on persons served, which is an orientation different from other "product" or "service to the consumer" quality management models. The other quality management frameworks include the Malcolm Baldrige National Quality Program (Baldrige), the International Organization for Standardization (ISO), and the European Foundation for Quality Management (EFQM).

EVOLUTIONARY PHASES IN ACCREDITATION

The evolutionary phases of accreditation as a rehabilitation industry–specific quality management framework can be illustrated against the dynamic characteristics of the broader health care environment (Figure 34.1). One characteristic is the degree to which the environment is closed or exclusive. In contrast, an inclusive environment would purposefully engage and optimize the involvement of diverse stakeholders or participants in its processes. Another characteristic is the degree to which an environment is transparent and therefore provides for an enhanced public accountability. A transparent environment often evolves in response to demands for greater accountability. As these environmental factors change, so do characteristics of the quality management framework. The continuum of these factors (exclusiveness to inclusiveness and low to high degrees of transparency) acts as reference points to the evolution of accreditation. Accreditation, as described through various eras, is influenced by environmental dynamics concurrent to the period of time or era. The described eras are not mutually exclusive and the features of one, in fact, can carry over to future eras. Over time, accreditation evolves to satisfy the demands of quality. As a unique quality framework and business orientation, accreditation is greatly positioned to optimize its effect on enhancing services to the lives of persons served (Stavert & Boon, 2003). Each of the following eras illustrates accreditation's evolutionary paths with specific reference to rehabilitation.

The Professions Era (1960–1980)

In its early evolutionary steps, accreditation began as the result of the exclusive activity of the rehabilitation professions seeking to provide a quality template and to pursue excellence in the delivery of service and care. Although certification, licensure, and various forms of regulation existed regarding the practice of care, these administrative requirements were not seen by rehabilitation professionals or regulators as guides to improving services or programs. As there existed no external benchmark for excellence, accreditation was sponsored as a guide to excellence from a supporting grant from the Vocational Rehabilitation Administration in 1966 (Galvin, 1999). Many of the professional rehabilitation and health care associations supported and promoted accreditation as an industry-based quality initiative. Until recently, CARF's governance model was comprised of a Board of Trustees of sponsoring members who represented many of the major professional organizations in the rehabilitation industry. The CARF Board can be traced back to these early days sourcing its board from the professions in health care.

During this era, quality standards were developed collegially, via expert consensus-based panels, and then endorsed by the community of providers. Accreditation processes

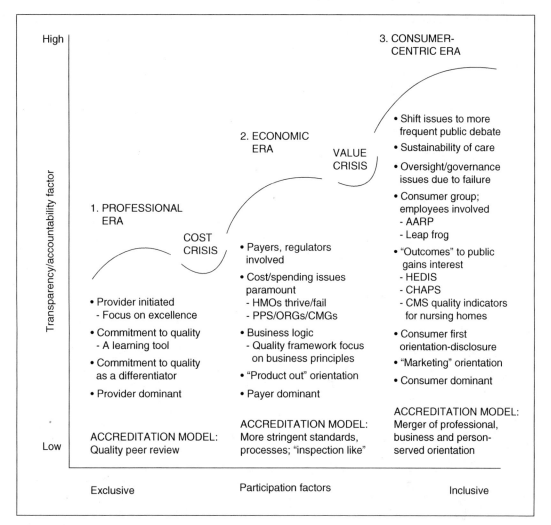

FIGURE 34.1 Evolutionary phases of accreditation.

took the form of on-site review visits or surveys of organizations to determine the degree of compliance/conformance to required standards. The act of preparing for and successfully completing accreditation demonstrated that an organization was committed to demonstrating its conformance to quality standards and continuous improvement for the benefit of consumers. This distinction was used to differentiate organizations from one another, sometimes allowing for those organizations that were accredited to claim specialty status. Being accredited by a neutral third party gave organizations the opportunity to proclaim that their organization met the standard of a quality-based organization. Accreditation was promoted as a voluntary initiative in rehabilitation, although it was also used as a supplement to regulation or rule requirements to receive certain payments. Peer-based accreditation maintained and advanced the privilege of the professions "regulating" themselves through this commitment to quality via accreditation.

The process of quality accreditation review by peers maintained provider autonomy and "control" over quality for a significant period of time. To some extent, during this period of provider dominance, consumers were, as a group, less organized or active and, to a degree, individually "passive" recipients of service or treatment. However, this apparent era of professional autonomy was soon challenged by the era of economics as costs began to challenge the collective system. Advances in the use of medical technology and pharmaceuticals, and a growing demand for more health care and specialized rehabilitation services, resulted in rising costs. The challenges associated with these trends shifted the dynamics of the system from one predominated by professional direction and influence, to one in which economics became a predominant factor in a changing and dynamic environment.

The Economic Era (1980–Present)

Cost-Containment Tactics

As health care costs dramatically increased, discussions and concerns regarding the long-term affordability of health care and its effect on the delivery of quality service became a paramount industry and public-policy concern. Although the rehabilitation industry continued to support accreditation, emerging environmental factors provided the opportunity for new management philosophies to be considered in the industry as it responded to the crisis in the "business" of health care. It was during this period that regulators and payers became more involved as service concerns and rapidly rising costs, specifically in rehabilitation, became more transparent to the public. Managed care approaches evolved to control costs during this period while trying to maintain access to appropriate care (Eccleston, 1995). In response to economic crisis, health care leadership shifted to employing and adopting business logic to its health industry problems. Payers looked to alternative payment schemes and contract-management approaches to control costs. Providers experienced lower reimbursement rates or deep discount contracts, which resulted in fewer dollars per case and was part of the "rehabilitation carve-out" cost-management effort. The mantra of "doing more with less" was and remains a predominant theme in health care, much like the oft-heard phrase "funding dictates form." With an increasing sensitivity to costs, accreditation was used as a vendor prequalification step in procurement of services by some payers. Some insurers used accreditation as a contract-management risk tool to ensure that quality rehabilitation service was embedded in their extended specialty-service provider networks (e.g., brain injury services). Insurers would only reimburse providers if they received third-party accreditation for their claimed specialty in rehabilitation. Insurers used accreditation to confirm that those claiming to provide specialty rehabilitation services were qualified and ran programs to known quality standards. Similar logic was also employed by regulators and policy makers who may have passed rules, declarations, mandates, or directives regarding the requirements of accreditation for reimbursement and "quality" oversight purposes.

Employees Enter as New Participants

In response to the cost crisis and the new business logic being employed, accreditation quality standards adjusted accordingly. Standards became longer, more stringent, and at times definitive or prescriptive. New programs/standards were added as outpatient rehabilitation or specialty services grew. By way of example, in response to the cost crisis in the workers compensation industry, the CARF created "work-hardening" standards to focus the provider, payer, and injured worker on the importance of return to work as an outcome of rehabilitation. The typical goals in rehabilitation, such as "improve strength" of the worker, included the demands to ensure the worker's return to work and ultimately contain costs. Quality rehabilitation standards relating to performance were also added, referencing measures of effectiveness, efficiency, or satisfaction. In an era of rising costs, results for dollars spent on quality standards relating to safety also became more of a priority with the increasing transparency of reported safety errors in the general health care system (Institute of Medicine, 1999). In partial response to the public-safety crisis, the accreditation process became a more rigorous or "inspective-like" quality-assurance exercise for organizations. The large, fragmented U.S. health care system, its structures and processes, lead to disrupted service delivery experiences, poor information flows, and misaligned incentives that degraded the quality and safety of care (Cebul, Rebitzer, Taylor, & Votruba, 2008).

It was also during this era that the employer community became a more vocal and influential participant in the industry, even a proxy representative of their employees' health care quality concerns. Examples of this include the National Business Group on Health (NBGH), formerly known as the Washington Business Group on Health, and The Leapfrog Group. The NBGH is a not-for-profit organization representing a large employer group dedicated to finding innovative and forward-thinking solutions to health care policy and practice issues such as cost control, patient safety, quality of care, and best practices (National Business Group on Health, 2009). It has most recently established a number of initiatives and institutes to advance its cause to improve outcomes, enhance quality, and manage costs. The Leapfrog Group (2009) is also a coalition of public and private organizations whose publicized priority tasks include improving safety of patient care or "saving lives," mobilizing employer purchasing power, recognizing and rewarding excellence in care through market-based incentives, and giving consumers information to make good choices about which hospital to use. The stated motivations of both of these groups are to advance safer health care practice, manage costs, and extend the value of service to the benefit of the employer and its employees. For some employers, health care benefit expenses are cause for concern as they increase infrastructure costs. Higher health benefits result in a higher cost of goods or services delivered, placing in jeopardy an employer's competitive position in a cost-conscious global environment.

It is also during this era that cost concerns and the effect of cost-containment strategies on quality led to public discussions and debates. The cost crisis therefore creates greater transparency in various forms, such as commissions, agencies, institutes, and "think tanks" to consider potential remedies and changes to improve the system. As one example, the President's Advisory Commission on Consumer Protection and Quality in the Health Care Industry (1998), established by President Clinton, studied health care quality and recommended improvement strategies to enhance the health system's responsiveness and effectiveness. Patient's rights legislation was one option considered from the report, the other being the established agency known as the National Forum for Quality Management and Reporting—an agency directed to establish common set performance indicators for the health system, such as public reporting of quality in systems of care (e.g., Nursing Home Compare). In a specific example of a cost-management strategy, even the Centers for Medicare and Medicaid Services (CMS) are trying to review and control costs related to reimbursement of intensive rehabilitation services provided to patients in inpatient rehabilitation hospital units—known as the "75% rule." All payers of services try to define and manage the cost parameters of health care, whether they are private insurance companies or a "government"-reimbursed service. An apparent universal truth in health care exists—demand always exceeds supply, a trend likely to continue. Significant public domain efforts signal collective unrest and potential changes in the environment, ultimately leading to a new era of health care delivery.

As the dynamics of the environment became more inclusive and open, and issues related to cost effectiveness, customer satisfaction, and safety became more prominent, the health care industry concurrently borrowed other industries' lessons and logic concerning quality. Health care/rehabilitation organizations began to employ quality frameworks (Counte & Meurer, 2001) such as ISO 9000, Baldrige, Total Quality Management (TQM), Continuous Quality Improvement (CQI), Quality Control Circles, Statistical Process Control (SPC), Balanced Scorecards/ Reports, Process Reengineering, Management by Results, and Outcome Management. The Disney Institute (2009) even ventured into providing its various programs to health care organizations that wished to advance their customer-service approach. A good organization will always challenge itself to discover cost-effective methods of delivering quality rehabilitation service. All of the above-noted techniques quality, if implemented effectively, to help organizations "to do more with less."

Cost containment is a predominant theme within the economic era, and the resulting service reality for the rehabilitation field was to "do more with less." An employed business logic that embraced quality frameworks from other industries created a gap between leadership and those who provided direct services to persons served. Essentially, a gap of cultures was created between management and practitioners in relation to the methods of delivering high-quality care in a reducing reimbursement environment.

A prevailing countertrend to the economically driven cost-containment era was a more vigilant, autonomous, and empowered collective of consumer groups. Consumers fought the apparent restrictions to access and care practices imposed by managed care techniques. Employers, too, continued to be concerned by rising health-benefit costs with no end in sight. Over time, as more costs shift to employers and their employees, and overall there is less access to services for the masses, the public debate will begin regarding the value for dollars spent in the emerging, "to be dominant" consumer-centric marketplace. The "crisis of value" will challenge the industry to once again reorient and adjust to a new circumstance of environment dynamics. Payers, regulators, and providers will need to embrace the shifting influence that persons served will have in reshaping the future delivery of health care and rehabilitation.

Consumer-Centric Era (2000 and Beyond)

The health and human services industry is beginning to experience the early signs of a fundamental change to their environment. Consumers or persons served are beginning to exercise choice, control, and, with greater frequency, bear the financial cost for services received. This period, referenced as the consumer-centric era, is that time when the economic and service challenges in the health care system are so great, that the apparent sustainability of the health service system is at stake. The current federal and state fiscal crises, an aging population with growing health demands, and other industry factors will likely conspire to create a service crisis. Costs will remain a critical variable for ongoing management. The crisis of service, cost, and sustainability will shift debate from the private boardrooms of companies to the broader and transparent public arena, where concerns regarding accountability for quality are at the forefront of that debate.

It is during this period that the Internet-knowledgeable consumer will demonstrate unprecedented influence and create new demands and channels (e.g., Facebook, Twitter) in the health care system. Consumers will transition from relatively uninformed, passive recipients of service to engaged and informed participants in their care and service plans. Consumers will be vigilant about timely access to affordable, high-quality service with expected outcomes commensurate with experienced risk. Informed consumers will begin to advocate for improvements in the dimensions of rehabilitation, such as timely and friendly access to care, practice patterns consistent with established guidelines, and outstanding clinical and functional outcomes (Goonan, 1994). This social shift in influence already can be observed in the growing number of consumer-directed health plans, spending accounts, and service options that have become instituted with greater frequency in the marketplace. Pharmaceutical companies have also recognized the power of consumer authority as they begin marketing directly to consumers, often via television commercials, supplementing the traditional physician-only sales channels: "the 'blue pill' will allow you to golf pain-free like Tiger Woods!"

In an era of greater transparency, consumers will want access to information with respect to quality indicators of rehabilitation service. They will also demand more information over time in the form of "public report cards." Signs of increasing transparency and, by extension, public accountability already exist, which are illustrated in a set of first-generation public reports. Examples of these public reports include, to name a few, the Health Plan Employers Data and Information Set (HEDIS), which is the tool used by the National Committee on Quality Assurance (2003, 2009) and which comprises a group of measures designed to evaluate health plans' key processes; the Consumer Assessment of Health Plans (CAHPS) developed and managed by a consortium of organizations (Aging for Health Care Research and Quality, American Institutes for Research, Harvard Medicine School, RAND, and Westat); the CMS Nursing Home Compare; and general satisfaction questionnaires such as Health Grades, Inc., conducted by J. D. Power and Associates (2004). Clearly, insurers/ payers, regulators, and health organizations are focused on indices of quality as they relate to the consumer. Outcomes for services rendered will drive consumers and payers to select and reinforce the high-performance provider. Further, with the growing influence of consumers and greater health care costs being paid directly by consumers (Organization for Economic Cooperation and Development [OECD], 2009), the dominant social forces that have an effect on human service systems will be consumer collectives. Consumer enclaves, in the traditional sense (e.g., American Association of Retired Persons) or via internet swarms (virtual collectives with common values and purpose) will create powerful social forces of significant magnitude to affect public policy, influence purchase trends, review quality, and ultimately assess the value of care via cost, service, and outcomes.

It is during this period of response to crises that key participants will reaffirm their primary focus on the task at hand—to organize systems, organizations, and services around persons served. If the explicit value of the system is to serve an engaged consumer, then services should be organized around the person served. A quality framework specific to rehabilitation should both support and advance this orientation. To be of value, quality frameworks must be inclusive and transparent to key participants in the system—provider, payer, and person served. With inclusive participation from key participants in the development of standards, rehabilitation accreditors can enhance their quality framework by importing the valuable knowledge from the rehabilitation field, and including input from persons served—the consumer.

Industries outside of human services incorporate the customer requirement in their production or manufacturing process, to meet the customers' specifications. Quality is built into the design of the product. In an inclusive environment, a rehabilitation accreditor must also incorporate multiple-party input into the process of designing and promoting quality standards. Providers, payers, regulators, and persons served should be "at the table" when accreditors develop quality standards and establish the process to assess quality. They all participate in the rehabilitation system. This approach is inclusive, transparent, and leads to advancing accountability in the system. In turn, quality rehabilitation standards should also prominently recognize the unique role that the person served plays in the design, delivery, and outputs of care. The emerging consumer-centric environment will require that organizational practices be consistent with the values in rehabilitation to fully and meaningfully engage persons served. Further, this quality framework should reestablish the link between process and outcome, which recognizes the important role that both clinicians and persons served play in contributing to a quality result. Accreditation will provide the architecture for organizational service design and quality assessment and will create an integrated, transparent, and value-based organization. In the consumer-driven era, a rehabilitation-specific accreditation quality framework will position organizations to shift their orientation by transitioning from pure business quality templates to accreditation quality templates to serve individuals better.

TRANSITION FROM A BUSINESS QUALITY MODEL TO AN ACCREDITATION QUALITY MODEL

Health care as an industry is a "big and complex business" in most developing countries. Internationally, health care spending continues to outpace economic growth in most industrialized countries, and in response, each country struggles with its own unique way to fund services through public, private, or variant hybrid payment systems. The magnitude of dollars spent on health care is poignantly reflected as a percentage of a country's gross domestic product (GDP). Utilizing data from OECD (2007), the proportion of GDP spent on health care in the United States reached 16.0%. In other countries, the numbers are almost as high: France at 11%, 10.8% for Switzerland, 10.4% for Germany, Belgium with 10.2%, and Canada and Australia each at 10.1%. In the United States, costs continue to escalate and outstrip other countries on many factors. In particular, total health spending per capita was $7,290 USD almost two-and-one-half times greater than the OECD average of $2,964. In the United States, health care spending reached $2.26 trillion in 2007 and is expected to increase at a growth rate of 6.7% (CMS, 2003). Health care is big business, and the cost and ability to access care for Americans has placed this topic as a priority for the Obama administration.

As previously noted, the overall environment of health care has recently and predominantly focused on cost relative to service. In an attempt to deal with the cost-to-quality issue, regulators, payers, and health care leaders in charge of health care plans or systems of care, including hospitals and rehabilitation settings, have tried to address the business complexity of health care by employing the logic necessary to survive in such a demanding environment. As a consequence, health care has employed and adapted a multitude of business-based quality tools, techniques, and principles. There exists some evidence that utilizing quality tools or techniques is perceived by management or organizational leadership as contributing to an organization's strategic or business goals (Yasin, Zimmerer, Miller, & Zimmerer, 2002). It is also interesting to note that the business-based quality frameworks are predated by accreditation-based quality framework methods (e.g., CARF accreditation—1966, ISO 9000—1987, Baldrige—1988). However, evolving quality management approaches found their way as, at times, a competing alternative or supplement to accreditation. It is plausible that accreditation business standards had not kept up with the business needs of organizations via its standards, and therefore were no longer felt to be relevant or of value. An equally plausible reason is that the accreditation process was seen as a professional validation effort by clinicians to affirm that their processes were of high quality, resulting in clinical/functional gains. However, during an "economic squeeze" cycle, pure functional gains appear to be less relevant to cost-focused administrators and payers. Perhaps accreditation was really never perceived by administrators as a "true quality framework," but rather a requirement for payment or a clinically focused exercise. Further, in larger human service systems, the accreditation of a rehabilitation program was rarely elevated to the attention of the President/CEO or Executive Director. In fact, if successful accreditation was realized repeatedly, it may have lost significance over time. Lastly, as the business challenges in health care grew, executives employed to lead health plans and hospitals had other management, industry, and educational experiences, and were more familiar with other quality models to advance the performance of their organization.

Since industry-based quality programs were known to help the competitiveness of industry globally, it was reasoned that these quality programs could help the health care industry to address its concerns. Industry quality frameworks were innovative, prestigious, and something new to many organizations. As a by-product of adopting the business quality techniques, it was hoped that these programs would create organizational spirit, trust, and renewal with staff. Undoubtedly, the opportunity for the clinician to become empowered in an organization to identify, discuss, and provide solutions to work problems can create a better service and work environment. However, although these quality programs were being introduced and business logic was employed, the greatest long-term result of these organizational efforts, even if it was not appropriately implemented, was to create organizations comprised of leadership and practitioners that were "two minded and culturally disintegrated" (Goldsmith, 1998). In essence, the leadership and staff became disengaged from one another. This gap relates to an "orientation gap" in which the actions of the business-based quality framework, such as business process improvement teams, at times disengaged from the reality of day-to-day interactions between clinicians and the treatment complexities of their patients. Often-heard statements from clinicians during such sessions were "...but my patients are not like those identified"; hence the tensions created by a lop-sided business-only quality management approach.

In the human services industry and particularly in rehabilitation there are unique issues that are foreign to the typical manufacturing or service environments in which quality frameworks operate. As an illustration (Figure 34.2), in the manufacturing industry quality is a function of many causal factors, including worker, material, method, measurement, and machine (Ishikawa, 1985). These collectives of causal factors constitute a process that can be controlled via standardization to create a quality effect. In manufacturing, the effect is targeted quality—a certain level of designed quality. Quality of conformance is an indication of how far the actual product conforms to its quality target or design. Let us translate this quality formula to the human services industry and, specifically, to rehabilitation. The worker providing the services is the clinician. The method employed is his or her clinical intervention and/or process. The material is the person served, and the machine could be pharmaceutical or a technology that helps with functional restoration (e.g., a weight machine for strengthening exercise). However, the formula is even more complex in rehabilitation since an engaged consumer, or person served, is both the material *and* part worker or producer of an outcome. This is a unique factor that differentiates an accreditation quality framework from those employed by business where customer needs or requirements are defined and a product is produced or service generated to meet those desired needs and features. In the case of rehabilitation, the person served is both the coproducer of service and the recipient of service with an associated outcome. The rehabilitation process makes accommodations for this complex variable in the equation, and therefore a quality framework must emphasize this

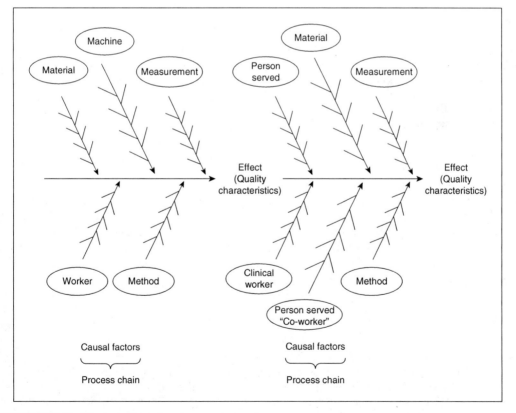

FIGURE 34.2 Cause–effect diagram.

distinct point if it is to be relevant and of value. It is this distinction that those who provide direct services in the health and rehabilitation environment recognize and the reason why most employed business-based quality programs in health care are perceived as "foreign" or force-fitted into the health and rehabilitation industry.

As an interesting note, despite the business philosophy employed during the economic era, health care and its delivery continued to remain fragmented, and escalating cost factors often outstripped inflation at a rate two or three times that of the consumer price index rate.

THE IMPORTANCE OF PROCESS MEASURES AND PERSONS SERVED

There exists the desire by leaders in health and rehabilitation to ensure that human service systems meet the highest standards with respect to both business and clinical service excellence. Much study specific to assessing quality in health care has already been conducted. One well-known approach is to assess quality via its structure, processes, and outcomes (Donabedian, 1978, 1996). Structural assumptions of quality identify the necessary and enabling conditions that must be present in the provision of care or service, such as infrastructure and staff. Structural elements are necessary conditions but alone do not ensure quality. Process measures focus on the activities delivered according to accepted and predetermined standards; that is, those standards related to care and the delivery of care within a program or organizational unit of analysis. Outcomes refer to the attainment of desired goals for the individual (e.g., return to work), at the level of the organization (e.g., reduced medical errors, patient satisfaction) or at a systems level (e.g., measures of community health, social participation). For organizational leadership, structure and outcomes factors are of more relevance and interest because they are more tangible for deliberation and debate. Administrative staff see "aggregate numbers"; therefore, they understand structure and outcome data such as unit costs, total paid staff time, profit margins, and patient satisfaction. Process measures typically fall under the primary domain of interest for providers of health services. Clinicians treat patients one person at a time and need to manage all the service intersect processes that occur during the rehabilitation continuum. This insight into the service continuum is a gap for some administrators. When outcomes can be linked to process, certainly providers are engaged as other parties in an evidence-based or a promising practices approach. Persons served are also concerned with outcomes and the processes that they must participate in as well as those risks and consequences.

The advantages and disadvantages of process measures relative to outcome measures have been well articulated in other articles (Mant, 2001; Rubin, Provonost, & Diette, 2001). Outcomes measures are of relevance to persons served. However, quality frameworks again fail to recognize the role of persons served in producing an outcome, and therefore process measures are also relevant to persons served. Process measures have immediate appeal to clinicians in the health and rehabilitation environment. These measures identify exactly which processes are followed that are believed to result in an effective output or outcome. Measures that relate to process, the "science and art of doing," provide information that is observable and therefore function as a frame of reference for what needs to be changed to improve outcomes. Process measures utilized as standards of quality also reflect the care of service delivered, and therefore clinicians feel accountable for them because they have face validity—"it is what we do." Although outcomes are the desired goals of any rehabilitation process, it is recognized that many factors affect health care outcomes beyond the control of the provider, such as patient involvement and commitment to treatment regimens, as well as many other external factors. There exists clinical comfort in using process measures. The challenge to a processes-only approach is confirming evidence that supports the relationship between a clinical process and outcome, which then puts the clinician and, by extension, persons served at risk in an environment where economics alone begins to influence the method, timing, and appropriateness of services. Where these links have been determined, all parties will focus on good process for expected outcomes. However, it is difficult to link the process to outcomes because of the necessity to provide for risk-adjusted outcomes to incorporate unique features of complex rehabilitation patient populations. Much research is needed to advance promising practices or the practice of evidence-based care and to advance the role of the person served as a critical resource in that process-outcome linkage analysis.

For an accreditation model to provide for a robust quality framework, it must appeal to the various key participants in the delivery system. Governance and executive leadership want a framework that is a template for the system of business (structure/process) and service performance (outcomes) of the organization that the excellence award programs typically provide. Clinical staff members desire a template to judge their care processes (process) and results (outcomes) achieved to some standard or benchmark. Persons served want input, participation (process), and assurances of quality (outcomes) results. The drive of the collective then is to ensure that organizations are assessed against the framework of structure, process, and outcomes. In relation to these dimensions, accreditation will be assessed in reference to three other respected business-quality frameworks (Baldridge, ISO, and EFQM) and then will be differentiated against these frameworks to demonstrate the best fit within the rehabilitation industry and in the consumer-centric era.

QUALITY IMPROVEMENT FRAMEWORKS AND THE ACCREDITATION MODEL OF QUALITY

Clearly the success of any business enterprise depends upon how an organization manages its resources to create effective and efficient delivery systems of service. In an effort to meet this challenge, health care organizations have implemented various respected quality frameworks referenced previously. Further, many organizations simultaneously pursue accreditation for purposes of "deemed status," mandates, or the extended philosophy of continuous improvement in the rehabilitation setting. The CARF accreditation model of quality will be compared to three predominant and respected business-quality frameworks: the Malcolm Baldrige National Quality Program—Health Care Criteria for Performance Excellence (2009), the International Organization for Standardization—ISO 9000: 2000 Quality Management Principles (2000), and the European Foundation for Quality Management (EFQM)—Excellence Model (1999). The accreditation model used is the Commission on Accreditation of Rehabilitation Facilities (CARF)—Medical Rehabilitation Standards (2009). In late 2009, the ISO 9001:2008 version of the certification process was released, and EFQM also released major revisions to their model. CARF releases updates every year on its standards, with a major review every 3 years. The comparison approach has been adapted from an international review of business excellence and award programs (Calingo, 2002). The author would also like to underscore that all these models are excellent for organizations that wish to advance their business and service practices. Further, all of these frameworks are complementary and can be employed as a holistic step-wise model to enhance business and service improvement.

All of the selected quality frameworks have a directional purpose, which is to advance the success of the organization employing the respective framework (Table 34.1). The Baldrige and EFQM models evolved in response to industry concerns regarding quality in an increasingly competitive national and global economy. The Baldrige approach was extended to health care in 1999, and the EFQM has been employed as a guide in the health industry via the EFQM International Health Sector Group. Since its inception, the oldest of the quality models namely the CARF model has been directed to "enhancing the lives of persons served" as a quality framework in the human services. To provide a sense of CARF's extended reach, CARF accredits more than 42,000 programs at more than 19,000 sites, all attributable to its

TABLE 34.1 *Purpose of Quality Framework*

Framework	Inception (Revisions)	Orientation	Percentage of Applicant Sites Visited	Outcome
Baldrige	1988, Health in 1999 (Annual revisions)	Recognition of organizational excellence and best practice promotion	15–20	Award
ISO 9000	1987, 1994, 2000 (Originated in 1947)	Requirements for quality management systems and guidance for performance improvement	100	Certification, follow-up surveillance audits on corrective actions, option for scheduled audits
EFQM	1991	Recognition of organizational excellence and best practice promotion	20	Award
CARF	1966 (Many)	Recognition that an organization demonstrates quality, value, and optimal outcomes of services through continuous improvement focused on enhancing lives of persons served	100	Accreditation, follow-up quality improvement plan and ongoing annual conformance to quality reports

42-year history of valued accreditation. ISO, like other quality frameworks, has been equally utilized in health along with many other industry sectors (Table 34.2). The orientations of these programs also differ. Both Baldrige and EFQM focus on advancing an organization's practices, capabilities, and results. The award process, which includes self-assessment and external scoring, could include a site visit if the potential of finalist status exists. An ISO outcome is the status of certification that demonstrates compliance with quality-management system principles via specific 9001 requirements, and thus requires that all organizations be assessed via site visit. In CARF accreditation, organizations must demonstrate their conformance to business and service/care standards, confirmed by site visit to receive an accreditation outcome. CARF requires ongoing conformance—the sustainability of quality. By far, ISO is the largest of the quality framework models comprising 157 national standards bodies and 3,183 technical bodies, reflecting the scope of this organization. As of December 2007, 951,486 ISO 9001:2000 conformity certificates were issued by more than 750 certification bodies in 170 countries (ISO, 2007).

Each of the quality frameworks also recognizes that there exist many pathways to performance improvement and operational excellence. The excellence benchmarks in Baldrige and EFQM are found both in their scoring structure and evaluative dimensions. A points system is employed in Baldrige and EFQM. Those exceeding a cumulative 700 points in Baldrige or a 750 cumulative point threshold in EFQM are typically eligible as finalists to receive a quality award (Table 34.3). The EFQM Excellence Model also provides gradients in the evolution of excellence via its stepwise approach: commitment to excellence, recognition of excellence status, and award status. The European Quality Award (EQA) signifies the best of excellent performing organizations. ISO 9000 compliance is audited on-site via a checklist guide reflecting the audit 9001 criteria. Compliance is either met or not met—the resulting outcome

TABLE 34.2 *Adaptation to Sectors*

Framework	Adaptation	Number of Sectors
Baldrige	Unique but equal criteria (process/results) for sectors: businesses—manufacturing, service and small organizations—education, health care, and nonprofit	6
ISO 9000	Multiple industries and increased depth (example: ISO 9001 criteria is applied)	Multiple Industry
EFQM	Unique but nine equal criteria for sectors: large commercial, subsidiary operating units, small to medium enterprise, public sector	4
CARF	Equal business criteria, multiple sector specific criteria—aging services, children and youth, employment and community, behavioral health, medical rehabilitation and increased depth by program within sector	Medical rehabilitation subsectors programs: Comprehensive integrated inpatient Spinal cord system of care Interdisciplinary pain Brain injury Outpatient medical Home and community Case management Health enhancement Pediatric family centered Occupational rehabilitation Residential Vocational Amputation specialty Stroke specialty Rehabilitation process for persons served

leading to a certificate of compliance that extends to 3 years. CARF accreditation has two determined outcomes, accreditation or nonaccreditation. The accreditation outcome is based on the degree of conformance (Table 34.4) to standards as determined by surveyor via checklist. However, there are levels of accreditation that are time-based.

A 1-year level of accreditation outcome signifies that there is organizational conformance to many standards; however, deficiencies are noted requiring correction, and therefore a return site visit in 1 year. A 3-year outcome is awarded if the organization exemplifies substantial conformance to standards—both in policy and practice. Both Baldrige and EFQM review their respective criteria of quality along the evaluative dimensions of whether an organization

TABLE 34.3 *Levels of Quality Recognition*

Framework	Number of Levels	Description
Baldrige	1	1,000 points; > 700 points usually trigger award
ISO 9000	1	Certification of compliance
EFQM	3	Commitment to excellence, recognition of excellence (350 points), European quality award (> 750 points)
CARF	3	Time-based—3 year, 1 year, or nonaccreditation

TABLE 34.4 *Evaluation Dimensions*

Framework	Dimension Structure
Baldrige	Process: Approach, deployment, learning, and integration. Results: Levels, trends, comparisons, and integration
ISO 9000	Compliance/noncompliance: Plan–do–check–act process improvement approach is endorsed
EFQM	For enablers and results criteria the following apply: Results, approach, deployment, assessment, and review
CARF	Conformance rating: Non-, partial, substantial, exemplary

plans and deploys improvement strategies in the organizations, links the results to action, and learns and integrates information to further improve organizational performance. The notion of this "approach, deployment, results, learning, and integration" sequence is embedded within the structure of CARF's Aspire to Excellence structure of standards, which are scorable because of their unidimensional and measurable design. In all four quality frameworks, the "review" is conducted by a third party or neutral agent to the organization seeking an award, certification, or accreditation (Table 34.5). In the case of Baldrige, EFQM, and CARF, awards or accreditation is provided by the quality organization that conducts and manages the reviews/accreditation process. In contrast, ISO utilizes its 157 national standard body organizations to accredit registration bodies that employ auditors to determine ISO compliance and certification. ISO does not directly certify ISO compliance.

Lastly, each quality framework also employs set criteria or standards. Although the scope of the chapter is not to review the details of each framework's criteria, there exist both notable high-level similarities and differences (Table 34.6). All frameworks recognize the importance of leadership, focus on customer, involvement of staff/human resources, continuous improvement utilizing information, and performance. The Baldrige, EFQM, and CARF frameworks have well-formulated Leadership/Strategic Planning standards that reinforce the need to set short-/long-term direction, and the deployment of plans with follow-up, comparison, and revision. Key organizational performance results are also well emphasized in Baldrige/EFQM, including results for patients, financial results, staff, and operating results. Baldrige, EFQM, and ISO focus on higher-order system measures (e.g., financial results, market share measures). EFQM also includes results for society, extending the notion of social responsibility to an outcome for the organization. The other quality frameworks also address results in similar ways. Again, Baldrige includes results for patient and stakeholder (e.g., payers), financial and marketplace performance results.

CARF also has a well-defined organizational performance section that requires an organization to focus on organizational metrics of efficiency, effectiveness, service access, and

TABLE 34.5 *Reviewer Categories*

Framework	Title of Reviewers	Number of Reviewers	Training Time
Baldrige	Examiner	≈560	3/4 days, inclusive of 35–50 hours pretraining
ISO 9000	Registrars—Auditor	–	–
EFQM	Assessor	≈169	2.5 days
CARF	Surveyor	1,400	3.5 days, 20 hours pretraining and intern program

TABLE 34.6 *Criteria of Quality Frameworks*

Baldrige: 2009	ISO 9000: 2000	EFQM—Excellence Model	CARF—Aspire to Excellence Model
Organizational profile	Customer focus	Leadership	Assess the environment
Leadership	Leadership	People	Set strategy
Strategic planning	Involvement of people	Policy and strategy	Persons served and other stakeholders—obtain input
Measurement, analysis, knowledge, and management	Process approach	Partnership and resources	Implement the plan Legal Finance Risk Technology Rights of persons served Accessibility Health and safety Human resources
Workforce	Systems approach management	Processes	Review results
Process management	Continued improvement	People results	Effect change
Results	Factual approach to decision making Mutually beneficial supplier relationship	Customer results Society results Key performance results	Rehabilitation process for persons served

satisfaction from the perspective of persons served and other stakeholders. CARF's accreditation focus looks at the business components of an organization and drills down to the organizational unit (program) delivering rehabilitation to persons served. CARF requires that effectiveness (e.g., work status at 1-month after discharge) to persons served also be measured at a point in time following service to measure true long-term effectiveness or the specific organizational outcomes related to persons served. CARF's other accreditation criteria, such as input from persons served, accessibility, and rights of persons served, also differentiate CARF from the other quality frameworks.

Other quality frameworks typically lack standards that detail the quality standards to protect the rights of persons served, such as requirements to demonstrate a commitment to recognize diversity (culture), to exceed policies to ensure confidentiality and privacy, and to provide access to information and ensure informed choice. The key stakeholders who have contributed to CARF's medical rehabilitation standards development have placed the persons served at the center of an organization's quality assessment. It has been this way since its inception almost 43 years ago. This approach affirms that, in rehabilitation, quality is influenced by the inclusiveness of persons served as key participants in the output or outcome of the process. Hence, service or treatment planning includes shared responsibility and commitment between provider and persons served. As an example of a measured substandard, treatment goals are to be written in the words of persons served in order that the person is engaged and understands the purpose and goals of service. Further, the rehabilitation practitioner is aware of the reasons why the person is seeking services, what goals he or she wants to achieve, and the activities in which they wish to participate.

The person-centric theme or approach has been similarly referenced in a publication written by the Institute of Medicine (2001), which identified that one of the aims for health care improvement is to include a patient-centered approach that is customized to patient needs/values, where the patient is the source of control and in a system that is transparent in its efforts. In the behavioral health sector of rehabilitation, a similar theme has also emerged in the final report of the President's New Freedom Commission on Mental Health (2003), which also affirmed that mental health services and treatment should be consumer and family centered to promote and ensure that individualized care plans are directed to enhancing full community participation. Social responsibility and value of rehabilitation also come to the forefront via CARF's focus on accessibility. Accessibility standards, which are directed to promoting access to services and removing barriers for persons with disability, such as attitudinal or environmental barriers to effect a positive outcome for persons served as active participants in society. This single feature differentiates CARF and its rehabilitation-industry values from the other reputable and noteworthy quality frameworks.

To further instill the person-served orientation, the organization and its leadership must also demonstrate that they promote and protect the rights of persons served as part of their business/service focus. The accreditation-based quality framework emphasizes that enhanced communication efforts to the consumer, the creation of programs and services appropriate to the diversity of the population served, and a demonstration of cultural competency will differentiate providers in the future. Accreditation standards focused on consumer input go beyond mere assessment of input forums of persons served, satisfaction surveys, or market analysis of customer requirements. These are all excellent exercises to better serve customers. Quality frameworks in rehabilitation should advance the orientation to persons served within the organizational business context to organizations that seek to provide high-quality service to people in an era where there will be no alternative to the benchmark of assessed value. Rehabilitation organizations of the future must embrace their responsibility to persons served to ensure value and quality in their privileged position of service. Those organizations, leadership and staff, that embrace this orientation will be well prepared for the consumer-centric era.

The last differentiator in the CARF quality framework is the standard related to the rehabilitation process—specific "process-based" standards often defined by the person served population (e.g., persons with brain injury). A quality framework in rehabilitation must outline process standards that are directed to effecting positive change in the functional ability of persons served. On the basis of the specific rehabilitation population served, the composition of the rehabilitation team, scope of services, program goals, assessment or diagnostic services rendered, establishing treatment plans and goals, and community reintegration planning all vary dramatically. CARF's accreditation quality model outlines specific quality protocols for such processes that do not exist in other quality frameworks (see Table 34.2).

A quality framework that also provides rehabilitation relevant consensus standards creates an additional point of reference for organizations to design new rehabilitation programs or to offer more services in their community. Further, a quality framework can serve as a reference point to experiment and assess outcomes when deviating from the designed rehabilitation standard or targeted quality. Standards can act as blueprints for design, as process controls, and as benchmarks for internal or external comparison. These kinds of standards have "face validity" for clinicians and persons served and/or their families in the rehabilitation community not offered by other quality frameworks. It is the accreditation-based quality framework with its unique orientation to persons served and sector specificity that differentiates it from other quality frameworks.

THE EXTENDED VALUE OF ACCREDITATION

All of the previously referenced quality frameworks, techniques, and philosophies offer the discipline of thought and action necessary to improve the performance of an organization.

Accreditation, with its unique history, depth of rehabilitation-specific standards, and persons-served orientation, offers an extended value beyond the accreditation site visit to the benefit of key participants in the system. The extended value of accreditation can be seen in the benefits to persons served, organizations, payers, regulators, and society (Table 34.7).

TABLE 34.7 *Extended Value in Accreditation*

Society

General
- Maintains the importance of quality in the "human services" in a world of competing interests
- Quality and excellence in systems lead to greater access for people
- Systems focused on people, perform well, create participation opportunities for persons with disabilities; these outcomes contribute to thriving communities/nations
- A well-performing rehabilitation sector reduces stigma of disability, enhances participation for persons
- Congruence with laws (e.g., ADA, Olmstead decision)

Regulators general
- Allows experts and public to determine quality indicators in "specialty" areas; done by a third-party accreditor
- Highest priority risks can be focused of quality oversight by regulator
- Accreditation template provides systems with quality benchmarks across a continuum of services
- Accreditation, with specificity built into programs, sets service standards expectation regardless of location, size, etc. All people deserve high-quality care regardless of location/site (standardize quality)
- Supports public's demand for enhanced quality

Payer
- Requirement that providers be accredited demonstrates commitment to quality on behalf of accounts/ lives covered
- Accreditation standards can be used for service protocols/management practices/cost models/etc.
- Accreditation used as external confirmation of declared specialty, ensuring best care/outcome/service expectation for all stakeholders
- Accreditation requirement of all providers to establish information and outcome management system could be leveraged to establish system improvement efforts; contribute to report cards
- Standards used to create quality continuum of service to better serve accounts/lives concerned

Organization

Governance/executive
- Another third-party review enhances accountability disclosure/quality assurance/risk management function
- Snapshot of human service/business competencies
- Maintains corporate vigilance to society/persons served
- Public demonstration of commitment to quality; can be used as promotional tool
- Bridges "the business with the care" to learn and improve
- May fulfill legal and regulatory requirements
- Balances long-term/short-term business and care priorities

Clinician
- Maintains prominence of persons served as cocreator of outcomes, helps to focus on person-based outcomes
- Program standards act as process templates (face validity), expedite program/service development
- Standards represent embedded knowledge of profession and service of those who participate, at different levels, in the service system
- Standards can be used to appropriately minimize or extinguish undesirable variations in service; enhance learning
- Standards can be translated to technology platform to enhance practice

Person served
- Reasonable assurance of quality, focus on person orientation
- Expectation of individualized approach, participation; that rights and dignity will be maintained
- In rehabilitation, designation of specialty states if program accredited (e.g., spinal cord injury)

To persons served, accreditation offers a reasonable assurance that the services they are to receive meet "current industry standards" with respect to quality and that they will be engaged in care processes and decisions that affect them. Organizations benefit by knowing that they practice their trade against known standards, endorsed by experts and consumers alike. Accreditation creates and confirms the "business and service to person served" alignment. Organizations that maintain their commitment to quality via third-party accreditation, specifically designed and conducted for their rehabilitation-specific business, commit to an accountability framework—both internal and external. In an era of transparency, post-Enron, public trust can be further fortified by organizations that undergo additional third-party review. The accreditation process also bridges the business with the clinical care of components of rehabilitation service delivery. Payers can participate in quality systems by endorsing the requirement of quality service via accreditation as part of their extended service strategy, rebuilding public confidence to well-run and well-intended health service organizations. The opportunity also extends beyond a public relations exercise if accreditation is used to employ service protocols and aid in contract-management practices inclusive of incentives for performance and the collection of data for system improvement opportunities.

Person served, providers, and payers must integrate their efforts in the long run if the system is to achieve a desired state of sustained performance and enhanced access. Regulators who utilize accreditation as a partial oversight function are also afforded the opportunity to focus on their highest priorities, relieving providers of administrative review processes that are duplicative to accreditation and outside their area of expertise. Most importantly, a hallmark differentiator of the value of accreditation specific to rehabilitation is confirmed in its social responsibility function, which links results for the individual served to the greater society. As one of many available quality frameworks, only accreditation maintains the importance of rehabilitation to broader society. With its intense focus on persons served, accreditation standards act as "reference grids" to create effective systems of service and set goals focused on enhancing community participation opportunities for persons with disabilities (e.g., work) to minimize the stigma and barriers associated with disabilities. This clarity of purpose afforded by accreditation is the extended thread of value from persons served to society as a whole.

CONCLUSIONS

Accreditation has evolved over many years in response to different trends in the health and rehabilitation industry. Many indicators suggest discontinuous change in the health care and rehabilitation field. The engaged and informed consumer will continue to challenge the entire service delivery system—its leadership and skilled health professionals. The internet will become of greater use to consumers as they make decisions about care and service options. Report cards will be accessed by the masses. Payers and employers are likely to facilitate the development of incentives to reward providers for quality and excellence. Excellence awards and accreditation models in principle will remain focused on their similar intent to improve and guide organizations to performance excellence. Quality frameworks utilized by organizations will be required to embrace the changing and unique features specific to the business of delivering health care and rehabilitation services. Valued quality frameworks will need to recognize the importance and role of persons served both as contributors to the health and rehabilitation process, and as recipients of the output or outcomes. This factor alone requires a unique quality framework that accreditation can provide. Further, the accreditor who builds a model of quality and standards through an inclusive process will create greater face validity and value within the broader community served—the community of citizenship.

To be of value and relevant, accreditation must also evolve to the needs of its customers. Accreditors are in a unique position of having many beneficiaries, such as accredited organizations, state agencies that mandate third-party accreditation, payers, and to some extent the general public. The general public will insist that accountability be created in our health system. One "check and balance" process that employs the necessary integrity is the accreditation process and the outcome or "seal of quality." As not-for-profit entities, accreditors must serve a higher purpose in view of the direct recipients of service, the persons served. That higher-order purpose is a moral obligation. In the collective sense, persons served are the community, the country, and the nation served. Since the wealth of any nation is no greater than its health, creating efficient and effective quality-based delivery systems is to the ultimate to the benefit of society. Efficiency, effectiveness, and satisfaction regardless of the quality framework employed create capacity in the human services system for greater access to those who may not be privileged to receive the best of care. It also stands to reason that the health of any nation and the quality of its health care is no greater than its access to that care. A commitment to quality, therefore, is a commitment to all persons served.

REFERENCES

Baldrige National Quality Program. (2009). *Health care criteria for performance excellence.* Gaithersburg, MD: National Institute of Standards and Technology.

Calingo, L. M. R. (2002). National quality and business excellence awards: Mapping the field and prospects for Asia. In L. M. R. Calingo (Ed.), *The quest for global competitiveness through national quality and business excellence awards* (pp. 21–40). Tokyo: Asia Productivity Organization.

Cebul, R. D., Rebitzer, J. B., Taylor, L. J. & Votruba, M. (2008). Organizational fragmentation and care quality in the U.S. healthcare system. *Journal of Economic Perspectives, 22,* 93–113.

Center for Medicare and Medicaid Services. (2003). Retrieved from http://cms.hhs.gov

Commission on Accreditation of Rehabilitation Facilities. (2009). *Medical rehabilitation standards manual.* Tucson, AZ: Author.

Counte, M. A. & Meurer, S. (2001). Issues in the assessment of continuous quality improvement implementation in health care organizations. *International Journal for Quality Health Care, 13,* 197–207.

Disney Institute. (2009). Retrieved from http://www.disneyinstitute.com

Donabedian, A. (1978). The quality of medical care. *Science, 200,* 856–864.

Donabedian, A. (1996). Evaluating quality of medical care. *Millbank Quarterly, 44,* 166–206.

Eccleston, S. M. (1995). *Managed care and medical cost containment in workers' compensation: A national inventory 1995–1996.* Cambridge, MA: Workers' Compensation Research Institute.

European Foundation for Quality Management. (1999). *The EFQM excellence model 1999.* Tilburg, Netherlands: Pabo Prestige Press.

Galvin, D. (1999). Accreditation as an accountability strategy. In L. R. McConnell (Ed.), *Accountability from several perspectives: A report on the 20th Mary E. Switzer Memorial Seminar* (pp. 44–51). Alexandria, VA: National Rehabilitation Association.

Goldsmith, J. (1998). Integration reconsidered: Five strategies for improved performance. *Health Care Strategist,* 1–8.

Goonan, K. J. (1994). Using quality assurance systems to change behaviour. In T. W. Granneman (Ed.), *Review, regulate or reform? What works to control workers' compensation medical costs* (pp. 247–267). Cambridge: Workers' Compensation Research Institute.

Institute of Medicine. (1999). *To err is human.* Washington, DC: National Academy Press.

Institute of Medicine. (2001). *Crossing the quality chasm. A new health system for the 21st century.* Washington, DC: National Academy Press.

International Organization for Standardization. (2000). *ISO 9000—2000 (E).* Geneva, Switzerland: Author.

Ishikawa, K. (1985). *What is total quality control. The Japanese way.* Englewood Cliffs, NJ: Prentice-Hall.

J. D. Power and Associates. (2004). Retrieved from http://www.jdpower.com Leapfrog Group. (2004). Retrieved from http://www.leapfroggroup.org

Mant, J. (2001). Process versus outcome indicators in the assessment of quality of health care. *International Journal of Quality Health Care, 13,* 475–480.

National Business Group on Health. (2009). Retrieved from http://www.businessgrouphealth.org

National Committee on Quality Assurance. (2003). *Achieving the promise: Transforming mental health care in America. Final Report.* Rockville, MD: Department of Health and Human Services.

National Committee on Quality Assurance. (2009). Retrieved from http:// www.ncqua.org

Organization for Economic Cooperation and Development *Health Data*. (2009). Retrieved from http://www.oedc.org

President's Advisory Commission on Consumer Protection and Quality in the Health Care Industry. (1998). *Quality first: Better care for all Americans*. Washington, DC: U.S. Government Printing Office.

Rubin, H. R., Provonost, P., & Diette, G. B. (2001). The advantages and disadvantages of process-based measures of health care quality. *International Journal for Quality in Health Care, 13*, 469–474.

Stavert, D. & Boon, B. J. (2003). Listening to consumers...Canada opens. *International Journal of Heath Care Quality Assurance Incorporating Leadership in Health Service, 16*, 1–9.

The Leapfrog Group. (2009). Retrieved from http://www.leapfroggroup.org

Yasin, M. M., Zimmerer, L. W., Miller, P., & Zimmerer, T. W. (2002). An empirical investigation of the effectiveness of contemporary management philosophies in a hospital operational setting. *International Journal of Health Care Quality Assurance, 15*, 268–276.

35

Challenges and Opportunities for Quality in Rehabilitation

Dale C. Strasser, MD

Evidence demonstrating significant numbers of medical errors and variations of services has propelled efforts to address quality deficits in U.S. health care (Schillie, 2007; Wachter, 2009). The need for effective quality improvement (QI) is well recognized by professional, regulatory, and accreditation groups (Agency for Healthcare Research and Quality [AHRQ] 2009; Commission on the Accreditation of Rehabilitation Hospitals [CARF] 2009; Center for Medicare and Medicaid Services [CMS], 2009a), and two reports from the Institute of Medicine (IOM) have provided catalysts for action (IOM, 1999, 2001). Nevertheless, the improvement of quality has been frustratingly modest. Multiple reasons are cited for the difficulties in addressing these issues, including the challenges of quality measurement, embedded financial and professional interests, poorly aligned incentives, and a culture of service delivery unfamiliar with coordination across medical specialties, heath professional disciplines, and organizations. In addition, there may be misconceptions of what quality means specifically, and these misconceptions may impede progress in the area.

The word "quality" has diverse and seemingly contradictory meanings and connotations. The term is frequently used to specify characteristics of a particular item, such as the quality of fabric in an item of clothing. The term is commonly linked with an adjective such as "high, superior," "low, inferior," or "average." In common usage, the term is used alone to imply a superior or desirable attribute, such as a quality individual or a quality service. In health service delivery, the term shares more in common with a third use, similar to its use in engineering and business. Quality in health care is usually linked with a process of problem identification, measurement, intervention to address the problem, feedback, and refinements in an iterative manner called continuous process improvement. The IOM (2001) has defined quality as "the degree to which health services for individuals and populations increase the likelihood of desired health outcomes and are consistent with the best available evidence." Although this definition seems straight forward, the day-to-day experience of many clinicians is that quality initiatives are imposed by others and may inadvertently hinder what is best for the patient or effective-service delivery (Casalino, 1999; Werner & Asch, 2007).

This chapter focuses on quality in inpatient rehabilitation settings in the United States. Initially, an overview of quality including quality measurement and the paradox of quality is presented. Then a framework using the Donabedian model of structure, process, and outcomes is offered. The current status of quality measures in rehabilitation medicine with a particular emphasis on the strengths and limitations of the Functional Independence Measure®

(FIMTM) is reviewed. Finally, suggestions are offered on how to address the quality paradox including rehabilitation-specific quality indicators and activities directed at rehabilitation structure, process, and outcomes.

OVERVIEW—QUALITY OF CARE IN HEALTH CARE

The evidence for inadequate health care is staggering (IOM, 2001; Wachter, 2009). Wide variations in the management of common conditions, high rates of medical errors, and improper treatments (both under and over treatment) have provided the impetus for more effective QI efforts. The emphasis on quality is evident in the regulatory and accreditation requirements of the CMS (2009a, 2009b), the Joint Commission on the Accreditation of Hospital Organizations (JCAHO, 2009), the CARF (2009a, 2009b), and the research and advocacy activities of the AHRQ (2009), and numerous private organizations. Although this chapter focuses on the United States, similar issues arise in other developed countries (Schillie, 2007; Wachter, 2009), which suggests that deficiencies in quality cannot be explained solely by specific economic or societal factors.

Significant variations in health care services have been well documented in various areas including the management of acute myocardial infarctions, hip fractures, colon cancer, strokes, diabetes, and depression along with surgical procedures such as coronary artery bypass graft, hysterectomies, and spinal procedures. For example, an individual in Boston is twice as likely to get elective spine surgery than a similar case in New Haven. Furthermore, patients in areas of higher utilization (and health care costs) do not have better outcomes. A recent article in *The New Yorker* (Gawande, 2009), which examines the difference in health care expenses between two similar cities in Texas, has been referenced by President Obama and others involved in the ongoing discussion on health care reform. In a similar vein, the service delivered is only consistent with published evidence a little over half the time (McGlynn et al., 2003). Although there are inappropriate amounts of health services, the service provided frequently does not match published evidence.

Extensive evidence exists of a high rate of medical errors and inappropriate care. An estimated 44,000–98,000 deaths a year occur because of medical errors, with medication errors alone accounting for more deaths (7,000) than workplace injuries (6,000) according to the IOM (1999, 2001) report, To Err is Human: Building a Safer Health System (IOM, 1999). Although data on medical errors and inappropriate care specific to inpatient rehabilitation settings are limited, it is reasonable to assume that comparable levels exist.

A subsequent IOM report (2001), Crossing the Quality Chasm, identified six aims for improvement in health care as follows:

1. Safe (freedom from medical errors)
2. Effective (treatments consistent with best available evidence)
3. Patient-centeredness (focus on a patient's needs and wishes)
4. Efficient (optimal use of scarce resources)
5. Timeliness (care delivery is as prompt as the situation dictates)
6. Equity (without disparities by funding source, socioeconomic class, and ethnicity)

Governmental, professional, and private organizations (AHRQ, 2009; CMS, 2009a, 2009b; JCAHO, 2009) have spearheaded a broad range of activities to address quality deficits in health care. A common theme involves identification of the problem, development of an action plan, monitoring results of the intervention, and using this information to design other interventions. A popular approach is the "Plan, Do, Study, Act" cycle associated with C. Edward Deming (Plsek, 1999). This method is usually diagrammed as a circle to underscore its iterative nature and to demonstrate the iterative nature of continuous process improvement.

MEASUREMENT OF QUALITY

The development and use of measureable items is pivotal to QI. Valid and reliable measures provide a yardstick to study the underpinnings of quality and to monitor the success of interventions to address deficits. Understandably, discrete items such as mortality, the use of a particular medication, and length of time to a specific intervention have proven easier to measure and associate with specific medical interventions than related issues of morbidity, complex interventions, and long-term outcomes. CMS now publishes quality measures on 20 items ranging in areas of acute myocardial infarction (e.g., β-blocker), heart failure (e.g., heart function evaluation), pneumonia (e.g., oxygenation assessment), and surgical care (e.g., prophylactic antibiotic use) (CMS, Hospital Compare, 2009b). Although the identification and publication of these quality indicators have been associated with improved care in particular areas, these improvements have not carried over to related areas. For example, although specific measures on postoperative infections have been associated with decreases in such infections, they have not resulted in decrease in hospital-acquired pneumonias.

THE QUALITY PARADOX

Clinicians experience a paradox about quality and QI efforts. We endorse the idea, but see organizational efforts to improve quality as a distraction from our own clinical experience (Casalino, 1999; Werner & Asch, 2007). Quality issues are presented at the macrolevel of medical errors and appropriateness of services. Clinicians treat individual patients at the microlevel, where patient-specific issues dominate in the context of community norms and financial considerations.

Many clinicians use the term "quality" in reference to a particular trait or characteristic of an entity (such as a restaurant) or a person. In contrast, its use in health service research refers to the extent to which health services can be associated with patient outcomes. Operationally, quality is linked to system issues of process improvement where hospital leadership indentifies a problem, implements intervention, monitors the effect, and modifies the intervention based on the data collected. Clinicians may view the specific issue selected as tangential to their concerns with individual patients. Hence, the health care approach to quality, the relevance of the identified issue, and the associated terminology may not resonate with busy clinicians treating individual patients. Clinicians have multiple and diverse demands on their time. When presented with yet another time request, many of us will look for ways to minimize the perceived intrusion on our work.

Quality initiatives can have unintended consequences of worsening of quality of care (Casalino, 1999; Werner, & Asch, 2007; Walter, Davidowitz, Heineken, & Covinsky, 2004). Much goes on in a patient–physician encounter and quality measures only capture a small fraction of the variables. By directing attention to a few easily measurable aspects, the subtext is that the rest of the patient encounter is not important. The proverbial baby is thrown out with the bathwater.

For example, in the past year, my hospital system has emphasized compliance with hand-washing guidelines and "call to order" and "time out" periods before invasive procedures including soft tissue and joint injections. Hand washing is clearly important to the reduction of hospital-acquired infections, and call to order procedures strive to reduce error in procedures such as operating on the wrong leg. However, on an inpatient rehabilitation unit where, for example, maintaining a scheduled toileting program or carryover of skills learned in therapy to the unit are ongoing challenges, an exclusive quality emphasis on hand washing and call to order procedures can be seen as a distraction from other clinical issues.

The causes of such disregard for identified quality issue are diverse. Professional arrogance plays a part, as does a naïveté concerning the extent of the problem and one's own contribution to it. In addition, this situation reveals a detachment between regulatory agencies and hospital leadership on the one hand and the clinician–patient relationship on the other.

Recent analyses of traffic safety may offer insights on quality in health care. Psychological factors exert a tremendous influence on traffic safety (Vanderbilt, 2008). Although suburban utility vehicles may seem safer than cars given their size and construction, drivers of such vehicles are more likely not to wear seat belts, to talk on cell phones, and to have accidents. Human behavior can easily mitigate well-intentioned safety efforts. Likewise, efforts to improve safety can have unintended consequences. Stop signs and concerns about speeding tickets can be a distraction from the driving process. The United States has 36% greater fatalities per mile than the United Kingdom, even though the former has better roads, safer cars, and greater traffic controls (Staddon, 2008).

Comparing approaches between the United States and the United Kingdom, it has been asserted that traffic management assumes a more distrustful attitude and imposes controls to reduce driver discretion in the United States, whereas more responsibility is placed on the drivers in the United Kingdom (Roach, 2008). The extent to which traffic safety offers insights to health care quality suggests that interventions to improve quality can be a distraction from an individual's effort to deal with the personal circumstances of a complex patient.

The excessive use of antibiotics may offer other clues to the challenges of QI. Clinicians acting on the perceived need for individual patients tend to over-prescribe antibiotic medications, which leads to multiresistant organisms. On the one hand, hospital leadership may be "over-prescribing" patient safety efforts. On the other hand, clinicians may be failing to take seriously their own roles in medicals errors and patient safety. These analogies (e.g., traffic control and antibiotic use) may help health care professionals and leaders to appreciate the complexities of the issues and the possibilities of unintended consequences when quality initiatives are initiated.

The resolution of this quality paradox involves a multifaceted effort among clinicians, hospital organizations, and accrediting and regulatory agencies. Clinicians do not appreciate how practices with individual patients contribute to systemic problems. Likewise, regulatory agencies and hospital leadership have not been able to factor in the complexity and nuances of the patient–physician interaction in devising quality measures. Clearly, further research is needed. In the meantime, quality initiatives should be relevant to the day-to-day experience of clinicians and framed such that clinicians see their clinical work as more effective when merged with quality. Physicians and other rehabilitation professionals will adopt quality approaches if it produces better outcomes or makes it easier to do their job.

QUALITY IN REHABILITATION—STRUCTURE, PROCESS, AND OUTCOMES

A conceptual model developed by Avedia Donabedian, a health service researcher at the University of Michigan, has proven helpful in the development of measures of quality (Donabedian, 1980, 1988; Wachter, 2009). The "Donabedian Triad" divides quality measures into structure, process, and outcomes. Although there are areas of overlap across these three areas, the model provides a useful framework for understanding quality measures. Each of the areas has strengths and limitations as a perspective on quality in rehabilitation.

Structural characteristics of rehabilitation affect quality. For example, the degree to which the physical facility and organizational structure promote functional independence of patients, family and caregiver education, discharge planning, and the interdisciplinary collaboration are potential quality measures. Examination on the influences of space and design on rehabilitation process and outcomes brings valuable insights on potential and modifiable determinants of stroke rehabilitation effectiveness (Connell, 1997). Likewise, the organization of clinical services such as discipline-specific units (e.g., occupational therapists, speech language pathologists) versus patient diagnostic categories (e.g., stroke or spinal cord injury unit) influence interdisciplinary collaboration among health care professionals. Generally, discrete, measureable structural variables have proven more difficult to link to changes in patient outcomes than process measures.

The process of rehabilitation refers to how services are delivered. Interventions are delivered by an interdisciplinary team of professionals to address the multifaceted determinants of function. In this respect, rehabilitation units resemble educational environments as much as traditional medical treatment. Positive outcomes occur when a patient and his or her family demonstrate new skills and functional abilities in contrast to other inpatient services where outcomes are measured in (usually passive) terms such as recovery from an infection or survival of a myocardial infarction. The nature of rehabilitation interventions and the underlying biopsychosocial approach creates challenges in the development of quality measures.

The process of rehabilitation has been called a black box because of the limited knowledge on how process influences outcomes. Nevertheless, extensive evidence exists to support the team approach in rehabilitation (Langhorne & Dennis, 2004). Working closely with a group of researchers supported by the Veterans Administration (VA), Judy Falconer and I developed and tested a model of rehabilitation treatment effectiveness consisting of inputs, transformational processes, and outcomes (Strasser & Falconer, 1997a, 1997b). Inputs consist of organizational characteristics (such as hospital culture), treatment/technology (specifics of therapy), and participants (patients, families, and staff). The model postulates that team functioning (process) plays a central role as a transformational variable between inputs (structural elements) and patient outcomes. Team functioning consists of team relations (social climate and interprofessional relations) and team actions (team leadership and managerial practices). The primary outcomes are functional gain, discharge destination, and length of stay. This model has guided a comprehensive study of stroke rehabilitation outcomes and VA rehabilitation teams (Strasser, Smits, Falconer, Herrin, & Bowen, 2005; Strasser et al., 2008). In addition, other research support the use of process measures to understand rehabilitation outcomes (DeJong, Horn, Conroy, Nichols, & Healton, 2005; Duncan et al., 2002).

Outcomes measures are the most advanced quality tools in rehabilitation. The FIMTM is the dominant functional outcomes measurement tool in the United States, and it is used extensively internationally. It is an 18-item measurement tool where rehabilitation staff rate the burden of care from a scale of 1 (total dependence) to 7 (complete independence) in 13 areas of activities of daily living and 5 areas of cognitive functioning. The 18 items contain six subscales and two domains (motor and cognition). The first 13 items (or four subscales) are commonly referred to as the motor FIMTM (mFIM), and the last 5 items (or two subscales) as the cognitive FIM (cFIM). For each item, staff rate the level of assistance required from 1 (total assistance) to 7 (complete independence). The FIMTM focuses on the amount of assistance needed (or burden of care) to perform particular activities. For example, a total FIMTM score of 60 (or an individual item rating of 3) equates to the individual needing the help of another for approximately 4 hours a day (Granger, 2008).

Although inpatient rehabilitation services in the United States have their roots in the care of injured soldiers in World War II, standardized tools of assessment and outcomes were slow to develop (Table 35.1). Because of the lack of such measurements, comparisons of outcomes across settings and providers were severely hindered for several decades. By the 1980s, this lack of standardized measurement was becoming increasingly problematic. In 1983, a joint task force of the American Academy of Physical Medicine and Rehabilitation and the American Congress of Rehabilitation Medicine was established to develop measurements of the severity of patient disability and outcomes of medical rehabilitation (Granger & Fiedler, 1997). The process expanded to include representatives from groups affiliated with specific disciplines (e.g., nursing, occupational therapy, physical therapy, and speech language pathology), diagnoses (e.g., spinal cord and head injury), and accreditation (e.g., American Hospital Association and the predecessor to CARF). Over the next several years, participants refined their ideas and built on earlier work including the Barthel index with the intent to develop a brief yet comprehensive measure of function that was reliable, valid, and feasible in clinical settings. In the mid-1980s, the FIMTM was tested in pilot, trial, and implementation phases. By 1987, the FIMTM was available for general use. Subsequent research has established

TABLE 35.1 *Functional Independence Measure (FIM)*®

FIM Items	FIM Levels
Self-care	No helper
A. Eating	
B. Grooming	7 Complete independence (Timely, Safely)
C. Bathing	6 Modified independence (Device)
D. Dressing—Upper	Helper—modified dependence
E. Dressing—Lower	
F. Toileting	5 Supervision (Subject = 100%)
Sphincter control	4 Minimal assistance (Subject = 75% or more)
	3 Moderate assistance (Subject = 50% or more)
G. Bladder	
H. Bowel	Helper—complete dependence
Transfers	
	2 Maximal assistance (Subject = 25% or more)
I. Bed, Chair, Wheelchair	1 Total assistance (Subject less than 25%)
J. Toilet	0 Activity does not occur; Use this code only at admission.
K. Tub, Shower	
Locomotion	
L. Walk/Wheelchair	
M. Stairs	
Communication	
N. Comprehension	
O. Expression	
Social cognition	
P. Social Interaction	
Q. Problem Solving	
R. Memory	

Modified from CMS Inpatient Rehabilitation Facility–Patient Assessment Instrument (IRF-PAI). http://www.cms.hhs.gov/ InpatientRehabFacPPS/downloads/CMS-10036.pdf

acceptable measurement properties of the FIMTM with respect to reliability, validity, precision, and feasibility (Granger & Fiedler, 1997).

Since the late 1980s, the utility of the FIMTM improved with advances in measurement and analysis. Stineman and others spearheaded efforts to develop functional related groups (FRGs) (Stineman et al., 1994; Stineman, Jette, Fiedler, & Granger, 1997), which allow quantitative comparisons across rehabilitation impairment groups, medical diagnoses for major areas in rehabilitation (e.g., stroke and amputation), and the extent of initial disability. The FIMTM-FRG system has been incorporated into the patient grouping and tracking mechanism of the U.S. federally mandated, inpatient rehabilitation facility–patient assessment instrument (IRF–PAI). In addition, the application of Rasch analysis converted the ordinal properties of the FIM measurements into more equal intervals, thus allowing more use of more sophisticated analytic tools. Making use of Rasch analysis, Heinemann, Linacre, Wright, Hamilton, and Granger (1993; Baker, Granger, & Fiedler, 1997) demonstrated that the 18-item FIMTM can be divided into the mFIM (initial 13 items) and the cFIM (last 5 items). With the FIMTM and subsequent refinements, the field had a common yardstick to compare outcomes and evaluate interventions. As of 2008, Granger estimates that there are more than 600 articles published concerning use of the FIMTM and related activities of Uniform Data Systems (UDS) (Granger, 2008).

In January 2002, the CMS implemented a congressional mandate that fundamentally changed the funding of inpatient rehabilitation services from a cost-based system to a prospective payment system (PPS) supported by Medicare Part A. While the earlier system paid hospitals proportional to their reported cost, the PPS reimbursed hospitals based on severity-adjusted averages. With the newer PPS, there were clear incentives for hospitals to deliver comparable services at lower costs (and shorter lengths of stay). Of note, physician reimbursement under Medicare Part B did not undergo such a dramatic shift.

Concurrent with the implementation of PPS, the CMS established the IRF–PAI (CMS, 2009c). With some relative minor modifications (Granger, Deutsch, Russell, Black, & Ottenbacher, 2007), the FIMTM served as the core functional assessment tool of IRF–PAI.

Although rehabilitation has clearly benefited from the FIMTM, this measure has limitations. Both floor and ceiling effects have been described. An individual with a severe stroke may make modest but significant functional gain so that when combined with caregiver education, it enables the individual to return to the community. Likewise, a high-functioning stroke survivor may make meaningful gains in the use of the affected upper extremity, which does not translate into major changes in the FIMTM score. The FIMTM measures the amount of assistance needed, and significant functional improvements can occur with little or no change in the FIMTM score.

The FIMTM is a brief measure of function (burden of care) and is used primarily for program evaluation and QI. The measure is too blunt for use by discipline-specific rehabilitation professionals, such as ambulation for physical therapists, transfers and toileting for occupational therapists, and cognitive functioning for speech language pathologists and neuropsychologists. The FIMTM does not address quality of life, medical stability, or appropriateness of medical interventions.

The FIMTM is a staff assessment of functional capabilities in the hospital setting. As a measurement tool, it does not take into account an individual's home environment, the availability of support in the community, and the perception of the patient or caregivers. The FIM does not measure either the patient-centeredness of rehabilitation or the congruence of patient–family goals with staff goals. The FIMTM is neutral with respect to the social or environmental resources of the patient, all of which are deemed critical to understanding and effectively intervening with a disabled individual.

DISCUSSION ON QI IN REHABILITATION

Quality assessment in medical rehabilitation should account for the multidimensionality of the interventions and desired outcomes. As with QI across health care settings, efforts to improve quality in rehabilitation are hampered by the measurement tools, and these tools need to be discrete measures that link treatment to outcomes (AHRQ, 2009). AHRQ goes on to define quality indicators operationally as readily available administrative data. Interested readers should review the AHRQ material to gain an appreciation of how the term is operationally defined. Here, I discuss current quality measures in rehabilitation and offer new approaches that build on existing research.

Outcome measurements are the only widely used quality measures in rehabilitation. The FIMTM is a valid and reliable measure of functional status, particularly in the context of caregiver burden. Aspects of patient outcomes not measured by the FIMTM include health status, quality of life, and functional abilities in particular settings. In addition to the FIMTM, the IRF–PAI (CMS, 2009d) lists four optional areas of quality indicators—admission and discharge ratings in respiratory status (#48–50), pain (#51), pressure ulcers (#52 A–E), and safety (#53 and 54). As quality indicators, each topic is measureable and has empirical support for their inclusion as quality measures. However as a group, these recommended quality indicators are far from being comprehensive.

The Donabedian model of "structure," "process," and "outcomes" provides a useful framework for health care quality initiatives and its use is advocated in rehabilitation (Duncan & Velozo, 2007; Eldar, 1999; Hoenig et al., 2002). The structure of medical rehabilitation includes the administrative organization, physical facilities, and personnel and patient-level characteristics. Variations in organizational structure include hospital versus free-standing units and discipline-specific (e.g., physical therapy) versus rehabilitation content (e.g., stroke unit) work groups. Personnel include not only the number of staff, but also their level of training, education, and experience with the particular patients served. Patient-level factors include medical and sociodemographic characteristics and the congruence of these attributes with the services offered.

In general, structure has not proven useful in assessing quality, in part, because structural variables are difficult to associate directly with patient outcomes. However, evidence exists that structure influences process. In a national study on stroke rehabilitation services (Strasser et al., 2002), our group found that hospital administrators perceived the hospital culture differently than rehabilitation team members, and that among rehabilitation team members, the perception of organizational culture predicted perceived quality of team functioning. In a follow-up study (Smits, Falconer, Herrin, Bowen, & Strasser, 2003), the degree of supervisor support for the rehabilitation team was associated with more cohesive teams. These studies support the notion that structure influences process, and suggest that further research could identify structural measures that could serve as quality indicators in rehabilitation.

In many areas of health care, process measures are the preferred approach in quality assessment as these measures can be associated with outcomes (Wachter, 2009). Examples of quality indicators based on process measures include the use of aspirin after an acute myocardial infarction and anticoagulation for individuals with atrial fibulation. In contrast to these discrete measures, process measures in rehabilitation present unique complexity and would need to account for the biopsychosocial framework of rehabilitation. The value of process measures in other areas of health care suggests that these measures could be useful in rehabilitation QI.

In stroke rehabilitation, one process measure, the adherence to a postacute stroke guideline, was associated with greater patient satisfaction (Duncan et al., 2002; Reker et al., 2002). More recently, a change in process of care, the comanagement of frail elderly patients with femur fractures, was associated with higher quality of care (Friedman, Mendelson, Kates, & McCann, 2008). In our work in stroke rehabilitation, patient outcomes were associated with characteristics of team functioning, and the specific outcomes (e.g., functional improvement and length of stay) varied by the particular aspect of team functioning (task orientation, order and organization, and team effectiveness) (Strasser et al., 2005). In a subsequent clinical trial, measures of team functioning provided useful feedback information in a successful trial of process improvement in stroke rehabilitation (Strasser et al., 2008).

Outcomes comprise the third Donabedian component, and are seen as changes in health status attributable to the interventions. In rehabilitation, measurements of functional status including subcategories of mobility, self-care, communication, and cognition are routinely assessed by the FIMTM. Case-mix adjustment is accomplished primarily with the FRGs, which permit more accurate comparisons across patient groups and treatment settings. While the FIMTM allows for calculation of rehabilitation efficiency by dividing the FIMTM gain by the length of stay, this efficiency measure has some limitations (Duncan, DeJong, Hoenig, & Vogel, 2005). Postacute rehabilitation discharge destination is also routinely recorded in the IRF–PAI. Important process and outcome considerations of quality in rehabilitation not covered by the IRF–PAI include team functioning, functional abilities at the discharge location (e.g., home environment with family caregivers), patient satisfaction, health promotion, and postacute medical stability, and care coordination.

Building on current knowledge, the VA Rehabilitation Teams Project (Strasser et al., 2005, 2008), and my own clinical experiences, some candidates for quality indicators emerge. With respect to structure, two potential indicators include perception of hospital culture and staff attendance at team conference. For process, measures of team leadership, physician involvement, and team functioning would be valuable. In addition, the use of established rehabilitation guidelines represent another measure and are associated with improved outcomes in stroke rehabilitation (Duncan et al., 2002; Reker et al., 2002). For outcomes, the FIMTM has established reliability and validity. The development and use of assessments in quality of life, functional abilities in the home environment, and postacute medical coordination of care measures would expand the quality indicators in outcomes.

Staff perception of hospital culture as more personal than bureaucratic predicts higher levels of team functioning (Strasser et al., 2002). In addition, the level of discipline-specific supervisor support for the interdisciplinary team correlates with team functioning (Smits et al., 2003). These findings suggest that clinical indicators that capture the organizational support for the interdisciplinary team would be useful. The degree of participation by hands-on providers in team conferences is an administrative and supervisor decision. Commonly, discipline representatives (e.g., nursing and rehabilitation therapies) will report for hands-on providers. Although this approach may allow more "efficient" use of the clinical resources, it deprives the team of valuable insights from the direct providers and inhibits creative team problem solving. Based on my own clinical experience and related research activities, team communication is enhanced when hands-on therapists and nurses attend team conferences as opposed to sending representatives. In particular, the participation of nurses in team conferences enhances team effectiveness. The influence of team conference participation by primary rehabilitation providers (e.g., registered nurse, physical therapist, speech-language pathologist) on team functioning and patient outcomes merits further study. Clinical experience suggests that it would be a reasonable quality indicator. Bowel and bladder management represent another potential quality indicator in stroke rehabilitation. Bowel and bladder continence predict discharge destination from acute inpatient rehabilitation, and effective management typically includes medical, nursing, and therapy input. It is reasonable to propose that more effective rehabilitation team functioning would be reflected in interdisciplinary approaches to bladder management and that coordinated medical and behavioral approaches to bladder management are more effective than single interventions. Support for such a quality indicator can be found in studies on predictors of stroke rehabilitation outcomes (Falconer, Naughton, Strasser, Dunlap, & Sinacore, 1994), our preliminary work on team functioning and bladder management (Strasser, Falconer, Herrin, & Bowen, 2001), and extensive research in related areas (Brittain, Peet, Potter, & Castleden, 1999).

Team functioning predicts patient outcomes in rehabilitation (Strassser, 2005) and similar associations of process and outcomes are supported in rehabilitation (DeJong et al., 2005) and other areas of health care (Friedman et al., 2008; Shortell et al., 1994; Young et al., 1994). In addition, measures of team functioning proved useful in a clinical trial of process improvement in stroke rehabilitation (Stevens, Strasser, Uomoto, Bowen, & Falconer, 2007). Although work on these measures is ongoing, there is good evidence that team leadership and staff perceptions of physician support predict team effectiveness (Smits et al., 2003). Hence, measures of team functioning hold potential as useful measures of rehabilitation process.

Medical stability is a prerequisite to patient participation in inpatient rehabilitation. In addition, CMS guidelines state that the need for 24-hour medical and nursing monitoring is a requirement for acute inpatient rehabilitation. QI issues for physicians and nurses in rehabilitation parallel those in other acute hospital settings. Examples of potential quality indicators for physicians and nurses with respect to medical stability are listed in Table 35.2. A detailed discussion of this aspect of quality in rehabilitation is beyond the scope of this chapter, but obviously relevant to quality in inpatient rehabilitation.

CLINICIANS AND QUALITY—A DISCONNECT?

QI in medical rehabilitation is hampered by a disconnect between how issues are defined at the organizational level and how they are experienced by hands-on providers. This tension

TABLE 35.2   *Proposed Quality Indicators*

Structure	Process	Outcomes
Medical issues		
Admission assessment	Venous thromboembolism prophylaxis	Communication with physicians
Computerized physician order entry	Pain management	Medical follow-up
Accuracy of admission medication list	Diabetic education	Medication compliance
Communication of medical information	Health promotion	Health
Rehabilitation issues		
Perception of hospital culture	Team functioning	Quality of life
Team meeting attendance	Bladder management	Functional abilities in the home environment
Speciality rehab unit	Team leadership—physician support	Patient and family satisfaction
Supervisor support for team activities	Practice guidelines	Life space

between macro- and microperspectives occurs across health care specialties and may explain some of the difficulties in addressing known quality deficits. As a clinician, if I see limited utility of quality measures in patient care activities and outcomes, I am not likely to devote much effort into the accuracy of data collection or the use of the reports generated from the data. This attitude is shared by others (Casalino, 1999; Werner, 2007).

The perceived limited relevance of indicators to direct patient care makes it easy to discount these initiatives as a distraction from other pressing needs. Of the four areas on the IRF–PAI (CMS, 2009d), the pressure sore indicator seems most useful and informative. Although appropriate pain management is relevant to quality of rehabilitation, the specific measure consists of an admission and discharge patient rating and does not assess how the pain was treated (pharmacological and nonpharmacological), side effects of treatment, or the relationship between pain and patient outcomes. In a similar manner, the specific indicators on respiratory status and safety provided may identify problem areas, but provide no information how to address the issues.

Overcoming this disconnect will not be easy. First, the poor alignment of incentives creates barriers. Physicians are generally reimbursed by volume with fewer, if any, financial incentives to improve coordination and to incorporate a macroperspective needed for QI. Likewise, the productivity of therapists and nurses are more likely measured by volume of patients and not care coordination and integration. Financial disincentives explain only part of the challenges with quality initiatives.

Clinicians deal with one person at a time and quality data are aggregate. Clinicians may be naïve to the relevance of aggregate data on their dealings with individual patients, perhaps similar to the blind spot that parents can have about the undesirable social influences on their children. Certainly, efforts to further educate clinicians on the well-documented discrepancies (service variations, medical errors, inappropriate services) are needed. In particular, the relevance of these trends to their own clinical work should be highlighted. In addition, there is a need for quality initiatives that directly affect the outcomes of individual providers.

In a national study, we asked rehabilitation team leaders at 16 VA hospitals to learn the basics of team functioning and to utilize this knowledge in clinical practice (Stevens et al., 2007). In general, we found that clinicians will incorporate new approaches in their busy clinical practice if they experience the effort as improving patient outcomes or in making them more effective clinicians. They will not utilize new approaches unless they simultaneously experience improved treatments and patient outcomes. The crucial issue is whether the quality initiative improves the patient outcomes of individual providers. Effective QI initiatives should be woven into the practice of clinical care. As part of the fabric of care, individuals will utilize the new approach.

SUGGESTED ACTIVITIES TO IMPROVE QUALITY

Here, I offer five activities likely to improve quality, which can be related to direct patient care (Table 35.3). First, regular case discussions among peers, particularly physicians, improves quality (see Gawande, 2009). Experts note that cost-effective care is associated with settings where peers discuss challenging cases and provide feedback to each other. Second, ample clinical experience suggests that role of nursing is less clearly defined and demonstrates wider variations than other core disciplines on rehabilitation teams. Activities to integrate nursing into the rehabilitation treatment process should improve quality, including carryover of skills learned in therapy to the nursing unit, proactive engagement of the patient and caregivers in bowel, bladder, and skin care, and optimizing the role of nursing in family and caregiver education. Third, as the medical acuity of rehabilitation inpatients increase, the involvement of rehabilitation therapies in the promotion of healthy behavior should improve quality. For example, the activities of physical therapists, occupational therapists, and speech language pathologists can incorporate salient issues of diet and exercise along with the management of chronic diseases such as blood pressure, diabetes, heart disease, and depression. Fourth, the provisions of timely process and outcome information to rehabilitation staff was associated with improved stroke outcomes (Stevens et al., 2007; Strasser et al., 2008). This experience suggests that the more relevant quality information increases the likelihood that it will be used to improve outcomes. And fifth, the team approach is a defining characteristic of inpatient rehabilitation. Team-building activities can improve patient outcomes as demonstrated in our national clinical trial on process improvement (Stevens et al., 2007).

CONCLUSIONS

"It does not count if it isn't counted." Variations of this mantra abound in health care and in rehabilitation. The idea behind this sentiment is sobering given the challenges to understand and measure the black box of rehabilitation. Some fear that our inability to measure the determinants of rehabilitation quality may relegate the field to the proverbial dustbin. And clearly as health care resources become more constrained, rehabilitation professionals must justify their interventions. For busy clinicians, gathering current findings to support

TABLE 35.3 *Quality Improvement Activities*

Team conference attendance

Regular case discussions among peers

Nursing involvement in rehabilitation process

Therapy involvement in medical and nursing issues

Process and outcomes information feedback

Staff training to improve team functioning

Use of model of rehabilitation effectiveness

care improvements along with conducting primary research in treatment effectiveness are daunting tasks.

Still, individual rehabilitation providers and services can make a difference. Atul Gawande's (2007) book, *Better: A Surgeon's Notes on Performance*, provides valuable insights on how individuals improve quality. He highlights themes of diligence, doing right, and ingenuity. He offers simple, yet profound advice including "count something" (pp. 254–255) and "write something" (pp. 255–256). The counting should be discrete issues where clinical experience suggests there are opportunities for improvement such as bladder programs and team conference attendance. The writing spans from in-house newsletters to family educational material to peer review publications. It is important for dedicated individuals to be engaged in the process of performance improvement.

The impetus on quality arises from the increasing evidence of suboptimal patient care and outcomes across a swath of settings and specialties. Wide variations in service provision combined with evidence of medical errors underscore the need to address quality. Given the magnitude of the issues, the difficulty in addressing established quality deficiencies speak of the challenges and complexities of these issues. Clearly, the development of quality indicators as discrete and readily available is vital to meaningful QI. However in some instances, I feel we are getting the cart before the horse. Quality indicators should arise from a knowledge base of the underpinnings of medical rehabilitation, particularly the processes by which inputs are translated into patient outcomes. In addition, quality as measured by indicators that are perceived as relevant to the activities of clinicians are more likely to be taken seriously by these providers.

The Donabedian triad of structure, process, and outcome has proven useful in the development of quality initiatives. The lack of valid, reliable, and readily available measures of structure and process severely hampers our ability to improve quality. The FIMTM represents a major achievement in understanding and evaluating outcomes in rehabilitation. With the FIMTM and subsequent improvements in measurement and case-mix adjustments, we now have a reliable and valid measure to compare outcomes across locations and type of interventions. Similar to the broad coalition of professional, governmental, accreditation, and citizen groups that spearheaded the development of the FIMTM, a major effort is warranted to understand and measure the structural and process elements that lead to desirable rehabilitation outcomes. From this knowledge base, assessment tools and quality indicators can be developed.

The IOM report on quality identified six aims—safe, effective, patient-centered, efficient, timeliness, and equity (IOM, 2001). The medical dimensions of Rehabilitation offer providers an opportunity to have an effect on health care quality in health promotion and chronic disease management where such issues can more effectively be addressed by an interdisciplinary team. "Provider and team-centered" as opposed to "administrative-centered" service delivery predicts better patient outcomes. The conceptual framework of rehabilitation treatment effectiveness developed by my colleagues may be helpful (Strasser, 1997a, 1997b) in developing QI initiatives. With a serious effort to improve quality, rehabilitation providers have the opportunity to achieve gains in the six identified areas of the IOM report.

QI is an iterative process of problem identification, action, reanalysis, and further action. Rehabilitation distinguishes itself by an emphasis on function. The field emphasizes active patient participation and the involvement of an interdisciplinary team of professionals. Over the past 60 years dedicated professionals have made tremendous strides and yet there remains much to do. Based on our record of creativity and innovation in improving the lives and functional abilities of our patients over the past 60 years, I believe the field has the capabilities to address these issues. In the process, our patients will be better served and we will offer valuable insights to others.

REFERENCES AND SELECTED BIBLIOGRAPHY

Agency for Healthcare Research and Quality (AHRQ). (2009). *Inpatient quality indicator overview.* Retrieved July 11, 2009, from http://www.qualityindicators.ahrq.gov/iqi_overview.htm

Baker, J. G., Granger, C. V., & Fiedler, R. C. (1997). A brief outpatient functional assessment measure: Validity using Rasch measures. *American Journal of Physical Medicine & Rehabilitation, 76*, 8–13.

Brittain, K. R., Peet, S. M., Potter, J. F., & Castleden, C. M. (1999). Prevalence and management of urinary incontinence in stroke survivors. *Age and Ageing, 28*, 509–511.

CARF Standards Manual, Medical Rehabilitation. (2009). Commission on Accreditation of Rehabilitation Facilities (CARF). Tucson, AZ. *Program description.* Retrieved July 11, 2009, from http://www.carf.org/pdf/MedProgDesc.pdf

Centers for Medicare and Medicaid Services (CMS). (2009a). *Quality of care concerns: What can your quality improvement organization address.* Retrieved July 11, 2009, from http://www.medicare.gov/Publications/Pubs/pdf/11362.pdf

Centers for Medicare and Medicaid Services (CMS). (2009b). *Hospital compare—A quality tool provided by Medicare.* Retrieved July 11, 2009, from www.hospitalcompare.hhs.gov

Centers for Medicare and Medicaid Services (CMS). (2009c). *Inpatient Rehabilitation Facility Classification.* CMS transmittal 347. Retrieved July 11, 2009, from http://www.cms.hhs.gov/InpatientRehabFacPPS/downloads/R347CP.pdf

Centers for Medicare and Medicaid Services (CMS). (2009d). Inpatient Facility Patient Assessment Instrument (IFPAI). Retrieved July 11, 2009, from http://www.cms.hhs.gov/InpatientRehabFacPPS/04_IRFPAI.asp#TopOfPage

Casalino, L. P. (1999). The unintended consequences of measuring quality on the quality of medical care. Sounding Board. *New England Journal of Medicine, 341*, 1147–1150.

Connell, B. R. (1997). The physical environment of inpatient stroke rehabilitation settings. *Topics in Stroke Rehabilitation, 4*, 40–58.

DeJong, G., Horn, S. D., Conroy, R., Nichols, D., & Healton, E. B. (2005). Opening the black box of post-stroke rehabilitation: Stroke rehabilitation patients, processes, and outcomes. *Archives of Physical Medicine and Rehabilitation, 86*(12, Suppl. 2), S1–S7.

Donabedian, A. (1980). *Explorations on quality assessment and monitoring: The definition of quality and approaches to its assessment* (Vol. 1). Ann Arbor, MI: Health Administration Press.

Donabedian, A. (1988). Quality assessment and assurance: Unity of purpose, diversity of means. *Inquiry, 25*, 173.

Duncan, P. W., Horner, R. D., Reker, D. M., Samsa, G. P., Hoenig, H., Hamilton, B. B., et al. (2002). Adherence to postacute rehabilitation guidelines is associated with functional recovery in stroke. *Journal of the American Heart Association, 33*, 167–178.

Duncan, P. W., DeJong, G., Hoenig, H., & Vogel, B. (2005). Letter to the editor. Length of stay, functional outcome, and mortality following medical rehabilitation. *Journal of the American Medical Association, 293*, 294–295.

Duncan, P. W., & Velozo, C. A. (2007). State-of-the-science on postacute rehabilitation: Measurement and methodologies for assessing quality and establishing policy for postacute care. *Archives of Physical Medicine and Rehabilitation, 88*, 1482–1487.

Eldar, R. (1999). Quality of care in rehabilitation medicine. *International Journal for Quality in Health Care, 11*, 73–79. Retrieved July 11, 2009, from http://intqhc.oxfordjournals.org/cgi/reprint/11/1/81.pdf

Falconer, J. A., Naughton, B. J., Strasser, D. C., Dunlap, D., & Sinacore, J. M. (1994). Predicting stroke inpatient rehabilitation outcome using a classification approach. *Archives of Physical Medicine and Rehabilitation, 75*, 177–182.

Friedman, S. M., Mendelson, D. A., Kates, S. L., & McCann, R. M. (2008). Geriatric co-management of proximal femur fractures: Total quality management and protocol-driven care result in better outcomes for a frail patient population. *Journal of the American Geriatrics Society, 56*, 1349–1356.

Gawande, A. (2009, June 1). The cost conundrum. *The New Yorker.* pp. 36–44.

Gawande, A. (2007). *Better: A surgeon's notes on performance.* New York: Metropolitan Books.

Granger, C. V., Deutsch, A., Russell, C., Black, T., & Ottenbacher, K. J. (2007). Modifications of the FIM instrument under the Inpatient Rehabilitation facility Prospective Payment System. *American Journal of Physical Medicine & Rehabilitation, 86*, 883–892.

Granger, C. V., & Fiedler, R. C. (1997). The measurement of disability. In M. J. Fuhrer (Ed.), *Assessing medical rehabilitation practices—The promise of outcomes research* (pp. 103–126). Baltimore, MD: Paul Bowles Publishing Co.

Granger, C. V. (2008). *Quality and outcome measures for rehabilitation programs.* Retrieved from http://emedicine.medscape.com/article/317865-overview

Heinemann, A. W., Linacre, J. M., Wright, B. D., Hamilton, B. B., & Granger, C. (1993). Relationships between impairment and physical disability as measured by the functional independence measure. *Archives of Physical Medicine and Rehabilitation, 74,* 566–573.

Hoeing, H., Duncan, P. W., Horner, R. D., Reker, D. M., Samsa, G. P., Dudley, T. K., et al. (2002). Structure, process, and outcomes in stroke rehabilitation. *Medical Care, 40,* 1036–1047.

Institute of Medicine. (1999). In L. Kohn, J. Corrigan, & M. Donaldson (Eds.), *To err is human: Building a safer health system.* Washington, DC: National Academies Press.

Institute of Medicine. (2001). *Crossing the quality chasm.* Washington, DC: National Academies Press.

The Joint Commission on the Accreditation of Hospital Organizations (JCAHO). (2009). *The Joint Commission. About quality check.* Retrieved July 13, 2009, from http://www.jointcommission.org/qualitycheck/06_about_qc.htm

Langhorne, P., & Dennis, M. S. (2004). Stroke units: The next 10 years. *Lancet, 363,* 834–835.

McGlynn, E. A., Asch, S. M., Adams, J., Keesey, J., Hicks, J., DeCristofaro, A., et al. (2003). The quality of health care delivered to adults in the United States. *New England Journal of Medicine, 348,* 2635–2645.

Plsek, P. E. (1999). Quality improvement methods in clinical medicine. *Pediatrics, 103,* 203S–214S.

Reker, D. M., Duncan, P. W., Horner, R. D., Hoenig, H., Samsa, G. P., Hamilton, B. B., et al. (2002). Post stroke guideline compliance is associated with greater patient satisfaction. *Archives of Physical Medicine and Rehabilitation, 83,* 750–756.

Roach, M. (2008, August 10). Book Review. Slow-Moving Vehicle. *The New York Times.*

Schillie, S. F. (2007). *Quality improvement in healthcare.* Retrieved July 11, 2009, from http://cme.medscape.com/viewarticle/561651

Shortell, S. M., Zimmerman, J. E., Rousseau, D. M., Gillies, R. R., Wagner, D. P., Draper, E. A., et al. (1994) The performance of intensive care units: Does good management make a difference? *Medical Care, 32,* 508–525.

Smits, S. J., Falconer, J. A., Herrin, J., Bowen, S. E., & Strasser, D. C. (2003). Patient focused rehabilitation team cohesiveness in Veterans Administration hospitals. *Archives of Physical Medicine and Rehabilitation, 84,* 1332–1338.

Staddon, J. (2008, July/August). Distracting Miss Daisy. *The Atlanta Monthly.* Retrieved July 11, 2009, from http://www.theatlantic.com/dolc/200807/traffic

Stevens, A. B., Strasser, D. C., Uomoto, J., Bowen, S. E., & Falconer, J. A. (2007). Utility of treatment implementation methods in a clinical trial with rehabilitation teams. *Journal of Rehabilitation Research and Development, 44,* 537–546.

Stineman, M. G., Escarce, J. J., Goin, J. E., Hamilton, B. B., Granger, C. V., & Williams, S. V. (1994). A casemix classification system for medical rehabilitation. *Medical Care, 32,* 366–379.

Stineman, M. G., Jette, A., Fiedler, R., & Granger, C. (1997). Impairment–specific dimensions within the functional independence measure. *Archives of Physical Medicine and Rehabilitation, 78,* 636–643.

Strasser, D. C., & Falconer, J. A. (1997a). Linking treatment to outcomes through teams: Building a conceptual model of rehabilitation effectiveness. *Topics in Stroke Rehabilitation, 4,* 15–27.

Strasser, D. C., & Falconer, J. A. (1997b). Rehabilitation team process. *Topics in Stroke Rehabilitation, 4,* 34–39.

Strasser, D. C., Falconer, J. A., Herrin, J. S., & Bowen, S. E. (2001). The relation of rehabilitation team functioning and urinary continence for Veterans Administration stroke patients (Poster). *Archives of Physical Medicine and Rehabilitation, 82,* 1491.

Strasser, D. C., Falconer, J. A., Herrin, J. S., Bowen, S. E., Uomoto, J. M., & Smits, S. J. (2002). The influence of hospital culture on rehabilitation team functioning in VA hospitals. *Journal of Rehabilitation Research and Development, 39,* 115–125.

Strasser, D. C., Smits, S. J., Falconer, J. A., Herrin, J. S., & Bowen, S. E. (2005). Team functioning and patient outcomes in stroke rehabilitation. *Archives of Physical Medicine and Rehabilitation, 86,* 403–409.

Strasser, D. C., Falconer, J. A., Stevens, A. B., Uomoto, J. M., Herrin, J., Bowen, S. E., et al. (2008). Team training and stroke rehabilitation outcomes: A cluster randomized trial. *Archives of Physical Medicine and Rehabilitation, 89,* 10–15.

Vanderbilt, T. (2008). *Traffic: Why we drive the way we do (and what it says about us)*. New York: Alfred E. Knopf.

Wachter, R. (2009). *The quality of healthcare—How to measure and improve it*. A knol by Robert Wachter. Retrieved July 11, 2009, from http://knol.google.com/k/robert-wachter/the-quality-of-healthcare/BL7br6-s/nIN3GA#

Walter, L. C., Davidowitz, N. P., Heineken, P. A., & Covinsky, K. E. (2004). Pitfalls of converting practice guidelines into quality measures: Lessons learned from a VA performance measure. *Journal of the American Medical Association, 291*, 2466–2470.

Werner, R. M., & Asch, D. A. (2007). Clinical concerns about clinical performance measurement. *Annals of Family Medicine, 5*, 159–163.

Young, G. J., Charns, M. P., Desai, K., Khuri, S. F., Forbes, M. G., Henderson, W., et al. (1994). Patterns of coordination and clinical outcomes: A study of surgical services. *Health Services Research, 33*(5, Pt. 1), 1211–1236.

36

Telerehabilitation: Solutions to Distant and International Care

Andrew J. Haig, MD*

Disruptive Innovation: Improving a system through radical and often external change. It's a good thing.

Glabman (2009) highlighted the need for health care to change in radical ways. She pointed to telemedicine as one of five important radicalizations of the future. Robert Litan quoted, "As much as $200 million could be saved over 25 years if patients communicated electronically with their providers." Paul Keckley claimed that "at least 60% of adult care living or skilled nursing facility residents could remain at home with electronic devices." Keckley's savings calculation for in-home technologies is $400 billion.

Telerehabilitation—rehabilitation management from a distance—is part of that radical change of disruptive innovation. Telerehabilitation includes assessment of patients, treatment of their disabling conditions, and ensuring compliance and understanding. It also involves education of clinicians, second opinions, multicenter research trials, and strategic business collaborations. Telerehabilitation clinicians and scientists have provided us with technology, demonstration projects, and validation studies. However, if Glabman is right, their work is not part of the medical mainstream yet. The real radical changes are yet to come. What changes? Are they as simple as "more people doing it"? Or will even the scientists and clinicians involved in telerehabilitation be taken by surprise? This chapter takes a look backwards at work to date in an attempt to allow all of us to be part of the solution for the future.

Table 36.1 shows the evolution of communication and the implication of these changes on rehabilitation. The huge leaps in communication technology have been driven by society's general need and are nearly universally accepted as a part of life in industrialized countries. But most of rehabilitation communication occurs at the basic level of observation and spoken word. New technology is used primarily for ancillary tasks such as appointment making and billing. The core of rehabilitation communication is at the least technologically sophisticated level, far below the day-to-day management of other business and social activities in society.

The concept of telemedicine has been around as long as there have been telephones. Changes in the health care landscape and technology over the last decade have made telerehabilitation more practical and more compelling. This chapter reviews some of the tools available in telerehabilitation and ways they have been used. However, one cannot assume that technology

* The author is president of Rehabilitation Team Assessments, LLC, a company that works with hospitals and clinics to develop rehabilitation programs.

TABLE 36.1 *Societal Drivers and Rehabilitation Uses of Historical Advances in Communication*

Communication	Societal Drivers	Rehabilitation Use
Observation	Survival	Physical examination
Gestures and noises	Collaboration	Physical examination
Speech	Direct and be directed	History
Written language	Accurate reproduction, spread, and retention of information	Records, patient instructions, clinician education, policy
Telegraph	Instant distant communication	No clear models
Radio	Rapid spread of information Marketing	Marketing and public education
Telephone	Rapid simple 1:1 communication	Clarification, scheduling, instructions
Television	Rapid one-way spread of graphic and moving information, marketing	Marketing and public relations
Cell phone	1:1 communication independent of wires	Urgent access
Fax	Rapid graphic communication Business-to-business	Primarily professional and business uses
E-mail	Instant distant access; instant simultaneous communication Spam advertising and information	Patient–clinician communication, scheduling, professional and client networks
Web video/chat	Rapid multidirectional, personalized communication Family and friend connectivity Distant group meetings	Distant assessment and management Distant team meetings
Portable computer/ communication devices iPod Blackberry Satellite phone Global positioning systems	Social, financial, political revolution with decreased cost and energy consumption	Assessment, monitoring, interventions, outcome measurement, safety assurance
Symbols again	Communication in a global community	Assessment and direction independent of language and literacy

improves care. Indeed, the initial assumption is that distance decreases accuracy of examination and imprecise treatment. Hence, it is important to evaluate the impact of telerehabilitation using sound research methodology. Validation through research is not sufficient to ensure that an effective tool is used. In addition, we need to explore the political, social, and financial factors that impact the growth of telerehabilitation.

TOOLS IN TELEREHABILITATION

Until recently, the actual act of communication was the most challenging aspect of telerehabilitation. However, communication has advanced exponentially. Telegraph is gone and landline telephones are not a requirement. Radio has been supplanted by television, and land-based television towers transmitting analog signals are transitioning to satellite-based digital media that can reach anywhere in the world. These advances permitted early telerehabilitation and are still used to some extent. However, the real advance in telerehabilitation has occurred as a result of rise of the Internet and computer technology. These new modalities have almost trivialized the challenge of communication for most telerehabilitation applications.

These days almost every teenager in the developed world has an email address, thanks to the rapid spread of the Internet and the associated software. They network via Facebook, access videos on YouTube, and educate each other using blogs. Basic laptops have capacity for audio recording, video cameras, and wireless broadcasting. Skype and other Web services provide audiovisual communication for fun. Web site development was a high-tech job only a decade ago; these days many pre-teens can build a quality Web site. In contrast to the technical challenges that were barriers to telerehabilitation a few years ago, these days many of our patients and their families are as competent in telecommunication as the clinical teams who serve them.

The huge storage and logic capacity of many devices has had another effect. Telerehabilitation or some components of telerehabilitation often do not involve communication with a person. In fact, the need for distant *communication* is often somewhat arbitrary. Virtual reality instruction or simulation might involve software contained in the user's computer or Web-connection to a server on the other side of the world. Podcasts carried on iPods, handheld telephones with computer capacity, and global positioning systems with internal maps blur barriers and definitions. It may be easier to define what is not telerehabilitation: The part of an interaction that is hands-on or face-to-face is not telerehabilitation.

Some applications require high Internet bandwidth and are affected by delays in transmission as may occur on the Internet. But most rehabilitation interventions are not so time critical. Phillips, Vesmarovich, Hauber, Wiggers, and Egner (2001) did not find a difference between telephone and video conferencing. Lemaire, Boudrias, and Greene (2001) found low-bandwidth video acceptable in transmitting rehabilitation information.

Typing skills remain a barrier to some persons who require help, especially the elderly, who typically have little typing or computer training. A Japanese group found good success in using a pen-type imaging sensor with home computers to provide social support to elderly clients served by a "home helper" office (Ogawa et al., 2003). This office transferred messages to helpers' mobile phones for timely responses.

There do remain some technical communication barriers. Many regions of the world are still not connected to the Internet or are connected at the speed of a telephone line. Bandwidth on the Internet is sometimes insufficient and always variable based on the traffic at any given time. Hence, real-time transmission of complex data is not straightforward. Still, the technical challenges of communication itself are now largely replaced with the technical challenges of designing-usable rehabilitation devices.

TELEREHABILITATION TECHNOLOGY

Aside from the communication alone, what advances have been made in rehabilitation-related technology? The distant measurement of many physiological parameters is now technologically feasible. Oxygen levels, blood pressure, electrocardiogram, pulse, temperature, and numerous other parameters can be measured from a distance and in ambulatory settings (Lymberis, 2004). Where therapy is to be applied from a distance, it is important to be able to measure motion and assess its quality from a distance. Numerous technologies have been proposed (Zheng, Black, & Harris, 2005).

One of the most exciting new advances is the electronic activity monitor (Grant, Ryan, Tigbe, & Granat, 2006). These lightweight devices can be worn for many days at home to measure distances walked and caloric expenditure, among other parameters. Now, for the first time, instead of surveying the patient regarding their integration into the community, clinicians and scientists have an objective measure. So, for instance, we now know that obese people do not just consume more than other people, they also walk less and thus burn fewer calories during their usual activity at home (Yamakawa, Tsai, Haig, Miner, & Harris, 2004).

The science of using at-home monitoring to determine the real level of disability and the objective effect of treatments ranging from joint replacement to multidisciplinary rehabilitation is just beginning.

The challenge for telerehabilitation advocates is to answer the "so what?" question. When a barrier to participation and quality of life exists, how is that barrier addressed as a result of the technology? There have been many examples of rehabilitation interventions from a distance.

Distant intervention for speech or cognitive problems typically involves technologies that are well established on the Internet, including voice-over-Internet and Internet transmission of video images. Baron, Hatfield, and Georgeadis (2005) review integration of face-to-face speech therapy with family coaching, group therapy, and telerehabilitation communication. Most of this literature demonstrates that distant intervention is a viable alternative to on-site treatment. However, a distinct clinical advantage is not clearly proven. This means that current arguments for telerehabilitation are related to improved access, convenience, and cost.

A unique strength of telerehabilitation technology is its ability to help the patient generalize behaviors or exercises to nonclinical settings. Fancy words like "prosthetic memory" are used to describe sophisticated software that reminds patients what to do, when to do, where to do, and how to do. And in fact, the advances in this software for brain-injured people have been amazing. However, the fact is that this is now a common aspect of life for all of us. We use cell phones to check our grocery list with the people back home before leaving the store. We keep schedules on computers rather than on paper. Rather than relying on our geographic memory, we use GPS devices to find our way through town. All of these augmentations of cognitive processes are chosen by the general public by a complex process of decision making involving an assessment of personal cognitive strengths in comparison to life tasks, cost, and convenience.

Many therapists in the community use this readily available and fairly inexpensive technology without any rehabilitation-specific software to get the job done. More than a prosthetic memory, portable communication may provide more situation-specific intervention and more timely feedback in the real world. Hence, the occupational therapist might send a pragmatically impaired brain-injured person alone into a grocery store, then call to remind him/her to thank the checkout clerk. The efficiencies and timeliness of mobile devices are clear, and the technology is available now almost everywhere.

Virtual reality games and training are increasingly common. Using strict definitions, a virtual reality rehabilitation exercise that resides on the patient's computer is not telerehabilitation, whereas the one that taps into a distant server or involves interaction with a distant clinician is telerehabilitation (Burdea, 2003). Regardless, this is an emerging important technology. Holden's review of 121 studies in virtual reality has four major conclusions: (1) people with disabilities appear capable of motor learning within virtual environments; (2) movements learned by people with disabilities in VR transfer to real-world equivalent motor tasks in most cases, and in some cases even generalize to other untrained tasks; (3) in the few studies ($n = 5$) that have compared motor learning in real versus virtual environments, some advantage for VR training has been found in all cases; and (4) no occurrences of cybersickness in impaired populations have been reported to date in experiments where VR has been used to train motor abilities (Holden, 2005). Our group's BackQUACK interactive video game intends to teach more than factual knowledge to patients and clinicians suffering from spinal disorders. Through humor, it encourages patients to become intelligent consumers and teaches the language that clinicians need to use to encourage patients to make these intelligent decisions. A trial of BackQUACK in two Michigan communities is about to begin. We can only speculate as to whether this type of education is superior to traditional continuing medical education and patient pamphlets.

Motor rehabilitation from a distance is not easy. While watching a simple exercise on the computer or recording the number of repetitions of a day-to-day exercise is not so hard, telerehabilitation is challenged to provide the kind of immediate feedback that occurs in hands-on physical therapy. Motion involves force, velocity, and direction, all of which need to be measured and transmitted accurately and rapidly if feedback is to be timely. The feedback loop involving a computer or a therapist operating a parallel device is complex as well, causing further delays. Depending on the rehabilitation task, these delays may result in feedback that is too late for the patient or the device to make a correction.

On the other hand, devices can often monitor physical activity that a clinician cannot. An electrocardiogram can monitor both effort by measuring the percentage of maximal heart rate with an activity and cardiac dysfunction by measuring cardiac arrhythmias or changes in wave form such as S-T segment depression that can indicate cardiac ischemia. Surface electromyography (EMG) can measure tremor, spasm, co-contraction, fatigue, and effort. Force plates can measure effort, speed, strain, and balance. Temperature and EMG biofeedback can measure and train relaxation. Note, however, that this paragraph is about technology, not telerehabilitation. These tools are not unique to telerehabilitation, and many of them are not routinely used in face-to-face therapy. One must come up with a compelling reason for their use in telerehabilitation. Where distant therapy is tried, however, they may provide a substitute for direct therapist observation.

VALIDATION OF TELEREHABILITATION

Jennet and colleagues (2003) performed a comprehensive review of 4,646 articles on telehealth. They concluded that telemedicine interventions offered "significant socio-economic benefit, to patients and families, health care providers and the health care system. The main benefits identified were: increased access to health services, cost-effectiveness, enhanced educational opportunities, improved health outcomes, better quality of care, better quality of life and enhanced social support."

van Dijk and Hermens (2004) reviewed quality research studies on rehabilitation interventions 4 years ago. They found that the EMG biofeedback literature was of relatively good quality, but research on newer concepts like virtual reality was poor, reflecting the immaturity of the concepts. As in every other area of medicine, validation will always lag far behind the technology, leaving the potential user in a vulnerable position of using common sense, rather than good evidence in adopting telerehabilitation techniques. Evidence-based guidelines typically weigh the quality of research methodology used to study an intervention more than the potential magnitude of change, common-sense practicality, or cost. Because these guidelines drive policy, practice, and reimbursement, it is critical for telerehabilitation research to meet the quality standards of evidence-based reviews.

Just as rehabilitation integrates many other aspects of health care, to understand telerehabilitation and its effects we can look to research on telemedicine for related problems. Reviews of telepsychiatry and telepsychology have shown surprisingly positive effects. Distant counseling may be as effective as face-to-face counseling for depression (Andersson, 2006). A computerized self-help program for obsessive compulsive disorders seems to be useful, and other programs for diseases ranging from bulimia to gambling addiction have been studied (Mataix-Cols & Marks, 2006).

Home health care comprises fields peripheral to rehabilitation, including medication compliance, wound management, and patient education. Many studies and demonstration projects in home health care have shown improved compliance and understanding, decreased complications, and sometimes decreased cost compared to traditional care. However, the research is not iron-clad. In a comprehensive review of 950 clinical trials, only 24 were felt to be of sufficient quality for a systematic review of telehealth interventions for chronic disease (Garcia-Lizana & Sarria-Santamera, 2007). These included monitoring and management of diabetes, hypertension, and heart disease. For example, Hoenig and colleagues (2006) used landline telephone and video to provide home evaluation and instruction to 13 home-based subjects. There was compliance with 60% of 12 recommendations per subject.

Patients generally respond favorably to telerehabilitation interventions, but it is not known if this is an artifact of the novelty of the intervention or the added attention, rather than actual improvement in quality of care. In the author's experience, caregivers on the receiving end of expert advice also are generally delighted with the help received. Specialists on the other end of the line seem less enthusiastic (Lemaire & Greene, 2002). This may be an artifact of technophobia or related to the lack of some cues that the physicians find useful. Smell, touch, and some physical aspects of the interpersonal interactions are not transmitted via cable. Whether these are critical components of the examination or simply irrelevant but hard habits to break is an important consideration. Logan and Radcliffe (2000) discussed the challenges of video conferencing between rehabilitation team members who are distant. Physical contact, transfer of physical objects between members, and cultural aspects of care are challenging.

PROJECTS IN TELEREHABILITATION

Telemedicine interventions can be differentiated into clinician–clinician interactions (e.g., a therapist consulting with a distant physiatrist) and clinician–patient interactions (e.g., a distant assessment or treatment of the patient by a therapist or physician), according to Huis in 't Veld, van Dijk, Hermens, and Vollenbroek-Hutten (2006). This review of evaluation methods for posture and movement disorders concludes that the methods are acceptable to patients and physicians.

The actual rehabilitation, rather than patient assessment, has been the focus of much of the telemedicine research. Innovations occur in both communication and protocol when telerehabilitation is attempted. There are opportunities for computerized learning and counseling, home-based assistive devices/training devices, telephone- or Internet-based counseling, biofeedback training, and more detailed charting of progress via Internet and computer use. Because the use of computers for communications involves a machine that is really designed to perform logical functions, it is natural that telemedicine projects often incorporate computer software that could be useful even in a face-to-face situation. For example, a computer-driven hand rehabilitation device designed by Popescu, Burdea, Bouzit, and Hentz (1999) and Popescu, Burdea, Bouzit, Girone, and Hentz (2000) is probably most valuable for its software and hardware design, rather than the fact that it can be used from the home versus the clinic. The barrier between telerehabilitation and computerized rehabilitation is blurred.

Numerous demonstration projects have shown feasibility of various rehabilitation techniques, but randomized trials are rare, and cost-effectiveness analysis is almost nonexistent. Pain rehabilitation has been the subject of some research. One study in patients with chronic pain showed that self-regulatory skills can be effectively taught via telephone or closed-circuit television (Appel, Bleiberg, & Noiseux, 2002). On the other hand, Andersson, Lundstrom, and Strom (2003) performed a randomized controlled trial of headache sufferers, in which half had frequent telephone contact initiated by the counselor, while the other half initiated contact on a schedule. Dropout rates were about 1/3 regardless of group, and the effectiveness of treatment was not improved by therapist-initiated contact. This study in a disorder commonly seen in rehabilitation practice raises questions about the relevance of patient compliance and motivation in telerehabilitation.

Using games, exercises, and information, Reinkensmeyer, Pang, Nessler, and Painter (2002) demonstrated the feasibility of a stroke rehabilitation program, including measurement of compliance and improvement. Burdea, Popescu, Hentz, and Colbert (2000) have designed an orthopedic telerehabilitation system that shows promise, but was only tested in one subject. A pediatric telerehabilitation program has been described (Conner, 1999).

In some cases, telerehabilitation is best considered in the context of social services changes. For example, in Japan, it has been proposed that the integration of occupational therapy telerehabilitation into community life centers for older patients will help the system to efficiently stretch occupational therapy resources (Tsuchisawa, Ono, Kanda, & Kelly, 2000).

It is quite realistic for persons with severe disability or reduced consciousness to be maintained at home, at great cost savings to society but with substantial stresses on the family

(Doble, Haig, Anderson, & Katz, 2003). A few randomized trials support the use of telemedicine to maintain patients at home. In 111 persons with spinal cord injuries, no difference was noted among those who received 9 weeks of telerehabilitation advice (either video or telephone contact) compared to others in terms of quality of life, but there was a trend toward shorter subsequent hospitalizations in the telerehabilitation group (Phillips et al., 2001). A small survey of persons with traumatic brain injury suggested that there was good acceptability for telerehabilitation services, notably for assistance in cognitive areas and activities of daily living (Ricker et al., 2002). For a small group of five persons with severe traumatic brain injuries, video conferencing during the first 2 months after discharge from home resulted in fewer ongoing family needs and more patients remaining at home at 6- to 9-month follow-up, compared with a control group (Hauber & Jones, 2002).

Education of practitioners is an important aim in telerehabilitation. Models have ranged from online courses to online peer support. The motivation to share information and the motivation to use it need to be explored. The University of Michigan medical school is spending over a million dollars to put its entire curriculum on line for free consumption. The university believes that this information will be available in the future regardless of its effort, but if it presents it early and in a very organized and accessible way, it will gain whatever advantages there are in the global "market" for education and reputation.

But what about practicing clinicians? In the world at large, there are few, if any, requirements for continuing professional education, and so practitioners may treat based on their training of 20, 30, or more years in the past. Because the occupational health services of global employers are financially at risk when a worker becomes disabled, a partnership was formed between a global employer and a university to develop telehealth educational programs including primarily issues related to musculoskeletal rehabilitation (Haig, Biggs, et al., 2009). The results showed that over half of the company's practitioners anonymously used the program, that they had a statistically significant increase in knowledge, and that simplification and brevity resulted in significant improvement in user satisfaction. In this demonstration project, the employer was motivated by the savings incurred with improved care and decreased cost of educational travel. A cascade of knowledge was observed. The physicians, often more affluent or in greater leadership positions than independent physicians, are often practice leaders for their medical communities.

ORGANIZATIONAL ASPECTS OF TELEREHABILITATION

Telerehabilitation is done by organizations that need it, see it as a financially viable solution, and have the technology and interpersonal strengths to succeed.

The need of an organization relates to the responsibilities that it has. So the United States military, a leader in telemedicine and telerehabilitation, is driven by the need to manage rehabilitation needs for people all over the world in diverse situations where the rehabilitation expertise may not exist. A national health service may have similar needs. A private hospital or clinic in a rural area may see its mission and its opportunity in care without transportation. Furthest down the hierarchy is the urban hospital or clinic. This kind of organization may feel that its patients are well taken care of and that transportation is a mere inconvenience.

In its current state telerehabilitation is still not driven by market forces. Programs are driven by an organization's interest in getting ahead (basically "research and development" funds), or by the marketing value of a token program, or by external funding for research, or by philanthropy. Often the real drive is to not disappoint a valuable clinician or researcher who is driven by a passion to work on telerehabilitation.

Sustainable telerehabilitation must be profitable or at least budget-neutral for an organization to use it in the long term. In the American fee-for-service model, payment for telerehabilitation care is not well established among insurers and the cost of malpractice liability is not well understood. Where health care systems have a defined budget or are "capitated," the equation balances the savings that may or may not occur with the cost and potential inefficiencies. In a system where the health care system is responsible for the overall functioning and quality of life of persons, the equation tips strongly toward telerehabilitation. For example, worker disability liability (worker's compensation) insurers loose hundreds of dollars a day when a worker is away from work receiving therapy. Governments that are able to track costs from the ministry of health versus benefits to the tax base or social productivity will have a different balance point.

Organizational competency is a key factor to the success of telerehabilitation. The ability to innovate is an obvious requirement. So is the financial ability to share profit and risk across a distance. However, any expert in telemedicine will point out that the human factors among the actual team are the most critical. In rehabilitation, work like that of Strasser and colleagues (2008) has shown that patient outcomes relate directly to the quality of team interaction. Hence, the need for telerehabilitation teams to work well together makes sense. However, the teams are often at a distance, and frequently the telerehabilitation team is not the core team in their lives. Telerehabilitation programs need to spend the face-to-face time or distant communication time to become a team and to maintain high-quality team interaction. Teamwork should be a formal agenda item at organizational meetings. Teams should consider taking time to actually play out teamwork games with each other, outside of the clinical problem. This helps them to separate issues of teamwork and communication from specific technical or medical issues.

TELEREHABILITATION TECHNOLOGY OF THE FUTURE

If there is to be a lesson from Table 36.1, it is this: Although need drives technology for society in general, rehabilitation need does not always drive development of highly accepted forms of telerehabilitation technology. Instead, rehabilitation happens to take advantage of technology designed for other purposes. Perhaps this will change. What rehabilitation-specific technology is on the horizon?

Carignan and Krebs (2006) view the use of robotics in telerehabilitation as an important path to the future. They discuss concepts of "unilateral" robotics in which the patient has a robot but the therapist does not and bilateral rehabilitation in which both sides have robotic devices. For example, a therapist monitoring a patient who is using a driving simulator is unilateral. Bilateral robotics allows the therapist to manipulate a device that is perceived by the patient and vice versa. This bilateral process looks more like individual therapy as one would receive in person; however, bandwidth and Internet delays are serious impediments to perfect interaction.

Dittmar, Axisa, Delhomme, and Gehin (2004) speculate on specific future technologies. They point out that clothing covers 90% of the body, and it can be designed as "health smart." Housing can be made more intelligent and personalized.

Interestingly, now that the world is easily connected, some of our most basic communication skills are seen as barriers. We can send instructions to almost anyone. However, a large proportion of the population is functionally illiterate. In public hospitals in Atlanta, 35% of English speakers and 62% of Spanish speakers were unable to read basic health information (Williams et al., 1995). The numbers increased to more than 80% illiteracy in persons aged 60 years and older in both language groups. We do have the technical capability to communicate around the world. However, there are more than 7,000 languages in the world and the speakers of these languages increasingly show up in clinics where the staff does not speak their language.

Advantages in communication and computer technology allow us to bypass language and literacy to return to the most basic symbolic and observational methods of communication. Recently, for instance, our group has developed the Language Independent Functional Evaluation (LIFE), a video-animated functional assessment scale (Haig, Jayarajan, et al., 2009). The LIFE includes gender and culture-neutral graphic figures performing, requiring assistance, or failing to perform various functional activities that are part of the written Barthel Index (Figure 36.1). In research in Ghana, Mongolia, the United States, and Colombia, the LIFE has demonstrated that computer graphic assessment can have good face validity, content validity, reproducibility, and construct validity. The LIFE relates well to the written Barthel Index and to perhaps be superior to the Barthel in terms of understandability and utility. It has potential as an epidemiological tool in multilingual countries as an outcome measure that allows equivalent measure of treatment effectiveness across continents.

CONCLUSIONS

Looking toward the future, much of the fascination is with the amazing possibilities in rehabilitation technology. There are fantastic opportunities here, but what have we learned from the past? The huge leap in telerehabilitation was not because of technological advances in the field. It came as an unforeseen consequence of society espousing the Internet and high-technology gadgets. Universal design, not rehabilitation technology, will be the technological driver.

Mostly, telerehabilitation is not happening. Despite all of the writing and all of the advances, the fact is that most people who could be served from a distance either receive no care or travel for their care. Telerehabilitation programs remain primarily demonstration projects. Few have been emulated by others. Most projects come about because of grants and not because of good business principles. The successes have come from visionary leadership, research grants, or close interpersonal relations. But visionary leaders are hard to come

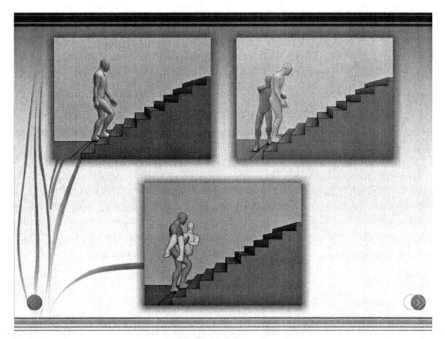

FIGURE 36.1 Still pictures from the video-animated Language Independent Functional Evaluation (LIFE). On a touch screen the subject chooses graphics meant to indicate independent stair climbing, assisted stair climbing, or dependence in stair climbing. Copyright 2007, The Regents of The University of Michigan, reproduced with permission.

by, and by definition research grants do not pay for the routine. Glabman's (2009) article in *Managed Care* draws this conclusion: Disruptive technology requires more than technology to succeed. It must be attached to a successful business model.

If telerehabilitation is to assume its rightful role as an effective part of the health care system, it will do so because its finances are aligned. Most health care payors are not currently exposed to the cost of travel and many have no real incentive to provide better care when distance impedes access to quality services. When payors reward efficiency and quality in caring for the whole person over a lifetime, telerehabilitation will flourish. When governments recognize that the new era of global communication requires removal of legal and financial barriers to distant practice, the door will be open. At this juncture, efforts to change government policy and payor reform are at least as important as research into technological advances and clinical efficacy.

REFERENCES

Andersson, G. (2006) Internet-based cognitive-behavioral self help for depression. *Expert Review of Neurotherapeutics, 6,* 1637–1642.

Andersson, G., Lundstrom, P., & Strom, L. (2003). Internet-based treatment of headache: Does telephone contact add anything? *Headache, 43,* 353–361.

Appel, P. R., Bleiberg, J., & Noiseux, J. (2002). Self-regulation training for chronic pain: Can it be done effectively by telemedicine? *Telemedicine Journal and E-Health, 8,* 361–368.

Baron, C., Hatfield, B., & Georgeadis, A. (2005). Management of communication disorders using family member input, group treatment, and telerehabilitation. *Topics in Stroke Rehabilitation, 12,* 49–56.

Burdea, G. C. (2003). Virtual rehabilitation—Benefits and challenges. *Methods of Information in Medicine, 42,* 519–523.

Burdea, G. C., Popescu, V., Hentz, V., & Colbert, K. (2000). Virtual reality-based orthopedic telerehabilitation. *IEEE Transactions on Rehabilitation Engineering, 8,* 430–432.

Carignan, C. R., & Krebs, H. I. (2006). Telerehabilitation robotics: Bright lights, big future? *Journal of Rehabilitation Research and Development, 43,* 695–710.

Conner, K. (1999). Technology through television. Pediatric telemedicine furthers rehab's continuum of care. *Rehab Management, 12,* 72–75.

Dittmar, A., Axisa, F., Delhomme, G., & Gehin, C. (2004). New concepts and technologies in home care and ambulatory monitoring. *Source Studies in Health Technology and Informatics, 108,* 9–35.

Doble, J. E., Haig, A. J., Anderson, C., & Katz, R. (2003). Impairment, activity, participation, life satisfaction and survival in persons with locked in syndrome for over a decade. Follow-up on a previously reported cohort. *Journal of Head Trauma Rehabilitation, 18,* 435–444.

Garcia-Lizana, F., & Sarria-Santamera, A. (2007). New technologies for chronic disease management and control: A systematic review. *Journal of Telemedicine and Telecare, 13,* 62–68.

Glabman, M. (2009, January). Disruptive innovations that will change your life in health care. *Managed Care,* 12–21.

Grant, P. M., Ryan, C. G., Tigbe, W. W., & Granat, M. H. (2006). The validation of a novel activity monitor in the measurement of posture and motion during everyday activities. *British Journal of Sports Medicine, 40,* 992–997.

Haig, A. J., Biggs, D., Comstock, M., Stern, D., Larez, E., & Woolliscroft, J. O. (2009). *International postgraduate education driven by the needs of a multinational corporation.* Proceedings of the International Society for Physical and Rehabilitation Medicine, Istanbul, Turkey.

Haig, A. J., Jayarajan, S., Maslowski, E., Yamakawa, K. S. J., Tinney, M., Beier, K. P., et al. (2009). Development of a Language Independent Functional Evaluation (L.I.F.E.). *Archives of Physical Medicine and Rehabilitation, 90,* 2074–2080.

Hauber, R. P., & Jones, M. L. (2002). Telerehabilitation support for families at home caring for individuals in prolonged states of reduced consciousness. *Journal of Head Trauma Rehabilitation, 17,* 535–541.

Hoenig, H., Sanford, J. A., Butterfield, T., Griffiths, P. C., Richardson, P., & Hargraves, K. (2006). Development of a teletechnology protocol for in-home rehabilitation. *Journal of Rehabilitation Research and Development, 43,* 287–298.

Holden, M. K. (2005). Virtual environments for motor rehabilitation: Review. *Cyberpsychology & Behavior, 8,* 187–211; discussion 212–219.

Huis in 't Veld, M. H., van Dijk, H., Hermens, H. J., & Vollenbroek-Hutten, M. M. (2006). A systematic review of the methodology of telemedicine evaluation in patients with postural and movement disorders. *Journal of Telemedicine and Telecare, 12*, 289–297.

Jennet, P. A., Affleck Hall, L., Hailey, D., Ohinmaa A., Anderson, C., Thomas, R., et al. (2003). The socio-economic impact of telehealth: A systematic review. *Journal of Telemedicine and Telecare, 9*, 311–320.

Lemaire, E. D., Boudrias, Y., & Greene, G. (2001). Low-bandwidth, Internet-based videoconferencing for physical rehabilitation consultations. *Journal of Telemedicine and Telecare, 7*, 82–89.

Lemaire, E. D., & Greene, G. (2002). Continuing education in physical rehabilitation using Internet-based modules. *Journal of Telemedicine and Telecare, 8*, 19–24.

Logan, G. D., & Radcliffe, D. F. (2000). Supporting communication in rehabilitation engineering teams. *Telemedicine Journal, 6*, 225–236.

Lymberis, A. (2004). Research and development of smart wearable health applications: The challenge ahead. *Studies in Health Technology and Informatics, 108*, 155–161.

Mataix-Cols, D., & Marks, I. M. (2006). Self-help with minimal therapist contact for obsessive-compulsive disorder: A review. *European Psychiatry: Journal of the Association of European Psychiatrists, 21*, 75–80.

Ogawa, H., Yonezawa, Y., Maki, H., Sato, H., Hahn, A. W., & Caldwell, W. M. (2003). A Web-based home welfare and care services support system using a pen type image sensor. *Biomedical Sciences Instrumentation, 39*, 199–203.

Phillips, V. L., Vesmarovich, S., Hauber, R., Wiggers, E., & Egner, A. (2001). Telehealth: Reaching out to newly injured spinal cord patients. *Public Health Reports, 116*(Suppl. 1), 94–102.

Popescu, V. G., Burdea, G. C., Bouzit, M., Girone, M., & Hentz, V. R. (1999). PC-based telerehabilitation system with force feedback. *Studies in Health Technology and Informatics, 62*, 261–267.

Popescu, V. G., Burdea, G. C., Bouzit, M., & Hentz, V. R. (2000). A virtual-reality-based telerehabilitation system with force feedback. *IEEE Transactions on Information Technology in Biomedicine, 4*, 45–51.

Reinkensmeyer, D. J., Pang, C. T., Nessler, J. A., & Painter, C. C. (2002). Web-based telerehabilitation for the upper extremity after stroke. *IEEE Transactions on Neural Systems and Rehabilitation Engineering, 10*, 102–108.

Ricker, J. H., Rosenthal, M., Garay, E., DeLuca, J., Germain, A., Abraham-Fuchs, K., et al. (2002). Telerehabilitation needs: A survey of persons with acquired brain injury. *Journal of Head Trauma Rehabilitation, 17*, 242–250.

Strasser, D. C., Falconer, J. A., Stevens, A. B., Uomoto, J. M., Herrin, J., Bowen, S. E., et al. (2008). Team training and stroke rehabilitation outcomes: A cluster randomized trial. *Archives of Physical Medicine and Rehabilitation, 89*, 10–15.

Tsuchisawa, K., Ono, K., Kanda, T., & Kelly, G. (2000). Japanese occupational therapy in community mental health and telehealth. *Journal of Telemedicine and Telecare, 6*(Suppl. 2), S79–S80.

van Dijk, H., & Hermens, H. J. (2004). Distance training for the restoration of motor function. *Journal of Telemedicine and Telecare, 10*, 63–71.

Williams, M. V., Parker, R. M., Baker, D. W., Parikh, K., Coates, W. C., Nurss, J. R. (1995). Inadequate functional health literacy among patients at two public hospitals. *Journal of the American Medical Association, 274*, 1677–1682.

Yamakawa, K., Tsai, C. K., Haig, A. J., Miner, J. A., & Harris, M. J. (2004). Relationship between ambulation and obesity in older persons with and without low back pain. *International Journal of Obesity and Related Metabolic Disorders, 28*, 137–143.

Zheng, H., Black, N. D., & Harris, N. D. (2005). Position-sensing technologies for movement analysis in stroke rehabilitation. *Medical & Biological Engineering & Computing, 43*, 413–420.

37

Future Directions of Rehabilitation Research

Tamara Bushnik, PhD

As in all other fields of medicine, rehabilitation service providers find themselves subject to outside pressures that influence the way in which rehabilitation medicine is practiced. Changes in health care policy at the federal and state levels, the complexity of health care insurance and the requirements of third-party payers, and the growing complexity of the world in which individuals with disability must navigate have created a situation in which rehabilitation research must play a proactive role in garnering the evidence needed to support current and future practice. This chapter begins with a brief history of rehabilitation and rehabilitation research, describes the key values that should be included in conducting rehabilitation research, introduces some common frameworks that can assist researchers in designing and describing their studies, describes the current status of rehabilitation research, discusses the need for knowledge translation at all stages of the research process, and concludes with future directions.

HISTORY OF REHABILITATION RESEARCH

It was not until the 20th century that modern-day rehabilitation centers were established to provide not only care for individuals with disabilities but also education and training to maximize the physical and mental functional abilities of the individual to participate in society. Physical, occupational, and vocational therapies were the first to develop into recognized fields to provide for the needs of those in federal service, primarily veterans in the armed services, to return to work following injury. By the 1940s, federal law had established the Veterans Administration and the Social Security Act to provide vocational and other services for military and civilian populations. In 1946, the first rehabilitation service in the United States with dedicated personnel and beds serving the civilian population was established by Dr. Howard Rusk at Bellevue Medical Center in New York City. The term "rehabilitation" was added to the Physical Medicine medical specialty in 1947 in response to two events: individuals returning from World War II and those who had contracted poliomyelitis during the 1945–1952 poliomyelitis epidemic.

Rehabilitation has continued to evolve to meet the needs of those with disabilities. The very nature of rehabilitation is to involve multiple disciplines working together to address the unique physical, mental, and psychosocial needs of each individual to optimize the ability of that person to function maximally within society. As centers and programs dedicated to rehabilitation were established, there was a concomitant growing pressure to document the benefits of specialized rehabilitation programs for the purposes of reimbursement, as well as to develop new interventions and strategies to balance the need to better serve the individual and to minimize costs. Rehabilitation is, by no means, the only specialty that has needed to provide evidence to support its practices; all of medicine is facing these requirements to provide better services and outcomes in the most cost-effective manner.

As a result, rehabilitation research has also evolved to meet these requirements and has followed other medical fields in adopting the premise of evidence-based medicine (EBM). Evidence-based medicine is defined as "the conscientious, explicit, and judicious use of current best evidence in making decisions about the care of individual patients" (Sackett, Rosenberg, Gray, Haynes, & Richardson, 1996). The goal of EBM is to produce standardized practice guidelines that are created from a well-constructed body of evidence to support those guidelines. As will be discussed later, there are particular challenges to the rehabilitation field in producing the kinds of evidence that are found in other medical specialties. Regardless, rehabilitation research is the essential bedrock on which rehabilitation clinical practice must rest, and researchers must be aware of the unique aspects of rehabilitation in designing and implementing research studies.

KEY VALUES GUIDING REHABILITATION RESEARCH

The very nature of rehabilitation is to involve multiple disciplines—physiatry; physical, occupational, and recreational therapies; speech and language pathology; (neuro)psychology; social work; nursing; and other medical disciplines as required—that work together as an interdisciplinary team to address all of the physical and cognitive needs of the individual with a disability. Consequently, rehabilitation research must embrace this interdisciplinary approach when conducting research. Other key tenets for conducting rehabilitation research are as follows:

- importance of theory,
- inclusion of clients and families in planning,
- incorporation of cultural context in planning,
- incorporation of the perspectives of all stakeholders—practitioners, payers, policy makers, and researchers, in addition to service recipients and families in research,
- investigation of all components of the International Classification of Functioning, Disability and Health (ICF) (World Health Organization [WHO], 2001) in research designs, and
- use of a broad range of research designs and analytical methods (Barlett et al., 2006).

EVIDENCE-BASED MEDICINE: COMMON FRAMEWORKS FOR RESEARCH

International Classification of Functioning, Disability, and Health

In 2001, the WHO endorsed the ICF as the international standard to describe and measure health and disability, and it has won increasing endorsement as the overarching framework in rehabilitation. It was developed to measure health and disability both at the individual and the population level and uses a common metric that can facilitate investigations into the rehabilitation process and recovery. It makes the assumption that anyone can experience a decrease in health that will result in some level of disability and shifts the emphasis away from "fixing the problem" to assessing the impact of the disability on the individual and trying to accommodate to maximize function. The ICF contains three major interacting areas: body functions and structures, activities, and participation. Disability can result from any of these areas being impacted: impairment of body functions and structures, restriction of activities, and limitation in participation. Moderating these three major areas are environmental factors such as the physical, social, and attitudinal milieus in which the individual lives and personal factors such as unique features of the individual and his or her background. By using the structure and language of the ICF, rehabilitation researchers can ensure that all aspects of disability are investigated.

As an example, a study may choose to examine an intervention to moderate the disability experienced after a motor and sensory complete cervical level 5 traumatic spinal cord injury. At the level of body function and structure, the study may address the effectiveness of inject-ing a compound into the spinal cord at the level of injury to decrease glial scarring, promote axonal growth across the injury, and lower the functional level of injury one level, thereby increasing upper extremity function. At the level of activities, the study may seek to inves-tigate how to improve the individual's independence in eating through the use of a novel orthotic device. At the level of participation, the study may investigate methods to decrease the individual's exclusion from social situations such as dining out. The moderating factors would include investigating environmental factors such as the attitudes of other people and personal factors such as the age of the individual with SCI.

Levels of Evidence

There are a number of classification systems that exist to provide grading algorithms of indi-vidual studies and facilitate the synthesis of research results. The Cochrane Collaboration (Higgins & Green, 2006) and the American Academy of Neurology (AAN; Edlund, Gronseth, So, & Franklin, 2004) are two of the more widely used systems for grading evidence based solely on research design. The Cochrane system only allows evidence from randomized clini-cal trials of interventions to be considered; if these studies are lacking, then no practice guide-line is created and "more research needed" is recommended. In the AAN system, minimum requirements for the number of studies of a particular design are set before a practice recom-mendation is created; if these requirements are not met, again no recommendation is made (Edlund et al., 2004).

For use in rehabilitation research, however, both of these systems are difficult. In many cases, it is difficult to design a randomized controlled trial (RCT) of the highest quality; for example, in a hypothetical study of a range of motion therapy, it is virtually impossible to "blind" the participant as to the therapy that he or she is receiving. Similarly, the therapist administering the therapy cannot be practically "blinded" either. In addition, the typical high-quality RCT compares an intervention against a control, or placebo, condition. In reha-bilitation, it is not ethical to withhold treatment to create a true control condition; therefore, comparisons must be made between standard of care therapy versus a novel intervention. Finally, interventions of interest in rehabilitation are not typically a single well-defined entity, such as a medication, but rather difficult to define interventions such as patient education and advocacy training, which do not lend themselves to a simple RCT framework. These natu-ral constraints within the practice of rehabilitation medicine make it exceedingly difficult to meet the "gold standard" of RCTs to build an evidence base for rehabilitation practice.

A more helpful example of a system of grading evidence that is appropriate for rehabilita-tion is the Grades of Recommendation, Assessment, Development and Evaluation (GRADE; GRADE Working Group, 2004; Guyatt, Oxman, Kunz, et al., 2008, Guyatt, Oxman, Vist, 2008). The GRADE approach specifies four levels of quality of the evidence: high, moderate, low, and very low. At the simplest level, the research design dictates the level, similar to Cochrane and AAN; randomized trials are high, observational trials are low, and case series/case reports are very low. However, the level of a study may be upgraded or downgraded because of the presence of factors that impact the quality of the evidence. The moderating factors that could increase the quality level of a study include a large magnitude of effect, demonstration of a dose-response gradient, or confounding factors would be expected to decrease the reported effect size. Factors that could decrease a study's quality level include limitations in the design and implementation of the study suggesting a high probability of bias, indirectness of the evidence, unexplained heterogeneity or inconsistency of results, imprecision of results, and high probability of publication bias. These factors are more subjective in nature and require an expert consensus of the reliability of the evidence among the reviewers to accurately classify each study. With these moderating factors, the GRADE levels of quality are as follows:

High: Sufficient confidence in the estimate of the effect that it is unlikely that further research will change the conclusion. Typical studies that support this level of evidence are randomized trials without serious limitations and/or observational studies with very large effects.

Moderate: The current estimate of the effect will probably be impacted by further research. Typical studies are randomized trials with serious limitations and/or observational studies with large effects.

Low: There is a high likelihood that further research will change the estimate of the effect; therefore, confidence is low. Typical studies are randomized trials with very serious limitations and/or observational studies with important limitations.

Very low: The estimate of effect is very uncertain. Typical studies are randomized trials with very serious limitations and inconsistent results, observational studies with serious limitations, and/or unsystematic clinical observations such as case series or case reports (Brozek, Akl, Alonso-Coello, et al., 2009a, 2009b).

As can be seen, this type of classification system allows for non-RCTs to be considered as a basis for making practice recommendations. Indeed, the Task Force on Systematic Reviews and Guidelines, convened by the National Center for the Dissemination of Disability Research (NCDDR), published a position paper that strongly cautioned against the absolute reliance on RCTs (Dijkers, 2009a, 2009b) and recommended that, for rehabilitation researchers, the most appropriate approach is to select a study design that will best answer the research question and not be forced into the oftentimes unnatural constraint of conducting an RCT. Indeed, if a number of very well-designed, large sample, nonrandomized trials with concurrent controls all point to the same conclusion that an intervention is effective, should it matter that an RCT has not been conducted? Many rehabilitation researchers would argue "no" and that it is more than sufficient to accept the evidence of all well-designed studies addressing the issue. As such, the GRADE system is far more appropriate for rehabilitation research and the construction of evidence-based recommendations for rehabilitation. For further reading, please see Brozek, Akl, Alonso-Coello, et al. (2009), Brozek, Akl, Jaeschke, (2009), and Dijkers (2009).

Current State of Rehabilitation Research

Rehabilitation research is driven, to a greater or lesser extent, by the organizations that provide funding to the institutions and investigators. Until about 2007, the major funding organizations for rehabilitation research were the National Institute on Disability and Rehabilitation Research (NIDRR) in the Office of Special Education and Rehabilitative Services of U.S. Department of Education, the National Center for Medical Rehabilitation Research (NCMRR) in the Eunice Kennedy Shriver National Institute of Child Health and Human Development of the National Institutes of Health, and the Veterans Affairs (VA) Rehabilitation Research and Development (RR&D) Service in the VA Office of Research and Development of the U.S. Department of Veterans Affairs.

Within the public domain, NIDRR is the pre-eminent organization to support rehabilitation research and, indeed, has the largest budget dedicated to supporting rehabilitation research. It was created in 1978 with the mission of generating, disseminating, and promoting new knowledge to improve the lives of individuals with disabilities. To that end, NIDRR has developed a wide variety of programs for fulfill this mission. These include coordinated programs of research focusing on research and training (Rehabilitation Research and Training Centers) and rehabilitation engineering (Rehabilitation Engineering Research Centers). In addition, research and development projects, advanced research training projects for postdoctoral students, field-initiated projects, and model systems of research have been established to further NIDRR's traditional areas of research focus: health and function, employment, technology for access and function, independent living and community integration, and other associated disability areas.

The model systems of research were the first large-scale collaborative projects that were tasked with developing a comprehensive system to care extending from the time of injury throughout the lifespan of the individual. The Spinal Cord Injury Model Systems of Care (SCIMS), in fact, were authorized by Congress in 1970 and funded in 1973, preceding the creation of NIDRR. The Traumatic Brain Injury Model Systems of Care (TBIMS) were funded in 1987, followed by the Burn Injury Rehabilitation Model Systems of Care (BIRMS) in 1994. The uniqueness and strength of the Model Systems (MS) programs are twofold. First, each program has established a national database, with set inclusion and exclusion criteria, into which information about individuals with the disability of interest is entered. This information has changed over the years but can be categorized into the following main groups: premorbid history, demographic characteristics, causes and severity of injury, nature of diagnoses, types of treatment/services, costs of treatment/services, and measurement and prediction of outcomes including impairment, disability, and participation. Both the SCIMS and TBIMS follow individuals longitudinally until the person withdraws, is lost to follow-up, or expires; thus, the SCIMS and TBIMS have information on individuals who are at least 30 years post-SCI and 20 years post-TBI, respectively, at the time of the writing of this chapter. The BIRMS is slightly different in that outcomes are captured up until 2 years postinjury. The richness of the information contained within the national databases has resulted in numerous seminal papers that have impacted and will continue to impact the rehabilitation field over the years. Second, the MS structure, bringing together rehabilitation programs with similar levels of clinical and research expertise, permits a level of collaboration that is extremely difficult to attain without explicit support from funding agencies. This has allowed monetary, intellectual, and, crucially, participant resources to be combined in such a way that research questions could be posed which could not have been answered in a single-site project.

NIDRR has fostered this collaborative synergy by funding MS collaborative projects that are multisite studies that must include a minimum of four MS sites. As an example, a 5-year, multicenter trial of the efficacy of amantadine in reducing post-TBI irritability and fatigue was funded in 2008; this trial includes six institutions, of which five are TBIMS and provide more than 4 million dollars in funding to enroll 168 individuals with post-TBI irritability. The probability of six institutions cooperating to such a level without such explicit programmatic support is unlikely, as is the likelihood of enrolling 168 individuals with post-TBI irritability at one or even two collaborating sites within a reasonable timeframe, in this case 5 years.

Other funding agencies have recognized the power of fostering this type of collaboration and attempted to emulate it. NCMRR funded the Traumatic Brain Injury Clinical Trials (TBI-CT) Network in 2002 with eight centers and a data coordinating center. The purpose was to provide the infrastructure in which multicenter, complex clinical trials for TBI rehabilitation could be efficiently developed and implemented. Since its inception, only two trials have been conducted, speaking to the difficulty in successfully implementing a research network. More recently, VA RR&D funded Centers of Excellence (CoE) for rehabilitation research; however, these CoE are primarily located in one city, fostering collaboration within a circumscribed geographic location. Finally, the U.S. Department of Defense, in 2007, created the Defense CoE focusing on returning soldiers with TBI and/or posttraumatic stress disorder and their families. The Defense CoE collaborates with the Department of Defense, Department of Veterans Affairs, and a network of military and civilian agencies across the United States.

Although NIDRR has clearly led the way in developing and fostering collaborative and cooperative rehabilitation research, it remains woefully underfunded when compared with other agencies. As an example, with the current level of funding for MS collaborative projects and assuming equal distribution of funds between institutions, each site would receive a maximum of $142,500 per year over the 5-year period to conduct these complex projects. This number includes both direct and indirect costs. In a recent analysis of the costs of the NIH program of clinical trials from 1977 to 2000 (expressed in 2004 dollars), 28 phase III clinical trials were funded at a total cost of $335 million dollars (Johnston, Rootenberg, Katrak, Smith, & Elkins, 2006). One randomized drug trial with 21 collaborative centers lasted 2 years and enrolled 365 individuals with subarachnoid hemorrhage; the total cost of the trial was $9.8 million dollars, which corresponds to each center receiving about $215,000 per year, although this is a low estimate because the research network was already established (Haley, Kassell, Torner, Truskowski, & Germanson, 1994). In a single-site RCT of a drug to prevent posttraumatic seizures, 312 patients were enrolled and followed for 2 years, and the 5 years of funding totaled $5.5 million dollars, which corresponds to $1 million dollars per year to conduct the trial (Temkin et al., 1999). Clearly, NIDRR by itself is not able to provide a feasible funding level for complex, multisite research studies. Efforts have been made to increase NIDRR's funding or to create a separate institute within NIH to fund rehabilitation research; unfortunately, neither has succeeded to date. The creation of a separate institute is attractive in that funding would be clearly designated for rehabilitation research and not subject to the vagaries of being a small program (rehabilitation research) within a larger funding organization (e.g., National Institutes on Neurological Disorders and Stroke). However, it is essential that the gestalt of the rehabilitation research funded by NIDRR, including medical, psychosocial, and vocational research, be maintained in any institute that is established.

All of the efforts described earlier emphasize the growing realization that isolationism, be it one agency or one institution, cannot effectively and efficiently conduct the caliber of research that is needed to advance the field. No one agency has the funding and no one institution has the participant pool and infrastructure to conduct the large-scale trials that are required to provide the basis for evidence-based guidelines for rehabilitation clinical practice. The continued support and funding of research networks, not only within the civilian and military realms but between them, is a critical component that will ensure that rehabilitation research continues to advance the field and improve the lives of individuals with disabilities and their families.

Knowledge Translation

The last consideration in this section is the concept of knowledge translation as another framework that rehabilitation researchers should use when conducting research. The term "knowledge translation" was first defined by the Canadian Institutes of Health Research (CIHR) in 2000 as "the exchange, synthesis and ethically-sound application of knowledge—within a complex system of interactions among researchers and users—to accelerate the capture of the benefits of research for Canadians through improved health, more effective services and products, and a strengthened health care system" (CIHR, 2005, para. 2). More recently, NIDRR created a working definition of knowledge translation as "the multidimensional, active process of ensuring that new knowledge gained through the course of research ultimately improves the lives of people with disabilities, and furthers their participation in society" (NIDRR, 2005).

The CIHR model details six opportunities during the research process where activities to foster and facilitate knowledge translation should occur (CIHR, 2005). The first two opportunities are in the process of defining the research question/methodology and conducting the research. Of particular importance for EBM are the remaining four opportunities: making the research results accessible in terms of format and language appropriate to the audience; placing the results in the context of other knowledge and sociocultural norms; using the results to make decisions; and influencing future research based on how the knowledge is used. What this effectively means is that conducting research without a plan to disseminate the results to the appropriate audience is no longer acceptable. Researchers must consider how the research may be used a priori when designing either a single research project or a research program. Although EBM calls for practice decisions being made using a body of research for justification, there continue to be significant impediments to this interactive process (Bennett et al., 2003; Meline & Paradiso, 2003).

How can knowledge translation be facilitated? Jacobson and colleagues (2003) proposed five domains that should be considered when planning for this interaction: the user group; the issue; the research; the researcher–user relationship; and the dissemination strategies. Essentially, each domain needs to be examined and characterized to better frame how the information should be presented. For example, the Brain Injury Association of America (BIAA) has partnered with a number of professional organizations, including the NIDRR-funded TBI Model Systems of Care, to produce consumer versions of professional peer-reviewed abstracts relevant to brain injury. The interaction between the professional, who produced the original research, and the BIAA, representing consumers and professionals, is an iterative process whereby information is made accessible to individuals and their family members in an appropriate format. Throughout rehabilitation research, knowledge translation needs to be implemented so that decisions informing practice and future research can be made on a solid evidence base. For a more in-depth examination of knowledge translation, please refer to Sudsawad (2007).

FUTURE DIRECTIONS FOR REHABILITATION RESEARCH

The multidisciplinary nature of rehabilitation must extend to the conduct of research as well. Although it has been suggested that all disciplines be involved during the many stages of a research project or program, this spirit of collaboration needs to be expanded to agencies that fund rehabilitation research. Rehabilitation is a complex process that involves all aspects of the physical, cognitive, and psychosocial characteristics of the individual; the research that is required to address this milieu spans federal and state agencies that currently fund rehabilitation research programs. Initiatives have begun at the federal level to facilitate interagency collaboration, including increased dialogue between civilian and military organizations that fund rehabilitation research. An excellent example of just such collaboration is the interagency agreement between NIDRR and the Department of Defense in which the TBIMS National Datacenter is providing expert advice and assistance in helping polytrauma research centers that have been so designated to develop a compatible longitudinal database to track long-term outcomes of soldiers who have incurred TBI. Hopefully such efforts will continue to expand to the betterment of rehabilitation research and ultimately to the provision of the most effective rehabilitation services.

The recognized need for interagency collaboration has also brought to light the wide range of outcome and assessment tools and measures that are used. It is frequently very difficult to compare a body of work in a particular area because the studies use different metrics for assessment and outcome. There are several initiatives that have begun to address this problem and to try and create a common measurement compendium that researchers can use. The Patient Reported Outcomes Measurement Information System (PROMIS) and the Neuro-QOL initiatives are both federally funded efforts to create scales that will be used in clinical trials and clinical practice and provide the cross-walk that is needed to compare and contrast interventions and treatment results across studies. In addition, researchers are working with the PROMIS and Neuro-QOL items as a basis for developing disability-specific scales, such as for TBI and SCI, which will not only provide information that is relevant to the disability, because original PROMIS and Neuro-QOL items are included, but also allow for comparison with other populations who have taken the PROMIS and/or Neuro-QOL. Another example of such an effort is the work conducted by the Interagency TBI and Psychological Health work groups that were convened by the National Institute of Neurological Disorders and Stroke, Department of Veterans Affairs, Department of Defense, and NIDRR to create recommendations for common data elements to support TBI and Psychological Health research studies.

The intent was to facilitate the selection of assessment and outcome tools by researchers in the field through provision of recommendations for "core" measures that must be included if appropriate, "supplemental" measures that should be included for specific topics or populations, and "emerging" measures, which are currently under development and may prove to be superior to current "core" or "supplemental" measures. All of these laudable efforts have the potential to create a common platform from which researchers and clinicians can "speak the same language." Within the next few years, it is hoped that the current lack of standardization of metrics will be a historical curiosity; the increase in knowledge generated by rehabilitation research should then be able to grow at a much greater rate.

As has been described earlier, rehabilitation research has started to embrace a number of common frameworks—interagency cooperation, collaborative research networks and consortia, and the development of common metrics—by which investigators can facilitate the establishment of a body of research on which practice can be based. However, these initiatives must continue to grow and expand. Rehabilitation research needs to involve *all persons* to whom that research may pertain—this must include individuals with disabilities and their families, as well as the community at large, all allied health care professionals, policy makers, and others—at every stage of the research cycle. When this process is effective, the resultant research is focused and has the greatest likelihood of addressing questions that are important to the intended recipient—be they researcher, clinician, or individual with a disability.

REFERENCES

Barlett, D. J., Macnab, J., Macarthur, C., Mandich, A., Magill-Evans, J., Young, N. L., et al. (2006). Advancing rehabilitation research: An interactionist perspective to guide question and design. *Disability and Rehabilitation, 28*, 1169–1176.

Bennett, S., Tooth, L., McKenna, K., Rodger, S., Strong, J., Ziviani, J., et al. (2003). Perceptions of evidence based practice: A survey of Australian occupational therapists. *Australian Occupational Therapy Journal, 50*, 13–22.

Brozek, J. L., Akl, E. A., Alonso-Coello, P., Lang, D., Jaeschke, R., Williams, J. W., et al. (2009a). Grading quality of evidence and strength of recommendations in clinical practice guidelines (Part 1 of 3): An overview of the GRADE approach and grading quality of evidence about interventions. *Allergy, 64*, 669–677.

Brozek, J. L., Akl, E. A., Jaeschke, R., Lang, D. M., Bossuyt, P., Glasziou, P., et al. (2009b). Grading quality of evidence and strength of recommendations in clinical practice guidelines (Part 2 of 3): The GRADE approach to grading quality of evidence about diagnostic tests and strategies. *Allergy, 64*, 1109–1116.

Canadian Institutes of Health Research (2005). *About knowledge translation*. Retrieved October 19, 2009, from http://www.cihr-irsc.gc.ca/e/29418.html

Dijkers, M. P. J. M.; for the NCDDR Task Force on Systematic Review and Guidelines. (2009a). *When the best is the enemy of the good: The nature of research evidence used in systematic reviews and guidelines*. Austin, TX: SEDL.

Dijkers, M. P. J. M., & The Task Force on Systematic Reviews and Guidelines. (2009b). The value of "traditional" reviews in the era of systematic reviewing. *American Journal of Physical Medicine and Rehabilitation, 88*, 423–430.

Edlund, W., Gronseth, G., So, Y., & Franklin, G. (2004). *Clinical practice guidelines process manual—2004 edition*. St. Paul, MN: American Academy of Neurology.

GRADE Working Group. (2004). Grading quality of evidence and strength of recommendations. *British Medical Journal, 328*, 1490–1494.

Guyatt, G. H., Oxman, A. D., Kunz, R., Vist, G. E., Falck-Ytter, Y., & Schunemann, H. J. (2008). What is 'quality of evidence' and why is it important to clinicians? *British Medical Journal, 26*, 995–998.

Guyatt, G. H., Oxman, A. D., Vist, G. E., Kunz, R., Falck-Ytter, Y., Alonso-Coello, P., et al. (2008). GRADE: An emerging consensus on rating quality of evidence and strength of recommendations. *British Medical Journal, 26*, 924–926.

Haley, E. C., Jr., Kassell, N. F., Torner, J. C., Truskowski, L. L., & Germanson, T. P. (1994). A randomized trial of two doses of nicardipine in aneurismal subarachnoid hemorrhage: A report of the Cooperative Aneurysm Study. *Journal of Neurosurgery, 80*, 788–796.

Higgins, J. P. T., & Green, S. (Eds.). (2006). *Cochrane handbook for systematic reviews of interventions 4.2.6* [updated September 2006]. Chichester, UK: John Wiley.

Jacobson, N., Butterill, D., & Goering, P. (2003). Development of a framework for knowledge translation: Understanding user context. *Journal of Health Services Research Policy, 8,* 94–99.

Johnston, S. C., Rootenberg, J. D., Katrak, S., Smith, W. S., & Elkins, J. S. (2006). Effect of a US National Institutes of Health programme of clinical trials on public health and costs. *Lancet, 367,* 1319–1327.

Meline, T., & Paradiso, T. (2003). Evidence-based practice in schools: Evaluation research and reducing barriers. *Language, Speech, and Hearing Services in Schools, 34,* 273–283.

National Institute on Disability and Rehabilitation Research. (2005). *Long-range plan for fiscal years 2005–2009.* Retrieved September 12, 2008, from http://www.ed.gov/legistation/FedRegister/other/2006–1/o21506.pdf

Sackett, D. L., Rosenberg, W. M., Gray, J. A., Haynes, R. B., & Richardson, W. S. (1996). Evidence-based medicine: What it is and what it isn't. *British Medical Journal, 312,* 71–72.

Sudsawad, P. (2007). *Knowledge translation: Introduction to models, strategies, and measures.* Austin, TX: SEDL. Retrieved from http://www.ncddr.org/kt/products/ktintro.pdf

Temkin, N. R., Dikmen, S. S., Anderson, G. D., Wilensky, A. J., Holmes, M. D., Cohen, W., et al. (1999). Valproate therapy for prevention of post-traumatic seizures: A randomized trial. *Journal of Neurosurgery, 91,* 593–600.

World Health Organization. (2001). *International Classification of Functioning, Disability and Health (ICF).* Geneva: WHO.

Index